D1581881

Reichel's Care of the Elderly

Clinical Aspects of Aging

Seventh Edition

Reichel's Care of the Elderly

Clinical Aspects of Aging

Seventh Edition

Editors-in-Chief:

Jan Busby-Whitehead, MD, CMD, AGSF, is Mary and Thomas Hudson Distinguished Professor and Chief, Division of Geriatric Medicine, and Director, Center for Aging and Health, University of North Carolina, Chapel Hill

Christine Arenson, MD, is Professor and Interim Chair, Department of Family and Community Medicine, Sidney Kimmel Medical College at Thomas Jefferson University, and Co-Director, Jefferson Center for Interprofessional Education, Thomas Jefferson University

Editors:

Samuel C. Durso, MD, MBA, AGSF, is Mason F. Lord Professor of Medicine and Director, Division of Geriatric Medicine and Gerontology, Johns Hopkins University School of Medicine

Daniel Swagerty, MD, MPH, AGSF, is Associate Professor, Department of Family Medicine, and Associate Director, Landon Center on Aging, University of Kansas School of Medicine

Laura Mosqueda, MD, AGSF, is Chair, Department of Family Medicine; Professor of Family Medicine and Geriatrics (Clinical Scholar); and Associate Dean of Primary Care, Keck School of Medicine of the University of Southern California

Maria Fiatarone Singh, MD, is John Sutton Chair of Exercise and Sports Science, and Professor of Medicine, Sydney Medical School, University of Sydney

Editor Emeritus:

William Reichel, MD, AGSF, is Affiliated Scholar, Pellegrino Center for Clinical Bioethics, Georgetown University Medical Center

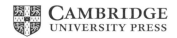

CAMBRIDGE
UNIVERSITY PRESS

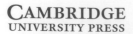

CAMBRIDGE
UNIVERSITY PRESS

University Printing House, Cambridge CB2 8BS, United Kingdom

Cambridge University Press is part of the University of Cambridge.

It furthers the University's mission by disseminating knowledge in the pursuit of education, learning and research at the highest international levels of excellence.

www.cambridge.org
Information on this title: www.cambridge.org/9781107054943

First published 2009

Seventh Edition 2016

Printed in the United Kingdom by TJ International Ltd. Padstow Cornwall

A catalogue record for this publication is available from the British Library

Library of Congress Cataloguing in Publication data
Busby-Whitehead, Jan, editor.
Reichel's care of the elderly : clinical aspects of aging / editors-in-chief, Jan Busby-Whitehead, Christine Arenson ; editors, Samuel C. Durso, Daniel Swagerty, Laura Mosqueda, Maria Fiatarone Singh ; editor emeritus, William Reichel.
Care of the elderly
Seventh edition. | Cambridge ; New York : Cambridge University Press, 2016. | Includes bibliographical references and index.
LCCN 2015045191 | ISBN 9781107054943 (hardback)
| MESH: Geriatrics – methods. | Aging – physiology. | Health Services for the Aged.
LCC RC952.55 | NLM WT 100 | DDC 618.97–dc23
LC record available at http://lccn.loc.gov/2015045191

ISBN 978-1-107-05494-3 Hardback

....

Contents

Color plates are situated between pp. 436 and 437

Editorial Advisory Committee

CO-CHAIRS:

Debra Bynum, MD, MMEL
Associate Professor
Internal Medicine Residency Program Director
Department of Medicine
Division of Geriatric Medicine
Center for Aging and Health
University of North Carolina School of Medicine
Chapel Hill, NC

Lauren R. Hersh, MD
Instructor
Department of Family and Community Medicine
Division of Geriatric Medicine and Palliative Care
Sidney Kimmel Medical College at Thomas
Jefferson University
Philadelphia, PA

MEMBERS:
Kathryn Beldowski, MD
Fellow
Department of Family and Community Medicine
Division of Geriatric Medicine and Palliative Care
Thomas Jefferson University Hospital
Philadelphia, PA

Justin H. Brown, J.D., LL.M
Flaster/Greenberg, PC
Philadelphia, PA

Edward M. Buchanan, MD
Assistant Professor
Department of Family and Community Medicine
Sidney Kimmel Medical College at Thomas
Jefferson University
Philadelphia, PA

Barbara Carroll, MD, CMD
Medical Director
Broadmead Retirement Community
Cockeysville, MD

Danielle Cayea, MD, MS
Assistant Professor
Department of Medicine
Director, Daniel and Jeannette Hendin Schapiro
Geriatric Medical Education Center
Johns Hopkins University School of Medicine
Baltimore, MD

Cristine Clarke, EdD
Coordinator, Carolina Geriatric Education Center
Center for Aging and Health
University of North Carolina at Chapel Hill
Chapel Hill, NC

Jeremy D. Close, MD
Assistant Professor
Director, Primary Care Sports Medicine Fellowship
Department of Family and Community Medicine
Sidney Kimmel Medical College at Thomas
Jefferson University
Philadelphia, PA

Jessica Colburn, MD
Assistant Professor
Department of Medicine
Division of Geriatric Medicine and Gerontology
Johns Hopkins University School of Medicine
Baltimore, MD

Jiadi Cook, MD
Fellow

Department of Family and Community Medicine
Division of Geriatric Medicine and Palliative Care
Thomas Jefferson University Hospital
Philadelphia, PA

Amanda Victoria Z. de la Paz, MD
Fellow
Department of Family and Community Medicine
Division of Geriatric Medicine and Palliative Care
Thomas Jefferson University Hospital
Philadelphia, PA

Veronica Deza, MD
Director, Geriatrics and Community Medicine
Department of Family Medicine
Franklin Square Medical Center
Baltimore, MD

Christine Downey, DDS, MS
Clinical Assistant Professor
Department of Dental Ecology
University of North Carolina School of Dentistry
Chapel Hill, NC

Stephanie Fleegle, MD
Department of Geriatrics
Kaiser Permanente Hawaii Region
Honolulu, HI

Mary Beth Friedel, PharmD
Clinical Pharmacist
IgG America, Inc.
Linthicum Heights, MD

Gregory J. Hanson, MD
Assistant Professor
Department of General Internal Medicine
Mayo Clinic
Rochester, MN

Laura Hanson, MD, MPH
Professor
Department of Medicine

Division of Geriatric Medicine
Center for Aging and Health
University of North Carolina School of Medicine
Chapel Hill, NC

Jennifer Hayashi, MD
Assistant Professor
Department of Medicine
Johns Hopkins University School of Medicine
Baltimore, MD

Kim Isaacs, MD
Professor
Department of Medicine
Division of Gastroenterology and Hepatology
University of North Carolina School of Medicine
Chapel Hill, NC

Deborah Lynn Kasman, MD, MA
Medical Bioethics Director
Kaiser Permanente
Baldwin Park, CA

Heidi Klepin, MD
Associate Professor
Department of Internal Medicine – Hematology
and Oncology
Comprehensive Cancer Center, Sticht Center on
Aging
Wake Forest University School of Medicine
Winston-Salem, NC

Jean Lee, MD, FACP
Professor
Department of Medicine – Nephrology,
Hypertension, and Kidney
Transplantation
Temple University School of Medicine
Philadelphia, PA

Sarah G. Lowman, MPH
Dental Student
University of North Carolina School of Dentistry
Chapel Hill, NC

P. Kay Lund, PhD
Professor
Department of Cell Biology and Physiology
University of North Carolina School of Medicine
Chapel Hill, NC

Amy MacKenzie, MD
Assistant Professor
Department of Medical Oncology
Division of Regional Cancer Care
Sidney Kimmel Cancer Center at Thomas Jefferson University
Philadelphia, PA

Yorgi Mavros, PhD, ESSAM AEP
Postdoctoral Research Associate/CRN in Advancing Exercise and Sports
Science
Exercise, Health, and Performance
Faculty Research Group Faculty of Health Sciences
The University of Sydney
Lidcombe, NSW, Australia

Matthew McNabney, MD
Associate Professor
Department of Medicine
Johns Hopkins University School of Medicine
Baltimore, MD

Geoffrey Mills, MD, PhD
Assistant Professor
Department of Family and Community Medicine and Department of Physiology
Sidney Kimmel Medical College at Thomas Jefferson University
Philadelphia, PA

Esther Oh, MD
Assistant Professor
Department of Medicine
Division of Geriatric Medicine and Gerontology
Johns Hopkins University School of Medicine
Baltimore, MD

Pikai Oh, MD
Clinical Instructor
Department of Physical Medicine and Rehabilitation
Sidney Kimmel Medical College at Thomas Jefferson University
Philadelphia, PA

Philip Panzarella, MD
Chair
Department of Internal Medicine
Franklin Square Medical Center
Baltimore, MD

Neesha Patel, MD
Geriatrics Fellow
Department of Family and Community Medicine
Division of Geriatric Medicine and Palliative Care
Thomas Jefferson University Hospital
Philadelphia, PA

Michael Reinhardt, MD
Department of Psychiatry and Behavioral Sciences
Division of Geriatric Psychiatry
SUNY Downstate Medical Center
Brooklyn, NY

Emily Richie, MD
Faculty in Family Medicine
Franklin Square Medical Center
Baltimore, MD

Ellen Roberts, MD, MPH
Research Associate Professor
Department of Medicine
Division of Geriatric Medicine
Center for Aging and Health
University of North Carolina School of Medicine
Chapel Hill, NC

Mandi Sehgal, MD
Clinical Associate Professor
Department of Family Medicine Division of Geriatrics and Palliative Medicine

Landon Center on Aging
University of Kansas Medical Center
Kansas City, KS

Danielle Snyderman, MD, CMD
Assistant Professor
Department of Family and Community Medicine
Division of Geriatric Medicine and Palliative Care
Sidney Kimmel Medical College at Thomas Jefferson University
Philadelphia, PA

James S. Studdiford, MD, FACP
Professor
Department of Family and Community Medicine
Sidney Kimmel Medical College at Thomas Jefferson University
Philadelphia, PA

Kathryn P. Trayes, MD
Assistant Professor
Department of Family and Community Medicine
Sidney Kimmel Medical College at Thomas Jefferson University
Philadelphia, PA

Amy M. Westcott, MD, CMD, FAAHPM
Associate Professor
Department of Medicine
The Pennsylvania State University College of Medicine
Hershey, PA

Michele Q. Zawora, MD
Chair
Department of Physician Assistant Studies
Jefferson College of Health Professions
Assistant Professor
Department of Family and Community Medicine
Division of Geriatric Medicine and Palliative Care
Sidney Kimmel Medical College at Thomas Jefferson University
Philadelphia, PA

Meng Zhang, MD
Assistant Professor
Department of Medicine, and Department of Geriatrics and Palliative
Medicine
Icahn School of Medicine at Mount Sinai
New York, NY

Contributors

Jowairiyya Ahmad, MD
Department of Geriatrics, Montefiore Medical Centre, New York, USA Rheumatology Fellow, Thomas Jefferson University Hospital, Philadelphia, Pennsylvania, USA

Matthew Alcusky, PharmD, MS
Jefferson School of Population Health, Thomas Jefferson University, Philadelphia, Pennsylvania, USA

Cathy Alessi, MD
Director, Geriatric Research, Education, and Clinical Center and Chief, Division of Geriatrics, Veterans Administration Greater Los Angeles Healthcare System, Professor at David Geffen School of Medicine at UCLA, Los Angeles, California, USA

Christine Arenson, MD
Professor, Division of Geriatric Medicine and Palliative Care, Department of Family and Community Medicine, Sidney Kimmel Medical College at Thomas Jefferson University, Philadelphia, Pennsylvania, USA

Christopher D. Askew, PhD
Adjunct Associate Professor, Faculty of Health, School of Exercise and Nutrition Sciences, Queensland University of Technology, Brisbane, Queensland, Australia

Charles A. Austin, MD
Fellow, Division of Pulmonary and Critical Care Medicine, Department of Medicine, Center for Aging and Health University of North Carolina School of Medicine, Chapel Hill, North Carolina, USA

Stacy Cooper Bailey, PhD, MPH
Assistant Professor, Division of Pharmaceutical Outcomes and Policy, University of North Carolina

Eshelman School of Pharmacy, Chapel Hill, North Carolina, USA

B. Lynn Beattie, MD, FRCP(C)
Professor Emeritus, Division of Geriatric Medicine, University of British Columbia, Vancouver, British Columbia, Canada

Michele F. Bellantoni, MD, CMD
Associate Professor and Clinical Director, Division of Geriatric Medicine and Gerontology, Johns Hopkins University School of Medicine, Baltimore, Maryland, USA

Shelley Bhattacharya, DO, MPH
Associate Professor, Division of Geriatrics and Palliative Care, Department of Family Medicine, Landon Center on Aging, University of Kansas School of Medicine, Kansas City, Kansas, USA

Neetu Bhola, MD
Fellow in Geriatrics, University of California, Irvine, California, USA

James T. Birch, Jr., MD, MSPH, CMD
Assistant Professor, Division of Geriatrics and Palliative Care, Department of Family Medicine, Landon Center on Aging, University of Kansas School of Medicine, Kansas City, Kansas, USA

Michelle R. Boyce, MD
Resident Physician, Department of Ophthalmology, University of Kansas Medical Center, Kansas City, Kansas, USA

Jan Busby-Whitehead, MD, CMD, AGSF
Mary and Thomas Hudson Distinguished Professor of Medicine, Chief of Division of Geriatric Medicine, Department of Medicine, Director of Center for Aging and Health,

University of North Carolina School of Medicine, Chapel Hill, North Carolina, USA

David B. Carr, MD
Professor, Division of Geriatrics and Nutritional Sciences, Washington University School of Medicine, St. Louis, Missouri, USA

Shannon S. Carson, MD
Professor of Medicine, Chief of Division of Pulmonary and Critical Care Medicine, Department of Medicine, University of North Carolina School of Medicine, Chapel Hill, North Carolina, USA

Lisa B. Caruso, MD, MPH
Assistant Professor of Medicine, Section of Geriatrics, Department of Medicine, Boston University School of Medicine/Boston Medical Center, Boston, Massachusetts, USA

Lauren Collins, MD
Associate Professor, Division of Geriatric Medicine, Department of Family and Community Medicine, Sidney Kimmel Medical College at Thomas Jefferson University, Philadelphia, Pennsylvania, USA

Kadesha Collins-Fletcher, MD
Assistant Professor of Medicine, Hofstra North Shore – Long Island Jewish School of Medicine, Division of Geriatric and Palliative Medicine, North Shore – LIJ Health System Department of Medicine, Great Neck, New York, USA

Albert G. Crawford, PhD, MBA, MSIS
Jefferson College of Population Health, Thomas Jefferson University, Philadelphia, Pennsylvania, USA

Natalie R. Danna, MD
Resident Physician, Department of Orthopaedic Surgery, New York University Hospital for Joint Diseases, New York University Langone Medical Center, New York, New York, USA

Lucia Loredana Dattoma, MD
Clinical Instructor of Medicine, David Geffen School of Medicine at UCLA, Division of Geriatric Medicine, Los Angeles, California, USA

G. Kevin Donovan, MD, MA
Director, Professor at Pellegrino Center for Clinical Bioethics, Professor at Georgetown University Medical Center, Washington, DC, USA

David J. Doukas, MD
William Ray Moore Endowed Chair of Family Medicine and Medical Humanism, Director in Division of Medical Humanism and Ethics, Department of Family and Geriatric Medicine, University of Louisville, Louisville, Kentucky, USA

Margaret Drickamer, MD
Clinical Professor of Medicine, Division of Geriatric Medicine, Department of Medicine, Center for Aging and Health UNC-Chapel Hill School of Medicine, Chapel Hill, North Carolina, USA

David van Duin, MD
Associate Professor of Medicine, Division of Infectious Diseases, University of North Carolina School of Medicine, Director of Immunocompromised Host Infectious Diseases Section, Chapel Hill, North Carolina, USA

Samuel C. Durso, MD, MBA
Mason F. Lord Professor of Medicine, Director of Division of Geriatric Medicine and Gerontology, Johns Hopkins University School of Medicine, Executive Vice Chairman of Department of Medicine, Johns Hopkins Bayview Medical Center, Baltimore, Maryland, USA

Joseph M. Dzierzewski, PhD
Assistant Professor, David Geffen School of Medicine, University of California, Los Angeles, Geriatric Research, Education, and Clinical Center, VA Greater Los Angeles Healthcare System, Los Angeles, California, USA

Rebecca D. Elon, MD, MPH
Chief Medical Officer, FutureCare Health and Management Corporation, Associate Professor of Medicine, Division of Geriatric Medicine, Johns Hopkins University School of Medicine, Pasadena, Maryland, USA

Jonathan Evans, MD, MPH
Adjunct Professor, School of Law, University of Virginia, Charlottesville, Virginia, USA

Mindy J. Fain, MD
Anne & Alden Hart Professor of Medicine, Chief of Division of Geriatrics, General Internal Medicine and Palliative Medicine, Co-Director of Arizona Center on Aging, University of Arizona College of Medicine, Tucson, Arizona, USA

Ana C. G. Felix, MBBCh
Assistant Professor, Department of Neurology, University of North Carolina School of Medicine, Chapel Hill, North Carolina, USA

Susan Gaylord, PhD
Director of Program on Integrative Medicine, Associate Professor in Department of Physical Medicine and Rehabilitation, University of North Carolina School of Medicine, Chapel Hill, North Carolina, USA

John D. Gazewood, MD, MSPH
Associate Professor and Residency Program Director, Department of Family Medicine, University of Virginia School of Medicine, Charlottesville, Virginia, USA

Jonathan Golledge, MChir, FRACS
Professor in Department of Surgery, Head of Vascular Biology Unit, James Cook University, Townsville, Queensland, Australia

Lisa Granville, MD
Professor and Associate Chair, Department of Geriatrics, Florida State University College of Medicine, Tallahassee, Florida, USA

Jan S. Greenberg, PhD
Professor, School of Social Work and Waisman Center, University of Wisconsin, Madison, Wisconsin, USA

Tomas L. Griebling, MD, MPH, FACS, FGSA, AGSF
Professor and Vice Chair, Department of Urology, Faculty Associate, Landon Center on Aging, University of Kansas School of Medicine, Kansas City, Kansas, USA

Emily R. Hajjar, PharmD, BCPS, BCACP, CGP
Associate Professor, Jefferson College of Pharmacy, Thomas Jefferson University, Philadelphia, Pennsylvania, USA

Karen E. Hall, MD, PhD
Clinical Professor, Department of Internal Medicine, Division of Geriatric and Palliative Medicine, University of Michigan Healthcare System, Medical Director at UM-SJMH Acute Care for Elders Unit, St. Joseph Mercy Health, Ann Arbor, Michigan, USA

Jung Hee Han, DO
Department of Family Medicine, Geriatrics, University of California, Irvine, California, USA

Molly M. Hanson, CRNP
Palliative Care Nurse Practitioner, Division of Geriatrics and Palliative Care, Department of Family and Community Medicine, Thomas Jefferson University Hospital, Philadelphia, Pennsylvania, USA

Stephen S. Hanson, PhD
Associate Professor, Department of Philosophy, University of Louisville, Louisville, Kentucky, USA

Déon Cox Hayley, DO
Associate Professor, Department of Internal Medicine, Division of General and Geriatric Medicine, University of Kansas School of Medicine, Kansas City, Kansas, USA

Lauren R. Hersh, MD
Instructor, Department of Family and Community Medicine, Sidney Kimmel Medical College at Thomas Jefferson University Hospital, Philadelphia, Pennsylvania, USA

Peter Hollmann MD
University Medicine, Chief Medical Officer, Rhode Island Hospital, Providence, Rhode Island, USA

Diana Homeier, MD
Associate Professor of Clinical Family and Internal Medicine, Keck School of Medicine of University of Southern California, Los Angeles, California, USA

Christine Hsieh, MD
Assistant Professor, Department of Family and Community Medicine, Jefferson Medical College, Sidney Kimmel Medical College at Thomas Jefferson University, Philadelphia, Pennsylvania

Myra Hyatt, LSCSW
Landon Center on Aging, University of Kansas, Kansas City, Kansas, USA

Theodore M. Johnson II, MD, MPH
Professor and Chief, Division of Medicine and
Geriatrics, Department of Veterans Affairs,
Birmingham/Atlanta Geriatric Research Education
and Clinical Center, Department of Medicine, Emory
University School of Medicine, Atlanta, Georgia

Jessica L. Kalender-Rich, MD
Associate Professor of Medicine, Division of General
and Geriatric Medicine, Department of Internal
Medicine, Landon Center on Aging, University of
Kansas Medical Center, Kansas City, Kansas, USA

Rebecca J. Kamil, BS
Medical Student, Pre-doctoral Research Fellow,
Center on Aging and Health, Albert Einstein College
of Medicine, Bronx, New York, USA

Marshall B. Kapp, JD, MPH
Director, Center for Innovative Collaboration in
Medicine and Law, Florida State University College of
Medicine and College of Law, Tallahassee, Florida,
USA

Aaron Kaufman, MD
Health Sciences Assistant Clinical Professor,
Department of Psychiatry and Biobehavioral Services,
David Geffen School of Medicine at UCLA, Los
Angeles, California, USA

Amber E. King, PharmD, BCPS
Assistant Professor, Jefferson College of Pharmacy,
Thomas Jefferson University, Philadelphia,
Pennsylvania, USA

James L. Kirkland, MD, PhD
Robert and Arlene Kogod Center on Aging, Mayo
Clinic, Rochester, Minnesota, USA

Deepika Koganti, MD
Department of Surgery, Thomas Jefferson University
Hospital, Philadelphia, Pennsylvania, USA

Alexis N. Kuerbis, LCSW, PhD
Assistant Professor, Silberman School of
Social Work, Hunter College of CUNY, New York,
New York, USA

Susan W. Lehmann, MD
Associate Professor, Director of Geriatric
Psychiatry Day Hospital, Department of
Psychiatry and Behavioral Sciences, Johns Hopkins

University School of Medicine, Baltimore, Maryland,
USA

Tsao-Wei Liang, MD
Associate Professor of Neurology, Sidney Kimmel
Medical College at Thomas Jefferson University,
Philadelphia, Pennsylvania, USA

Frank R. Lin, MD, PhD
Associate Professor of Otolaryngology – Head and
Neck Surgery, Geriatric Medicine, Epidemiology, and
Mental Health, Johns Hopkins University School of
Medicine, Baltimore, Maryland, USA

Angela Lipscomb-Hudson, MD
Clinical Assistant Professor, Department of Physical
Medicine and Rehabilitation, University of North
Carolina School of Medicine, Chapel Hill, North
Carolina, USA

Marsha R. Mailick, PhD
Vice Chancellor for Research and Graduate
Education, Vaughan Bascom and Elizabeth M. Boggs
Professor, School of Social Work and Waisman
Center, University of Wisconsin, Madison,
Wisconsin, USA

Caroline Mariano, MD, FRCPC
Medical Oncology, Royal Columbian Hospital, Clinical
Assistant Professor, University of British Columbia,
New Westminster, British Columbia, Canada

Alayne D. Markland, DO, MSc
Chief of Geriatrics, Department of Veterans Affairs,
Birmingham VA Medical Center, Birmingham/
Atlanta Geriatric Research, Education and Clinical
Center, Associate Professor of Medicine, Department
of Medicine, Division of Gerontology, Geriatrics, and
Palliative Care at the University of Alabama,
Birmingham, Alabama, USA

Rachel Mason, MD
Assistant Professor of Medicine, Division of General
Medicine and Geriatrics, Department of Internal
Medicine, Faculty Associate in Landon Center on
Aging, University of Kansas School of Medicine,
Kansas City, Kansas, USA

John F. McAna, PhD
Jefferson College of Population Health, Thomas
Jefferson University, Philadelphia,
Pennsylvania, USA

Christopher B. McFadden, MD
Associate Professor, Division of Nephrology, Department of Medicine, Cooper Medical College of Rowan University, Camden, New Jersey, USA

Phil Mendys, PharmD, FAHA, CPP
Adjunct Professor of Medicine and Pharmacotherapy, University of North Carolina Heart and Vascular Center, Chapel Hill, North Carolina, USA

Barret Michalec, PhD
Associate Professor, Department of Sociology, University of Delaware, Newark, Delaware, USA

M. Jane Mohler, NP-C, MPH, PhD
Professor of Medicine, Public Health, Pharmacy, and Nursing, Associate Director of Arizona Center on Aging, University of Arizona College of Medicine, Tucson, Arizona, USA

Alison A. Moore, MD, MPH
Professor of Medicine and Psychiatry, David Geffen School of Medicine at UCLA, Division of Geriatric Medicine, Los Angeles, California, USA

Kendall F. Moseley, MD
Assistant Professor, Division of Endocrinology, Johns Hopkins University School of Medicine, Baltimore, Maryland, USA

Laura Mosqueda, MD, AGSF
Associate Dean of Primary Care, Chair and Professor of Family Medicine and Geriatrics, Keck School of Medicine of University of Southern California, Los Angeles, California, USA

Hyman Muss, MD
Mary Hudson Distinguished Professor of Medicine, Division of Hematology and Oncology, Department of Medicine University of North Carolina School of Medicine, Chapel Hill, North Carolina, USA

Rakhi Naik, MD, MHS
Assistant Professor of Medicine and Oncology, Johns Hopkins University School of Medicine, Baltimore, Maryland, USA

Eun Ha Namkung, MSW
PhD candidate, School of Social Work and the Waisman Center, University of Wisconsin, Madison, Wisconsin, USA

David Newman-Toker, MD, PhD
Associate Professor of Medicine, Department of Neurology, Johns Hopkins University School of Medicine, Baltimore, Maryland, USA

Carrie Nieman, MD, MPH
Resident, postdoctoral research fellow, Center on Aging and Health, Department of Otolaryngology – Head and Neck Surgery, Johns Hopkins University School of Medicine, Baltimore, Maryland, USA

Elizabeth O'Toole, MSPH
Project Manager, Department of Family Medicine and Geriatrics, Keck School of Medicine of University of Southern California, Los Angeles, California, USA

Allyson K. Palmer, BA MD/PhD
candidate, Mayo Medical School and Mayo Graduate School, Robert and Arlene Kogod Center on Aging, Mayo Clinic, Rochester, Minnesota, USA

Mary H. Palmer, PhD, RN-C, FAAN
Helen W. and Thomas L. Umphlet Distinguished Professor in Aging, School of Nursing, University of North Carolina at Chapel Hill, North Carolina, USA

Susan Parks, MD
Associate Professor, Director in Division of Geriatric Medicine and Palliative Care, Department of Family and Community Medicine, Sidney Kimmel Medical College at Thomas Jefferson University, Philadelphia, Pennsylvania, USA

Belinda J. Parmenter, PhD, AEP
Exercise Physiology Unit, School of Medical Sciences, Faculty of Medicine, University of New South Wales, Sydney, New South Wales, Australia

Alice K. Pomidor, MD, MPH, AGSF
Professor, Department of Geriatrics, Florida State University College of Medicine, Tallahassee, Florida, USA

Christina Prather, MD
Assistant Professor of Medicine, Division of Geriatrics and Palliative Medicine, George Washington University School of Medicine, Washington, DC, USA

Peter V. Rabins, MD, MPH
Professor of Psychiatry and Behavioral Sciences, Johns Hopkins University School of Medicine, Baltimore, Maryland, USA

William Reichel, MD, AGSF
Affiliated scholar, Center for Clinical Bioethics, Georgetown University School of Medicine, Washington, DC, USA

Michael W. Rich, MD
Professor of Medicine, Washington University School of Medicine, St. Louis, Missouri, USA

David W. Rittenhouse, MD
Division of Acute Care Surgery: Trauma, Critical Care, and Emergency Surgery, Department of Surgery, Sidney Kimmel Medical College at Thomas Jefferson University, Philadelphia, Pennsylvania, USA

Juan C. Rodriguez, MD
Instructor of Medicine at Pontificia Universidad Catolica de Chile, Research Fellow in Geriatric Medicine at University of California, Los Angeles, Geriatric Research, Education, and Clinical Center, VA Greater Los Angeles Healthcare System, Los Angeles, California, USA

Barry W. Rovner, MD
Professor, Departments of Neurology and Psychiatry and Human Behavior, Sidney Kimmel Medical College at Thomas Jefferson University, Jefferson Hospital for Neurosciences, Philadelphia, Pennsylvania, USA

Murrium I Sadaf, MD
Student researcher, Cambridge, Ontario, Canada

Brooke Salzman, MD
Associate Professor, Division of Geriatric Medicine and Palliative Care, Department of Family and Community Medicine, Sidney Kimmel Medical College at Thomas Jefferson University, Philadelphia, Pennsylvania, USA

Allen D. Samuelson, DDS
Clinical Associate Professor, Department of Dental Ecology, UNC School of Dentistry, Chapel Hill, North Carolina, USA

Mihai Cosmin Sandulescu, MD
Neurology resident, Einstein Healthcare Network, Philadelphia, Pennsylvania, USA

Christopher J. Sayed, MD
Department of Dermatology, University of North Carolina School of Medicine, Chapel Hill, North Carolina, USA

Joanne G. Schwartzberg, MD
Scholar-in-residence, Accreditation Council for Graduate Medical Education, Chicago, Illinois, USA

Laura Scorr, MD
Senior Associate, Movement Disorder Program, Department of Neurology, Emory University School of Medicine, Atlanta, Georgia, USA

Sonia Sehgal, MD
Associate Professor, Division of Geriatrics and Gerontology, University of California, Irvine, California, USA

Satish Shanbhag, MBBS, MPH
Assistant Professor of Medicine and Oncology, Division of Hematology, Department of Medicine, Johns Hopkins University School of Medicine, Baltimore, Maryland, USA

Fatima Sheikh, MD, MPH
Medical Director at FutureCare Health and Management Corporation, Instructor in Division of Geriatric Medicine, Johns Hopkins University School of Medicine, Baltimore, Maryland, USA

Catherine Sherrington
Professorial Research Fellow, The George Institute for Global Health, Sydney Medical School, University of Sydney, Sydney, New South Wales, Australia

Ross J. Simpson, Jr. MD, PhD
Professor of Medicine and Epidemiology, Division of Cardiology, University of North Carolina School of Medicine, Chapel Hill, North Carolina, USA

Maria A. Fiatarone Singh, MD, FRACP
John Sutton Chair of Exercise and Sport Science, Professor, Sydney Medical School, University of Sydney, Lidcombe, New South Wales, Australia

William D. Sirover, MD
Assistant Professor, Division of Nephrology, Department of Medicine, Cooper Medical College of Rowan University, Camden, New Jersey, USA

Jennifer Sloane, MD
Assistant Professor, Division of Rheumatology, Department of Medicine, Sidney Kimmel Medical College at Thomas Jefferson University, Philadelphia, Pennsylvania, USA

Danielle Snyderman, MD CMD
Assistant Professor, Department of Family and Community Medicine, Sidney Kimmel Medical College at Thomas Jefferson University, Philadelphia, Pennsylvania, USA

Jason A. Sokol
Associate Professor of Ophthalmology, Department of Ophthalmology, University of Kansas Medical Center, Kansas City, Kansas

Joshua M. Stolker, MD
Adjunct Associate Professor, St. Louis University School of Medicine, St. Louis, Missouri, USA

Daina L. Sturnieks
Research Fellow, Neuroscience Research Australia and School of Medical Sciences, University of New South Wales, Sydney, New South Wales, Australia

Daniel Swagerty, MD, MPH, AGSF
Professor of Family Medicine and Internal Medicine, Associate Chair for Geriatrics and Palliative Care, Department of Family Medicine, Associate Director for Education, Landon Center on Aging, University of Kansas School of Medicine, Kansas City, Kansas, USA

Kristine Swartz, MD
Assistant Professor, Division of Geriatric Medicine and Palliative Care, Department of Family and Community Medicine, Sidney Kimmel Medical College at Thomas Jefferson University, Philadelphia, Pennsylvania, USA

Laila S. Tabatabai, MD
Houston Methodist Specialty Physician Group, Houston, Texas, USA

Steven Tam, MD
Assistant Clinical Professor, Division of Geriatrics, Department of Family Medicine, Department of Internal Medicine, University of California, Irvine, California, USA

Paul Thananopavarn, MD
Clinical Assistant Professor, Department of Physical Medicine and Rehabilitation,

University of North Carolina, Chapel Hill, North Carolina, USA

Katherine M. Varman, MD
Department of Dermatology, University of North Carolina at Chapel Hill, North Carolina, USA

Diane Villanyi, MD
Clinical Instructor, Division of Geriatric Medicine, University of British Columbia, Vancouver, British Columbia, Canada

Michael S. Weinstein, MD, FACS, FCCM
Associate Professor of Surgery, Division of Acute Care Surgery: Trauma, Critical Care, and Emergency Surgery, Department of Surgery, Sidney Kimmel Medical College at Thomas Jefferson University, Philadelphia, Pennsylvania, USA

Lindsay A. Wilson, MD, MPH
Assistant Clinical Professor, Division of Geriatric Medicine, Department of Internal Medicine, University of North Carolina School of Medicine, Chapel Hill, North Carolina, USA

Laraine Winter, PhD
Research Psychologist, Philadelphia Research and Education Foundation, Philadelphia VA Medical Center, Philadelphia, Pennsylvania, USA

David Alain Wohl, MD
Associate Professor of Medicine, Division of Infectious Diseases, University of North Carolina School of Medicine, Site Leader – UNC AIDS Clinical Trials Unit at Chapel Hill, Director at NC AIDS Training and Education Center, Co-Director at HIV Services for the North Carolina Department of Public Safety (Department of Corrections), Chapel Hill, North Carolina, USA

Brooke K. Worster, MD
Assistant Professor of Medicine, Division of Geriatric Medicine and Palliative Care, Department of Family and Community Medicine, Sidney Kimmel Medical College at Thomas Jefferson University, Philadelphia, Pennsylvania, USA

Swaytha Yalamanchi, MD
Research and Clinical Fellow, Division of Endocrinology, Johns Hopkins University School of Medicine, Baltimore, Maryland

Louise Ye, DO, LAc
Fellow in Geriatric Medicine, University of Southern California / Los Angeles County + USC Medical Center, Los Angeles, California, USA

Gwen Yeo, PhD, AGSF
Director Emerita and Senior Ethnogeriatric Specialist, Stanford Geriatric Education Center, Stanford University School of Medicine, Stanford, California, USA

Michele Q. Zawora, MD
Chair, Department of Physician Assistant Studies, Jefferson College of Health Professions, Assistant Professor, Department of Family and Community Medicine, Division of

Geriatric Medicine and Palliative Care, Sidney Kimmel Medical College at Thomas Jefferson University, Philadelphia, Pennsylvania, USA

Tanya Zinner, MD
Clinical Assistant Professor, Department of Physical Medicine and Rehabilitation, University of North Carolina, Chapel Hill, North Carolina, USA

Joseph D. Zuckerman, MD
Professor and Chairman, Department of Orthopaedic Surgery, New York University Hospital for Joint Diseases, New York, New York, USA

Acknowledgments

The editors wish to gratefully acknowledge the support and contributions of our many colleagues who made this book possible, and our families, without whose support we could not do this work. We especially thank our mentor and friend, William Reichel, MD, Editor Emeritus, whose vision and leadership continues to inspire us. Lastly, we dedicate this book to our patients, who remind us daily of the joy and privilege of geriatric medicine.

Chapter

Essential principles in the care of the elderly

William Reichel, MD, AGSF, Christine Arenson, MD, and
Jan Busby-Whitehead, MD

The world is aging. Already in 2012, the US Census Bureau reported that 43.1 million people in the United States – 13.7% of the population – were 65 years or older.[1] The first baby boomers turned 65 in 2011, and 79.7 million Americans will be over the age of 65 by 2040. The oldest old – those 85 and older – are the fastest growing segment of the American population, and their number will reach 14.1 million in 2040. Further, 21% of those 65 and older are members of racial or ethnic minorities. Twenty-eight percent of those over 65 reported some earned income in 2012, while 9.1% lived below the proverty level. However, as calculated by the new Supplemental Poverty Measure, which takes into account regional variations in living costs, noncash benefits received, and nondiscretionary expenditures such as out-of-pocket medical expenses, 14.8% of those over 65 lived in poverty.[1]

The aging of the population, coupled with advances in chronic disease management; diffusion of "best practices"; increased attention to maintaining physical, cognitive, and psychological function; and availability of improved treatments for the most common causes of death and disability is likely to continue to extend both average life expectancy and years of active life. However, it must be noted that fully 35.9% of those over 65 reported at least one disability in 2012.[1] Moreover, an increasing awareness of persistent inequalities in our health-care system, a decreasing number of working adults to support dependent children and retirees, and an increasing burden on family caregivers are just some of the countervailing forces that continue to limit the promise of healthy, productive aging.

We certainly want good health care waiting for us in our golden years. But what is good care? In the care of the elderly patient, eleven essential principles

should be considered: (1) the role of the physician as the integrator of the biopsychosocial-spiritual model; (2) continuity of care; (3) the bolstering of the family and home; (4) good communication skills; (5) a sound doctor-patient relationship; (6) the need for appropriate evaluation and assessment; (7) disease prevention and health maintenance; (8) intelligent treatment with attention to ethical decision making; (9) interprofessional collaboration; (10) respect for the usefulness and value of the aged individual; and (11) compassionate care. These essentials are closely related to the six health system redesign imperatives identified by the Institute of Medicine in its landmark 2001 report, *Crossing the Quality Chasm*.[2] More recently, Donald Berwick articulated the Triple Aim: improving the patient experience of care, improving the health of populations, and reducing the per capita cost of health care.[3] The embodiment of these eleven principles, along with the Triple Aim, represents a standard of excellence to which we can all aspire.

The physician as integrator of the biopsychosocial-spiritual model

The past 50 years have witnessed enormous growth in technology and options to cure acute illness and manage chronic conditions. However, one result of these changes has been increasingly complex, specialized care. Good care requires having a physician who provides leadership in the integration and coordination of the health care of the elderly patient. The current generation of older adults has witnessed amazing advances in research and great accomplishments in diagnostic and curative medicine, but we have also realized that scientific reductionism is not enough.

Reichel's Care of the Elderly, 7th Edition, ed. Jan Busby-Whitehead *et al*. Published by Cambridge University Press.
© Cambridge University Press 2016.

The reforms in medical education, care, and research over the past century have too often resulted in fragmentation of medical thought and care. It is imperative that the health-care professional responsible for the care of older adults keeps the "big picture" firmly in mind – we must never forget that the patient is so much more than the sum of his or her organ systems.[4, 5]

What society is calling for are physicians who are committed to the person, and not just to a specific disease state or mechanism. The person is part of a family and a larger community (sadly, there are some elders who have no family and are isolated from the community). The first essential for the physician who cares for the elder is to act as an integrator of the biopsychosocial, and one may add, spiritual, model. To accomplish this, the physician must know the patient thoroughly. This is not to denigrate the excellence of the specialties and subspecialties that have achieved so much during the past few decades. But the ideal model of health care will exist only when the patient is seen not from a single specialty point of view, but with the full appreciation of other organ systems, emotional or psychosocial factors, information based on continuity over a period of time, and knowledge of the patient's family and community.

In recent years, medical specialty organizations, purchasers of care, and even third-party payers have begun to recognize the need to reintegrate coordinated, person-centered, comprehensive primary care as the foundation for an effective health-care system. The patient-centered medical home model for primary care practice redesign has been embraced by family medicine, internal medicine, and geriatric medicine as a framework for "continuous, caring relationships" and to restore a robust primary care infrastructure in the United States.[6] At the same time, it is clear that effective primary care must recognize and begin to address the social determinants of health as critical to achieving overall health for individuals and populations.[7]

Fortunately, important efforts are underway to reintegrate a fragmented health system and incorporate the goals of prioritizing patients and families in care plans. The palliative care and hospice movement, public calls for independence and dignity in aging and during the dying process, and enhanced focus on shared decision making are all enhancing the autonomy and supporting the values of patients. Other developed nations such as Canada, the United Kingdom, and Australia have already made significant strides in reinvigorating primary care and generalist practice. No population will benefit more from effective, coordinated, well-resourced primary care than older adults.

The primary care provider also must ensure the coordination, supervision, and interpretation that is vital for the older patient to navigate a complex system that often provides conflicting recommendations, and in which the vested self-interest of the "system" is not always secondary to the needs of the individual patient. The primary physician, then, acts as an advocate to obtain needed services, but also as an advisor and confidant. At times, the best advice is to avoid tests or treatments that have little or no potential benefit, and which pose significant potential to harm. Perhaps most important, this physician will come to know the patient as an individual, within a family and a community, with particular values, beliefs, and priorities. Thus, the physician comes to serve as interpreter and integrator, helping patients obtain health care that is most consistent with their own preferences and needs. This will most often be the role of a family physician, general internist, geriatrician, or nurse practitioner. However, for some patients, the role may be filled by a trusted oncologist, cardiologist, or other specialist. The key factors are the health-care provider's interest in and ability to see the patient as a whole person, not simply the sum of his or her organ systems, as well as the clinician's time and expertise to serve in this critical role.

We can expect more evidence in coming years that will clarify interventions that address the relationship of biological, psychological, social, and spiritual components to health. Already we know that clinical distrust, chronic stress, and depression have been linked with increased inflammatory markers that may result in higher rates of cardiovascular disease.[8] There is now overwhelming evidence that depression coexisting with diabetes leads to poor outcomes, including increased mortality.[9] In addition, one study has demonstrated that social support may have a protective effect with respect to interleukin-6 (IL-6) elevation and thus, potentially, result in a survival benefit in ovarian cancer patients.[10] The clinician in practice today is aware of the higher mortality in the first year after widowhood (more pronounced in the surviving widower than in the widow) and the higher morbidity and mortality seen

2

in the elderly person on relocation.[11] Thus, we still have much to learn about the dynamic relationship among wellness and disease, psychosocial factors, and the spiritual state.

Continuity of care

The ideal situation for the older adult may be a warm and supportive relationship with the same personal physician serving as advisor, advocate, and friend as the patient moves throughout the labyrinth of medical care. And yet, the realities of today's complex medical environment – that is, patients moving between office, home, hospital, specialized care units (coronary care units, intensive care units, stroke units, or oncology centers), nursing home, and hospice care – often make this ideal impossible. So, in many instances, patients receive the better care from physicians and other health professionals who instead focus their practice in these specialized environments. Thus, the medical intensivist provides the most up-to-date, skilled care in the ICU, and the physician in regular nursing home practice is more available to patients, staff, and families than the one who has a few nursing home patients scattered among several facilities.

The failure of physicians in the United States to make visits as necessary in the home and in long-term care facilities is related to several factors, including training, physician attitudes, and reimbursement systems. Our medical schools and residencies for generalist physicians continue to struggle with incorporating excellence in house calls and nursing home care as part of their educational program. Although reimbursement for visits to the home and nursing home have generally improved in recent years, high office overhead and productivity expectations have continued to limit the ability of physicians to practice in these relatively time-efficient sites. Physician attitudes have also been a problem; doctors in the health-care system of the past few decades have been more interested in the acute aspects of care rather than in chronic and long-term care. These attitudes have been reinforced by the educational and reimbursement systems in place. Recent years have witnessed a marked increase in research and education initiatives designed to address the gap in chronic care knowledge as well as the attitudes of our students and residents.[12, 13]

Nevertheless, continuity of care remains an essential principle in the care of the older patient.[14] Recently, a wealth of literature documenting the critical importance of adequate communication among health professionals around transitions in care lends support to the notion that safe, effective, efficient, and patient-centered care can only occur when the in-depth knowledge and understanding of the personal physician is communicated to and incorporated by the specialized teams in the ICU, general hospital setting, long-term care facility, and even hospice setting.[15–17] Although electronic health records offer the promise of more effective and efficient communication within and across care teams and settings, that vision has not yet been fully realized.

We must recognize that optimum health care can only be provided to the older adult by an ever expanding team of professionals, including primary care and specialty physicians, hospitalists, nurses, therapists, social workers, and others. This does not mean we can abandon the concept of continuity. Rather, we must pay even more attention. Physicians, nurse practitioners, and others with a long-term relationship with a patient may remain active advocates and sounding boards, even when they are not the "provider of record" at a given point in time. Equally important, indeed critical, to the safety of our patients is increased attention to continuity at transition points in the care of the older patient – from home to hospital, from hospital to rehab unit or nursing home. The physician responsible for the care of patients at each of these junctures must communicate fully and accurately with the patient, family, and receiving health-care team to ensure that the patient's treatment plan, values, expectations, and preferences are known and honored every step of the way.

Bolstering family and home

Every physician should enlist whatever means are necessary to keep an elderly person either in the individual's home or in an extended family setting. It should certainly be our goal to keep elderly persons functioning independently, preserving their lifestyles and self-respect as long as possible. The physician should use the prescription for a nursing home as specifically as a prescription for an antibiotic or an antihypertensive medication.

A number of forces have resulted in patients going to institutional settings when other alternatives might have been possible. Between 1960 and 1975, a massive push toward institutionalization took place, creating

3

hundreds of thousands of nursing home beds. What are the forces that contributed to excessive institutional care? Funding mechanisms have been disproportionately directed toward reimbursement for institutional care rather than for other alternatives. With the increased mobility of families, there simply may not be family members available in the community to participate in the elderly person's care. Homes are architecturally based on a small, nuclear family and do not permit housing an elderly patient. Finally, the movement of women into the workforce has meant that fewer family members are available to remain at home with the impaired or disabled elderly person. In spite of these forces, rates of institutionalization have actually declined slightly in recent years; older adults and their families have overcome amazing obstacles to keep loved ones at home whenever possible. Additionally, a rapid growth in largely privately funded assisted-living facilities has provided an option for older adults with less extensive care needs and the financial resources to pay for a lower acuity, more homelike living situation.[18]

What alternative resources can the physician recommend to these caregivers of older adults? A simple list includes homemakers, home health aides, other types of home care, day care, aftercare, specialized housing settings, visiting nurses, friendly visitors, foster home care, chore services, home renovation and repair services, congregate and home-delivered meal programs, transportation programs, and shopping services. Personal physicians should also understand and utilize legal and protective services for the elderly whenever indicated.

Publicly financed programs such as the Program for All Inclusive Care of the Elderly (PACE) and home-based Medicaid waiver programs that support nursing home–eligible elders to remain in their homes have increased in recent years, as federal and state governments have recognized that supporting seniors' desire to stay in their own homes translates into better, less expensive care.[19] States have explored options to provide services in the homes of nursing home–eligible patients through a combination of medical assistance waivers and other programs. In addition, a growing body of research demonstrates the benefits of home-based interventions that target patient and caregiver priorities and teach problem-solving skills to maintain physically frail and demented individuals in their homes.[20, 21]

In spite of the pressure to contain institutional long-term care costs, funds have not been available for adequate expansion of publicly funded programs to support frail older adults in their own home. Further, many of the evidence-based interventions that might provide cost-effective strategies for supporting older persons in the community are not reimbursed by insurance. Thus, resources remain limited and disjointed. The role of health-care providers is to facilitate referrals, coordinate services, and become knowledgeable about general resources available and appropriate referral sources (i.e., care manager, area agency on aging) with expertise to help patients and their families navigate the system effectively.

Who are the caregivers in American society? Data from the Family Caregiver Alliance National Center on Caregiving document that 43.5 million Americans are providing care to someone who is 50 plus years old; 14.9 million care for someone who has Alzheimer's disease or other dementia.[21] Family/informal caregiver services were valued at $450 billion per year in 2009 (nearly equivalent to the total Medicaid spend [$509 billion] and similar to Walmart sales [$408 billion]) and continue to be the largest source of long-term care services to the population 65 and older. More women than men are caregivers, and women continue to shoulder more of the most difficult personal care tasks, such as bathing. The majority of caregivers have provided care for three years or more and spend an average of 20.4 hours per week on caregiving tasks. That increases to 39.3 hours per week when the caregiver lives with the care recipient. The average age of the caregiver providing care to someone over age 65 is 63 years, and one-third of these caregivers rate their own health as fair to poor. Forty to 70 percent of caregivers experience symptoms of depression, and caring for a person with dementia may negatively impact the caregiver's immune function for up to three years after the experience ends. Caregivers continue to experience adverse economic impacts, with many having to reduce their work hours or even stop working. Those caring for older adults lost an estimated $13 trillion in lost wages, pensions, retirement funds, and benefits. Employers of caregivers experience an average of 6.6 lost workdays and an 18.5% reduction in worker productivity.

Today, many families feel the burden of caregiving; the adults are sandwiched between the demands of their parents and of their children and grandchildren. It has been said that the empty nest syndrome has been replaced by a crowded nest syndrome. Many caregivers experience extreme burden and stress, and sometimes the question is, Who is the real patient – the patient or the caregiver? The physician will often see that the caregiver is in more distress than the patient, and in fact develops serious physical and emotional problems as a result of the burden and stress encountered.[22, 23]

The belief that old people are rejected by their families is a much exploited social myth. Many families are struggling to cope with the needs of parents who are frail and debilitated. The family member, friend, or neighbor is often the crucial link in guaranteeing that the dependent elder will remain in the community. In repeated studies, the characteristics of the caregiver, more than those of the elderly patient, are essential in predicting institutional placement. Even when adult children and elderly parents are separated by distance, their quality of relationship may be unaffected, maintaining cohesion despite limited face-to-face contact.

Communication skills

Specific communication skills are critical in managing well the care of elderly patients. Most important to good communication are listening and allowing patients to express themselves. The physician should use an open-ended approach, interpreting what the patient is saying and reading between the lines. The physician can utilize intuition in deciding what the patient truly means. Why did the patient really come to see the physician? The elderly patient complaining of a headache or backache may be expressing depression or grief. We should not miss important verbal clues when the patient tells us, "Doctor, I really think these headaches started when I lost my husband."

It is helpful to leave the door open for other questions or comments by the patient, both at the conclusion of the visit and in the future. It is always helpful to say, "Are there other questions or concerns that you have at this time?" A physician anticipating a specific problem can make it easier for the patient to discuss the issue. For example, "You are doing well, but I know that you are concerned about your arthritis and whether or not you will be able to climb the stairs in your home. At some point, we may want to discuss the various alternatives that are open to you."

One important aspect of the aging American is the increasing diversity of older adults.[1] In the past, white English-speaking individuals comprised the vast majority of our older population. However, healthcare providers will increasingly need to be prepared to care for a racially, ethnically, and linguistically diverse population of elders. Physicians and other professionals caring for older patients need to provide culturally sensitive care, recognizing the unique and varied cultural contexts of their patients. Further, groups including the federal government have started to recognize the critical role of appropriate health translators in order to provide appropriate care to patients who are not proficient in English. All of these issues may be magnified in the care of older patients.

Just as the physician providing care to pediatric patients must deal with the children's parents, the physician providing care to elderly patients must be able to deal with their adult children. These children play a vital role in making decisions and providing support, and the physician, therefore, must possess skills in communicating with them and also in dealing with their emotional reactions, such as guilt or grief. The physician taking care of an elderly patient with cancer must be prepared when the adult daughter tells him: "Whatever you do, please don't tell my father that he has cancer," especially when it is apparent that the parent is totally and fully aware of all aspects of his illness.

The physician should be careful when meeting with an elderly patient who discusses his absent spouse or child, or when dealing with adult children or grandchildren who are discussing the parent or grandparent who is not present. The physician should not necessarily accept the assumptions that are stated about the absent family member. Physicians must be able to listen carefully, ask questions, and collect information; our opinion of the situation might be entirely different if we had an opportunity to hear the view of the absent family member.

Peabody, in 1927, said: "The good physician knows his patients through and through, and his knowledge is bought dearly. Time, sympathy and understanding must be lavishly dispensed, but the reward is to be found in that personal bond that forms the greatest satisfaction of the practice of medicine."[24] The physician who enters the patient's universe and understands the patient's perceptions, assumptions, values, and religious beliefs is a tremendous advantage. Frankl, in *Man's Search for Meaning*, demonstrated how physicians can help patients understand the meaning and value of their lives.[25] Of course, how elders find meaning in their lives is related to how they found meaning during other stages in their lives. It is therapeutic for the patient to feel that the physician cares enough about that individual to understand his or her life, particularly the meaning and purposes of the patient's present existence. Frankl stated in *The Doctor and the Soul* that human life can be fulfilled, not only in creating and enjoying, but also in suffering.[26] He provides examples in which suffering becomes an opportunity for growth, an achievement, a means for ennoblement. Frankl's existential psychiatry or logotherapy is a useful psychologic method that helps the elderly patient appreciate the positive attributes, meanings, and purposes of his or her life.

Yalom defines existential psychotherapy as "a dynamic approach to therapy which focuses on concerns that are rooted in the individual's existence."[27] Many individuals are tormented by a crisis of meaning.[28] They may suffer an existential vacuum, experiencing a lack of meaning in life. [25–29] The patient experiencing an existential vacuum may demonstrate symptoms that will rush to fill it, in the form of somatization, depression, alcoholism, and hypochondriasis. The physician recognizing an existential vacuum can help the patient find meaning. Engagement or involvement in life's activities is a therapeutic answer to a lack of meaning in life. The physician can help guide the patient toward engagement with life, life's activities, other people, and other satisfactions.

Frankl provides advice to all physicians in utilizing hope as a therapeutic tool.[25, 26] The physician dealing with elderly patients must focus on the significant role of hope in daily practice. As physicians, we must eventually understand the biologic basis of hope. We do not yet comprehend sufficiently the biochemical, neurophysiologic, and immunologic concomitants of different attitudes and emotions, and how they are affected by what is communicated from the physician. Physicians have an opportunity to worsen panic and fear; physicians also have an opportunity to create a state of confidence, calm, relaxation, and hope.

In this day and age of increasing technology and subspecialization, the patient's recovery may still depend on the physician's ability to reduce panic and fear, and to raise the prospect of hope. Cousins describes the "quality beyond pure medical competence that patients need and look for in their physicians. They want reassurance. They want to be looked after and not just over. They want to be listened to. They want to feel that it makes a difference to the physician, a very big difference, whether they live or die. They want to feel that they are in the physician's thoughts."[30] For example, in building the doctor–elderly patient relationship, nothing is more effective than the physician's picking up the phone and calling the patient and saying: "I was thinking about your problem. How are you doing?" This expression of interest by telephone represents a potent method for cementing the relationship between doctor and patient.

Jules Pfeiffer's cartoon character, the "modern Diogenes," carries on the following discourse upon meeting an inquisitive fellow traveler through the sands of time.

"What are you doing with the lantern?" asks the traveler.
"I'm searching," replies Diogenes.
"For an honest man?" he asks.
"I gave that up long ago!" exclaims Diogenes.
"For hope?"
"Lots of luck."
"For love?"
"Forget it!"
"For tranquility?"
"No way."
"For happiness?"
"Fat chance."
"For justice?"
"Are you kidding?"
"Then what are you looking for?" he implores of Diogenes.
"Someone to talk to."
Help comes from feeling that one has been heard and understood.[31]

Doctor–patient relationship: what the doctor and patient bring to each encounter

The physician must understand what both he or she and the patient bring to each interaction, including positive and negative feelings. The patient may view old age negatively and fearfully, believing illness signifies misery, approaching death, loss of self-esteem, loneliness, and dependency. The physician's own fears about aging and death may color the interview as well. The doctor may simply not view helping the older, impaired patient as worthwhile. The physician may have low expectations for success of treatment, writing off the elderly patient as senile or mentally ill, or as a hypochondriac. The doctor may have significant conflicts in his or her own relationship with parent figures or may feel threatened that the patient will die.

Knowing the patient

Several steps are recommended in building a sound doctor–patient relationship, particularly applicable to the elderly patient.[24] The first step toward building that relationship is for the physician to know the patient thoroughly; the second step is for the physician to know the patient thoroughly; and the third step is for the physician to know the patient thoroughly. The interested physician performs the first step in building a sound doctor–patient relationship by gathering a complete history – including the personal and social history – and doing a complete physical. Ideally, the physician should be a good listener, warm and sensitive, providing the patient ample opportunity to express multiple problems and reflect upon his or her life history and current life situation. Thus, the physician will be able to understand the meanings and purposes of the patient's present existence. But forces in the health-care industry oftentimes prevent the physician from being a good listener or warm and sensitive. The physician may not be listening as he or she is inputting information into an electronic health record system. The physician sadly may not be present for his or her patient.[32]

As stated earlier, family and friends represent the principal support system for the elderly and usually call for nursing home placement only as a last resort, after all alternatives have failed. However, the physician must be able to recognize the dysfunctional family. There are elderly people who have been rejected by their children. There are elderly people who have rejected a child for a variety of reasons. There are families with members estranged from each other for many years. The patient may have had a stable and supportive marriage, but increasingly older adults have had multiple marriages, or may be divorced, or partnered in a same-sex relationship. It is critical for the practitioner to have an accurate understanding of family dynamics and history in order to appropriately rally family support, and also to recognize when family dysfunction is harming the patient.

Creating a partnership with the patient

In all dealings with the patient, the physician should be frank and honest and share information truthfully. The patient should feel a sense of partnership with the physician. In this partnership, the doctor first reviews his or her perception of the patient's problems. Then, for each problem, alternative choices are considered, and decision making is shared with the patient. Although there are situations in which frankness is counterproductive, with most patients, frankness is helpful. There are also situations in which the elderly patient does not want to share in the decision making, but simply wants to surrender his or her autonomy to a relative such as spouse or adult child, or to the physician. Again, in most cases, the physician should attempt to enter a partnership with the patient and share as much of the decision making as possible.

As a society, we are beginning to realize that dying in America is often not optimal, and there is a crying-out for end-of-life care to be improved. The negative aspects of how the dying process is handled by the medical profession and by families and their community has created a demand for assisted suicide. But there are many alternatives to assisted suicide that can improve the care of the dying patient. The greatest danger of assisted suicide or euthanasia in the era of cost-cutting is that society or patients themselves will decide that a patient's life is not worth living. To paraphrase a line from Woody Allen's *Love and Death* (1975), think of death as cutting down on your expenses. At a time when cost-containment is paramount, we must fear for frail, debilitated elderly persons, those who have been marginalized as a result of Alzheimer's disease and other major disorders.

Some might consider physician-assisted suicide as the ultimate act of patient autonomy – the opportunity to define the conditions and time of one's own death. However, it is critical that discussions with the patient or family members be presented in a hopeful manner. As noted earlier, it is important for the physician to offer a positive approach whenever possible. His or her infusion of optimism and cheerfulness is therapeutic. The physician should help patients appreciate such positive attributes or purposes in their lives as the role of religion and their religious community, relationships with children and grandchildren, the enjoyment of friends, or the enjoyment of the relationship with doctors, nurses, and other health professionals in the immediate therapeutic environment.

The physician should be cautious that discussions with family members be held with the patient's consent. If the patient is sufficiently mentally impaired, then it might be appropriate to deal with the closest relative or identified surrogate decision maker. Complex ethical and legal questions arise in the matter of confidentiality and decision making in regard to the elderly patient with partial mental impairment.

Need for thorough evaluation and assessment

The physician must avoid prejudging the patient. We must not allow preconceived notions of common patterns of illness to preclude the most careful individualized assessment of each patient. Conscientious history and physical examination are essential. Treatment choices should be considered only following a thorough evaluation. Judicious consideration of all factors may result in a decision to treat or not to treat certain problems in certain patients. Attention to lesser problems may be postponed according to the priorities of the moment, rather than complicate an already complex therapeutic program.

Physicians must avoid wastebasket diagnoses. The past concept of "chronic brain syndrome" or "senile dementia" is one such example. Not all mental disturbance in the elderly represents dementia; not all dementias in older people are Alzheimer's disease. Neuropsychiatric disturbance in the elderly might be placed into a wastebasket and casually accepted as both inevitable and untreatable when, in reality, a very treatable cause may be present. The physician must consider and seek out treatable disease.

For example, neuropsychiatric disturbance, including a dementia syndrome, may be caused by severe depression that is a very treatable disorder. Neuropsychiatric disturbance may also include delirium secondary to many types of medical illness or drug toxicity. Such delirious states can be helped if the primary disorder is recognized and treated; failure

to do so may in fact lead to the hastened death of the patient.

It is often difficult to disentangle the physical from the emotional. Emotional disorder may present in the elderly as a physical problem, such as musculoskeletal tension being the principal manifestation of depression. Conversely, physical disease in the elderly might present as a mental disorder with confusion, disorientation, or delirium often being the first sign of many common medical ailments including myocardial infarction, pulmonary embolism, occult cancer, pneumonia, urinary tract infection, and dehydration. For this reason, it cannot be emphasized too many times that proper diagnosis is essential in order to make specific treatment plans, such as the treatment of urinary tract infection in the case of an acute delirious state, or the treatment of thyroid deficiency in the treatment of depression. Each of these is very specific. Treatment in each case would be irrational if a specific diagnosis were not known.

It is often not sufficient to know the organic or anatomic or psychiatric diagnosis; rather, we should seek a total understanding of the elderly patient. Many times, it is more important to assess the elderly patient's functional status, which might have greater significance than the diagnostic or anatomic label. For example, in the case of a cerebrovascular accident, knowledge of the precise anatomic lesion via MRI angiography may not help the patient as much as understanding the patient's functional state. It may be more important to know whether the patient can walk or climb stairs; can handle his or her own bathing, eating, and dressing; can get out of bed and sit in a chair, handle a wheelchair, or be in need of a cane or walker. All of these functional concerns must be considered in evaluating an elderly patient.

Affecting our diagnostic thinking in evaluating an elderly patient would be the consideration of what is physiologic versus what is pathologic. Aging itself can be defined as the progressive deterioration or loss of functional capacity that takes place in an organism after a period of reproductive maturity. The Baltimore Longitudinal Study of Aging since 1958 has studied this decline in each of several specific functional capacities, such as glucose tolerance and creatinine clearance.[33] There is a progressive deterioration of glucose tolerance with each decade of life. Indeed, hyperglycemia is so common in the elderly that to avoid labeling a disquietly high proportion of people as diabetics, Elahi, Clark, and Andres have formulated a percentile system that ranks a subject with age-matched cohorts.[34] (Some individuals, however, show no evidence of deterioration of glucose tolerance or insulin tolerance to glucose with aging.) Although currently the accepted definitions allow the same diagnostic criteria to be applied at any age, it is recognized that treatment decisions must be individualized, especially for the frail or very old person.[35]

In fact, two major conclusions from the Baltimore Longitudinal Study of Aging emerge. Even when specific functional capacities change with age, health problems need not be a consequence of aging. Many of the most common disorders of old age result from pathological processes and not from normal aging. The second important finding is that no single chronological timetable of normal aging exists. Even within one individual, the physiological capacities of organs show aging at different rates. Between individuals, more difference is noted in older people than in younger people.[33]

Polypharmacy is a major problem in the care of the elderly patient. Many medications considered benign in younger individuals may cause significant delirium in elders. Altered renal and hepatic functions may affect drug elimination. In general, older individuals demonstrate greater variability and idiosyncrasy in drug response in comparison to younger persons. Prudence, therefore, is extremely important in prescribing drugs for the elderly individual. The physician must determine if the patient's overall function will be enhanced or harmed with pharmacologic treatment. Is this medication absolutely necessary? Might the new symptom in fact be an adverse drug reaction caused by a current medication? The skill of the physician is required in weighing benefit versus risk. The benefit–risk balance is more crucial and often more narrowly defined in the elderly patient than in younger people. The physician must attempt to keep the total number of medications to as small a number as possible. Tools such as the Beers Criteria for Potentially Inappropriate Medications in the Elderly are available to assist the clinician.[36]

Also affecting our diagnostic ability in the elderly is that signs and symptoms of disease in the aged may be slight or hidden. Pain, white blood cell response, and fever and chills are examples of defense mechanisms that may be diminished in older persons. The aged person may have pneumonia or pyelnephritis without chills or a rise in temperature.[37] Myocardial infarction, ruptured abdominal aorta, perforated appendix, or mesenteric infarction may be present without pain in the elderly patient.[38]

Multiple clinical, psychological, and social problems are characteristic of older people. Clinically and pathologically, an elderly patient may have 10 or 15 problems. Geriatric patients should benefit from the use of a problem-oriented approach to medical records. Medical records should include not only the medical problem, but they should demonstrate an understanding of functional, psychological, social, and family problems as well. The key feature of the problem-oriented record is the problem list, which serves as a table of contents to the patient's total medical history. Current electronic health records provide structured formats for the problem list, but it falls to the clinical care team to develop a comprehensive list of current and past conditions and concerns. Without a detailed problem list, we can easily lose track over time of the elderly patient's multiple problems – for example, that the patient in 1975 was hospitalized for a psychiatric problem or that, in 1995, the patient suffered a compression fracture of the T10 vertebra secondary to slipping on ice. These problems may be lost to memory without some form of problem-oriented system. In addition, care is enhanced by maintaining a medication list that is kept current at each patient visit.

Prevention and health maintenance

A tremendous revolution is taking place in the United States with emphasis on prevention, health maintenance, and wellness. Unfortunately, evidence for the care of frail or extremely old people is lacking. For example, less is known about primary and secondary prevention for heart disease and stroke for elderly patients than for younger adults. Clinicians caring for these patients need to be prepared to discuss the relative risks and benefits of screening tests and preventive medicine in the context of the patient's overall health status and preferences.

More and more physicians and nurses are emphasizing health maintenance and wellness in their practice and in their community educational programs. However, the drive for wellness is coming not only from the health professionals, but also from the public itself. The personal physician has an opportunity to encourage preventive medicine and health maintenance at every age level and at each level of functional ability or disability.

A remarkable amount of new information is being discovered about the role of exercise and strength training in the prevention or reversibility of frailty and physiologic decline.[39] The health of many elders might be improved by regular prescriptions of exercise and physical activity. The next decade will see more advances in nutrition, exercise, and therapeutic measures to retard the aging process.

How do physicians and health professionals determine the standard for health screening and health promotion? *The Guide to Clinical Preventive Services* represents one standard for health screening guidelines.[40] However, evidence for screening and prevention in older adults is still often lacking, or controversial. For instance, the 2014 guide recommends against screening for prostate cancer, in spite of clear recommendations from the American Cancer Society that shared decision making between providers and patients should inform prostate cancer screening decisions.[41] It is clear that each practicing physician must follow the medical literature and evaluate the algorithms and guidelines that unfold in the decade ahead. For each question, new evidence is being generated and existing evidence is being reevaluated in light of changing professional and public understanding and new treatment options.

At any time, with the state of evidence-based knowledge that we do have in preventive medicine and health screening, there remains the differential between the physician's intellectual acceptance and awareness of these guidelines and the actual use of these guidelines on a regular, consistent basis. Increasingly, geriatric practice will rely on technology, such as electronic health records, to ensure consistent application of prevention and wellness guidelines. Adoption of quality improvement strategies to ensure consistent practice will continue to be driven both by the demands of our patients and, increasingly, the use of pay-for-performance strategies by insurers, including Medicare.

Intelligent treatment with attention to ethical decision making: choosing wisely

The common aphorism "First, do no harm" paraphrases the Hippocratic oath and provides a guidepost

to the practice of medicine. It is particularly important in the care of older adults, where interventions may easily cause more harm than benefit without careful consideration of the whole patient. A similar concept was articulated more than 50 years ago by Seegal as the "principle of minimal interference" in the management of the elderly patient.[42] "First, do no harm" and the "principle of minimal interference" should be remembered when one reviews the abundant examples of iatrogenic problems that elderly patients experience.[43, 44]

The principle of minimal interference can be applied to many diagnostic and treatment decisions, including the use of diagnostic tests (the principle of diagnostic parsimony), surgical intervention, and decision making in regard to hospitalization or placement in a long-term care facility. The principle of minimal interference may result in decisions that are both humanistic and cost-effective: for example, a decision that a patient should remain in his or her own home, despite limited access to medical therapy, rather than reside in a long-term care facility; or a decision not to do a gastrointestinal workup in the evaluation of anemia when the patient is terminal as a result of a malignant brain tumor.

In the care of older people, there are times for minimal interference, and there are times for maximal intervention. Certainly the patient with dementia caused by myxedema deserves every effort to replace thyroid hormone carefully. The elderly patient with severe congestive heart failure secondary to rheumatic or congenital heart disease deserves full consideration for definitive treatment, including surgery, for his or her cardiac problems. The elderly patient with depression deserves specific treatment for this very treatable disorder.

Increasing national attention has been focused on these challenging decisions at the interface of clinical and ethical decision making. The Triple Aim (improving the experience of care, improving the health of populations, and reducing the per capita cost of care) has become widely accepted as a definition of successful health system redesign.[45] The Choosing Wisely initiative of the American Board of Internal Medicine Foundation has leveraged the concept of the Triple Aim and encouraged specialty societies to define key opportunities "to promote conversations between providers and patients by helping patients choose care that is supported by evidence, not duplicative of other tests or procedures already received, free from harm, and truly necessary."[46] To date, at least 15 organizations have adopted and publicized Choosing Wisely guidelines that specifically address issues of importance to older adults. For instance, the American Geriatrics Society advises against use of percutaneous feeding tubes in advanced dementia patients due to an excess of harm with no evidence of meaningful benefit: it also recommends a goal hemoglobin A1c of less than 7.5% in most adults aged 65 and older due to evidence that moderate control results in overall better functional benefit with reduced risk of harm compared to tight control in older adults.[47] Organizations as diverse as the American Academy of Family Physicians, the Society of General Internal Medicine, the Society for Hospital Medicine, the American Medical Directors Association, American Cancer Society, American Physical Therapy Association, American Academy of Nursing, and specialty societies such as the American Academy of Hospice and Palliative Medicine, American College of Emergency Physicians, American Society of Nephrology, and Infectious Disease Society of America among others have responded to the ABIM Foundation's call to adopt more evidence-based, cost-effective, and patient-centered practice for all patients, including elders.

In the future, health-care providers will be faced with more and more difficult decisions of an ethical nature. For example, an 80-year old man may present with a past history of resection of an abdominal aneurysm 15 years ago, multiple myocardial infarctions, and multiple strokes causing severe dementia. His main problem in the current hospitalization is pneumonia, causing a worsening of his confused state. Because of periods of sinus arrest, a pacemaker is considered. Should a pacemaker be utilized in patients with significant dementia? Should pneumonia be treated in patients with severe dementia or terminal carcinoma? Difficult and ambiguous clinical problems such as these will face the personal physician with increasing frequency. The physician in the future will be called upon to make complex decisions according to the accepted traditions and values of a specific society, culture, religion, or nation, with major guidance from the patient's stated wishes that were affirmed at a time when the patient was fully competent.

In regard to all therapeutic decisions, a personal physician is at an advantage if his or her understanding of the patient is based on continuity of care. The physician then can consider the patient in totality, including psychological, spiritual, social, family, and environmental factors. To recommend intelligently any treatment plan, it is beneficial to have the knowledge of home or institutional environment, the family constellation, the availability of friends, access to transportation, and the economic situation of the patient. Also, as the physician grapples with complex decisions of an ethical nature, specific knowledge of the patient's value systems and beliefs is critically important.

Interprofessional collaboration

The physician must understand when to call upon other health professionals. He or she must know when to call upon nutrition education, visiting home nurses, social workers, psychologists, or representatives of community agencies. He or she must know when to call for legal or financial counseling. All physicians would do well to work in closer harmony with their patient's or family's clergy.

The physician should know when to recommend specific rehabilitative therapies. Specific use of physical, occupational, recreational, and speech therapies are vital for the proper care of certain problems. For example, the elderly patient with diabetic neuropathy and flapping gait might benefit from bilateral leg braces. Another patient recovering from stroke might benefit from occupational therapy that should be used as a reintroduction of the patient to the activities of normal daily living, and not simply as a recreational or diversionary therapy.

The improvement of health care of the chronically ill elderly patient requires that health professionals work together for the best interest of the patient. What is required is a genuine collaborative effort to act in a unified fashion in order to bring about a system that will best meet the needs of frail elders. There is increasing evidence that effective collaborative practice improves patient outcomes,[48] and competencies for effective collaborative practice have been defined and are actively being promoted in health professions education.[49]

Respect for the usefulness and value of the aged individual

Much in our society works to reject or devalue the aged person. We are certainly living in a youth-oriented era, and a physician must guard against viewing the elderly patient as useless, insignificant, or worthless. This lack of respect and devaluation occurs in society at large – in the workplace, in the family, in the entertainment media – but it should not occur in the doctor's office or other clinical settings. The anthropologist knows other cultures and societies where the elders of the community are most valued. An hour of watching Western television is instructive to witness the youth orientation of our society. It is unfortunate that many elderly patients report that previous physicians treated them poorly because the patient was old.

An exceptional book, although not actively directed to the elderly, is *Respectful Treatment: A Practical Handbook of Patient Care*.[50] The author, Martin Lipp, describes the therapeutic benefit of respect in the doctor–patient relationship, especially in dealing with those we consider problem patients: the angry patient; the dependent, passive patient; the complaining, demanding patient; the denying patient; the overly affectionate patient; the mentally ill patient; etc. Respect is therapeutic. Many patients feel weak and vulnerable, and demonstrate a low self-esteem by virtue of age, illness, and various psychological and personality factors. Respect is a message to the patient that quickly brings about a more sound doctor–patient relationship.

Most countries are witnessing an unprecedented growth in their aging populations, especially in the cohort over 85. We hope that social and economic changes will allow elders to function as a continuing resource in our society. We can expect to see reduced restrictions on older workers with particular reference to mandatory retirement. We can also expect to see more educational programs that will provide skilled training, job counseling, and placement for older men and women in order to initiate, enhance, and continue their voluntary participation in the workforce. We should anticipate the breakdown of stereotypes and greater recognition of the value of the elderly person as a human resource.

There are many social forces at play. Already, more and more older adults are choosing to remain in the workforce. In 1930, 54% of males aged 65 and over were in the workforce. By 1985, only 15.8% of older men were working. Compare this to 2013, when 23.5% of men and 14.9% of women were working, representing 5% of the US labor force. Interestingly, participation in the workforce by men aged 65 and over declined steadily from 1900 through the 1980s. After remaining level for nearly two decades, participation of older adults in the workforce has been steadily increasing since 2002.[1]

Evaluation of workers aged 51 to 56 in 1992 and 2004 as part of the Health and Retirement Study suggests that lower rates of retiree health insurance from employers, higher levels of educational attainment, and lower rates of defined benefit pension coverage have led significantly more workers from the 2004 cohort to expect to work past age 65, compared to the 1992 cohort.[51] Many older workers indicate that they would prefer phasing down – that is, continuing to do some paid work when they retire. Others approaching or in retirement opt for a retirement career. There are many in good health and who have financial stability or a satisfactory pension who would prefer to pursue a retirement career with passion. This may be part-time or full-time. The person retiring today at age 65 or younger may enjoy a retirement career that might span 10–20 years. Society must allow elders to fulfill such roles, and to retain the wisdom that has accumulated with time. Then again, there are those approaching retirement who would not want or be able to continue employment, whether in their former role or in new roles that could be created. All of these variations need to be considered in counseling our patients.

Compassionate care

In an increasingly technological society, caring and compassion must be foremost in the practice of medicine. We must avoid the possible dehumanization that takes place when patients simply become subjects for study and treatment. Every year in the United States, we are seeing new accomplishments in medical technology and specialization. Every increasing sophistication of diagnostic testing, including computerized tomography, computerized nuclear medicine, magnetic resonance imaging, positron emission tomography, organ transplants, and achievements in cardiovascular surgery, hemodialysis, intensive and critical care along with the increased impact of genomics, proteinomics, and personalized medicine all have become part of our routine medical environment. In such a medical world, it is imperative that compassionate care not be lost in daily encounters between health professionals and elderly patients.

In all the great religions, various forms of a Golden Rule are stated; many religions teach: "You must love your neighbor as you do yourself" and "What you do not want done to yourself, do not do to others." Surpassing new technical achievements and new specialized knowledge is the need to express compassion. Hippocrates reminds us that the physician's duty is "to cure sometimes, treat often, comfort always."

Critically important is the attitude of the doctor toward the elderly patient. Is the physician willing to spend time with the patient? Is the physician willing to be involved in the chronic and long-term aspects of the patient as well as in the acute illness? Is the physician concerned with the social, psychological, and family aspects of the patient, in addition to clinical and organic aspects?

Care and compassion mean that the physician must dispense sufficient time with elderly patients. There is evidence in one study that physicians spent less time with elderly patients than with younger ones, even before current pressures on clinical productivity drove down the time physicians spend with patients. [52] Fifteen to twenty minutes may be minimal time to carry out a visit in the office, home, hospital, or long-term care facility. One and one-half hours, not necessarily in one sitting, may be required to complete an examination of a new patient, particularly in the presence of multiple complex problems. More time will be required in each encounter or more frequent encounters scheduled if the various functions of counseling, psychologic support, health maintenance, and prevention are to be carried out, in addition to making decisions about treatment and possible rehabilitation.

The physician should be a good listener and read between the lines when the patient is speaking. Often, by nonverbal means, the physician can express warmth, understanding, and empathy. Staying close to the patient and maintaining eye contact is helpful. Sitting adjacent to the patient's bed or sitting on the edge of the bed in the hospital or long-term care facility brings the doctor right into the patient's small universe. The physician might put a hand on the patient's shoulder and pat or touch the patient or hold hands at appropriate points during the visit. But, as previously stated, the physician, faced with increasing pressures, may not be present for the patient. As primary care practices transition to patient-centered medical homes, one benefit will be the expanded team available to contribute to the care of older patients and their families, bringing not only additional skills and expertise but additional time to get to know the patient and understand the context and priorities for his or her care.

As the revered physician, Eugene Stead, Jr., would say: "What this patient needs is a doctor."[53] Our elderly patients – and in fact all of our patients – are yearning for a physician who will listen and understand. Again, we remember Peabody's words: "One of the essential qualities of the clinician is interest in humanity, where the secret of the care of the patient is in caring for the patient."[24]

Changing times in health care

In the performance of these essential aspects of care of the elderly patient, the physician may be distraught that these are difficult times, when the delivery and payment models are changing rapidly and not always predictably. Physicians and other health professionals may feel discouraged during this period of cost-containment, evolving pay-for-performance rules, increased competition, threats of malpractice, and other forces in health-care reform taking place today. The physician may be disheartened by a system that frequently rewards doing a procedure over talking to a patient, that scrutinizes and profiles the physician in the hospital, and that often seems to emphasize the financial bottom line rather than excellence of patient care. Despite this tug of war, the physician must simply have faith that excellence of patient care that is compassionate and humane, care that is characterized by continuity, care that is sensitive to psychosocial and family issues, and care that is characterized by all the other essential principles will endure. As mentioned previously, the promise of the Triple Aim, that better care is actually less expensive, is informing current reform efforts.[45] In the long run, these trends promise to reward physicians who engage with these fundamental principles.

Although the organization of health-care delivery will undoubtedly change, we can expect society to ultimately demand a quality of care that we would each want for ourselves. The authors can visualize social pressure enforcing the maintenance of quality of care, patient satisfaction, and the fulfillment of the professional ethic of medicine and the other health-care professions. The example of the Federal Aviation

Agency to the aviation industry (which is characterized in the United States by high standards of safety and quality) has been cited as one model that the current changing health-care system might follow.

We have already discussed the work of Frankl and Yalom, and the presence of an existential vacuum.[25–27] The physician caring for 80- and 90-year-old patients must be prepared to hear the patient utter, "I don't know why I'm still here" or "I don't know why God doesn't take me away. I have lived long enough." The physician must be alert to the presence of depression and suicidal ideation. But if the physician's assessment is that these statements do not represent suicidal thoughts, then the physician must be prepared to respond to ruminations about death that are heard commonly in the oldest old. Without entering too much into the world of theology, it is certainly appropriate for the physician to remind the patient of relationships and activities that he or she still enjoys, and to reinforce hope in the future. For instance, the physician can point to his or her own relationship with the patient, or that of a dear friend or favorite relative. Many older patients are eager to participate in life events of younger generations: a graduation, a wedding, the birth of a new child. Further, in the absence of significant dementia, most elders continue to engage in and enjoy lifelong or new hobbies, such as listening to music, creating art, reading, and watching movies.

What about the extraordinarily independent patient who is feisty and maybe a bit eccentric? This patient will not accept what seems to be needed treatment or will refuse home health aides or day care. Others have divorced themselves from the medical system, at least for the present time, because of a past experience that was burdensome, expensive, and seemingly unnecessary. Some will refuse supports such as having health aides because they do not want the burden of strangers in their home or the expense of this assistance (even though they can afford it). They do not want to divert their savings in case they need it in the future or in order not to reduce an inheritance to a loved one. They may recall bad experiences when health-care bills amounted to thousands of dollars. Or the patient may be wary of the medical system, remembering that each time she suffered a fractured vertebra related to her osteoporosis, she was kept in the hospital emergency room for 12–36 hours and underwent repeated bone scans and other seemingly needless tests. It would seem

prudent to state the case for what is reasonable, but to allow as much self-determination and autonomous action as possible. This respect for the patient's autonomy may help cement or enhance the doctor–patient relationship. Many elderly people who exhibit extraordinary independence appear to do well despite their selective lack of participation in medical care or other support systems. Segerberg, in *Living to Be 100*, describes anecdotally manifestations of exceptional independence in 1,200 centenarians.[54] Extraordinary independence needs to be studied more as a positive factor in successful aging, at least in some individuals. More recently, self-rated health and cognitive function have been shown to correlate with the Positive Attitude Towards Life domain on the Personality Outlook Profile Scale.[55] Clearly, traits of independence and positive personality have some impact on the length and quality of life.

References

1. Administration on Aging. A profile of older Americans: 2013. US Department of Health and Human Services. Available at: www.aoa.acl.gov/Aging_Statistics/Profile/2013/docs/2013_Profile.pdf (accessed on April 12, 2015).

2. Institute of Medicine. *Crossing the Quality Chasm: A New Health System for the 21st Century*. Washington, DC: National Academy Press, 2001.

3. Berwick D. The IHI Triple Aim. Institute for Healthcare Improvement. Available at: www.ihi.org/Engage/Initiatives/TripleAim/pages/default.aspx (accessed on April 12, 2015).

4. Engel GL. The need for a new medical model: a challenge for biomedicine. *Science*. 1977; **196**:129–136.

5. Fava GA, Sonino N. The biopsychosocial model thirty years later. *Psychother Psychosom*. 2008; **77**:1–2.

6. American Academy of Family Physicians. Joint principles of the patient-centered medical home. Available at: www.aafp.org/dam/AAFP/documents/practice_management/pcmh/initiatives/PCMHJoint.pdf (accessed on December 2, 2015).

7. Braveman P, Egerter S, Williams DR. The social determinants of health: coming of age. *Annual Review of Public Health*. 2011; **32**:381–398.

8. Ranjit N, Diez-Roux AV, Shea S, Cushman M, Seeman T, Jackson SA, Ni H. Psychosocial factors and inflammation in the multi-ethnic study of atherosclerosis. *Arch Intern Med*. 2007; **167**:174–181.

9. Park M, Katon WJ, Wolf FW. Depression and risk of mortality in individuals with diabetes: a meta-analysis and systematic review. *Gen Hosp Psychiatry*. 2013; **35**(3):217–225.

10. Costanzo ES, Lutgendorf SK, Sood AK, Anderson B, Sorosky J, Lubaroff DM. Psychosocial factors and interleukin-6 among women with advanced ovarian cancer. *Cancer.* 2005; **104**(2):305–313.

11. Holmes TH, Rahe RH. The social readjustment rating scale. *J. Psychosomatic Research.* 1967; **11**:213–218.

12. Wagner EH, Coleman K, Reid RJ, Phillips K, Abrams MK, Sugarman JR. The changes involved in patient-centered medical home transformation. *Prim Care.* 2012; **39**(2):241–259.

13. Fulmer T. Gaines M. Partnering with patients, families, and communities to link interprofessional practice and education. Proceedings of a conference sponsored by the Josiah Macy Jr. Foundation in April 2014. New York: Josiah Macy Jr. Foundation, 2014.

14. Reichel W. The continuity imperative. *JAMA.* 1981; **246**:2065.

15. Jones CD, Vu MB, O'Donnell CM, Anderson ME, Patel S, Wald HL, Coleman EA, DeWalt DA. A failure to communicate: a qualitative exploration of care coordination between hospitalists and primary care providers around patient hospitalizations. *JGIM.* 2014; **30**(4):417–424.

16. Coleman EA, Smith JD, Frank JC, Min SJ, Parry C, Dramer AM. Preparing patients and caregivers to participate in care delivered across settings: the care transitions intervention. *JAGS.* 2004; **52**(11):1817–1825.

17. Clancy CM. Care transitions: a threat and an opportunity for patient safety. *Am J of Med Qual.* 2006; **21**:415–417.

18. Grabowski DC, Stevenson DG, Cornell PY. Assisted living expansion and the market for nursing home care. *Health Services Research.* 2012; **47**(6):2296–2315.

19. Meret-Hanke LA. Effects of the program of all-inclusive care for the elderly on hospital use. *Gerontologist.* 2011; **51**(6): 774–785.

20. Belle SH, Burgio L, Burns R, Coon D, Czaja SJ, Gallagher-Thompson D, et al. Resources for Enhancing Alzheimer's Caregiver Health (REACH) II Investigators. Enhancing the quality of life of dementia caregivers from different ethnic or racial groups: a randomized, controlled trial. *Ann of Int Med.* 2006; **145**(10): 727–738.

21. Family Caregiver Alliance National Center on Caregiving. Available at: https://caregiver.org/selected-caregiver-statistics (accessed on April 18, 2015).

22. Pinuart M, Sorensen S. Correlates of physical health of informal caregivers: a meta-analysis. *J Gerontology Series B-Psych Sci & Social Sci.* 2007; **62**(2):126–137.

23. Parks SM, Novielli KD. A practical guide to caring for caregivers. *Am Fam Physician.* 2000; **62**(12):2613–2622.

24. Peabody FW. The care of the patient. *JAMA.* 1927; **88**: 877–882.

25. Frankl VE. *Man's Search for Meaning.* Boston: Beacon Press, 1959.

26. Frankl VE. *The Doctor and the Soul.* New York: Knopf, 1955.

27. Yalom ID. *Existential Psychotherapy.* New York: Basic Books, Inc., 1980.

28. Cassel EJ. The nature of suffering and the goals of medicine. *NEJM.* 1982; **306**: 639–645.

29. Kushner H. *When All You've Ever Wanted Isn't Enough.* New York: Summit Books, 1986.

30. Cousins N. The physician as communicator. *JAMA.* 1982; **248**:587–589.

31. Frank JD, Frank JB. *Persuasion and Healing: A Comparative Study of Psychotherapy.* 3rd edition. Baltimore: Johns Hopkins University Press, 1991.

32. Elon, R. Personal communication.

33. National Institute on Aging. Baltimore longitudinal study of aging. Available at: www.blsa.nih.gov (accessed on April 17, 2015).

34. Elahi D, Clark B, Andres R. Glucose tolerance, insulin sensitivity and age. In: Armbracht HJ, Coe RM, Wongsurawat N. eds. *Endocrine Function and Aging.* New York: Springer-Verlag, 1990: 48–63.

35. American Geriatrics Society Expert Panel on the Care of Older Adults with Diabetes Mellitus. Guidelines abstracted from the American Geriatric Society Guidelines for improving the care of older adults with diabetes mellitus: 2013 update. *JAGS.* 2013; **61**(11): 2020–2026.

36. Campanelli, C. M. for the American Geriatrics Society 2012 Beers Criteria Update Expert Panel. American Geriatrics Society updated Beers criteria for potentially inappropriate medication use in older adults. *JAGS.* 2012; **60**(4):616–631.

37. Norman DC. Fever in the elderly. *Clinical Infectious Disesases.* 2000; **31**(1):148–151.

38. Gibson SJ, Helme RD. Age-related differences in pain perception and report. *Clinics in Geriatric Medicine.* 2001; **17**(3):433–456.

39. Chou C-H, Hwang C-L, and Wu Y-T. Effect of exercise on physical function, daily living activities, and quality of life in the frail older adults: a meta-analysis. *Archives of Physical Medicine and Rehabilitation.* 2012; **93**(2):237–244.

40. US Preventive Services Task Force. *The Guide to Clinical Preventive Services 2014.* Washington, DC: Agency for Healthcare Research and Quality, 2014.

41. American Cancer Society. Recommendations for prostate cancer early detection. Available at: www.cancer.org/cancer/prostatecancer/moreinformation/prostatecancerearlydetection/prostate-cancer-early-detection-acs-recommendations (accessed on April 17, 2015).

42. Seegal D. The principle of minimal interference in the management of the elderly patient. *J Chron Dis.* 1964; **17**:299–300.

43. Reichel W. Complications in the care of 500 elderly hospitalized patients. *JAGS.* 1965; **13**:973–981.

44. Long SJ, Brown KF, Ames D, Vincent C. What is known about adverse events in older medical hospital inpatients? A systematic review of the literature. *International Journal for Quality in Health Care.* 2013; **25**(5):542–554.

45. Berwick DM, Nolan TW, Whittington J. The Triple Aim: care, health, and cost. *Health Affairs.* 2008; **27**(3):759–769.

46. ABIM Foundation. Choosing Wisely: An initiative of the ABIM Foundation. Available at: www.choosingwisely.org (accessed on April 18 2015).

47. American Geriatrics Society. Ten things physicians and patients should question. Choosing Wisely: An Initiative of the ABIM Foundation. Available at: www.choosingwisely.org/doctor-patient-lists/american-geriatrics-society (accessed on April 18, 2015).

48. Zwarenstein M, Goldman J, Reeves S. Interprofessional collaboration: effects of practice-based interventions on professional practice and healthcare outcomes. *Cochrane Database of Systematic Reviews.* 2009; **3**:CD000072. DOI:10.1002/14651858.CD000072.pub2.

49. Hopkins D (ed). *Framework for Action on Interprofessional Education & Collaborative Practice* (WHO/HRH/HPN/10.3). Geneva, Switzerland: Health Professions Network Nursing and Midwifery Office, Department of Human Resources for Health, World Health Organization. 2010.

50. Lipp MR. *Respectful Treatment: A Practical Handbook of Patient Care.* 2nd edition. New York: Elsevier, 1986.

51. Mermin GB, Johnson RW, Murphy DP. Why do boomers plan to work longer? *J Gerontology Series B-Psych Sci & Social Sci.* 2007; **625**:S286–S294.

52. Keeler EB, Solomon DH, Beck JC, Mendenhall RC, Kane RL. Effect of patient age on duration of medical encounters with physicians. *Med Care.* 1982; **20**:1101–1108.

53. Wagner GS, Cebe B, Rozear MP (eds). *E. A. Stead, Jr.: What This Patient Needs Is a Doctor.* Durham, NC: Carolina Academic Press, 1978.

54. Segerberg O. *Living to Be 100.* New York: Charles Scribners Sons, 1982.

55. Kato K, Zweig R, Schechter CB, Verghese J, Barzilai N, Atzmon G. Personality, self-rated health, and cognition in centenarians: do personality and self-rated health relate to cognitive function in advanced age? *Aging.* 2013; **5**(3):183–191.

Chapter

2

The biology of aging

Allyson K. Palmer, BA, and James L. Kirkland, MD, PhD

Introduction

The term "aging" refers not only to humans progressing chronologically from conception to death; it also refers to the molecular, physiologic, and functional changes that occur during the lifespan. Aging processes are universal within a species, intrinsic, and progressive. Aging is "universal" because all individuals in a species exhibit the particular aging changes if they live long enough. It is "intrinsic" because aging changes occur despite environmental cues, although environmental cues can influence the timing of the aging change. "Progressive" refers to the time-dependent development of aging processes. Age-related changes or diseases are phenotypes of fundamental aging processes that occur globally or locally at particular stages in life – for example, development of dementia or certain cancers, such as prostate cancer. These age-related changes are heterogeneous, with varied effects across tissues of the body, and cause pathology at different times across individuals. Aging is generally associated with a decline in tissue and global function, loss of reproductive capacity, and waning resilience, or ability to adapt to environmental stressors.

The biology of aging is deeply rooted in the study of lifespan and the identification of factors that allow certain individuals – for example, centenarians, within the human population, or entire species, such as naked mole rats – to live exceptionally long lives. Lifespan is arguably the best biomarker for following effects of interventions that alter fundamental aging processes. While these investigations are ongoing and important for understanding the basis and limitations of lifespan, the aging research community has shifted its focus in part to improving human "healthspan," or the amount of time lived without significant disease or debilitation. The common risk factor for cognitive decline,

metabolic syndrome, cardiovascular disease, cancer, and many other ailments is age. By targeting mechanisms shared by age-related diseases and aging itself, biological and aging researchers hope to delay these diseases as a group instead of one at a time, thus extending healthspan, improving the quality of life of the population, and perhaps also increasing maximum lifespan.[1, 2]

Fundamental aging mechanisms are generally conserved across species; therefore findings related to aging in lower species are more likely to be translatable than is the case for many other areas of research (i.e., disease-specific investigation). It is beneficial to have reliable animal models with short lifespans, since investigation of modulators of the human lifespan is generally impractical. While disease-specific therapeutic strategies might allow risk to shift from one disease (e.g., heart disease) to another (e.g., cancer), a delay of aging processes could slow the development of diseases as a group and extend human healthspan by allowing longer disease-free survival.[1] This potential for translation to humans underscores the importance of basic aging biology research. This research will lead to interventions that could transform geriatrics clinical practice from one that aims to treat age-related pathologies and maintain activities of daily living in the context of preexisting conditions, to a dynamic practice that specifically targets fundamental aging processes in order to slow or prevent the initial occurrence of disease, dysfunction, and loss of resilience.

Theories of aging

Why do people age, and how did the aging process evolve? Why is there such a wide range of lifespan

Reichel's Care of the Elderly, 7th Edition, ed. Jan Busby-Whitehead *et al.* Published by Cambridge University Press.
© Cambridge University Press 2016.

within the animal kingdom? What is the limit to human lifespan? Are aging mechanisms modifiable, reversible, or preventable? The complex process of aging has prompted the development of many theories to explain it, once reported to exceed 300.[3] These include many proximal hypotheses – for example, the telomere erosion theory or the neuroendocrine theory – which ultimately collapse into several broader conceptual theories that attempt to explain the purpose or origins of aging. The following is one system of categorizing these theories.

Evolutionary senescence

The earliest theories of aging and death held that limited lifespan creates room for upcoming generations, therefore helping the species as a whole. This would also allow natural selection for the fittest individuals to occur faster, with more individuals being born per unit of time. However, in nature, mortality usually has little to do with aging, and is more commonly associated with environmental, or extrinsic, factors, such as predation, infectious disease, or starvation.[4] An evolutionary theory of aging rose from the work of J. B. S. Haldane, Peter Medawar, and George Williams, based on the idea that natural selection acts at an individual level, not a species level, and that only genes involved in survival and health preceding the reproductive period would be acted upon by natural selection.[5] There is less need to maintain integrity of processes such as macromolecular repair and tight control of molecular pathways as organisms progress beyond sexual maturity, when the fitness of the organism is no longer evolutionarily relevant. Therefore natural selection's effects would decline with age, and mutations that are deleterious in older age will be passed on before they are able to negatively affect the organism. Later in life these deleterious mutations would give rise to aging phenotypes. This became known as the mutation accumulation theory.

A related theory, that of antagonistic pleiotropy, states that genes responsible for aging processes may not have been passively allowed, as in the mutation accumulation theory, but that they may have actually undergone positive selection due to some benefit they confer to individuals in early life.[5] These benefits would outweigh deleterious pro-aging effects past reproductive age, which are less subject to evolutionary pressures. Cellular senescence, which will be discussed later in the chapter, is considered to be an

example of antagonistic pleiotropy because it defends against malignancy in early life but contributes to disease and tissue dysfunction later in life.

A third evolutionary theory of aging is that of the disposable soma, proposed by Thomas Kirkwood.[6, 7] Because an organism has a finite amount of resources and energy, it must choose to allocate them among the processes of growth, repair, and reproduction. Enough resources must be allocated to repair in order to prevent what has been called "error catastrophe," or the accumulation of so many units of damage or error that the organism can no longer survive.[8] However, some basal level of error must be allowed because energy must be allocated to the essential processes of reproduction and metabolism. It follows that species threatened by predation should allocate more energy to reaching reproductive capacity rather than repairing damage, and may thus have an increased rate of aging. Therefore, safer environments should favor a reduced rate of aging, and organisms that reproduce later in life should have a reduced rate of aging, since selective pressure would persist longer into the lifespan.

Programmed aging

The programmed aging theory rejects the possibility that aging is a stochastic process of wear and tear on an organism, and suggests that aging is programmed just as development is. Subsets of this theory propose genetic, hormonal, or immunologic control of aging and longevity.

The idea that genes evolved to modulate longevity has been mostly discounted based on the idea that natural selection has most of its effects before the reproductive stage of life. However, it is plausible that certain gene variants may confer lifespan advantages, or that gene expression may change to favor deleterious processes later in life. Many pathways have been implicated in a genetic basis for aging in model systems such as yeast and the nematode $C.$ $elegans$, most notably the growth hormone/insulin-like growth factor (IGF-1) pathway, as will be discussed.[9] In humans, the link between genetics and a long and healthy life is more elusive, although familial clustering of longevity has been reported. [10, 11] Many studies of centenarians hinge on the idea that genes having increased prevalence with age should confer benefits to lifespan. Several variants have been identified that seem to correlate with longer life – for example variants in the apolipoprotein E (APO-E) and IGF-1 signaling pathways – but these studies have yet to find a smoking gun for the longevity phenotype.

Hormones modulate metabolic activity and insulin sensitivity regulate oxidative stress, drive maturation, and direct processes such as bone formation and remodeling that have huge impacts on organismal health.[12] Thus, there is much interest in the possibility that hormones influence aging by a sort of biological clock, and that changes in hormone levels over the lifespan cause age-related phenotypes. The longest-lived mouse is the Ames dwarf mouse, which has a 70% greater maximum lifespan than nonmutant mice.[13] These dwarf mice are deficient in growth hormone as well as prolactin and thyroid-stimulating hormone. Growth hormone receptor knockout mice also have increased maximum lifespan [14] as do other vertebrates and invertebrate species with reduced growth hormone/IGF-1 action. Interestingly, humans with Laron dwarfism lacking the growth hormone receptor have essentially no risk of diabetes or cancer, even in old age.[15] Female children of centenarians with an IGF receptor mutation, in addition to having a longer life expectancy than their spouses, have shorter stature than their spouses.[16] Furthermore, smaller individuals within a species live longer on average than larger members (e.g., small versus large dogs). This, in turn, has been linked to reduced growth hormone/IGF-1 signaling.[17]

The immunosenescence theory of aging points to a decline in immunity with age that can cause increased susceptibility to infection and therefore increased mortality. Immune cells, in addition to having a limited replication capacity, undergo a decline in function in aging organisms – for example, decreased activation potential of T cells in older individuals.[18] In addition, it has been proposed that anti-inflammatory pathways may also decline in function with age, allowing the development of a chronic, low-grade sterile inflammatory state that causes tissue damage. This imbalance between pro- and anti-inflammatory pathways has been termed "inflammaging."[19]

Somatic inevitability

The somatic inevitability theory, also known as the wear-and-tear theory, addresses the practical concern that organisms simply cannot have normal function indefinitely, due to environmental and metabolic damage as well as a limit to regenerative mechanisms. Aging is therefore an accumulation of damage and an exhaustion of regenerative potential.

One version of this theory is called the rate-of-living hypothesis, which is based on the work of Max Rubner and Raymond Pearl and postulates that lifespan should have an inverse relationship to metabolic rate. Denham Harman later linked this theory to free radicals and oxidative stress.[20] However, it has since been determined that the rate of living of an organism cannot alone account for its lifespan potential. For example, naked mole rats and mice are approximately the same size, and although naked mole rats have a tenfold longer lifespan than mice, they have an increased metabolic rate and free radical generation compared to mice.[21] Other components of the wear-and-tear theory are the cross-linking theory, in which the accumulation of protein cross-links and glycation of macromolecules slow down metabolic processes and cause age-related dysfunction, and the DNA damage theory, in which accumulated DNA damage during the lifespan causes cellular and mitochondrial dysfunction that lead to age-related pathology.

Tissue-level changes with age

Regardless of the validity of global aging theories, there are many processes at the cellular and tissue level that manifest change, or wane with age. These age-related changes can be grouped into four main interrelated pathways in aging and age-related diseases, which are outlined as follows. Each category represents an important component of age-related disease and offers potential targets for the development of therapies for aging and age-related diseases. The onset of human diseases, which often occur as a group, represents the intersection of these aging changes over time.

Chronic, "sterile" inflammation

Low-level, chronic inflammation is detected in many tissues with increasing age and is associated with age-related disease states such as diabetes, Alzheimer's disease, sarcopenia, and atherosclerosis.[19] Age-related sterile inflammation is frequently associated with the infiltration of immune cells as well as the release of pro-inflammatory cytokines such as interleukin 6 (IL-6) and interleukin 8 (IL-8). This chronic inflammation is known as sterile inflammation due to the lack of detectable pathogens or the characteristic redness, pain, heat, or swelling seen in local, acute inflammation. The source of this chronic inflammation has not been well defined, although candidate sources include diminished regulation of the immune system, oxidative stress, chronic antigenic stress, and senescent cell accumulation.[19, 22]

In humans, the inflammatory factors IL-6 and C-reactive protein have been implicated as predictors of mortality, independent of age, sex, body mass index (BMI), smoking status, diabetes, or cardiovascular disease.[23] IL-6 alone has been shown to be a correlate of frailty and a predictor of functional disability in older adults.[24, 25] With enough evidence and reliable measurement strategies, immunologic biomarkers may help us to predict which individuals are more likely to experience disability, frailty, or morbidity in the near future. This could allow preventative measures to be taken before the onset of disease or disability, and perhaps these biomarkers can even be used to follow response to interventions.

Cellular senescence

Cellular senescence is an essentially irreversible growth arrest that can be triggered by a host of stimuli – including but not limited to oncogene activation, oxidative stress, metabolic stress, and telomere erosion – that evolved as a defense against tumor formation. Cells that undergo senescence adopt a characteristic enlarged shape, accumulate tumor suppressor proteins such as p21 and p16, exhibit a senescence-associated increase in beta galactosidase activity, and begin to secrete a variety of growth factors, cytokines, and matrix remodeling factors, collectively termed the senescence-associated secretory phenotype (SASP).[26] Often cited as an example of antagonistic pleiotropy, senescent cells protect organisms against malignancy in early life but can have detrimental effects as they accumulate in tissues with age, paradoxically including the promotion of pro-tumor environments.[27]

The burden of senescent cells in human skin correlates with age.[28] They also accumulate in adipose tissue with advancing age in wild-type mice, but at a slower rate in long-lived Ames and growth hormone receptor deficient mice.[29] Cellular

senescence and the resulting SASP are thought to produce a chronic, low-level inflammatory state in the body and have been implicated in a variety of age-related pathologies.[27, 30] Recent work in genetic mouse models allowing clearance of senescent cells has established a causal link between cellular senescence and age-related disease by showing that removal of senescent cells from progeroid mice can extend healthspan and delay age-related phenotypes, such as subcutaneous fat tissue loss, cataract formation, and sarcopenia. In addition, senescent cell removal later in life stalled progression of age-related pathology, even after it had emerged.[31] These studies support a causal link of senescent cells to age-related disease pathologies and establish senescent cells and their secretory phenotype as promising targets for developing agents to delay, prevent, ameliorate, or treat age-related diseases and dysfunction.[22]

Macromolecular dysfunction

At the most fundamental level, aging has profound effects on macromolecules, including protein, DNA, RNA, and lipids. These changes can fall into two categories: processes that decline or become defective with age, such as DNA damage repair or autophagy, or processes that are less common early in life but which occur more frequently with age, such as advanced glycation end product formation and lipotoxicity.

Organisms acquire genomic damage over time through exposure to the environment and metabolic byproducts, and they require the action of DNA repair mechanisms to deal with these insults. Accordingly, a positive correlation between DNA repair and longevity has been shown, as well as premature aging phenotypes in mice with genetic ablation of genome repair mechanisms.[32] Accumulation of mitochondrial DNA damage, thought to be mainly caused by reactive oxygen species (ROS), could cause mitochondrial dysfunction with age, leading to less efficient adenosine triphosphate (ATP) production. This age-related mitochondrial dysfunction might play a major role in cardiovascular, metabolic, skeletal, and other age-related pathologies.[33] Other levels of genetic regulation can also be compromised with aging (e.g., at the level of noncoding RNA). Dysregulation of cellular processes can occur in part because of an age-related decline in Dicer protein, which processes microRNA.[34]

Alteration of proteins, including increased glycation, oxidation, and cross-linking, paired with reduced turnover of proteins, or autophagy, can cause cellular dysfunction and protein aggregation with age. Aggregation of proteins is known to play a role in many diseases, such as Alzheimer's, Parkinson's, insulin-dependent diabetes, dilated cardiomyopathy, and glomerulosclerosis.[35] Rates of autophagy decline with age, and conversely, genetic inhibition of autophagy mimics aging pathology.[36]

In addition to proteins, glycation can affect phospholipids and nucleic acids to form what are known as advanced glycation end products (AGEs). With age, defenses against the formation of these glycation adducts is reduced. AGEs can activate to pro-inflammatory signaling cascades by input through a cell surface receptor-mediated mechanism (RAGE).[37] AGEs are known to accumulate in normal aging brains, but have also been implicated in cultured neuron toxicity as well as amyloid beta ($A\beta$) aggregation.[38, 39] AGEs have been implicated in the pathogenesis of diabetes and its complications.[40]

With age, even lean individuals acquire ectopic lipid deposition in non-adipose tissues such as muscle, liver, and pancreatic beta cells. This can lead to lipotoxicity, which contributes to metabolic dysfunction, especially in the setting of overnutrition.[41] Defenses against lipotoxicity at both the cellular and organismal level are also blunted with age, exacerbating lipotoxic effects on tissues.[42, 43]

In sum, the accumulation of damage paired with a loss of regulatory mechanisms causes increased stochasticity with age, which results in tissue dysfunction and disease. Because the repair and regulatory mechanisms that control these processes are so fundamental, and because their failure with age is implicated in many age-related diseases, these mechanisms represent possible targets for the development of clinical interventions with potentially transformative impact.

Progenitor cell function decline

Stem cell and progenitor pools are not unlimited and may become depleted with age and increased need for tissue repair. In addition, intrinsic stem cell function declines with age. Aged stem cells may fail to self-renew, fail to respond to growth and differentiation signals in their environment, or may undergo senescence.[44] Even if they are able to differentiate, stem cells may produce a skewed population of progeny cells – for example, a skew toward the myeloid

lineage with age in the context of the hematopoietic system.[45]

The aging microenvironment, both local and systemic, also plays a large role in the dysfunction of stem cells with aging. The chronic, sterile inflammation of aging may contribute to a toxic or suppressive environment that does not allow proper stem cell function. In addition, crosstalk between organ systems – for example, between adipose tissue and bone – is known to affect progenitor cell function and could serve as a mechanism for the propagation of aging signals. [46] Heterochronic parabiosis experiments, in which an experimental animal is exposed to the systemic circulation of a separate animal, have shown that exposure to a young circulating environment can rejuvenate stem cells from aging animals.[47] This suggests that aging progenitor cells may have at least some preservation of function, but their replicative capacity is suppressed by the aging microenvironment.

The human lifespan

Centenarians

At the 2010 census, there were 1.74 centenarians for every 10,000 people in the United States. Notably, those individuals living more than 100 years often experience a "compression of morbidity," developing cancer, heart disease, and other common ailments much later in life than the population at large.[48, 49] This effect becomes more apparent in supercentenarians, or those living more than 110 years, exemplified in a 2012 study classifying 69% of people older than 110 as "escapers" who had experienced onset of only one age-related disease after the age of 100.[50]

There has been a longstanding interest in determining characteristics that differentiate centenarians from the general population. Genome-wide association studies have been conducted to compare the genetic makeup of centenarians' children with the spouses of those children, presumably not descendants of centenarians. These studies have struggled to find strong correlations between any single nucleotide polymorphism and exceptional lifespan.[51] A 1994 study found that ApoE4 mutations predisposing to atherosclerosis were less common in centenarians as compared to a general population of age 20 to 70.[52] Polymorphisms in insulin signaling pathway genes (e.g., FOXO3A) have also been implicated in human longevity, consistent with work showing that inhibition of insulin signaling extends lifespan in *C. elegans* and mice. [53–55]

Premature aging in HIV patients and survivors of childhood cancers

Treatments that prolong life in patients with human immunodeficiency virus (HIV) and cancer have recently been implicated in premature aging. Patients with HIV, even well controlled, seem to develop age-related diseases prematurely. This may be partially due to residual infection, coinfection (e.g., viral hepatitis), and chronic activation of the immune system that leads to exhaustion of immune cells and inflammation. However, antiretroviral (HAART) therapy has also been implicated as a source of oxidative and mitochondrial damage that may contribute to premature aging, and has been linked to dysfunction of multiple organ systems as well as increased deposition of Tau protein, a neurodegenerative marker.[56]

Individuals who underwent treatment for childhood cancers are another population in which premature aging syndrome has been observed. Frailty phenotypes have been found to be more prevalent in survivors of childhood cancer, especially in females, compared to an age-matched control group.[57] These individuals have also started to show early incidence of diseases such as coronary artery disease, which are normally associated with aging and therefore not usually screened for until later in life.[58] These findings have implications for the long-term care of this emerging cohort, which continues to be rigorously studied.

Gender differences in longevity

It has long been observed that human females have a longer life expectancy than males. Eighty-two percent of centenarians in the 2010 census were female.[59] As noted earlier, pharmacologic lifespan extension strategies in basic research have shown differential effects on male and female experimental animals, as do some single gene mutations such as IGF-1 receptor deficiency. These observations introduce a new wrinkle into aging research by suggesting that lifespan- or healthspan-extending strategies may not have similar effects in males and females. On the other hand, this observation presents an opportunity. If we can discover the pathways responsible for greater female longevity, we may be able to target that pathway pharmacologically to the benefit of both older men and women.

Disparities in US lifespan

Disparities in longevity exist within the United States that cannot be easily attributed to metabolism, genetics, or other basic biological processes. Nearly 83% of centenarians in 2010 were white, whereas only 5.8% were Hispanic, compared to 72.4% and 16.3% in the general population, respectively.[59] In regard to ordinary longevity, Native Americans have a life expectancy that is 4.1 years lower than that of the general population, and in Hawaii, Native Hawaiians have close to 10 years lower life expectancy than the longest-lived ethnic group in the state, the Japanese.[60] African-American males and females are expected to live 4.7 and 3.3 years less than their white counterparts, based on the CDC's 2014 life tables.[61] These differences in life expectancy are a direct reflection of health disparities that exist in the United States, and the underlying public health issues deserve as much attention and research as the limits of human lifespan.

Clinical translation of aging biology research

Healthspan interventions

Decades of aging research conducted in worms, flies, rodents, and nonhuman primates have laid a solid foundation for translation of basic aging biology to humans. Efforts are underway to exploit fundamental aging mechanisms elucidated through basic research to develop therapeutic strategies to improve healthspan and delay age-related disease. It is impractical to study the success of experimental strategies to extend lifespan and healthspan in humans, but the effectiveness of a new therapy cannot be approved without clinical data. Therefore, logical and useful parameters must be established to allow researchers to track success of lifespan and healthspan interventions as they are translated to humans. These parameters may be measures of frailty or resilience (e.g., recovery after elective surgery, chemotherapy, myocardial infarction, etc.). They might also include multiple age-related chronic disease outcomes in patients with comorbidities. Symptoms of progeria might also serve as markers of success. In addition, short-term studies may be appropriate for agents that are expected to reverse age-related pathology in older individuals.

Factors that are known to affect maximum lifespan are caloric restriction, several hundred single-gene mutations across species, and an increasing number of pharmacologic agents. There are currently at least 12 drugs known to increase lifespan in various model organisms; some of the studies are still to be published. These drugs include rapamycin,[62, 63] curcumin (effective in *Drosophila*),[64] metformin,[65] and several drugs that have preferential effects on male mice: aspirin (which affects median but perhaps not maximum lifespan),[66] 17a-estradiol,[67] acarbose,[67] and nordihydroguaiaretic acid (NDGA).[67] In addition to efforts by individual research programs, the Interventions Testing Program (ITP), funded by the National Institute on Aging, is a collaborative effort to find treatments that extend lifespan or healthspan in mice, based on basic aging research in lower organisms or smaller studies in mammals, that may be amenable to clinical translation.

Caloric restriction

Caloric restriction (CR) is known to extend lifespan in yeast, worms, flies, and rodents and has been shown to affect a large number of downstream metabolic and post-transcriptional pathways.[68] More limited data in primates has been unable to clearly link CR with lifespan extension; however, delayed onset of age-related disease has been shown in calorie-restricted rhesus monkeys.[69,70] Although humans practicing caloric restriction exhibit a range of improved metabolic phenotypes – including decreased body weight and fasting glucose, increased insulin sensitivity, and low prevalence of metabolic syndrome – CR has also been shown to have negative effects on quality of life. These effects can include irritability, slow wound healing, decreased libido, and reduced body temperature.[71]

Senolytic therapy

Cellular senescence has been implicated in chronic sterile inflammation, age-related diseases, and the promotion of tumor spread. As previously mentioned, clearance of senescent cells in mice has

beneficial effects in both the amelioration of preexisting disease phenotypes and in the prevention of onset of age-related disease phenotypes. Therefore, there is great interest in translating these results into the prevention and treatment of human disease.[22] This requires selective targeting of senescent cells without disruption of surrounding normal cells and preservation of tissue architecture, which is no small feat. Another strategy to prevent the detrimental effects of senescent cells is to target SASP components, either one by one or as a group, and either locally or systemically, depending on the disease process being treated.

Conclusion

Many theories exist to explain why we age, but the common biological mechanisms underlying the aging process are becoming clearer through aging biology research, a field that has been moving rapidly in the past decade. By understanding the basic mechanisms of aging – such as cellular senescence, inflammation, decline of regenerative potential, and immunosenescence – as well as understanding the basis for heterogeneity of longevity, we can exploit these pathways in the development of strategies to reverse or prevent age-related processes. The development of therapeutics that target aging mechanisms has the potential to treat or prevent age-related pathologies as a whole rather than individually. We are at the point where it seems increasingly likely that interventions that target fundamental aging mechanisms could start to be integrated into clinical applications for diseases and disabilities that affect the elderly population.

References

1. Goldman DP, Cutler D, Rowe JW, Michaud PC, Sullivan J, Peneva D, et al. Substantial health and economic returns from delayed aging may warrant a new focus for medical research. *Health Affairs*. 2013 Oct; 32(10):1698–705. PubMed PMID: 24101058. Pubmed Central PMCID: 3938188.

2. Kirkland JL. Translating advances from the basic biology of aging into clinical application. *Experimental Gerontology*. 2013 Jan;48(1):1–5. PubMed PMID: 23237984. Pubmed Central PMCID: 3543864.

3. Medvedev ZA. An attempt at a rational classification of theories of aging. *Biological Reviews*. 1990 August 1990;65(3):375–98.

4. Kirkwood TB, Austad SN. Why do we age? *Nature.* 2000 Nov 9;**408**(6809):233–8. PubMed PMID: 11089980.

5. Williams GC. Pleiotropy, natural selection, and the evolution of senescence. *Evolution; International Journal of Organic Evolution.* 1957;**11**(4):398–411.

6. Kirkwood TB. Evolution of ageing. *Nature.* 1977 Nov 24;**270**(5635):301–4. PubMed PMID: 593350.

7. Kirkwood TB, Holliday R. The evolution of ageing and longevity. *Proceedings of the Royal Society of London Series B, Containing papers of a Biological Character Royal Society.* 1979 Sep 21;**205**(1161):531–46. PubMed PMID: 42059.

8. Orgel LE. The maintenance of the accuracy of protein synthesis and its relevance to ageing: a correction. *Proceedings of the National Academy of Sciences of the United States of America.* 1970 Nov;**67**(3):1476. PubMed PMID: 5274472. Pubmed Central PMCID: 283377.

9. Guarente L, Kenyon C. Genetic pathways that regulate ageing in model organisms. *Nature.* 2000 Nov 9;**408**(6809):255–62. PubMed PMID: 11089983.

10. Perls TT, Wilmoth J, Levenson R, Drinkwater M, Cohen M, Bogan H, et al. Life-long sustained mortality advantage of siblings of centenarians. *Proceedings of the National Academy of Sciences of the United States of America.* 2002 Jun 11;**99**(12):8442–7. PubMed PMID: 12060785. Pubmed Central PMCID: 123086.

11. Schoenmaker M, de Craen AJ, de Meijer PH, Beekman M, Blauw GJ, Slagboom PE, et al. Evidence of genetic enrichment for exceptional survival using a family approach: the Leiden Longevity Study. *European Journal of Human Genetics: EJHG.* 2006 Jan;**14**(1):79–84. PubMed PMID: 16251894.

12. Brown-Borg HM. Hormonal regulation of longevity in mammals. *Ageing Research Reviews.* 2007 May;**6**(1):28–45. PubMed PMID: 17360245. Pubmed Central PMCID: 1978093.

13. Brown-Borg HM, Borg KE, Meliska CJ, Bartke A. Dwarf mice and the ageing process. *Nature.* 1996 Nov 7;**384**(6604):33. PubMed PMID: 8900272.

14. Coschigano KT, Clemmons D, Bellush LL, Kopchick JJ. Assessment of growth parameters and lifespan of GHR/BP gene-disrupted mice. *Endocrinology.* 2000 Jul;**141**(7):2608–13. PubMed PMID: 10875265.

15. Guevara-Aguirre J, Balasubramanian P, Guevara-Aguirre M, Wei M, Madia F, Cheng CW, et al. Growth hormone receptor deficiency is associated with a major reduction in pro-aging signaling, cancer, and diabetes in humans. *Science Translational Medicine.* 2011 Feb 16;**3**(70):70ra13. PubMed PMID: 21325617. Pubmed Central PMCID: 3357623.

16. Suh Y, Atzmon G, Cho MO, Hwang D, Liu B, Leahy DJ, et al. Functionally significant insulin-like growth factor I receptor mutations in centenarians. *Proceedings of the National Academy of Sciences of the United States of America.* 2008 Mar 4;**105**(9):3438–42. PubMed PMID: 18316725. Pubmed Central PMCID: 2265137.

17. Sutter NB, Bustamante CD, Chase K, Gray MM, Zhao K, Zhu L, et al. A single IGF1 allele is a major determinant of small size in dogs. *Science.* 2007 Apr 6;**316**(5821):112–5. PubMed PMID: 17412960. Pubmed Central PMCID: 2789551.

18. Jackola DR, Ruger JK, Miller RA. Age-associated changes in human T cell phenotype and function. *Aging.* 1994 Feb;**6**(1):25–34. PubMed PMID: 8043623.

19. Franceschi C, Capri M, Monti D, Giunta S, Olivieri F, Sevini F, et al. Inflammaging and anti-inflammaging: a systemic perspective on aging and longevity emerged from studies in humans. *Mechanisms of Ageing and Development.* 2007 Jan;**128**(1):92–105. PubMed PMID: 17116321.

20. Harman D. Aging: a theory based on free radical and radiation chemistry. *Journal of Gerontology.* 1956 Jul;**11**(3):298–300. PubMed PMID: 13332224.

21. Edrey YH, Hanes M, Pinto M, Mele J, Buffenstein R. Successful aging and sustained good health in the naked mole rat: a long-lived mammalian model for biogerontology and biomedical research. *ILAR Journal / National Research Council, Institute of Laboratory Animal Resources.* 2011;**52**(1):41–53. PubMed PMID: 21411857.

22. Tchkonia T, Zhu Y, van Deursen J, Campisi J, Kirkland JL. Cellular senescence and the senescent secretory phenotype: therapeutic opportunities. *J Clin Invest.* 2013 Mar 1;**123**(3):966–72. PubMed PMID: 23454759. Pubmed Central PMCID: 3582125.

23. Harris TB, Ferrucci L, Tracy RP, Corti MC, Wacholder S, Ettinger WH, Jr., et al. Associations of elevated interleukin-6 and C-reactive protein levels with mortality in the elderly. *American Journal of Medicine.* 1999 May;**106**(5):506–12. PubMed PMID: 10335721.

24. Cohen HJ, Pieper CF, Harris T, Rao KMK, Currie MS. The association of plasma IL-6 levels with functional disability in community-dwelling elderly. *J Gerontol A Biol.* 1997 Jul;**52**(4):M201–M8. PubMed PMID: WOS:A1997XK46700011. English.

25. Leng S, Chaves P, Koenig K, Walston J. Serum interleukin-6 and hemoglobin as physiological correlates in the geriatric syndrome of frailty: a pilot study. *Journal of the American Geriatrics Society.* 2002 Jul;**50**(7):1268–71. PubMed PMID: 12133023.

26. Coppe JP, Patil CK, Rodier F, Sun Y, Munoz DP, Goldstein J, et al. Senescence-associated secretory phenotypes reveal cell-nonautonomous functions of

oncogenic RAS and the p53 tumor suppressor. PLoS Biology. 2008 Dec 2;6(12):2853–68. PubMed PMID: 19053174. Pubmed Central PMCID: 2592359.

27. Campisi J. Senescent cells, tumor suppression, and organismal aging: good citizens, bad neighbors. *Cell.* 2005 Feb 25;120(4):513–22. PubMed PMID: 15734683. Epub 2005/03/01. eng.

28. Dimri GP, Lee X, Basile G, Acosta M, Scott G, Roskelley C, et al. A biomarker that identifies senescent human cells in culture and in aging skin in vivo. *Proceedings of the National Academy of Sciences of the United States of America.* 1995 Sep 26;92(20):9363–7. PubMed PMID: 7568133. Pubmed Central PMCID: 40985.

29. Stout MB, Tchkonia T, Pirtskhalava T, Palmer AK, List EO, Berryman DE, et al. Growth hormone action predicts age-related white adipose tissue dysfunction and senescent cell burden in mice. *Aging.* 2014 Jul; 6 (7):575–86. Pubmed Central PMCID: 4153624.

30. Jeyapalan JC, Sedivy JM. Cellular senescence and organismal aging. *Mechanisms of Ageing and Development.* 2008 Jul–Aug;129(7–8):467–74. PubMed PMID: 18502472. Pubmed Central PMCID: PMC3297662. Epub 2008/05/27. eng.

31. Baker DJ, Wijshake T, Tchkonia T, LeBrasseur NK, Childs BG, van de Sluis B, et al. Clearance of p16Ink4a-positive senescent cells delays ageing-associated disorders. *Nature.* 2011 Nov 10;479(7372):232–6. PubMed PMID: 22048312. Epub 2011/11/04. eng.

32. Garinis GA, van der Horst GT, Vijg J, Hoeijmakers JH. DNA damage and ageing: new-age ideas for an age-old problem. *Nature Cell Biology.* 2008 Nov;10(11):1241–7. PubMed PMID: 18978832.

33. Dai DF, Chiao YA, Marcinek DJ, Szeto HH, Rabinovitch PS. Mitochondrial oxidative stress in aging and healthspan. *Longevity & Healthspan.* 2014;3:6. PubMed PMID: 24860647. Pubmed Central PMCID: 4013820.

34. Morin P, Jr., Dubuc A, Storey KB. Differential expression of microRNA species in organs of hibernating ground squirrels: a role in translational suppression during torpor. *Biochimica et Biophysica Acta.* 2008 Oct;1779(10):628–33. PubMed PMID: 18723136.

35. Rubinsztein DC, Marino G, Kroemer G. Autophagy and aging. *Cell.* 2011 Sep 2;146(5):682–95. PubMed PMID: 21884931.

36. Madeo F, Tavernarakis N, Kroemer G. Can autophagy promote longevity? *Nature Cell Biology.* 2010 Sep;12 (9):842–6. PubMed PMID: 20811357.

37. Ramasamy R, Vannucci SJ, Yan SS, Herold K, Yan SF, Schmidt AM. Advanced glycation end products and RAGE: a common thread in aging, diabetes, neurodegeneration, and inflammation. *Glycobiology.* 2005 Jul;15(7):16R–28R. PubMed PMID: 15764591.

38. Takeuchi M, Bucala R, Suzuki T, Ohkubo T, Yamazaki M, Koike T, et al. Neurotoxicity of advanced glycation end-products for cultured cortical neurons. *Journal of Neuropathology and Experimental Neurology.* 2000 Dec;59(12):1094–105. PubMed PMID: 11138929.

39. Woltjer RL, Maezawa I, Ou JJ, Montine KS, Montine TJ. Advanced glycation endproduct precursor alters intracellular amyloid-beta/A beta PP carboxy-terminal fragment aggregation and cytotoxicity. *Journal of Alzheimer's Disease.* 2003 Dec;5(6):467–76. PubMed PMID: 14757937.

40. Goh SY, Cooper ME. Clinical review: the role of advanced glycation end products in progression and complications of diabetes. *Journal of Clinical Endocrinology and Metabolism.* 2008 Apr;93(4): 1143–52. PubMed PMID: 18182449.

41. Slawik M, Vidal-Puig AJ. Lipotoxicity, overnutrition and energy metabolism in aging. *Ageing Research Reviews.* 2006 May;5(2):144–64. PubMed PMID: 16630750.

42. Guo W, Pirtskhalava T, Tchkonia T, Xie W, Thomou T, Han J, et al. Aging results in paradoxical susceptibility of fat cell progenitors to lipotoxicity. *American Journal of Physiology Endocrinology and Metabolism.* 2007 Apr;292(4):E1041–51. PubMed PMID: 17148751.

43. Wang ZW, Pan WT, Lee Y, Kakuma T, Zhou YT, Unger RH. The role of leptin resistance in the lipid abnormalities of aging. *FASEB Journal.* 2001 Jan;15(1):108–14. PubMed PMID: 11149898.

44. Jones DL, Rando TA. Emerging models and paradigms for stem cell ageing. *Nature Cell Biology.* 2011 May;13(5):506–12. PubMed PMID: 21540846. Pubmed Central PMCID: 3257978.

45. Rossi DJ, Bryder D, Zahn JM, Ahlenius H, Sonu R, Wagers AJ, et al. Cell intrinsic alterations underlie hematopoietic stem cell aging. *Proceedings of the National Academy of Sciences of the United States of America.* 2005 Jun 28;102(26):9194–9. PubMed PMID: 15967997. Pubmed Central PMCID: 1153718.

46. Gimble JM, Nuttall ME. The relationship between adipose tissue and bone metabolism. *Clinical Biochemistry.* 2012 Aug;45(12):874–9. PubMed PMID: 22429519.

47. Conboy IM, Conboy MJ, Wagers AJ, Girma ER, Weissman IL, Rando TA. Rejuvenation of aged progenitor cells by exposure to a young systemic environment. *Nature.* 2005 Feb 17;433(7027):760–4. PubMed PMID: 15716955. Epub 2005/02/18. eng.

48. Fries JF. Aging, natural death, and the compression of morbidity. *New England Journal of Medicine.* 1980 Jul 17;303(3):130–5. PubMed PMID: 7383070.

49. Fries JF, Bruce B, Chakravarty E. Compression of morbidity 1980–2011: a focused review of paradigms and progress. *Journal of Aging Research*. 2011;**2011**:1–10. PubMed PMID: 21876805. Pubmed Central PMCID: 3163136.

50. Andersen SL, Sebastiani P, Dworkis DA, Feldman L, Perls TT. Healthspan approximates lifespan among many supercentenarians: compression of morbidity at the approximate limit of lifespan. *Journals of Gerontology: Series A, Biological Sciences and Medical Sciences*. 2012 Apr;**67**(4):395–405. PubMed PMID: 22219514. Pubmed Central PMCID: 3309876.

51. Sebastiani P, Solovieff N, Dewan AT, Walsh KM, Puca A, Hartley SW, et al. Genetic signatures of exceptional longevity in humans. *PloS One*. 2012;**7**(1):e29848. PubMed PMID: 22279548. Pubmed Central PMCID: 3261167.

52. Schachter F, Faure-Delanef L, Guenot F, Rouger H, Froguel P, Lesueur-Ginot L, et al. Genetic associations with human longevity at the APOE and ACE loci. *Nature Genetics*. 1994 Jan;**6**(1):29–32. PubMed PMID: 8136829.

53. Kenyon NS, Russell TR, Xu XM, Knapp J, Ricordi C. Enrichment of hematopoietic stem cells from human vertebral body marrow. *Transplantation Proceedings*. 1997 Jun;**29**(4):1951. PubMed PMID: 9193467.

54. Willcox BJ, Donlon TA, He Q, Chen R, Grove JS, Yano K, et al. FOXO3A genotype is strongly associated with human longevity. *Proceedings of the National Academy of Sciences of the United States of America*. 2008 Sep 16;**105**(37):13987–92. PubMed PMID: 18765803. Pubmed Central PMCID: 2544566.

55. Bluher M, Kahn BB, Kahn CR. Extended longevity in mice lacking the insulin receptor in adipose tissue. *Science*. 2003 Jan 24;**299**(5606):572–4. PubMed PMID: 12543978.

56. Smith RL, de Boer R, Brul S, Budovskaya Y, van Spek H. Premature and accelerated aging: HIV or HAART? *Frontiers in Genetics*. 2012;**3**:328. PubMed PMID: 23372574. Pubmed Central PMCID: 3556597.

57. Ness KK, Krull KR, Jones KE, Mulrooney DA, Armstrong GT, Green DM, et al. Physiologic frailty as a sign of accelerated aging among adult survivors of childhood cancer: a report from the St. Jude Lifetime Cohort Study. *Journal of Clinical Oncology*. 2013 Dec 20;**31**(36):4496–503. PubMed PMID: 24248696. Pubmed Central PMCID: 3871511.

58. Meeske KA, Nelson MB. The role of the long-term follow-up clinic in discovering new emerging late effects in adult survivors of childhood cancer. *Journal of Pediatric Oncology Nursing*. 2008 Jul–Aug;**25**(4):213–9. PubMed PMID: 18539912.

59. Meyer J. *Centenarians: 2010*. Washington, DC: United States Census Bureau Special Reports 2010, No. C2010SR-03; 2012.

60. Ka'opua LS, Braun KL, Browne CV, Mokuau N, Park CB. Why are Native Hawaiians underrepresented in Hawai'i's older adult population? Exploring social and behavioral factors of longevity. *Journal of Aging Research*. 2011;**2011**:701232. PubMed PMID: 21966592. Pubmed Central PMCID: 3182069.

61. Arias, E. United States Life Tables, 2010. *National Vital Statistics Reports*. 2014;**63**(7):1–63. Pubmed PMID: 25383611.

62. Harrison DE, Strong R, Sharp ZD, Nelson JF, Astle CM, Flurkey K, et al. Rapamycin fed late in life extends lifespan in genetically heterogeneous mice. *Nature*. 2009 Jul 16;**460**(7253):392–5. PubMed PMID: 19587680. Pubmed Central PMCID: 2786175.

63. Miller RA, Harrison DE, Astle CM, Baur JA, Boyd AR, de Cabo R, et al. Rapamycin, but not resveratrol or simvastatin, extends lifespan of genetically heterogeneous mice. *Journals of Gerontology: Series A, Biological Sciences and Medical Sciences*. 2011 Feb;**66**(2):191–201. PubMed PMID: 20974732. Pubmed Central PMCID: 3021372.

64. Strong R, Miller RA, Astle CM, Baur JA, de Cabo R, Fernandez E, et al. Evaluation of resveratrol, green tea extract, curcumin, oxaloacetic acid, and medium-chain triglyceride oil on lifespan of genetically heterogeneous mice. *Journals of Gerontology: Series A, Biological Sciences and Medical Sciences*. 2013 Jan;**68**(1):6–16. PubMed PMID: 22451473. Pubmed Central PMCID: 3598361.

65. Martin-Montalvo A, Mercken EM, Mitchell SJ, Palacios HH, Mote PL, Scheibye-Knudsen M, et al. Metformin improves healthspan and lifespan in mice. *Nature Communications*. 2013;**4**:2192. PubMed PMID: 23900241. Pubmed Central PMCID: 3736576.

66. Strong R, Miller RA, Astle CM, Floyd RA, Flurkey K, Hensley KL, et al. Nordihydroguaiaretic acid and aspirin increase lifespan of genetically heterogeneous male mice. *Aging Cell*. 2008 Oct;**7**(5):641–50. PubMed PMID: 18631321. Pubmed Central PMCID: 2695675.

67. Harrison DE, Strong R, Allison DB, Ames BN, Astle CM, Atamna H, et al. Acarbose, 17-alpha-estradiol, and nordihydroguaiaretic acid extend mouse lifespan preferentially in males. *Aging Cell*. 2014 Apr;**13**(2):273–82. PubMed PMID: 24245565. Pubmed Central PMCID: 3954939.

68. Fontana L, Partridge L, Longo VD. Extending healthy lifespan – from yeast to humans. *Science*. 2010 Apr 16;**328**(5976):321–6. PubMed PMID: 20395504. Pubmed Central PMCID: 3607354.

69. Mattison JA, Roth GS, Beasley TM, Tilmont EM, Handy AM, Herbert RL, et al. Impact of caloric restriction on health and survival in rhesus monkeys from the NIA study. *Nature*. 2012 Sep 13;**489**(7415):318–21. PubMed PMID: 22932268. Pubmed Central PMCID: 3832985.

70. Colman RJ, Anderson RM, Johnson SC, Kastman EK, Kosmatka KJ, Beasley TM, et al. Caloric restriction delays disease onset and mortality in rhesus monkeys. *Science.* 2009 Jul 10;**325**(5937):201–4. PubMed PMID: 19590001. Pubmed Central PMCID: 2812811.

71. Dirks AJ, Leeuwenburgh C. Caloric restriction in humans: potential pitfalls and health concerns. *Mechanisms of Ageing and Development.* 2006 Jan;**127**(1):1–7. PubMed PMID: 16226298.

Chapter 3

Comprehensive geriatric assessment

Rachel Mason, MD, and John D. Gazewood, MD, MSPH

Geriatric providers must evaluate and manage their patients with a focus on function in order to provide optimal care. Assessing function is necessary for a number of reasons: older adults are more heterogeneous in their functional capacities than younger adults; functional capacity correlates highly with quality of life,[1] and function, itself, is an important outcome in older patients. Functional status is also an important predictor of mortality and institutionalization in a variety of settings,[2, 3] and changes in functional capacity frequently signal changes in an individual's health. Unfortunately, physicians are frequently unaware of or underestimate their patients' functional limitations.[4] The care of the older adult, therefore, must go beyond a focus on medical disease to address the psychological, social, and cognitive issues that shape the functioning, quality of life, and overall health of the patient (Figure 3.1).

Comprehensive geriatric assessment (CGA) is "a multidimensional, interdisciplinary diagnostic process to determine the medical, psychological and functional capabilities of a frail elderly person in order to develop a co-ordinated and integrated plan

for treatment and long-term follow up."[6] The goals of CGA are to improve diagnostic accuracy, optimize medical treatment and outcomes, improve functional status, recommend the most appropriate living environment, and minimize unnecessary use of services.[7] Although investigators continue to refine the CGA, principles of geriatric care garnered from this model have become more widely adopted in a variety of clinical settings.

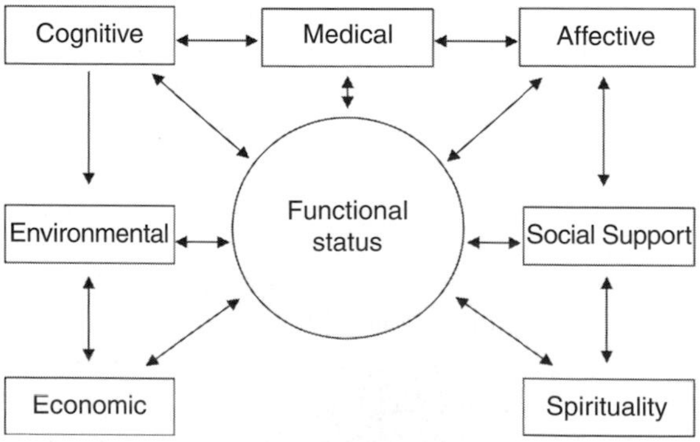

The process of CGA involves a team of health-care providers, often a geriatrician, a nurse practitioner, and a medical social worker. Geriatric psychiatry, pharmacy, nutrition, and physical and occupational therapy are other disciplines that may participate in CGA in some settings. This interprofessional (previously termed "multidisciplinary") team uses a systematic approach that incorporates validated assessment tools to assess multiple domains of function, including the physical, mental, social, functional, and environmental.[8] The team meets and develops recommendations based on results of the evaluation; the integration of information and the interprofessional perspectives brought to bear on this information facilitate its translation into a rational plan of care.[8] The efficacy of CGA has been difficult to study due to the inherent heterogeneity when caring for frail adults with multimorbidity. However, the interprofessional approach to CGA has been rigorously evaluated in a variety of settings, including the home, outpatient clinic, inpatient consultation services, and inpatient geriatric units.[7] In the early 1990s, Stuck et al. performed a meta-analysis of CGA, combining original data from 28 randomized controlled trials with a total of 5,000 control and 5,000 intervention patients.[9] Overall, at 12 months, the outcomes in patients with CGA were as follows: mortality was 14% less likely, hospital admission was

Figure 3.1 Interacting dimensions of geriatric assessment.[5]

Reichel's Care of the Elderly, 7th Edition, ed. Jan Busby-Whitehead *et al.* Published by Cambridge University Press.
© Cambridge University Press 2016.

12% less likely, institutionalization was 26% less likely, and there was no statistically significant effect on functional status. Stuck and associates examined the effects of characteristics of the various interventions on outcomes and found that four covariates influenced effectiveness. Programs that excluded either the very healthy or the very ill were more likely to show benefit, as were programs that maintained control over implementation of recommendations and programs that provided long-term ambulatory follow-up of patients.[9] A Cochrane review in 2011 further confirmed these findings for hospitalized patients; in particular, patients who received CGA were significantly more likely to be alive at home up to a year following the intervention (as compared to usual care).[6]

Evidence supporting functional assessment in primary care settings

Several CGA trials were performed in primary care settings or incorporated into their design delivery of interventions in primary care settings. A CGA trial in community-dwelling elders included an intervention to promote patient communication with their primary care physician, as well as close communication of the CGA team with the primary care doctor. These interventions improved mortality, function, emotional well-being, mental health, and pain outcomes. This study demonstrated that treatment recommendations provided in primary care settings can be effective.[10] A two-year randomized trial of interprofessional primary care in a group of veterans showed that an interprofessional intervention which included an interdisciplinary assessment improved functional status, health perception, social activity, life satisfaction, and cognitive function, and lessened depression and clinic visits.[11]

Several groups have investigated coupling brief functional screenings with focused recommendations to the physician. In a study conducted in a general medicine training practice, patients completed a brief functional assessment tool, and computer-generated feedback reports were provided to physicians; these reports listed functional deficits, linked them to the patient's medical problems, and suggested management interventions. After six months, patients in the intervention group had better emotional well-being and fewer limitations in social activities.[12] Moore et al. studied the effectiveness of a 10-minute office

staff–administered screening.[13] Physicians received brief, written evidence-based intervention recommendations for patients with identified conditions. At six months, patients in the study group were more likely to have hearing impairment identified and evaluated, but there were no differences in health status. Both office staff and physicians found the brief screening instrument useful and feasible.

In a large trial in Great Britain, community-dwelling elders were randomized to a universal in-depth in-home evaluation or to a brief screening coupled with an in-depth evaluation if targeting criteria were met. Participants were then randomized to follow-up by their general practitioner or a geriatrician. The study showed basically equivalent outcomes between the general practitioner and geriatrician groups, which suggests that general practitioners are capable of managing functional deficits and medical problems in patients once these problems have been identified.[14]

Patient selection for comprehensive geriatric assessment

Using CGA for the appropriate patient is key to its effectiveness,[7, 9] and no benefit has been shown in studies that have included elders who were too well or too ill.[17] CGA is most effective when targeted at older patients *at risk for*, but not already suffering from, progressive disability. These individuals exhibit decline in physiological reserve in a number of organ systems, making it harder for them to respond to intrinsic (disease) or extrinsic (environmental) challenges to their physiological or functional status.

Many of the elderly at risk for frailty and functional decline oscillate between states of functional impairment and disability,[18] where longer or more frequent episodes of disability indicate greater risk for recurrent, prolonged, or inevitable functional decline.[19] If individuals suffer progressive physiological and functional decline, they may pass a "point of no return" leading to disability and death. It is therefore imperative to intervene before continuous decline is inevitable. On the other hand, individuals who are not frail may be too healthy to garner benefit from CGA.

Targeting criteria, tested empirically in a number of studies, include diseases that serve as markers for physiological impairment, evidence of functional impairment or disability, and geriatric syndromes

Table 3.1 Targeting criteria

Age: ≥75 years

Functional status: ≥1 ADL deficiency; falls; poor self-rated health

Medical utilization: ≥1 hospital admission in past year; ≥6 physician visits in past year; ≥ 5 prescription medications

Medical conditions: coronary artery disease, diabetes mellitus, depression, urinary incontinence

Social: absence of a caregiver

that may be markers for underlying frailty (Table 3.1). Targeting criteria include exclusionary criteria that identify individuals who are too ill or too severely impaired to benefit from a comprehensive multidimensional assessment.[11, 20, 21]

What happens during a CGA?

A few studies provide some insight into the CGA process. In a pilot study in which outpatient CGA was assessed, 528 interventions were developed for 139 patients. Prioritization of these interventions by the geriatrician of the CGA team resulted in identification of a "most important" recommendation for each patient. These fell into the following categories: general medical problems (30%); depression (21%); incontinence (19%); musculoskeletal problems (12%); hypertension (8%); functional impairment (6%); and falls, visual and hearing problems, and other problems (5% or less).[22] In a three-year study of home-based CGA, geriatric nurse practitioners identified an average of 19.2 problems per patient and made 5,694 specific recommendations. Approximately 66% of patients had a medical problem, 23% a mental health problem, 19.8% a social problem, and 17% a functional problem. Slightly more than half the recommendations involved self-care activities, such as performing Kegel exercises or increasing fluid intake; 29% involved referral to a physician, most commonly to change a medication, discuss an examination finding or functional problem, or to request a treatment or procedure; and 20% involved referral to a nonphysician health professional or community service.[23]

Another important consideration in achieving success in CGA settings is the degree of adherence to the recommendations generated in the process.[10] Physicians, family members, and patients often have widely divergent goals.[24] A cohort study of caregivers of patients who underwent CGA found higher rates of adherence to treatment recommendations if the caregivers agreed with them.[25]

Making functional assessment work: picking an instrument

There are a plethora of instruments available to assess functional domains. Characteristics to consider in selecting an instrument include its validity, reliability, responsiveness, and ease of administration. Of course, the most important consideration in choosing an instrument is that its use will lead to improved outcomes for patients. Because all CGA trials use assessment instruments, it is reasonable to believe that their use leads to better patient outcomes.[9, 26]

Validity is typically assessed using content, construct, and criterion validity. A measure with content validity makes sense to experts and to patients who take it: it looks like it addresses the area of concern. Construct validity refers to how well the instrument measures what it intends to measure. Criterion validity measures how well an instrument compares with a criterion or gold standard. Sensitivity, specificity, and predictive value are how criterion validity is typically measured in the clinical literature. Diagnostic accuracy of instruments is also measured and compared by using a receiver-operating curve. By plotting the true-positive rate (sensitivity) against the false-positive rate (1 – specificity) a curve is constructed. Instruments with a larger area under the curve (AUC) are more accurate.

A reliable instrument measures in a reproducible fashion. Reliability requires internal consistency and reproducibility. Internal consistency is a measure of how closely different items in an instrument relate to each other. A reproducible measure shows good interrater, intrarater, and test–retest reliability; that is, results within and between observers and results for the same patient when a test is repeated over a short period of time are stable.

Responsiveness indicates how well an instrument can determine meaningful changes over time. Ceiling and floor effects, which indicate the upper and lower limits of an instrument's measurement range, limit instrument responsiveness. For example, a scale of activities of daily living (ADLs) is not likely to give a

Table 3.2 Mobile applications for geriatric assessment

Mobile Application	Assessment Tool	Subject
American Geriatrics Society	2012 Beers Criteria	Medication management
Geriatric Depression Scale	GDS (15-question version)	Depression Screening
Depression Test	PHQ-9	Depression Screening
Health Measuring Tools	Katz Index	ADL assessment
	Barthel Index	ADL assessment
	Cornell Scale for Depression	Depression Screening in dementia patients
MNA	MNA-SF	Nutritional status
Echelle Doloplus	DOLOPLUS-2	Pain assessment in dementia patients

meaningful picture of a functionally independent person, as this person's function is above the ability of the instrument to discriminate meaningful changes (ceiling effect).

The properties of functional assessment instruments can be affected by characteristics of the population in which they are developed. Language, culture, education, socioeconomic status, and severity of a condition can all affect the performance of an assessment tool, either changing the scoring or rendering the instrument altogether useless in a given population. In general, it is best to use only instruments that have been validated in a population that is similar to the intended target population (grade D).*

It is also important to consider more practical aspects of instrument administration. Functional assessment tools can be completed by the patient or a proxy, or through direct observation. Patients overestimate their functional capacity in comparison to proxy measures or direct measurement.[27] It may

sometimes be necessary to assess certain aspects of function with multiple instruments or sources of information, particularly if an individual's reported functional status is incongruent with other measures or one's general clinical impression. Ease of use is, from a practical standpoint, one of the most important considerations in selecting a functional assessment instrument. Instruments should not take too much time to administer, be too burdensome on a patient or caregiver, or be difficult to score. Many instruments are available that can be filled out by the patient or caregiver. Office staff or other health personnel can complete others. None requires a physician to administer them, although clinicians can find observation of the patient during instrument completion helpful in formulating clinical impressions. Many instruments are now available in electronic format for mobile devices or via the Internet. These programs allow for automated scoring and make some instruments easier to use (Table 3.2).

Functional assessment in primary care settings: making it work

Comprehensive geriatric assessment is not widely available, and there will not be enough geriatricians to provide care to an aging populace.[28, 29] The evidence presented thus far allows for some broad recommendations to be made on how to perform a comprehensive evaluation in a busy primary care setting. First, not all patients require a comprehensive

---

* Grades of recommendation are those developed by the Centre for Evidence-Based Medicine, Oxford, and are available at www.cebm.net/levels_of_evidence.asp:

Grade A: consistent level 1 studies

Grade B: consistent level 2 or 3 studies or extrapolations from level 1 studies

Grade C: level 4 studies or extrapolations from level 2 or 3 studies

Grade D: level 5 evidence or troublingly inconsistent or inconclusive studies of any level

evaluation. Using a brief screening tool based on targeting criteria can identify patients who may benefit from a more comprehensive evaluation and will help practices to focus limited resources toward patients most likely to benefit (grade A). Second, a systematic process should be used when performing either a screening assessment or a comprehensive assessment (grade A). This will ensure that important aspects of the evaluation are not overlooked. Third, validated instruments should be used whenever available (grade A). Fourth, the physician does not have to directly obtain all of the information needed to complete either a screening evaluation or a comprehensive evaluation. Patients and their caregivers can complete some instruments, medical assistants or nurses can complete other assessment instruments, and the physician can use outside resources for other parts of the assessment (grade B). For example, a referral to a home health agency can help the physician in obtaining an assessment from a home health nurse, a physical therapist, and a social worker. Finally, working with the patient, family, and caregivers, physicians and patients should develop a prioritized list of goals that will make patient and family adherence to interventions more likely (grade A).

The Patient Protection and Affordable Care Act passed by the US Congress in 2010 now provides for an annual wellness visit, which incorporates many elements of a traditional CGA. As described earlier, the screening tools can be administered by a non-physician health professional with recommendations then developed by the physician based upon relevant findings. Currently there is no outcome data available with regard to this new service, but as practices develop implementation models, this information will hopefully become available.

Making geriatric assessment work: putting it together

The components of geriatric assessment are listed in Table 3.3. Because the presence of known functional or other deficits may influence the examination process, exploring this information before performing the history and physical examination will increase efficiency (grade D). Much of the information can be obtained prior to the physician encounter via questionnaires or having non-physician (or even nonmedical) staff administer part of the assessment.

Table 3.3 Domains of geriatric assessment

Physical health
Traditional history and physical examination
Hearing and vision screen
Oral and dental health
Continence assessment
Gait, mobility, and falls risk assessment
Nutrition assessment
Functional ability
ADLs
IADLs
Performance measures
Mental status
Cognitive function
Depression screening
Social support
Social history
Advanced directive
Caregiver burden
Finances
Environment

For example, in one family medicine office, a 22-minute assessment performed by an office assistant identified at least one new or incompletely treated geriatric problem in 68% of patients.[30]

History and physical examination

History

A thorough history is necessary to ensure diagnostic accuracy. Accommodations must be made for barriers to communication. Having a pocket talker available and speaking clearly in a low-pitched voice while looking directly at the patient will improve communication with a hearing impaired person. Many older patients will be accompanied by a caregiver, and incorporating this third party into the encounter while maintaining primary focus on the patient is a necessary skill. The caregiver can corroborate and expand on a patient's report and will provide important history when the patient has cognitive impairment. Establishing rapport and a good working relationship with the caregiver will also be helpful in maximizing the therapeutic effect of your relationship with the patient.

The history should explore acute and subacute problems, with a particular focus on problems that affect function. In the patient with a recent functional decline, delineating the impairments contributing to the decline will help determine prognosis and therapy. For example, difficulty dressing could result from cognitive impairment, weakness secondary to a stroke, or a frozen shoulder. The history includes a review of chronic medical conditions (including complications), and the medical, surgical, and psychiatric history, including immunizations. The history should also review episodes of disability and length of disability because both increase future risk of disability.[19]

A substance use history, including tobacco, alcohol, and other drugs should be obtained. Inquire about all forms of tobacco use, not just cigarettes. Components of the AUDIT tool, a more detailed screen than the CAGE questionnaire developed by the World Health Organization, should be used to screen for alcohol abuse (grade A). The first question of the AUDIT-C is "How often did you have a drink containing alcohol in the past year?" Follow-up questions are (1) "In the past year, how many drinks did you typically have when you drank?" and (2) "How often did you have six or more drinks on one occasion in the past year?" Answers to the questions are scored, with higher scores indicative of hazardous drinking. [31, 32]

A thorough evaluation of the patient's medications may be one of the most important components of the assessment. Medication review and reconciliation in outpatient CGA programs have been found to reduce the risk of serious adverse drug reactions. In one trial, the most commonly implicated classes of medications were cardiovascular, central nervous system, antimicrobials, hormones, and blood modifying agents.[33] Patients should be asked to bring all of their medications, including vitamins, supplements,

and over-the-counter medications. Every medication should have an appropriate indication and dose, and potential drug interactions should be identified. Several tools are available to help identify potentially inappropriate medications (PIMs) in older adults, the most frequently used of which are the Beers Criteria and the Screening Tool of Older Person's Potentially Inappropriate Prescriptions (STOPP). A recent cross-sectional study of 407 patients demonstrated that the 2012 update of the Beers Criteria identified PIMs in 42% of patients, while STOPP did so in 35.4% of patients. The degree of agreement between STOPP and the 2012 Beers Criteria was low, suggesting that the tools identify different PIMs and therefore are likely complementary.[34]

The social history should elucidate the patient's sources of support, including emotional, spiritual, physical, and financial sources. Understanding the patient's educational, occupational, and avocational history will provide a richer picture of the patient. The family history, although perhaps less important than in younger patients, can still provide useful information regarding the longevity and late-life health of the patient's parents and siblings, as well as information that may influence screening decisions for certain cancers.

The review of systems should address changes in hearing as well as vision, oral, and dental problems. It should also include questions targeting geriatric syndromes. The review of systems is one aspect of the history that could be efficiently obtained in questionnaire format, assuming that the patient or caregiver is functionally literate.

Physical examination

Vital signs should include supine and standing pulse and blood pressure, weight and height, and determination of body mass index (BMI). If a patient is unable to stand, height can be estimated using the length of the patient's lower leg.*[35] Office staff can assess vision using a Snellen or handheld chart. Hearing is best assessed using a handheld audiometer, the

---

* Alternative height calculations using knee-to-heel measurements: with knee at 90-degree angle (foot flexed or flat on floor or bed board), measure from bottom of heel to top of knee.

Men: Ht (cm) = (2.02 × knee height, cm) − (0.04 × age) + 64.19

Women: Ht (cm) = (1.83 × knee height, cm) − (0.24 × age) + 84.8834.

Audio-Scope (Welch Allyn, Inc., Skaneateles Falls, NY). The audio-scope is easy to use, and office staff can screen the patient for hearing loss by setting the sound intensity to 40 dB. Alternatively, a brief self-response questionnaire, the Hearing Handicap Inventory for the Elderly-Screening version can be used. With a cut-off of 10 points, the sensitivity ranges from 63% to 80%. The whisper test, although easy to perform, has uncertain reliability and accuracy.[36]

Examination of the head and neck should include an assessment of oral and dental health. Oral and dental problems are highly predictive of poor outcomes. Poorly fitting dentures, broken teeth, missing teeth, carious teeth, gingivitis, and periodontitis can all contribute to poor oral intake, and the latter three may produce inflammatory mediators that can lead to functional decline.[37] Thorough musculoskeletal and neurological examinations are especially important in the presence of functional impairment.

A comprehensive geriatric assessment should always include systematic assessment of cognition, affect, functional status, falls, continence, nutrition, environment, and social support, based on assessment of these domains in multiple CGA trials (grade A).

Cognitive assessment

Cognitive impairment can be secondary to dementia, delirium, depression, and aphasia, among others. A complete assessment of mental status includes evaluation of attention, executive function, memory, orientation, language, visuospatial abilities, psychomotor speed, and intelligence. There are more than 25 brief screening instruments used in clinical practice, and none of the instruments used in primary care office settings addresses all of these domains. Consequently, many of the instruments used for mental status testing in the office setting have low sensitivities and high specificities, meaning that in a population of older patients in whom dementia is prevalent, a positive test is likely to be true, and a negative test may frequently miss a patient with cognitive impairment. Everything considered, no ideal screening test has emerged from the many available, but the benefits and drawbacks of several are described in the following paragraphs. The widely used and well-validated Mini-Mental Status Examination (MMSE) evaluates orientation, memory, calculation, language, and visuospatial orientation. It has 30 items and takes approximately 10 minutes to administer. The cut-off score is 24, the sensitivity

ranges from 0.7 to 0.9, and the specificity ranges from 0.56 to 0.96.[38] Sensitivity is lower for mild dementia, and the score must be adjusted for age and education level.[39] A low score on the MMSE reliably identifies patients with cognitive impairment, but a normal score does not rule out cognitive impairment. In patients or populations where dementia is more likely, the Montreal Cognitive Assessment (MoCA) and St. Louis University Mental Status Exam (SLUMS) are more sensitive screening tests that should be considered; both are available in the public domain.[40, 41]

Very brief screening tests have been developed in an effort to lessen the burden of dementia screening. The Time and Change test requires the patient to tell the time given on a large clockface diagram and make one dollar's worth of change from a standard amount of change. An individual who fails either is positive for dementia. The Time and Change test has a sensitivity of 0.86 and a specificity of 0.71, and takes 23 seconds to complete.[42] The Mini-Cog combines three-item recall with a clock-drawing test. Individuals are given three items to remember, are asked to draw a clock, and then are asked to recall the three items. A positive test is either failure to recall all three items, or failure to recall one or two items and failure on the clock-drawing test.[43] In a large, population-based cohort study, the Mini-Cog had a sensitivity of 0.76 and a specificity of 0.84. The MMSE in this same study had a sensitivity of 0.71 and a specificity of 0.94.[44]

Several informant-based tests for cognitive impairment may be more sensitive than the MMSE for detection of dementia. The Informant Questionnaire for Cognitive Decline in the Elderly (IQCODE) is filled out by an informant, who compares the patient's current functional state to 10 years ago by using a Likert scale. The long time scale may cause difficulties for some respondents.[38] When cognitive impairment is identified by an MMSE score less than 24 and an IQCODE score greater than 4, the sensitivity of this combination is 0.93 with a specificity of 0.81.[45]

Assessment of affect

The US Preventive Services Task Force recommends screening for depression in all adults when staff-assisted depression care supports are available (grade B).[47] Many older adults suffering from depression do not display classic symptoms, and instruments can be helpful in identifying these patients. There are a number of validated instruments available for screening and diagnosis of depression, although only a few have been adequately validated in older individuals.

A systematic review identified three instruments with proven validity for diagnosis of major depression in the elderly: the Geriatric Depression Scale (GDS), the Center of Epidemiologic Studies Depression Scale (CES-D), and the SelfCARE questionnaire. Each instrument takes two to three minutes to administer and performed similarly in studies.[46] The 15-question GDS is widely used, can be administered in questionnaire or interview format, and has the benefit of a simple yes/no format in question responses. The CES-D is a 20-item self-report depression scale that requires respondents to rate how frequently they experienced depressive symptoms during the past week. The SelfCARE (D) consists of 12 questions, with scoring based on a Likert scale, asking respondents to answer based on symptoms during the past month. In a large cohort study, the 10-item CES-D was found to have the best sensitivity in the outpatient setting, and the 15-item GDS was best in a nursing home population.[47]

Two studies have established validity of the Patient Health Questionaire-9 (PHQ-9) in diagnosing depression in elderly outpatients.[48, 49] In these studies, the PHQ-9 had similar performance to the GDS. The advantage of this tool is that it can screen and diagnose major depression without additional evaluation because it is derived from the *Diagnostic and Statistical Manual for Mental Disorders*. The drawback is more complex scoring than the GDS. The Cornell Scale for Depression was validated for identification of depression among patients with dementia and relies on patient observation and caregiver report. In hospital and outpatient settings, it has a reported sensitivity of 0.9 and a specificity of 0.75.[46]

Functional assessment

Assessing functional status requires evaluation of the domains of physical activity necessary for independent living in modern society. These domains include basic activities of daily living (ADLs), instrumental activities of daily living (IADLs), and mobility. Typical facets of these domains are listed in Table 3.4. These measures typically scale responses from complete independence in an

Table 3.4 Functional assessment domains

ADLs	Bathing
	Dressing
	Grooming
	Toileting
	Transferring
	Eating
	Continence
IADLs	Food preparation
	Housekeeping
	Laundry
	Shopping
	Managing personal finances
	Administration of medications
	Use of transportation
	Use of telephone
Mobility	Walking
	Transferring
	Balance
	Stairs

activity to complete dependence. In the clinical setting, these scales are used to identify specific functional deficits in order to develop specific interventions. All of these instruments suffer from both floor and ceiling effects. Supplementing these largely self-reported measures of function with physical performance measures can help identify those highly functioning individuals at risk for functional decline.[50]

Activities of daily living

ADL instruments measure basic functioning and in the outpatient setting are typically completed by patient and caregiver report. In home, inpatient, or rehabilitation settings, they can also be completed by direct observation. The Katz Index of Independence in Activities of Daily Living is the prototypic ADL scale, assessing function in the basic activities noted in Table 3.4.[51] The Katz index is a hierarchical scale where more advanced functions such as bathing are lost before the most basic function, eating. The Katz index, although frequently used in clinical settings, lacks the validity and reliability for use in research or health administration.[52] The Barthel Index is frequently used in rehabilitation settings.[53] It was designed to use observation (as opposed to patient report) to establish a level of ADL independence.

Instrumental activities of daily living

IADL scales measure more advanced functions that require intact cognitive and executive function, in addition to intact physical function. Impairment in IADLs can be an early indicator of conditions affecting cognitive function, such as dementia. In the outpatient setting, these are almost always completed by self- or informant-report. Lawton and Brody's IADL scale asks about the respondent's ability to perform eight items necessary for independent living in the community.[54]

Physical performance measures can identify individuals at risk of functional decline and other poor outcomes who are not identified by ADL and IADL measures.[55] These instruments typically require direct observation of the patient performing a simple task and may require timing, subjective assessment by the observer, or more sophisticated measurement using calibrated instruments of subject performance. [56] For example, the get-up-and-go test is a widely used physical performance measure that requires the observer to evaluate subjectively the patient's ability to rise from a chair, walk three meters, turn around, walk back, and sit down.[66] It can identify patients at risk for falls and can indicate specific physical impairments, such as proximal muscle weakness. The timed version of this test has been extensively studied, and although it has varying ability to predict falls,[57] it does predict general disability in ADLs and IADLs, and in particular the ability to prepare a hot meal (AUC 0.8) and manage money (AUC 0.91).[58]

Table 3.5 Determination of gait speed

Test administration	
Patient instructed to "walk at your own speed"	
1-meter start up	
4-meter timed distance	
Test interpretation	
<0.06 meter/second	High risk
0.06 meter/second to 1 meter/second	Intermediate risk
>1 meter/second	Low risk

Source: Cutler LJ. Assessment of physical environments of older adults. In: Kane RL, Kane RA, editors. *Assessing Older Persons: Measures, Meaning, and Practical Applications.* Oxford: Oxford University Press; 2000. pp. 360–79.

Gait speed has been studied to evaluate many outcomes in older adults and has even been found to predict survival in older adults.[59] Regarding functional decline, gait speed demonstrated AUC values for identification of highly functioning older adults at risk of functional decline that are comparable to the AUC of the well-validated EPESE (Established Populations for Epidemiologic Studies of the Elderly) physical performance test battery in a large and ethnically diverse group of older patients.[55]

There is also growing evidence that even perception of difficulty can identify highly functioning individuals at risk of functional decline and disability.[60] In a study of independent older women, a report of slowed walking was associated with new onset of difficulty walking at one year.[61] Patients who used a cane and reported no walking difficulty were more likely to develop new mobility problems at two years than patients who did not use a cane. [62] Asking highly functioning patients about task modification, as manifested by slower walking or use of assistive devices, is recommended to identify a subset at increased risk of functional decline (grade B).

Falls

Falls are an important cause of morbidity and mortality in older adults; they are also associated with poor function and earlier admission to long-term care facilities. As they can be prevented, all elderly patients should be asked about the occurrence of falls in the past year, frequency of falls, and difficulties with gait or balance.[63] Patients who present for evaluation after a fall, have recurrent falls, or have an abnormal get-up-and-go test require a multifactorial fall risk assessment addressing all potential intrinsic (i.e., sensory, strength, and balance deficits) and extrinsic factors (i.e., medications, footwear, and environmental hazards); much of this evaluation would be included in a typical CGA.

Incontinence

Although incontinence can have a marked impact on ADLs and socialization, older adults are often hesitant to report it either due to embarrassment or belief that is a normal part of aging. Therefore, the CGA includes an assessment of continence, and routine use of questionnaires is recommended (grade D).[64] A systematic review has identified that the King's Health Questionnaire and Urinary Distress Inventory are both well validated.[65] However, the King's Health Questionnaire is 29 items, and the short form of the Urinary Distress Inventory is not in the public domain. Alternatively, two simple questions can be used to identify incontinence: "In the last year, have you lost urine and gotten wet?" and "Have you lost urine on six separate days?"[5] Evaluation of patients with incontinence includes defining the type of incontinence and the effect incontinence has on quality of life because patients can have marked differences in tolerance for incontinence.

Nutrition

Malnutrition in older patients is associated with increased risk of functional decline, hospitalization, and death. Rates of malnutrition vary in the elderly population: 1% to 5% of community-dwelling elders are malnourished, compared to at least 20% of those admitted to the hospital and 37% of those residing in long-term care facilities.[66] The Mini-Nutritional Assessment Short Form (MNA-SF) is a six-item instrument derived from the well-validated full-length version. It correlates very well with the longer version, with an AUC of 0.96, a sensitivity of 0.979, and specificity of 1.00 for patients with malnutrition. [67] In hospital settings, the Subjective Global Assessment predicts poor outcomes.[68] This instrument has been used in randomized trials of patients undergoing elective surgery, and, in combination with nutritional interventions, has resulted in improved outcomes.[69]

Environment

The goals of environmental assessment in the geriatric evaluation are to ensure that an older person lives safely in a home that maximizes functional independence.[70] Many trials to prevent falls in older persons include interventions to improve home safety, and these interventions are effective in reducing falls. [71, 72] Common fall-related hazards in homes include low ambient lighting, slippery surfaces in bathrooms, throw rugs, stairs, absence of railings, and trailing cords.[73–75] Safety assessment also includes attention to fire safety, such as the presence of smoke detectors, fire extinguishers, carbon monoxide detectors, and use of portable heaters.[76, 77] Assessing the presence and storage of firearms, as well as crime safety, is also necessary. Assessment of accessibility includes queries about the use of adaptive

equipment, such as grab bars, in the home, and how readily patients who require a mobility aid, such as a wheelchair or walker, can access and move about in their home.

Some successful randomized trials of geriatric assessment have not included a home visit.[10, 11, 78, 79] However, fall-reduction trials typically include an in-home environmental assessment,[80] as do a number of successful trials of geriatric assessment.[26, 81, 82] A study examining the effectiveness of providing home safety checklists showed no difference between the intervention and control groups in the rate of home safety improvements, [83] so if an elderly patient is at risk for falling, an in-home environmental assessment should be a part of the evaluation (grade A). This assessment could be conducted by a variety of health-care professionals, including home health nurses, physical or occupational therapists, and social service workers.

Social assessment

Assessing an elder's social situation includes assessment of social support, caregiver stress, and risk for elder abuse. Social support refers to friends, family, and other persons who are available to provide care for the elderly person, and includes an assessment of the number available for crises and long-term care. [84] The Lubben Social Network Scale-6 is an abbreviated version of the widely used Lubben Social Network Scale that has been shown to have good internal reliability and validity.[85] Evaluation of financial resources can help older patients and their caregivers plan for in-home or institutional long-term care needs.

Caring for an ill or disabled elderly person can be stressful, and caregiver burden has been associated with increased mortality[86] and with institutionalization of patients with dementia.[98, 99] The Zarit Burden Interview has good reliability and validity and has been widely used. It consists of 22 items scored from "never" to "nearly always" that can be self-administered or completed during an interview. [87] The seven-item version of the Screen for Caregiver Burden also has good reliability and validity and is easy to administer, but it has not been widely used.[88]

Elder mistreatment encompasses elder abuse, neglect, exploitation, and abandonment, and affects up to 5% of older Americans. Frail elders, who are more likely to undergo comprehensive geriatric assessment, are at increased risk of elder mistreatment. Because older adults are unlikely to report mistreatment, clinicians must ask older adults about mistreatment and should do so without the caregiver present. A systematic review of instruments to screen for elder mistreatment recommend three instruments for clinical use (grade B). The Brief Abuse Screen for the Elderly is a five-item questionnaire that takes one minute to complete by a health-care provider. The Conflict Tactics Scale is a 19-item self-report or interview instrument that assesses physical and verbal abuse. It has good psychometric properties and has been the most widely used.[89]

Optional assessment

Systematic assessments of health literacy, spirituality, driving ability, and pain have not been routinely included in CGA trials. Although the available evidence does not require their inclusion in the comprehensive assessment of an older patient, many geriatricians include assessment of these domains (grade D).

Health literacy

Health literacy describes a basic mathematical, reading, and communication skill set that allows patients to function in the health-care system and to use health information.[90] Low levels of health literacy are associated with lower functional status,[91] more comorbidities and poorer access to health care,[92] and higher health-care costs.[93] Low health literacy is common, affecting 30% of well-educated community-dwelling elders.[94] Understanding the ability of an elderly patient or the primary caregiver to use health information is important to help provide appropriate health education and supporting materials.

One question, "How often do you have someone help you read hospital materials?" (responses – never, occasionally, sometimes, often, always) had an AUC of 0.87, in comparison to a version of the Test of Functional Health Literacy in Adults (a well-validated, but long instrument), and a sensitivity of 0.8 and specificity of 0.77 for low health literacy with a response of "sometimes" as the cut-off point.[95] In another clinic population, the question "How confident are you filling out medical forms by yourself?" (responses – extremely, quite a bit, somewhat,

a little bit, not at all) had an AUC of 0.82, in comparison to the Rapid Estimate of Adult Literacy in Medicine (five- to six-minute screening tool), and a sensitivity of 0.83 and specificity of 0.65 for impaired health literacy with a cut-off point of "somewhat."[96] Using one of these questions is a quick and reasonably accurate way to screen for impaired health literacy.

Spirituality and religiosity

Religious beliefs and practice become more important as people age.[97] Religiosity and spirituality are also associated with improved psychosocial and cognitive function and better health.[98] Patients' desire to have physicians ask about their spiritual or religious beliefs seems to depend on their health status: in one multicenter study, only 33% felt that their physician should routinely inquire about spiritual beliefs, but fully 70% responded that they would want their physicians to ask about spiritual beliefs if they were seriously ill.[99]

Because older patients are likely to turn to spiritual or religious beliefs to make sense of the many losses they experience, physicians have a responsibility, derived from the principles of beneficence and fidelity to the patient, to assess spirituality.[100, 101] Appropriate times to assess spirituality include during a discussion of support systems, advanced directive discussions, discussions of coping with chronic pain and illness, new diagnoses of serious or terminal illness, and end-of-life care planning.[102] There are no brief instruments that have been validated for use in clinical settings, although several have been developed and validated for research purposes.[103] A common sense approach to spiritual assessment involves informal exploration of patients' sources of hope, belief, support, and meaning in their lives. Further exploration of a patient's spirituality or religiosity can be guided by their initial response to these queries.

Driving ability

Most elderly patients continue to rely on driving for transportation. Unfortunately, they have the highest fatality rate per mile driven of any age group, other than drivers younger than 25.[104] Older drivers are more likely to have accidents, and their increased frailty increases their susceptibility to fatal injury. [104] A number of factors are associated with increased accident risk, including age, medical conditions, dementia, and polypharmacy.[104] All older patients should be asked if they drive, as well as about accidents, near misses, or driving citations (grade D). Driving errors most frequently associated with unsafe driving include problems negotiating an intersection, poor gap estimate in lane change or merging, and failure to maintain appropriate speed.[105]

In the outpatient setting, assessments normally included in a geriatric assessment can identify patients requiring further evaluation. Patients with decreased visual acuity; strength less than 4/5 in either the upper or the right lower extremity, and a decreased range of motion or with a full range of motion performed slowly or with pain, and those patients who walk three meters up and back in more than 7 seconds are more likely to have motor vehicle accidents.[104] A score of 4 or less on the clock-drawing test when using the Freund scoring system was 0.64 sensitive and 0.98 specific for identifying individual's who were unsafe drivers (Table 3.6). [123] The trail-making part B test also predicts unsafe driving because it evaluates skills such as visual scanning, selective and divided attention, task switching, and working memory.[104] If individuals at risk for unsafe driving want to continue to drive, they should be referred for formal driving assessment. This can be done by an occupational therapist in a driver rehabilitation program. However, these programs are not typically covered by insurance. In many cases, these patients must be tested through a governmental agency that conducts driver testing.

Table 3.6 Freund method of scoring the clock-drawing test

Characteristic	Points
One hand points to 2 (or symbol representative of 2)	1
Exactly two hands	1
Absence or intrusive marks	1
Numbers are inside the clock circle	1
All numbers 1–12 are present; no duplicates or omissions	1
Numbers spaced equally or nearly equally from each other	1
Numbers spaced equally, or nearly equally from edge of circle	1
Cut-off score	**4**

Pain

The prevalence of significant pain in community-dwelling elderly ranges from 25% to 50%.[124] Evaluation of pain includes assessment of its intensity, duration, frequency, location, quality, and alleviating and precipitating factors. Older patients may deny the presence of "pain" but acknowledge discomfort, hurting, or aching. The interaction of pain with performance of ADLs and IADLs should be assessed, as should the use of analgesic medications and the patient's and caregiver's attitudes and beliefs regarding pain.[106]

A validated scale should be used to measure pain intensity.[106] A number of scales are available, including visual analog scales (VAS), numeric rating scales, verbal descriptor scales (VDS), face pain scales, and combinations of these. Several studies have compared the performance of these scales directly and found that the VDS may be the best scale for use in the elderly population, although all of these scales, apart from the VAS, are acceptable.[52, 107] The VDS consists of seven adjectival descriptions ranging from "no pain" to "moderate pain" to "the most intense pain imaginable."[108]

Pain assessment in patients with dementia is more difficult, as patients have less cognitive capability to process and communicate their experience of pain. For patients with advanced dementia who are unable to communicate, a number of pain-rating scales that use observable behaviors, such as grimacing and moaning, have been developed.[109] A systematic review of available instruments rated them using comprehensive, validated criteria.[110] The three highest scoring instruments in this review that are suitable for clinical use are the DOLOPLUS-2,[111] the Pain Assessment Checklist for Seniors with Limited Ability to Communicate (PACSLAC),[112] and the Pain Assessment in Advanced Dementia (PAINEAD). Of these, the DOLOPLUS-2 has been the most widely used,[110] although in studies the PAINEAD and PACSLAC have been found to be clinically useful.[113]

Geriatric assessment in various settings

Home visits offer insights important for the care of the older patient. In a study of dementia patients evaluated in both the home and the clinic, 81% had a problem identified at home, but not in the clinic.[114] Home visits are also effective; a meta-analysis of 18 trials with 13,347 older adults showed that geriatric assessment in the home improved function and decreased mortality among those younger than 80 and decreased nursing home admission if the home visit program included comprehensive geriatric assessment and multiple visits.[115] Videoconferencing is a promising use of technology for extending the reach of geriatricians to isolated rural elders, but the data of its use remains scarce at this point in time.[116] Assessment instruments used in outpatient settings can be readily used in the home setting as well.

CGA in the hospital can be done by an inpatient geriatric consult team or on a unit designed for the care of the older patient. Inpatient consultations teams are effective if they have control over implementation of management recommendations.[9] Geriatric evaluation and management (GEM) units utilize an interprofessional approach and assessment of functional domains, including assessment of caregiver capabilities and the patient's social situation.[117] These units have been shown to reduce functional decline at discharge[117] and can improve long-term function and reduce institutionalization if coupled with long-term follow-up.[9] Acute care for the elderly units combine environmental modifications with protocol-driven functional interventions and a geriatrician-led review of medications and care aimed at minimizing harm. They have multiple benefits, including fewer cases of falls and delirium, less decline in functional status, shorter lengths of stay, and fewer discharges to nursing homes.[118] As is true in the outpatient setting, targeting these interventions to the appropriate patient is important for their success. The assessment instruments used in outpatient settings can also be used in hospital settings.

All patients cared for in nursing homes that receive Medicare or Medicaid payments undergo assessment using the Minimum Data Set (MDS).[119] The MDS addresses multiple domains of function in the frail elderly. The MDS was revised to a 3.0 version in 2010 in an effort to make it more clinically relevant and to add more resident "voice." It has good interrater reliability[120] and includes many valid screening instruments for geriatric syndromes, including the PHQ-9 for depression, the Confusion Assessment Method for delirium, a numeric or verbal descriptor scale for pain, and the Brief Inventory of Mental Status for cognition.[121] Although the tools included in this assessment are not always the "gold standard" screening items, the development of the MDS 3.0 marks a major improvement from previous versions.[122]

Conclusion

Because evidence demonstrates efficacy of the CGA for patients at risk for decline, physicians who want to provide optimal care for their older patients must find ways to incorporate a systematic approach to functional assessment into their practice. Although few trials of CGA have been done in circumstances identical to the busy outpatient settings in which most primary care physicians find themselves, various approaches have provided guidance to make CGA feasible. In brief, assessments should be comprehensive, employ validated instruments that are easy to use, and involve the patient and caregivers in goal setting. The assessment can be spread out over several visits, and the process is more practical and enjoyable if done in collaboration with other health-care professionals. By developing a process of functional assessment that works in their practice, physicians can improve the quality of care and, in turn, the quality of life for their older patients.

References

1. Ferrucci L, Baldasseroni S, Bandinelli S, et al. Disease severity and health-related quality of life across different chronic conditions. *J Am Geriatr Soc.* 2000;**48**:1490–5.

2. Reuben D, Rubenstein LV, Hirsch SH, Hays RD. Value of functional status as a predictor of mortality: Results of a prospective study. *Am J Med.* 1992;**93**:663–9.

3. Satish S, Winograd CH, Chavez C, Bloch DA. Geriatric targeting criteria as predictors of survival and health care utilization. *J Am Geriatr Soc.* 1996;**44**(8):914–21.

4. Nelson E, Conger B, Douglass R, Gephart D, Kirk J, Page R, et al. Functional health status levels of primary care patients. *JAMA.* 1983;**249**(24):3331–8.

5. Rosen SL, Reuben DB. Geriatric assessment tools. *Mt Sinai J Med.* 2011;**78**(4):489–97.

6. Ellis G, Whitehead MA, O'Neill D, Langhorne P, Robinson D. Comprehensive geriatric assessment for older adults admitted to hospital. *Cochrane Database Syst Rev.* 2011(7):Cd006211.

7. Rubenstein LZ. Joseph T. Freeman award lecture: comprehensive geriatric assessment: from miracle to reality. *Journals of Gerontology Series A-Biological Sciences & Medical Sciences.* 2004;**59**(5):473–7.

8. Anonymous. National Institutes of Health Consensus Development Conference Statement: geriatric assessment methods for clinical decision-making. *J Am Geriatr Soc.* 1988;**36**(4):342–7.

9. Stuck AE, Siu AL, Wieland GD, Adams J, Rubenstein LZ. Comprehensive geriatric assessment: a meta-analysis of controlled trials. *Lancet.* 1993;**342**(8878):1032–6.

10. Reuben DB, Frank JC, Hirsch SH, McGuigan KA, Maly RC. A randomized clinical trial of outpatient comprehensive geriatric assessment coupled with an intervention to increase adherence to recommendations [see comments]. *J Am Geriatr Soc.* 1999;**47**(3):269–76.

11. Burns R, Nichols LO, Martindale-Adams J, Graney MJ. Interdisciplinary geriatric primary care evaluation and management: two-year outcomes. *J Am Geriatr Soc.* 2000;**48**:8–13.

12. Rubenstein LV, McCoy JM, Cope DW, Barrett PA, Hirsch SH, Messer KS, et al. Improving patient quality of life with feedback to physicians about functional status. *Journal of General Internal Medicine.* 1995;**10**(11):607–14.

13. Moore AA, Siu A, Partridge JM, Hays RD, Adams J. A randomized trial of office-based screening for common problems in older persons. *American Journal of Medicine.* 1997;**102**(4):371–8.

14. Fletcher AE, Price GM, Ng ESW, Stirling SL, Bulpitt CJ, Breeze E, et al. Population-based multidimensional assessment of older people in UK general practice: a cluster-randomised factorial trial. *Lancet.* 2004;**364**(9446):1667–77.

15. Stuck AE, Beck JC, Egger M. Preventing disability in elderly people.[comment]. *Lancet.* 2004;**364** (9446):1641–2.

16. Hughes C. What you need to know about the Medicare preventive services expansion. *Fam Pract Manag.* 2011;**18**(1):22–5.

17. Reuben DB, Borok GM, Wolde-Tsadik G, Ershoff DH, Fishman LK, Ambrosini VL, et al. A randomized trial of comprehensive geriatric assessment in the care of hospitalized patients. *N Engl J Med.* 1995;**332** (20):1345–50.

18. Gill TM, Allore HG, Hardy SE, Guo Z. The dynamic nature of mobility disability in older persons. *J Am Geriatr Soc.* 2006;**54**(2):248–54.

19. Hardy SE, Allore HG, Guo Z, Dubin JA, Gill TM. The effect of prior disability history on subsequent functional transitions. *Journals of Gerontology Series A-Biological Sciences & Medical Sciences.* 2006;**61**(3):272–7.

20. Pacala JT, Boult C, Boult L. Predictive validity of a questionnaire that identifies older persons at risk for hospital admission. *J Am Geriatr Soc.* 1995;**43**(4):374–7.

21. Rubenstein LZ, Goodwin M, Hadley E, Patten SK, Rempusheski VF, Reuben D, et al. Working group recommendations: targeting criteria for geriatric evaluation and management research. *J Am Geriatr Soc.* 1991;**39**(9 Pt 2):37S–41S.

22. Reuben DB, Maly RC, Hirsch SH, Frank JC, Oakes AM, Siu AL, et al. Physician implementation of and patient adherence to recommendations from comprehensive geriatric assessment [see comments]. *American Journal of Medicine.* 1996;**100**(4):444–51.

23. Alessi CA, Stuck AE, Aronow HU, Yuhas KE, Bula CJ, Madison R, et al. The process of care in preventive in-home comprehensive geriatric assessment. *J Am Geriatr Soc.* 1997;**45**(9):1044–50.

24. Glazier SR, Schuman J, Keltz E, Vally A, Glazier RH. Taking the next steps in goal ascertainment: a prospective study of patient, team, and family perspectives using a comprehensive standardized menu in a geriatric assessment and treatment unit. *J Am Geriatr Soc.* 2004;**52**(2):284–9.

25. Bogardus ST, Jr., Bradley EH, Williams CS, Maciejewski PK, Gallo WT, Inouye SK. Achieving goals in geriatric assessment: role of caregiver agreement and adherence to recommendations. *J Am Geriatr Soc.* 2004;**52**(1):99–105.

26. Stuck AE, Aronow HU, Steiner A, Alessi CA, Bula CJ, Gold MN, et al. A trial of annual in-home comprehensive geriatric assessments for elderly people living in the community. *N Engl J Med.* 1995;**333**(18):1184–9.

27. Rubenstein LZ, Schairer C, Wieland GD, Kane R. Systematic biases in functional status assessment of elderly adults: effects of different data sources. *Journal of Gerontology.* 1984;**39**(6):686–91.

28. Reuben DB, Zwanziger J, Bradley TB, Fink A, Hirsch SH, Williams AP, et al. How many physicians will be needed to provide medical care for older persons? Physician manpower needs for the twenty-first century. *J Am Geriatr Soc.* 1993;**41**(4):444–53.

29. Besdine R, Boult C, Brangman S, Coleman EA, Fried LP, Gerety M, et al. Caring for older Americans: the future of geriatric medicine. *J Am Geriatr Soc.* 2005;**53**(6 Suppl):S245–56.

30. Miller DK, Brunworth D, Brunworth DS, Hagan R, Morley JE. Efficiency of geriatric case-finding in a private practitioner's office. *J Am Geriatr Soc.* 1995;**43**(5):533–7.

31. Bush K, Kivlahan DR, McDonell MB, Fihn SD, Bradley KA. The AUDIT alcohol consumption questions (AUDIT-C): an effective brief screening test for problem drinking. Ambulatory Care Quality Improvement Project (ACQUIP). Alcohol Use Disorders Identification Test. *Arch Intern Med.* 1998;**158**(16):1789–95.

32. Perkins NA, Murphy JE, Malone DC, Armstrong EP. Performance of drug–drug interaction software for personal digital assistants. *Annals of Pharmacotherapy.* 2006;**40**(5):850–5.

33. Schmader KE, Hanlon JT, Pieper CF, Sloane R, Ruby CM, Twersky J, et al. Effects of geriatric evaluation and management on adverse drug reactions and suboptimal prescribing in the frail elderly. *American Journal of Medicine.* 2004;**116**(6):394–401.

34. Blanco-Reina E, Ariza-Zafra G, Ocana-Riola R, Leon-Ortiz M. 2012 American Geriatrics Society Beers Criteria: enhanced Applicability for Detecting Potentially Inappropriate Medications in European Older Adults? A Comparison with the Screening Tool of Older Person's Potentially Inappropriate Prescriptions. *J Am Geriatr Soc.* 2014;**62**(7):1217–23.

35. Chumlea WC, Roche AF, Steinbaugh ML. Estimating stature from knee height for persons 60 to 90 years of age. *J Am Geriatr Soc.* 1985;**33**:116–20.

36. Yueh B, Shapiro N, Maclean CH, Shekelle PG. Screenning and management of adult hearing loss in primary care: scientific review. *JAMA.* 2003;**289**(15):1976–85.

37. Hamalainen P, Rantanen T, Keskinen M, Meurman JH. Oral health status and change in handgrip strength over a 5-year period in 80-year-old people. *Gerotontology.* 2004;**21**(3):155–60.

38. Boustani M, Peterson B, Hanson L, Harris R, Lohr KN; US Preventive Services Task Force. Screening for dementia in primary care: a summary of the evidence for the US preventive services task force. *Ann Int Med.* 2003;**138**:927–37.

39. Tombaugh TN, McIntyre NJ. The Mini-mental State Examination: a comprehensive review. *J Am Geriatr Soc.* 1992;**40**(9):922–35.

40. Mitchell AJ, Malladi S. Screening and case finding tools for the detection of dementia. Part I: evidence-based meta-analysis of multidomain tests. *Am J Geriatr Psychiatry.* 2010;**18**(9):759–82.

41. Cummings-Vaughn LA, Chavakula NN, Malmstrom TK, Tumosa N, Morley JE, Cruz-Oliver DM. Veterans affairs Saint Louis University mental status examination compared with the Montreal Cognitive Assessment and the short test of mental status. *J Am Geriatr Soc.* 2014;**62**(7):1341–6.

42. Inouye SK, Robison JT, Froehlich TE, Richardson ED. The Time and Change Test: a simple screening test for dementia. *J Gerontol: Med Sci.* 1998;**53A**(4):M281–M6.

43. Borson S, Scanlan J, Brush M, Vitaliano P, Dokmak A. The Mini-Cog: a cognitive "vital signs" measure for dementia screening in multi-lingual elderly. *Int J Geriatr Psychiatry.* 2000;**15**:1021–7.

44. Borson S, Scanlan JM, Chen P, Ganguli M. The Mini-Cog as a screen for dementia: validation in a population-based sample. *J Am Geriatr Soc.* 2003;**51**:1451–4.

45. MacKinnon A, Mulligan R. Combining cognitive testing and informant report to increase accuracy in screening for dementia. *Am J Psych.* 1998;**155**:1529–35.

46. Watson LC, Pignone MP. Screening accuracy for late-life depression in primary care: a systematic review [see comment]. *Journal of Family Practice.* 2003;**52**(12):956–64.

47. Blank K, Gruman C, Robison JT. Case-finding for depression in elderly people: balancing ease of administration with validity in varied treatment settings. *Journals of Gerontology Series A-Biological Sciences & Medical Sciences.* 2004;**59**(4):378–84.

48. Phelan E, Williams B, Meeker K, Bonn K, Frederick J, Logerfo J, et al. A study of the diagnostic accuracy of the PHQ-9 in primary care elderly. *BMC Fam Pract.* 2010;**11**:63.

49. Lamers F, Jonkers CC, Bosma H, Penninx BW, Knottnerus JA, van Eijk JT. Summed score of the Patient Health Questionnaire-9 was a reliable and valid method for depression screening in chronically ill elderly patients. *J Clin Epidemiol.* 2008;**61**(7):679–87.

50. Reuben DB, Seeman TE, Keeler E, Hayes RP, Bowman L, Sewall A, et al. Refining the categorization of physical functional status: the added value of combining self-reported and performance-based measures. *Journals of Gerontology Series A-Biological Sciences & Medical Sciences.* 2004;**59**(10):1056–61.

51. Katz S, Akpom CA. A measure of primary sociobiological functions. *Int J Health Serv.* 1976;**6**:493–507.

52. McDowell I. *Measuring Health: A Guide to Rating Scales and Questionnaires.* 3rd ed. New York: Oxford University Press; 2006.

53. Mahoney F, Barthel D. Functional evaluation: the Barthel Index. *Maryland State Med J.* 1965;**14**(2):61–5.

54. Lawton MP, Brody EM. Assessment of older people: self-maintaining and instrumental activities of daily living. *Gerontologist.* 1969;**9**(3):179–86.

55. Guralnik JM, Ferrucci L, Pieper CF, Leveille SG, Markides KS, Ostir GV, et al. Lower extremity function and subsequent disability: consistency across studies, predictive models, and value of gait speed alone compared with the short physical performance battery. *Journals of Gerontology Series A-Biological Sciences & Medical Sciences.* 2000;**55**(4):M221–31.

56. Curb JD, Ceria-Ulep CD, Rodriguez BL, Grove J, Guralnik JM, Willcox BJ, et al. Performance-based measures of physical function for high-function populations. *J Am Geriatr Soc.* 2006;**54**:737–42.

57. Barry E, Galvin R, Keogh C, Horgan F, Fahey T. Is the timed up and go test a useful predictor of risk of falls in community dwelling older adults: a systematic review and meta-analysis. *BMC Geriatr.* 2014;14:14.

58. Donoghue OA, Savva GM, Cronin H, Kenny RA, Horgan NF. Using timed up and go and usual gait speed to predict incident difficulty in daily activities among community-dwelling adults aged 65 and older. *Arch Phys Med Rehabil.* 2014 Oct;95(10):1954–61.

59. Studenski S, Perera S, Patel K, Rosano C, Faulkner K, Inzitari M, et al. Gait speed and survival in older adults. *JAMA.* 2011;305(1):50–8.

60. Chaves PH, Garrett ES, Fried LP. Predicting the risk of mobility difficulty in older women with screening nomograms: the Women's Health and Aging Study II. *Archives of Internal Medicine.* 2000;160(16):2525–33.

61. Pine ZM, Gurland B, Chren MM. Report of having slowed down: evidence for the validity of a new way to inquire about mild disability in elders. *Journals of Gerontology Series A-Biological Sciences & Medical Sciences.* 2000;55(7):M378–83.

62. Pine ZM, Gurland B, Chren MM. Use of a cane for ambulation: marker and mitigator of impairment in older people who report no difficulty walking. *J Am Geriatr Soc.* 2002;50(2):263–8.

63. Summary of the Updated American Geriatrics Society/ British Geriatrics Society clinical practice guideline for prevention of falls in older persons. *J Am Geriatr Soc.* 2011;59(1):148–57.

64. *Management of Urinary Incontinence in Primary Care: A National Clinical Guideline.* Edinburgh: Scottish Intercollegia Guidelines Network, Royal College of Physicians; 2004 [cited 2006].

65. Donovan JL, Badia X, Corcos J, Gotoh M, Kelleher C, Naughton M, et al. Symptom and quality of life assessment. In: Abrams P, Cardozo L, Khoury S, Wein A, editors. *Incontinence: 2nd International Consultation on Incontinence, Paris, July 1–3, 2001.* Plymouth: Health Publications, Ltd; 2002: 267–314.

66. Guigoz Y, Lauque S, Vellas B. Identifying the elderly at risk for malnutrition: the Mini Nutritional Assessment. *Clin Ger Med.* 2002;18(4):737–57.

67. Rubenstein LZ, Harker JO, Salva A, Guigoz Y, Vellas B. Screening for undernutrition in geriatric practice: developing the short-form mini-nutritional assessment (MNA-SF). *Journals of Gerontology Series A-Biological Sciences & Medical Sciences.* 2001;56(6): M366–72.

68. Covinsky KE, Martin GE, Beyth RJ, Justice AC, Sehgal AR, Landefeld CS. The relationship between clinical assessments of nutritional status and adverse outcomes in older hospitalized medical patients. *J Am Geriatr Soc.* 1999;47(5):532–8.

69. Detsky AS, Smalley PS, Chang J. The rational clinical examination. Is this patient malnourished? *JAMA.* 1994;271(1):54–8.

70. Cutler LJ. Assessment of physical environments of older adults. In: Kane RL, Kane RA, editors. *Assessing Older Persons: Measures, Meaning, and Practical Applications.* Oxford: Oxford University Press; 2000: 360–79.

71. Close J, Ellis M, Hooper R, Glucksman E, Jackson S, Swift C. Prevention of falls in the elderly trial (PROFET): a randomised controlled trial. *Lancet.* 1999;353(9147):93–7.

72. Nikolaus T, Bach M. Preventing falls in community-dwelling frail older people using a home intervention team (HIT): results from the randomized Falls-HIT trial. *J Am Geriatr Soc.* 2003;51(3):300–5.

73. Stevens M, Holman CD, Bennett N. Preventing falls in older people: impact of an intervention to reduce environmental hazards in the home. *J Am Geriatr Soc.* 2001;49(11):1442–7.

74. Van Bemmel T, Vandenbroucke JP, Westendorp RGJ, Gussekloo J. In an observational study elderly patients had an increased risk of falling due to home hazards. *Journal of Clinical Epidemiology.* 2005;58(1):63–7.

75. Marshall SW, Runyan CW, Yang J, Coyne-Beasley T, Waller AE, Johnson RM, et al. Prevalence of selected risk and protective factors for falls in the home. *American Journal of Preventive Medicine.* 2005;28(1):95–101.

76. Runyan CW, Johnson RM, Yang J, Waller AE, Perkis D, Marshall SW, et al. Risk and protective factors for fires, burns, and carbon monoxide poisoning in US households. *American Journal of Preventive Medicine.* 2005;28(1):102–8.

77. Tanner EK. Assessing home safety in homebound older adults. *Geriatric Nursing.* 2002;24(4):250–4.

78. Burns R, Nichols LO, Graney MJ, Cloar FT. Impact of continued geriatric outpatient management on health outcomes of older veterans. *Archives of Internal Medicine.* 1995;155(12):1313–8.

79. Engelhardt JB, Toseland RW, O'Donnell JC, Richie JT, Jue D, Banks S. The effectiveness and efficiency of outpatient geriatric evaluation and management [see comments]. *J Am Geriatr Soc.* 1996;44(7):847–56.

80. Gillespie LD, Gillespie WJ, Robertson MC, Lamb SE, Cumming RG, Rowe BH. Interventions for preventing falls in elderly people. *Cochrane Database Syst Rev.* 2006;4:CD000340.

81. Fabacher D, Josephson K, Pietruszka F, Linderborn K, Morley JE, Rubenstein LZ. An in-home preventive assessment program for independent older adults: a randomized controlled trial. *J Am Geriatr Soc.* 1994;42(6):630–8.

82. Boult C, Boult L, Murphy C, Ebbitt B, Luptak M, Kane RL. A controlled trial of outpatient geriatric evaluation and management. *J Am Geriatr Soc.* 1994;**42**(5):465–70.

83. Gerson LW, Camargo CA, Jr., Wilber ST. Home modification to prevent falls by older ED patients. *American Journal of Emergency Medicine.* 2005;**23**(3):295–8.

84. Lubben JE, Gironda M. Social support networks. In: Osterweil D, Brummel-Smith K, Beck JC, editors. *Comprehensive Geriatric Assessment.* New York: McGraw-Hill; 2000: 121–38.

85. Lubben J, Blozik E, Gillmann G, Iliffe S, von Renteln Kruse W, Beck JC, et al. Performance of an abbreviated version of the Lubben Social Network Scale among three European community-dwelling older adult populations. *Gerontologist.* 2006;**46**(4):503–13.

86. Schulz R, Beach SR. Caregiving as a risk factor for mortality: the Caregiver Health Effects Study. *JAMA.* 1999;**282**(23):2215–9.

87. Zarit SH, Reever KE, Bach-Peterson J. Relatives of the impaired elderly: Correlates of feelings of burden. *Gerontologist.* 1980;**20**:649–55.

88. Hirschman KB, Shea JA, Xie SX, Karlawish JHT. The development of a rapid screen for caregiver burden. *J Am Geriatr Soc.* 2004;**52**(10):1724–9.

89. Fulmer T, Guadagno L, Bitondo Dyer C, Connolly MT. Progress in elder abuse screening and assessment instruments. *J Am Geriatr Soc.* 2004;**52**(2):297–304.

90. Berkman ND, DeWalt DA, Pignone MP, Sheridan S, Lohr KN, Lux L, et al. *Literacy and Health Outcomes. Summary, Evidence Report/Technology Assessment No. 87.* Rockville, MD: Agency for Healthcare Research and Quality; 2004 January. Report No.: AHRQ Publication No. 04-E007-1.

91. Wolf MS, Gazmararian JA, Baker DW. Health literacy and functional health status among older adults [see comment]. *Archives of Internal Medicine.* 2005;**165**(17):1946–52.

92. Howard DH, Sentell T, Gazmararian JA. Impact of health literacy on socioeconomic and racial differences in health in an elderly population. *Journal of General Internal Medicine.* 2006;**21**(8):857–61.

93. Howard DH, Gazmararian J, Parker RM. The impact of low health literacy on the medical costs of Medicare managed care enrollees [erratum appears in *Am J Med.* 2005 Aug;118(8):933]. *Am J Med.* 2005;**118**(4):371–7.

94. Gausman Benson J, Forman WB. Comprehension of written health care information in an affluent geriatric retirement community: use of the Test of Functional Health Literacy. *Gerontology.* 2002;**48**(2):93–7.

95. Chew LD, Bradley KA, Boyko EJ. Brief questions to identify patients with inadequate health literacy. *Family Medicine.* 2004;**36**(8):588–94.

96. Wallace LS, Rogers ES, Roskos SE, Holiday DB, Weiss BD. Brief report: screening items to identify patients with limited health literacy skills. *Journal of General Internal Medicine.* 2006;**21**(8):874–7.

97. Saad L. Religion is very important to majority of Americans: Gallup News Service; 2003 [updated December 5, 2003; cited 2006 October 23, 2006]. Available from: http://brain.gallup.com/content/default.aspx?ci=9853.

98. Koenig HG, George LK, Titus P. Religion, spirituality, and health in medically ill hospitalized older patients. *J Am Geriatr Soc.* 2004;**52**(4):554–62.

99. MacLean CD, Susi B, Phifer N, Schultz L, Bynum D, Franco M, et al. Patient preference for physician discussion and practice of spirituality. *Journal of General Internal Medicine.* 2003;**18**(1):38–43.

100. Post SG, Puchalski CM, Larson DB. Physicians and patient spirituality: professional boundaries, competency, and ethics [see comment]. *Annals of Internal Medicine.* 2000;**132**(7):578–83.

101. Daaleman TP. Religion, spirituality, and the practice of medicine. *Journal of the American Board of Family Practice.* 2004;**17**(5):370–6.

102. Anandarajah G, Hight E. Spirituality and medical practice: using the HOPE questions as a practical tool for spiritual assessment [see comment]. *American Family Physician.* 2001;**63**(1):81–9.

103. Daaleman TP, Frey BB. The Spirituality Index of Well-Being: a new instrument for health-related quality-of-life research. *Annals of Family Medicine.* 2004;**2**(5):499–503.

104. Wang CC, Kosinski CJ, Schwartzberg JG, Shanklin AV. *Physician's Guide to Assessing Counseling Older Drivers.* Washington, DC: National Highway Traffic Safety Administration; 2003.

105. Di Stefano M, Macdonald W. Assessment of older drivers: relationships among on-road errors, medical conditions and test outcome. *Journal of Safety Research.* 2003;**34**(4):415–29.

106. AGS Panel on Chronic Pain in Older Persons. The management of persistent pain in older persons. *J Am Geriatr Soc.* 2002;**50**:S205–24.

107. Herr KA, Spratt K, Mobily PR, Richardson G. Pain intensity assessment in older adults: use of experimental pain to compare psychometric properties and usability of selected pain scales with younger adults. *Clinical Journal of Pain.* 2004;**20**(4):207–19.

108. Herr KA, Garand L. Assessment and measurement of pain in older adults. *Clinics in Geriatric Medicine.* 2001;**17**(3):457–78.

109. Stolee P, Hillier LM, Esbaugh J, Bol N, McKellar L, Gauthier N. Instruments for the assessment of pain in

older persons with cognitive impairment. *J Am Geriatr Soc.* 2005;**53**(2):319–26.

110. Zwakhalen SMG, Hamers JPH, Abu-Saad HH, Berger MPF. Pain in elderly people with severe dementia: A systematic review of behavioural pain assessment tools. *BMC Geriatrics.* 2006;**6**(3).

111. DOLOPLUS-2: Behavioral pain assessment scale for elderly subjects with verbal communication disorders 2004 [updated March, 2004; cited 2006 November 24]. Available from: www.doloplus.com/versiongb/index.htm.

112. Fuchs-Lacelle S, Hadjistavropoulos T. Development and preliminary validation of the pain assessment checklist for seniors with limited ability to communicate (PACSLAC). *Pain Manag Nurs.* 2004;**5**(1):37–49.

113. Zwakhalen SMG, Hamers JPH, Berger MPF. The psychometric quality and clinical usefulness of three pain assessment tools for elderly people with dementia. *Pain.* 2006;**126**(1–3):210–20.

114. Ramsdell JW, Jackson JE, Guy HJB, Renvall MJ. Comparison of clinic-based home assessment to a home visit in demented elderly patients. *Alzheimer Disease & Associated Disorders.* 2004;**18**(3):145–53.

115. Stuck AE, Egger M, Hammer A, Minder CE, Beck JC. Home visits to prevent nursing home admission and functional decline in elderly people: systematic review and meta-regression analysis. *JAMA.* 2002;**287**(8):1022–8.

116. Brignell M, Wootton R, Gray L. The application of telemedicine to geriatric medicine. *Age Ageing.* 2007;**36**(4):369–74.

117. Cohen HJ, Feussner JR, Weinberger M, Carnes M, Hamdy RC, Hsieh F, et al. A controlled trial of inpatient and outpatient geriatric evaluation and management. *N Engl J Med.* 2002;**346**(12):905–12.

118. Fox MT, Persaud M, Maimets I, O'Brien K, Brooks D, Tregunno D, et al. Effectiveness of acute geriatric unit care using acute care for elders components: a systematic review and meta-analysis. *J Am Geriatr Soc.* 2012;**60**(12):2237–45.

119. Mor V. A comprehensive clinical assessment tool to inform policy and practice: applications of the minimum data set. *Medical Care.* 2004;**42**(4 Suppl): III50–9.

120. Saliba D, Buchanan J. Making the investment count: revision of the Minimum Data Set for nursing homes, MDS 3.0. *J Am Med Dir Assoc.* 2012;**13**(7):602–10.

121. Saliba D, Buchanan J, Edelen MO, Streim J, Ouslander J, Berlowitz D, et al. MDS 3.0: brief interview for mental status. *J Am Med Dir Assoc.* 2012;**13**(7):611–7.

122. Steinberg K. Minimum Data Set 3.0: a big step forward. *J Am Med Dir Assoc.* 2013;**14**(2):139–40.

Chapter

4

Prevention and screening

James T. Birch, Jr., MD, MSPH, CMD, and Shelley Bhattacharya, DO, MPH

Introduction

In most developed countries of the world, prevention and screening for preventable disease have been a sustained priority for local and national health organizations as well as the health-care and insurance industries. The benefits of primary and secondary prevention are well known and well documented. However, the risk-benefit for screening procedures in the elderly population, and particularly the oldest old, has recently come into question.[1] Given the multiple comorbidities and polypharmacy issues that are common in the older adult population, complications of screening procedures can also have a negative impact on the quality of life of an individual who already has a limited number of years of lifespan remaining. Therefore it becomes extremely important when engaging in the practice of prevention and screening in older adults to individualize the approach based upon age, functional status, additional comorbidities, and the potential for harm that may occur as a result of implementing treatment or diagnostic procedures.[1] Having recognized these concerns, the American Cancer Society and the US Preventive Services Task Force have modified their guidelines to recommendations that convey a more conservative approach.[1] The purpose of this chapter is to provide updates on prevention and screening as they relate to common conditions encountered in the older adult population.

Infectious disease

Infection is the leading cause of death in one-third of adults aged 65 and older. For prevention of common infections, such as influenza and streptococcal pneumonia, immunization is the most important preventive strategy.

Pneumococcal vaccine

Although pneumococcal vaccination may not prevent pneumonia in older adults, rates of bacteremia and invasive pneumococcal disease are decreased in immunized patients, and mortality is lower for patients who were vaccinated prior to admission.[2] Pneumococcal vaccine is recommended for all persons 65 years and older (also under age 65) with comorbid conditions. Two vaccines are available: a 23-valent polysaccharide vaccine (PPSV23) and a 13-valent pneumococcal conjugate vaccine (PCV13). In 2014, the Advisory Committee on Immunization Practices (ACIP) revised the recommendations for pneumococcal vaccination in older adults so that currently, both PCV13 and PPSV23 are to be given sequentially to all adults aged 65 and older. (See Figure 4.1.)

Influenza vaccine

The influenza vaccine reduces the severity of disease, subsequent hospitalization, and mortality by about 70%–90%.[3] A "high-dose" inactivated influenza vaccine is available for adults older than 65. A recent study showed that among persons 65 years of age or older, high-dose vaccine induced significantly higher antibody responses and provided better protection against laboratory-confirmed influenza illness than did the standard dose.[4] During outbreaks, chemoprophylaxis with amantadine, rimantadine, zanamivir, and oseltamavir are effective for protection during the two weeks immediately after immunization until an antibody response provides protection.

Shingles vaccine

Herpes zoster (shingles) is a painful and sometimes pruritic vesicular skin eruption that occurs with reactivation of the varicella zoster virus in the dorsal root ganglia or cranial nerves.[5] Postherpetic neuralgia

---

Reichel's Care of the Elderly, 7th Edition, ed. Jan Busby-Whitehead *et al.* Published by Cambridge University Press.
© Cambridge University Press 2016.

Pneumococcal vaccine-naïve persons aged ≥65 years

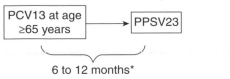

Persons who previously received PPSV23 at age ≥65 years

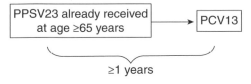

Persons who previously received PPSV23 before age 65 years who are now aged ≥65 years

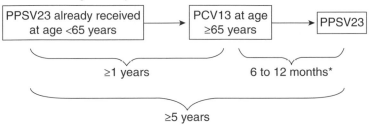

Figure 4.1 Sequential administration and recommended intervals for PCV13 and PPSV23 for adults aged ≥65 years – ACIP, United States.[13]
PCV13: 13-valent pneumococcal conjugate vaccine; PPSV23: 23-valent pneumococcal polysaccharide vaccine.

* Minimum interval between sequential administration of PCV13 and PPSV23 is 8 weeks; PPSV23 can be given later than 6–12 months after PCV13 if this window is missed.

(PHN) is the major and most common complication of herpes zoster.[5] Both shingles and PHN are preventable conditions. The Centers for Disease Control and Prevention (CDC) recommends one single dose of the herpes vaccine (Zostavax) for persons aged 60 and over.[5, 6]

Hypertension

The aging process is a known dominant risk factor in the progression of hypertension and in some cases for its onset in later life.[7] Active screening for hypertension can take place only when the blood pressure of an individual is measured. In early 2014, the Eighth Joint National Committee (JNC8) published an evidence-based guideline for the management of high blood pressure in adults. With regards to the elderly patient, most of the national and international guidelines recommend treatment targets for patients ≥60 years of age toward systolic BP less than 150/90 [SOR=A]. [8–10] Controversy exists as to whether there is any additional benefit to target systolic less than 140/90 mmHg due to the potential development of increasing frailty or further decline in quality of life

or in end-organ function.[9, 10] Prevention of hypertension continues to include the recommendation for a low salt diet and moderate exercise three or four times per week.[8]

Lipid disorders

Recent new evidence-based guidelines on the treatment of blood cholesterol were developed and published by the American College of Cardiology (ACC) and the American Heart Association (AHA). [11] These new guidelines place less emphasis on specific low-density lipoprotein (LDL) targets and are developed to address more specific issues such as the optimal LDL and high-density lipoprotein (HDL) goals of treatment for both primary and secondary prevention. At this point in time, the evidence does not support the continuation of statin drugs for persons ≥75 years of age who are already taking and tolerating these drugs.[11] However, the use of moderate-intensity statin therapy for secondary prevention in individuals with atherosclerotic cardiovascular disease (ASCVD) in this age group is supported by a larger amount of data.[11] There is no support for high-intensity therapy for purposes of secondary prevention.[11] Furthermore there is insufficient data supporting a reduction benefit in primary prevention of ASCVD events for patients ≥75 years of age without clinical ASCVD.[11] There is also a lack of strong evidence of health benefits supporting recommendations for any of the other drug classes for primary treatment of LDL cholesterol (fibrates, niacin, bile acid sequestrants, ezetimibe, and omega-3 fatty acids). The clinical decision to initiate statin therapy for primary prevention of hyperlipidemia in patients ≥75 years of age involves the consideration of present comorbidities (as well as the potential of their increasing in number), safety concerns (drug interactions, polypharmacy, organ transplantation, etc.), and goals of care[11]. Calculation of the 10-year risk of ASCVD might also be helpful for clinical decision making (http://tools.cardiosource.org/ASCVD-Risk-Estimator).

In summary, four groups of individuals were identified through a rigorous review of randomized clinical trials, as demonstrating evidence of reduction in ASCVD events, with a good margin of safety, from the use of moderate- or high-intensive statin therapy:[11]

1   Individuals with clinical ASCVD
2   Individuals with primary elevation of LDL-C ≥190 mg/dL
3   Individuals 40–75 years of age with diabetes and LDL-C of 70–189 mg/dL, without evidence of ASCVD
4   Individuals without diabetes or clinical ASCVD who are 40–79 years of age and have LDL-C of 70–189 mg/dL and an estimated ASCVD 10-year risk of greater than 7.5%; a clinician-patient discussion is required

Osteoporosis

Osteoporosis is not an inevitable consequence of aging; it is a preventable disease. Osteoporotic fractures are a substantial contributor to mortality and morbidity in older adults and have a remarkable burden on the health-care system.[12] Prevention strategies are aimed at maximizing peak bone mass and minimizing bone loss with aging.

Screening and primary prevention form the core of most of the clinical guidelines for osteoporosis.[12] The Fracture Risk Assessment Tool (FRAX; www.shef.ac.uk/FRAX) is utilized to estimate the 10-year risk of hip and other osteoporotic fractures by assessing risk factors and bone mineral density (BMD)

measurement.[12, 13] BMD testing can be utilized for both screening and diagnosis of osteoporosis. The findings of BMD testing can be entered into the FRAX tool to further refine the risk of osteoporotic fracture.[13] FRAX is designed to estimate osteoporotic fracture risk in postmenopausal women and men over the age of 50.[13] It is not validated for use with individuals who have received any treatment for osteoporosis unless there has been cessation of therapy for an interval of one to two years. Another screening tool, the Osteoporosis Self-Assessment Screening Tool (OST) was found in a recent study to be slightly better than FRAX at identifying individuals at low risk of osteoporosis for whom BMD screening can be omitted.[12] Further information on diagnostic criteria can be found in the National Osteoporosis Foundation guidelines for 2013.[13, 14]

Prevention of osteoporosis requires application of multiple intervention strategies, which include specifications on oral calcium intake, oral vitamin D intake, weight-bearing and muscle strengthening exercise, smoking cessation, and alcohol intake.[13–18]

Weight and physical activity

The American Heart Association (AHA) and the American College of Sports Medicine (ACSM) provide recommendations for adults over age 65 for various types of activity and guidance for implementing weight bearing and muscle strengthening exercise programs.[19] Exceeding the minimum amount will lead to greater health benefits; however it is recommended that the patient always consult a health-care provider prior to beginning any exercise program. Some of the minimum recommendations include:

1   Aerobic exercise involving use of large muscle groups for 30 minutes duration five days per week, 20 minutes duration three days per week, or a combination of the two.
2   Muscle strengthening activities targeting major muscle groups such as arms, shoulders, legs, hips, back, chest, and abdomen on two or more nonconsecutive days per week.
3   To sustain the flexibility and range of motion needed for regular activity and activities of daily living, it is recommended that older adults participate in such exercises two days each week for at least 10 minutes every day.

4 The preferred types, frequency, and duration of balance exercise have not been ascertained in the clinical guidelines; however, balance exercise three times weekly was effective in several fall prevention studies.[20]

The National Institute on Aging has an exercise and physical activity guide that is free to individuals or can be ordered in bulk for selected purposes (http://go4life.niapublications.org).

Hearing loss

It is a well-known fact that the prevalence of hearing loss increases with age.[21] Hearing loss can be divided into two categories: conductive and sensorineural. Conductive hearing loss is caused by the inability to mechanically transmit sound vibrations from the environment to the inner ear.[22] The majority of sensorineural hearing loss is a result of disorders of the inner ear itself and is not directly related to dysfunction of the vestibulocochlear nerve.[22]

The US Preventive Services Task Force (USPSTF) finds insufficient evidence for or against screening for hearing loss in asymptomatic adults 50 years or older.[23] However, the effectiveness of screening questionnaires and clinical tools are validated for use in the primary care clinic.[23] Examples of physical examination tools to screen for hearing loss include the whisper test, finger rub, and watch tick tests.[23, 24] Pure tone audiometry can be performed with a hand-held audiometer.[23] Pure-tone audiometry requires a quiet testing environment with low levels of background noise because hearing loss is worsened with competing background noise. [23, 24]

Visual impairment

Persons over the age of 65 should be screened for vision problems every one to two years.[25] Most causes of vision loss are either preventable or treatable. The USPSTF recommends that visual acuity screening should be a part of the periodic health examination of individuals over the age of 65.[25] Disease-specific screening for diabetic retinopathy, cataracts, glaucoma, and macular degeneration, as well as screening for ophthalmological adverse effects of medications, is best conducted by an ophthalmologist.[25] The Early Treatment of Diabetic Retinopathy (ETDRS) chart or the Snellen Chart (hand-held or wall fixture) are useful for in-office screening of refractory errors.[25]

Cancer

Screening for the common causes of cancer death is controversial for the older adult. The USPSTF and other guideline panels by national medical specialty organizations all have separate and sometimes congruent recommendations for when to initiate and when to discontinue screening. For the older adult, decisions about screening for cancer should be individualized and centered on the current evidence-based guidelines, the patients' life expectancy, the benefits and harms of screening, and integration of the values and preferences of the patient into the screening decisions.[26, 27] The following is a list of recommendations for the *age of cessation* for specific types of cancer screening and a summation of the conditions or exceptions to be followed:[27]*

Cervical cancer: 65–70 years of age if not at high risk and with adequate recent screening with normal Pap smears (AAFP, USPSTF); screening determined on an individual basis to include such factors as the patient's medical history and the physician's ability to monitor the patient in the future (ACOG); three or more normal Pap tests in a row and no abnormal Pap smear tests in the past 10 years (ACS); there is little evidence for or against screening women beyond age 70 who have been regularly screened in previous years (AGS).

Breast cancer: The decision to stop screening should be individualized on the basis of the potential benefits and risks of screening in the context of overall health status and longevity (ACS); screening may continue in women with an estimated life expectancy of four or more years (AGS); women with comorbid conditions that limited life expectancy are unlikely to benefit from screening (USPSTF).

Colon cancer: The USPSTF recommends against the routine screening in adults 76–85 years of age; it recommends against screening in adults older than 85 years of age.

Prostate cancer: Screening for prostate cancer is not recommended in men aged 75 years and older (AAFP/USPSTF); screening for prostate cancer should be offered annually beginning at 50 years of age to men who have a life expectancy of at least 10 years (ACS/AUA).

---

* AAFP – American Academy of Family Physicians; ACOG – American College of Obstetricians and Gynecologists; ACS – American Cancer Society; AGS – American Geriatrics Society; AUA – American Urological Association; USPSTF – United States Preventive Services Task Force

It is important to note that cessation of cancer screening is primarily done to prevent harm and not to ignore problems or suspicious symptoms. A two-way dialogue based on evidence-based guidelines and individual preferences is pertinent in making a decision to continue or stop cancer screening.[26, 27] These are core principles of good medical practice and should be applied to cancer screening decisions. [27] Although some patients may be relieved with the thought of not undergoing further testing, others may feel discrimination on the basis of perceived ageism by the physician and/or the medical community.[26]

Depression

Depression is very common in older adults and frequently unrecognized by clinicians and patients alike. [28] Elderly patients with depression often present with vague symptoms such as fatigue, anorexia, insomnia, and weight loss.[28] Inadequate treatment of depression is known to contribute to higher risk of morbidity and poorer outcomes.[29]

The definition of major depressive disorder (MDD) has recently been modified in the fifth edition of the *Diagnostic and Statistical Manual of Mental Disorders* (DSM-5) by the removal of the bereavement and the persistent depressive disorder category.[30] Major depressive disorder is defined by a patient having one or more depressive episodes (MDE) and the lifetime absence of mania and hypomania.[30]

The USPSTF recommends screening adults for depression in clinical practices that have systems in place to ensure accurate diagnosis, effective treatment, and follow-up.[29] There is minimal benefit for screening if these systems are not in place. The USPSTF found no evidence of harms of screening for depression in adults and reports good evidence that treatment with antidepressants, psychotherapy, or both decreases clinical morbidity and improves outcomes in adults with depression, which is verified through screening in the primary care setting.[29]

For screening of depression, many different instruments are available. The USPSTF found no significant evidence that one instrument is superior to another, but positive results on any screening test should provide the impetus to move on to full diagnostic testing tools that use criteria at minimum from the DSM-IV.[29]

Screening tools for older adults include:[29, 31]

- PHQ-2: Patient Health Questionnaire with two simple questions about mood and anhedonia.

Sensitivity = 100% and specificity = 77% in older adults. If positive on initial screening, the American Geriatrics Society recommends follow-up testing with either the PHQ-9 or the Geriatric Depression Scale (GDS).
- PHQ-9: Patient Health Questionnaire with nine questions. Sensitivity = 61% and specificity = 94% in adults.
- GDS: Five-item and 15-item questionnaires are available. The 15-item screening tool has sensitivity = 74%–100% and specificity = 53%–98%. It is also a well-validated screening instrument for older adults.
- Longer screening instruments include the Beck Depression Inventory and the Zung Depression Scale.
- Hamilton Rating Scale for Depression takes somatic symptoms into account in screening for depression; it was initially published in 1960.[31]

When results of screening tests indicate that depression is or could be present, the diagnosis needs to be confirmed according to DSM-IV or DSM-5 diagnostic criteria. If the diagnostic criteria are not met, the depressive symptoms could be due to other psychological syndromes. Be mindful when screening that several different medical conditions can also contribute to depressive symptoms in older adults.[29]

Hypothyroidism

Hypothyroidism is very common in older adults, with women being 10 times more likely to be affected than men.[32] In older adults, fatigue and weakness are the most common symptoms, and many of the classic signs and symptoms of hypothyroidism may be mistakenly assumed to be associated with normal aging. [32, 33]

There is no consensus among many medical professional organizations to guide screening for thyroid disease.[33] The USPSTF and the Canadian Task Force do not find enough evidence to recommend for or against screening in asymptomatic elderly women; however, a high index of suspicion and low threshold for evaluating thyroid function should be maintained in the at-risk population.[33, 34] Included in this category are those elderly patients who present with vague, nonspecific symptoms, persons older than 60, women, and persons with concomitant autoimmune disease.[33, 35] The American Academy of

Family Physicians (AAFP) and the American Association of Clinical Endocrinologists (AACE) recommend measurement of thyroid function "periodically" in older, postmenopausal women.[35]

The most common tests that are ordered for screening of thyroid disease are the total thyroxine (TT4), free thyroxine index (FT4I), and the sensitive thyrotropin (sensitive-TSH).[36] Tests for triiodothyronine and anti-thyroid antibodies may be used as follow-up tests in some situations, but they have no utility as screening tests.[36] Patients who have low or undetectable TSH levels and an elevated free thyroxine level have overt hyperthyroidism, and patients who have a TSH level that is elevated (≥ 10 mU/L) and a low free thyroxine level have overt hypothyroidism.[34] A formal system to identify these patients with arrangement for follow-up evaluation should be a part of any screening program.[34]

Subclinical hypothyroidism (SCH) is a commonly encountered laboratory finding in clinical practice.[37] Lab results will often demonstrate an elevated TSH level in the serum and normal levels of free thyroxine based on the reported reference ranges.[37] The prevalence of SCH is difficult to determine, although it is thought to be more prevalent than overt thyroid disease.[33, 37] A percentage of individuals with SCH will progress to clinical or overt hypothyroidism with a variable incidence in research studies ranging from 2% to 26.2% after about two years.[37] A diagnosis of SCH, however, does not always merit treatment, especially if the TSH elevations are transient (persists less than three to six months) and the patient does not have risk factors for developing overt hypothyroidism.[37] Treatment should be individualized and restricted to high-risk patients.[33]

Dementia

Dementia is a debilitating and degenerative neurologic condition for which there is no cure.[38] Alzheimer's disease, the most common form of dementia, causes the destruction of brain cells, which creates problems with memory, attention, language, decision making, and behavior. These problems are severe enough to negatively impact family, social, and occupational functioning, and eventually the most basic activities of daily living (BADLS).[39–41] There are many different types of dementia, and Alzheimer's disease accounts for

approximately 60% of all cases.[39] Mild cognitive impairment (MCI) is a different condition because patients are able to maintain independence with BADLS and instrumental activities of daily living, but detection may be useful for predicting the eventual development of dementia.[41]

The USPSTF in 2003 concluded that there was insufficient evidence to recommend for or against routine screening for dementia in older adults.[38, 41, 42] This is due to a lack of studies that evaluate the efficacy, benefits, and harms of dementia screening in primary care.[38]

Individuals with dementia usually present to their family physician first, who is also often the first physician to observe patients with possible dementia and the only physician to make the diagnosis.[39] Cognitive impairment might not be recognized with routine history and physical examination, and despite the benefits of early intervention, dementia continues to be underdiagnosed.[41] The Centers for Medicare and Medicaid Services (CMS) provides coverage for the costs of an annual wellness visit for Medicare beneficiaries; the visit includes, among its nine elements, detection for cognitive impairment.[38]

There are two primary methods of screening a patient for dementia.[39] One approach is to use a performance measure or screening tool, which is a test administered and scored.[39] A second approach is to interview an informant or someone close to the patient who can report how the cognition has changed and how the change has impacted the patient's ability to perform everyday activities.[39]

With regards to performance-based tools, the Mini-Mental Status Examination (MMSE) has been used frequently and is the best study instrument, but it has inherent biases according to age, race, education, and socioeconomic status.[39] Several other screening tools are now available and are updated regularly to provide primary care physicians with effective diagnostic tools that are easy to administer. The Mini-Cognitive Assessment Instrument (Mini-Cog) is briefer and not associated with the same language or education biases as the MMSE.[39] Although more complex than the MMSE or Mini-Cog, the Montréal Cognitive Assessment (MoCA) has the advantage of testing multiple cognitive domains with an easy scoring system and is free for clinical use.[39] It was also developed to assist physicians with MCI.[39] Other screening tools that have been commonly utilized include the clock-drawing test (CDT), Word Fluency-Animal Naming, Sweet 16, Trail Making B, Kingston Standardized Cognitive Assessment-Revised (mini-KSCAr), and the Short Portable Mental Status Questionnaire (SPMSQ).[41, 43]

Informant-based screening tools include the Ascertain Dementia (AD-8), which is an eight-item, brief screening interview, and the short or full Informant Questionnaire on Cognitive Decline in the Elderly (IQCODE).[39, 41]

Screening for dementia by itself does not automatically lead to better clinical care.[40] Screening tools can sometimes lead to a wrong conclusion, particularly when relying on simple, single cut-off scores.[43] Corrections need to be made for age and intelligence or educational level.[43] Minor deviations while administering screening tools can alter results.[43] It also equally important to use cognitive screening tools with "updated norms" that reflect cohort differences to avoid compromising the screening accuracy.[43]

Elder mistreatment

There are 450,000 new cases of elder abuse annually, and unfortunately this statistic is considered to be an inaccurate underestimation because for every case of elder abuse or neglect that is reported, there are five cases that are not reported.[44] Elder abuse is a very complex problem and takes on many forms. This includes physical abuse, emotional abuse, verbal abuse, financial abuse, sexual abuse, neglect, and so on.[44] Elders at highest risk are those who are ill, frail, disabled, mentally impaired, or depressed, but high-risk individuals are not restricted to these categories.[44] Physicians and extended caregivers need to be better educated to recognize the signs of elder abuse and neglect as well as develop familiarity with the reporting requirements and the resources available for assistance.[44]

Several screening tools have been developed to facilitate the detection of elder abuse. The USPSTF concluded that current evidence for screening of elder abuse and neglect is insufficient to assess its potential benefits or harm.[45] Given the known association between elder abuse, adverse health outcomes, and increased utilization of health services, efforts are being made to develop and assess the validity of screening tools in multiple settings while developing an evidence-based evaluation of their effectiveness. [46] The elder abuse suspicion index (EASI) consists

Table 4.1 Screening tools for detecting elder abuse

HALF	Health, Attitudes towards Aging, Living Arrangements, and Finances; consists of a 37-item checklist requiring an interview and a period of observation
EAI	Elder Assessment Instrument; a 42-item checklist of selected common presentations of elder mistreatment
BASE	Brief Abuse Screen for the Elderly; contains five brief questions that take only a minute to complete
IOA	Indicators of Abuse Screen; a 40-item checklist
CTS	Conflict Tactics Scale; a 19-item self-report or interview

of six questions and can be administered in two minutes.[44] Another tool created by the AMA consists of nine questions.[44] An answer of "yes" to any question in either screening tool should initiate a more thorough evaluation. Additional screening tools are listed in Table 4.1.[47]

One way to approach detection of elder mistreatment is to obtain a portion of the history in private without family members or caregivers present so that the screening tools can be administered at that time. [44] This should be followed by a thorough physical examination. The findings of bruises or lacerations in various stages of healing, burns, or injuries not consistent with the history should be alerts to the medical provider of possible physical abuse. Findings that should raise concerns about neglect include decubitus ulcers, sores, dehydration, and poor hygiene. It is very important to keep in mind that the same findings also occur in cases of self-neglect.

In spite of the magnitude of elder abuse around the world, there is a paucity of knowledge about how to prevent it before it occurs or how to stop it once it starts.[46] The local Adult Protective Services is the first line of intervention and investigation when elder abuse is suspected. In order to make a report, one only needs a legitimate concern to prompt a more thorough evaluation of the patient and his or her living situation by local authorities. Accusations should be avoided in reports and should be focused on the provider's physical or emotional findings that raise concerns about abuse.[44]

Falls

Falls are common in older adults and impact their independence and quality of life, and increase the likelihood of nursing home placement. This is a multifactorial geriatric syndrome usually precipitated by impairment in multiple domains resulting in compensatory compromise.[48]

One of the first steps to take toward the prevention of falls is to identify the patient's fall risk(s), many of which are inherent in his or her chronic medical conditions. It is important for clinicians to ask about a previous history of falls and the circumstances of the fall.[28] Additional pertinent history includes lower extremity weakness, age, gender, the presence of cognitive impairment, gait instability from any cause, history of stroke, Parkinson's disease, orthostasis, diabetes, dizziness, visual disturbances, current use of an ambulatory assist device, anemia, and a "fear of falling," to mention a few.[49–51] A medication review should be completed to identify high-risk medications.[52] Judicious alcohol use, low-heeled footwear, and a home safety evaluation are preventative interventions that have been supported by research studies.[53–55]

Additional physical examination tools that can be used to screen for high fall risk include the Tinetti Balance and Gait evaluation and the Get Up and Go Test (or Timed Up and Go Test [TUG]).[56, 57] Assessment of scores of these tools and attention to specific abnormalities of components of either test can lead to further evaluation and placement of interventions such as physical therapy, occupational therapy, and an ambulatory assist device that can reduce fall risk as well as allow patients to maintain independence and quality of life.[49]

Alcohol and substance abuse/misuse

The older adult population experiences the greatest proportion of chronic illness and functional limitations.[58] Now that the "baby boom" cohort approaches the age of 65 and older, the number of older adults who misuse alcohol, psychoactive prescription drugs, and other substances is steadily increasing at a higher rate than previous generations.[59] The attitudes and beliefs about the use of substances and the more widespread exposure to alcohol, tobacco, and illegal drugs during their youth contribute to the observed differences.[60] The use of psychoactive medications to manage anxiety, stress, sleep, and pain to cope with daily life and its pressures has also become more prevalent.[59, 60] Chronic illnesses are more challenging to treat or are worsened by the use of alcohol and other substances.[58] Alcohol can exaggerate or reduce the pharmacologic effects of many different medications, as well as precipitate adverse drug events, falls, accidental injuries, and premature death.[58] Older adults often under report their drinking habits.[59] They have less social contact than their younger counterparts, which makes the alcohol use less noticeable, and the stigma associated with alcohol use is a barrier itself to reaching out for help.[61]

There are a few tools available to facilitate screening of alcohol misuse and related disorders in the older adult. Some common instruments are not ideal for the older adult patient because there are some criteria that may not apply to the older adult (work performance, social interaction, and measurement of alcohol tolerance).[60] The validated instruments that have been used successfully with older adults are:[58–60]

CAGE (cut down, annoyed, guilty, eye opener) questionnaire

AUDIT (Alcohol Use Disorders Identification Test)

SMAST-G (Short Michigan Alcoholism Screening Test – Geriatric Version)

ASSIST (Alcohol, Smoking, and Substance Involvement Screening Test)

ARPS (Alcohol-Related Problems Survey)

The AUDIT is a brief screening tool for excessive drinking that is well validated and was developed by the World Health Organization.[59] It is also recommended to cross-culturally screen for the use of alcohol.[60] The AUDIT-C is a three-item questionnaire than can be utilized in the primary care setting and is thought to be a more efficient tool for identifying heavy drinkers that might benefit from brief interventions.[62]

The ARPS is a tool to facilitate alcohol-related health risk identification and a system for health risk education in screening older patients for the more dangerous categories of alcohol consumption such as *harmful* (consumption that may exacerbate or complicate existing alcohol-related problems), *hazardous* (consumption that possesses risk of future harm for individuals with specific medical condition[s], functional status, or symptoms; taking specific medication[s]; or engaging in risky behaviors such as smoking), and *healthwise* (neither harmful nor hazardous and potentially beneficial).[58]

As the population of older adults in the world increases, so will the number of alcohol misuse and substance abuse problems. Screening for these particular issues can take place in many different healthcare settings.[59] With successful implementation of innovative screening, intervention, and treatment methods for older adults, current and future generations with substance misuse problems will have the opportunity for improved physical and emotional quality in their lives.[59]

Driving safety

The purpose of assessing driving safety in older adults is to ensure their driving physical fitness while maintaining their independence. Functional decline, rather than chronological age, correlates with diminished driving fitness. The decline is usually due to a combination of physiologic, age, and disease state severity.

Screening tests for an at-risk driver involve performing a focused physical examination of vision, hearing, the musculoskeletal system, and cognition. [63] Certain characteristics associated with adverse driving events, driving cessation, and self-limited driving by the patient include dementia, being unable to draw intersecting pentagons on the MMSE, heart disease, one or more accidents in the previous year, vision impairment, and limited range of motion of the neck, feet, or ambulation in general.[63] Other screening tests that can be predictive of driving safety on the road include the Trails A and B tests and the Snellgrove Maze test.[64] A recent study suggests that the results of Trails A should be stratified according to age and education.[65]

A behind-the-wheel driving evaluation is the most efficacious form of driving evaluation. It is usually operated by certified occupational therapist.[63] This type of evaluation measures the impact of the multifactorial aspects of the patient's cognition and physical impairments on driving ability.[63] Based on the results of the evaluation, the occupational therapist recommends either that the patient resume driving with no restrictions, have adaptive equipment installed in the vehicle, undergo a specified number of hours of driving rehabilitation, or refrain from driving.[63] Recommendations should be documented in writing for the patient.[63] The impact of "no driving" news can lead to depression, isolation, and

feelings of helplessness, resulting in major lifestyle changes for the older adult.[63]

Smoking cessation

Smoking cessation and prevention primarily involve the use of counseling and encouragement to induce behavior change and different therapeutic modalities to reduce and ultimately to discontinue use. Approximately two-thirds of smokers have visited a physician at some point in time, providing an opportunity for counseling and cessation.[66] Counseling in combination with pharmacotherapy appears more effective for smoking cessation. It can include individual or group therapy; audio, video, or CD formats; and behavioral therapies such as setting a quit date, identifying strategies to reduce cravings, and dealing with stress. In addition, smokers learn to manage withdrawal symptoms and prevent relapse. [66] Choices need to be individualized, and clinicians need to remind patients of the benefits of quitting, regardless of age.

Nicotine replacement therapy is effective when utilized cautiously, in combination with the options previously mentioned. Replacement therapies are available in the form of chewing gum, transdermal patch, sprays, and inhalers.[67] Smoking cessation rate at one year is about 20% in older adults.[68]

Non-nicotine preparations to facilitate smoking cessation include bupropion, clonidine, and nortriptyline. The sustained release bupropion alone or in combination with the nicotine patch has shown a higher abstinence rate at one year.[67] The usual duration of treatment is eight weeks to six months.

Summary

Given the complexity of comorbidities that are common in older adults, it becomes extremely important when engaging in the practice of prevention and screening in older adults to individualize the approach based upon age, functional status, comorbidities, and the potential for harm that may occur as a result of implementing treatment or diagnostic procedures. The purpose of this chapter has been to provide updates on prevention and screening as they relate to common conditions encountered in older adults. Please refer to other references for in-depth discussions about screening instruments and treatment as they relate to prevention or positive results of screening procedures.

References

1. Clarfield AM. Screening in frail older people: an ounce of prevention or a pound of trouble? *Journal of the American Geriatrics Society*. 2010;**58**(10):2016–21.

2. Vila-Corcoles A, Ochoa-Gondar O, Hospital I, Ansa X, Vilanova A, Rodriguez T, et al. Protective effects of the 23-valent pneumococcal polysaccharide vaccine in the elderly population: the EVAN-65 study. *Clinical Infectious Diseases: an Official Publication of the Infectious Diseases Society of America*. 2006;**43**(7): 860–8.

3. Rivetti D, Jefferson T, Thomas R, Rudin M, Rivetti A, Di Pietrantonj C, et al. Vaccines for preventing influenza in the elderly. *Cochrane Database of Systematic Reviews*. 2006(3):CD004876.

4. DiazGranados CA, Dunning AJ, Kimmel M, Kirby D, Treanor J, Collins A, et al. Efficacy of high-dose versus standard-dose influenza vaccine in older adults. *New England Journal of Medicine*. 2014;**371**(7):635–45.

5. Fashner J, Bell AL. Herpes zoster and postherpetic neuralgia: prevention and management. *American Family Physician*. 2011;**83**(12):1432–7.

6. Wilson JF. Herpes zoster. *Annals of Internal Medicine*. 2011;**154**(5):ITC31–15; quiz ITC316.

7. Fukutomi M, Kario K. Aging and hypertension. *Expert Review of Cardiovascular Therapy*. 2010;**8**(11):1531–9.

8. Mahvan TD, Mlodinow SG. JNC 8: what's covered, what's not, and what else to consider. *Journal of Family Practice*. 2014;**63**(10):574 84.

9. Kjeldsen S, Feldman RD, Lisheng L, Mourad JJ, Chiang CE, Zhang W, et al. Updated national and international hypertension guidelines: a review of current recommendations. *Drugs*. 2014;**74**(17): 2033–51.

10. James PA, Oparil S, Carter BL, Cushman WC, Dennison-Himmelfarb C, Handler J, et al. 2014 evidence based guideline for the management of high blood pressure in adults: report from the panel members appointed to the Eighth Joint National Committee (JNC 8). *JAMA*. 2014;**311**(5):507–20.

11. Stone NJ, Robinson JG, Lichtenstein AH, Bairey Merz CN, Blum CB, Eckel RH, et al. 2013 ACC/AHA guideline on the treatment of blood cholesterol to reduce atherosclerotic cardiovascular risk in adults: a report of the American College of Cardiology/ American Heart Association Task Force on Practice Guidelines. *Circulation*. 2014;**129**(25 Suppl 2):S1–45.

12. Pang WY, Inderjeeth CA. FRAX without bone mineral density versus osteoporosis self-assessment screening tool as predictors of osteoporosis in primary screening of individuals aged 70 and older. *Journal of the American Geriatrics Society*. 2014;**62**(3):442–6.

13. Cosman F, de Beur SJ, LeBoff MS, Lewiecki EM, Tanner B, Randall S, et al. Clinician's guide to prevention and treatment of osteoporosis. *Osteoporosis International: a Journal Established as Result of Cooperation between the European Foundation for Osteoporosis and the National Osteoporosis Foundation of the USA*. 2014;**25**(10):2359–81.

14. Foundation No. 2013 Clinician's Guide to Prevention and Treatment of Osteoporosis 2013 [cited 2015 January 15, 2015]. Available at: http://nof.org/fil es/nof/public/content/file/917/upload/481.pdf.

15. Recommendations abstracted from the American Geriatrics Society Consensus Statement on vitamin D for Prevention of Falls and Their Consequences. *Journal of the American Geriatrics Society*. 2014;**62**(1):147–52.

16. Institute of Medicine Committee to Review Dietary Reference Intakes for Vitamin D, Calcium. The National Academies Collection: reports funded by National Institutes of Health. In: Ross AC, Taylor CL, Yaktine AL, Del Valle HB (eds). *Dietary Reference Intakes for Calcium and Vitamin D*. Washington, DC: National Academies Press (US) National Academy of Sciences.; 2011.

17. Kanis JA, Johnell O, Oden A, Johansson H, De Laet C, Eisman JA, et al. Smoking and fracture risk: a meta-analysis. *Osteoporosis International: a Journal Established as Result of Cooperation between the European Foundation for Osteoporosis and the National Osteoporosis Foundation of the USA*. 2005;**16**(2): 155–62.

18. Kanis JA, Johansson H, Johnell O, Oden A, De Laet C, Eisman JA, et al. Alcohol intake as a risk factor for fracture. *Osteoporosis International: a Journal Established as Result of Cooperation between the European Foundation for Osteoporosis and the National Osteoporosis Foundation of the USA*. 2005;**16**(7): 737–42.

19. Nelson ME, Rejeski WJ, Blair SN, Duncan PW, Judge JO, King AC, et al. Physical activity and public health in older adults: recommendation from the American College of Sports Medicine and the American Heart Association. *Circulation*. 2007;**116**(9):1094–105.

20. Robertson MC, Campbell AJ, Gardner MM, Devlin N. Preventing injuries in older people by preventing falls: a meta-analysis of individual-level data. *Journal of the American Geriatrics Society*. 2002;**50**(5):905–11.

21. Nash SD, Cruickshanks KJ, Klein R, Klein BE, Nieto FJ, Huang GH, et al. The prevalence of hearing impairment and associated risk factors: the Beaver Dam Offspring Study. *Arch Otolaryngol Head Neck Surg*. 2011;**137**(5):432–9.

22. Gates GA, Mills JH. Presbycusis. *Lancet*. 2005;**366**(9491):1111–20.

23. Walker JJ, Cleveland LM, Davis JL, Seales JS. Audiometry screening and interpretation. *American Family Physician*. 2013;**87**(1):41–7.

24. Arlinger S. Negative consequences of uncorrected hearing loss – a review. *Int J Audiol*. 2003;**42** Suppl 2:2S17–20.

25. Pelletier AL, Thomas J, Shaw FR. Vision loss in older persons. *American Family Physician*. 2009;**79**(11): 963–70.

26. Albert RH, Clark MM. Cancer screening in the older patient. *American Family Physician*. 2008;**78**(12): 1369–74.

27. Walter LC, Covinsky KE. Cancer screening in elderly patients: a framework for individualized decision making. *JAMA*. 2001;**285**(21):2750–6.

28. Rosen SL, Reuben DB. Geriatric assessment tools. *Mt Sinai J Med*. 2011;**78**(4):489–97.

29. Maurer DM. Screening for depression. *American Family Physician*. 2012;**85**(2):139–44.

30. Uher R, Payne JL, Pavlova B, Perlis RH. Major depressive disorder in DSM-5: implications for clinical practice and research of changes from DSM-IV. *Depress Anxiety*. 2014;**31**(6):459–71.

31. Cahoon CG. Depression in older adults. *American Journal of Nursing*. 2012;**112**(11):22–30; quiz 1.

32. Mauk KL. Rooting out hypothyroidism in the elderly. *Nursing*. 2005;**35**(12):65–6.

33. Mohandas R, Gupta KL. Managing thyroid dysfunction in the elderly: answers to seven common questions. *Postgraduate Medicine*. 2003;**113**(5):54–6, 65–8, 100.

34. American College of Physicians. Clinical guideline, part 1: screening for thyroid disease. *Annals of Internal Medicine*. 1998;**129**(2):141–3.

35. Felz MW. Who should be screened for thyroid disease? *Postgraduate Medicine*. 2005;**118**(3):9–10.

36. Helfand M, Crapo LM. Screening for thyroid disease. *Annals of Internal Medicine*. 1990;**112**(11):840–9.

37. Hennessey JV, Espaillat R. Subclinical hypothyroidism: a historical view and shifting prevalence. *International Journal of Clinical Practice*. 2015 Jul;**69**(7):771–82.

38. Fowler NR, Boustani MA, Frame A, Perkins AJ, Monahan P, Gao S, et al. Effect of patient perceptions on dementia screening in primary care. *Journal of the American Geriatrics Society*. 2012;**60**(6):1037–43.

39. Galvin JE, Sadowsky CH. Practical guidelines for the recognition and diagnosis of dementia. *J Am Board Fam Med*. 2012;**25**(3):367–82.

40. Borson S, Frank L, Bayley PJ, Boustani M, Dean M, Lin PJ, et al. Improving dementia care: the role of screening and detection of cognitive impairment. *Alzheimers Dement*. 2013;**9**(2):151–9.

41. Lin JS, O'Connor E, Rossom RC, Perdue LA, Eckstrom E. Screening for cognitive impairment in older adults: a systematic review for the US Preventive Services Task Force. *Annals of Internal Medicine*. 2013;**159**(9):601–12.

42. Boustani M. Dementia screening in primary care: not too fast! *Journal of the American Geriatrics Society*. 2013;**61**(7):1205–7.

43. Kilik LA, Hopkins RW, Prince CR. How to avoid 3 common errors in dementia screening. *Journal of Family Practice*. 2014;**63**(8):E1–7.

44. Bond MC, Butler KH. Elder abuse and neglect: definitions, epidemiology, and approaches to emergency department screening. *Clinics in Geriatric Medicine*. 2013;**29**(1):257–73.

45. Forum on Global Violence P, Board on Global H, Institute of M, National Research C. The National Academies Collection: Reports funded by National Institutes of Health. *Elder Abuse and Its Prevention: Workshop Summary*. Washington, DC: National Academies Press (US). Copyright 2014 by the National Academy of Sciences. All rights reserved; 2014.

46. *Elder Abuse and Its Prevention: Workshop Summary*. Washington, DC: National Academy of Sciences; 2014 Mar 18.

47. Fulmer T, Guadagno L, Bitondo Dyer C, Connolly MT. Progress in elder abuse screening and assessment instruments. *Journal of the American Geriatrics Society*. 2004;**52**(2):297–304.

48. Tinetti ME, Inouye SK, Gill TM, Doucette JT. Shared risk factors for falls, incontinence, and functional dependence: unifying the approach to geriatric syndromes. *JAMA*. 1995;**273**(17):1348–53.

49. Vaught SL. Gait, balance, and fall prevention. *Ochsner J*. 2001;**3**(2):94–7.

50. Nevitt MC, Cummings SR, Hudes ES. Risk factors for injurious falls: a prospective study. *J Gerontol*. 1991;**46**(5):M164–70.

51. Penninx BW, Pluijm SM, Lips P, Woodman R, Miedema K, Guralnik JM, et al. Late-life anemia is associated with increased risk of recurrent falls. *Journal of the American Geriatrics Society*. 2005;**53**(12): 2106–11.

52. Woolcott JC, Richardson KJ, Wiens MO, Patel B, Marin J, Khan KM, et al. Meta-analysis of the impact of 9 medication classes on falls in elderly persons. *Archives of Internal Medicine*. 2009;**169**(21):1952–60.

53. Cumming RG, Thomas M, Szonyi G, Salkeld G, O'Neill E, Westbury C, et al. Home visits by an occupational therapist for assessment and modification of environmental hazards: a randomized trial of falls prevention. *Journal of the American Geriatrics Society*. 1999;**47**(12):1397–402.

54. Cawthon PM, Harrison SL, Barrett-Connor E, Fink HA, Cauley JA, Lewis CE, et al. Alcohol intake and its relationship with bone mineral density, falls, and fracture risk in older men. *Journal of the American Geriatrics Society.* 2006;**54**(11):1649–57.

55. Tenccr AF, Koepsell TD, Wolf ME, Frankenfeld CL, Buchner DM, Kukull WA, et al. Biomechanical properties of shoes and risk of falls in older adults. *Journal of the American Geriatrics Society.* 2004;**52**(11): 1840–6.

56. Tinetti ME. Performance-oriented assessment of mobility problems in elderly patients. *Journal of the American Geriatrics Society.* 1986;**34**(2):119–26.

57. Mathias S, Nayak US, Isaacs B. Balance in elderly patients: the "get-up and go" test. *Arch Phys Med Rehabil.* 1986;**67**(6):387–9.

58. Wilson SR, Knowles SB, Huang Q, Fink A. The prevalence of harmful and hazardous alcohol consumption in older US adults: data from the 2005–2008 National Health and Nutrition Examination Survey (NHANES). *J Gen Intern Med.* 2014;**29**(2):312–9.

59. Blow FC, Barry KL. Alcohol and substance misuse in older adults. *Curr Psychiatry Rep.* 2012;**14**(4):310–9.

60. Wang YP, Andrade LH. Epidemiology of alcohol and drug use in the elderly. *Curr Opin Psychiatry.* 2013;**26**(4):343–8.

61. Bakhshi S, While AE. Older people and alcohol use. *Br J Community Nurs.* 2014;**19**(8):370–4.

62. Bush K, Kivlahan DR, McDonell MB, Fihn SD, Bradley KA. The AUDIT alcohol consumption questions (AUDIT-C): an effective brief screening test for problem drinking. Ambulatory Care Quality Improvement Project (ACQUIP). Alcohol Use Disorders Identification Test. *Archives of Internal Medicine.* 1998;**158**(16):1789–95.

63. Messinger-Rapport BJ. How to assess and counsel the older driver. *Cleve Clin J Med.* 2002;**69**(3):184–5, 9–90, 92.

64. Ott BR, Davis JD, Papandonatos GD, Hewitt S, Festa EK, Heindel WC, et al. Assessment of driving-related skills prediction of unsafe driving in older adults in the office setting. *Journal of the American Geriatrics Society.* 2013;**61**(7):1164–9.

65. Tombaugh TN. Trail making Test A and B: normative data stratified by age and education. *Arch Clin Neuropsychol.* 2004;**19**(2):203–14.

66. Rigotti NA. Clinical practice: treatment of tobacco use and dependence. *New England Journal of Medicine.* 2002;**346**(7):506–12.

67. Helge TD, Denelsky GY. Pharmacologic aids to smoking cessation. *Cleve Clin J Med.* 2000;**67**(11):818, 21–4.

68. Connolly MJ. Smoking cessation in old age: closing the stable door? *Age and ageing.* 2000;**29**(3):193–5.

Chapter

5

Appropriate use of medications in the elderly

Emily R. Hajjar, PharmD, BCPS, BCACP, CGP, Amber E. King, PharmD, BCPS, and Lauren R. Hersh, MD

Introduction

In 2010, 40 million people, 13% percent of the US population, were over the age of 65 years.[1] Approximately 47% of these individuals consumed five or more prescription medications.[2] The number of prescription medications used and the increased risk of adverse drug reactions (ADRs) from their use requires heightened diligence in prescribing. Reasons for the increased attention to prescribing in the elderly population include an increased sensitivity to drug effects secondary to pharmacokinetic and pharmacodynamic changes that occur with aging, complexity of medication regimens and issues with medication adherence, lack of guidance from treatment guidelines for older adults, and a high incidence of inappropriate prescribing and polypharmacy. Older adult patients are often medically and socially complex, with multiple disease states and varying levels of functional ability and psychosocial and financial support. Addressing these issues, using an interdisciplinary team-based approach, will help optimize drug therapy in this population.

Pharmacokinetic and pharmacodynamic changes in the elderly

There are a number of age-related changes in drug pharmacokinetics (Table 5.1) and pharmacodynamics that occur in the elderly population. "Pharmacokinetics" describes drug absorption, distribution, metabolism, and elimination. "Pharmacodynamics" refers to the effects that a drug has on the body. Although all of the changes that will be described may occur in the elderly, it is important to remember that these age-related

Table 5.1 Potential age-related physiologic changes that can affect drug pharmacokinetics in the elderly[3]

Absorption	Metabolism
↑ gastric pH	↓ hepatic mass/ hepatic blood flow
↓ gastric motility	
↓ surface area of small intestine	↓ activity of CYP1A2, CYP2C9, CYP2C19, and CYP3A4 enzymes
↓ gastrointestinal blood flow	
↓ hepatic mass/hepatic blood flow	

Distribution	Elimination
↑ total body fat	↓ kidney size
↓ lean body mass and total body water	↓ renal blood flow
↓ albumin concentrations	↓ glomerular filtration
↑ α-1 acid glycoprotein concentrations	↓ tubular secretion

physiologic changes do not occur uniformly in every patient. Although many of these changes may be attributed to the aging process alone, many may be due to the combined effects of age with other factors such as concomitant disease states, polypharmacy, genetics, and environment.

Pharmacokinetic changes

Absorption and bioavailability

Absorption appears to be the least affected of the pharmacokinetic processes in the elderly. Most medications are absorbed through passive diffusion, so age-related changes in physiology only minimally alter absorption.[3] However, the absorption of drugs can be affected by several physiologic changes such as

---

Reichel's Care of the Elderly, 7th Edition, ed. Jan Busby-Whitehead *et al.* Published by Cambridge University Press. © Cambridge University Press 2016.

increase in gastric pH and reductions in gastric motility, mucosal absorptive surface area in the small intestine, and gastrointestinal blood flow.[4–6] These potential alterations are more likely to cause a slight delay in the rate of drug absorption, and usually do not significantly impact the overall extent of absorption.

Bioavailability of drugs may be affected by age-related physiologic changes. Clearance of drugs that would normally be subject to extensive first-pass metabolism (e.g., propranolol, morphine) may be impaired due to a reduction in liver mass and hepatic blood flow.[7, 8] Consequently, there may be an increase in bioavailability of these drugs. The function of P-glycoprotein, which normally acts as an efflux pump and serves as a barrier for drug absorption, does not appear to be significantly altered by the aging process.[9] Additionally, the bioavailability of drugs administered via the transdermal route does not appear to be affected by age.[10]

Distribution

Age-related changes in body composition and protein binding may affect drug distribution. The elderly population generally exhibits an increase in total body fat and reduction in lean body mass and total body water. It is estimated that lean body mass may be reduced by as much as 15% and total body fat may be increased by as much as 40%.[11] Consequently, drugs that are more water soluble (hydrophilic) or that distribute primarily to muscle (e.g., digoxin, aminoglycosides, theophylline) may have a reduced volume of distribution, resulting in increased plasma concentrations.[12] In contrast, drugs that are more fat soluble (lipophilic) may have an increased volume of distribution (e.g., diazepam, oxazepam), leading to an increase in tissue concentration and duration of action.[3]

In the elderly, plasma albumin concentration is reduced by 15%–20%.[13] Although this reduction in albumin may be attributed in part to age-related physiologic changes, it may also be a result of malnutrition and/or comorbid disease states (e.g., heart failure, chronic kidney disease, rheumatoid arthritis, cancer).[13] Acidic drugs (e.g., phenytoin, sulfonylureas, warfarin, levothyroxine) primarily bind to albumin. Reduction in plasma albumin concentration causes an increase in the free (unbound) concentration of these drugs, which may increase risk of toxicity.[14] Basic drugs, such as propranolol, primarily bind to α-1 acid glycoprotein, which is an acute phase reactant protein. Concentrations of this protein are believed to increase with aging, in chronic inflammatory disease states, malignancies, or in reaction to stress, such as post-myocardial infarction.[14] Consequently, plasma binding of these basic drugs may be increased, leading to a reduction in free plasma concentrations. Alterations in drug distribution that occur secondary to changes in protein concentration are less clinically significant for basic than for acidic drugs.

Metabolism

Drug metabolism primarily takes place in the liver. Age-related declines in liver mass and hepatic blood flow may account for a decline in drug clearance, which could lead to an increased risk of drug toxicity. In fact, it is estimated that hepatic blood flow decreases by up to 40% in the older adult population.[8] Consequently, hepatic clearance of drugs that have a high hepatic extraction ratio (e.g., morphine, propranolol, verapamil) may be decreased, resulting in increased plasma concentrations.[15]

Age-related hepatic changes affect liver enzymes responsible for metabolism. In general, drug metabolism can be categorized into phase I and phase II reactions. Only phase I reactions appear to be significantly affected by age.[15–17] Phase I reactions include the processes of oxidation, reduction, and hydrolysis. Most oxidative reactions involve the cytochrome P-450 (CYP) enzyme system. Drugs that induce or inhibit certain isoenzymes act to decrease or increase, respectively, the plasma concentration of certain drugs (substrates) metabolized by a particular isoenzyme. Although the results of various studies have shown inconsistent effects of age on CYP isoenzyme activity, in general it appears that a decline in the activity of the CYP1A2, CYP2C9, CYP2C19, and CYP3A4 enzymes can occur.[18] Because of the complexity of potential drug interactions that can occur via the CYP enzyme system, it is essential for practitioners to become familiar with common drugs that serve as substrates, inhibitors, or inducers of this system. Phase II reactions, which involve the processes of glucuronidation, acetylation, and sulfation, are not significantly affected by age.[15, 17] Certain benzodiazepines such as oxazepam, lorazepam, and temazepam are subject only to phase II metabolism; therefore, the metabolism of these drugs is unchanged. Other benzodiazepines, such as chlordiazepoxide and diazepam, undergo both phase I and phase II metabolism, and may have impaired clearance in the elderly.[19] Consequently, selecting a benzodiazepine that exclusively undergoes phase II metabolism may be more prudent in the older patient.

Renal elimination

Age-related reductions in kidney size, renal blood flow, glomerular filtration, and tubular secretion may contribute to a decline in drug clearance.[17] Renal blood flow decreases by approximately 10% each decade after the age of 40.[20] These changes may be compounded by disease states such as hypertension and diabetes, which are frequently present in the older adult population and which may further impair renal function. As a result, clearance of drugs that are primarily excreted unchanged by the kidneys may be significantly reduced.

Serum creatinine alone should not be used to estimate the patient's renal function, as the amount of lean body mass decreases with aging.[21] Instead, to provide a more accurate approximation for medication dosing, calculation of the creatinine clearance (CrCl) is used. Creatinine is a by-product of muscle breakdown; age-related reduction in muscle mass leads to a decrease in production of creatinine. Therefore, even in the presence of renal dysfunction, an elderly patient's SCr may appear to be "normal" (i.e., <1 mg/dL). The Cockcroft-Gault formula, which incorporates SCr as well as age and weight to estimate CrCl, can be used in elderly patients:

$$CrCl\ (ml/min) = \frac{(140 - age) \times weight\ (kg)}{72 \times serum\ creatinine\ (mg/dL)}$$
$$\times\ 0.85\ for\ females$$

In elderly patients with a SCr less than 1 mg/dL, a value of "1" should be used for the SCr in this equation to avoid overestimating CrCl. Although the Cockcroft-Gault formula is frequently used to both assess renal function and to make dosage adjustments of renally excreted drugs, it is important for clinicians to be aware that this equation tends to underestimate the glomerular filtration rate (GFR) of older adults. [21] Most recently, the Modification of Diet in Renal Disease (MDRD) equation is being advocated as an alternative method for assessing renal function because it appears to have a better correlation with GFR when compared with the Cockcroft-Gault formula.[22, 23] Moreover, although the MDRD

equation was derived from patients with chronic kidney disease, it has been shown to provide a more accurate estimate of renal function in the elderly when compared to the Cockcroft-Gault formula.[24] However, because the MDRD equation has not been validated for use in adjusting drug dosages, health-care providers should continue to use the Cockcroft-Gault formula for this purpose.

Pharmacodynamic changes

A number of age-related physiologic changes may occur that increase or decrease sensitivity to a drug. Mechanisms for altered age-related pharmacodynamics include changes in receptor number and affinity, changes in drug concentrations at the receptor, alterations in postreceptor signaling, and alterations in homeostatic mechanisms.[25] In the cardiovascular system, because of the decline in β-receptor activity that occurs with age, a decline in β-adrenergic responsiveness may occur which could minimize heart rate response to both β-agonists and β-blockers.[26] Older adults also have a lessened reduction in blood pressure from β-blockers.[25] Additionally, blunting of the baroreceptor reflex can occur with aging, resulting in the development of exaggerated postural hypotensive effects during therapy with drugs such as nitrates, diuretics, calcium channel blockers, and α_1 blockers.[27, 28] Changes in the pharmacodynamics of central nervous system agents may also occur, including alterations in the permeability of the blood brain barrier and changes in brain size and alterations of neurotransmitters.[25] The overall result of these changes is an increased sensitivity to central nervous system agents. Although no significant differences in the pharmacokinetics of warfarin have been demonstrated between younger and older patients, the pharmacodynamics of this drug may be altered in the elderly population, potentially resulting in an enhanced anticoagulant effect and an increased risk of bleeding.[25, 28] Consequently, it may be prudent for health-care providers to use lower initial and maintenance doses of warfarin in this population.

Beers Criteria

Older adults are particularly susceptible to inappropriate prescribing due to age-related pharmacokinetic and pharmacodynamic changes, increased comorbidities, increased risk of drug interactions, polypharmacy, and adverse drug reactions. The use of medication is considered potentially inappropriate when the possible risk outweighs the expected clinical benefit. The Beers Criteria, initially developed by an expert panel in 1991 to target nursing home residents, are the most widely cited criteria used to identify high risk, or "potentially inappropriate," medication in older adults.[29] The Beers Criteria are now in a fourth permutation, having been most recently updated in 2012, and are intended for use by clinicians in both inpatient and community settings. The current criteria include three groups of medications: medications to avoid in older adults regardless of disease or condition (e.g., barbiturates, megestrol, glyburide, and sliding scale insulin); medications to avoid when used in older adults with certain diseases or conditions (e.g., avoidance of medications with anticholinergic properties in patients with cognitive impairment); and a new, third group of medications that should be prescribed with universal caution (dabigatran, SSRIs).[30] Numerous studies have evaluated health-care outcomes associated with the use of the potentially inappropriate drugs included in the Beers Criteria. There is clear evidence that inappropriate medication use is associated with adverse drug reactions and increased costs across all health-care settings (ambulatory, acute, and long term care).[31]

Although the Beers Criteria have been increasingly used as a quality-of-care measure (as evidenced by the Beers-like list of inappropriate drugs adopted by the 2006 Health Plan Employer and Data and Information Set [HEDIS]), the criteria have been criticized for using an explicit method that may not take clinical application into account for assessing drug therapy appropriateness.[32, 33] In an effort to highlight the possibility of criteria misuse or misinterpretation, the American Medical Directors Association and the American Society of Consultant Pharmacists have released a position statement identifying the Beers Criteria as a "helpful general guide."[34] Clinicians are warned against inappropriately using the criteria as an absolute prohibition against specific medications in older adults. Instead, clinicians are encouraged to make prescribing decisions in the context of a complete clinical picture that includes the entire medication regimen, history of medication use, comorbidities, functional status, and prognosis.

STOPP/START criteria

The STOPP (Screening Tool of Older People's potentially inappropriate Prescriptions) and START (Screening Tool to Alert doctors to the Right Treatment) criteria were developed to address limitations observed in the Beers Criteria. STOPP is comprised of clinically significant criteria for potentially inappropriate prescribing. Each criterion is supported by a concise explanation as to why the prescribing practice is potentially inappropriate and includes consideration of drug–drug interactions and duplication of therapy. START consists of evidence-based prescribing indicators for commonly encountered diseases.[35] In two studies, the STOPP critiera identified a significantly higher percentage of older patients requiring hospitalization as a result of an adverse drug event (ADE) than did the 2003 Beers Criteria.[36, 37]

Adverse drug reactions in the elderly: an overview

Adverse drug reactions (ADRs) are noxious responses to medications used in usual doses that require treatment of the effect, modification of the drug regimen, or cessation of treatment.[38] The incidence of hospital admissions caused by ADRs in older adults, many of which are avoidable, ranges from 3% to 10%.[33, 39] The prevalence of ADRs in older outpatients ranges from 5% to 35%. [40] The consequences associated with ADRs are not insignificant; studies have demonstrated that the cost of ADRs adds a financial burden to an already overspent health-care system.[41, 42]

ADRs in older adults are frequently exaggerated responses to expected pharmokinetic and pharmacodynamic shifts. Polypharmacy, a common occurrence in this population, increases the risk of ADRs due to drug interactions, synergistic toxic effects, and non-adherence to complicated or expensive medication regimens. Decreased mobility, multiple disease states, low body weight, renal and/or hepatic dysfunction, female sex, and a prior history of ADRs further increase the risk for the development of ADRs.[40]

Common ADRs in the elderly include an increased risk of falls, changes in mental status, and effects on urinary continence. Table 5.2 identifies some of the common pharmacologic agents that may cause each of these ADRs.

61

Table 5.2 Adverse drug reactions in the elderly[30, 43]

	Increased fall risk	Delirium	Cognitive impairment	Chronic constipation
Prescription agents (by class)	Antidepressants	Anticholinergics	Anticholinergics	Anticholinergics
	Anticonvulsants	Benzodiazepines	Antipsychotics	Antispasmodics
	Antipsychotics	Corticosteroids	Benzodiazepines	Antihistamines
	Sedative/hypnotics	Histamine-2 receptor antagonists	Antispasmodics	Antimuscarinics for urinary incontinence
	Benzodiazepines	Meperidne	Histamine-2 receptor antagonists	Non-dihydropyridine calcium channel blockers
	Type Ia antiarrhythmics	Sedative hypnotics	Zolpidem	
	Digoxin	Tricyclic antidepressants		
	Diuretics			
	Antihypertensives			
	Opioid analgesics			
	Hypoglycemics			
	α_1 blockers			

Adverse drug reactions: falls

Falls are of significant concern because of their associated morbidity and mortality. Nearly one-third of adults over the age of 65 fall at least once per year.[43] Approximately 10% of such falls result in serious injury, most notably hip fractures, with up to 75% of hip fracture patients failing to regain their prior level of function.[44, 45] Fall-related injuries are associated with a decline in functional status and an increased likelihood of nursing home placement.[46] In one study, 20% of elderly patients who experienced a hip fracture died within a year of the fracture.[46]

Medication use is one of the most modifiable risk factors for falls.[45] Polypharmacy may be a marker of underlying comorbidity and frailty, rendering a patient more susceptible to falling. Regardless of whether agents are considered to be high risk, falls are more common in elderly patients who take more than four drugs per day.[47] Risk of medication-related falls can be mitigated through

patient education, slow dose titration, and avoidance of polypharmacy and high-risk medication when possible. Certain medication classes, when used alone or in combination with other medications, can increase fall risk.[47] Psychotropic and antidepressant medications are frequently prescribed in the elderly to treat depression, psychosis, and insomnia and may increase fall risk when taken with other medications that carry a high-risk profile. Antipsychotic medications can cause many adverse effects, including extrapyramidal symptoms, orthostasis, and cognitive impairment.[48] These effects are more commonly associated with the typical antipsychotics (e.g., haloperidol, thiothixine, droperidol), but they have also been documented with the newer atypical agents (quetiapine, risperidone, olanzapine).[48, 49] The anticholinergic properties of sedation, orthostatic hypotension, and confusion associated with tricyclic antidepressants (TCAs) were one of the original perceived barriers to prescribing in older adults. Although selective serotonin reuptake inhibitors

(SSRIs) cause markedly less sedation, studies suggest that SSRIs are associated with fall rates similar to the TCAs.[50, 51]

Benzodiazepines have been implicated in increasing fall risk. It is frequently stated that short-acting benzodiazepines are safer than long-acting benzodiazepines for the elderly. However, this distinction may be blurred, as the pharmacokinetic half-life of benzodiazepines in the blood may be misleadingly short compared with the duration of pharmacodynamic effects on the nervous system. [52] It is likely that risk increases with increasing dose; therefore, if benzodiazepines must be used, the lowest dose should be used for the shortest duration possible.[48, 50]

The use of opioid analgesics, with proper monitoring, is increasingly recognized as a reasonable option for treating pain in older patients, despite persistent misconceptions about addictive potential and the real concern for sedation and fall risk.[53] The risk of addiction in patients using opioids appropriately for pain is low.[53] Although there is contradicting data on whether opioids cause falls, adequate pain control may be warranted for patients with regard to quality of life. Careful selection of agent and dose, titration, and use of adjunct agents should be considered to minimize risk.[54, 55]

Any agent that causes hypotension or dizziness may increase fall risk. Agents such as α_1 blockers, which are used to treat benign prostatic hypertrophy, commonly cause dizziness.[56] Evidence linking fall risk with antihypertensive agents, however, is mixed. Some studies show that patients have an increased risk with these agents whereas others do not.[54] It has been demonstrated in observational studies that type Ia antiarrhythmics, digoxin, and diuretics are associated with increased fall rates.[54] Because these agents are commonly used in the older adult population, it is important to educate patients about the risk of falls due to hypotension or dizziness and preventative measures that can be taken. Whenever possible, antihypertensives and other agents known to cause dizziness should be dosed at bedtime in order to decrease risk.[57]

Adverse drug reactions: cognitive impairment

Patients with an acute illness, such as a urinary tract infection, or a worsening chronic condition, such as heart failure, can present with cognitive dysfunction in the form of confusion or mental status changes. [58, 59] Many commonly used medications can also precipitate or contribute to the development of cognitive disturbances. It can be challenging for the practitioner to distinguish between cognitive impairment secondary to a disease process versus a medication. It is, therefore, appropriate to consider the possibility that changes in cognitive function may be partially or wholly due to medications. [60]

Any medication with central nervous system (CNS) effects has the potential to cause cognitive dysfunction. Opioid analgesics can cause sedation, confusion, and even hallucinations.[61] Amphetamines cause CNS stimulation and excitation, effects that are often exaggerated in the elderly.[61] Antipsychotics, used to treat behavioral problems as well as psychotic disorders, can cause anticholinergic-associated cognitive impairment.[49] A small observational trial demonstrated significant cognitive decline in patients with dementia who used neuroleptic agents compared with those who did not.[62] Anticholinergic agents are frequently responsible for causing CNS disturbances such as confusion, excitement, disorientation, and delirium.[56] Many commonly used medications, including over-the-counter antihistamines (diphenhydramine, chlorpheniramine), as well as prescription-only antidepressants (e.g., amitriptyline, doxepin, imipramine), skeletal muscle relaxants (cyclobenzaprine, orphenadrine), and bronchodilators (atropine and ipratropium) have anticholinergic actions.[49, 63, 64] Risk of cognitive impairment increases with the number of medications used, especially anticholinergic agents.[49, 61] Anticholinergic-associated cognitive dysfunction may also potentiate preexisting cognitive impairment.[49, 63] Physicians must be aware of an agent's potential to cause cognitive dysfunction and must consider the "anticholinergic burden" of a patient's entire medication regimen when prescribing. Whereas a single medication may not result in anticholinergic-associated cognitive changes, the use of multiple drugs with such effects may increase that risk.[63]

Drug prescribing patterns: underutilization of drug therapy

Whereas extensive research has focused on overprescribing for older adults; underprescribing appropriate medications is increasingly recognized as a potential clinical pitfall. In fact, clinicians may avoid overprescribing inappropriate drug therapies while underprescribing indicated therapies.[65] The interconnectedness of polypharmacy and undertreatment has been repeatedly illustrated, and studies have demonstrated that the probability of underprescribing increases as the size of a patient's drug regimen increases.[66, 67] Undertreatment of medical conditions has been observed to occur in 64%–83% of elderly patients receiving more than five medications.[66, 67]

The highest incidence of undertreatment has been observed with laxatives used to prevent constipation in patients receiving chronic opioids, and with ACE inhibitor and β-blocker use in cardiovascular disease.[66, 68] Other agents underused in the geriatric population include antihypertensives, aspirin, antihyperlipidemics, oral hypoglycemic agents, and calcium supplements.[67, 68] In a study of patients with coronary artery disease in an academic nursing home, only 62% received aspirin, 58% received an ACE-inhibitor or an angiotensin II receptor blocker, 57% received a β-blocker, 27% received a calcium channel blocker, and 21% received a statin.[68] None of these patients had a contraindication to the agents with which they were not treated.

In evaluating ways to minimize both polypharmacy and the underutilization of well-studied and supported therapeutic initiatives, a collaborative approach has been observed.[69] When the addition of a clinical pharmacist to the geriatric team (Geriatric Evaluation and Management [GEM] care) was compared to the use of the GEM alone, intervention patients (stratified by age and number of medications) were more likely to benefit from a clinically appropriate medication regimen.[69]

Drug adherence

The true rate of medication adherence is estimated to be 50%, with a range of 26%–59% in patients aged 60 and older.[70] As many as 10% of hospital admissions and 23% of nursing home admissions may be attributed to medication nonadherence.[70] Seventy-five percent of hospital admissions related to nonadherence involved cardiovascular and CNS medications. Falls, postural hypotension, heart failure, and delirium were the most common manifestations of nonadherence.[70]

Factors affecting drug adherence

Once an optimal therapeutic regimen is determined for a patient, adherence becomes a key component to therapeutic success. "Adherence" is a preferred term to "compliance" as it implies a collaborative relationship between the patient and/or caregiver and the health-care provider. "Compliance," in comparison, implies a one-way relationship wherein the health-care provider makes all decisions and provides "directions" independent of the wants and needs of the patient.[71]

Factors that affect medication adherence include demographics (e.g., occupation, level of education, and health literacy), medical parameters (type, severity, and duration of disease), medication profile (complexity of regimen and side-effect profile), behavioral factors (patient-provider communication and patient health beliefs), and economic constraints (type of insurance, cost of medication, and patient income). The elderly are at high risk of nonadherence.[72]

Improving drug adherence

Patients who self-administer medications typically take less than half of what is prescribed; therefore efforts to improve adherence assume high impact.[73] Increasing patient communication and discussing the importance of following the drug regimen is one of the few simple interventions that can improve adherence. Involvement of caregivers, supplementation with written material, simplified dosing schedules, and dosing aids to organize medications (e.g., pillboxes) have demonstrated additional benefits. Patients who miss medical appointments are more likely to be nonadherent; assistance with scheduling and more frequent visits may provide additional benefit. Minimizing polypharmacy and mindfulness of financial burden to the patient also improve adherence rates.[74–76]

Fixed-dose medication combinations also have a positive impact on adherence. These products typically contain two active agents, each at a specific dose. Fixed-dose agents currently exist for the disease states of hypertension, human immunodeficiency virus, tuberculosis, and diabetes. A meta-analysis showed that the use of these products resulted in a significant 26% decrease in the risk of noncompliance compared to single-drug component regimens. A 24% reduction in the risk of noncompliance was noted for hypertension alone.[77]

Strategies for improving medication use

A thorough medication history that includes prescription, nonprescription, and alternative agents is the first step to improving medication use. Having patients bring in all medications at each health-care visit can help ensure that providers are making clinical decisions with complete medication information. Asking patients about nonprescription or alternative therapy use is necessary as these agents are frequently omitted from medication lists.

Once a complete list of medications has been obtained, each medication should be evaluated to determine its necessity for the patient at that point in time. Each medication should have an indication, and if no indication exists, the medication should be evaluated for taper or discontinuation. Each medication should also be evaluated for efficacy, especially if a specific symptom is being treated. Medications prescribed for the purpose of treating the adverse effects of other medications should be carefully assessed. Although prescribing cascades may be unavoidable, medication complexity must be taken into account. Undertreated medical conditions should be assessed to determine if the addition of medication is warranted.

If a medication is deemed necessary, its use, therapeutic goals, and response should be monitored regularly as medical conditions and patient pharmacokinetic and pharmacodynamic responses may change with time. Medication reconciliation should be performed for all transitions in care to ensure no medication omissions have occurred. Risk-benefit assessments should be performed for each medication to see if benefits outweigh potential risks. Duplicate medications should be tapered and discontinued. Drug–drug and drug–disease interactions, medication regimen complexity, prescription formulary information, and financial burden must also be considered to alleviate medication burden to the patient. Consideration should be shown to those medications that can be given on a regular basis as few times per day as possible to increase patient adherence. Medication counseling should be provided to both patient and caregiver verbally and in print.

Medication necessity should be considered at end of life. Goals of care, time to benefit, and remaining life expectancy are important factors to assess, and they may render certain medications irrelevant.[78]

Conclusion

The safe, effective, and optimal use of medications in the elderly requires heightened diligence in comparison to other patient populations. The issues of increased sensitivity to drug effects (both desired and adverse), the underuse of proven drug therapies, and a high incidence of medication nonadherence increase the need for due diligence in prescribing and monitoring drug therapy in this population. The employment of a multidisciplinary approach to patient care as well as the use of known methods for improving medication adherence are key to long-term success in the medical management of the elderly patient.

References

1. Federal Interagency Forum on Aging-Related Statistics. *Older Americans Update 2010: Key Indicators of Well-Being. Federal Interagency Forum on Aging-Related Statistics.* Washington, DC: US Government Printing Office; July 2010. Available at: www.agingstats.gov.

2. www.cdc.gov/nchs/data/hus/hus13.pdf#092 (accessed on December 2, 2015).

3. Corsonello A, Pedone C, Incalzi RA. Age-related pharmacokinetic and pharmacodynamic changes and related risk of adverse drug reactions. *Curr Med Chem* 2010;**17**:571–84.

4. Kekki M, Samloff IM, Ihamaki T, et al. Age- and sex-related behaviour of gastric acid secretion at the population level. *Scand J Gastroenterol* 1982;**17**:737–43.

5. Orr WC, Chen CL. Aging and neural control of the GI tract: IV. Clinical and physiological aspects of gastrointestinal motility and aging. *Am J Physiol* 2002;**283**:G1226–31.

6. Corazza GR, Frazzoni M, Gatto MR, et al. Aging and small bowel mucosa: a morphometric study. *Gerontology* 1986;**32**:60–5.

7. Anantharaju A, Feller A, Chedid A. Aging liver: a review. *Gerontology* 2002;**48**:343–53.

8. Le Couteur DG, McLean AJ. The aging liver: drug clearance and an oxygen diffusion barrier hypothesis. *Clin Pharmacokinet* 1998;**34**:359–73.

9. Brenner SS, Klotz U. P-glycoprotein function in the elderly. *Eur J Clin Pharmacol* 2004;**60**:97–102.

10. Kaestli LZ, Wasilewski-Rasca AF, Bonnabry P, Vogt-Ferrier N. Use of transdermal formulations in the elderly. *Drugs Aging* 2008;**25**:269–80.

11. Beaufrere B, Morio B. Fat and protein redistribution with aging: metabolic considerations. *Eur J Clin Nutr* 2000;**54**:S48–53.

12. Cusack B, Kelly J, O'Malley K, et al. Digoxin in the elderly: pharmacokinetic consequences of old age. *Clin Pharmacol Ther* 1979;**25**:772–6.

13. Campion EW, deLabry LO, Glynn RJ. The effect of age on serum albumin in healthy males: report from the Normative Aging Study. *J Gerontol* 1988;**43**:M18–20.

14. Verbeeck RK, Cardinal JA, Wallace SM. Effect of age and sex on the plasma binding of acidic and basic drugs. *Eur J Clin Pharmacol* 1984;**27**:91–7.

15. Woodhouse KW, James OF. Hepatic drug metabolism and ageing. *British Medical Bulletin.* 1990;**46**:22–35.

16. Schmucker DL. Liver function and phase I drug metabolism in the elderly: a paradox. *Drugs Aging* 2001;**18**:837–51.

17. Hammerlein A, Derendorf H, Lowenthal DT. Pharmacokinetic and pharmacodynamic changes in the elderly: clinical implications. *Clin Pharmacokinet* 1998;**35**:49–64.

18. Benedetti MS, Whomsley R, Canning M. Drug metabolism in the pediatric population and in the elderly. *Drug Discov Today* 2007;**12**:599–610.

19. Bressler R, Bahl JJ. Principles of drug therapy for the elderly patient. *Mayo Clin Proc* 2003;**78**:1564–77.

20. Muhlberg W, Platt D. Age-dependent changes of the kidneys: pharmacological implications. *Gerontology* 1999;**45**:243–53.

21. Fliser D. Assessment of renal function in elderly patients. *Curr Opin Nephrol Hypertens* 2008;**17**:604–8.

22. Stevens LA, Coresh J, Greene T, Levey AS. Assessing kidney function: measured and estimated glomerular filtration rate. *N Engl J Med* 2006;**354**:2473–83.

23. Levey AS, Bosch JP, Lewis JB, et al. A more accurate method to estimate glomerular filtration rate from serum creatinine: a new prediction equation. Modification of Diet in Renal Disease Study Group. *Ann Intern Med* 1999;**130**:461–70.

24. Verhave JC, Fesler P, Ribstein J, du Cailar G, Mimran A. Estimation of renal function in subjects with normal serum creatinine levels: influence of age and body mass index. *Am J Kidney Dis* 2005;**46**:233–41.

25. Bowie MW, Slattum PW. Pharmacodynamics in older adults: a review. *Am J Geriatr Pharmacother* 2007;**5**:263–303.

26. Abernethy DR, Schwartz JB, Plachetka JR, Todd EL, Egan JM. Comparison in young and elderly patients of pharmacodynamics and disposition of labetalol in systemic hypertension. *Am J Cardiol* 1987;**60**:697–702.

27. Schwartz JB, Gibb WJ, Tran T. Aging effects on heart rate variation. *J Gerontol* 1991;**46**:M99–106.

28. Trifior G, Spina E. Age-related changes in pharmacodynamics: focus on drugs acting on central nervous and cardiovascular systems. *Curr Drug Metab* 2011;**12**:611–20.

29. Beers MH, Ouslander JG, Rollingher J, Reuben DB, Beck JC. Explicit criteria for determining inappropriate medication use in nursing home residents. *Arch Intern Med* 1991;**151**:1825–32.

30. American Geriatrics Society 2012 Beers Criteria Update Expert Panel. American Geriatrics Society updated Beers Criteria for potentially inappropriate medication use in older adults. *J Am Geriatri Soc.* 2012 Apr;**60**(4):616–31.

31. Jano E, Aparasu RR. Healthcare outcomes associated with Beers' criteria: a systematic overview. *Ann Pharmacother* 2007;**41**:438–48.

32. Fialova D, Onder G. Medication errors in elderly people: contributing factors and future perspectives. *Br J Clin Pharmacol* 2009;**67**:641–5.

33. Onder G, Pedone C, Landi F, Cesari M, Della Vedova C, Bernabei, Gambassi G. Adverse drug reactions as a cause of hospital admissions: results from the Italian Group of Pharmacoepidemiology in the Elderly (GIFA). *J Am Geriatr Soc* 2002;**50**:1962–8.

34. Swagerty D, Brickley R. American Medical Directors Association and American Society of Consultant Pharmacists joint position statement on the Beers list of potentially inappropriate medications in older adults. *J Am Med Dir Assoc* 2005;**6**:80–6.

35. Gallagher P, Ryan C, Byrne S, Kennedy J, O'Mahony D. STOPP (Screening Tool of Older Person's Prescriptions) and START (Screening Tool to Alert doctors to Right Treatment). Consensus validation. *Int J Clin Pharmacol Ther* 2008 Feb;**46**(2):72–83.

36. Gallagher P, O'Mahony D. STOPP (Screening Tool of Older Persons' potentially inappropriate Prescriptions): application to acutely ill elderly patients and comparison with Beers' criteria. *Ageing* 2008;**37**(6):673–79.

37. Hamilton H, Gallagher P, Ryan C, Byrne S, O'Mahony D. Potentially inappropriate medications defined by STOPP criteria and the risk of adverse drug events in older hospitalized patients. *Arch Intern Med* 2011;**171**(11):1013.

38. Edwards IR, Aronson JK. Adverse drug reactions: definitions, diagnosis, and management. *Lancet* 2000;**356**:1255–9.

39. Kongkaew C, Noyce PR, Ashcroft DM. Hospital admissions associated with adverse drug reactions: a systematic review of prospective observational studies. *Ann Pharmacother* 2008;**42**:1017–25.

40. Hanlon JT, Artz MB, Lindblad CI, Pieper CF, Sloane RJ, Ruby CM, Schmader KE. Adverse drug reaction risk factors in older outpatients. *Am J Geriatr Pharmacother* 2003;**1**:82–9.

41. Ernst FR, Grizzle AJ. Drug-related morbidity and mortality: updating the cost-of-illness model. *J Am Pharm Assoc (Wash)* 2001 Mar–Apr;**41**(2):192–9.

42. Bootman JL, Harrison DL, Cox E. The health care cost of drug-related morbidity and mortality in nursing facilities. *Arch Intern Med* 1997 Oct 13;**157**(18): 2089–96.

43. Tinetti ME, Speechley M, Ginter SF. Risk factors for falls among elderly persons living in the community. *N Engl J Med* 1988;**319**:1701–7.

44. Tinetti ME. Clinical practice: preventing falls in elderly persons. *N Engl J Med* 2003;**348**:42–9.

45. Moylan, KC, Binder EF. Falls in older adults: risk assessment, management and prevention. *American Journal of Medicine* 2007; **120**(6):493 e1–e6.

46. US Department of Health and Human Services. Bone health and osteoporosis a report of the surgeon general – 2004. Available at: www.surgeongeneral.gov /library/bonehealth/content.html (accessed October 5, 2007).

47. Zeire G, Dieleman JP, Hofman A, et al. Polypharmacy and falls in the middle age and elderly population. *Br J Clin Pharmacol* 2005;**61**:218–23.

48. Leipzig RM, Cumming RG, Tinetti ME. Drugs and falls in older people: a systematic review and meta-analysis: I. Psychotropic drugs. *J Am Geriatr Soc* 1999;**47**:30–9.

49. Maixner SM, Mellow AM, Tandon R. The efficacy safety and tolerability of antipsychotics in the elderly. *J Clin Psychiatry* 1999;**60**:29–41.

50. Ensrud DE, Blackwell TL, Mangione CM, et al. Central nervous system-active medications and risk for falls in older women. *J Am Geriatr Soc* 2002;**50**:1629–37.

51. Thapa PB, Gideon P, Cost TW, Milam AB, Ray WA. Antidepressants and the risk of falls among nursing home residents. *N Engl J Med* 1998;**339**:875–82.

52. Cook PJ. Benzodiazepine hypnotics in the elderly. *Acta Psychiatr Scand* 1986;**73**(Suppl 332):149–58.

53. Hayes BD, Klein-Schwartz W, Barrueto Jr., F. Polypharmacy and the geriatric patient. *Clinics in Geriatric Medicine* 2007; **23**(2):371–90.

54. Leipzig RM, Cumming RG, Tinetti ME. Drugs and falls in older people: a systematic review and meta-analysis: II. Cardiac and analgesic drugs. *J Am Geriatr Soc* 1999;**47**:40–50.

55. Buckeridge D, Huang A, Hanley J, Kelome A, Reidel K, Verma A, et al. Risk of injury associated with opioid use in older adults. *J Am Geriatr Soc* 2010;**58**(9):1664–70.

56. McEvoy GK, ed. *AHFS Drug Information 2007.* Bethesda, MD: ASHP; 2007.

57. Carruthers SG. Adverse effects of alpha 1-adrenergic blocking drugs. *Drug Saf* 1994;**11**:12–20.

58. Liang SY, Mackowiak PA. Infections in the elderly. *Clin Geriatr Med* 2007;**23**:441–56.

59. Cohen MB, Mather PJ. A review of the association between congestive heart failure and cognitive impairment. *Am J Geriatr Cardiol* 2007;**16**:171–4.

60. Knopman DS, Peterson RC. Mild cognitive impairement and mild dementia: a clinical perspective. *Mayo Clin Proc* 2014;**89**:1452–9.

61. Fick DM, Cooper JW, Wade WE, Waller JL, Maclean JR, Beers MH. Updating the Beers criteria for potentially inappropriate medication use in older adults: results of a US consensus panel of experts. *Arch Intern Med* 2003;**163**:2716–24.

62. McShane R, Keene J, Gedling K, Fairburn C, Jacoby R, Hope T. Do neuroleptic drugs hasten cognitive decline in dementia? *Br Med J* 1997;**314**:266–70.

63. Mintzer J, Burns A. Anticholinergic side-effects of drugs in elderly people. *J R Soc Med* 2000;**93**:457–62.

64. Ancelin ML, Artero S, Portet F, et al. Non-degenerative mild cognitive impairment in elderly people and use of anticholinergic drugs: longitudinal cohort study. *Br Med J* 2006;**332**:455–9.

65. Higashi T, Shekelle PG, Solomon DH, Knight EL, Roth C, Chang JT, Kamberg CJ, MacLean CH, Young RT, Adams J, Reuben DB, Avorn J, Wenger NS. The quality of pharmacologic care for vulnerable older patients. *Ann Intern Med* 2004;**140**(9):714–20.

66. Kuijpers MAJ, vanMarum RJ, Egberts ACG, Jansen PAF. Relationship between polypharmacy and underprescribing. *Br J Clin Pharmacol* 2008;**65**:130–3.

67. Steinman MA, Landefeld CS, Rosenthal GE, et al. Polypharmacy and prescribing quality in older people. *J Am Geriatr Soc* 2006;**54**:1516–23.

68. Ghosh S, Ziesmer V, Aronow WS. Underutilization of aspirin, beta blockers, angiotensin-converting enzyme inhibitors, and lipid-lowering drugs and overutilization of calcium channel blockers in older persons with coronary artery disease in an academic nursing home. *J Gerontol* 2002;**57A**:M398–400.

69. Spinewine A, Swine C, Dhillon S, et al. Effect of a collaborative approach on the quality of prescribing for geriatric inpatients: a randomized, controlled trial. *J Am Geriatr Soc* 2007;**55**:658–65.

70. MacLaughlin EJ, Raehl CL, Treadway AK, et al. Assessing medication adherence in the elderly – which tools to use in clinical practice? *Drugs Aging* 2005;**22**:231–55.

71. Bisonette JM. Adherence: a concept analysis. *J Ad Nurs* 2008;**63**:634–43.

72. Marzec LN, Maddox TM. Medication adherence in patients with diabetes and dyslipidemia: associated factors and strategies for improvement. *Curr Cardiol Rep* 2013;**15**:418.

73. Haynes RB, Ackloo E, Sahota N, McDonald HP, Yao X. Interventions for enhancing medication adherence.

Cochrane Database Syst Rev 2008:2:CD000011. DOI: 10.1002/14651858.CD000011.pub3.

74. Viswanathan M, Golin CE, Jones CD, et al. Interventions to improve adherence to self-administered medications for chronic diseases in the United States: a systematic review. *Ann Intern Med* 2012;**157**:785–95.

75. McDonald HP, Garg AX, Haynes RB. Interventions to enhance patient adherence to medication prescriptions: scientific review. *JAMA* 2002;**288**: 2868–79.

76. Kripalani S, Yao X, Haynes RB. Interventions to enhance medication adherence in chronic medical conditions: a systematic review. *Arch Intern Med* 2007;**167**:540–50.

77. Bangalore S, Kamalakkannan G, Parkar S, et al. Fixed-dose combinations improve medication compliance: a meta-analysis. *Am J Med* 2007;**120**:713–9.

78. Holmes HM, Hayley DC, Alexander GC, Sachs GA. Reconsidering medication appropriateness for patients late in life. *Arch Intern Med* 2006;**166**:605–9.

Chapter

6

Healthy aging: exercise and nutrition as medicine for older adults

Diane Villanyi, MD, Maria A. Fiatarone Singh, MD, FRACP, and B. Lynn Beattie, MD, FRCP(C)

Clinicians in the ambulatory or hospital setting traditionally focus on diagnosis and treatment of specific diseases. However, it is clear that effective exercise and nutrition prescriptions, adequate counseling, and support of healthy lifestyle choices are at least as important if older adults are to achieve healthy aging.

Exercise

Aging and physical activity goals

Currently, disparities exist among population groups in habitual physical activity patterns that exaggerate the negative health consequences of a sedentary lifestyle. Unchanged from the 1996 Surgeon General's Report on Physical Activity and Health,[1] demographic groups still at highest risk for suboptimal activity levels are older adults, women, minorities, those with low income or educational background, and those with disabilities or chronic health conditions.[2] As might be expected, these are the same demographic groups that both bear a large burden of the diseases amenable to prevention and treatment with exercise, and yet often have the least access and opportunity for health promotion efforts related to physical activity. Therefore, health-care providers should identify and understand barriers to physical activity and incorporate theoretically grounded behavioral programs and strategies that address these barriers into their practice, particularly for such vulnerable individuals. If exercise is truly to be viewed as medicine, then it requires the same attention to specific indications, evidence-based application, prescriptive elements, assessment of risks and benefits, and monitoring and promotion of adherence

and outcomes, such as applied to other medical treatments.

Objectives for middle-aged and older adults have traditionally focused on physical activities designed to improve cardiorespiratory fitness and thus potentially prolong life, as well as prevent and treat cardiovascular and other chronic disease.[3] However, it is increasingly recognized that older adults can benefit substantially from physical activities designed to maintain or improve functional independence, by addressing age-related changes in physiology and geriatric syndromes, and thus enhancing quality of life.[4] The specific physical fitness components that optimize physical function as individuals age include muscle strength and power, cardiovascular and muscular endurance, balance, and flexibility.[5, 6] The prevalent problems of mobility impairment, falls, arthritis, osteoporotic fractures, and functional status are clearly related in part to sarcopenia (loss of muscle mass and function),[7] a feature of aging that is amenable to intervention even in frail elders.[8] Additionally, the metabolic benefits of retention and activation of muscle mass are now increasingly recognized as an important facet of the epidemic of age and obesity-related insulin resistance and type 2 diabetes.[9, 10] The Physical Activity Guidelines Advisory Committee Report, 2008 suggests the following minimum goals for older adults:[2]

(1) 150 minutes of moderate or 75 minutes of vigorous aerobic leisure time physical activity per week or an equivalent combination

(2) muscle-strengthening activities at moderate or higher intensity for all major muscle groups two times per week

(3) exercises that maintain or improve balance for those at risk of falling

---

Reichel's Care of the Elderly, 7th Edition, ed. Jan Busby-Whitehead *et al.* Published by Cambridge University Press.
© Cambridge University Press 2016.

69

These guidelines recognize that modification may be needed for those with chronic conditions and low fitness, and such individuals should be as physically active as their abilities and conditions allow. Additionally, the guidelines state that higher levels of activity (e.g., 300 minutes per week of moderate intensity aerobic activity or more) will provide additional health and functional benefits. These guidelines have recently been examined for their relationship to mortality in the National Health Interview Survey cohort of 242,397 adults, demonstrating that adherence to the aerobic or combined aerobic and strength training guidelines significantly reduced mortality, with the greatest benefits in older adults with at least one chronic condition, where adherence reduced adjusted mortality risk by 48%.[11]

Unfortunately, US survey and other data indicate that women in general (who are at higher risk of sarcopenia-related morbidity) report lower than average adult participation levels, particularly for strength training (11% vs. 16%).[12] Additionally, despite the evidence on safety and efficacy in even frail elders, the prevalence rate for resistive exercise is even lower among the old (6% at ages 65–74) and the very old (4% above age 75).[13, 14] Individuals in this latter age group, particularly over the age of 85, are primarily women, making an understanding of the risks and benefits of exercise in this population a priority.[15]

Rationale for the integration of exercise prescription into geriatric care

The rationale for the integration of a physical activity prescription into geriatric health care is based on four essential concepts.[16] First, there is a great similarity between the physiologic changes that are attributable to disuse (sarcopenia, osteopenia, central and generalized adiposity, low fitness, insulin resistance, etc.) and those that have been typically observed in aging populations, leading to the speculation that the way in which we age may in fact be greatly modulated with attention to activity levels.[17] Second, chronic diseases increase with age, and exercise has now been shown to be an independent risk factor and/or potential treatment for most of the major causes of morbidity and mortality in industrialized societies (see Table 6.1), a potential which is currently vastly underutilized. Third, traditional medical interventions don't typically address disuse syndromes

accompanying chronic disease, which may be responsible for much of their associated disability. Exercise is particularly good at targeting these syndromes of disuse. Finally, many pathophysiologic aberrations that are central to a disease or its treatment may be equally or better addressed by exercise than by pharmacologic therapy (e.g., the visceral adiposity and insulin resistance of metabolic syndrome), which therefore deserves a place in the mainstream of medical care, not as an optional adjunct.

It is clear that the optimum approach to "successful aging" or to health care in the older population cannot ignore the overlap of these areas. In some cases, exercise can be used to avert "age-related" decrements in physiologic function and thereby maximize function and quality of life in the elderly. On the other hand, the combination of exercise and sound nutrition, particularly in relation to favorable alterations in body composition, will have numerous important effects on risk factors for chronic disease as well as the disability that accompanies such conditions. Therefore, understanding the effects of aging on exercise capacity and how habitual physical activity can modify this relationship in the older adult, including its specific utility in treating medical diseases, is critical for health-care practitioners of all disciplines.

Monitoring the benefits of exercise

Many health outcomes appear to be related to the accumulated volume and/or intensity of exercise, and so simply monitoring adherence to the physical activity recommendations will theoretically provide evidence that the targeted benefits are occurring, in addition to the role exercise plays in promoting adherence to the prescription.[18] However, there may be benefits also in monitoring the actual physiological improvements from training. For example, aerobic capacity itself has an even stronger relationship to mortality than level of physical activity,[19] and increase in muscle mass after resistance training is directly linked to improved metabolic and inflammatory profile in older adults with type 2 diabetes.[10, 20] Documenting improvements in fitness, function, or body composition may have a reinforcing effect on long-term behavioral adaptations as well. Improved fitness/function across the multiple domains of exercise capacity may be shown, for example, by:

Table 6.1 Major benefits of exercise in older adults for optimal aging and disease prevention and treatment

Physiological structure or functional capacity	Effect of aging/disuse/inactivity	Major associated geriatric syndrome(s) or disease (s)	Exercise effective as preventive strategy?	Exercise effective as treatment strategy?	Comments
Adipose tissue mass; central and visceral redistribution including intrahepatic, pancreatic, and intramuscular lipid infiltration	Increase	Obesity CVD, HTN, FVC Stroke Diabetes Osteoarthritis Depression Dementia Cancer of esophagus, breast, endometrium, colon and rectum, kidney, pancreas, thyroid, and gallbladder Mobility impairment Disability	Yes	Yes	Both aerobic and resistive exercise effective; for treatment best combined with diet
Aerobic capacity, maximal stroke volume and cardiac contractility, oxygen extraction and utilization in skeletal muscle	Decrease	Low fitness Disability CVD	Yes	Yes	Aerobic and interval training most effective; resistance exercise with modest benefits; exercise effects on cardiac contractility not seen in women
Atherosclerosis	Increase	CAD, MI, CHF Renal failure Stroke PVD Dementia	Yes	Yes	Both aerobic and resistance exercise beneficial for prevention and treatment
Autonomic nervous system function, heart rate variability, baroreceptor function	Decrease	Postural hypotension Cardiac arrhythmias CVD mortality	Yes	Yes	Aerobic and resistive exercise beneficia

Table 6.1 (cont.)

Physiological structure or functional capacity	Effect of aging/disuse/inactivity	Major associated geriatric syndrome(s) or disease (s)	Exercise effective as preventive strategy?	Exercise effective as treatment strategy?	Comments
Balance and gait stability	Decrease	Falls Mobility impairment Disability Fear of falling	Yes	Yes	Balance and resistance exercise beneficial; tai chi and yoga also effective
Bone density and mass	Decrease	Osteoporosis, osteoporotic fracture	Yes	Yes	High-impact, weight-bearing, resistance training most effective
Brain volume, neurogenesis, synaptic connectivity, cognitive performance	Decrease	Cognitive impairment Dementia Disability	Yes	Yes (structural changes variable; executive function benefits greater than memory enhancement)	Both aerobic and resistance exercise beneficial
Cartilage degeneration, thinning, tears	Increase	Osteoarthritis Tendinopathy, tears Disability Mobility impairment	Yes	Yes	Both aerobic and resistance training beneficial; strengthening may need to precede weight-bearing exercise
Central and peripheral blood pressure; arterial stiffness	Increase	HTN CVD, PVD Stroke Dementia Renal failure Type 2 diabetes Macular degeneration, retinopathy	Yes	Yes	Both aerobic and resistance exercise beneficial for BP, only aerobic exercise improves arterial stiffness

Connective tissue elasticity, flexibility	Decrease	Mobility impairment	Yes	Stretching exercise recommended after tissues warmed up with other exercise modalities; resistance exercise also beneficial
Glucose homeostasis, insulin sensitivity and signaling, glycogen storage, glycolytic enzyme capacity	Decrease	Insulin resistance, glucose intolerance, type 2 diabetes	Yes	Both aerobic and resistance exercise beneficial
Hemodynamic stability in face of stressors (postural, volumetric, hormonal, pharmacologic)	Decrease	Postural hypotension Post-prandial hypotension Mobility impairment, falls Fear of falling	Yes	Aerobic exercise and lower extremity contractions helpful; avoid Valsalva which may decrease venous return
Immune function, resistance to infection, suppression of malignant cell proliferation	Decrease	Cancer Infectious disease Autoimmune diseases AIDS Chronic inflammation	Yes, obesity-related cancers; variable for infectious diseases such as acute respiratory infections	Most evidence for aerobic in prevention and resistance exercise in treatment of cancer Immune function may be impaired by excessive exercise/overtraining Yes (cancer survival and recurrence, management of treatment side effects, cancer cachexia and fatigue, AIDS symptoms and survival, RA survival and function)
Lipid metabolism	Increased LDL, TG, total cholesterol Decreased HDL cholesterol	Atherosclerosis CVD PVD Stroke Dementia	Yes	Aerobic and resistance exercise beneficial
Muscle mass and function (strength, power, endurance)	Decrease	Sarcopenia Mobility impairment CVD Type 2 diabetes Dementia Disability Osteoporosis, fracture	Yes	Progressive resistance training primary effective modality

Table 6.1 (cont.)

Physiological structure or functional capacity	Effect of aging/disuse/inactivity	Major associated geriatric syndrome(s) or disease (s)	Exercise effective as preventive strategy?	Exercise effective as treatment strategy?	Comments
Neural reaction time, motor coordination	Decrease	Falls Mobility impairment	Yes	Yes	Aerobic, resistance, and balance training all beneficial
Positive affect and mood, psychological well-being	Decrease	Anxiety Negative affect Depression, suicide attempts Low self-esteem Poor quality of life	Yes	Yes	Both aerobic and resistance exercise beneficial
Pulmonary structure (alveolar number), airway function (flow rates and volumes)	Decrease	Asthma Bronchitis Chronic obstructive pulmonary disease	Variable (may prevent asthma via prevention of obesity, maintain pulmonary function)	Yes (outside of acute exacerbations)	Both aerobic and resistance exercise beneficial in chronic lung disease; inspiratory muscle training also beneficial; resistance training needed to counteract chronic corticosteroid therapy
Renal function	Decrease	Renal failure (dialysis, organ transplant)	Yes (via prevention of HTN and type 2 diabetes)	Yes (treatment of sarcopenia accompanying CRF, dialysis, and organ transplant)	Aerobic and resistive exercise with complementary benefits
Sleep quality and quantity	Decrease	Insomnia Obstructive sleep apnea Obesity; metabolic abnormalities	Yes	Yes	Both aerobic and resistance exercise beneficial; obesity reduction key for OSA

- improved measurements of peak aerobic capacity
- decreased heart rate and blood pressure response to a fixed submaximal workload
- decreased rating of perceived exertion for a fixed submaximal workload
- improved muscle strength, endurance, or power
- ability to lift a submaximal load more times
- ability to withstand postural stress or negotiate obstacles without losing balance
- improved joint range of motion
- improved functional performance (e.g., gait speed, chair stand time, stair climbing, six-minute walk distance, etc.).

Exercise testing for older adults

Cardiovascular endurance

Since treadmill testing and indirect calorimetry are not always available or feasible, particularly in frail older adults over 75, field estimates of aerobic capacity and cardiovascular responses are often substituted. A simple way to do this in clinical practice that requires minimal equipment is the six-minute walk test.[21] This test has been used as an index of rehabilitation in cardiac, pulmonary, and other patients, and it is known to predict outcomes and improve with effective interventions. With training, pulse and blood pressure at six minutes should decrease, and distance covered should increase by at least 25 m–50 m. Alternatives to the six-minute walk are walking a fixed distance (e.g., 400 m), climbing multiple flights of stairs as rapidly as possible, or stepping up and down a single step for several minutes, followed by the preceding measurements. However, availability of stairs and the potential for musculoskeletal injury due to balance, hip and knee arthritis, or vision problems make rapid stepping tests less desirable in the older adult. The six-minute walk test reflects not only aerobic capacity, but also contributions from gait stability, muscle strength, pain, body composition, and neuropsychological function, and thus is a good overall index of exercise capacity (not simply aerobic capacity), and has direct clinical relevance to ambulatory function in daily life.[22]

Strength testing

If maximal strength itself cannot be measured, or is not considered safe or feasible in an elderly individual, there is an option that is commonly used to rate effort during a lift, using a scale of perceived exertion, such as Borg's Rating of Perceived Exertion (RPE) scale. [23] On this scale from 6 to 20, a rating of 15 to 18 (hard to very hard) is equivalent to 70%–80% of maximum lifting capacity in studies conducted in young and older adults, and is therefore an appropriate training goal for a robust and safe resistance training prescription.[9, 15] In addition, functional tests that may be used as an index of muscle strength and power include multiple chair stand time and stair climb time, although lower extremity arthritis or poor balance may distort the relationship between muscle capacity and performance on these tests. Although in epidemiological studies, grip strength is often used as a general index of muscle function or nutritional status in older adults and does predict mortality, morbidity, and disability,[24, 25] measures of lower extremity muscle strength and power, if obtainable, are more directly applicable to mobility impairment, fall risk, and specific exercise recommendations for relevant muscle groups of the hip, knee, and ankle.[4, 26]

Pre-exercise assessment in older adults

Most older adults, despite the presence of chronic diseases and disabilities, are able to undertake and benefit from an exercise prescription that is tailored to their physiological capacities, comorbidities, and neuropsychological and behavioral needs.[2, 16] The relatively few permanent exclusions to any structured exercise are generally for severe, irreversible conditions that are obvious exclusions because of the nature of the specific exercise prescription under consideration or the risk the exercise would impose upon the health status of the individual. There may be some forms of exercise that even permanently bed-bound patients, or those with severe behavioral problems, may engage in, even if such individuals are not able to participate in the usual aerobic, resistive, or balance exercises that will be described shortly. For some older adults, such as those with critical aortic stenosis, cardiac or peripheral vascular ischemia at rest, or an enlarging aortic aneurysm or known cerebral aneurysm (when surgery is not an option due to other medical considerations or very advanced age), any exercise that significantly elevates cardiac workload or blood pressure is considered high risk, and therefore not recommended.[9, 15] It is anticipated that relatively few older adults (even those in long-term care) would be excluded from all exercise programs

75

based on items in this category (see Table 6.2) other than those with severe forms of dementia or terminal illness.

The majority of questions about exercise prescription eligibility will be because of items in the "temporary exclusion" or WAIT category (see Table 6.2), so judgments must be made based on the severity of the diagnosis, timing of the event in question, and re-evaluation after a diagnostic workup or an adjustment of medications is made. Most older adults in this category will be able to be reclassified as appropriate for exercise once their condition has been treated or stabilized. Notably, these are all conditions that require stabilization or medical attention *regardless* of the intent to begin exercise, so a review of exercise eligibility also serves as a check for optimal control of most acute and chronic health conditions.

Table 6.2 Screening older adults for an exercise program

I. STOP! Permanent exclusion	II. WAIT! Temporary exclusion	III. GO! Exercise recommended
If any boxes in this column are checked, individual is ineligible for any moderate to vigorous exercise prescription at this time but may undertake certain low intensity activites as tolerated under supervision.	If any boxes in this column are checked, follow protocols for further evaluation of these concerns with medical personnel prior to reevaluating for appropriateness/ modification of exercise prescription.	If only boxes in this column are checked, individual is suited for an exercise prescription with input from allied health staff to tailor program to specific needs or impairments to prevent injuries
☐ End-stage congestive heart failure	☐ Acute change in mental status or delirium, psychosis	☐ Arthritis, stable
☐ Permanent bed-bound status	☐ Cerebral hemorrhage within the past three months	☐ Chronic obstructive pulmonary disease, asthma
☐ Severe cognitive impairment or behavioral disturbance	☐ Exacerbation of chronic inflammatory joint disease or osteoarthritis	☐ Congestive heart failure, stable
☐ Unstable abdominal, thoracic, or cerebral aneurysm	☐ Eye surgery within the past two weeks	☐ Coronary artery disease, stable
☐ Untreated severe aortic stenosis	☐ Fracture in healing stage	☐ Chronic renal failure
☐ Other _____	☐ Hernia, symptomatic (abdominal or inguinal) or bleeding hemorrhoids	☐ Cancer (history or current)
	☐ Myocardial infarction or cardiac surgery within past three months	☐ Chronic liver disease
	☐ Other acute illness or change in symptoms	☐ Chronic venous stasis
	☐ Proliferative diabetic retinopathy or severe nonproliferative retinopathy	☐ Dementia, cognitive impairment

Table 6.2 (cont.)

I. STOP! Permanent exclusion	II. WAIT! Temporary exclusion	III. GO! Exercise recommended
	☐ Pulmonary embolism or deep venous thrombosis within three months	☐ Depression, anxiety, low morale
	☐ Soft tissue injury, healing	☐ Diabetes
	☐ Active suicidality or suicidal ideation	☐ Drugs causing muscle wasting (steroids)
	☐ Systemic infection	☐ Frailty
	☐ Uncontrolled blood pressure (>160/100)	☐ Falls, history of hip fracture
	☐ Uncontrolled diabetes mellitus (FBS >200mg/dL)	☐ Gait and balance disorders, mobility impairment
	☐ Uncontrolled malignant cardiac arrhythmia (ventricular tachycardia, complete heart block, atrial flutter, symptomatic bradycardia)	
	☐ Unstable angina (at rest or crescendo pattern, ECG changes)	☐ Hypertension
		☐ HIV infection
	☐ Other	☐ Hyperlipidemia
		☐ Malnutrition, poor appetite
		☐ Neuromuscular disease
		☐ Obesity
		☐ Osteoporosis
		☐ Parkinson's disease
		☐ Peripheral vascular disease
		☐ Stroke, stable

Notably, the vast majority of chronic illnesses (GO category, Table 6.2) are *indications for*, rather than *contraindications to*, regular exercise. For example, if a patient with osteoporosis, chronic renal failure, osteoarthritis, and depression is *not* exercising, his or her medical management can be seen as suboptimal, as regular exercise is in fact additive to the benefits of usual medical care in these and all of the other chronic conditions listed. Therefore, screening a patient for exercise should be seen as an opportunity to "screen in" those sedentary adults who have exercise-responsive diseases, rather than primarily as a task of "screening out" those few adults with conditions which absolutely preclude exercise of any sort.

Exercise prescription in older adults

It is quite likely that after initial screening, many barriers and difficulties with adherence will be identified in the typically sedentary older individual. Therefore, it becomes important to know how to deliver the prescription in logical stages that are palatable and feasible, and have some likelihood of successful implementation. Current position stands and consensus guidelines for physical activity in older adults generally recommend a multi-modal exercise prescription including aerobic, strengthening, balance, and flexibility training, via a combination of structured and incidental (lifestyle–integrated) activities.[5, 6] However, it is usually best to start with only one mode of exercise and let the older adult get used to the new routine of exercise before adding other components, or optimal adherence and adaptation may be compromised.[27] This approach obviously requires attention to risk factors, medical history, physical exam findings, and personal preferences in order to prioritize prescriptive elements, and will be different for each individual. However, there are a few generalizations that can be made.

- If significant deficits in muscle strength or balance are identified, then these should be addressed prior to the initiation of aerobic training. Prescribing progressive aerobic training in the absence of sufficient balance or strength is likely to result in knee pain, fear of falling, falls, and limited ability to progress aerobically, and is not recommended. Attempting to ambulate those who cannot lift their body weight out of a chair or maintain standing balance is likely to fail.

- Paying attention to the physiological determinants of transfer ability and ambulation, and targeting these specifically with the appropriate exercise prescription when reversible deficits are uncovered is most likely to succeed.

- In some cases, a chronic health condition may benefit equally from resistance or aerobic training (as in the treatment of depression, for example [28]), but the decision is made based on ability to tolerate one form of exercise over another. Severe osteoarthritis of the knee, recurrent falls, and a low threshold for ischemia may make resistance training safer than aerobic training as an antidepressant treatment in this case.

- Prioritization requires careful consideration of the risks and benefits of each mode of activity, as well as the current health status and physical fitness level.

- Patient preference for group vs. individual exercise, structured vs. lifestyle physical activity, level of supervision desired, and attraction or aversion to specific modalities of exercise must be considered to optimize behavioral change and long-term adherence.

Aerobic activity

Aerobic or cardiovascular endurance training refers to exercise in which large muscle groups contract many times (thousands of times at a single session) against little or no resistance other than that imposed by gravity.[9] The purpose of this type of training is to increase the maximal amount of aerobic work that can be carried out, as well as to decrease the physiologic response and perceived difficulty of submaximal aerobic workloads. Extensive adaptations in the cardiopulmonary system, peripheral skeletal muscle, circulation, and metabolism are responsible for these changes in exercise capacity and tolerance. Many different kinds of exercise fall into this category, including walking and its derivatives (hiking, running, dancing, stair climbing, biking, swimming, ball sports, etc.). The key distinguishing feature between activities that are primarily aerobic vs. resistive in nature is the much lesser degree of overload to the muscle in aerobic training as well as the higher number of contractions compared to resistance training. Obviously, there may be some overlap if aerobic activities are altered to increase the loading to muscle, as in resisted stationary cycling or stair climbing machines. However, such activities are still primarily aerobic in nature, as they do not cause fatigue within a very few contractions the way resistance training does, and they therefore do not cause the kinds of adaptations in the nervous system and muscle which lead to marked strength gain and hypertrophy.

Modes of aerobic exercise

There are many more kinds of cardiovascular exercise available than is the case for strengthening exercise. The decision about how to train aerobically depends on factors such as preference, access, likelihood of injury, and health-related restrictions or desired benefits. In general, although there are differences in oxygen consumption among various kinds of aerobic exercise, unless one is training for a particular sport, personal preference can provide much of the direction in this regard, as long-term compliance will require that an enjoyable pursuit has been selected. Given attention to the following intensity and volume requirements, most activities can contribute to improvements in cardiovascular efficiency, a reduction of metabolic risk factors, and reduced risk of many chronic diseases.

Two other factors assume importance in older adults, and older women in particular. The first is the beneficial effect of weight-bearing aerobic activities on bone density.[29] The loading of bone is critical to this outcome; thus, non-weight-bearing aerobic activities (such as swimming and biking) have not been shown to maintain or increase bone density, but aerobics, jogging, and stepping have positive effects in cross-sectional and longitudinal studies. Secondly, isolated high-impact activities such as skipping rope, hopping, and plyometrics (jumping), although exceptionally beneficial for bone formation in animal models, children, and premenopausal women,[30, 31] particularly at the hip, have been associated with significant rates of knee and ankle injuries, even in healthy older adults, and have generally not been shown to increase bone density by themselves in postmenopausal women.[32] In older adults with preexisting arthritis or fall risk, such high-impact activities are neither feasible nor recommended, as they are even more likely to result in injuries and exacerbations of arthritis in this cohort. Balancing the skeletal need for weight-bearing or mixed loading and the safety requirements of the joints and connective tissues for low-impact loading, one would favor exercises such as walking, dancing,

hiking, and stair climbing over running, step aerobics, and jumping rope in most very old or frail adults. By contrast, men and women without underlying arthritis or balance disorders may generally perform higher impact activities safely as long as muscle and ligament strength and joint structure is normal, and such exercise should improve muscle power and associated functional outcomes as well as bone strength. [26, 33]

Overall, walking and its derivations surface as the most widely studied, feasible, safe, accessible, and economical mode of aerobic training for men and women of most ages and states of health. This does not require special equipment or locations, and it does not need to be taught or supervised (except in the cognitively impaired, very frail, or medically unstable individual). Walking bears a natural relationship to ordinary activities of daily living, making it easier to integrate into lifestyle and functional tasks than any other mode of exercise. Therefore, it is theoretically more likely to translate into improved functional independence and mobility than other types of aerobic exercise.

Intensity

The intensity of aerobic exercise refers to the amount of oxygen consumed (VO_2), or energy expended, per minute while performing the activity, which will vary from about 5 kcal/min for light activities; 7.5 kcal/minute for moderate activities, and 10–12 kcal/min for very heavy activities.[9] Energy expenditure increases with increasing body weight for weight-bearing aerobic activities, as well as with inclusion of larger muscle mass, and increased work (force × distance) and power output (work/time) demands of the activity. Therefore, the most intensive activities are those that involve the muscles of the arms, legs, and trunk simultaneously, necessitate moving the full body weight through space, and are done at a rapid pace (e.g., cross-country skiing). Adding extra loading to the body weight (backpack, weight belt, wrist weights) increases the force needed to move the body part through space, and therefore increases the aerobic intensity of the work performed. Biomechanical inefficiency (e.g., gait disorder, arthritis pain, use of an assistive device) increases the oxygen demands of a given task, which must be considered when prescribing aerobic exercise to adults with such impairments.

The rise in heart rate is directly proportional in normal individuals in sinus rhythm to the increasing oxygen consumption or aerobic workload. Thus, monitoring heart rate has traditionally been a primary means of both prescribing appropriate intensity levels as well as following training adaptations when direct measurements of oxygen consumption are not available. The heart rate reserve (HRR) method is the most useful estimate of intensity based on heart rate[5], calculated as:

$$HRR = relative\ percent \times [maximal\ HR$$
$$-resting\ HR] + resting\ HR$$

Maximal HR can be taken from a maximal treadmill test or very roughly estimated as [220 – age]. Training intensity is normally recommended at a moderate (40%–59% HRR) level,[5, 34] although vigorous (60%–84% HRR) training levels may be used in selected individuals, and may provide increased adaptation or health benefits for some disease outcomes. High-intensity interval training (HIIT), using short bouts (most commonly 4 minutes) of near-maximal (approximately 90% peak HR) effort interspersed with rest periods of several minutes, has been demonsrated to be a more time-efficient and effective way to increase aerobic capacity and some health outcomes in recent years,[35, 36] although the long-term safety and benefits of HIIT, particularly outside of supervised clinical trials, requires more study in older and clinical cohorts before it can be generally recommended.

Difficulties with an intensity prescription based on heart rate in the older adult include inaccurate pulse recording during exercise and the presence of arrhythmias, pacemakers, or beta-blockers (systemic or ophthalmologic) that will alter the heart rate response to exercise. Therefore, a more easily obtainable and reliable estimate of aerobic intensity is to prescribe a moderate level as 12–14, or a vigorous level as 15–17 on the rating of perceived exertion (RPE) scale, which runs from 6 to 20.[34] At a moderate level, the exerciser should note increased pulse and respiratory rate, but still be able to talk. This scale has been validated for use in men and women, young and old, those with coronary disease as well as healthy adults, and is therefore of widespread applicability. It is easy to teach and is a way to "supervise" training intensity from afar, by means of written or electronic diaries or telephone calls, making it cost-effective in community programs

and health-care or e-health settings. Usually a visual representation of the RPE scale is used to increase accuracy, but assessment can even be done without this prop in patients who are blind or cannot read.

As is the case with all other forms of exercise, in order to maintain the same relative training intensity over time, the absolute training load must be increased as fitness improves. In younger individuals, typically walking may be changed to jogging and then running to increase intensity as needed. More appropriate in older or frail adults are progressive alterations in workload that increase energy expenditure without converting to a high-impact form of activity. Examples of how to prescribe such progression for various modes of aerobic exercise are given in Table 6.3. The workloads should be progressed based on ratings of effort at each training session.

Table 6.3 Increasing the intensity of aerobic exercise

Mode of exercise	Ways to increase intensity
Walking	Add small weights around wrists Swing arms Use "race walking" style Add inclines, hills, stairs Carry weighted backpack or waist belt* Push a wheelchair or stroller (with someone in it)
Cycling	Increase pedaling speed Increase resistance to pedals Add hills Add backpack* Add child carrier to back of bike
Water activities	Use arms and legs in strokes Add resistive equipment for water Increase pace
Tennis	Convert from doubles to singles game
Golf	Carry clubs* Eliminate golf cart
Dance	Increase pace of movements Add more arm and leg movements

* Avoid flexing the spine when doing this to prevent excessive compressive forces on the thoracic spine

Once the perceived exertion slips below 12 on the RPE scale, the workload should be increased to maintain the physiologic stimulus for continued cardiovascular adaptation. As with resistance training, the most common error in aerobic training is *failure to progress*, which results in an early suboptimal plateau in cardiovascular and metabolic improvement. In very frail adults, the workloads that elicit a moderate rating of based on perceived exertion, rated subjectively or objectively.

Volume

In most older adults, 150 minutes of moderate intensity or 75 minutes of vigorous intensity aerobic exercise each week will be sufficient to provide benefits in the domains of improved maximal and submaximal cardiovascular efficiency, psychological well-being, and control of chronic diseases such as arthritis, diabetes, peripheral vascular disease, chronic lung disease, coronary artery disease, and congestive heart failure, for example, and even lower amounts of exercise (60 minutes moderate intensity) will provide benefit in the initially sedentary. Higher volumes of exercise generally result in greater fitness adaptations [37] and health and mortality benefits,[11, 38] and up to 420 minutes per week are recommended for the treatment of obesity.[39] It should be noted, however, that very little research on aerobic training in very old or frail adults has actually been conducted, and most recommendations are simply extrapolated from studies in younger individuals.

It has been shown that aerobic exercise does not need to be carried out at a single session to provide training effects, and may be broken up into bouts of 10 minutes at a time to reach the desired volume of training.[9] Shorter duration sessions of moderate intensity have not been evaluated for efficacy, although public health recommendations for integrating short bouts of even five minutes into the daily routine have been made recently. As mentioned, high-intensity interval training bouts may be even shorter (ranging from one to four minutes in most studies), [36] although the feasibility of such prescriptions requires further study. Very frail adults may only tolerate two to five minutes of walking or other aerobic activities initially, and a reasonable goal is to increase tolerance for longer workloads until 10 to 20 minutes of exercise can be sustained without resting. This would provide substantial functional benefit

in the nursing home, as walking for 20 minutes would likely enable the older adults to get to almost any location in the home without having to stop and rest.

Overall, a session or sessions of aerobic exercise carried out at least once every three days adding up to at least 60 minutes a week appears to be the minimal prescription for health and longevity and justifiable based on the currently available literature. Higher volumes of exercise than this (e.g., 30–60 minutes per day, 5 days per week, or 150–300 minutes per week), or short bouts of higher-intensity activity are generally associated with greater health-related outcomes and improvements in fitness.[9, 36] It is not recommended to exercise in very long bouts once or twice a week as an alternative to several shorter sessions, as this is likely to result in overuse muscle soreness and injuries. The risk of sudden death during physical activity appears to be concentrated in those who do not exercise on a regular basis (at least one hour per week), which is another reason for advocating regular, moderate doses of exercise rather than periodic high volume training.

Benefits

The benefits of aerobic exercise have been extensively studied over the past 50 years, and the most important benefits for older adults are listed in Table 6.1. They include a broad range of physiological adaptations that are in general opposite to the effects of aging on most body systems, as well as major health-related clinical outcomes.[40] The health conditions that are responsive to aerobic exercise include most of those of concern to older adults: osteoporosis, heart disease, stroke, breast cancer, diabetes, obesity, hypertension, arthritis, depression, memory loss, and insomnia.[38] These physiological and clinical benefits form the basis for the inclusion of aerobic exercise as an essential component of the overall physical activity prescription for healthy aging.[41]

Risks

The major potential risks of exercise are listed in Table 6.4. Most of these adverse events are preventable by paying attention to the underlying medical conditions present, making appropriate choices regarding the modality of exercise used, avoiding exercise during extreme environmental conditions, wearing proper footwear and clothing, and minimizing or avoiding exercise during acute illness or in the presence of new, undefined symptoms. Most fluid

Table 6.4 The risks of exercise in older adults

Musculoskeletal	Cardiovascular	Metabolic
Falls	Arrhythmia	Dehydration
Foot ulceration or laceration	Cardiac failure	Electrolyte imbalance
Fracture, osteoporotic or traumatic	Hypertension	Energy imbalance
Hemorrhoids*	Hypotension	Heat stroke
Hernia*	Ischemia	Hyperglycemia
Joint or bursa inflammation, exacerbation of arthritis	Pulmonary embolism	Hypoglycemia
Ligament or tendon strain or rupture	Retinal hemorrhage or detachment, lens detachment	Hypothermia
Muscle soreness or tear	Ruptured cerebral or other aneurysm	Seizures
Stress incontinence	Syncope or postural symptoms	

* Primarily associated with increased intra-abdominal pressure during resistive exercise, but may occur if Valsalva maneuver occurs during aerobic activities

balance problems can be handled by exercising in reasonable temperature and humidity only and drinking extra fluid on exercise days.

All older adults should have yearly ophthalmologic exams for glaucoma and retinal changes, and the initiation of an exercise regimen is a good time to reinforce this preventive health measure, particularly in those with hypertension or diabetes. Retinopathy is not a contraindication to exercise, except in the case of proliferative retinopathy or an acute bleed or retinal tear/detachment until stabilized. If someone has had recent ophthalmologic surgery, exercise is contraindicated for several weeks to avoid raising intraocular pressure, and the exact recommendations should be obtained from the ophthalmologist in these cases.

Metabolic complications are rare unless diabetes is out of control at the time exercise is initiated, or dehydration, fever, or acute illnesses are present. The improvement in insulin sensitivity at the initiation of regular exercise may require modification of insulin and oral hypoglycemic medications to prevent hypoglycemia. Exercising in the one to two hours after meals should both prevent hypoglycemia as well as minimize the post-prandial rise in serum glucose, which is an independent risk factor for cardiovascular events, even in those who are not diabetic.[42] This cardiovascular toxicity is mediated by oxidant stress, which triggers inflammation, endothelial dysfunction,

hypercoagulability, sympathetic hyperactivity, and other atherogenic changes. Exercise has been shown to attenuate this post-prandial dysmetabolism, which may mediate some of the cardio protective effects of exercise.[42, 43]

Cardiovascular complications are most likely if ischemic heart disease is not well controlled medically or surgically prior to exercise initiation, if warning signs are ignored, or if sudden, vigorous exercise is tried in a previously completely sedentary individual. When properly prescribed and monitored, both aerobic and resistance training have been shown to reduce the incidence of angina and medication use in cardiac rehabilitation settings, and are indicated as part of standard medical management of coronary artery disease.[15] Although claudication is mentioned as a possible adverse side effect of exercise in those with peripheral vascular disease, there is an important treatment caveat here. It has been shown that aerobic exercise (even arm ergometry) significantly increases exercise tolerance in patients with peripheral vascular disease (i.e., time to claudication), and resistance training has some benefit as well.[44] However, exercise has been intentionally continued for about 30–90 seconds if possible after the onset of claudication in some trials ("exercise to maximal pain"). This remains the recommendation of the TASC-II consensus group,[45] although the most recent meta-analysis suggests that inducing moderate to severe claudication may attenuate fitness benefits in this cohort.[46] Recommendations to continue exercise in the face of peripheral ischemic pain stands in contrast to angina or any of the other symptoms listed in Table 6.4, for which exercise should be stopped immediately if they occur.

Musculoskeletal problems are more common than any other risk of aerobic or resistive exercise, particularly in the novice exerciser or very frail adult, and those with underlying joint disease. Often if significant weakness or balance impairment is present, it is best to avoid aerobic exercise altogether until strength and balance have been improved sufficiently with specific training, so as to allow safe weight-bearing exercise such as walking. If this is not done, falls, arthritis pain, fear of falling, and muscle fatigue will be so limiting that effective aerobic training is precluded. Warming up muscles gently with slow movements prior to aerobic routines is important to avoid soft tissue injury. The most important point is to avoid high-impact activities (such as jumping, step aerobics, jogging) in those with pre-existing arthritis or weak muscles and ligaments, as this is a principal cause of sports-related injury.

Strength training

Progressive resistance training (PRT), or strength training, is one of the four basic modalities of exercise that are recommended for older adults as part of a balanced physical activity program, whether this is formalized as an exercise prescription or integrated into lifestyle changes.[41] PRT is the process of challenging the skeletal muscle with an unaccustomed stimulus, or load, such that neural and muscle tissue adaptations take place, leading ultimately to increased muscle force producing capacity (strength) and muscle mass.[9] In this kind of exercise, the muscle is contracted slowly just a few times in each session against a relatively heavy load. Any muscle may be trained in this way, although usually 8 to 10 major muscle groups with clinical relevance are trained, for a balanced and functional outcome.

Equipment

There are many ways to carry out PRT. Equipment may range from only body weight to technologically sophisticated pneumatic or hydraulic resistance training machines. In general, in the older adult, machine-based training allows the most robust adaptations to be achieved, offers maximum safety, and requires less technique to be learned. Free weights, on the other hand, offer significant advantages in terms of cost and flexibility in programming, and may provide a better stimulus for motor coordination and balance and functional outcomes, and are the only option in most home and limited-space clinical or residential care settings.

Intensity

Virtually all of the randomized controlled trials of resistance training in the elderly that have resulted in large gains in strength have used an intensity of approximately 70%–80% of maximum strength as the training intensity (a level of 15–17 on the RPE scale can be used to prescribe the proper intensity if strength cannot be measured [47]). There is no evidence that this intensity is unsafe or poorly tolerated in men and women, healthy or frail, even those over 100 years of age, or in early outpatient cardiac rehabilitation, for example. By contrast, low-intensity training results in negligible or modest gains in strength and associated physical, functional, and neuropsychological benefits, and therefore cannot be recommended if the primary intent of training is to prevent or treat sarcopenia and its clinical sequelae.[48] The exception is low-intensity, high-velocity power training, which may improve power and balance via changes in muscle contraction velocity rather than torque capacity.

Volume

The volume of resistance training refers to the frequency of sessions, and the number of sets and repetitions (lifts) performed during each session for each muscle group. It is most effective to recommend training frequencies of two to three days per week in the older adult, with at least a day of rest between sessions. There is no consistent evidence that multiple sets (two to three) are substantially superior to one set (of 8 to 10 repetitions) in terms of strength gain, so if time is a barrier to implementation, one high-intensity set will provide good clinical benefits most efficiently. [41] Increased volume of low-intensity repetitions will not provide the musculoskeletal adaptations associated with high-intensity training.

Velocity

Generally, recommendations have been to perform the concentric (shortening or lifting) and eccentric (lengthening or lowering) contractions slowly over

83

three to four seconds each, to maximize strength and hypertrophic adaptations to PRT. However, there is growing evidence that power training (high-velocity concentric contractions performed at maximal velocity) may improve power and function, as well as bone density and balance, better than slow velocity training, while preserving strength gains seen with traditional training.[49] Notably, the applicability of such high-velocity (ballistic) movements to older adults with rotator cuff, medial meniscus, gluteus minimus, and other common degenerative tears is in some cases limited or contraindicated, and much more data in these and other frail clinical cohorts is needed.

Benefits

Robust increases in muscle size and strength following appropriate PRT are not seen with other forms of exercise, and are also not obtainable with low-intensity nonprogressive resistance training. Therefore, if a primary goal of exercise is to prevent or treat sarcopenia, then there is no effective substitute for this modality of exercise. The hypertrophic response to training does appear to be affected by health status, anabolic hormonal milieu, nutritional substrate availability, changes in protein synthesis with age, genetic profile, and other factors yet to be identified. Although exogenous anabolic steroids can augment the hypertrophic response to resistive exercise in young men, their usage in older men is complicated by the risk of coronary artery disease, prostatic hypertrophy, and cancer. Trials with growth hormone or its secretagogues, or estrogen, have thus far been variably effective in terms of muscle mass or strength gains in older adults when given alone or in combination with resistance training. Given that most studies now show that low levels and accelerated losses of muscle strength and power are more predictive of disability and mobility impairment than low or decreasing muscle mass,[26] the need to enhance muscle hypertrophy pharmacologically beyond that achievable by PRT alone, given the potential adverse effects of such agents, is not clear.

The benefits of PRT extend far beyond the prevention and treatment of sarcopenia itself, as shown in Table 6.1.[30, 50] Resistance training has now been shown to have benefit for the treatment of type 2 diabetes, obesity, depression, osteoporosis, frailty, falls, hip fracture, joint replacement, arthritis, insomnia, coronary artery disease, peripheral vascular disease, congestive heart failure, chronic obstructive pulmonary disease (COPD), cancer cachexia, HIV wasting, end stage renal failure, cognitive impairment and neuromuscular disease, and efficacy in other conditions is emerging as well.[15, 51] Resistance training has also been shown to lower the risk for cardiovascular and metabolic disease as well as all cause mortality.[52] This broad spectrum of benefit places PRT within the mainstream of treatment options for older adults.

Risks

Progressive resistance training has been thought of as a risky form of exercise in the past, and therefore has been sometimes avoided by health-care professionals in their counseling of older adults. However, a wealth of literature over several decades indicates that this modality of exercise is in fact quite safe, and is more feasible in many groups of patients and frail elders than is cardiovascular exercise.[15] There are relatively few absolute medical contraindications to progressive resistance training, such as unstable coronary disease, unrepaired aneurysms, malignant arrhythmias, symptomatic hernias, or critical aortic stenosis (see Table 6.2). Apart from these specific circumstances, resistance training is a realistic option even in very frail elderly individuals. *Frailty is not a contraindication to strength training; conversely it is one of the most important reasons to prescribe it.*[16]

The potential risks of resistance training are primarily musculoskeletal injury and cardiovascular events, as shown in Table 6.4. Musculoskeletal injury is largely preventable with attention to the following points:

- adherence to proper form
- isolation of the targeted muscle group
- slow velocity of lifting in those with underlying or suspected degenerative joint or tendon disease
- limitation of range of motion to the pain-free arc of movement
- avoidance of use of momentum to complete a lift
- use of machines or chairs with good back support
- observation of rest periods between sets and rest days between sessions

In patients with preexisting arthritis, there may be intermittent exacerbation of joint symptoms or inflammation with the initiation of PRT. However, the overall effect of training is to moderately decrease chronic arthritis pain and disability over time.[53] During periods of disease flare-up, it may be necessary to switch to isometric contractions, lower the weight lifted, limit the range of motion through which the load is lifted, or insert additional days of rest between training sessions. It is advisable to continue isometric contractions if nothing else, as this will prevent loss of strength, and will not further increase pain. Once the symptoms have lessened, normal exercise sessions may resume.

Blood pressure changes are difficult to measure during PRT because of the transient nature of the rises, and the fact that blood pressure falls almost immediately after a repetition is completed. This makes monitoring of intra-arterial pressure the only accurate way to gather such information. The heart rate response to PRT is in general lower than that due to aerobic exercise such as walking up an incline or stair climbing, whereas the increase in systolic blood pressure tends to be intermediate between walking and stair climbing. Diastolic pressure elevations are greater with PRT than aerobic exercise, thus increasing mean arterial pressure to a greater degree. The double product (the product of systolic blood pressure and heart rate), which is felt to be representative of myocardial oxygen demand, is greatest for stair climbing, followed by weight lifting and walking.

In the largest series of maximum strength tests yet reported, in 26,000 individuals undergoing testing, not a single cardiovascular event occurred.[54] Additionally, the literature suggests a reduction in ischemic signs and symptoms after PRT in cardiac patients, attesting to the safety of this form of exercise even in individuals with heart disease.

Patients with unstable cardiovascular signs and symptoms should not begin any exercise regimen, including weight lifting, without medical evaluation. Cardiovascular stress is minimized with attention to the factors listed in Box 6.1.

Balance exercises for individuals at fall risk or with mobility impairment

Balance training is probably the least standardized of the various exercise modalities. Despite the use of balance-enhancing modalities for decades by physical therapists and others working with adults and children with developmental or degenerative neurological diseases affecting balance, only recently have there been well-controlled formalized studies of theoretically grounded techniques and outcomes. The recognition that balance impairment is a risk factor for falls and hip fracture even in adults without identifiable neurological disease has expanded the potential target population for balance training to the general aging cohort. The pressing need for definitive outcome data on feasibility and efficacy of various intervention techniques has stimulated quantitative research that will assist in the development of clinical protocols. In the meantime, the balance prescription must be formulated from a variety of evidence collected in epidemiological studies, experimental trials, and clinical practice. It should be noted that in many cases, it is difficult to compare the results across trials, as investigators have used unique training interventions as well as different outcome measures.[55, 56]

Any activity that increases one's ability to maintain balance in the face of a threat to stability may be considered a balance-enhancing activity. Common stressors include:

- narrowing of the base of support
- perturbation of the ground support
- decrease in proprioceptive sensation
- diminished or misleading visual inputs
- disturbed vestibular system input
- increased compliance of the support surface

BOX 6.1 Factors related to increased circulatory stress during resistance training

- Higher relative intensity of load lifted
- Static contractions
- Early phase of concentric contraction
- Greater muscle mass used
- Performance of a Valsalva maneuver during lifts
- Increasing number of repetitions
- Fatigue of muscles (performing a set "to failure")

Circulatory stress = increase of heart rate and blood pressure in response to resistive exercise

- movement of the center of mass of the body away from the vertical
- addition of a cognitive distractor or "dual tasking" while practicing balance

In real life, stressors may also include things such as environmental hazards to traverse, postural hypotension, and drugs that affect central nervous system function, for example. The plethora of conditions that contribute to gait and balance abnormalities in older adults requires a multifactorial approach to balance enhancement and falls prevention.[57, 58] What is presented in the following discussion is a summary of exercise techniques that have favorable effects on this physiological capacity, and therefore form an important part of the exercise prescription for older adults.

General technique

Balance-enhancing activities improve the central nervous system control of balance and coordination of movement, or augment the peripheral neuromuscular system response to signals that balance is threatened. The general approach to the enhancement of balance should rely on theoretical principles that are designed to elicit adaptations in the central neurological control of posture and equilibrium. The basic idea is to progressively challenge the system with stressors of increasing difficulty in four different domains:

1. narrowing the base of support for the body
2. displacing the center of mass to the limits of tolerance
3. removing or minimizing contributions of visual, vestibular, and proprioceptive pathways to balance
4. adding simultaneous cognitive tasks (dual-tasking) such as verbal fluency (e.g., animal naming) or calculations (serial 7s, etc.) during balance exercises

All balance movements should be done slowly and with deliberation, as this stresses the control systems more and produces better physiologic adaptation. It can be seen, for example, that an exercise such as heel walking is actually easier when done rapidly rather than slowly, so the challenge and adaptation will be greater when the slow speed is practiced. Balance training may also be prescribed as structured exercise forms such as tai chi [59] or yoga, or may be incorporated into resistance training during one legged standing movements,[60] or integrated directly into daily activities,[61] which has been shown to be superior to structured balance/strength training sessions for fall prevention.

Intensity

Intensity in balance training refers to the degree of difficulty of the postures, movements, or routines practiced. *The appropriate level of difficulty or "intensity" for any balance-enhancing exercise is the highest level that can be tolerated without inducing a fall or near fall.* In a supervised session, the individual can be pushed to the limits of such tolerance, as safety is assured by the physical presence of the trainer. In an unsupervised setting, the person should be told to try movements only up to the level that they fail to master completely. For example, if the goal is to hold the heel-to-toe stand for 15 seconds, then if someone can only hold the posture for 10 seconds before grabbing the wall for support, this is the appropriate initial training intensity. Progression in intensity is the key to improvement,[56] as in other exercise domains, but this concept of mastery of the previous level before progression must be adhered to for safety. This is particularly important in frail elders, who are at highest risk of falls, osteoporotic fractures, and other injuries.

Volume and frequency

No definite statement can be made at this time about optimal or minimum effective dose of balance-training techniques described earlier. Regimens have ranged from one to seven days per week, and from once a day to several times per day. A recent systematic review of 54 trials has classified high dose as greater than 50 hours of training, and suggested that 2 hours per week of home and/or supervised training is the minimum recommended best practice dose for falls prevention at this stage,[62] while acknowledging the limited robust dose-response trials in this regard. It is likely that as with other forms of training, a dose-response relationship exists, although thresholds have not been defined. There is no evidence that any negative effects are seen with high volume training. Therefore, for adults with significant balance impairments and/or recurrent falls that require intervention, training up to seven days per week may be advantageous, particularly if the exercises are to be integrated into daily life.[61] On the other hand, healthy adults may require only preventive practice one day a week for maintenance of mobility and function. Many more studies are needed in this area to define the recommendation further.

Benefits

Balance training has been shown to result in improved balance performance, decreased fear of falling, decreased incidence of falls, and increased ability to participate in other activities that may have been limited by gait and balance difficulties.[58] It is expected, although not proven, that such changes would ultimately lead to improvements in functional independence, reduced hip fractures and other serious injuries, and improved overall quality of life. Such long-term outcomes will require larger studies of longer duration than those that have been reported to date. In particular, there is a need for data on the feasibility and efficacy of balance training in the very old and frail, in whom deficits are larger, fall risk is usually multifactorial, and cognitive impairments or degenerative neurological diseases exist, although exercise (generally balance and strength training) has been shown in a small literature to reduce fall risk in those with cognitive impairment and in nursing home residents.[63, 64]

Balance training does not generally result in increased strength or aerobic capacity by itself, whereas resistance training in some cases may improve balance.[60] However, there may be some maintenance of muscle strength from the isometric contractions that occur during many of the balance-enhancing and one-legged postures and the bent knee stance during tai chi.[59] In addition, to the extent that balance training results in increased overall physical activity and mobility, these other activities may lead to improvements in strength and endurance. Generally, mobility impairment and falls risk mandates prescription of both balance and strength training, not either in isolation, whereas simple walking programs have not been shown to enhance falls prevention outcomes.[62]

Risks

The only real risk of balance training is actual or threat of loss of balance, resulting in a fall or injury or increased fear of falling. This is preventable with attention to the factors governing progression, intensity, setting, and supervision described earlier. There is little or no elevation in pulse or blood pressure during these kinds of exercises, so cardiovascular events are not an expected or reported consequence.

Musculoskeletal injury, other than that resulting from a fall, would also be unlikely.

There might be exacerbation of preexisting arthritic pain or inflammation of the knee during prolonged one-legged standing or tai chi or yoga postures requiring a semicrouched stance. These positions may have to be adapted or avoided entirely in those with significant weight-bearing pain in the joint. However, once quadriceps muscle strength improves with appropriate resistive exercises (see earlier), these kinds of movements may be tolerable. Impaired flexibility may also limit some tai chi or yoga postures initially, and may lead to injury if range of motion is forced in the beginning. Gradual progression over time in the complexity of postures should prevent most injuries to soft tissues.

Summary

Exercise is integral to the prevention, treatment, and rehabilitation strategies necessary for the care of the geriatric patient. Exercise should be prescribed, as is all other medical treatment, with consideration of patient risks and benefits, knowledge of appropriate modality and dose (intensity, frequency, volume), monitoring for drug interactions, benefits and adverse events, and utilization of the strongest possible behavioral medicine techniques known to optimize adoption and adherence. The emerging recommendations to reduce overall sitting time or length of uninterrupted sitting bouts[65] will likely not be sufficient to oppose the significant age-related changes in physiology and function outlined earlier, although linked to mortality, obesity, and cardio-metabolic risk in some studies. It is likely that reductions in sedentary time will prevent chronic diseases to some degree, although such empirical data are just emerging. However, recommendations focusing on simply reducing sedentary behavior are unlikely to emerge as robust *treatment* of established disease, such as depression, diabetes, cardiovascular disease, sarcopenia/wasting syndromes, osteoporosis, arthritis, chronic lung disease, Parkinson's disease, stroke, and so on, whereas the evidence for the benefits of targeted exercise prescription and adherence for treatment of these and many other conditions is very strong.[61] There is no age above which physical activity ceases to have benefits across a wide range of diseases and disabilities. *Insufficient physical activity and excess sedentary behavior are lethal conditions; physical activity is the antidote*, and health care practitioners should be well-educated leaders and role models in the effort to enhance functional independence, psychological well-being, and quality of life through promotion of exercise for the aged, both fit and frail.

Nutrition

Sufficient intake of energy and nutrients is key for the human body's ability to optimize physiology and organ function as well as contribute to overall health. Consequences of undernutrition include an increase in morbidity and mortality: more specifically, decreased bone mass, impaired muscle function, immune system dysfunction, poor wound healing, and prolonged postoperative recovery.[66] Different segments of the geriatric population have been found to have various prevalence of malnutrition: 5% of community-living elderly, 14% of nursing home residents, 39% of geriatric patients in acute care, and 51% in geriatric rehabilitation are suboptimally nourished.[67]

Older adults may have a decreased desire to eat and drink as a result of a multitude of risk factors that interact with an older adult's changing physiology, one's environment, and the burden of comorbid illness. There is reduced olfactory and gustatory function, along with a decrease in the density of taste buds. The threshold for recognizing a particular taste is increased for all of the basic tastes: salty, sweet, bitter, and sour.[68] Diminished taste alters the pleasure of eating, which can culminate in protein-energy undernutrition. Other changes with aging include diminished central orexigenic signals and a relative increase in gastrointestinal satiety. These physiological changes can be looked upon as a balancing act: an adaptation to decreasing energy requirements with advancing age, which may have potential for malnutrition if the reduction in food intake is excessive.

The response to hunger hormones such as ghrelin and cholecystokinin is blunted in the elderly. A fatty meal increases GLP-1, which increases insulin sensitivity in the hypothalamus, causing a dysregulated energy homeostasis, leading to decreased food intake.[69] Pro-inflammatory cytokines activate pro-opiomelanocortin neurons and inhibit neuropeptide Y neurons, which are involved in mediating hunger and satiety.

Often, the integrity of the oral cavity, which is key to ingestion and the initiation of digestion, is overlooked. For optimal chewing function, one must maintain good oral health and hygiene.[70] Important oral considerations include the status of the patient's teeth, specifically whether the patient has untreated caries, is edentulous/wearing dentures/missing teeth, and the existence of periodontal disease. If an individual has experienced recent weight loss, the dentures may be ill-fitting and result in gingival and buccal irritation, further compounding potential weight loss by adversely impacting a person's desire to eat. In addition to tooth considerations, mouth hydration impacts oral health. Saliva, composed of over 99% water, also contains electrolytes, minerals, mucus, antibacterials (IgA and lysozyme), and enzymes. The enzymes are critical to the initiation of digestion and serve a role in minimizing bacterial decay and cary formation. Saliva serves a lubricative function, which facilitates swallowing and prevents drying of the oral cavity. Xerostomia (dry mouth) can hinder chewing, taste perception, and swallowing. This condition is not a consequence of normal aging; rather it can be secondary to medications, comorbidities, and decreased oral fluid intake. For all these reasons, attention to oral health is paramount.

Malnutrition in the elderly also has diverse social causes including social isolation, loneliness, financial challenges, and mood disorder. An older adult may have superimposed health issues such that the acute and chronic illnesses and the associated medications required for treatment can adversely affect appetite and simultaneously create a setting of increased caloric requirement as a result of cachexia or malabsorption.

Malnutrition syndromes

Anorexia

With aging, food choice starts to change secondary to the influences of biological factors, palatability, financial status, social determinants, and psychological factors. Anorexia of aging can be subdivided into physiologic, pathologic, environmental, and psychological.[71] Physiological changes include impaired chewing, decreased action of salivary glands, impaired esophageal motility, reduced gastric secretions, and decreased sensitivity of taste and smell. In contrast, pathological anorexia is the consequence of acute or chronic illnesses such as malignancy, stroke, COPD, dementia, and mood disorder. The negative effect of many classes of medications on appetite should not be overlooked.

Cachexia

Cachexia is defined as a "complex metabolic syndrome associated with underlying illness and characterized by loss of muscle with or without loss of fat mass. The prominent feature of cachexia is weight loss in adults."[72] The illnesses associated with cachexia include cancer, COPD, chronic kidney disease (CKD), chronic liver failure (CLF), chronic infections, and congestive heart failure (CHF).[73] Cachexia is the result of complex interactions between chronic disease, host metabolism (insulin resistance, increased lipolysis and lipid oxidation, increased protein breakdown), and an imbalance between pro-inflammatory and anti-inflammatory cytokines. Progressive muscle loss is accompanied by a decrease in function and a decline in quality of life, and is predictive of increased morbidity and mortality.[74, 75] As stated by Muscaritoli et al., "[T]hough not all malnourished patients are cachectic, all cachectic patients are invariably malnourished."[76] The Society of Sarcopenia, Cachexia and Wasting Disorders (SCWD) developed a set of diagnostic criteria for cachexia, helping differentiate late stage cachexia from pre-cachexia, in an effort to identify conditions that cause cachexia as well as focus on earlier initiation of interventions.[77]

Sarcopenia

Sarcopenia is characterized by progressive and generalized loss of skeletal muscle mass and strength with a risk of adverse outcomes such as physical disability, poor quality of life, and death.[78, 79] This loss of muscle mass compromises strength, immunocompetence, and the body's metabolic homeostasis.[80] With the associated functional impairment resulting from a decrease in muscle mass, there is increased likelihood of falls and associated loss of autonomy. [81] Consensus papers with a goal of defining sarcopenia have been published. Walking speed, hand grip, and muscle mass are the common parameters used for assessment.

Importantly, it is recognized that in some conditions, such as malignancy, rheumatoid arthritis, and aging, lean body mass can be lost while fat mass remains unchanged or increases. This imbalance between a loss of muscle mass and an increase in body fat results in marked weakness. In the elderly, skeletal muscle protein synthesis is resistant to the anabolic action of insulin. This resistance may lead to age-related muscle loss. As adipose tissue is recognized to be metabolically active, it is thought that an increase in visceral fat may lead to an increase in secretion of pro-inflammatory cytokines (IL-6, TNF-a), which in turn have a catabolic effect on muscles, further contributing to sarcopenia.[81]

Nutritional requirements of older adults

A revised *Dietary Guidelines for Americans* was published in 2010 by the US Department of Agriculture and the US Department of Health and Human Services on a mandated five-year cycle.[82] The two main concepts in the document are (1) to maintain calorie balance over time to achieve and sustain a healthy weight and (2) to focus on consuming nutrient-dense foods and beverages. A healthy diet includes vegetables, fruits, whole grains, fat-free or low-fat milk and milk products, seafood, lean meats and poultry, eggs, beans and peas, and nuts and seeds, while limiting intake of sodium, solid fats, added sugars, and refined grains.

These are based on the premise that the goal is to meet one's nutritional needs through food consumption rather than relying too heavily on supplements or fortified foods. A balanced diet that incorporates the Institute of Medicine of the US National Academy of Sciences Dietary Reference Intakes (DRIs) considers an individual's age, gender, and activity level. The DRIs are nutrient reference values, encompassing more than 40 nutrient substances, that provide a scientific basis for the development of food guidelines in the United States and Canada.[83, 84] Multiple reference values are provided by the DRIs including:

1. Recommended dietary allowances (RDAs): This represents the daily dietary intake level of a nutrient considered sufficient to meet the requirements of 97.5% of healthy individuals in each life stage and gender group.

2. Adequate intake (AI): For these nutrients, there is insufficient scientific evidence to establish an Estimated Average Requirement (EAR) or to set an RDA. It is a recommended average daily nutrient intake level based on observed or experimentally determined approximations or estimates of nutrient intake by a group of apparently healthy people who are assumed to be maintaining an adequate nutritional state.

3. Estimated average requirement (EAR): This is the median value that is estimated to meet the requirement of half the healthy individuals in a life stage and gender group. The EAR is used to calculate the RDA: (EAR + 2 standard deviations = RDA).

4. Tolerable upper intake level (UL): This is the maximum level of daily nutrient intake that is likely to pose no risk of adverse health effects. In general there is no established benefit to healthy individuals of ingesting nutrients in amounts exceeding the RDA or AI. Folate use in pregnant women for the prevention of neural tube defects represents an exception.

There are recommendations for the percentage of calories in the diet that should be derived from carbohydrate, protein, and fat. The Institute of Medicine established the Acceptable Macronutrient Distribution Range (AMDR), which considers both chronic disease risk reduction and intake of essential nutrients. For adults (19 years and older), the diet should contain a mixture of 45%–65% carbohydrates, 10%–35% protein, and 20%–35% fat.

There are only a few points in the document that pertain specifically to the older adult:

1. Adults 50 years and older are advised to include foods fortified with vitamin B12 or take vitamin B12 dietary supplements due to the recognition that older adults may not have optimal vitamin B12 absorption.

2. Estimated calorie needs per day are broken down by age, gender, and physical activity level and are based on estimated energy requirements (EER) equations. The graded levels of physical activity are sedentary, moderately active, and active. Moderately active males over the age of 75 have an estimated requirement of 2,200 calories per day, and a moderately active female over the age of 75 requires 1,800 calories per day. Physical activity is the counterweight to calorie intake. The US Department of Health and Human Sciences published a set of physical activity recommendations entitled *2008 Physical Activity Guidelines for Americans*.[85] Those 65 and older should still follow the adult guidelines; however, it is recognized that not all older adults can meet those recommendations. In that case, they should be as physically active as their abilities and conditions allow. It is important to focus on balance exercises to decrease the risk of falls.

We must help older adults to understand how their chronic medical conditions may affect their ability to do regular physical activity safely.

Micronutrients

Older adults may have micronutrient deficiency in addition to macronutrient deficiency. Micronutrients include vitamins, minerals, and trace elements. The requirement for micronutrients does not diminish with age; thus, with the encroachment of malnutrition, the elderly can become deficient, particularly in vitamin D, calcium, folic acid, and vitamin B12.[86] After menopause, a woman's need for iron diminishes to the level that is required by men. Antioxidants such as beta-carotene, alpha-tocopherol, and ascorbic acid are important parts of the body's response to oxidative stress against free radicals. Trace elements, such as zinc, selenium, and iron as well as vitamins A, C, and E exhibit antioxidant properties in the process of cell replication and protect the immune cells from oxygen free radicals. The latter is important to support an immune system that is recognized to weaken with advancing age due to declining production of antibodies by B cells and lower cytokine production by T cells.[86]

Vitamin B12

There is a 10%–20% prevalence of vitamin B12 deficiency in older adults as shown by low or low normal serum cobalamin levels and elevations in serum methylmalonic acid and homocysteine.[87] It is important to recognize that although someone's cobalamin level may be in the low normal range, they may be deficient and manifest neurologic, psychological, and/or hematologic abnormalities. Traditionally, a deficiency of intrinsic factor was thought to account for vitamin B12 deficiency; however, more is now understood about the pathophysiology. About 15% of older adults absorb protein-bound vitamin B12 poorly, as a result of gastric achlorhydria or atrophic gastritis. This process of chronic inflammation of the stomach mucosa results in decreased secretion of intrinsic factor and a concomitant lowered absorption of the food-protein-B12 complex.[88] In addition, the prevalent and prolonged use of potent acid blockers for reflux or prophylaxis of gastroesophogeal bleeding has been associated with B12 deficiency, and such individuals should be considered at higher risk of deficiency. There may be some association with *H. pylori* infection. Given the high prevalence of vitamin B12 deficiency and the safety of its treatment, there are some proponents of routine vitamin B12 screening in those over age 65. This is not yet incorporated into any screening guideline. Rather, older adults should take supplements containing vitamin B12 or eat fortified food products. Of course, those with malabsorption-related vitamin B12 deficiency need a higher vitamin B12 dose of 1,000 mcg daily to optimize the serum vitamin B12 level and correct any hematological abnormality.

Vitamin D and calcium

With advancing age, there is age-related decrease of vitamin D and calcium receptor expression in the duodenum in women. This, combined with impaired skin synthesis of previtamin D and decreased hydroxylation in the kidneys, can result in vitamin D deficiency in many older adults.[89] Nutritional intake of vitamin D is also often low in older adults. The consequences of low vitamin D status in the older adult are significant: muscle weakness, low mood, increased risk of falls with resultant fractures, and an overall decrease in functional status.[90] Low vitamin D status has been linked to other chronic comorbidities such as hypertension, diabetes, dyslipidemia, and peripheral vascular disease.[91] Interestingly, in individuals who had severe vitamin D deficiency but did not have cardiovascular risk factors, the risk of developing diabetes, hypertension, and dyslipidemia was increased. Universal screening for vitamin D is not part of any guideline. Rather, it is important to recognize those who may be at greater risk for being vitamin D deficient (less than 20 nmol/L or 8 ng/ml) or insufficient (less than 75 nmol/L or 30 ng/ml): institutionalized older adults and people who are housebound, have limited sun exposure, have dark skin, osteoporosis, liver or renal impairment, chronic use of drugs which impair vitamin D status (e.g., anticonvulsants, prednisone, or methotrexate), or malabsorption.

The Institute of Medicine released a report in 2010 on dietary intake of vitamin D. For those over age 70, the RDA is 800 international units daily. At baseline, increased dietary consumption of vitamin D from foods such as salmon, mackerel, snapper, egg yolk, milk, and fortified soy milk should be encouraged. It is recognized that older adults may not spend enough time outdoors and that skin synthesis is reduced, so supplementing with vitamin D 600 to 800 international units daily is suggested.

With advancing age, calcium absorption diminishes, such that individuals who are 80 years old only absorb about two-thirds of the calcium compared to a younger adult. Calcium supplementation has become controversial due to its possible risk of increasing cardiovascular disease. Two meta-analyses assessing calcium or calcium with or without vitamin D brought forth concern about an increased risk of myocardial infarction in those patients assigned to calcium versus placebo.[92, 93] The criticism of the trials in these meta-analyses was that they were not designed to assess cardiovascular outcomes a priori. Yet other meta-analyses have not shown an increase in cardiovascular events with calcium. Prospective studies have subsequently been done, and, interestingly, when comparing dietary calcium to calcium supplements, dietary calcium intake was associated with no relationship or even reduction in heart disease, myocardial infarction risk, and death. Thus, when possible, dietary sources of calcium form the basis of most recommendations.

Nutrition screening tools

Recognizing undernutrition can be a challenge as there is no gold standard for diagnosis. One must also consider the setting of the patient, as not all tools are validated in a general geriatric population. Consideration must be given to whether the patient is community dwelling or is in residential care or acute hospital care. Commonly used nutrition screening tools include the Mini-Nutritional Assessment (MNA), the Malnutrition Universal Screening Tool (MUST), and the Subjective Global Assessment. A more detailed assessment follows the use of a screening tool and can include anthropometric measurements, quantifying weight loss, food intake, and medication history, as well as laboratory investigations comprising serum albumin, lymphocyte count, and total cholesterol.

The two screening tools that exhibit greater than 80% sensitivity and specificity are the Mini-Nutritional Assessment Short Form (MNA-SF) and Malnutrition Screening Tool (MST). The MUST is also frequently used and is quick to administer.

MNA-SF

The MNA-SF uses six questions from the MNA covering the following areas: survey of food intake in the past three months, weight loss in the past three

91

months, mobility, psychological stress or acute medical illness in the past three months, neuropsychological problems, and BMI (calf circumference can be substituted if BMI not available). A score of 12–14 reflects normal nutritional status, whereas a score of 8–11 suggests a person is at risk of malnutrition, and a score of less than 7 is concerning for malnutrition. This tool can be used in the acute care setting as well as in residential care and in the community. The MNA-SF demonstrates good sensitivity when compared to the full 12-item MNA, and offers the advantage of being a rapid screening tool for nutritional assessment.[94]

MST

The MST has been validated for use in acute care, ambulatory care settings, and residential care.[95] It consists of two questions related to recent unintentional weight loss, quantifying the weight loss and screening for poor eating because of a decreased appetite.

MUST

The MUST was developed in England in 2003 and is used worldwide. It is comprised of five steps including gathering nutritional assessment (weight, height, BMI), checking for recent unplanned weight loss, establishing recent acute illness of more than five days during which there has been no nutritional intake, determining the overall risk score of malnutrition (based on adding the scores from the first three steps) yielding a score of 0 (low risk) to 2 (high risk), and finally, implementing management guidelines for patients. The MUST takes less than five minutes to complete.

Weight Loss and BMI

Body weight generally increases through adulthood until the sixth to seventh decade of life, at which point it begins to decline. Cross-sectional studies have shown that the finding of a decline in body weight is at least partially due to the premature death of obese individuals. Both intentional and unintentional weight loss is associated with adverse outcomes. Between 20 and 80 years of age, muscle mass decreases by about 30%. After age 50, approximately 1%–2% of muscle mass is lost each year thereafter. Muscle remodeling ensues, consisting of intramuscular fat accumulation, muscle atrophy (type IIA fibers), decreased

satellite cell proliferation, and a decrease in the number of motor units.[76] Any illness that results in bedrest or immoblization for a period of 10 days results in a loss of 1 kg of muscle mass.[96]

There is uncertainty as to the optimal body mass index for an elderly person. Based on World Health Organization guidelines, suggested BMI to maintain good health is 18.5–24.9 kg/m2. Interestingly, a meta-analysis by Flegal showed that being overweight (BMI 25–<30) was, in fact, significantly associated with lower all-cause mortality.[97] Mortality risk in the low BMI group is increased and, as a result, mortality rates in the higher BMI groups may be falsely low.[98] This was not exclusive to the elderly. The "obesity paradox," which describes the improved survival associated with obesity, is seen in patient populations (advanced malignancies, CHF, ESRD) that have protein-calorie malnutrition, whereby those who started off with a higher BMI may have some protection conferred to them in the form of nutritional reserve. Alternatively, it has been argued that the low mortality rates in the higher BMI groups are artificially low given that the mortality risk in the low BMI group is increased due to prevalence of chronic disease. Another consideration among the elderly is that BMI may not be as valid a measure as in the younger population because of the disproportionate loss of muscle mass associated with aging. BMI is now sometimes used as a prognosticator for various disease states. In a study assessing optimal treatment strategies for STEMI, BMI (along with serum troponin level) was found to be predictive of failure to discharge home.[99]

Nutritional supplements and other interventions

Nutritional supplements are often invoked when an elderly person screens positive for malnutrition; however, there is limited evidence supporting the effectiveness of nutritional supplements. A Cochrane Database systematic review in 2009 comprising 62 trials and 10,187 participants examined whether oral protein and energy supplementation showed a benefit in terms of weight gain, mortality, risk of complications, and any change in functional status in older people.[100] Results showed that supplementation produced a 2.2% weight change and a signal toward a mortality benefit in undernourished individuals – overall limited gains.

The concept of tailoring food offered based on the cause of anorexia is emerging.[71] For the individual with early satiety, one could offer a more nutrient-dense meal; alternatively for someone with diminished taste and/or smell, flavor-enriched foods would be preferred, and in those with an increased inflammatory state, a diet higher in polyunsaturated fats may prove beneficial. These specific, tailored interventions are more likely to be effective once routine screening for malnutrition is in place and there is a better understanding of the particular cause of a specific individual's malnutrition.

References

1. US Dept of Health and Human Services. *Physical activity and health: A report of the surgeon general.* Atlanta: US Dept of Health and Human Services, Centers for Disease Control and Prevention, National Center for Chronic Disease Prevention and Health Promotion; 1996.

2. Physical Activity Guidelines Advisory Committee report, 2008. To the Secretary of Health and Human Services. Part A: executive summary. *Nutrition reviews* 2009;**67**:114–20.

3. Sui X, LaMonte MJ, Laditka JN, et al. Cardiorespiratory fitness and adiposity as mortality predictors in older adults. *JAMA* 2007;**298**:2507–16.

4. Pahor M, Guralnik JM, Ambrosius WT, et al. Effect of structured physical activity on prevention of major mobility disability in older adults: the LIFE study randomized clinical trial. *JAMA* 2014;**311**:2387–96.

5. Nelson ME, Rejeski WJ, Blair SN, et al. Physical activity and public health in older adults: recommendation from the American College of Sports Medicine and the American Heart Association. *Med Sci Sports Exerc* 2007;**39**:1435–45.

6. Chodzko-Zajko W, Proctor D, Fiatarone Singh M, et al. American College of Sports Medicine position stand. Exercise and physical activity for older adults. *Med Sci Sports Exerc* 2009;**41**(7):1510–30.

7. Morley JE, Anker SD, von Haehling S. Prevalence, incidence, and clinical impact of sarcopenia: facts, numbers, and epidemiology-update 2014. *Journal of Cachexia, Sarcopenia and Muscle* 2014;**5**:253–9.

8. Fiatarone MA, Marks EC, Ryan ND, Meredith CN, Lipsitz LA, Evans WJ. High-intensity strength training in nonagenarians: Effects on skeletal muscle. *JAMA* 1990;**263**(22):3029–34.

9. Haskell WL, Lee IM, Pate RR, et al. Physical activity and public health: updated recommendation for adults from the American College of Sports Medicine and the American Heart Association. *Med Sci Sports Exerc* 2007;**39**:1423–34.

10. Mavros Y, Kay S, Anderberg KA, et al. Changes in insulin resistance and HbA1 c are related to exercise-mediated changes in body composition in older adults with type 2 diabetes: interim outcomes from the GREAT2DO trial. *Diabetes Care* 2013;**36**:2372–9.

11. Schoenborn CA, Stommel M. Adherence to the 2008 adult physical activity guidelines and mortality risk. *American Journal of Preventive Medicine* 2011;**40**: 514–21.

12. Azevedo MR, Araujo CL, Reichert FF, Siqueira FV, da Silva MC, Hallal PC. Gender differences in leisure-time physical activity. *Int J Public Health* 2007;**52**:8–15.

13. Fiatarone MA, O'Neill EF, Ryan ND, et al. Exercise training and nutritional supplementation for physical frailty in very elderly people. *N Engl J Med* 1994;**330** (25):1769–75.

14. Morris J, Fiatarone M, Kiely D, et al. Nursing rehabilitation and exercise strategies in the nursing home. *Journals of Gerontology Series A – Biological Sciences and Medical Sciences* 1999;**54**:M494–500.

15. Williams MA, Haskell WL, Ades PA, et al. Resistance exercise in individuals with and without cardiovascular disease: 2007 update: a scientific statement from the American Heart Association Council on Clinical Cardiology and Council on Nutrition, Physical Activity, and Metabolism. *Circulation* 2007;**116**:572–84.

16. Fiatarone Singh M. Exercise comes of age: Rationale and recommendations for a geriatric exercise prescription *Journal of Gerontology, Medical Sciences* 2002;**57**:M262–82.

17. Bortz WM. Redefining human aging. *J Am Geriatr Soc* 1989;**37**:1092–6.

18. Ainsworth B, Cahalin L, Buman M, Ross R. The current state of physical activity assessment tools. *Progress in Cardiovascular Diseases* 2015;**57**:387–95.

19. Blair SN, Kampert JB, Kohn HW, et al. Influences of Cardiovascular Fitness and Other Precursors on Cardiovascular Disease and All-Cause Mortality in Men and Women. *JAMA* 1996;**276**:205–10.

20. Mavros Y, Kay S, Simpson KA, et al. Reductions in C-reactive protein in older adults with type 2 diabetes are related to improvements in body composition following a randomized controlled trial of resistance training. *Journal of Cachexia, Sarcopenia and Muscle* 2014;**5**:111–20.

21. Guyatt G, Thompson P, Berman L, et al. How should we measure function in patients with chronic heart and lung disease? *J Chronic Dis* 1985;**38**:517–28.

22. Boxer RS, Wang Z, Walsh SJ, Hager D, Kenny AM. The utility of the 6-minute walk test as a measure of frailty in older adults with heart failure. *Am J Geriatr Cardiol* 2008;**17**:7–12.

23. Borg G, Linderholm H. Perceived exertion and pulse rate during graded exercise in various age group. *Acta Med Scand* 1970;**472**(Supp l):194–206.

24. Yorke AM, Curtis AB, Shoemaker M, Vangsnes E. Grip strength values stratified by age, gender, and chronic disease status in adults aged 50 years and older. *Journal of Geriatric Physical Therapy* 2015;**38**(3):115–21.

25. Legrand D, Vaes B, Mathei C, Adriaensen W, Van Pottelbergh G, Degryse JM. Muscle strength and physical performance as predictors of mortality, hospitalization, and disability in the oldest old. *J Am Geriatr Soc* 2014;**62**:1030–8.

26. Reid KF, Fielding RA. Skeletal muscle power: a critical determinant of physical functioning in older adults. *Exercise and Sport Sciences Reviews* 2012;**40**:4–12.

27. Baker MK, Atlantis E, Fiatarone Singh MA. Multi-modal exercise programs for older adults. *Age Ageing* 2007;**36**:375–81.

28. Singh NA, Stavrinos TM, Scarbek Y, Galambos G, Liber C, Fiatarone Singh MA. A randomized controlled trial of high versus low intensity weight training versus general practitioner care for clinical depression in older adults. *J Gerontol A Biol Sci Med Sci* 2005;**60**:768–76.

29. Marques EA, Mota J, Carvalho J. Exercise effects on bone mineral density in older adults: a meta-analysis of randomized controlled trials. *Age* 2012;**34**:1493–515.

30. Suominen H. Muscle training for bone strength. *Aging Clin Exp Res* 2006;**18**:85–93.

31. Zhao R, Zhao M, Zhang L. Efficiency of jumping exercise in improving bone mineral density among premenopausal women: a meta-analysis. *Sports Medicine* 2014;**44**:1393–402.

32. Martyn-St James M, Carroll S. A meta-analysis of impact exercise on postmenopausal bone loss: the case for mixed loading exercise programmes. *British Journal of Sports Medicine* 2009;**43**:898–908.

33. Pojednic RM, Clark DJ, Patten C, Reid K, Phillips EM, Fielding RA. The specific contributions of force and velocity to muscle power in older adults. *Experimental Gerontology* 2012;**47**:608–13.

34. Borg G, Linderholme H. Exercise performance and perceived exertion in patients with coronary insufficiency, arterial hypertension and vasoregulatory asthenia. *Acta Med Scand* 1970;**187**:17–26.

35. Aamot IL, Karlsen T, Dalen H, Stoylen A. Long-term exercise adherence after high-intensity interval training in cardiac rehabilitation: a randomized study. *Physiotherapy Research International: the Journal for Researchers and Clinicians in Physical Therapy* 2015 Feb 16. DOI: 10.1002/pri.1619. [Epub ahead of print.]

36. Weston KS, Wisloff U, Coombes JS. High-intensity interval training in patients with lifestyle-induced cardiometabolic disease: a systematic review and meta-analysis. *British Journal of Sports Medicine* 2014;**48**:1227–34.

37. Church TS, Earnest CP, Skinner JS, Blair SN. Effects of different doses of physical activity on cardiorespiratory fitness among sedentary, overweight or obese postmenopausal women with elevated blood pressure: a randomized controlled trial. *JAMA* 2007;**297**: 2081–91.

38. Pedersen BK, Saltin B. Evidence for prescribing exercise as therapy in chronic disease. *Scandinavian Journal of Medicine & Science in Sports* 2006;**16**:3–63.

39. Jakicic JM, Clark K, Coleman E, et al. American College of Sports Medicine position stand: appropriate intervention strategies for weight loss and prevention of weight regain for adults. *Med Sci Sports Exerc* 2001;**33**:2145–56.

40. Paterson DH, Jones GR, Rice CL. Ageing and physical activity: evidence to develop exercise recommendations for older adults. *Can J Public Health* 2007;**98**(Suppl 2):S69–108.

41. Nelson ME, Rejeski WJ, Blair SN, et al. Physical activity and public health in older adults: recommendation from the American College of Sports Medicine and the American Heart Association. *Circulation* 2007;**116**: 1094–105.

42. O'Keefe JH, Bell DS. Postprandial hyperglycemia/ hyperlipidemia (postprandial dysmetabolism) is a cardiovascular risk factor. *Am J Cardiol* 2007;**100**:899–904.

43. Rizvi AA. Management of diabetes in older adults. *Am J Med Sci* 2007;**333**:35–47.

44. Parmenter B, Raymond J, Dinnen P, Fiatarone Singh M. A systematic review of randomized controlled trials: walking versus alternative exercise prescription as treatment for intermittent claudication. *Atherosclerosis* 2011;**218**:1–12.

45. Norgren L, Hiatt WR, Dormandy JA, et al. Inter-society consensus for the management of peripheral arterial disease (TASC II). *Journal of Vascular Surgery* 2007;**45** (Suppl S):S5–67.

46. Parmenter BJ, Dieberg G, Smart NA. Exercise training for management of peripheral arterial disease: a systematic review and meta-analysis. *Sports Medicine* 2015;**45**:231–44.

47. Lagally KM, Amorose AJ. The validity of using prior ratings of perceive exertion to regulate resistance exercise intensity. *Percept Mot Skills* 2007;**104**:534–42.

48. Seynnes O, Fiatarone Singh M. Relationship between resistance training intensity and physiological and functional adaptation in frail elders. *J Gerontol (Biol Sci Med Sci)* 2004;**59**(A):3–9.

49. Reid KF, Doros G, Clark DJ, et al. Muscle power failure in mobility-limited older adults: preserved single fiber function despite lower whole muscle size, quality and

rate of neuromuscular activation. *European Journal of Applied Physiology* 2012;**112**:2289–301.

50. Taaffe DR. Sarcopenia – exercise as a treatment strategy. *Aust Fam Physician* 2006;**35**:130–4.

51. Umpierre D, Ribeiro PA, Kramer CK, et al. Physical activity advice only or structured exercise training and association with HbA1c levels in type 2 diabetes: a systematic review and meta-analysis. *JAMA* 2011;**305**:1790–9.

52. Tanasescu M, Leitzmann MF, Rimm EB, Willett WC, Stampfer MJ, Hu FB. Exercise type and intensity in relation to coronary heart disease in men. *JAMA* 2002;**288**:1994–2000.

53. Conn VS, Hafdahl AR, Minor MA, Nielsen PJ. Physical activity interventions among adults with arthritis: meta-analysis of outcomes. *Semin Arthritis Rheum* 2007;**0**(0):307–16.

54. Gordon N, Kohl H, Pollock M, Vaandrager H, Gibbons S, Blair S. Cardiovascular safety of maximal strength testing in healthy adults. *Am J Cardiol* 1995;**76**:851–3.

55. Cadore EL, Rodriguez-Manas L, Sinclair A, Izquierdo M. Effects of different exercise interventions on risk of falls, gait ability, and balance in physically frail older adults: a systematic review. *Rejuvenation research* 2013;**16**:105–14.

56. Sherrington C, Tiedemann A, Fairhall N, Close JC, Lord SR. Exercise to prevent falls in older adults: an updated meta-analysis and best practice recommendations. *New South Wales Public Health Bulletin* 2011;**22**:78–83.

57. Oliver D, Connelly JB, Victor CR, et al. Strategies to prevent falls and fractures in hospitals and care homes and effect of cognitive impairment: systematic review and meta-analyses. *BMJ* 2007;**334**:82.

58. Rubenstein LZ. Falls in older people: epidemiology, risk factors and strategies for prevention. *Age Ageing* 2006;**35**(Suppl 2):ii37–41.

59. Tsang WW, Hui-Chan CW. Comparison of muscle torque, balance, and confidence in older tai chi and healthy adults. *Med Sci Sports Exerc* 2005;**37**:280–9.

60. Orr R, Raymond J, Fiatarone Singh M. Efficacy of progressive resistance training on balance performance in older adults: a systematic review of randomized controlled trials. *Sports Med* 2008;**38**:1–51.

61. Clemson L, Fiatarone Singh MA, Bundy A, et al. Integration of balance and strength training into daily life activity to reduce rate of falls in older people (the LiFE study): randomised parallel trial. *BMJ* 2012;**345**: e4547.

62. Sherrington C, Tiedemann A, Fairhall N, Close JC, Lord SR. Exercise to prevent falls in older adults: an updated meta-analysis and best practice

recommendations. *New South Wales Public Health Bulletin* 2011;**22**:78–83.

63. Chan WC, Fai Yeung JW, Man Wong CS, et al. Efficacy of physical exercise in preventing falls in older adults with cognitive impairment: a systematic review and meta-analysis. *Journal of the American Medical Directors Association* 2015;**16**:149–54.

64. Silva RB, Eslick GD, Duque G. Exercise for falls and fracture prevention in long term care facilities: a systematic review and meta-analysis. *Journal of the American Medical Directors Association* 2013;**14**: 685–9 e2.

65. Thorp AA, Owen N, Neuhaus M, Dunstan DW. Sedentary behaviors and subsequent health outcomes in adults a systematic review of longitudinal studies, 1996–2011. *American Journal of Preventive Medicine* 2011;**41**:207–15.

66. Visvanathan R, Chapman I. Undernutrition and anorexia in the older person. *Gastroenterol Clin N Am* 2009;**38**:393–409.

67. Kaiser MJ, Bauer JM, Ramsch C, et al. Frequency of malnutrition perspective using the Mini Nutritional Assessment. *J Am Geriatr Soc* 2010;**58**:1734–8.

68. Nordin S, Bamerson A, Bringlov E, et al. Substance and tongue-specific loss in specific taste quality identification in elderly adults. *Eur Arch Otorhinolaryngol* 2007;**264**:285–89.

69. Di Francesco V, Barazzoni R, Bissoli L, et al. The quantity of meal fat influences the profile of postprandial hormones as well as hunger sensation in healthy elderly people. *J Am Med Dir Assoc* 2010;**11**: 188–93.

70. Walls AW, Steele JG. The relationship between oral health and nutrition in older people. *Mech Ageing Dev* 2004;**125**(12):853–7.

71. Donini LM, Poggiogalle E, Piredda M, et al. Anorexia and eating patterns in the elderly. *PLoS One* 2013;**8**: e63539.

72. Evans WJ, Morley JE, Argiles J, et al. Cachexia: a new definition. *Clin Nutr* 2008; **27**:793.

73. Von Haehling S, Anker SD. Cachexia as a major underestimated and unmet medical need: facts and numbers. *J Cachex Sarcopenia Muscle* 2010;**1**(1):1–5.

74. Krasnow SM, Marks DL. Neuropeptides in the pathophysiology and treatment of cachexia. *Curr Opin Support Palliat Care* 2010;**4**(4):266–71.

75. Tisdale MJ. Cancer cachexia. *Curr Opin Gastroenterol* 2010;**26**(2):146–51.

76. Muscaritoli M, Lucia S, Molfino A, et al. Muscle atrophy in aging and chronic diseases: is it sarcopenia or cachexia? *Internal and Emergency Medicine* 2013;**8**: 553–60.

77. Morely JE, Abbatecola AM, Argiles JM, et al. Sarcopenia with limited mobility: an international consensus. *J Am Med Dir Assoc* 2011;**12**(6):403–9.

78. Evans WJ. Skeletal muscle loss: cachexia, sarcopenia, and inactivity. *Am J Clin Nutr* 2010;**91**: 1123S–1127S.

79. Goodpaster BH, Park SW, Harris TB, et al. The loss of skeletal muscle strength, mass, and quality in older adults: the health, aging and body composition study. *J Gerontol A Biol Med Sci* 2006;**61**:1059–64.

80. Muller MJ, Geisler C, Pourhassan M, et al. Assessment and definition of lean body mass deficiency in the elderly. *European Journal of Clinical Nutrition* 2014;**68**: 1220–27; doi: 10.1038/ejcn.2014.169 published online August 2014.

81. Santilli V, Bernetti A, Mangone M, et al. Clinical definition of sarcopenia. *Clin Cases Miner Bone Metab* 2014; **11**(3): 177–80.

82. US Department of Agriculture. Dietary guidelines for Americans 2010: executive summary. Available at: www.cnpp.usda.gov/sites/default/files/dietary_guidelines_for_americans/ExecSumm.pdf (accessed February 23, 2015).

83. Institute of Medicine. Dietary reference intakes tables and application. Available at: www.iom.edu/Activities/Nutrition/SummaryDRIs/DRI-Tables.aspx (accessed February 25, 2015).

84. Health Canada. The DRI values: definitions. Available at: www.hc-sc.gc.ca/fn-an/nutrition/reference/dri_ques-ques_anref-eng.php#a5a (accessed February 25, 2015).

85. 2008 physical activity guidelines for Americans. Available at: www.cdc.gov/physicalactivity/downloads/pa_fact_sheet_adults.pdf (accessed February 20, 2015).

86. Elmafa I, Meyer AL. Body composition, changing physiological functions and nutrient requirements of the elderly. *Ann Nutr Metab* 2008;**52**(1):2–5.

87. Pennypacker LC, Allen RH, Kelly JP, et al. High prevalence of cobalamin deficiency in elderly outpatients. *J Am Geriatr Soc* 1992;**40**(12):1997–204.

88. Van Asselt DZ, de Groot LC, van Staveren WA, et al. Role of cobalamin intake and atrophic gastritis in mild cobalamin deficiency in older Dutch subjects. *Am J Clin Nutr.* 1998;**68**:328–334.

89. Walters JR, Balesaria S, Chavele KM, et al. Calcium channel TRPV6 expression in human duodenum: different relationships to the vitamin D system and aging in men and women. *J Bone Miner Res* 2006;**21**: 1770–7.

90. Bischoff-Ferrari HA, Dawson-Hughes B, Willett WC, et al. Effect of Vitamin D on falls: a meta-analysis. *JAMA* 2004;**291**(16):1999–2006.

91. Anderson JL, May HT, Horne BD, et al. Relation of vitamin D deficiency to cardiovascular risk factors, disease status, and incident events in a general healthcare population. *Am J Cardiol* 2010;**106**(7): 963–8.

92. Bolland MJ, Avenell A, Baron JA, et al. Effect of calcium supplements on risk of myocardial infarction and cardiovascular events: meta-analysis. *BMJ* 2010;**341**:c3691.

93. Bolland MJ, Grey A, Avenell A, et al. Calcium supplements with or without vitamin D and risk of cardiovascular events: reanalysis of the Women's Health Initiative limited access dataset and meta-analysis. *BMJ* 2011;**342**:d2040.

94. Kaiser M, Bauer J, Ramsch C, et al. Validation of the nutritional assessment short-form (MNA-SF): a practical tool for identification of nutritional status. *J Nutr Health Aging* 2009;**13**(9):782–8.

95. Isenring EA, Bauer JD, Banks MD, et al. The malnutrition screening tool is a useful tool for identifying malnutrition risk in residential aged care. *Journal of Human Nutrition and Dietetics* 2009;**22**(6): 545–50.

96. Kortebein P, Ferrando A, Lombeida J, et al. Effect of 10 days bedrest on skeletal muscle in healthy older adults. *JAMA* 2007;**297**:1772–4.

97. Flegal KM, Kit BK, Orpana H, et al. Association of all-cause mortality with overweight and obesity using standard body mass index categories: a systematic review and meta-analysis. *JAMA* 2013;**309**(1):71–82.

98. Fontana L, Hu F. Optimal body weight for health and longevity: bridging basic, clinical, and population research. *Aging Cell* 2014;**13**(3):391–400.

99. Sujino Y, Tanno J, Nakano S, et al. Impact of hypoalbuminemia, frailty, and body mass index on early prognosis in older patients (>/= 85 years) with ST-elevation myocardial infarction. *Journal of Cardiology* 2014; http://dx.doi.org/10.1016/j.jjcc.2014.12.001.

100. Milne AC, Potter J, Vivanti A, et al. Protein and energy supplementation in elderly people at risk from malnutrition. *Cochrane Database Syst Rev* 2009 Apr 15;(2):CD003288.

Frailty

Mindy J. Fain, MD, and M. Jane Mohler, NP-C, MPH, PhD

Introduction

Many older adults appear frail, and a common impression is that the thin, stooped, and slow-moving elder represents normal aging. Decades of research, however, have illuminated the differences between normal aging and frailty, and frailty is now recognized as an important geriatric syndrome characterized by diminished physiologic reserves and function and a decreased capacity to withstand stressors.[1, 2] More than a third of people older than 85 are estimated to be frail,[1, 3] and frail adults are at higher risk of adverse health outcomes, including dependency, institutionalization, and death.[4] The recognition of frailty, especially in its early stages, may help to prevent or mitigate many of the potentially adverse clinical outcomes. However, the lack of consensus regarding the definition of frailty creates challenges in advancing clinical care and research. This chapter will provide an overview of the frailty syndrome.

> Frailty is an important geriatric syndrome that is associated with high morbidity and mortality.

Definition

Frailty is a clinical state of age-related vulnerability to stressors due to multiple organ system declines in physiologic reserve and function.[2] These cumulative and accelerated declines in reserves can trigger disproportionate changes in health status resulting from even minor stressful events, and place the individual at risk for increased dependency and/or accelerated trajectory leading to death. Frailty is characterized by diminished strength and endurance, and impaired physiologic function in many interrelated organ systems (including the musculoskeletal, neuroendocrine, and immune systems) and includes nutritional, cognitive, and psychosocial dimensions. Although advanced age, multimorbidity, and disability are associated with frailty, there is strong evidence that frailty is a distinct entity.[1] It is a dynamic condition along a clinical spectrum that can improve or worsen over time.

> Frailty is a clinical state of age-related vulnerability to stressors due to multi-organ system declines in physiologic reserve and function.

The two main frailty constructs are (1) a biological syndrome model and (2) an accumulation of deficits model; both are associated with the same adverse outcomes.[5] However, there is no consensus for a single operational definition of frailty,[6] and the numerous scales include combinations of nutritional status, physical activity, mobility, energy, strength, cognition, mood, and social relations and support. Most operational definitions fall into two approaches.

The phenotype model

The phenotype model, described by Fried and colleagues, conceptualizes frailty as a clinical syndrome with strong biological underpinnings.[1] Based upon a secondary analysis of data from the Cardiovascular Health Study (CHS), the frailty syndrome consists of at least three of the following five criteria: weight loss, exhaustion, weakness, slowness, and reduced physical activity. This definition was validated in a community-dwelling population from the Women's Health and Aging Studies.[7] It is the most commonly used model in research, and it correlates with increased risk of adverse outcomes in a variety of settings. It is

Reichel's Care of the Elderly, *7th Edition*, ed. Jan Busby-Whitehead *et al.* Published by Cambridge University Press.
© Cambridge University Press 2016.

challenging for clinicians to use this model routinely because the components are not typically evaluated in geriatric assessments,[8] and the measurement of gait speed requires mobility.

The deficit model

The deficit model, described by Rockwood and colleagues, is based on risk accumulation.[5] It considers symptoms, diseases, geriatric syndromes, physical and cognitive impairments, psychosocial risk factors, and disabilities; the sum generates a frailty index. The greater the number of deficits, the higher the frailty index score. The deficit index is a more sensitive predictor of adverse health outcomes than the phenotype model because of its wider range of possible scores and its closer connection to real world clinical conditions, including disability itself. It does not require gait speed and can be assessed using administrative data. However, it is not easily used in clinical settings due to its complexity and the difficulty in accessing all necessary data.

Screening tools

There are numerous frailty scales in use based upon the phenotype and deficit models, with substantial differences in their content validity, feasibility in clinical settings, and predictive ability. The intention of the screening is a key consideration when choosing a tool. There is an inherent tradeoff between achieving the most accurate risk prediction versus selecting a tool that allows for the best timing and targeting of an intervention.[9, 2]

The phenotype of frailty scale is shown in Table 7.1.[10] Other scales include the Rockwood Frailty Index and the Study of Osteoporotic Fractures. The FRAIL scale (using questions on fatigue, resistance, aerobic, illness, and loss of weight) utilizes findings from the African-American Health cohort and incorporates functional, deficit, and biological models in an interview-based tool.[11, 12]

Epidemiology

Frailty is a recognized risk factor for older adults. According to the CHS, the overall prevalence of frailty in the United States in community-dwelling older adults aged 65 or older ranges from 7% to 12%. Similar findings are reported for older adults in Europe and Latin America. In 2013, a systematic literature review examined the association of frailty with survival in community-dwelling older adults.[13] For studies using the phenotype model, the pooled prevalence in older adults aged 65 and older was 14%, and studies using the deficit model demonstrated a pooled prevalence of 24%. Although the prevalence of frailty in long-term care settings has not been examined in depth, it is higher than in community dwellers, carrying much higher mortality rates.

Prevalence by age, race/ethnicity, and gender

The prevalence of frailty increases with age and stratifies within subgroups. Using the phenotype definition, the prevalence of frailty for 65- to 70-year-olds ranges from 3% to 6%, and increases to 5% to 15% using the deficit definition. For those over age 80, the prevalence of frailty is more than 16% for either definition used. For the phenotype definition, prevalence

Table 7.1

Cardiovascular Health Study (CHS) Index – Fried criteria [1]
Frail = 3 of the following findings present
Pre-frail = 1 or 2 of the following findings present
Weight loss (≥5% of body weight in last year)
Exhaustion (positive response to questions regarding effort required for activity)
Weakness (decreased grip strength)
Slow walking speed (>6–7 sec to walk 15 ft)
Decreased physical activity. Males expending <383 kcals/week and females <270 kcal/week in physical activity. (For reference: walking 4 mi in 1 hr = 300 kcal)

increased from 16% for those aged 80 to 85, to 26% in those aged 85 and over. Using the deficit accumulation model, more than half of the people over the age of 85 are frail.[13] The different operational definitions of frailty may identify different groups of older adults.

The prevalence of frailty differs among ethnic/racial groups, and it is important to employ ethnically sensitive measures. African Americans have a high prevalence of frailty. According to two studies, and using both accumulation and phenotype definitions, more than half of older African Americans were frail. [14, 15] The prevalence of frailty in Hispanic older adults ranged from 8% to 20%, depending upon the scale used.[16] Among Caucasians, the prevalence of frailty ranged from 6% to 12% using the phenotype definition, and from 15% to 40% using the deficit accumulation criteria.[13]

Frailty appears to be higher among women than among men. In older women, the prevalence of frailty defined by phenotype is 13%, and defined by deficit accumulation it is 26%. For older men, the prevalence by phenotype is 7%, rising to 24% utilizing the deficit definition. Among African-American women over the age of 85, the prevalence of frailty is highest, at 60%.[1, 13]

Association with survival

Frailty is associated with poor survival in both men and women.[13] When comparing frail with non-frail older adults, the relative increase in mortality risk averages 50% when using the phenotype definition and 15% when using the deficit definition. In a study of the course of disability in the last year of life, frailty was the most common condition leading to death.[17]

Association with comorbidities and disability

Comorbidity is defined by having two or more chronic conditions. Disability refers to chronic limitations or dependence in activities of daily living, instrumental activities of daily living, and/or mobility. The phenotype model distinguishes frailty from disability and comorbidity, and considers disability to be a frailty outcome. The deficit construct includes measures of disability and comorbidity in the model.

Frailty is associated with multiple comorbidities, including an increased rate of cognitive decline.[18]

Frail patients who are also cognitively impaired suffer from an increased likelihood of adverse health outcomes. Frailty is related to cardiovascular disease, with a 25% to 50% prevalence rate, and frail patients undergoing cardiovascular interventions have worse outcomes than non-frail patients.[19]

The recognition of sarcopenic obesity is important because of the increasing prevalence of obesity in older adults. Approximately 20% of US adults over the age of 65 are obese, and obesity is associated with impaired physical functioning and frailty. The commonly held stereotype of a thin frail elder may soon be replaced by the obese and disabled frail older adult.[A]

Pathogenesis

The clinical manifestations of frailty are postulated to be due to an interrelated and self-perpetuating cycle of negative energy balance, generalized weakness, diminished strength, reduced exertional tolerance, and sarcopenia. The underlying molecular, cellular, physiological, and functional changes of frailty are likely impacted by genetic and environmental factors, in combination with epigenetic mechanisms (see Figure 7.1).

Natural history of frailty

The cycle concept raises the question as to whether an individual can enter at any point, or if there is an ordered pattern of development of signs and symptoms. Longitudinal studies indicate some hierarchical order despite heterogeneity in initial symptoms.[20] Different patterns may represent different causative pathways linked to specific systemic physiologic dysregulation. Elucidating the common patterns of

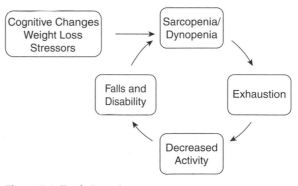

Figure 7.1 The frailty cycle.
Source: Adapted from elder care provider sheet, "Frailty – Elders at Risk," http://aging.arizona.edu/sites/default/files/frailty.pdf

clinical onset might lead to early identification and intervention.

Transitions across frailty stages (e.g., non-frail, pre-frail, frail) are of clinical and research interest. In a longitudinal study of community-living older adults,[21] more than half had at least one transition, and nearly a quarter had two transitions, although regression from frail to non-frail was extremely unlikely.

Immune system

Abnormal inflammation appears to have a major role in the development of frailty, and an accumulation of pro-inflammatory responses is one of the fundamental findings in frailty syndrome.[22] These responses are unlike typical acute inflammatory responses; rather, they are characterized by high levels of pro-inflammatory cytokines.[23] An expanding number of pro-inflammatory cytokines has been independently associated with the frailty syndrome, including interleukin 6,[24] C-reactive protein (CRP), and tumor necrosis factor-alpha (TNFα). Since inflammation is associated with catabolism of skeletal muscle and adiposity and shares several core features of frailty – such as malnutrition, anorexia, sarcopenia, weight loss, and cognitive changes – assigning inflammation a major causative role in frailty is very attractive. However, the elevation of pro-inflammatory cytokines as a root cause is not well understood. Additionally, there is an association between frailty and several clotting markers (factor VIII, fibrinogen, and D-dimer) as well as evidence that immune system activation may generate the clotting cascade. Lastly, white blood cell and monocyte counts are elevated in frail older adults living in the community, which provides further evidence for immune activation.[25]

> Abnormal inflammation appears to have a major role in the development of frailty.

Endocrine pathways

Aging is associated with changes in the hypothalamo-pituitary axis, which have an impact on metabolism and energy through several hormones. There is a decrease in growth hormone synthesis, which results in a reduction in insulin-like growth factor-1 (IGF-1). IGF-1 is involved in anabolic activity, specifically skeletal muscle strength. There are reductions in estradiol and testosterone secretion, reduction in the activity of adrenocortical cells that produce the sex steroid precursors such as adrenal dehydroepiandrosterone sulfate (DHEA-S), and a slow rise in cortisol levels. The impact of these changes in IGF-1, sex hormones, steroid precursors, and cortisol secretion, and their association with frailty are not well understood. Although levels of IGF-1 are significantly lower in frail than non-frail older women,[26] trials of IGF-1 supplementation in older adults have not shown benefit. There is mixed evidence that lower levels of reproductive hormones are linked to frailty.[27, 28] Similarly, the link between frailty and elevated cortisol concentrations that was demonstrated in one cross-sectional study is under investigation.[29, 30]

Musculoskeletal system

Sarcopenia, the progressive and generalized age-related loss of skeletal muscle mass and either low muscle strength and/or low physical performance, is an important physiologic contributor to frailty.[31, 32] It begins between the ages of 20 and 30, accelerates after age 50, and is a major cause of disability, poor quality of life, and death. Skeletal muscle mass measurements alone do not capture functionality, and thus do not define sarcopenia. The societal and economic costs of sarcopenia are significant. Direct health-care costs due to the associated physical disability were estimated to be approximately $18.5 billion in 2000 in the United States, and is expected to rise with our aging population.[B]

With aging, there is a delicate balance between muscle formation and loss coordinated by hormonal and immune systems, the brain, nutritional factors, and physical activity.[29] Usual age-related musculoskeletal changes include declines in skeletal muscle fibers, satellite cells, and neuromuscular junctions; infiltration by fibrous and adipose tissue, and an increase in apoptosis. There is evidence for alterations in mitochondrial function and the renin-angiotensin axis affecting muscle quality. The physiologic changes in frailty, including inflammatory cytokines and lower levels of growth hormone and sex steroids, and higher levels of cortisol, accelerate the decline in muscle mass and strength. With sarcopenic obesity, fatty infiltration is associated with lower muscle quality, a hyper-inflammatory state, and an accelerated loss of lean body mass, despite a high body mass index.

Clinical applications

Clinicians encounter frail individuals in a wide variety of stages and settings. Some may be able to recover after a stressful event, and others may never regain full function. An older patient may appear vigorous yet be unable to tolerate the stress of elective surgery. An individual at home may experience an apparent minor insult, such as a mild infection or a new medication, and decline rapidly, quickly transitioning from independent to dependent, from ambulatory to immobile.

The inaccurate identification of a patient as frail may limit appropriate interventions, resulting in denial of elective surgery, or may, alternatively, expose an unrecognized frail patient to unrealistic and invasive interventions that are not aligned with the patient's and/or family's goals, preferences, or values. Especially in the early stages, frailty is often overlooked. Thus a systematic approach to frailty assessment is recommended.

> Recognition of frailty is important to guide clinical care and decision making.

Clinical settings

Frailty is recognized as an important syndrome to guide clinical care and decision making. Screening is recommended by the American College of Surgeons, as frailty independently predicts postoperative complications, length of stay, and need for transition to a skilled or assisted living facility in older adults undergoing surgery.[33] A comprehensive frailty score has been shown to be more predictive for adverse postoperative outcomes in older surgical patients than traditional assessment tools.[C] For geriatric trauma patients, the Frailty Index has been shown to be an independent predictor of in-hospital complications and adverse discharge disposition, and superior to age for clinical risk stratification.[D]

Frailty risk assessment is important in caring for older patients with cardiovascular conditions; it predicts increased morbidity and mortality.[19] It can help in risk stratification for older adults with cancer. Frail patients may fail to launch an adequate immune response to the influenza and pneumococcal vaccines. [34, 35] As more conditions are studied, the expectation is that frailty will emerge as a core measure for risk assessment.

Common related signs and symptoms

Weakness is a frequent complaint among older adults and a common symptom of frailty. It is strongly associated with impaired function and disability as well as increased risk for future mobility disability. Studies into the relationships among weakness, muscle mass, muscle quality, muscle strength, and function have demonstrated that although low muscle mass is associated with weakness, low muscle mass alone is poorly or not associated with impaired function and disability. Dynopenia refers to muscle weakness, emphasizing the difference between low muscle mass and impaired performance. A recent national consensus project proposed screening based on mobility performance (e.g., gait speed), strength testing (e.g., grip strength), and adjusted body composition assessment to guide research to identify individuals who will benefit from interventions.[36] Most frail people suffer from sarcopenia.

Other syndromes, such as cachexia, are associated with prominent muscle wasting and may be confused with sarcopenia. Cachexia is a severe wasting condition accompanying disease states such as cancer or end-stage renal disease, and is characterized by loss of muscle with or without loss of fat mass. It is frequently associated with inflammation and anorexia and breakdown of muscles. It is distinct from starvation, malabsorption, and age-related loss of muscle mass. Most sarcopenic individuals are not cachectic.

Malnutrition occurs in approximately 5% of older community dwellers, 35% of hospitalized older adults, and ~50% of patients in rehabilitation settings. It implies a mechanism of protein-energy status imbalance, does not imply wasting, and should be applied to conditions that clearly respond to feeding. The nutritional needs of older adults are determined by multiple factors – including specific acute or chronic medical problems; their activity level, energy expenditures, and caloric needs; and their ability to access, prepare, and digest food – and criteria have been established to diagnose malnutrition.[37, 38] Additionally, the six-question Mini-Nutritional Assessment – Short Form (MNA-SF) is easy to administer, validated with high sensitivity and specificity, and predictive of poor outcomes.

Older individuals are at greater risk for undernutrition and involuntary weight loss than younger adults. Older adults are less able to adapt to periods of low food intake that may occur due to illness or other medical, psychological, or socioeconomic conditions. Clinically important weight loss is the loss of 4%–5% of total body weight over 6–12 months, though recommendations vary depending upon the amount of weight lost and the period of time involved. The recommended clinical approach to weight loss is beyond the scope of this review.

Interventions

Goals for interventions include reduced prevalence and severity of frailty, and improved clinical outcomes aligned with patient and family goals of care. Currently there are no available curative treatments for frailty.

Physical activity: aerobic and resistance exercise

Exercise is currently the most effective intervention to improve function and quality of life among frail elders. The many demonstrated benefits of exercise in older adults include increased muscle strength, decreased falls, enhanced gait and mobility, reduced inflammation, enhanced cognition, and improved well-being. Several studies have demonstrated that even the frailest adults can benefit from physical activity that includes resistance training and aerobic activity.[39–41] Obese frail elders also benefit from a weight loss and exercise. A randomized clinical trial comparing the independent and combined effects of weight loss and exercise demonstrated that a combination program resulted in the greatest improvement in physical function.[A]

> Exercise is currently the most effective intervention to improve function and quality of life among frail elders.

The Health, Aging, and Body Composition observational study demonstrated that participation in self-selected exercise could both prevent the onset of frailty and delay the progression of frailty.[42] A randomized clinical trial of a home-based physical activity program for frail elders reduced the progression of functional decline among those with moderate frailty, but not those with severe frailty.[43] A systematic review demonstrated that long-term multicomponent exercise interventions performed several times per week for 30–45 minutes may be helpful for the management of frail elders.[40] There

is growing evidence that frail adults in a wide variety of settings can improve their functional performance, activity of living performance, and quality of life by regular exercise training, but more high-quality trials are still needed.

Nutritional intervention

Despite the belief that the core components of frailty, including weight loss and weakness, would be amenable to nutritional interventions, evidence supporting the efficacy of this approach is scarce. According to a Cochrane review, nutritional supplementation with extra protein and energy produced a small but consistent weight gain in older people, and a small reduction in mortality for undernourished elders, but yielded no improvement in function.[44] Although there is some indication that high protein supplements produce clinical benefits to counteract the catabolic effects of disease and recovery from illness, strong evidence for its use in frail elders has not been demonstrated.[45] For frail elders, facilitating access to food, optimizing food preparation, and encouraging socialization at meals can be helpful in improving nutritional status. Appetite stimulants and micronutrient supplements are not currently recommended.

Hormonal intervention

Various hormonal therapies have been proposed, but the benefits and risks are currently unknown. Testosterone improves muscle mass by increasing protein synthesis and muscle strength, and although there may be a role for low dose testosterone in combination with nutritional supplementation in frail older men who are hypogonadal, testosterone therapy brings significant systemic side effects and is not recommended.[46]

Vitamin D prescription for elderly people who are deficient might reduce the number of falls. Vitamin D supplements along with calcium can improve muscle strength and balance.[47] Despite the evidence that low vitamin D levels are strongly associated with frailty,[48] the benefits of vitamin D to treat frailty in nondeficient elders have not been demonstrated.[2] Further studies are indicated.

Growth hormone therapy results in an increase in muscle mass in normal elderly, but there is no increase in strength unless exercise is also added to the intervention. Since there is no demonstrated clinical benefit, and the short- and long-term safety is not known, supplementation is not recommended.[49]

Other pharmacological approaches

Polypharmacy contributes to frailty, and avoidance of inappropriate medications is highly recommended. Several guidelines are helpful in reducing unnecessary or potentially harmful medications in this vulnerable group.[50] Other areas of investigation include angiotensin-converting enzyme inhibitors because of their impact on the structure and function of skeletal muscle.[51] The use of systemic anti-inflammatory agents, although not formally evaluated in frail elders, carries significant adverse effects.[4]

Comprehensive geriatric evaluation and specialized clinical programs

Comprehensive geriatric evaluation by a skilled interprofessional team is commonly considered to be the gold standard for developing and implementing a plan of care that is consistent with the patient's goals, values, and preferences. A targeted approach to prevent the range of biological, socioeconomic, and environmental stressors to improve clinical outcomes is appealing. However, the evidence for improved outcomes, especially among frail elders, is still emerging.

> Interprofessional clinical programs targeted to the frail elderly have been shown to improve clinical outcomes in a variety of settings.

Clinical programs targeted to the frail elderly have been shown to improve clinical outcomes in a variety of settings.[29] Frail patients cared for in specialized inpatient units are more likely to return to their homes, are less likely to suffer functional or cognitive decline, and have lower mortality rates than usual ward care.[52] A recent small study examined the impact of frailty on rehabilitation outcomes in a geriatric evaluation and management unit, and although all patients experienced functional improvement, the frailest patients experienced greater improvement than those who were less frail.[53] The results of community-based care demonstrate mixed results, indicating the complexity of the task and the need for more research.[52]

Conclusion

Frailty is an important geriatric syndrome associated with high morbidity and mortality. The prevention, early diagnosis, and management across the spectrum of frailty represent crucial areas in the clinical care of older adults. Early risk assessment, implementation of exercise programs, and access to geriatric interprofessional assessment and management represent the most effective ways to improve health outcomes. However, more research is needed. An understanding of the underlying mechanisms of frailty at the level of molecules, cells, and tissues may open the door to pharmacologic prevention and treatment strategies.[23] Objective, easily administered assessment tools, including biomarkers and biosensors, are sorely needed. High-value team-based models of care linked with community resources are required for this rapidly growing, vulnerable population.

References

1. Fried LP, Tangen CM, Walston J, Newman AB, Hirsch C, Gottdiener J, et al. Frailty in older adults evidence for a phenotype. *Journals of Gerontology Series A, Biological Sciences and Medical Sciences.* 2001;**56**(3): 146–57.

2. Morley JE, Vellas B, van Kan GA, Anker SD, Bauer JM, Bernabei R, et al. Frailty consensus: a call to action. *Journal of the American Medical Directors Association.* 2013;**14**(6):392–7.

3. Song X, Mitnitski A, Rockwood K. Prevalence and 10-year outcomes of frailty in older adults in relation to deficit accumulation. *Journal of the American Geriatrics Society.* 2010;**58**(4):681–7.

4. Chen X, Mao G, Leng SX. Frailty syndrome: an overview. *Clinical Interventions in Aging.* 2014;**9**:433–41.

5. Rockwood K, Andrew M, Mitnitski A. A comparison of two approaches to measuring frailty in elderly people. *Journals of Gerontology Series A, Biological Sciences and Medical Sciences.* 2007;**62**(7):738–43.

6. Rodriguez-Manas L, Feart C, Mann G, Vina J, Chatterji S, Chodzko-Zajko W, et al. Searching for an operational definition of frailty: a Delphi method based consensus statement: the frailty operative definition-consensus conference project. *Journals of Gerontology Series A, Biological Sciences and Medical Sciences.* 2013;**68**(1):62–7.

7. Bandeen-Roche K, Xue QL, Ferrucci L, Walston J, Guralnik JM, Chaves P, et al. Phenotype of frailty: characterization in the women's health and aging studies. *Journals of Gerontology Series A, Biological Sciences and Medical Sciences.* 2006;**61**(3):262–6.

8. Xue QL. The frailty syndrome: definition and natural history. *Clinics in Geriatric Medicine.* 2011;**27**(1):1–15.

9. Theou O, Brothers TD, Mitnitski A, Rockwood K. Operationalization of frailty using eight commonly used scales and comparison of their ability to predict all-cause mortality. *Journal of the American Geriatrics Society.* 2013;**61**(9):1537–51.

10. Bouillon K, Kivimaki M, Hamer M, Sabia S, Fransson EI, Singh-Manoux A, et al. Measures of frailty in population-based studies: an overview. *BMC Geriatrics.* 2013;**13**:64.

11. Abellan van Kan G, Rolland Y, Houles M, Gillette-Guyonnet S, Soto M, Vellas B. The assessment of frailty in older adults. *Clinics in Geriatric Medicine.* 2010;**26**(2):275–86.

12. Malmstrom TK, Miller DK, Morley JE. A comparison of four frailty models. *Journal of the American Geriatrics Society.* 2014;**62**(4):721–6.

13. Shamliyan T, Talley KM, Ramakrishnan R, Kane RL. Association of frailty with survival: a systematic literature review. *Ageing Research Reviews.* 2013;**12**(2):719–36.

14. Cigolle CT, Ofstedal MB, Tian Z, Blaum CS. Comparing models of frailty: the Health and Retirement Study. *Journal of the American Geriatrics Society.* 2009;**57**(5):830–9.

15. Bowles J, Brooks T, Hayes-Reams P, Butts T, Myers H, Allen W, et al. Frailty, family, and church support among urban African American elderly. *Journal of Health Care for the Poor and Underserved.* 2000;**11**(1):87–99.

16. Ottenbacher KJ, Ostir GV, Peek MK, Snih SA, Raji MA, Markides KS. Frailty in older Mexican Americans. *Journal of the American Geriatrics Society.* 2005;**53**(9):1524–31.

17. Gill TM, Gahbauer EA, Han L, Allore HG. Trajectories of disability in the last year of life. *New England Journal of Medicine.* 2010;**362**(13):1173–80.

18. Robertson DA, Savva GM, Kenny RA. Frailty and cognitive impairment–a review of the evidence and causal mechanisms. *Ageing Research Reviews.* 2013;**12**(4):840–51.

19. Afilalo J, Alexander KP, Mack MJ, Maurer MS, Green P, Allen LA, et al. Frailty assessment in the cardiovascular care of older adults. *Journal of the American College of Cardiology.* 2014;**63**(8):747–62.

20. Xue QL, Bandeen-Roche K, Varadhan R, Zhou J, Fried LP. Initial manifestations of frailty criteria and the development of frailty phenotype in the Women's Health and Aging Study II. *Journals of Gerontology Series A, Biological Sciences and Medical Sciences.* 2008;**63**(9):984–90.

21. Gill TM, Gahbauer EA, Allore HG, Han L. Transitions between frailty states among community-living older persons. *Archives of Internal Medicine.* 2006;**166**(4):418–23.

22. Leng S, Chaves P, Koenig K, Walston J. Serum interleukin-6 and hemoglobin as physiological correlates in the geriatric syndrome of frailty: a pilot study. *Journal of the American Geriatrics Society.* 2002;**50**(7):1268–71.

23. Mohler MJ, Fain MJ, Wertheimer AM, Najafi B, Nikolich-Žugich J. The Frailty Syndrome: Clinical measurements and basic underpinnings in humans and animals. *Experimental Gerontology.* 2014;**54**:6–13.

24. Ershler WB, Keller ET. Age-associated increased interleukin-6 gene expression, late-life diseases, and frailty. *Annual Review of Medicine.* 2000;**51**:245–70.

25. Leng SX, Xue QL, Tian J, Huang Y, Yeh SH, Fried LP. Associations of neutrophil and monocyte counts with frailty in community-dwelling disabled older women: results from the Women's Health and Aging Studies I. *Experimental Gerontology.* 2009;**44**(8):511–6.

26. Leng SX, Cappola AR, Andersen RE, Blackman MR, Koenig K, Blair M, et al. Serum levels of insulin-like growth factor-I (IGF-I) and dehydroepiandrosterone sulfate (DHEA-S), and their relationships with serum interleukin-6, in the geriatric syndrome of frailty. *Aging Clinical and Experimental Research.* 2004;**16**(2):153–7.

27. Travison TG, Nguyen AH, Naganathan V, Stanaway FF, Blyth FM, Cumming RG, et al. Changes in reproductive hormone concentrations predict the prevalence and progression of the frailty syndrome in older men: the concord health and ageing in men project. *Journal of Clinical Endocrinology and Metabolism.* 2011;**96**(8):2464–74.

28. Poehlman ET, Toth MJ, Fishman PS, Vaitkevicius P, Gottlieb SS, Fisher ML, et al. Sarcopenia in aging humans: the impact of menopause and disease. *Journals of Gerontology Series A, Biological Sciences and Medical Sciences.* 1995;**50**(Spec No):73–7.

29. Clegg A, Young J, Iliffe S, Rikkert MO, Rockwood K. Frailty in elderly people. *Lancet.* 2013;**381**(9868):752–62.

30. Varadhan R, Walston J, Cappola AR, Carlson MC, Wand GS, Fried LP. Higher levels and blunted diurnal variation of cortisol in frail older women. *Journals of Gerontology Series A, Biological Sciences and Medical Sciences.* 2008;**63**(2):190–5.

31. Ko FC. The clinical care of frail, older adults. *Clinics in Geriatric Medicine.* 2011;**27**(1):89–100.

32. Cruz-Jentoft AJ, Baeyens JP, Bauer JM, Boirie Y, Cederholm T, Landi F, et al. Sarcopenia: European consensus on definition and diagnosis: report of the European Working Group on Sarcopenia in Older People. *Age and Ageing.* 2010;**39**(4):412–23.

33. Makary MA, Segev DL, Pronovost PJ, Syin D, Bandeen-Roche K, Patel P, et al. Frailty as a predictor of surgical outcomes in older patients. *Journal of the American College of Surgeons.* 2010;**210**(6):901–8.

34. Yao X, Hamilton RG, Weng NP, Xue QL, Bream JH, Li H, et al. Frailty is associated with impairment of vaccine-induced antibody response and increase in post-vaccination influenza infection in community-dwelling older adults. *Vaccine.* 2011;**29**(31): 5015–21.

35. Ridda I, Macintyre CR, Lindley R, Gao Z, Sullivan JS, Yuan FF, et al. Immunological responses to pneumococcal vaccine in frail older people. *Vaccine.* 2009;**27**(10):1628–36.

36. Studenski SA, Peters KW, Alley DE, Cawthon PM, McLean RR, Harris TB, et al. The FNIH sarcopenia project: rationale, study description, conference recommendations, and final estimates. *Journals of Gerontology Series A, Biological Sciences and Medical Sciences.* 2014;**69**(5):547–58.

37. Bales CW, Ritchie CS. Sarcopenia, weight loss, and nutritional frailty in the elderly. *Annual Review of Nutrition.* 2002;**22**:309–23.

38. White JV, Guenter P, Jensen G, Malone A, Schofield M. Consensus statement of the Academy of Nutrition and Dietetics/American Society for Parenteral and Enteral Nutrition: characteristics recommended for the identification and documentation of adult malnutrition (undernutrition). *Journal of the Academy of Nutrition and Dietetics.* 2012;**112**(5):730–8.

39. Weening-Dijksterhuis E, de Greef MH, Scherder EJ, Slaets JP, van der Schans CP. Frail institutionalized older persons: A comprehensive review on physical exercise, physical fitness, activities of daily living, and quality-of-life. *American Journal of Physical Medicine & Rehabilitation / Association of Academic Physiatrists.* 2011;**90**(2):156–68.

40. Theou O, Stathokostas L, Roland KP, Jakobi JM, Patterson C, Vandervoort AA, et al. The effectiveness of exercise interventions for the management of frailty: a systematic review. *Journal of Aging Research.* 2011;**2011**:569194.

41. De Vries NM, van Ravensberg CD, Hobbelen JS, Olde Rikkert MG, Staal JB, Nijhuis-van der Sanden MW. Effects of physical exercise therapy on mobility, physical functioning, physical activity and quality of life in community-dwelling older adults with impaired mobility, physical disability and/or multi-morbidity: a meta-analysis. *Ageing Research Reviews.* 2012;**11**(1): 136–49.

42. Peterson MJ, Giuliani C, Morey MC, Pieper CF, Evenson KR, Mercer V, et al. Physical activity as a preventative factor for frailty: the health, aging, and body composition study. *Journals of Gerontology Series A, Biological Sciences and Medical Sciences.* 2009;**64**(1):61–8.

43. Gill TM, Baker DI, Gottschalk M, Peduzzi PN, Allore H, Byers A. A program to prevent functional decline in physically frail, elderly persons who live at home. *New England Journal of Medicine.* 2002;**347**(14): 1068–74.

44. Milne AC, Potter J, Vivanti A, Avenell A. Protein and energy supplementation in elderly people at risk from malnutrition. *Cochrane Database of Systematic Reviews.* 2009;**2**:CD003288.

45. Cawood AL, Elia M, Stratton RJ. Systematic review and meta-analysis of the effects of high protein oral nutritional supplements. *Ageing Research Reviews.* 2012;**11**(2):278–96.

46. Morley JE. Should frailty be treated with testosterone? *Aging Male: the Official Journal of the International Society for the Study of the Aging Male.* 2011;**14**(1):1–3.

47. Muir SW, Montero-Odasso M. Effect of vitamin D supplementation on muscle strength, gait and balance in older adults: a systematic review and meta-analysis. *Journal of the American Geriatrics Society.* 2011;**59**(12):2291–300.

48. Wong YY, McCaul KA, Yeap BB, Hankey GJ, Flicker L. Low vitamin D status is an independent predictor of increased frailty and all-cause mortality in older men: the Health in Men Study. *Journal of Clinical Endocrinology and Metabolism.* 2013;**98**(9): 3821–8.

49. Lamberts SW. The somatopause: to treat or not to treat? *Hormone Research.* 2000;**53**(Suppl 3):42–3.

50. Gallagher P, Ryan C, Byrne S, Kennedy J, O'Mahony D. STOPP (Screening Tool of Older Person's Prescriptions) and START (Screening Tool to Alert doctors to Right Treatment). Consensus validation. *International Journal of Clinical Pharmacology and Therapeutics.* 2008;**46**(2):72–83.

51. Onder G, Penninx BW, Balkrishnan R, Fried LP, Chaves PH, Williamson J, et al. Relation between use of angiotensin-converting enzyme inhibitors and muscle strength and physical function in older women: an observational study. *Lancet.* 2002;**359**(9310):926–30.

52. Ellis G, Whitehead MA, Robinson D, O'Neill D, Langhorne P. Comprehensive geriatric assessment for older adults admitted to hospital: meta-analysis of randomised controlled trials. *BMJ (Clinical research ed).* 2011;**343**:d6553.

53. Kawryshanker S, Raymond W, Ingram K. Effect of frailty on functional gain, resource utilisation, and discharge destination: an observational prospective study in a GEM ward. *Current Gerontology and Geriatric Research.* 2014;**2014**:357857.

Additional references

A. Villareal DT, Chode S, Parimi N, Sinacore DR, et al. Weight loss, exercise, or both and physical function in obese older adults. *N Engl J Med.* 2011;**364**:1218–29.

B. Janssen I, Shepard DS, Katzmarzyk PT, Roubenoff R. The healthcare costs of sarcopenia in the United States. *J Am Geriatr Soc.* 2004;**52**(1):80–5.

C. Kim SW. Multidimensional frailty score for the prediction of post-operative mortality risk. *JAMA Surgery.* 2014;**149**(7):633–40.

D. Joseph B, Pandit V, Zangbar B, Kulvatunyou N, Hashmi A, et al. Superiority of frailty over age in predicting outcomes among geriatric trauma patients. *JAMA Surg.* 2014;**149**(8):766–72.

Chapter 8

Gait impairment and falls

Daina L. Sturnieks and Catherine Sherrington

Key messages

1. The problem of falls and gait impairment
   - Falls are a common problem for older people.
   - Balance and mobility problems are important fall risk factors.
   - Gait impairment is prevalent in older people and is associated with poor health outcomes.
   - Gait impairments are central to common clinical conditions in older people.

2. Understanding gait impairment
   - One in three older people are classified as having abnormal gait.
   - Gait changes with age are due to declining physiological and cognitive functions.
   - Gait slowness can predict falls, physical health, cognitive health and death.
   - Up to half of the falls in older people are due to trips while walking.

3. Interventions to enhance gait and prevent falls
   - Exercise interventions can prevent falls in the general older community.
   - Exercise interventions can enhance gait in certain clinical groups.
   - The effectiveness of exercise-based fall prevention interventions in people with health conditions requires further investigation.

The problem of falls and gait impairment

Falls are a common problem for older people

Falls are a common problem for older populations, with considerable consequences for the individual and health-care systems. One in three people over the age of 65 will fall each year, with higher rates in older age groups, residents of aged care facilities, and clinical populations, such as those with Parkinson's disease.[1] Falls are the leading cause of injury-related hospitalization in people aged over 65 years, and they account for 14% of emergency admissions in this age group.[2] Falls can result in restriction of activity and fear of falling, decreased mobility, reduced quality of life, and loss of independence. Falls also account for about 40% of injury-related deaths in older people.[3]

Half of the falls reported by community-dwelling older people occur within their homes and surrounding areas. Most occur on level surfaces in commonly used rooms such as the kitchen, living room, and bedroom. With increasing age and frailty, fewer falls occur outside the home, reflecting the increased time spent indoors. Whereas some falls involve an external trigger such as a slippery floor or cracked pavement, many do not involve obvious environmental hazards. [4] Falls in older people most often occur during tasks of locomotion or transfer.[5, 6] Community-dwelling older people report that up to 75% of falls occur due to trips, slips, or loss of balance.[7]

Risk factors for falls

Falls were once considered to be random unavoidable events, but it is now known that falls can be predicted to a certain extent. As falls are often the result of a complex interaction between an individual's physical functioning, their behavior, and the environment, perfect prediction of falls is unlikely. However, a range of demographic, psychosocial, physiological, and medical risk factors for falls have been identified. [1] Demographic and psychosocial factors associated with an increased risk of falling include advanced age, limitations in activities of daily living, fear of falling,

Reichel's Care of the Elderly, 7th Edition, ed. Jan Busby-Whitehead *et al.* Published by Cambridge University Press.
© Cambridge University Press 2016.

depression, and a history of previous falls. Impaired vision and impaired cardiovascular function also increase the risk of falls.

Balance and mobility problems are particularly strong risk factors for falling in older people.[8] People with neurodegenerative and musculoskeletal conditions affecting balance and mobility such as stroke, Parkinson's disease, cognitive impairment, arthritis, foot problems, and chronic pain have higher rates of falling.[1] Other physiological risk factors for falls include impaired muscle strength, poor reaction time, impaired lower limb sensation, and poor vision,[1] so people with conditions affecting these such as cataracts and diabetes are also at a high risk of falling. Furthermore, declines in sensorimotor function or hemodynamic stability associated with age, inactivity, medication use, or minor pathology increase the risk of falls in older people without documented medical illness.

Gait impairment is prevalent in older people and associated with poor outcomes

Walking difficulties are highly prevalent in older people. One in three people in the United States, aged 65 and older, report difficulty walking three city blocks or climbing one flight of stairs.[9] The prevalence of observed gait impairment increases with age. The incidence of abnormal gait, defined by clinicians following visual inspection, was found to be 25% in people aged 70–74 and increased to almost 60% in those aged 80–84.[10]

Abnormal gait has been associated with greater risk for adverse outcomes in older people, including immobility, falls, dementia, morbidity, institutionalization, and mortality,[10–12] with greater impairment associated with increased risk. Abnormal gait patterns may be an early indicator of subclinical disease, as they are associated with an increased risk of cardiovascular disease, dementia, musculoskeletal and other diseases.[10, 13] For example, gait disorders have been shown to predict the onset of non-Alzheimer's dementia with a hazard ratio of 3.5.[14] However, abnormal gait is not an inevitable part of aging as approximately 20% of very old people show completely normal gait.[13]

The spinal cord executes rhythmical and sequential activation of muscles for locomotion, which is influenced by afferent information from multiple sensory channels for modulation of the motor output.

Appropriate integration of afferent input and coordination of force generation is important for steady and efficient locomotion. Since aging is associated with declines in sensory acuity and neuromuscular function, it is not surprising that gait changes with increasing age. Furthermore, central processes are important for initiation, termination, and adaptation of gait. Indeed, the control of gait seems to become more cognitively demanding with age. Older adults tend to walk slower and more cautiously than younger people, differences interpreted as adaptations for improved stability and safety. These patterns are more evident in older people who have previously fallen.

Gait impairments are central to common clinical conditions

Gait difficulties are commonly experienced by people with cognitive impairment and dementia and medical conditions including neurological, musculoskeletal, cardiac, and respiratory conditions. Gait disorders are also more common in older people in acute hospital and residential aged care facilities.[11]

Neurological conditions

Gait is one of the most affected motor characteristics of Parkinson's disease and contributes greatly to the high rate of falls in this population.[15–18] Parkinsonian gait is often slow, with reduced step length and height (shuffling), increased cadence and double-support time, and no arm swing. Some patients have difficulty initiating, adjusting, or terminating gait, leading to stumbles and falls. Increased age, disease duration and severity are strong predictors of falls in people with Parkinson's disease. [15, 17, 19]

Previous stroke is associated with an almost six-fold increased risk of falling,[20–26] with falls often attributed to loss of balance, misjudgment, poor concentration, or foot drag causing tripping.[27] Although the changes in gait depend largely on the brain region affected,[28] following stroke, people often have poor generation of muscle forces and muscle shortening, leading to an inability to efficiently drive gait.[29, 30] A reduced ability to generate joint powers and control of the swinging leg may increase the risk of tripping and recovering from gait perturbations. A reduced ability to generate sufficient extensor muscle force in the stance leg is also likely to increase the risk of falling.[31]

Gait disorders are common in people with cognitive impairment and dementia.[32, 33] Poorer performance in the cognitive domains of attention, executive function, and working memory are associated with slowing of gait in people with mild cognitive impairment, suggesting that these cognitive functions are related to the control of gait, particularly when under increased cognitive load.[34] Poorer performance in tests of cognitive function are also associated with falls in cognitively impaired and healthy older people. Poorer speed/executive attention is associated with increased falls, whereas memory is not.[35, 36] Older adults with cognitive impairment are twice as likely to fall than cognitively intact older people, and they have more severe consequences from falling such as fractures, institutionalization, and death.[37–39]

Musculoskeletal conditions

Arthritis is highly prevalent among older people and is a major cause of disability in this population.[40] The primary joints affected are the weight-bearing joints (hips, knees, ankle, spine) and hands. Arthritis has a detrimental effect on gait due to loss of joint range of motion, reduced muscle strength, and pain. Compared to healthy controls, people with arthritis tend to walk slower, with longer double support time, reduced joint range of motion, and altered lower limb joint moments and work.[41] To minimize pain and to account for decreased range of motion and muscle strength, people with arthritis and other joint problems are likely to modify their gait in an attempt to redistribute the loading to less painful joints. For example, people with hip osteoarthritis have increased ankle plantarflexion power generation and reduced hip moments, and people with medial knee osteoarthritis walk with increased toe out angle to reduce load on medial tibiofemoral compartment.[42]

Diagnosed arthritis is a significant risk factor for falling.[23–25, 43–47] In the United States, the age-adjusted median prevalence of two or more falls was found to be 137% higher among adults with arthritis compared with adults without arthritis.[48] Furthermore, self-reported symptoms associated with arthritic conditions, such as pain and reduced range of motion, are also associated with increased falls risk.[24, 25, 49]

Foot problems are common, affecting one in four people over the age of 45[50] and up to 85% of older people in long-term care facilities.[51, 52] Foot problems (including bunions, hammertoes, ulcers, hallux valgus, reduced ankle flexibility, reduced plantar tactile sensitivity, and toe muscle weakness) contribute to gait and mobility impairment in older people.[53] Older people with foot pain walk with reduced velocity and step length [54–56] and have an increased risk of falling.[37, 57, 58]

Understanding gait impairment

Observational gait analysis

Observational assessment of gait can be used in clinical settings and includes observation of walking at a natural and fast pace, walking in tandem (heel-to-toe), gait initiation behavior, and turning. An example is the Tinetti Performance-Oriented Assessment of Gait, designed to assist in clinical gait analysis, consists of nine areas of gait observation: gait initiation, step height, step length, step symmetry, step continuity, path deviation, trunk stability, walking stance (step width), and turning while walking.[59]

The Einstein Aging Study (EAS) conducted clinical examinations in almost 500 community volunteers aged 70–99 years, during which gait was observed. [10] Study clinicians determined that 35% of people had "abnormal gait," with approximately half being further subtyped as neurological in nature and the other half considered non-neurological. Neurological gait impairments commonly included unsteady/ataxic gait (almost half showed marked swaying or losing balance while walking, tandem walking, or turning); hemiparetic (one-quarter showed a leg swinging outward), frontal (one in eight people had short steps, wide base, and difficulty with foot lift), and parkinsonian (one in ten people demonstrated shuffling steps, stooped posture, absent arm swing, en bloc turns, and/or festination), found to be due to nervous system lesions, including neuropathies and stroke. Non-neurological gait impairments were commonly due to joint (85%), cardiac (10%), or respiratory (6%) problems. The features of non-neurological gait abnormalities were not described, but they are likely to have included slowed walking speed, step length asymmetry, and reduced range of motion.

Biomechanics of aging gait and falls

With increased age is a tendency to walk slower, with shorter step length, wider step width, and increased time in double-support.[60] Prospective studies also show significantly slower velocity and increased proportion of stride time spent in double-support in people who subsequently fall, compared with those who did not fall in the following year.[61] Prospective fallers are likely to have physical limitations, such as muscular weakness, that result in gait changes, or they may adapt their gait pattern with an awareness of their unsteadiness and fear of falling. Some early gait changes with aging may be compensated for in order to maintain walking speed. For example, some older people walk with reduced step length, but increase their cadence (rate of stepping) to maintain gait velocity.

It is likely that the control of gait in older adulthood declines due not only to deterioration in physical capacities, but also to the deterioration of cognitive efficiency in integrating sensory information for the precise regulation of the motor pattern. Walking can be an attention-demanding task, as evidenced by dual task studies that show gait to be adversely affected while simultaneously performing a cognitive task. Older age and poorer cognitive function are both associated with slowed walking while conducting a concurrent cognitive task.[62] Increased variability in gait parameters has also been shown with increased age,[63] and fall risk, including stride and swing time [64] and foot-lift asymmetries.[65] A more variable gait may indicate poorer neuromuscular control and might increase the risk of falling due to inaccuracies in foot trajectories.

Gait slowness has been shown to predict fall risk, cognitive health, physical health, and even death in older people;[66–69] therefore, gait speed is an important clinical measure in the aged care setting. Gait speed is easily measured by timing a walk over a known distance. The instructions (either walk comfortably or as fast as you can), the length of the walk, and the type of the gait measured (e.g., constant velocity walking) are important considerations.

Changes with age in kinematic (movement) and kinetic (force) gait parameters are numerous and include reduced hip and ankle motion,[70–74] reduced ankle power generation,[73, 75, 76] increased mechanical energy demands of lower limb musculature,[77–79] poorer control of footstrike;[66, 80] and a larger toe-out angle.[70, 75, 81] However, many of these are related to a slower walking velocity and shorter stride length in older, compared with younger people. Independent of walking speed, reduced hip extension angles [64] and increased anteroposterior heel contact velocity in older people [80] have been identified, which may increase the propensity to slip. [75, 82]

A prospective study of older people showed differences in kinematic and kinetic gait parameters in those who subsequently fell. Kemoun et al. examined gait patterns in 54 healthy older adults who had not previously experienced a fall. [61] Those who fell in the following 12 months walked with significantly reduced ankle range of motion and delayed dorsiflexion prior to heel strike, which might predispose to tripping. Indeed, the floor-toe clearance at mid-swing is reduced in older people, 11 mm for older adults compared with an average 13 mm for young adults, [60] increasing the risk of tripping. At the hip, future fallers, compared with nonfallers, had significantly reduced range of motion, a reduced flexion moment, and less power absorbed for energy return during the swing phase. Kerrigan et al. also found previous fallers exhibited reduced peak hip extension, compared with nonfallers.[83] These differences are likely to be related to slower walking speeds. Similarly Lee et al. measured walking kinetics in previous fallers and nonfallers.[84] Despite the fact that the fallers walked at half the speed, significant increases were found in their peak moments for hip flexion, hip adduction, knee extension, knee adduction, ankle dorsiflexion, and ankle eversion. Reduced power absorption at the knee and associated increased power absorption at the ankle indicates a poorer ability to efficiently control motion at these joints.

Biomechanics of trips and slips

Up to half of the falls in older people are attributed to tripping.[26, 43, 85–87] A trip induces a forward rotation of the body over the base of support, requiring a response to arrest the forward angular momentum of the body. Numerous studies have induced trips in the laboratory to study appropriate behaviors and limiting factors to successful recovery following a trip (for review, see [88]). Two different strategies to compensate for an induced trip have been identified.[89, 90] When the trip occurs in early swing phase, a lowering strategy is predominantly used, in which the tripped foot is quickly lowered to the ground and the contralateral foot initiates a recovery step. When the trip occurs in late swing phase, an elevating strategy is seen, in which the tripped limb is subsequently elevated over the obstacle in an attempt to continue the step. A slower walking speed is associated with an improved recovery following a trip [91] and may be one reason why older adults adopt a slower gait pattern for enhanced safety.[75]

The support limb is of great importance for successful recovery of balance following a trip.[31] A strong push-off reaction, prior to the recovery (stepping) limb contacting the ground enables time and clearance for correct positioning of the recovery limb. Furthermore, appropriate generation of joint moments in the support limb can help to arrest the angular momentum of the body. When properly placed, the recovery limb can also generate a force and moment that counteract the body angular momentum.[91] A slower development of mechanical responses seems to be a major factor limiting older adult's recovery from trips and other balance perturbations. Furthermore, older adults are less capable of adapting their gait (turning, sidestepping, stopping) to avoid an obstacle. Compared with young adults, they slow down, take more steps, and are less successful with shorter response times,[92] which is likely to lead to trips and falls.

Slips are another common gait-related mechanism of falls in older people that often result in injury due to the large impact forces. A slip occurs when the base of support moves relative to the body (forward translation of the foot), reducing the foot contact deceleration forces, leading to a backward rotation of the body. The incidence of slip initiation may be similar between young and older adults, yet older adults seem to have slower and less effective recovery responses than young adults; they slip longer and faster, and fall more often,[82] which may be due to age-related changes in vision, reaction time, and muscle strength.[93] Falling is more likely to occur with increased gait speed, increased forward heel displacement, increased posterior displacement of the body's center of mass relative to the base of support, and a larger angle of the leg relative to the ground (representative of a longer step length prior to the slip).[94]

Interventions to prevent falls and enhance gait

Interventions to prevent falls in community-dwelling older people

There is now strong evidence from randomized controlled trials that falls in older people living in the community can be prevented by well-designed intervention programs.[95] Effective interventions include targeted risk factor assessment and modification as well as a number of single interventions directed at the general community (exercise), high-risk individuals (home safety assessment and modification), and those with particular risk factors (removal of cataracts, reduction of psychoactive medication use, and podiatry intervention for those with foot pain).

Exercise programs have been found to prevent falls when delivered in group or home-based settings,[95] and exercise that targets balance has been found to have a greater fall prevention effect.[96] In the general community, falls can be prevented by exercise among people with identified risk factors for falls as well as in people without identified risk factors (i.e., from programs simply targeting the general older community).[95]

Exercise interventions can enhance gait in certain clinical groups

It is known that exercise interventions can improve gait for people with a range of clinical conditions. Systematic reviews of randomized trials show us that physiotherapy interventions and treadmill training can enhance gait in people with Parkinson's disease, [97, 98] and that a circuit class approach to therapy delivery and the use of treadmill training can enhance gait soon after stroke.[99] Findings of systematic reviews of trials of interventions to improve gait, and mobility more broadly, after hip fracture and stroke have been more mixed but individual trials have had promising findings.[100, 101] For example, a circuit class using "task-related" exercises (such as stepping, standing up, and reaching outside the base of support while standing) improved gait speed in long-term stroke survivors.[102] Gait speed and the need for walking aid use after hip fracture was improved by intensive outpatient physiotherapy and exercise training.[103] Further investigation is needed to establish optimal approaches to gait enhancement

111

in people with different clinical conditions, keeping in mind the relative costs and benefits of different approaches.

The effectiveness of exercise-based fall prevention interventions in people with health conditions requires further investigation

Unfortunately, the prevention of falls in older people with particular health conditions known to increase the risk of falls is less clear. For example, the Otago exercise program involves the tailored prescription of home exercises that challenge balance and strength. It is an effective falls prevention program and, importantly, falls injury prevention strategy in older people recruited through general practices but does not appear to have similar fall prevention effects in people with severe visual impairment.[104, 105] Similarly, although they enhanced mobility, a circuit-based exercise program did not prevent falls in stroke survivors,[102] and a home exercise program did not prevent falls in frail older people or those with recent hospital stays.[106, 107] However, in those with milder neurological disease, who are probably more similar to the general community dwellers, subgroup analysis has found that exercise as a single intervention strategy does appear to prevent falls.[102, 108]

Conclusion

Falls are a major problem for older people, our health systems, and our aging societies. Balance, gait, and mobility are strong risk factors for falls, with up to 75% of falls occurring due to trips, slips, or loss of balance. Gait problems, such as slow walking speed, also predict adverse outcomes in older people, including dementia, institutionalization, and death. Abnormal gait patterns have been identified in a number of clinical groups, including many neurological and musculoskeletal diseases. A range of intervention strategies has been found to prevent falls. In particular, exercise programs can reduce falls in older people as well as improve gait in particular clinical groups

References

1. Lord S, Sherrington C, Menz H, et al. *Falls in Older People: Risk Factors and Strategies for Prevention.* Cambridge: Cambridge University Press; 2007.

2. Close J, Ellis M, Hooper R, et al. Prevention of falls in the elderly trial (PROFET): a randomised controlled trial. *Lancet* 1999;**353**:93–7.

3. Centers for Disease Control and Prevention, National Center for Injury Prevention and Control. Web -based Injury Statistics Query and Reporting System (WISQARS) [online]. Accessed September 2, 2014.

4. Campbell AJ, Borrie MJ, Spears GF, et al. Circumstances and consequences of falls experienced by a community population 70 years and over during a prospective study. *Age Ageing* 1990;**19**:136–41.

5. Berg WP, Alessio HM, Mills EM, et al. Circumstances and consequences of falls in independent community-dwelling older adults. *Age Ageing* 1997;**26**:261–8.

6. Cali CM, Kiel DP. An epidemiologic study of fall-related fractures among institutionalized older people. *JAGS* 1995;**43**:1336–40.

7. Lord SR, Ward JA, Williams P, et al. An epidemiological study of falls in older community-dwelling women: the Randwick falls and fractures study. *Aust J Public Health* 1993;**17**:240–5.

8. Ganz DA, Bao Y, Shekelle PG, et al. Will my patient fall? *JAMA* 2007;**297**:77–86.

9. Brault MW, Hootman J, Helmick CG, et al. Prevalence and most common causes of disability among adults, United States, 2005. *MMWR* 2009;**58**:421–6.

10. Verghese J, LeValley A, Hall CB, et al. Epidemiology of gait disorders in community-residing older adults. *J Am Geriatr Soc* 2006;**54**:255–61.

11. Salzman B. Gait and balance disorders in older adults. *Am Fam Physician* 2010;**82**:61–8.

12. Waite LM, Grayson DA, Piguet O, et al. Gait slowing as a predictor of incident dementia: 6-year longitudinal data from the Sydney Older Persons Study. *J Neurol Sci* 2005;**229–230**:89–93.

13. Bloem BR, Haan J, Lagaay AM, et al. Investigation of gait in elderly subjects over 88 years of age. *J Geriatr Psychiatry Neurol* 1992;**5**:78–84.

14. Verghese J, Lipton RB, Hall CB, et al. Abnormality of gait as a predictor of non-Alzheimer's dementia. *N Engl J Med* 2002;**347**:1761–8.

15. Ashburn A, Stack E, Pickering RM, et al. A community-dwelling sample of people with Parkinson's disease: characteristics of fallers and non-fallers. *Age Ageing* 2001;**30**:47–52.

16. Burns R. Falling and getting up again. *Parkinson Report* 1994;**XV**:18.

17. Koller WC, Glatt S, Vetere-Overfield B, et al. Falls and Parkinson's disease. *Clin Neuropharmacol* 1989;**12**:98–105.

18. Paulson GW, Schaefer K, Hallum B. Avoiding mental changes and falls in older Parkinsons' patients. *Geriatrics* 1986;**41**:59–62.

19. Paul SS, Sherrington C, Canning CG, et al. The relative contribution of physical and cognitive fall risk factors in people with Parkinson's disease: a large prospective cohort study. *Neurorehabil Neural Repair* 2014;**28**:282–90.

20. Salgado R, Lord SR, Packer J, et al. Factors associated with falling in elderly hospital patients. *Gerontology* 1994;**40**:325–31.

21. O'Loughlin JL, Robitaille Y, Boivin JF, et al. Incidence of and risk factors for falls and injurious falls among the community-dwelling elderly. *Am J Epidemiol* 1993;**137**:342–54.

22. Herndon JG, Helmick CG, Sattin RW, et al. Chronic medical conditions and risk of fall injury events at home in older adults. *JAGS* 1997;**45**:739–43.

23. Dolinis J, Harrison JE. Factors associated with falling in older Adelaide residents. *Aust N Z J Public Health* 1997;**21**:462–8.

24. Campbell AJ, Borrie MJ, Spears GF. Risk factors for falls in a community-based prospective study of people 70 years and older. *J Gerontol* 1989;**44**:M112–7.

25. Nevitt MC, Cummings SR, Kidd S, et al. Risk factors for recurrent nonsyncopal falls: a prospective study. *JAMA* 1989;**261**:2663–8.

26. Prudham D, Evans JG. Factors associated with falls in the elderly: a community study. *Age Ageing* 1981;**10**:141–6.

27. Hyndman D, Ashburn A, Stack E. Fall events among people with stroke living in the community: Circumstances of falls and characteristics of fallers. *Arch Phys Med Rehabil* 2002;**83**:165–70.

28. Mitoma H, Hayashi R, Yanagisawa N, et al. Gait disturbances in patients with pontine medial tegmental lesions: clinical characteristics and gait analysis. *Arch Neurol* 2000;**57**:1048–57.

29. Moseley A, Wales A, Herbert R, et al. Observation and analysis of hemiplegic gait: stance phase. *Aust J Physiother* 1993;**39**:259–67.

30. Moore S, Schurr K, Wales A, et al. Observation and analysis of hemiplegic gait: swing phase. *Aust J Physiother* 1993;**39**:271–8.

31. Pijnappels M, Bobbert MF, van Dieen JH. Contribution of the support limb in control of angular momentum after tripping. *J Biomech* 2004;**37**:1811–18.

32. Taylor ME, Delbaere K, Mikolaizak AS, et al. Gait parameter risk factors for falls under simple and dual task conditions in cognitively impaired older people. *Gait Posture* 2013;**37**:126–30.

33. Verghese J, Robbins M, Holtzer R, et al. Gait dysfunction in mild cognitive impairment syndromes. *JAGS* 2008;**56**:1244–51.

34. Montero-Odasso M, Verghese J, Beauchet O, et al. Gait and cognition: a complementary approach to understanding brain function and the risk of falling. *JAGS* 2012;**60**:2127–36.

35. Herman T, Mirelman A, Giladi N, et al. Executive control deficits as a prodrome to falls in healthy older adults: a prospective study linking thinking, walking, and falling. *J Gerontol* 2010;**65**:1086–92.

36. Holtzer R, Friedman R, Lipton RB, et al. The relationship between specific cognitive functions and falls in aging. *Neuropsychology* 2007;**21**:540–8.

37. Tinetti ME, Speechley M, Ginter SF. Risk factors for falls among elderly persons living in the community. *N Engl J Med* 1988;**319**:1701–7.

38. Morris JC, Rubin EH, Morris EJ, et al. Senile dementia of the Alzheimer's type: an important risk factor for serious falls. *J Gerontol* 1987;**42**:412–17.

39. Laird RD, Studenski S, Perera S, et al. Fall history is an independent predictor of adverse health outcomes and utilization in the elderly. *Am J Manag Care* 2001;**7**:1133–8.

40. Prevalence of doctor-diagnosed arthritis and arthritis-attributable activity limitation–United States, 2010–2012. *MMWR* 2013;**62**:869–73.

41. Baan H, Dubbeldam R, Nene AV, et al. Gait analysis of the lower limb in patients with rheumatoid arthritis: a systematic review. *Semin Arthritis Rheum* 2012;**41**:768–88 e8.

42. Broström EW, Esbjörnsson A-C, von Heideken J, et al. Gait deviations in individuals with inflammatory joint diseases and osteoarthritis and the usage of three-dimensional gait analysis. *Best Pract Res Clin Rheumatol* 2012;**26**:409–22.

43. Blake A, Morgan K, Bendall M, et al. Falls by elderly people at home – prevalence and associated factors. *Age Ageing* 1988;**17**:365–72.

44. Buchner DM, Larson EB. Falls and fractures in patients with Alzheimer-type dementia. *JAMA* 1987;**257**:1492–5.

45. Robbins AS, Rubenstein LZ, Josephson KR, et al. Predictors of falls among elderly people – results of two population-based studies. *Arch Int Med* 1989;**149**:1628–33.

46. Tinetti ME, Williams TF, Mayewski R. Fall risk index for elderly patients based on number of chronic disabilities *Am J Med* 1986;**80**:429–34.

47. Torgerson DJ, Garton MJ, Reid DM. Falling and perimenopausal women. *Age Ageing* 1993;**22**:59–64.

48. Barbour KE, Stevens JA, Helmick CG, et al. Falls and fall injuries among adults with arthritis – United States, 2012. *MMWR* 2014;**63**:379–83.

49. Gabell A, Simons MA, Nayak USL. Falls in the healthy elderly: predisposing causes. *Ergonomics* 1985;**28**:965–75.

50. Thomas MJ, Roddy E, Zhang W, et al. The population prevalence of foot and ankle pain in middle and old age: a systematic review. *Pain* 2011;**152**:2870–80.

51. Hung L, Ho Y, Leung P. Survey of foot deformities among 166 geriatric inpatients. *Foot Ankle* 1985;**5**: 156–64.

52. Helfand AE, Cooke HL, Walinsky MD, et al. Foot problems associated with older patients – a focused podogeriatric study. *J Am Podiatr Med Assoc* 1998;**88**: 237–41.

53. Black JR, Hale WE. Prevalence of foot complaints in the elderly. *J Am Podiatr Med Assoc* 1987;**77**:308–11.

54. Guralnik J, Simonsick E, Ferrucci L, et al. A short physical performance battery assessing lower extremity function: association with self-reported disability and prediction of mortality and nursing home admission. *J Gerontol* 1994;**49**:M85–94.

55. Benvenuti F, Ferrucci L, Guralnik JM, et al. Foot pain and disability in older persons: an epidemiologic survey. *JAGS* 1995;**43**:479–84.

56. Menz HB, Lord SR. Gait instability in older people with hallux valgus. *Foot Ankle Int* 2005;**26**:483–9.

57. Menz HB, Morris ME, Lord SR. Foot and ankle risk factors for falls in older people: a prospective study. *J Gerontol* 2006;**61**:866–70.

58. Mickle KJ, Munro BJ, Lord SR, et al. Foot pain, plantar pressures, and falls in older people: a prospective study. *JAGS* 2010;**58**:1936–40.

59. Tinetti ME. Performance-oriented assessment of mobility problems in elderly patients. *JAGS* 1986;**34**: 119–26.

60. Winter DA. *The Biomechanics and Motor Control of Human Gait: Normal, Elderly and Pathological.* Waterloo, Ontario: University of Waterloo Press; 1991.

61. Kemoun G, Thoumie P, Boisson D, et al. Ankle dorsiflexion delay can predict falls in the elderly. *J Rehabil Med* 2002;**34**:278–83.

62. Al-Yahya E, Dawes H, Smith L, et al. Cognitive motor interference while walking: a systematic review and meta-analysis. *Neurosci Biobehav Rev* 2011;**35**:715–28.

63. Owings TM, Grabiner MD. Variability of step kinematics in young and older adults. *Gait Posture* 2004;**20**:26–9.

64. Hausdorff J, Rios D, Edelberg H. Gait variability and fall risk in community-living older adults: a 1-year prospective study. *Arch Phys Med Rehabi* 2001;**82**: 1050–6.

65. Di Fabio RP, Kurszewski WM, Jorgenson EE, et al. Footlift asymmetry during obstacle avoidance in high-risk elderly. *JAGS* 2004;**52**:2088–93.

66. Verghese J, Holtzer R, Lipton RB, et al. Quantitative gait markers and incident fall risk in older adults. *J Gerontol* 2009;**64**:896–901.

67. Abellan van Kan G, Rolland Y, Andrieu S, et al. Gait speed at usual pace as a predictor of adverse outcomes in community-dwelling older people an International Academy on Nutrition and Aging (IANA) Task Force. *J Nutr Health Aging* 2009;**13**:881–9.

68. Hardy SE, Perera S, Roumani YF, et al. Improvement in usual gait speed predicts better survival in older adults. *JAGS* 2007;**55**:1727–34.

69. Studenski S, Perera S, Patel K, et al. Gait speed and survival in older adults. *JAMA* 2011;**305**:50–8.

70. Murray MP, Kory RC, Clarkson BH. Walking patterns in healthy old men. *J Gerontol* 1969;**24**:169–78.

71. Crowinshield RD, Brand RA, Johnston RC. The effects of walking velocity and age on hip kinematics and kinetics. *Clin Orthop Rel Res* 1978;**132**:140–4.

72. Elble RJ, Thomas SS, Higgins C, et al. Stride-dependent changes in gait of older people. *J Neurol* 1991;**238**:1–5.

73. Kerrigan DC, Todd MK, Croce UD, et al. Biomechanical gait alterations independent of speed in the healthy elderly: evidence for specific limiting impairments. *Arch Phys Med Rehabil* 1998;**79**:317–22.

74. Hageman PA, Blanke DJ. Comparison of gait of young women and elderly women. *Phys Ther* 1986;**66**:1382–7.

75. Winter DA, Patla AE, Frank JS, et al. Biomechanical walking pattern changes in the fit and healthy elderly. *Phys Ther* 1990;**70**:340–7.

76. Judge JO, Davis RB, 3rd, Ounpuu S. Step length reductions in advanced age: the role of ankle and hip kinetics. *J Gerontol* 1996;**51**:M303–12.

77. McGibbon C, Krebs D. Age-related changes in lower trunk coordination and energy transfer during gait. *J Neurophysiol* 2001;**85**:1923–31.

78. McGibbon C, Puniello M, Krebs D. Mechanical energy transfer during gait in relation to strength impairment and pathology in elderly women. *Clin Biomech* 2001;**16**:324–33.

79. McGibbon CA, Krebs DE, Puniello MS. Mechanical energy analysis identifies compensatory strategies in disabled elders' gait. *J Biomech* 2001;**34**:481–90.

80. Mills PM, Barrett RS. Swing phase mechanics of healthy young and elderly men. *Hum Mov Sci* 2001;**20**: 427–46.

81. Murray MP, Drought AB, Kory RC. Walking patterns of normal men. *Journal of Bone and Joint Surgery* 1964;**46A**:335–60.

82. Lockhart TE, Woldstad JC, Smith JL. Effects of age-related gait changes on the biomechanics of slips and falls. *Ergonomics* 2003;**46**:1136–60.

83. Kerrigan DC, Lee LW, Collins JJ, et al. Reduced hip extension during walking: Healthy elderly and fallers versus young adults. *Arch Phys Med Rehabil* 2001;**82**:26–30.

84. Lee LW, Kerrigan DC. Identification of kinetic differences between fallers and nonfallers in the elderly. *Am J Phys Med Rehabil* 1999;**78**:242–6.

85. Campbell AJ, Reinken J, Allan BC, et al. Falls in old age: a study of frequency and related clinical factors. *Age and ageing* 1981;**10**:264–70.

86. Tinetti ME, Speechley M, Ginter SF. Risk factors for falls among elderly persons living in the community. *N Engl J Med* 1988;**319**:1701–7.

87. Lord SR, Ward JA, Williams P, et al. An epidemiological study of falls in older community-dwelling women: the Randwick falls and fractures study. *Aust J Pub Health* 1993;**17**:240–54.

88. Van Dieen JH, Pijnappels M, Bobbert MF. Age-related intrinsic limitations in preventing a trip and regaining balance after a trip. *Safety Science* 2005;**43**:437–53.

89. Pavol MJ, Owings TM, Foley KT, et al. Gait characteristics as risk factors for falling from trips induced in older adults. *J Gerontol* 1999;**54**:M583–90.

90. Pavol MJ, Owings TM, Foley KT, et al. Mechanisms leading to a fall from an induced trip in healthy older adults. *J Gerontol* 2001;**56**:M428–37.

91. Grabiner MD, Koh TJ, Lundin TM, et al. Kinematics of recovery from a stumble. *J Gerontol* 1993;**48**:M97–102.

92. Cao C, Ashton-Miller JA, Schultz AB, et al. Abilities to turn suddenly while walking: effects of age, gender, and available response time. *J Gerontol* 1997;**52**:M88–93.

93. Lockhart TE, Smith JL, Woldstad JC. Effects of aging on the biomechanics of slips and falls. *Hum Factors* 2005;**47**:708–29.

94. Brady RA, Pavol MJ, Owings TM, et al. Foot displacement but not velocity predicts the outcome of a slip induced in young subjects while walking. *J Biomech* 2000;**33**.803–8.

95. Gillespie LD, Robertson MC, Gillespie WJ, et al. Interventions for preventing falls in older people living in the community. *Cochrane Database Syst Rev* 2012;**9**: CD007146.

96. Sherrington C, Tiedemann A, Fairhall N, et al. Exercise to prevent falls in older adults: an updated meta-analysis and best practice recommendations. *NSW Public Health Bull* 2011;**22**:78–83.

97. Tomlinson CL, Patel S, Meek C, et al. Physiotherapy versus placebo or no intervention in Parkinson's disease. *Cochrane Database Syst Rev* 2013. DOI: 10.1002/14651858.CD002817.pub4.

98. Mehrholz J, Friis R, Kugler J, et al. Treadmill training for patients with Parkinson's disease. *Cochrane Database Syst Rev* 2010. DOI: 10.1002/14651858. CD007830.pub2.

99. English C, Hillier SL. Circuit class therapy for improving mobility after stroke. *Cochrane Database Syst Rev* 2010. DOI: 10.1002/14651858.CD007513.pub2.

100. Handoll HHG, Sherrington C, Mak JCS. Interventions for improving mobility after hip fracture surgery in adults. *Cochrane Database Syst Rev* 2011. DOI: 10.1002/14651858.CD001704.pub4.

101. States RA, Pappas E, Salem Y. Overground physical therapy gait training for chronic stroke patients with mobility deficits. *Cochrane Database Syst Rev* 2009. DOI: 10.1002/14651858.CD006075.pub2.

102. Dean CM, Rissel C, Sherrington C, et al. Exercise to enhance mobility and prevent falls after stroke: the Community Stroke Club Randomized Trial. *Neurorehabil Neural Repair* 2012;**26**:1046–57.

103. Binder EF, Brown M, Sinacore DR, et al. Effects of extended outpatient rehabilitation after hip fracture: a randomized controlled trial. *JAMA* 2004;**292**: 837–46.

104. Robertson MC, Campbell AJ, Gardner MM, et al. Preventing injuries in older people by preventing falls: a meta-analysis of individual-level data. *JAGS* 2002;**50**:905–11.

105. Campbell A, Robertson M, La Grow S, et al. Randomised controlled trial of prevention of falls in people aged 75 with severe visual impairment: the VIP trial. *BMJ* 2005;**331**:817–925.

106. Fairhall N, Sherrington C, Lord SR, et al. Effect of a multifactorial, interdisciplinary intervention on risk factors for falls and fall rate in frail older people: a randomised controlled trial. *Age Ageing* 2014;**43**:616–22.

107. Sherrington C, Lord SR, Vogler CM, et al. A post-hospital home exercise program improved mobility but increased falls in older people: a randomised controlled trial. *PloS one* 2014;**9**:e104412.

108. Canning C, Sherrington C, Lord S, et al. Exercise for falls prevention in Parkinson's disease: a randomized controlled trial. *Neurology* 2015 Jan 20;**84**(3):304–12.

Evaluation and management of dizziness

Samuel C. Durso, MD, MBA, and David Newman-Toker, MD, PhD

Introduction

Dizziness is a common symptom of the elderly. Patients may use a variety of terms such as "woozy," "lightheaded," "off-balance," or "spinning" to describe the phenomenon of dizziness, which is sometimes used interchangeably with "vertigo." However, dizziness, which is characterized by a distorted sense of spatial orientation, lacks the illusion of self-motion that is a feature of vertigo.[1] Either dizziness or vertigo may present as a primary complaint. Alternatively, they may accompany another primary symptom such as chest pain, dyspnea, or nausea. For the purpose of this chapter, "dizziness" will denote both terms unless otherwise specified.

Spatial orientation is governed by multiple sensory inputs from and affecting a wide array of physiological systems, including vestibular, visual, cerebellar, motor, and sensory systems. Dizziness (spatial disorientation without a false sense of self-motion) tends to occur when distorted input to the vestibular system is relatively symmetrical, whereas vertigo often occurs when the input is relatively asymmetrical. As a result, whether an individual experiences dizziness or vertigo is less a function of the cause for the spatial disorientation than the balance of inputs to the vestibular system. Furthermore, because the sensation of dizziness is necessarily subjective, individuals from different cultures, those with different languages, or those with cognitive impairment may describe the experience of dizziness resulting from similar mechanisms in different terms.[2]

Presyncope and unsteadiness may evoke descriptions by patients that overlap with those used to describe dizziness or vertigo.[2] Either can produce symptoms that encompass sensations of dizziness or vertigo, yet are distinguished from both. Presyncope is the sensation of impending faint without actual loss of consciousness. Syncope, which is a transient loss of consciousness due to transient global cerebral hypoperfusion, usually leads to a fall and full recovery of consciousness within 30 seconds. While many causes of presyncope (sensation of impending faint) overlap with causes of dizziness or vertigo and causes of loss of consciousness, true syncope begets a differential diagnosis that usually differs from presyncope and dizziness. Unsteadiness and directional pulsion, as can occur with sensory-motor disorders and Parkinson's disease, are balance disorders that sometimes produce dizziness or vertigo, though either can occur without head sensations.

Dizziness leads to more than five million primary care visits each year in the United States, disproportionately among the elderly,[3] and is one of the top three reported primary care symptoms.[4] Prevalence is age-dependent, ranging from about 30% at age 65 to 50% in those over 85.[5] In addition, dizziness is a major risk for falls and hip fractures.[6, 7] Because dysfunction of multiple physiological systems (e.g., visual, cardiovascular, neurological) with input to and from the vestibular system is common in the elderly, the description of the experience of dizziness often varies by individual irrespective of the precipitating cause (e.g., postural hypotension, medication side effect, benign positional vertigo). Furthermore, many older adults have more than one condition that produces or predisposes to dizziness. For example, an older adult may have dizziness caused by impaired balance due to Parkinson's disease and have dizziness related to side effects of the drugs used to treat that condition. For this reason, some propose thinking of dizziness as a geriatric syndrome.[8] Still, the elderly, like younger patients, can have discrete causes for

Reichel's Care of the Elderly, 7th Edition, ed. Jan Busby-Whitehead *et al.* Published by Cambridge University Press. © Cambridge University Press 2016.

dizziness. Although it may be useful to consider dizziness as a syndrome in the elderly, it is nevertheless important to accurately identify the underlying cause-(s) when possible to differentiate emergencies from less urgent causes, and for determining treatment and prognosis.

Classification

To diagnose the cause of dizziness, physicians have traditionally focused on asking the patient "What do you mean by dizziness?" It has been widely taught that accurate characterization of quality of dizziness is one of four types – vertigo, presyncope, disequilibrium (unsteadiness of gait), or nonspecific sensations not captured by the first three types – can guide the clinician to the cause.[9] As a result, characterizing dizziness accurately as "vertigo" is felt to reliably indicate a peripheral or central vestibular disturbance; similarly, identifying dizziness as "presyncope" is felt to point to global cerebral hypoperfusion from cardiac causes and "nonspecific dizziness" to result from a cerebral metabolic disorder such as hypoglycemia or psychiatric conditions.[10] However, research during the last decade has shown that characterizing the type of dizziness qualitatively is not sufficiently specific to identify the cause.[11] For one thing, patients often use qualitative descriptions inconsistently when describing an episode of dizziness.[2] Furthermore, cardiac arrhythmia, orthostatic hypotension, stroke, and panic attacks may cause frank vertigo, and dizziness without vertigo may occur with a full range of vestibular diseases.[2, 12] Studies have shown that more helpful than determining the type (quality) of dizziness is identification of the "timing," "triggers," and "associated symptoms" in the context of the complete medical history and physical exam.[11] "Timing" refers to the continuity and duration of symptoms. Dizziness may be discretely episodic

without symptoms between episodes or continuous with or without fluctuations in intensity. "Triggers" refers to maneuvers or actions that initiate an episode of dizziness (e.g., specific head movements, standing posture, or exercise). Associated symptoms, such as chest pain, weakness, headache, or hearing loss, can provide more specific clues to the underlying cause.

> "What do you mean by dizzy?" should not be your first question. Focus on timing and triggers, rather than type.

Therefore, more important than determining whether the sensation can be classified as dizziness or vertigo, the first step in diagnosis is to accurately assess the "timing," which allows one to characterize the phenomenon as episodic vestibular syndrome (EVS), acute vestibular syndrome (AVS), or chronic vestibular syndrome (CVS). "Triggers" such as reproduction of the dizziness sensation with specific head movements or with postural change can help localize the cause or uncover the abnormal physiological mechanism (e.g., otoliths in a semicircular canal or drop in blood pressure on standing). These three timing categories result in largely mutually exclusive differential diagnoses (Tables 9.1–9.3). However, it is not uncommon for the elderly to experience more than one cause of dizziness, either concurrently or sequentially over time. Concurrent causes (e.g., simultaneous presence of vestibular disease, medication side effect, and balance disorder) may cause overlapping dizziness syndromes. For example, a patient with CVS associated with unsteadiness that is always present when standing or walking may develop EVS due to a drop in postural blood pressure. A new postural cause of dizziness (EVS) may be hard to recognize against a background of chronic dizziness that occurs in the context of standing or walking. Therefore,

Table 9.1 Core differential diagnosis of episodic vestibular syndrome

(*Episode duration*: seconds–hours)	
Nonspontaneous (triggered)	**Spontaneous**
Position/posture: BPPV, orthostatic hypotension *Valsalva*: situational presyncope, inner ear fistula *Exertion*: valvular heart disease, myocardial ischemia, or cardiac insufficiency	*Less urgent*: vestibular migraine, Menière's disease, panic disorder, vasovagal presyncope *More urgent*: TIA, cardiac arrhythmia, hypoglycemia, pheochromocytoma, occult carbon monoxide exposure

Abbreviations: BPPV – benign paroxysmal positional vertigo; TIA – transient ischemic attack
Source: Modified from Newman-Toker.[24]

Table 9.2 Core differential diagnosis of acute vestibular syndrome

(*Illness duration*: days–weeks)	
Nonspontaneous (postexposure)	Spontaneous
Treatments: anticonvulsants, intra-tympanic gentamicin *Trauma*: acute traumatic brain injury, surgery (e.g., cochlear implantation) *Toxins*: chemicals (e.g., toluene), biotoxins	*Less urgent*: vestibular neuritis, labyrinthitis *More urgent*: stroke, cerebellar hemorrhage, bacterial mastoiditis, herpes zoster oticus (Ramsay-Hunt syndrome), brainstem encephalitis, Wernicke's syndrome (thiamine deficiency)

Source: Modified from Newman-Toker.[24]

Table 9.3 Tests to evaluate for stroke in the acute vestibular syndrome

Test	Sensitivity for stroke
Focal findings on general neurologic exam	~19% [17]
Brain CT scan	~16% [18]
Brain MRI MRI-DWI (first 48 hours)	~80%–85% [20]
HINTS to INFARCT	~99%* [20]

* The point estimate for sensitivity is 99% with 97% specificity in acute vestibular syndrome without hearing symptoms. Sensitivity is slightly lower (96%) when loss of hearing accompanies the AVS.[20]
Abbreviations: CT – computed tomography; HINTS– head impulse, nystagmus, test of skew; INFARCT –impulse normal, fast phase alternating, refixation on cover test; MRI-DWI – magnetic resonance imaging with diffusion weighted images

accurate assessment of timing and triggers, and heightened vigilance for associated conditions such as change in function, relationship to medication change, or illness is necessary.

Different causes producing the same dizziness syndrome may also occur over time. For instance, an older adult who has experienced EVS in the past due to benign paroxysmal positional vertigo (BPPV) may present with a new cause for episodic symptoms that is qualitatively similar (producing vertigo) but is due to a new underlying mechanism such as postural hypotension, cardiac arrhythmia, or transient ischemic attacks. Although the diagnosis may be straightforward when associated symptoms are present (i.e., temporal relation to starting a new medication, obvious anemia, new neurological findings), the diagnosis might be missed when associated

symptoms are absent and attention is paid only to the qualitative similarity to the previous episode. Assessing for the presence or absence of triggers (i.e., dizziness produced with upright posture, not head movement in the case of postural hypotension) is the principal task in such situations.

Although the diagnostic challenge created by multiple causes of dizziness producing qualitatively similar symptoms or overlapping syndromes does not negate the utility of assessing timing, triggers, and accompanying symptoms, it makes diagnosis and treatment of older adults more challenging than in younger patients who are more likely to have one underlying condition. In spite of this complexity, it is valuable to delineate the three timing syndromes when possible. Also it is important to note that in addition to inherently dangerous causes of dizziness such as stroke, even so called "benign" causes (e.g., BPPV, self-limited drug reactions, mild volume depletion) can be dangerous when they result in injurious falls or other harm. Likewise mild chronic dizziness can be debilitating and lead to deconditioning if it prevents the patient from staying physically active. Therefore, any complaint of dizziness must be addressed comprehensively.

Intermittent, brief episodes of dizziness lasting seconds to hours

Episodic vestibular syndrome (EVS) is characterized by intermittent, brief episodes of dizziness or vertigo lasting seconds to hours. Episodic vestibular syndrome is the most common pattern of dizziness. Because symptoms typically resolve quickly and are not associated with severe nausea or vomiting, most patients seek evaluation in the ambulatory care setting.

Differential diagnosis

The differential diagnosis of EVS is broad, and timing and triggers are particularly helpful for uncovering the etiology. BPPV and orthostatic hypotension are the most common etiologies, although this category includes a number of cardiac and central nervous system causes that are less common but which must be considered (Table 9.1). Arising from a recumbent position will trigger both BPPV and orthostatic hypotension, although BPPV will also be triggered by lying back down and by turning while supine, whereas orthostatic hypotension should not. Dangerous mimics of BPPV include central nervous system disease (e.g., posterior fossa tumors) and orthostatic hypotension due to bleeding, sepsis, or other acute disorders. Symptoms triggered by exertion raise the concern for dangerous cardiac and pulmonary causes. Unprovoked episodes with increasing frequency raise concern for transient ischemic attacks.[13]

> In those with episodic symptoms, worry when spells are spontaneous or triggered by exertion. When symptoms are positional, do test maneuvers for BPPV.

If the history suggests that the symptoms are triggered, then the dizziness should be reproduced by provocation at the bedside. For positional symptoms that are brief and postural, this is done by measuring the orthostatic blood pressure and by performing provocative positional testing for BPPV. The Dix-Hallpike maneuver (Figure 9.1) tests for posterior canal otoliths, which is the most common cause of BPPV. A positive test produces mixed upbeat and torsional nystagmus with the 12 o'clock portion of the eye beating toward the affected (tested) ear. The supine roll maneuver tests for horizontal canal BPPV, the second most common form. (See the Internet links listed at the end of this chapter.) A positive test produces horizontal nystagmus that beats either away or toward the affected ear. Horizontal canal BPPV is more likely to be mimicked by central disorders, so the patient should be referred for further evaluation if there is any doubt as to the diagnosis or response to therapy.

Spontaneous EVS (episodes lacking a clear, reproducible trigger) may occur with reflex presyncope, vestibular migraine, Menière's disease, and panic disorder. The diagnosis may be straightforward when the underlying condition is accompanied by typical features or accompanying symptoms, such as headache with vestibular migraine or fear and palpitations with panic disorder. In the absence of discriminating features, one must be careful to consider transient ischemic attacks, cardiac arrhythmias without palpitations, and hypoglycemia. If chest pain, dyspnea, or syncope is associated with a spontaneous episode, then a cardiovascular cause or pulmonary embolus is more likely than a neurological cause. Furthermore,

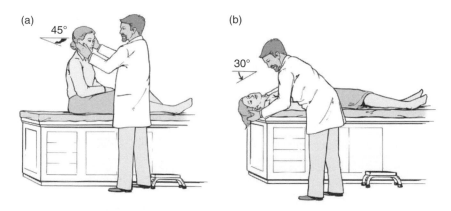

Figure 9.1 Dix-Hallpike maneuver (right ear).[25] The patient is seated and positioned so that the head will extend over the top edge of the table when supine. The head is turned 45° toward the ear being tested (position A). The patient is quickly lowered into the supine position with the head extending about 30° below the horizontal (position B). The patient's head is held in this position, and the examiner observes the patient's eyes for nystagmus. In this case with the right side being tested, the physician should expect to see a fast-phase counter-clockwise nystagmus. To complete the maneuver, the patient is returned to the seated position (position A) and the eyes are observed for reversal nystagmus, in this case a fast-phase clockwise nystagmus.

it is important to note (and not widely recognized) that cardiac causes may produce spinning-type vertigo.[14] Similarly, TIA may present with dizziness or vertigo in the absence of neurological signs in 10%–20% of individuals before proceeding to major stroke.[13] Therefore, a high index of suspicion is necessary when encountering recurring, spontaneous EVS, particularly if the symptoms are new in the prior six months and the frequency of attacks is increasing.

As noted earlier, it is important to differentiate truly episodic symptoms (brief episodes separated by asymptomatic intervals) from dizziness that is persistent but exacerbated by intolerance for head movement or dizziness that his always present with standing or walking in patient with unsteadiness.

Treatment

Patients with BPPV usually benefit from physical maneuvers to reposition canal otoliths (Figure 9.2).[15] Dizziness typically lasts only seconds and becomes progressively less intense with each episode.

Antihistamines are not helpful in BPPV and may produce side effects, including drowsiness, that increase the risk of falls. Vestibular migraine is probably more common than previously imagined; treatment is generally by a combination of lifestyle modification and prophylactic medication.[16]

Acute, continuous episodes of dizziness lasting days to weeks

Acute Vestibular Syndrome (AVS) is characterized by acute, continuous dizziness or vertigo lasting days to weeks associated with nausea or vomiting, intolerance to head movement, and gait unsteadiness. Nystagmus is typically present at the time of symptoms, although sometimes it is partially suppressed by normal vision, making it more difficult to detect. During an attack, most patients seek help in an emergency department or urgent care setting. Uncommonly, bouts of AVS may occur as part of a relapsing and remitting illness (usually multiple sclerosis) that results in chronic residual dizziness. Accurate assessment of the

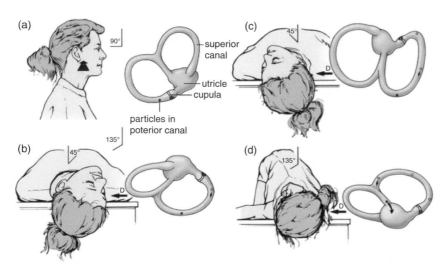

Figure 9.2 Particle repositioning maneuver (right ear): schema of patient and concurrent movement of posterior/superior semicircular canals and utricle.[25] The patient is seated on a table as viewed from the right side (A); (B)–(D) show the sequential head and body positions of a patient lying down as viewed from the top. Before moving the patient into position B, turn the head 45° to the side being treated (in this case it would be the right side): patient is in normal Dix-Hallpike head-hanging position (B). Particles gravitate in an ampullofugal direction and induce utriculofugal cupular displacement and subsequent counter-clockwise rotatory nystagmus. This position is maintained for 1–2 minutes. The patient's head is then rotated toward the opposite side with the neck in full extension through position C and into position D in a steady motion by rolling the patient onto the opposite lateral side. The change from position B to D should take no longer than 3–5 seconds. Particles continue gravitating in an ampullofugal direction through the common crus into the utricle. The patient's eyes are immediately observed for nystagmus. Position D is maintained for another 1–2 minutes, and then the patient sits back up to position A. (D) = direction of view of labyrinth, dark circle = position of particle conglomerate, open circle = previous position.

Source: Adapted from LS Parnes and J Robichaud. Further observations during the practice repositioning maneuver for benign paroxysmal positional vertigo. *Otolaryngol Head Neck Surg* 1997;116: 238–43.

"timing" characteristic depends on recognition of *continuous* symptoms over days to weeks, unlike EVS, which consists of brief episodes lasting seconds to hours even if they *recur* over days or weeks. When symptoms are present at the time of assessment, a physical exam can be useful for localizing the cause (e.g., focal neurological deficits, otitis media, or herpes zoster rash of Ramsey-Hunt syndrome). It is important to note, however, that a provocative test such as the Dix-Hallpike maneuver used to detect posterior semicircular canal otoliths will predictably exacerbate dizziness in an AVS patient who is experiencing head movement intolerance, and this exacerbating feature is commonly misinterpreted as a trigger. Likewise, the history may reveal a toxic drug exposure (i.e., phenytoin or gentamicin) or head trauma. One must be careful not to prematurely ascribe AVS to a peripheral labyrinth disorder as a result of exposure to a recent viral upper respiratory infection before an appropriate evaluation has excluded dangerous causes such as stroke.

> In acute, continuous dizziness, patients will feel worse when their head is moved, but this exacerbating feature has no diagnostic value. All AVS patients, whether due to stroke or vestibular neuritis, will feel worse when moved. Do not perform the Dix-Hallpike test in these patients.

Differential diagnosis

It is critical when a patient presents with AVS to differentiate between urgent and less urgent causes. An abridged differential diagnosis is provided in Table 9.2. Head trauma and medication are the most common exposures causing AVS. When the onset of AVS is spontaneous (i.e., lacking an obvious antecedent exposure), then acute unilateral peripheral vestibular neuritis (dizziness or vertigo only) or labyrinthitis (dizziness or vertigo with hearing loss) is likely. However, vestibular neuritis and labyrinthitis are diagnoses of exclusion, and stroke (particularly of the posterior fossa) can mimic either very closely. Note that focal neurologic signs and symptoms may be absent in approximately 80% of patients with stroke presenting with AVS.[17] Computed tomography (CT) has extremely low sensitivity (16%) for acute ischemic stroke,[18] so unless the patient has severe headache, lethargy, or hemiparesis (signs of cerebellar hemorrhage), CT should not be performed when

imaging is required.[19] Magnetic resonance (MRI) with diffusion-weighted imaging (DWI) misses approximately 15%–20% in the first 24 to 48 hours after onset of continuous symptoms, but it is our current gold standard test when obtained from 72 hours to seven days.[20] When encountering a patient with isolated AVS, strong evidence indicates that a careful eye exam (HINTS to INFARCT) outperforms MRI in ruling out stroke (Table 9.3).[20, 21] A central stroke, usually in the posterior fossa, is very likely when the patient has any one of three dangerous eye movement signs: (1) normal head impulse test of the vestibular ocular reflex, (2) fast-phase alternating nystagmus, or (3) vertical ocular misalignment (i.e., vertical skew deviation of eyes). Note that, paradoxically, a *normal* head impulse test is not good (that is *normal*, in the context of AVS, supports stroke).

In contrast, vestibular neuritis without hearing loss is likely when the bedside head impulse test of the vestibular ocular reflex is abnormal; there is predominantly horizontal, "direction-fixed" nystagmus consistently beating the opposite direction of the head impulse abnormality, regardless of the gaze position; and there is normal ocular vertical alignment with alternating cover test (absence of skew). Presence of all three findings has a tenfold greater power to rule out stroke than early MRI (negative likelihood ratio of 0.02 (CI: 0.01–0.09) vs. 0.21 (CI: 0.16 – 0.26).[22] Although this approach is now well validated in expert hands, it has not been tested when applied by nonspecialists. New portable video oculography devices may eventually make testing for these signs in primary or urgent care more readily available.[23]

> In acute, continuous dizziness, eye movement exams (HINTS) outperform our current gold standard, MRI, to look for ischemic stroke. New devices may eventually make it easier for primary care physicians to test these eye movements. Do not bother with CT unless a rare case of cerebellar hemorrhage is suspected.

Treatment

After stroke or other dangerous causes are ruled out, young patients with AVS due to vestibular neuritis and labyrinthitis are often able to be sent home from the emergency department with medication to suppress nausea and dizziness. Frail older adults, by

121

contrast, may require hospitalization to ensure that symptoms are controlled and hydration is maintained.

Chronic dizziness lasting from months to years

Many older adults have chronic vestibular syndrome (CVS). This category of dizziness is usually related to a chronic, progressive neurological or vestibular condition with pathological findings that are present at the time of examination that often suggest the diagnosis. Symptoms may be stable or progressive over months to years, even though they may fluctuate in severity over time. Dizziness is often context dependent, such as when the patient reports feeling dizzy only or always when walking. This should not be interpreted as "episodic" or as "triggered" by an upright posture. Because dizziness typically develops gradually with the progression of the underlying neurological or vestibular condition, patients most often seek evaluation in an outpatient setting.

In the elderly, common causes of CVS that are associated with unsteadiness are sensory peripheral neuropathy (e.g., diabetes, B12 and thyroid deficiency) and dizziness related to the gait disorder resulting from Parkinson's disease, degenerative joint disease of the lower extremities with instability, or dementia. Other causes are listed in Table 9.4. A thorough assessment of the patient includes bedside examination of musculoskeletal function and testing for upper motor neuron and extrapyramidal motor abnormalities; autonomic system dysfunction; peripheral sensory abnormalities; and vestibular, ocular, and cerebellar impairment. Depending on the patient's general health and preferences, neuroimaging may be indicated to rule out treatable conditions such as hydrocephalus.

Treatment

Chronic vestibular syndrome associated with gait unsteadiness may improve, depending on the cause, with physical conditioning and gait training, and with the use of an appropriate assistive device (e.g., cane, walker, or wheelchair). Correctable causes of dizziness may be uncovered by a careful history and physical exam, as well as targeted laboratory tests. Medications, whether recently started or long-standing, are common causes of dizziness. Careful medication assessment and reduction should be considered whenever possible. Correcting electrolyte and metabolic abnormalities such as hyponatremia, hyperglycemia, hypothyroidism, and B12 deficiency may also lead to resolution or improvement.

> Dizziness in the elderly is often multifactorial. Fix everything that is "fixable," emphasizing treatable neurologic and iatrogenic conditions (e.g., medication toxicity).

List of relevant web pages

American Academy of Neurology (Treatment Guidelines and Videos for BPPV Maneuvers):
www.aan.com/guidelines
www.neurology.org/content/70/22/2067/suppl/DC2
Dizziness and Balance (Timothy Hain):
www.dizziness-and-balance.com/index.html
Journal of Vestibular Research – Barany Society International Classification of Vestibular Disorders page (consensus criteria and definitions for vestibular disorders):
www.jvr-web.org/Barany.html

Table 9.4 Core differential diagnosis of chronic vestibular syndrome

(*Illness onset*: months–years)	
Nonspontaneous (context-dependent)	Spontaneous
While walking: Parkinson's disease, multisensory dizziness *While head moving:* chronic uni- or bilateral vestibulopathy *While eyes open:* visual dizziness (e.g., diplopia, new glasses)	*Less urgent:* cerebellar degeneration, post-concussive dizziness, presbylibrium, PPPD *More urgent:* cerebellar tumor, hydrocephalus, metabolic deficiency (e.g., Wilson's, B12, E), autoimmune or paraneoplastic cerebellopathy

PPPD – Persistent, Perceptual Postural Dizziness
Source: Modified from Newman-Toker.[24]

Neuro-Ophthalmology Virtual Education Library (NOVEL) (Newman-Toker Collection):

http://novel.utah.edu/Newman-Toker

References

1. Bisdorff A, Von Brevern M, Lempert T, Newman-Toker DE. Classification of vestibular symptoms: towards an international classification of vestibular disorders. *J Vestib Res.* 2009;**19**(1–2):1–13.

2. Newman-Toker DE, Cannon LM, Stofferahn ME, Rothman RE, Hsieh YH, Zee DS. Imprecision in patient reports of dizziness symptom quality: a cross-sectional study conducted in an acute care setting. *Mayo Clin Proc.* 2007 Nov;**82**(11):1329–40.

3. Sloane PD. Dizziness in primary care: results from the National Ambulatory Medical Care Survey. *J Fam Pract.* 1989;**29**(1):33–8.

4. Kroenke K, Mangelsdorff AD. Common symptoms in ambulatory care: incidence, evaluation, therapy, and outcome. *Am J Med.* 1989;**86**(3):262–6.

5. Jonsson R, Sixt E, Landahl S, Rosenhall U. Prevalence of dizziness and vertigo in an urban elderly population. *J Vestib Res.* 2004;**14**(1):47–52.

6. Wolinsky FD, Fitzgerald JF. The risk of hip fracture among noninstitutionalized older adults. *J Gerontol.* 1994;**49**(4):165–75.

7. Wolinsky FD, Fitzgerald JF. Subsequent hip fracture among older adults. *Am J Public Health.* 1994;**84**(8):1316–18.

8. Kao AC, Nanda A, Williams CS, Tinetti ME. Validation of dizziness as a possible geriatric syndrome. *J Am Geriatr Soc.* 2001;**49**(1):72–5.

9. Newman-Toker DE. *Diagnosing Dizziness In the Emergency Department – Why "What do you mean by 'dizzy'?" Should Not Be the First Question You Ask.* [Doctoral Dissertation, Clinical Investigation, Bloomberg School of Public Health] [PhD Clinical Investigation]. Baltimore, MD: The Johns Hopkins University; 2007.

10. Drachman DA. A 69-year-old man with chronic dizziness. *JAMA.* 1998;**280**(24):2111–8.

11. Newman-Toker DE. Symptoms and signs of neuro-otologic disorders. *Continuum (Minneap Minn).* 2012 Oct;**18**(5 Neuro-otology):1016–40.

12. Newman-Toker DE, Dy FJ, Stanton VA, Zee DS, Calkins H, Robinson KA. Primary cardiovascular disease causes true vertigo – a systematic review. Abstracts of the Bárány Society XXV International Congress, Kyoto, Japan, Mar 31–Apr 3, 2008. *J Vestib Res.* 2008.

13. Paul NL, Simoni M, Rothwell PM. Transient isolated brainstem symptoms preceding posterior circulation stroke: a population-based study. *Lancet Neurology.* 2013 Jan;**12**(1):65–71.

14. Newman-Toker DE, Dy FJ, Stanton VA, Zee DS, Calkins H, Robinson KA. How often is dizziness from primary cardiovascular disease true vertigo? A systematic review. *J Gen Intern Med.* 2008 Dec;**23**(12):2087–94.

15. Fife TD, Iverson DJ, Lempert T, Furman JM, Baloh RW, Tusa RJ, et al. Practice parameter: therapies for benign paroxysmal positional vertigo (an evidence-based review): report of the Quality Standards Subcommittee of the American Academy of Neurology. *Neurology.* 2008;**70**(22):2067–74.

16. Lempert T, Neuhauser H, Daroff RB. Vertigo as a symptom of migraine. *Annals of the New York Academy of Sciences.* 2009 May;**1164**:242–51.

17. Kattah JC, Talkad AV, Wang DZ, Hsieh YH, Newman-Toker DE. HINTS to diagnose stroke in the acute vestibular syndrome: three-step bedside oculomotor examination more sensitive than early MRI diffusion-weighted imaging. *Stroke.* 2009 Nov;**40**(11):3504–10.

18. Chalela JA, Kidwell CS, Nentwich LM, Luby M, Butman JA, Demchuk AM, et al. Magnetic resonance imaging and computed tomography in emergency assessment of patients with suspected acute stroke: a prospective comparison. *Lancet.* 2007;**369**(9558):293–8.

19. Edlow JA, Newman-Toker DE, Savitz SI. Diagnosis and initial management of cerebellar infarction. *Lancet Neurol.* 2008 Oct;7(10):951–64.

20. Newman-Toker DE, Kerber KA, Hsieh YH, Pula JH, Omron R, Saber Tehrani AS, et al. HINTS outperforms ABCD2 to screen for stroke in acute continuous vertigo and dizziness. *Academic Emergency Medicine: Official Journal of the Society for Academic Emergency Medicine.* 2013 Oct;**20**(10):986–96.

21. Saber Tehrani AS, Kattah JC, Mantokoudis G, Pula JH, Nair D, Blitz A, et al. Small strokes causing severe vertigo: frequency of false-negative MRIs and nonlacunar mechanisms. *Neurology.* 2014 Jul 8;**83**(2):169–73.

22. Tarnutzer AA, Berkowitz AL, Robinson KA, Hsieh YH, Newman-Toker DE. Does my dizzy patient have a stroke? A systematic review of bedside diagnosis in acute vestibular syndrome. *CMAJ: Canadian Medical Association Journal [Journal de l'Association medicale canadienne].* [Research Support, Non-US Gov't Research Support, US Gov't, PHS Review]. 2011 Jun 14;**183**(9):E571–92.

23. Newman-Toker DE, Saber Tehrani AS, Mantokoudis G, Pula JH, Guede CI, Kerber KA, et al.

Quantitative video-oculography to help diagnose stroke in acute vertigo and dizziness: toward an ECG for the eyes. *Stroke: A Journal of Cerebral Circulation*. [Research Support, N.I.H., Extramural Research Support, Non-US Gov't Research Support, US Gov't, PHS]. 2013 Apr;**44**(4):1158–61.

24. Newman-Toker DE. Vertigo and dizziness. In: Aminoff MJ, Daroff RB, editors. *Encyclopedia of the Neurological Sciences*. 2nd ed. Oxford: Elsevier; 2014: 629–37.

25. Parnes LS, Agrawal SK, Atlas J. Diagnosis and management of benign paroxysmal positional vertigo (BPPV). *CMAJ*. 2003;**169**(7):681–93.

Chapter 10

Evaluation and management of dementia

Lauren Collins, MD, Barry W. Rovner, MD, and
Kadesha Collins-Fletcher, MD

Key clinical points/pearls

- Diagnostic criteria for dementia are now separated into major and minor neurocognitive disorder and are based on severity of decline from a previous level of functioning (DSM-5).[1]
- Alzheimer's dementia remains the most common form of dementia in the elderly, accounting for 60%–80% of all cases;[2] however, "mixed" dementia representing a combination of Alzheimer's plus vascular and/or or Lewy body pathology is increasingly recognized.
- Although a definitive diagnosis of a particular dementia syndrome often requires a postmortem examination, a comprehensive approach with a thorough history taking, physical examination, tailored laboratory work and imaging studies, and neuropsychiatric testing when appropriate permit a probable diagnosis in the majority of cases.
- Multidimensional, tailored interventions have been shown to be effective in reducing caregiver burden as well as decreasing behavioral and psychological disturbances in patients with dementia.[2, 3]

Definition

The American Psychiatric Association released the fifth edition of *Diagnostic and Statistical Manual of Mental Disorders* (DSM-5) in 2013. Diagnostic criteria for dementia are now separated into major and minor neurocognitive disorders. The diagnostic criteria for "major neurocognitive disorder" are characterized by cognitive symptoms representing a significant decline from a previous level of functioning in at least one cognitive domain. These include memory and learning impairment, impairment in processing speed (i.e.,

the rate at which a task is completed), inability to recall the days of the week in reverse (complex attention), impairment in accuracy (perceptual-motor), and impairment in handling complex tasks (executive function). These cognitive symptoms must interfere with an aspect of instrumental activities of daily living and compromise independence. The singular criterion for mild neurocognitive disorder is moderate decline in cognition not affecting the ability to perform daily complex tasks. For both major and minor neurocognitive disorders, the disturbances are self-reported or detection is the result of informant concerns; in addition, the impairment is captured on clinical cognitive assessment or neuropsychological testing. The disturbances must be insidious in onset and progressive, and must not be better accounted for by another psychiatric diagnosis, such as delirium, or systemic disease.[1]

Epidemiology

The prevalence of dementia has been estimated to be approximately 11% of individuals aged 65 or older. The prevalence of dementia increases with age, rising from 15% among those aged 65–74 to more than 38% of those 85 years and older.[2] Incidence rates of Alzheimer's disease (AD) demonstrate exponential growth, doubling every five years after the age of 65, at least until the age of 90. The cost of caring for people with dementia is substantial. Current annual economic cost of dementia is estimated to be $214 billion. With the anticipated doubling of the population aged 65 and older by 2050, the financial impact of dementia on our society will be even more dramatic at an estimated $1.2 trillion.[2, 5]

Risk factors

Determining risk factors for dementia has been an area of intense study (see Table 10.1). The prevalence of AD

Reichel's Care of the Elderly, *7th Edition*, ed. Jan Busby-Whitehead *et al.* Published by Cambridge University Press.
© Cambridge University Press 2016.

Table 10.1 Risk factors for dementia

Identified risk factors	Additional potential risk factors
Age	Mild cognitive impairment (MCI)
Family history	Cardiovascular risk factors
APOE genetic endowment	Hypertension
Down syndrome	Diabetes mellitus
Traumatic brain injury (TBI)	Hyperlipidemia
	Elevated plasma homocysteine level
	High dietary fat intake
	Smoking Midlife and late-life depression Limited social and cognitive engagement Fewer years of formal education Vitamin D deficiency

Source: Adapted from references 2, 8, 9, 10, and 18.

and other dementias appears to be higher in African Americans and Hispanics. Many risk factors for dementia are not modifiable; thus, the search for ways to prevent dementia has garnered much attention. An observational study reported an association between vitamin D deficiency and decline in cognition,[6] and a prospective study found an increased risk of dementia in primary caregivers of spouses with dementia.[7] Other studies have shown that social, mental, and physical activity appear to be inversely associated with the risk for dementia, but these data come from large observational studies and meta-analyses that require additional validation.[8–12] It remains unclear if adopting these lifestyle characteristics will attenuate the risk for developing dementia.

Dementia subtypes

There are several different subtypes of dementia, with Alzheimer's dementia (AD) being the most common form. Definitive diagnosis for dementia requires pathological evaluation. However, recent dementia

research has demonstrated significant overlap between the various dementia syndromes, particularly between AD and vascular dementia (VaD).[13, 14] The etiology of certain dementia syndromes may be traced to a common pathophysiology. For example, it appears that the neurodegenerative dementias, such as AD, frontotemporal dementia (FTD), dementia with Lewy bodies (DLB), and prion disorders may actually be linked mechanistically to the conversion of normal proteins into insoluble aggregates. These aggregates form cerebral deposits or neuronal inclusions prompting neurotoxic cascades that attempt to remove the misfolded proteins.[15]

Alzheimer's disease

In 2011, the National Institute on Aging and the Alzheimer's Association Workgroup revised the diagnostic criteria for AD. The revision identified three distinct stages of AD: preclinical AD (no clinical application; diagnosed using cerebral spinal fluid and neuroimaging as biomarkers and intended to guide research); mild cognitive impairment attributed to AD without functional deficits; and dementia due to AD with cognitive impairment severe enough to cause deficits in activities of daily living.[16]

Alzheimer's dementia is the most common form of dementia in the elderly, accounting for 60%– 80% of all cases.[2] It is estimated that approximately 5 million adults over the age of 65 are currently living with AD in the United States.[2, 17] The cost of caring for one patient with AD is $47,000 per year, primarily as a result of hospitalization, long-term care, and hospice.[2] The economic burden of this disease is surpassed only by the tremendous social and emotional burden on patients, families, and caregivers.

Epidemiological research has identified the following risk factors for AD: age, presence of the apolipoprotein E epsilon 4 (APO E4) genotype, family history, Down syndrome, and head trauma. Cardiovascular risk factors, including diabetes, hypertension, and lipid abnormalities, have also been associated with AD.[8–10] It appears that "what is good for the heart is good for the brain."

Higher education has been found to be a protective risk factor for AD. Experts believe that individual differences in how tasks are processed may allow for a degree of "cognitive reserve" from brain pathology. Participation in both leisure and physical activity may also be protective for development of AD.[2]

Brain pathology consistent with AD includes the presence of extracellular amyloid-β protein-42 ($A\beta_{42}$) deposition, intracellular neurofibrillary tangles (NFTs), and dystrophic neuritis.[19, 20] AD is characterized by accumulation of an abnormal form of the protein tau inside neurons, leading to neuronal loss, especially among neurons that release the neurotransmitter acetylcholine.[19, 21]

The etiology of neuronal damage in the brains in AD patients is believed to be related to misfolded proteins that trigger oxidative and inflammatory damage to the neurons. The pathophysiology of AD likely traces back to a family of amyloid precursor proteins that are cleaved by specific secretases. When amyloid precursor protein is cleaved by a γ-secretase on one end and a β-secretase on the other end, a highly amyloidogenic Abeta42 protein is released. This protein appears to aggregate in diffuse plaques, which evolve into dense neuritic plaques.[22] Abeta oligomers, therefore, are probable mediators of neurotoxicity.[23] Once the neuritic plaque has formed, secondary cascades of inflammation, excitotoxicity, and apoptosis may trigger additional damage.[19]

The formation of NFTs and their role in the pathophysiology of AD remains controversial. NFTs consist of a hyperphosphorylated form of the microtubule-associated protein, tau. Severity of cognitive decline correlates with NFT burden more so than with amyloid deposition, suggesting that a mutant tau protein, rather than the NFT, may be the primary neurotoxic mediator.[24, 25] Cleavage of tau, a critical step in NFT formation, appears to be triggered by accumulation of Abeta42 protein through activation of caspases. Interestingly, brain changes may accumulate for more than 20 years before clinical symptoms are observed, leading experts to recognize that there may be a "continuum" of AD in which individuals are initially able to function without impairment but may progress as neuronal damage escalates.[2]

Clinically, AD is characterized by an insidious onset, and early detection is often the result of informant concerns. Early symptoms include loss of short-term memory, repeating statements, and apathy or depression. Later symptoms include difficulty with communication, confusion, poor judgment, and behavior changes. More advanced symptoms include difficulty speaking, swallowing, and walking. In late stages of AD, patients frequently become dependent on others for activities of daily living (ADLs), such as bathing and toileting.

AD is marked by a gradually progressive course and a shortened life expectancy. The sixth leading cause of death in the United Sates and the fifth leading of all-cause mortality in individuals aged 65 and older is AD. Median survival time from time of diagnosis is four to eight years.[2] Mortality predictors include dementia severity at time of diagnosis, abnormal neurological findings, and the presence of comorbidities, such as heart disease and diabetes.[26] Pneumonia is the most common terminal event in patients with progressive dementia.

Vascular dementia and vascular cognitive impairment

Cerebrovascular disease (CVD) is a heterogeneous group of disorders characterized by brain infarct, cerebral hemorrhage, white matter lesions, atherosclerosis, cerebral amyloid angiopathy, and genetic disorders.[27, 31, 32] Cerebrovascular disease is implicated in and contributes to various subtypes of dementia.[29] Due to a lack of consensus on the diagnostic criteria for vascular dementia (VaD), identification of VaD has been challenging for clinicians, and estimates of prevalence are harder to identify.[27, 29, 30] The American Heart Association (AHA) and American Stroke Association (ASA) recently proposed the terminology vascular cognitive impairment (VCI) to include syndromes of cognitive impairment with evidence of either clinical or subclinical vascular brain injury, spanning a spectrum from least severe to most severe.[27]

Vascular dementia (or VCI) is currently believed to be the second most common etiology for dementia, with risk doubling every 5.3 years after the age of 65. [27, 31, 33] Prevalence increases with both age and male gender.[27] Risk factors are similar to those for CVD and include hypertension, diabetes mellitus, smoking, hyperlipidemia, and atrial fibrillation.[27, 31, 33]

Diffuse hypoxia, disruption of the blood brain barrier, inflammation, and oxidative stress alter the neuronal networks involved in cognition, behavior, memory, and execution.[13, 27] Studies have shown that both AD and vascular lesions often coexist in approximately 25%–80% of subjects with dementia, confirming an overlap in these syndromes.[13] Increasingly experts agree that "mixed" dementia with AD plus VCI is far more common than previously recognized.[13]

Despite suffering from a lack of uniform diagnostic criteria, clinical features that may suggest the diagnosis VCI include onset of temporal cognitive deficit in two or more cognitive domains particularly in complex attention and frontal-executive function, abrupt onset of symptoms followed by a stepwise deterioration, and findings on physical examination that are consistent with a previous stroke.[1, 27, 29] Neuropathology in VCI shows focal, multifocal, or diffuse lesions, including white matter lesions (WMLs), lacunar and other cerebral microbleeds (CMBs), and hippocampal atrophy.[13, 27]

Frontotemporal dementia

Pathologically, frontotemporal dementia (FTD) is characterized by focal atrophy of the frontal and temporal lobes, in the absence of findings consistent with AD.[34] Specific regions of atrophy correlate with the clinical and neuropathological syndrome. [35] These regions often show decreased perfusion on single photon emission computed tomography, fluoro-deoxyglucose positron emission tomography (FDG-PET), and perfusion MRI.[36, 37, 38] Although mutations in the tau gene on chromosome 17 have been implicated in familial FTD, the pathogenesis of nonfamilial FTD remains unclear. [39, 40] Autopsy, neuroimaging, and cerebrospinal fluid studies suggest that FTD is characterized by a serotonergic deficit, which likely contributes to the behavioral abnormalities associated with FTD.[41]

There are three distinct clinical subtypes of FTD: behavioral, language, and motor.[42, 43] The behavioral subtype is the most common form of FTD, with 90% of patients developing personality changes during the course of their illness. The personality change is often dramatic and is characterized by social inappropriateness, poor judgment, and disinhibition.[44] Impairment of executive function, insight, and memory are also common features in behavioral FTD.[45, 46] Individuals affected by the behavioral-variant FTD often develop symptoms around age 60, younger than many patients typically diagnosed with dementia syndromes. Findings on perfusion imaging studies often correlate with behavioral symptoms. For example, prominent frontal hypoperfusion is associated with apathy and poor hygiene and self-care, and prominent temporal hypoperfusion is associated with hypomania and compulsive behaviors.[37]

Early progressive language dysfunction or "primary progressive aphasia" is the second most common phenotype in FTD and is characterized by three subtypes: progressive nonfluent aphasia (or nonfluent/agrammatic aphasia); progressive fluent aphasia (or semantic dementia); and progressive mixed aphasia (or logopenic aphasia). Progressive nonfluent aphasia is characterized pathologically by prominent inferior lobe atrophy and clinically by difficulty with interruption in speech. With progression, logorrhea (abundant unfocused speech) may develop. Progressive fluent aphasia is associated with marked anterior temporal lobe atrophy that may lead to white matter tract enervation, thereby inhibiting communication. Patients often present with difficulty in naming and in understanding words (secondary to involvement of the left temporal lobe) or with difficulty in face and object recognition but with normal speech (secondary to involvement of right temporal lobe). Progressive mixed aphasia is characterized pathologically by prominent parietal lobe atrophy and clinically by word-finding difficulty and inability to produce meaningful use (phonemic paraphasia). [47] Further studies are needed regarding the sensitivity of this new subtyping criteria.

The third type of FTD involves a prominent motor component on presentation. Patients demonstrate extra pyramidal motor symptoms or signs of bulbar or spinal motor neuron disease. Patients with bulbar or spinal motor neuron disease (FTD–motor neuron disease) often have motor symptoms within 12 months of disease onset and generally have a rapidly progressive disease course.[45]

Dementia with parkinsonism

A number of parkinsonian disorders are associated with dementia. The two most common forms of dementia with parkinsonism are dementia with Lewy bodies (DLB) and Parkinson's disease dementia (PDD). Atypical parkinsonian syndromes such as progressive supranuclear palsy (PSP), multisystem atrophy, and corticobasilar ganglionic degeneration also produce dementia syndromes.

Dementia with Lewy bodies

Dementia with Lewy bodies (DLB) now appears to be the second most common form of neurodegenerative dementia in older adults, with prevalence estimates ranging from 15% to 20% of all cases.[48, 49] A population study observed that the incidence rate was 3.5 per 100,000 person-years. DLB is associated with a younger onset and male sex, and increases exponentially with age.[50]

Pathologically, numerous Lewy bodies characterize DLB, but plaques and NFTs, often seen in AD, may also be present.[49] New immunocytochemical staining for ubiquitin, α-synuclein and NFTs has aided greatly in the detection of cortical Lewy bodies and significantly improved the detection of the disorder in postmortem studies.[51–55] Neuroimaging with (123I)beta-CIT SPECT and 18FDG-PET demonstrated high sensitivity for differentiating DLB from non-DLB via the decreased uptake of dopamine transporter at the presynaptic cleft in the basal ganglia. Pathologically, DLB is believed to be a consequence of α-synuclein aggregation.[56–58]

Despite improved pathological detection, the clinical diagnosis of DLB is still challenging. Patients with DLB can be distinguished from those with AD and VaD by parkinsonian features (including slowness and gait impairment) as well as marked cognitive fluctuations, persistent well-formed hallucinations, and coexisting sleep disturbances.[14, 49] With the inclusion of REM sleep behavior disorder (RBD) into the clinical diagnostic criteria for DLB in 2005, the likelihood of autopsy-confirmed DLB has increased.[59] DLB should be suspected in patients with signs of parkinsonism such as bradykinesia, muscular rigidity, and tremor. Supportive features for the diagnosis include a history of repeated falls, syncope, sensitivity to neuroleptic medications, delusions, hallucinations in nonvisual modes, and depression.[49] Of note, distinguishing DLB from AD and other dementias may be particularly important because of the risk of adverse events with antipsychotic medications in affected patients.[48] Also, patients with DLB may benefit from a trial of levodopa therapy, making early detection even more valuable. Prognosis for DLB appears to be slightly worse than that for AD, with some patients having a rapidly progressive course.[14]

Parkinson's disease dementia

Patients with Parkinson's disease (PD) have a significantly increased risk of developing associated dementia.[60] In one prospective cohort study, 30% of patients developed dementia within five years.[61] Patients with PD have gray matter atrophy in the limbic, paralimbic, and prefrontal regions. On pathological examination, Parkinson's disease dementia (PDD) demonstrates accumulation of α-synuclein aggregates in the substantia nigra, as well as accumulation of Lewy bodies in the cortex and other findings consistent with AD such as B-amyloid clumping and the presence of tau tangles throughout the brain.[62, 63]

Although PDD shares features of DLB pathologically, its clinical presentation differs from that of DLB in that it is defined by the onset of dementia in the setting of PD within one year. The dementia associated with PD is characterized by executive dysfunction, attention impairment, and memory impairment.[63]

Progressive supranuclear palsy

Progressive supranuclear palsy (PSP) mimics PD in its early stages, and patients are often found to have postural instability, bradykinesia, and rigidity. PSP is distinguished from PD by the presence of vertical supranuclear palsy with downward gaze abnormalities. Also, in contrast to PD, the bradykinesia and rigidity are often symmetrical.[64] Patients with PSP generally have a poor response to levodopa and frequently develop a pseudobulbar palsy with dysarthria and dysphagia.[65, 66]

Pathologically, patients with PSP have globose NFTs made up of hyperphosphorylated tau proteins. These lesions with associated neuronal loss are found in the substantia nigra, subthalamic nucleus, globus pallidus, superior colliculus, midbrain, and pons. Cortical involvement generally involves the frontal lobe as well.

Not surprisingly, the dementia associated with PSP is frequently a frontal lobe syndrome; however, it is more rapidly progressive than many other neurodegenerative dementias, with a median time to death following diagnosis of only six years.[67]

Creutzfeldt-Jakob disease

Human prion disease consists of a rare group of neurodegenerative diseases resulting from a misfolded protein (prion) that causes the brain to malfunction. Subtypes include Creutzfeldt-Jakob disease (sporadic CJD), variant Creutzfeldt-Jakob disease, Gerstmann-Sträussler-Scheinker syndrome, Kuru, and fatal insomnia.[68, 69] However, Creutzfeldt-Jakob disease (sporadic CJD) accounts for approximately 85% of prion disease.

Clinically, sporadic CJD presents with a rapid onset of cognitive impairment as well as motor deficits and seizures; mean age of onset is approximately 65 years old.[69] It should be suspected in any patient presenting with a rapidly progressive dementia, visual disturbance, change in personality, and ataxia.[69, 70] Mean duration of illness is eight months.[69]

Variant Creutzfeldt-Jakob disease is the second common type of prion disease and usually affects young adults. The primary risk factor is consumption of contaminated cattle affected by "mad cow" disease. Clinical presentation is a gradual onset associated with psychiatric and neurological manifestations.[68, 69] Electroencephalography, cerebrospinal fluid studies, and gray matter abnormalities on diffusion MRI can be helpful in determining the diagnosis.[71–73]

Reversible dementia

Although potentially reversible causes of dementia account for less than 10% of cases of dementia, identifying and treating these disorders remain a top priority.[74–76] Vitamin deficiencies, thyroid dysfunction, depression, and normal-pressure hydrocephalus (NPH) have all been identified as more common reversible causes of dementia to consider in the initial differential diagnosis (see Table 10.2) of a patient presenting with cognitive impairment, but there are numerous causes of potentially reversible dementias in an expanded differential (see Table 10.3). Although these syndromes are considered "potentially" reversible, it is important to note that the majority of patients with these syndromes do not improve even when these disorders are promptly discovered and treated. Rates of reversal range from only 0.6% to 11% of cases.[76, 77]

Normal-pressure hydrocephalus

Patients with NPH often present with a triad of gait disturbance ("magnetic gait"), urinary incontinence, and cognitive dysfunction. Although NPH should be considered in patients with these symptoms, it is also important to recognize that many older adults have one or more of these symptoms in the absence of NPH. Nevertheless, NPH is amenable to treatment with a surgical shunt and, therefore, should still be considered in patients who fit the clinical scenario. Risk factors include patients with a history of brain hemorrhage and meningitis. Confirmatory studies include imaging studies, radioisotope diffusion studies, and the Fisher test, which involves gait

Table 10.2 Differential diagnosis of cognitive impairment

Alzheimer's dementia (AD)
Vascular dementia (VaD)
Frontotemporal dementia (FTD)
Parkinson's disease dementia (PDD)
Dementia with Lewy bodies (DLB)
Creutzfeldt-Jakob disease (CJD)
Progressive supranuclear palsy (PSP)
Normal-pressure hydrocephalus
Alcohol-related dementia
Medication-induced dementia
AIDS dementia
Delirium
Major depressive disorder with cognitive impairment
Mild cognitive impairment (MCI)
Metabolic disorders

Source: Adapted from reference 211.

assessment before and after the removal of 30 mL of cerebrospinal fluid. The Fisher test is also useful in predicting a response to ventriculoperitoneal shunting, the treatment of choice.[14, 77, 78]

Delirium

Delirium, a condition characterized by fluctuating levels of consciousness and inattention, must also be distinguished from dementia. Whereas dementia is characterized by an insidious onset, the onset of delirium is usually abrupt and often precipitated by illness, intoxication, or medication. Delirium is associated with a high morbidity and mortality, but unlike dementia, delirium typically resolves if the underlying cause is addressed.[80, 81] Still, recovery from delirium may be protracted in older adults, and delirium may even become chronic in some patients, making it difficult to distinguish from dementia. (See Chapter 11 for more details.)

Mild cognitive impairment

Mild cognitive impairment (MCI) is a more recent research construct that attempts to define cognitive

Table 10.3 Potentially reversible dementias

Medication induced:
- Analgesics
- Anticholinergics
- Psychotropic medications
- Sedative hypnotics
- Steroids

Alcohol related:
- Intoxication
- Withdrawal

Metabolic disorders:
- Thyroid disease
- Vitamin B12 deficiency
- Hyponatremia
- Hypercalcemia

Hepatic dysfunction

Renal dysfunction

Depression ("pseudodementia")

Central nervous system neoplasm

Chronic subdural hematoma

Chronic meningitis

Normal-pressure hydrocephalus (NPH)

Human immunodeficiency virus

Creutzfeldt-Jakob disease (CJD)

Source: Adapted from references 75, 76.

impairment that does not significantly affect function, a hallmark of dementia. Most experts agree that MCI is a known risk factor for dementia, but studies have demonstrated that progression from MCI into dementia is variable. The prevalence of MCI observed in the Mayo Clinic Study of Aging (MCSA), a prospective study of community-dwelling adults 70–89 years of age without dementia, was 16% with a higher prevalence among men.[82] In another recent study, the incidence of MCI was 64 per 1,000 person-years, with a higher incidence in men.[83]

Neuropsychological testing further categorizes MCI into subtypes – amnestic (aMCI) or nonamestic (naMCI) – and as single-domain (sdMCI) or multiple-domain (mdMCI), dependent on the number of cognitive domain impairments on testing.[82, 83]

Patients with aMCI present with subjective or objective concerns regarding memory impairment with or without any cognitive domain deficit on exam and are most likely to transition to AD. Risk factors for aMCI include male gender, lower education level, social inactivity, and increasing age.[82–84] Patients with naMCI present clinically without memory impairment and may progress to dementia not due to AD.[83] A prospective population-based study observed that cardiac risk factors increase the likelihood of naMCI by threefold in women.[82, 85]

Progression of MCI to dementia varies, with an observed annual conversion rate of 5%–10%.[86] Predictors for progression to dementia include APOE epsilon4 allele carriers, amyloid deposition, CSF biomarkers, cerebral glucose hypometabolism, temporal lobe atrophy, and clinical severity of cognitive impairment.[87–93]

Diagnostic approach

Although a definitive diagnosis of a particular dementia syndrome often requires a postmortem examination, a comprehensive approach with a thorough history taking, physical examination, tailored laboratory work and imaging studies, and neuropsychiatric testing when appropriate permit a probable diagnosis in the majority of cases. In fact, in studies of AD, a diagnosis of "probable" AD was accurate in 90% of cases based on history from the patient and family members in combination with a clinical examination.[94]

History

Most patients with dementia do not present with a subjective complaint of memory loss. Rather, a caregiver or family member often raises the concern of memory loss or behavioral change to the practitioner. For example, informants may report that the patient has had trouble remembering events and preparing finances, has gotten lost in familiar settings, cannot find appropriate words, or has been demonstrating unusual behaviors. Informants play an integral role in helping providers understand the onset, nature, and progression of symptoms.

A thorough history also hinges on a systematic review of prescription and over-the-counter medication use. Use of medications that may impair cognition, such as anticholinergics, psychotropics, and sedative hypnotics, should be determined. Performing a functional assessment is another key step in the evaluation of patients with dementia. Functional impairment is often assessed by asking the patient and family members or informants about instrumental ADLs (i.e., managing finances, household chores, and taking medications) and ADLs (i.e., dressing, grooming, and toileting). The Global Deterioration Scale and Functional Assessment Staging is another standardized tool that can be used to measure dementia-related dependency.[65]

Physical examination

A comprehensive history and functional assessment should be followed by a complete physical examination. During the physical exam, special attention should be given to the neurologic examination to evaluate other possible causes of memory impairment. Focal neurological deficits consistent with previous stroke, signs of parkinsonism, and abnormal gait and eye movements may be particularly revealing.

Cognitive assessment

Although agreement between history and physical examination is suggestive of a diagnosis of dementia, a cognitive assessment is necessary to diagnose and differentiate dementia syndromes. Cognitive performance, however, is influenced by numerous factors, not all of which are indicative of dementia. For example, inefficient learning strategies, slowed processing, decreased attention, and sensory deficits may affect the results of cognitive testing. Age, education, and demographic factors may alter performance and must be incorporated into the analyses of test results.[96]

The Mini-Mental Status Examination (MMSE) is the most commonly used screening test for dementia. The examination tests orientation, registration, attention, and calculation, and it is used to diagnose and stratify patients into mild, moderate, and severe dementia. Traditionally, a perfect score is 30; scores of 25–29 suggest MCI; scores of 19–24 indicate mild dementia; scores of 15–19 indicate moderate dementia; and scores of 14 or less are consistent with severe dementia. Using a cut-off of 23/24, the MMSE has a sensitivity of 79% and a specificity of 95%.[97] Studies assessing the use of the MMSE have been done with relatively small sample sizes, and the MMSE is not as sensitive for mild dementia as it is for more moderate or sever impairment. In addition, the MMSE is influenced by age, education, language,

and motor and/or visual impairments. Tools that incorporate age, sex, and educational attainment are now available to help correct the interpretation of these results.[98, 99] For example, in patients with less than nine years of education, a score of 17 or less is consistent with mild, not moderate, impairment.

MMSE testing can be used not only to diagnose cognitive impairment or dementia, but also to follow its progression. Over time, most patients will display a steady deterioration in their MMSE testing scores. For example, in patients with AD, the average decline in MMSE is two to four points per year. More recently, the MMSE has also been used to assess decision-making competency. Studies suggest that scores higher than 23 or scores lower than 19 are reliable in distinguishing competency from incompetency. Intermediate scores may require a more complete evaluation.[100, 101]

The clock-drawing test (CDT) is a quick screen for cognitive impairment, taking less than five minutes to perform. During this test, the patient is asked to draw a clock face with all of the numbers and label the face with a specified time, such as "10 minutes to 2 o'clock." The person is given one point for labeling all 12 numbers, three points for placing the 12 at the top, one point for drawing two hands, and one point for the correct identification of the time. A score of fewer than four points indicates impairment.[102] The CDT is appealing because of ease of administration, but like the MMSE, it is not sensitive to mild impairment.[103]

The Mini-Cog is another brief screening test that combines the CDT and the three-item recall from the MMSE. Patients who recall none of the three words are classified as demented, those who recall all of the three words are nondemented, and those who recall one or two of the three words are classified as either demented or nondemented based on the results of their CDT.[104] A retrospective analysis and a post-hoc examination suggests that the sensitivity and specificity of the Mini-Cog is similar to that of the MMSE.[104, 105] The advantage of the Mini-Cog is its high sensitivity, ease of administration, and lack of influence by the patient's education level.

The Montreal Cognitive Assessment (MoCA) was designed to screen for mild cognitive impairment. The MoCA takes approximately 10 minutes to administer, and it is used to evaluate memory, attention, concentration, executive functions, language, visuospatial skills, and orientation. Similar to the MMSE, a perfect score is 30, adjusting for education; a cut-off score of 25/26 had 100% sensitivity and 87% specificity for detecting MCI.[106] The tool is freely available online with instructions for use and interpretation of results, including normative data (www.mocatest.org). Further research is needed to validate the use of MoCA as a screening tool in primary care. Studies comparing MoCA to MMSE demonstrated good sensitivity and moderate specificity in detecting MCI.[107, 108] MoCA may also be particularly helpful in detecting vascular dementia.[109–111]

Neuropsychological testing encompasses a wide array of tests and involves a more extensive evaluation of multiple cognitive domains. In a practice parameter from 2001, the American Academy of Neurology (AAN) concluded that neuropsychological testing is useful in distinguishing MCI from dementia in patients presenting with memory loss and in distinguishing different dementia syndromes. The five instruments deemed most reliable by the AAN were the animal naming test, the Modified Boston Naming test, the MMSE, Constructional Praxis, and Word List Memory.[112] An aggregate total score from these five tests has been shown to differentiate accurately patients undergoing normal aging from patients with AD.[113]

Finally, an assessment of premorbid literacy is crucial to determining the extent of dementia in a patient. The National Adult Reading Test involves the pronunciation of 50 English words and has been validated as an estimator of premorbid ability in a study of 80-year-olds.[114] This test is often administered prior to a full neuropsychiatric evaluation.

Laboratory evaluation

The only laboratory evaluation recommended for all patients with suspected dementia includes screening for hypothyroidism and B12 deficiency.[14] Tailored laboratory evaluation is otherwise guided by clinical findings and may include assessment of the complete blood count, liver function studies, electrolytes, syphilis and Lyme serology, and human immunodeficiency virus status. The cost-effectiveness of obtaining multiple laboratory studies has been called into question because of the low likelihood of detecting a reversible dementia.[115]

Recently, plasma phospholipids have been identified as a possible biomarker for the diagnosis of preclinical AD. Accuracy is approximately 90% for predicating progression to MCI or AD within two to three years in individuals without cognitive impairment.[116] Currently biomarker testing is not recommended as part of a routine laboratory evaluation, but extensive research in this area is underway.

Genetic testing

Genetic testing for most patients with dementia is not recommended. However, the American College of Medical Genetics and the National Society of Genetic Counselors do recommend genetic testing when familial AD is suspected (e.g., individuals or multiple family members have a history of early onset AD or have a relative with a known history for a mutated gene associated with early onset AD).[117] Although screening for the presence of the APO E4 allele has garnered much research interest because it is a known risk factor for AD, its utility as a diagnostic test is limited because not all persons who are homozygote for the allele develop AD.[118] Until more research is available in this area, the potential for harm based on over-diagnosis of the disease is tremendous.[119]

Neuroimaging

The role of neuroimaging in patients with suspected dementia is in evolution. Although many clinical prediction rules do not recommend routine screening with neuroimaging, the AAN recommends neuroimaging in the initial evaluation of all patients with dementia.[14] The Alzheimer's Association Position Statement recommends the use of MRI in clinical diagnosis of dementia and cognitive impairment to identify small lacunar infarcts, white matter ischemic changes, hippocampal atrophy, and volumetric changes.[120] MRI findings can lend support to a presumed diagnosis; for example, generalized or focal atrophy may be suggestive of AD, and white matter lesions may indicate ischemic disease.[14] Several studies suggest that hippocampal atrophy might allow for early detection of AD, may help in following the course of the disease, and may guide future treatment decisions.[121, 122] The Alzheimer's Disease Neuroimaging Initiative is a large, multisite study that is now underway and is designed to evaluate the specific role of neuroimaging in the diagnosis of AD and in monitoring the progression of MCI.[123]

The use of functional imaging studies, such as PET, single photon emission computerized tomography, and functional MRI (fMRI) in the diagnosis of dementia is currently being studied.[123] Fluorodeoxyglucose (FDG)-PET preliminary findings suggest that functional studies may detect temporoparietal deficits in early AD that shift to the frontal region with progression of AD.[123, 124] In 2005, the Centers for Medicare and Medicaid (CMS) approved reimbursement for FDG-PET as an adjunctive diagnostic tool for dementia. There is no evidence, however, that the additional diagnostic accuracy provided by PET leads to improved patient outcomes or cost-effective medical care. At present, The Alzheimer's Association and the National Institute on Aging (NIA) do not advocate routine use of PET imaging for a presumed diagnosis of dementia and cognitive impairment; however, PET usage is recommended for research in preclinical AD.[125]

Molecular neuroimaging using amyloid imaging tracers is a primary research focus to improve detection of AD before changes in brain structures occur. This may help to assess disease progression as well as efficacy of disease modifying medications in the future.[2] One agent, the Pittsburgh Compound-B (PIB), has demonstrated good binding to amyloid B peptide in areas with significant amyloid deposition in postmortem studies of the human brain.[126] A longitudinal study with PIB observed that amyloid deposition independent of brain atrophy does not accurately identify AD; however, it might be useful in conjunction with MRI to improve diagnostic accuracy of dementia.[126, 127]

Brain biopsy

The brain biopsy as a diagnostic tool has become nearly obsolete. It is rarely used in younger patients with acute onset of cognitive impairment or those with an atypical clinical presentation suggesting a reversible disorder. Brain biopsy is invasive, carries a low diagnostic yield, and rarely leads to specific treatment interventions.

Screening guidelines

Despite the availability of guidelines for the diagnosis of dementia, routine screening of all older adults is not widely recommended. In 2010, the Alzheimer's Association and Medicare Detection of Cognitive Impairment recommended that cognitive impairment assessment should be included in the annual wellness visit (AWV).[128] However, the US Preventive Services Task Forces has concluded that there is insufficient evidence (I recommendation) to support routine screening for dementia in older adults.[129] There are currently insufficient data to support a beneficial effect of early diagnosis and treatment. Also, the feasibility, cost-effectiveness, and potential harms of routine screening of all older adults are largely unknown.

Treatment of dementia

Advances in understanding the pathophysiology of dementia have allowed for development of more targeted pharmacological therapies; however, the cornerstone of the management of dementia is still symptomatic and geared largely toward minimizing functional disability, addressing behavioral disturbances, and preventing injury. Despite a number of setbacks, the search for effective disease-specific and disease-modifying therapies holds promise.

Pharmacological management

Acetylcholinesterase inhibitors

Destruction of neurons that release the neurotransmitter acetylcholine appears to play a role in the pathogenesis of AD and other dementias. By blocking the enzyme that breaks down acetylcholine, medications that inhibit cholinesterase raise acetylcholine levels in the brain. There are currently three FDA-approved acetylcholinesterase inhibitors (ChIs): donepezil, rivastigmine, and galantamine. Tacrine was the first agent used in the treatment of AD, but it carries a risk of hepatotoxicity and has been discontinued in the United States. Efficacy of the medications appears to be similar, but adverse effect profiles vary.[130]

The clinical benefit and cost-effectiveness of the ChIs is somewhat controversial, although these medications remain first-line agents in the treatment of AD. The average benefit of patients taking ChIs is a short-term improvement in cognition and ADLs. [131, 132] In a meta-analysis of 29 randomized, controlled trials, patients on ChIs improved only 0.1 standard deviation on ADL scales and 0.9 standard deviations on instrumental ADL scales, a change comparable to preventing a two-month per year decline in a typical patient with AD.[130] The long-term benefit of these medications, such as a delay in nursing home placement, is still unclear.[133, 134] In one nonindustry study, AD2000, ChIs showed no effect on timing of nursing home placement or progression of disability. [135] Additional evidence suggests that response to ChIs is variable, with 30%–50% of patients experiencing no benefit and a smaller percentage experiencing a significantly greater than average benefit. ChIs appear to be most effective early in the course of dementia, and, in the absence of other options, many patients and their families may opt for a trial of one of these medications.

The most common side effects of these medications are nausea, diarrhea, vomiting, dizziness, cardiac arrhythmia, and insomnia occurring in 10%–30% of patients. Syncope and hip fracture have been identified as additional adverse drug events, with a hazard ratio of 1.76 and 1.18, respectively.[136] Generally, the medications are titrated for two to four weeks to reach the maximum tolerated dose. Benefits may extend to one to three years; although little clinically symptomatic improvement may be noted, treated patients may function better than they otherwise would have without treatment. However, if the patient, family, and provider do not see a response, it is reasonable to discontinue the medication after a six-to-eight-week trial. These medications are often discontinued when patients progress to more advanced dementia, with the exception of donepezil (which is often used in conjunction with memantine for the treatment of moderate to severe dementia), and are only reintroduced if there is a deterioration following removal.

NMDA receptor antagonist

Memantine (Namenda®) is an N-methyl-D aspartate (NMDA) receptor antagonist that blocks pathological stimulation of N-methyl-D-aspartate receptors by glutamate and may protect against excitatory neurotoxicity in patients with moderate to severe dementia. A Cochrane review concluded that memantine has a small benefit on cognition, ability to perform ADLs, and agitation in patients with moderate or severe AD. This benefit, however, was not seen in patients with mild to moderate AD or in patients with VaD.[137, 138]

Memantine may also be helpful when used in combination with ChIs. One study suggests that patients taking memantine plus donepezil had better outcomes than those taking donepezil plus placebo on scales measuring cognition, ADLs, global outcome, and behavior.[139] In general, memantine is well tolerated, but adherence has been challenging since it is taken up to twice a day. In 2010, the FDA approved a once-daily extended-release version. The most common side effect of memantine is dizziness. Confusion, headache, diarrhea, and vomiting have also been noted. Withdrawal of the medication should be considered if a patient worsens shortly after starting it.[140]

Other

The search for disease-modifying agents to help slow or stop the progression of AD has been disappointing. [141, 142] Although vitamin E had some positive results at high doses, a recent meta-analysis revealed an increased risk of all-cause mortality, especially with high doses, leading many to abandon vitamin E supplementation.[143, 144] Investigation into nonsteroidal anti-inflammatory drugs (NSAIDs), statins, and estrogen replacement therapy for the prevention and treatment of dementia has also yielded disappointing outcomes.[145] The side-effect profile of NSAIDs led to significant withdrawal rates from studies.[16, 146, 147] Similarly, studies have shown that estrogen replacement therapy does not improve cognitive or functional outcomes in patients with dementia.[148, 149]

Despite attracting public interest, ginkgo biloba is also not recommended in the treatment of dementia. A 2009 Cochrane review of 36 trials found that ginkgo was not associated with a consistent clinically significant improvement in patients with dementia.[150] A large randomized, controlled trial, also conducted in 2009, found that ginkgo biloba at 120 mg twice daily did not decrease the rate of cognitive decline in cognitively intact older adults or in adults with mild cognitive impairment.[151] Lack of regulation of the herbal extract, including variability in the dosing and contents, as well as the risk of bleeding for patients who are also on aspirin, NSAIDs, or anticoagulants, has led experts to discourage its use.[152]

More recently, an interest in vitamin D supplementation has gained attention. In vivo research with vitamin D has demonstrated a decrease in amyloid burden and tau hyperphosphorylation with age-related cognitive decline associated with improving learning and memory. [153, 154] Preliminary results from two independent studies regarding the use of intranasal insulin therapy and transdermal nicotine therapy in nonsmokers showed an improvement in cognition with amnestic MCI. Further studies are to be undertaken.[155, 156] Pharmacological research using immunotherapy is being actively pursued. Two phase 3 trials with bapineuzumab and solanezumab, humanized monoclonal antibodies, demonstrated no improvement in cognitive or functional ability in patients with mild to moderate AD.[141, 157] Although both forms of immunotherapy had a positive impact on CSF biomarkers,[158, 159] adverse events included brain edema in both studies and hemorrhage with solanezumab only.[141, 157] A multicenter phase 2 trial investigating intravenous immunoglobulin reported a promising safety profile, but the effect on cognitive function remains to be demonstrated.[160]

Clinical trials with active immunization for AD with an amyloid-beta peptide AN1792 were suspended after several participants developed meningoencephalitis; however, a second-generation vaccine, CAD106, is currently under study.[161] Preliminary data have not reported meningoencephalitis as an adverse event with this agent; the most common adverse event reported is nasopharyngitis. Morever, 67%–82% of participants developed Aβ antibodies, and in vivo studies have demonstrated a reduction of amyloid accumulation.[162, 163] Additional clinical trials are needed to confirm safety, dose response, and efficacy.

Nonpharmacological management

Many nonpharmacologic interventions have been studied for the treatment of individuals with dementia. Cochrane reviews of 25 categories of nonpharmacologic therapies found evidence to support a beneficial effect for cognitive training, cognitive stimulation, and ADL training for patients with dementia.

Lifestyle

In several small studies, mental activities such as reading, playing games or puzzles, and playing a musical instrument have been associated with a decreased risk of cognitive impairment.[164–166] Better cognitive function has been demonstrated in both men and women who pursued high levels of long-term physical activity.[167–168] Physical activity also appears to promote functional autonomy as well as nutritional and cognitive status in those with AD.[169–171]

Nutrition

Inadequate nutrition is common in patients with dementia and is associated with increased morbidity and mortality. Oral nutritional supplements may help to offset this risk by increasing weight and fat-free mass.[172] A prospective, population-based cohort study concluded that adherence to a Mediterranean-type diet may reduce the risk for AD.[173]

Risk factor reduction

Aggressive identification and treatment of modifiable risk factors, including cardiovascular risk factors, may also help to slow cognitive decline. [12] In an early analysis of a 2014 multidomain prevention trial, diet, physical exercise, cognitive training, social activities, and control of vascular risk factors showed early promise for prevention of dementia, but further validation in a larger study is needed.[174]

Other management issues

Behavioral disturbances

The prevalence of neuropsychiatric symptoms in patients with dementia is common, occurring in nearly 60% of patients. This often accounts for significant caregiver burden.[175–177] Behavioral and psychological symptoms are often the most challenging management issue for caregivers and are predictive of nursing home placement;[176] therefore, attention to these behaviors is paramount in the care of patients with dementia. Longitudinal interventions tailored to the needs of the patient and the caregiver (including activity planning and environmental redesign as well as skills training, education, and support for caregivers) can help to decrease these symptoms.[178]

Improving communication and patient perception is one strategy to reduce behavioral disturbances. Reduction of sensory impairment is imperative in communicating with patients with dementia; glasses and hearing aids should always be available and environmental noise and visual disturbances should be minimized. Caregivers should be encouraged to interact with the patient at eye level, avoid threatening stances or gestures, and to speak softly and slowly.

Caregiver training to identify antecedents, response, and consequences of a problematic behavior may also be helpful. Using an "ABC" method, caregivers are asked first to identify the antecedents (A) or triggers for certain behavior such as a change in schedule, interpersonal conflict, or physical stressor; once identified, these antecedents can be avoided or minimized. The caregiver is then asked to describe the behavior (B) elicited by the antecedent and to understand when, where, and how often it occurs. Finally, the caregiver notes the consequences (C) of the behavior, such as how the caregivers reinforce or deter the activity and what happens after the behavioral disturbance.[179]

Another strategy to address behavioral disturbance is to approach the patient from a social, environmental, and medical perspective.[180] Tailored behavioral strategies in a randomized study of 272 caregivers and people with dementia demonstrated a 68% improvement in behavioral symptoms as well as alleviating depressive symptoms in a majority of caregivers.[181] A meta-analysis of 23 high-quality trials for multipronged caregiver intervention studies revealed a significant reduction in patient behavioral issues as well as caregiver stress reduction.[178]

Affective symptoms, such as apathy, depression, anxiety, and sleep disturbance occur in up to one-quarter of all demented patients.[182] Depressive symptoms may be modified by increasing time spent at pleasant events, increasing social interaction, and increasing activity level. Behavioral interventions to minimize sleep disturbance include improving sleep hygiene as well as addressing nighttime pain and nocturia.

Verbally disruptive behaviors, such as screaming, abusive language, and repetition, may result from cortical disinhibition, but may also signal untreated pain, sensory deprivation, or social isolation. Social interaction and sensory stimulation may improve this behavior. Sundowning, or confusion that increases at nighttime, is common among many elderly patients with dementia, especially in the acute care setting. Food, brief personal contact, music, improved hearing and vision, aromatherapy, light therapy, physical activity, and maintenance of a daily routine have been shown to reduce sundowning.[183, 184]

Aggressive behavior particularly during personal care is also common in patients with dementia; this behavior is often a self-protective response and may be secondary to confusion or misunderstanding.

Helping caregivers to understand that this behavior is not intended to be harmful may be beneficial. Also, employing assistance during bathing and other personal care efforts has been shown to be successful.[185]

Wandering and pacing can pose safety issues for many patients with dementia because of the associated potential for getting lost and for injury. Addressing unmet needs such as hunger, pain, and toileting may minimize pacing. Also, engaging the patient in low-risk exercise or structured physical therapy may help to reduce wandering. Finally, continuous supervision may be necessary to ensure patient safety.

Assessment of the etiology of agitation should be evaluated and treated initially. In the absence of other effective therapies, medications may be needed to address certain behavioral disturbances. In one large multicenter, randomized clinical trial (CitAD), adding citalopram 30 mg daily and a psychosocial intervention improved agitation in patients as well as decreased caregiver distress. However, adverse effects of citalopram include QT prolongation and worsening cognition and may limit use.[186] In the absence of other effective therapies, antipsychotic medications may be needed to address certain behavioral disturbances. In the setting of acute agitation or aggression that is not responsive to behavioral interventions, haloperidol has often been considered the drug of choice; however, recent studies have shown an increased risk of QT prolongation and torsade de pointes with intravenous and high dose haloperidol. Many experts now recommend an atypical antipsychotic agent as first line when an antipsychotic is indicated.[187, 188]

Atypical antipsychotic agents include clozapine, olanzapine, risperidone, aripiprazole, risperidone, and quetiapine.[188] For acute management of behavioral and psychological disturbances, a trial of atypical antipsychotics including clozapine, olanzapine, risperidone, and quetiapine may be warranted. Several reviews suggest that these agents have, at most, modest efficacy.[189–191] The 2006 Clinical Antipsychotic Trial of Intervention Effectiveness (CATIE) study suggests that adverse effects leading to intolerability may offset advantages in the efficacy of atypical antipsychotic drugs for the treatment of psychosis, aggression, or agitation in patients with AD.[189]

Despite higher expense, atypical antipsychotic agents do have a lower risk of extrapyramidal side effects than traditional antipsychotic medications. Still, adverse effects are common with these medications and include extrapyramidal symptoms, somnolence, and gait dysfunction. To offset some of these adverse effects, low doses are recommended. Olanzapine is started at 2.5 mg daily and titrated to a maximum of 5 mg twice a day. Of note, olanzapine has been associated with significant weight gain and insulin resistance and requires monitoring of fasting blood glucose. Quetiapine is started at 25 mg at bedtime and titrated to a maximum of 100 mg or 125 mg daily. Risperidone is started at 0.5 mg a day and titrated to 1 mg a day. At higher doses, significant extrapyramidal side effects may become a problem with risperidone. Clozapine is rarely used now because it carries a risk of agranulocytosis and requires frequent blood monitoring.

Despite frequent clinical use, atypical antipsychotic agents are not FDA approved for management of behavioral disorders, and these medications carry an associated mortality risk and increased risk of stroke. In April 2005, the FDA issued a public health advisory about the use of second-generation atypical antipsychotic agents because of increased mortality found in elderly patients taking these medications.[192] A subsequent meta-analysis confirmed these results and concerns have since been raised about the mortality risk of conventional antipsychotics as well.[193, 194]

Given the valid safety concerns associated with antipsychotic medications, they should be reserved for patients who are at imminent risk of harming themselves or others or have delusions and hallucinations that are distressing or that disrupt the patients' care. Practitioners must explain the risks and benefits of these medications and obtain informed consent from the patients and/or family members prior to use. Patients with DLB may be particularly sensitive to the extrapyramidal side effects of antipsychotics, so use by these patients should be avoided.

Depression

Depression, presenting with symptoms of low mood, apathy, social withdrawal, and sleep impairment, is seen in many patients with dementia. An estimate of prevalence for major depression in patients with dementia ranges from 5% to 40%, and depression adds to increased risk for disability, suicide, functional impairment, and mortality.[195]

However, overall performance of using antidepressants to treat patients with dementia and depression has been relatively disappointing.[196, 197] In a 2011 meta-analysis of seven trials, researchers were unable to confirm efficacy of antidepressant usage for patients with depression and dementia. [195] Patients with a history of antecedent recurrent depression appeared to have the greatest response to pharmacologic therapy, but further study is still needed in this area.

When an antidepressant trial is warranted, selective serotonin reuptake inhibitors (SSRIs) are considered first-line agents for treating depression in patients with dementia. Despite a paucity of studies comparing specific agents, longer-acting SSRIs, such as fluoxetine (Prozac*), are usually avoided in the elderly because of an increased risk of side effects. Paroxetine (Paxil*) is the most anticholinergic of the SSRIs and is also generally avoided. Adverse effects of SSRIs are not insignificant, and further research confirming efficacy of these medications is warranted.[198, 199]

Tricyclic antidepressants (TCAs) are second-line agents for treatment of depression in this population. Despite moderate efficacy in treating depression, TCAs are associated with confusion and additional anticholinergic side effects, carrying a significant risk of adverse events in an older population.

In certain instances, other classes of antidepressants may be considered to address individual patient characteristics. Bupropion (75 mg–150 mg twice daily) can be used in patients who cannot tolerate side effects of other medications or to augment patients who respond only modestly to SSRIs. Side-effect profiles of some antidepressants may also make them appealing choices in certain cases. For example, mirtazapine (7.5 mg–30 mg) may improve both sleep and appetite and potentially helping patients who suffer from insomnia and weight loss.[200] In a randomized controlled study from 2014, trazodone 50 mg daily demonstrated an increase in sleep by approximately 40 minutes per night.[201] Methylphenidate (5 mg–15 mg after meals) is a rapid-onset stimulant that may be useful in apathetic or somnolent depressed patients. Despite their anxiolytic properties, benzodiazepines are generally avoided in this population because of increased cognitive impairment, sedation, and risk of falls.

Safety

One of the most important safety issues to address in patients with dementia is driving. Patients with AD have been shown to have an increased risk of motor vehicle accidents, a risk that increases each year following diagnosis.[202] Early in the disease, many patients are able to drive safely, but with disease progression, it often becomes unsafe to drive. Discussion of driving cessation is often challenging for patients. Losing a driver's license may equate to loss of independence and may signal progression of disability. Many patients are unaware of their deficits and have difficulty accepting the potential danger associated with continued driving. The majority of states do not mandate physician reporting of patients with dementia to the Department of Motor Vehicles. Still, a majority of physicians refer patients to driver safety evaluations when family members express concern or if an office evaluation indicates significant cognitive impairment. Direct reporting of patients to the Department of Motor Vehicles will also enact a system for evaluating the patient's safety to drive, which includes roadside testing with retesting at regular intervals if the patient passes the test. In 2010, the American Academy of Neurology (AAN) issued guidelines to assist providers in identifying patients at increased risk for unsafe driving. These guidelines incorporate findings from the Clinical Dementia Rating (CDR) (level A); a caregiver's rating of patient's driving ability as marginal or unsafe (level B); a history of crashes, reduced driving mileage, or self-reported situational avoidance; MMSE score ≤ 24; and aggressive or impulsive personality characteristics (level C).[203]

In addition to driving, cooking may pose a significant safety hazard to patients with dementia because of distractibility, forgetfulness, and impaired judgment. Early use of microwave ovens may help to maintain independence while minimizing risk for injury or fire.

Advance care planning

Comprehensive care for the patient with dementia is not complete without addressing advance care planning. The first step in advance care planning involves education of the family or caregiver as to the natural history of the disease. Many families are not aware that dementia carries an average time to death from time of diagnosis of four to eight years.[2] Preparing patients, families, and caregivers for the progressive and terminal nature of the disease can help to set expectations and focus discussions around end-of-life wishes and goals of care. Early referral to supportive services may also help to allay the stress on the family and/or caregivers. Opening the discussion of end-of-life issues early in the course of disease can give patients the opportunity to designate a health-care power of attorney and complete an advance directive or values history if they have not already done so. Discussion of specific wishes of the patient or the proxy decision maker regarding cardiac resuscitation, future hospitalization, antibiotic use, and artificial nutrition are extremely important, often take place over multiple visits, and need to be readdressed regularly.

Placement of feeding tubes in patients with dementia has been an area of intense controversy and deserves special attention. A Cochrane review of enteral tube feeding did not find evidence to support its efficacy in prolonging life for patients with advanced dementia. National organizations, including the American Geriatric Society, do not recommend the use of feeding tubes in patients with advanced dementia; instead, careful hand feeding should be offered.[204] Difficulty with feeding is seen in more than 85% of patients with severe or advanced dementia and is a marker for a terminal prognosis.[205] Recognizing the progression of feeding difficulty and discussing this finding with family members may help family members to better understand a patient's prognosis and make informed decisions about his or her goals of care. In addition, artificial hydration and nutrition in patients with advanced dementia has not been shown to prolong life or reduce patient suffering and should be discussed in family meetings regarding end-of-life care.[206]

Caregivers

Caregivers play a pivotal role in the well-being of persons with dementia. The value of unpaid caregiving provided by family and other caregivers is estimated at $220 billion.[2] Caregiver stress, however, is nearly universal. This stress has been associated with increased rates of depressive symptoms and sense of burden. One large trial has shown that primary family caregivers have a high rate of developing clinical depression while caring for both hospitalized and nonhospitalized family members (63% and 44%,

Table 10.4 Community resources

Alzheimer's Organization
www.alz.org
800-621-0379

Administration on Aging
www.aoa.gov

National Association of Home Care
www.nahc.org
202-547-7424

ABA Commission of Legal Problems of the Elderly
www.abanet.org
202-662-8690

National Institute on Aging
Preventing Alzheimer's Disease: What Do We Know?
www.nia.nih.gov

respectively).[207] In addition, the presence of depression in the caregiver is one of the strongest predictors for nursing home placement.[207]

Providing caregiver support is a critical component of caring for a patient with dementia. Teaching caregivers techniques for handling patients with behavioral disturbance has been shown to lessen depressive symptoms in caregivers.[134, 181] Caregiver support programs, respite care, case management, and adult day services may also relieve caregiver stress and enhance caregiver quality of life.[208–210] Multidimensional interventions characterized by family sessions and support, individual consultation, and ongoing training for caregivers to manage behavioral symptoms have been shown to be effective in reducing caregiver burden and possibly decreasing behavioral problems in care recipients.[2, 3] Resources for caregivers (see Table 10.4) are widely available and can provide valuable information for caregivers. These resources include information about local support groups and respite and home care, case management, driving and personal safety, legal counsel, research, and information on finding missing individuals with dementia. The US Administration on Aging (www.aoa.gov) also provides information on state and local area agencies on aging.

References

1. American Psychiatric Association. *Diagnostic and Statistical Manual of Mental Disorders*. 5th ed. Arlington, VA: American Psychiatric Publishing; 2013.

2. Alzheimer's Association. 2014 Alzheimer's disease facts and figures. *Alzheimer's & Dementia*. 2014;1–46.

3. Elliott AF, Burgio LD, Decoster J. Enhancing caregiver health: findings from the resources for enhancing Alzheimer's caregiver health II intervention. *J Am Geriatr Soc*. 2010;**58**:30–7.

4. Corrada MM, Brookmeyer R, Paganini-Hill A, et al. Dementia incidence continues to increase with age in the oldest old: the 90+ study. *Ann Neurol*. 2010; **67**: 114–21.

5. Vincent GK, Velkoff VA. *The next four decades: The older population in the united sates: 2010–2050*. Current Population Reports. Washington, DC: US Department of Commerce Economics and Statistics Administration. 2010.

6. Llewellyn DJ, Lang IA, Langa KM, et al. Vitamin D and risk of cognitive decline in elderly persons. *Arch Intern Med*. 2010;**170**:1135–41.

7. Norton MC, Smith KR, Ostbye T, et al. Greater risk of dementia when spouse has dementia? The cache county study. *J Am Geriatr Soc*. 2010;**58**:895–900.

8. Fratiglioni L, Paillard-Borg S, Winblad B. An active and socially integrated lifestyle in late life might protect against dementia. *Lancet Neurol*. 2004;**3**:343–53.

9. Simonsick EM. Fitness and cognition: encouraging findings and methodological considerations for future work. *J Am Geriatr Soc*. 2003;**51**:570–1.

10. Coyle JT. Use it or lose it – do effortful mental activities protect against dementia? *NEJM*. 2003;**348**:2489–90.

11. Buchman AS, Boyle PA, Yu L, et al. Total daily physical activity and the risk of AD and cognitive decline in older adults. *Neurology*. 2012;**78**:1323–9.

12. Yaffe K, Fiocco AJ, Lindquist K, et al. Predictors of maintaining cognitive function in older adults: the health ABC study. *Neurology*. 2009;**72**:2029–35

13. Jellinger KA. Morphologic diagnosis of "vascular dementia" – a critical update. *Journal of the Neurological Sciences*.2008;**270**: 1–12.

14. Knopman DS, Boeve BF, Petersen RC. Essential of the proper diagnoses of mild cognitive impairment, dementia, and major subtypes of dementia. *Mayo Clin Proc*. 2003;**78**:1290–1308.

15. Snowden JS. Semantic dysfunction in frontotemporal lobar degeneration. *Dement Geriatr Cogn Disord*. 1999;**10**(Suppl 1):33–6.

16. Morris JC. Dementia update 2005. *Alzheimer Dis Assoc Disord*. 2005;**19**:100–17.

17. Jack Jr CR, Albert MS, Knopman DS, et al. Introduction to the recommendations from the national institute on aging – Alzheimer's Association workgroups on diagnostic guidelines for Alzheimer's disease. *Alzheimers Dement*. 2011;**7**:257–62.

18. Hebert LE, Weuve J, Scherr PA, Evans DA. Alzheimer disease in the United States (2010–2050) estimated using the 2010 census. *Neurology.* 2013;**80**:1778–83.

19. Barnes DE, Yaffe K, Byers AL, et al. Midlife vs late-life depressive symptoms and risk of dementia: Differential effects for Alzheimer disease and vascular dementia. *Arch Gen Psychiatry.* 2012;**69**:493–8.

20. Querfurth HW, Laferla FM. Mechanisms of disease: Alzheimer's disease. *NEJM.* 2010;**362**:1844–5.

21. Cummings JL, Vinters HV, Cole GM, et al. Alzheimer's disease: etiologies, pathophysiology, cognitive reserve, and treatment opportunities. *Neurology.* 1998;**51** (Suppl 1):S2–S17.

22. Mash DC, Flynn DD, Potter LT. Loss of M2 muscarine receptors in the cerebral cortex in Alzheimer's disease and experimental cholinergic degeneration. *Science.* 1985;**228**:1115–17.

23. Cummings JL. Alzheimer's disease. *NEJM.* 2004;**351**:56–67.

24. Gandy S. The role of cerebral amyloid beta accumulation in common forms of Alzheimer disease. *J Clin Invest.* 2005;**115**(5):1121–9.

25. Tanzi RE. Tangles and neurodegenerative disease – a surprising twist. *NEJM.* 2005;**353**:1853–5.

26. Santacruz K, Lewis J, Spires T, et al. Tau suppression in a neuro-degenerative mouse model improves memory function. *Science.* 2005;**309**:476–81.

27. Gorelick PB, Scuteri A, Black SE, et al. Vascular contributions to cognitive impairment and dementia: a statement for healthcare professionals from the American Heart Association/American Stroke. *Stroke.* 2011;**42**:2672–713.

28. Larson EB, Shadlen MF, Wang L, et al. Survival after initial diagnosis of Alzheimer disease. *Ann Intern Med.* 2004;**140**:501–9.

29. Román GC. Vascular neurocognitive disorder. In: *Gabbard's Treatments of Psychiatric Disorders*, 5th ed. Arlington, VA: American Psychiatric Publishing; 2014

30. Duthie EH, Glatt SL. Understanding and treating multi-infarct dementia. *Clin Geriatr Med.* 1988;**4**: 749–66.

31. Moorhouse P, Rockwood K. Vascular cognitive impairment: current concepts and clinical developments. *Lancet Neurol.* 2008;**7**:246–55.

32. Rincon F, Wright CB. Vascular cognitive impairment. *Curr Opin Neurol.* 2013;**26**:29–36.

33. Dichgans M, Zietemann V. Prevention of vascular cognitive impairment. *Stroke.* 2012;**43**:3137–46.

34. The Lund and Manchester Groups. Clinical and neuropathological criteria for frontotemporal dementia. *J Neurol Neurosurg Psychiatry.* 1994;**57**:416–18.

35. Whitwell JL, Jack Jr CR, Senjem ML, Josephs, KA. Patterns of atrophy in pathologically confirmed FTLD with and without motor neuron degeneration. *Neurology.* 2006;**66**:102–4.

36. Rabinovici GD, Miller BL. Frontotemporal lobar degeneration epidemiology, pathophysiology, diagnosis and management. *CNS Drugs.* 2010;**24**: 375–98.

37. McMurtray AM, Chen AK, Shapira JS, et al. Variations in regional SPECT hypoperfusion and clinical features in frontotemporal dementia. *Neurology.*2006;**66**: 517–22.

38. Mendez MF, McMurtray A, Chen, AK, et al. Functional neuroimaging and presenting psychiatric features in frontotemporal dementia. *J Neurol Neurosurg Psychiatry.* 2006;**77**:4–7.

39. Vanderzee J, Rademakers R, Engelborghs S, et al. A Belgian ancestral haplotype harbours a highly prevalent mutation for 17q21-linked tau-negative FTLD. *Brain.* 2006;**129**:841–52.

40. Mackenzie IR, Baker M, West G, et al. A family with tau-negative frontotemporal dementia and neuronal intranuclear inclusions linked to chromosome 17. *Brain.* 2006;**129**:853–67.

41. Huey ED, Putnam KT, Grafman J. A systematic review of neurotransmitter deficits and treatments in frontotemporal dementia. *Neurology.* 2006;**66**:17–22.

42. McKhann GM, Albert MS, Grossman M, et al. Clinical and pathological diagnosis of frontotemporal dementia: report of the Work Group on Frontotemporal Dementia and Pick's Disease. *Arch Neurol.* 2001;**58**:1803–9.

43. Neary D, Snowden JS, Northen B, et al. Dementia of frontal lobe type. *J Neurol Neurosurg Psychiatry.* 1988;**51**:353–61.

44. Chare L, Hodges JR, Leyton CE, et al. New criteria for frontotemporal dementia syndromes: Clinical and pathological diagnostic implications. *Journal of Neurology, Neurosurgery & Psychiatry.* 2014;**85**:865–70.

45. Hodges JR, Davies RR, Xuereb JH, et al. Clinicopathological correlates in frontotemporal dementia. *Ann Neurol.* 2004;**56**:399–406.

46. Eslinger PJ, Dennis K, Moore P, et al. Metacognitive deficits in frontotemporal dementia. *J Neurol Neurosurg Psychiatry.* 2005;**76**:1630–5.

47. Bonner MF, Ash S, Grossman M. The new classification of primary progressive aphasia into semantic, logopenic, or nonfluent/agrammatic variants. *Current Neurology & Neuroscience Reports.* 2010;**10**:484–90.

48. Campbell S, Stephens S, Ballard C. Dementia with Lewy bodies: clinical features and treatment. *Drugs Aging.* 2001;**18**:397–407.

49. McKeith IG. Spectrum of Parkinson's disease, Parkinson's dementia, and Lewy body dementia. *Neurol Clin.* 2000;**18**:865–902.

50. Savica R, Grossardt BR, Bower JH, et al. Incidence of dementia with Lewy bodies and Parkinson disease dementia. *JAMA Neurology.* 2013;**70**:1396–402.

51. Halliday GM, Song YJ, Harding AJ. Striatal beta-amyloid in dementia with Lewy bodies but not parkinson's disease. *J Neural Transm.* 2011;**118**:713–9.

52. Kalaitzakis ME, Walls AJ, Pearce RK, et al. Striatal abeta peptide deposition mirrors dementia and differentiates DLB and PDD from other parkinsonian syndromes. *Neurobiol Dis.* 2011;**41**:377–84.

53. Kantarci K, Lowe VJ, Boeve BF, et al. Multimodality imaging characteristics of dementia with Lewy bodies. *Neurobiol Aging.* 2012;**33**:2091–105.

54. Klein JC, Eggers C, Kalbe E, et al. Neurotransmitter changes in dementia with Lewy bodies and parkinson disease dementia in vivo. *Neurology.* 2010;**74**:885–92.

55. Shimada H, Shinotoh H, Hirano S, et al. Beta-amyloid in Lewy body disease is related to Alzheimer's disease-like atrophy. *Movement Disorders.* 2013;**28**:169–75.

56. Kupsch AR, Bajaj N, Weiland F, et al. Impact of DaTscan SPECT imaging on clinical management, diagnosis, confidence of diagnosis, quality of life, health resource use and safety in patients with clinically uncertain parkinsonian syndromes: A prospective 1-year follow-up of an open-label controlled study. *J Neurol Neurosurg Psychiatry.* 2012;**83**:620–8.

57. Lim SM, Katsifis A, Villemagne VL, et al. The 18 F-FDG PET cingulate island sign and comparison to 123I-beta-CIT SPECT for diagnosis of dementia with Lewy bodies. *Journal of Nuclear Medicine.* 2009;**50**:1638–45.

58. O'Brien JT, McKeith IG, Walker Z, et al. Diagnostic accuracy of 123I-FP-CIT SPECT in possible dementia with Lewy bodies. *British Journal of Psychiatry.* 2009;**194**:34–9.

59. Ferman TJ, Boeve BF, Smith GE, et al. Inclusion of RBD improves the diagnostic classification of dementia with Lewy bodies. *Neurology.* 2011;**77**: 875–82.

60. Aarsland D, Andersen K, Larsen JP, et al. Risk of dementia in Parkinson's disease: a community-based, prospective study. *Neurology.* 2001;**56**:730–6.

61. Stern Y, Marder K, Tang MX, Mayeux R. Antecedent clinical features associated with dementia in Parkinson's disease. *Neurology.*1993;**43**:1690–2.

62. Emre M. Dementia in Parkinson's disease: cause and treatment. *Curr Opin Neurol.* 2004;**17**:399–404.

63. Aarsland D, Perry R, Brown A, et al. Neuropathology of dementia in Parkinson's disease: a prospective, community-based study. *Ann Neurol.* 2005;**58**:773–6.

64. Quinn N. Parkinsonism–recognition and differential diagnosis. *BMJ.* 1995; **310**:447–52.

65. Litvan I, Campbell G, Mangone CA, et al. Which clinical features differentiate progressive supranuclear palsy (Steele-Richardson-Olszewski syndrome) from related disorders? A clinicopathological study. *Brain.* 1997;**120**(Pt 1):65–74.

66. Verny M, Jellinger KA, Hauw JJ, et al. Progressive supranuclear palsy: a clinicopathological study of 21 cases. *Acta Neuropathol (Berl).* 1996;**91**:427–31.

67. Maher ER, Lees AJ. The clinical features and natural history of the Steele-Richardson-Olszewski syndrome (progressive supranuclear palsy). *Neurology.* 1986;**36**: 1005–8.

68. Centers for Disease Control. Creutzfeldt-Jakob disease (CJD). Available at: www.cdc.gov/ncidod/dvrd/cjd (accessed April 28, 2015).

69. World Health Organization (WHO). *WHO manual for surveillance of human transmissible spongiform encephalopathies including variant Creutzfeldt-Jakob disease,* 2003. Available at: www.who.int/bloodproducts/ TSE-manual2003.pdf (accessed December 2, 2015).

70. Rinne ML, McGinnis SM, Samuels MA, et al. Clinical problem-solving: a startling decline. *N Engl J Med.* 2012;**366**:836–42.

71. Chohan G, Pennington C, Mackenzie JM, et al. The role of cerebrospinal fluid 14–3-3 and other proteins in the diagnosis of sporadic Creutzfeldt-Jakob disease in the UK: a 10-year review. *Journal of Neurology, Neurosurgery & Psychiatry.* 2010;**81**: 1243–8.

72. Heath CA, Cooper SA, Murray K, et al. Validation of diagnostic criteria for variant Creutzfeldt-Jakob disease. *Ann Neurol.* 2010;**67**:761–70.

73. Vitali P, Maccagnano E, Caverzasi E, et al. Diffusion-weighted MRI hyperintensity patterns differentiate CJD from other rapid dementias. *Neurology.* 2011 May;**76**:1711–19.

74. Chapman DP, Williams SM, Strine TW, et al. Dementia and its implications for public health. Available at: www.cdc.gov/pcd/issues/2006/apr/05_01 67.htm (accessed May 25, 2008).

75. Wivel ME. NIMH report: NIH consensus conference stresses need to identify reversible causes of dementia. *Hosp Community Psychiatry.* 1988;**39**:22–3.

76. Clarfield AM. The decreasing prevalence of reversible dementias: an updated meta-analysis. *Arch Intern Med.* 2003;**163**:2219–29.

77. Clarfield, AM. The reversible dementias: do they reverse? *Ann Intern Med.* 1988;**109**:476–86.

78. Williams MA, Relkin NR. Diagnosis and management of idiopathic normal-pressure hydrocephalus. *Neurol Clin Pract.* 2013;**3**:375–85.

79. Kiefer M, Unterberg A. The differential diagnosis and treatment of normal-pressure hydrocephalus. *Dtsch Arztebl Int.* 2012;**109**:15–25.

80. Tueth MJ, Cheong JA. Delirium: diagnosis and treatment in the older patient. *Geriatrics.* 1993;**48**:75–80.

81. Inouye SK, Westendorp RG, Saczynski JS. Delirium in elderly people. *Lancet.* 2014;**8**(383):911–22.

82. Petersen RC, Roberts RO, Knopman DS, et al. Prevalence of mild cognitive impairment is higher in men: the Mayo Clinic study of aging. *Neurology.* 2010;**75**:889–97.

83. Sachdev PS, Lipnicki DM, Crawford J, et al. Risk profiles of subtypes of mild cognitive impairment: the Sydney memory and ageing study. *J Am Geriatr Soc.* 2012;**60**:24–33.

84. Roberts RO, Geda YE, Knopman DS, et al. The incidence of MCI differs by subtype and is higher in men: the Mayo Clinic study of aging. *Neurology.* 2012;**78**:342–51.

85. Roberts RO, Geda YE, Knopman DS, et al. Cardiac disease associated with increased risk of nonamnestic cognitive impairment: stronger effect on women. *JAMA Neurology.* 2013;**70**:374–82.

86. Mitchell AJ, Shiri-Feshki M. Rate of progression of mild cognitive impairment to dementia – meta-analysis of 41 robust inception cohort studies. *Acta Psychiatr Scand.* 2009;**119**:252–65.

87. Boyle PA, Buchman AS, Wilson RS, et al. The APOE epsilon4 allele is associated with incident mild cognitive impairment among community-dwelling older persons. *Neuroepidemiology.* 2010;**34**:43–9.

88. De Meyer G, Shapiro F, Vanderstichele H, et al. Diagnosis-independent Alzheimer disease biomarker signature in cognitively normal elderly people. *Arch Neurol.* 2010;**67**:949–56.

89. Heister D, Brewer JB, Magda S, et al. for the Alzheimer's Disease Neuroimaging Initiative. Predicting MCI outcome with clinically available MRI and CSF biomarkers. *Neurology.* 2011;**77**:1619–28.

90. Landau SM, Harvey D, Madison CM, et al. Comparing predictors of conversion and decline in mild cognitive impairment. *Neurology.* 2010;**75**:230–8.

91. Lo RY, Hubbard AE, Shaw LM, et al. Longitudinal change of biomarkers in cognitive decline. *Arch Neurol.* 2011;**68**:1257–66.

92. Van Rossum IA, Vos SJ, Burns L, et al. Injury markers predict time to dementia in subjects with MCI and amyloid pathology. *Neurology.* 2012;**79**:1809–16.

93. Vemuri P, Wiste HJ, Weigand SD, et al. Serial MRI and CSF biomarkers in normal aging, MCI, and AD. *Neurology.* 2010;**75**:143–51.

94. Small GW, Rabins PV, Barry PP, et al. Diagnosis and treatment of Alzheimer's disease and related disorders. *JAMA.* 1997;**278**:1363–71.

95. Auer S, Reisberg B. The GDS/FAST system. *Int Psychogeriatr.* 1997;**9**:167–71.

96. Folstein M, Anthony JC, Parchad I, et al. The meaning of cognitive impairment in the elderly. *J Am Geriatr Soc.* 1985;**33**:228–35.

97. Hancock P, Larner AJ. Test your memory test: diagnostic utility in a memory clinic population. *Int J Geriatr Psychiatry.* 2011;**26**:976–80.

98. Grigoletto F, Zappala G, Anderson DW, et al. Norms for the mini-mental state examination in a healthy population. *Neurology.* 1999;**53**:315–20.

99. Dufouil C, Clayton D, Brayne C, et al. Population norms for the MMSE in the very old: estimates based on longitudinal data. *Neurology.* 2000;**55**:1609–13.

100. Karlawish JH, Casarett DJ, James, BD, et al. The ability of persons with Alzheimer disease (AD) to make a decision about taking an AD treatment. *Neurology.* 2005;**64**:1514–19.

101. Pruchno RA, Smyer MA, Rose MS, et al. Competence of long-term care residents to participate in decisions about their medical care: a brief, objective assessment. *Gerontologist.* 1995;**35**: 622–9.

102. Stahelin HB, Monsch AU, Spiegel R. Early diagnosis of dementia via a two-step screening and diagnostic procedure. *Int Pyschogeriatr.* 1997;**9**:123–30.

103. Powlishta KK, Von Dras DD, Stanford A, et al. The clock drawing test is a poor screen for very mild dementia. *Neurology.* 2002;**59**:898–903.

104. Borson S, Scanlan J, Brush M, et al. The Mini-Cog: a cognitive "vital signs" measure for dementia screening in multi-lingual elderly. *Int J Geriatr Psychiatry.* 2000;**15**:1021–7.

105. Borson S, Scanlan J, Chen P, et al. The Mini-Cog as a screen for dementia: validation in a population-based sample. *J Am Geriatr Soc.* 2003;**51**: 1451–4.

106. Nasreddine Z, Phillips N, Bédirian V, et al. The Montreal Cognitive Assessment, MoCA: a brief screening tool for mild cognitive impairment. *J Am Geriatr Soc.* 2005; **53**:695–9.

107. Fujiwara Y, Suzuki H, Yasunaga M, et al. Brief screening tool for mild cognitive impairment in older Japanese: validation of the Japanese version of the Montreal Cognitive Assessment. *Geriatrics & Gerontology International.* 2010;**10**:225–32.

108. Larner AJ. Screening utility of the Montreal Cognitive Assessment (MoCA): in place of – or as well as – the MMSE? *International Psychogeriatrics.* 2012;**24**:391–6.

109. Dong Y, Sharma VK, Venketasubramanian N, et al. The Montreal Cognitive Assessment (MoCA) is superior to the Mini-Mental State Examination (MMSE) for the detection of vascular cognitive

impairment after acute stroke. *J. Neurol. Sci.* 2010;**299**:15–18.

110. Godefroy O, Fickl A, Roussel M, et al. Is the Montreal Cognitive Assessment superior to the Mini-Mental State Examination to detect poststroke cognitive impairment? A study with neuropsychological evaluation. *Stroke.* 2011;**42**:1712–16.

111. Pendlebury ST, Cuthbertson FC, Welch SJ, et al. Underestimation of cognitive impairment by Mini-Mental State Examination versus the Montreal Cognitive Assessment in patients with transient ischemic attack and stroke: a population-based study. *Stroke.* 2010;**41**:1290–3.

112. Petersen RC, Smith GE, Ivnik RJ, et al. *Apolipoprotein E* status as a predictor of the development of Alzheimer's disease in memory-impaired individuals. *JAMA.* 1995;**273**:1274–8.

113. Chandler MJ, Lacritz LH, Hynan LS, et al. A total score for the CERAD neuropsychological battery. *Neurology.* 2005;**65**:102–6.

114. McGurn B, Starr JM, Topfer JA, et al. Pronunciation of irregular words is preserved in dementia, validating premorbid IQ estimation. *Neurology.* 2004;**62**:1184–6

115. Weyting MD, Bossuyt PM, van Crevel H. Reversible dementia: more than 10% or less than 1%? A quantitative review. *J Neurol.* 1995;**242**:466–71.

116. Mapstone M, Cheema AK, Fiandaca MS, et al. Plasma phospholipids identify antecedent memory impairment in older adults. *Nat Med.* 2014;**20**:415–18.

117. Goldman JS, Hahn SE, Catania JW, et al. Genetic counseling and testing for Alzheimer disease: joint practice guidelines of the American College of Medical Genetics and the National Society of Genetic Counselors. *Genet Med.* 2011;**13**:597–605.

118. Henderson AS, Easteal S, Jorm AF. *Apolipoprotein E* allele epsilon 4, dementia, and cognitive decline in a population sample. *Lancet.* 1995;**346**:1387–90.

119. Galasko D. Cerebrospinal fluid biomarkers in Alzheimer disease: a fractional improvement? *Arch Neurol.* 2003;**60**:1195–6.

120. Albert M, DeCarli C, DeKosky S, et al. The use of MRI and PET for the clinical diagnosis of dementia and investigation of cognitive impairment: consensus report. Available at: www.alz.org/national/documents/Imaging_consensus_report.pdf (accessed May 25, 2008).

121. Killiany RJ, Gomez-Isla T, Moss M, et al. Use of structural magnetic resonance imaging to predict who will get Alzheimer's disease. *Ann Neurol.* 2000;**47**:430–9.

122. Adak S, Illouz K, Gorman W, et al. Predicting the rate of cognitive decline in aging and early Alzheimer disease. *Neurology.* 2004;**63**:108–14.

123. Weiner MW, Veitch DP, Aisen PS, et al. The Alzheimer's disease neuroimaging initiative: a review of papers published since its inception. *Alzheimer's & Dementia.* 2012;**8**(1 Suppl):S1–68.

124. Wu X, Chen K, Yao L, et al. Assessing the reliability to detect cerebral hypometabolism in probable Alzheimer's disease and amnestic mild cognitive impairment. *J Neurosci Methods.* 2010;**192**:277–85.

125. McKhann GM, Knopman DS, Chertkow H, et al. The diagnosis of dementia due to Alzheimer's disease: recommendations from the National Institute on Aging – Alzheimer's Association workgroups on diagnostic guidelines for Alzheimer's disease. *Alzheimers Dement.* 2011;**7**:263–9.

126. Klunk WE, Engler H, Nordberg A, et al. Imaging brain amyloid in Alzheimer's disease with Pittsburgh Compound-B. *Ann Neurol.* 2004;**55**:306–19.

127. Jack Jr CR, Lowe VJ, Weigand SD, et al. Serial PIB and MRI in normal, mild cognitive impairment and Alzheimer's disease: implications for sequence of pathological events in Alzheimer's disease. *Brain.* 2009;**132**:1355–65.

128. Cordell CB, Borson S, Boustani M, et al. Alzheimer's Association recommendations for operationalizing the detection of cognitive impairment during the Medicare annual wellness visit in a primary care setting. *Alzheimers Dement.* 2013;**9**:141–50.

129. Lin JS, O'Connor E, Rossom RC, et al. Screening for cognitive impairment in older adults: a systematic review for the US Preventive Services Task Force. *Annals of Internal Medicine.* 2013;**159**(9)601–12.

130. Trinh NH, Hoblyn J, Mohanty S, et al. Efficacy of cholinesterase inhibitors in the treatment of neuropsychiatric symptoms and functional impairment in Alzheimer disease: a meta-analysis. *JAMA.* 2003;**289**(2):210–16.

131. Kaduszkiewicz H, Zimmermann T, Beck-Bornhold HP, et al. Cholinesterase inhibitors for patients with Alzheimer's disease: systematic review of randomised clinical trials. *BMJ.* 2005;**331**:321–7.

132. Doody RS, Stevens JC, Beck C, et al. Practice parameter: management of dementia (an evidence-based review): report of the Quality Standards Subcommittee of the American Academy of Neurology. *Neurology.* 2001;**56**:1154–66.

133. Geldmacher DS, Provenzano G, McRae T, et al. Donepezil is associated with delayed nursing home placement in patients with Alzheimer's disease. *J Am Geriatr Soc.* 2003;**51**:937–44.

134. Grossberg GT. The ABC of Alzheimer's disease: behavioral symptoms and their treatment. *Int Psychogeriatr.* 2002;**14**(Suppl 1):27–49.

135. Courtney C, Farrell D, Gray R, et al. Long-term donepezil treatment in 565 patients with Alzheimer's

disease (AD2000): randomized double-blind trial. *Lancet.* 2004;**363**:2105–15.

136. Gill SS, Anderson GM, Fischer HD, et al. Syncope and its consequences in patients with dementia receiving cholinesterase inhibitors: a population-based cohort study. *Arch Intern Med.* 2009;**169**:867–73.

137. Schneider LS, Dagerman KS, Higgins JP, et al. Lack of evidence for the efficacy of memantine in mild Alzheimer disease. *Arch Neurol.* 2011;**68**:991–8.

138. McShane R, Areosa Sastre A, Miakaran N. Memantine for dementia. *Cochrane Database Syst Rev.* 2006;**2**:CD003154.

139. Ridha BH, Josephs KA, Rossor MN. Delusions and hallucinations in dementia with Lewy bodies: worsening with memantine. *Neurology.* 2005;**65**: 481–2.

140. Reisberg B, Doody R, Stoffler A, et al. Memantine in moderate-to-severe Alzheimer's disease. *NEJM.* 2003;**348**:1333–41.

141. Doody RS, Farlow M, Aisen PS, Alzheimer's Disease Cooperative Study Data Analysis and Publication Committee. Phase 3 trials of solanezumab and bapineuzumab for Alzheimer's disease. *N Engl J Med.* 2014;**370**:1460.

142. Salloway S, Sperling R, Fox NC, et al. Two phase 3 trials of bapineuzumab in mild-to-moderate Alzheimer's disease. *N Engl J Med.* 2014;**370**:322–33.

143. Miller ER, Pastor-Barriuso R, Dalal D, et al. Meta-analysis: high dosage vitamin E supplementation may increase all-cause mortality. *Ann Intern Med.* 2005;**142**:37–46.

144. Dysken MW, Sano M, Asthana S, et al. Effect of vitamin E and memantine on functional decline in Alzheimer disease: the TEAM-AD VA cooperative randomized trial. *JAMA.* 2014;**1**;311:33–44.

145. Aisen PS, Saumier D, Briand R, et al. A phase II study targeting amyloid-B with 3-APS in mild-to-moderate Alzheimer disease. *Neurology.* 2006;**67**:1757–63.

146. Scharf S, Mander A, Ugoni A, et al. A double-blind, placebo-controlled trial of diclofenac/misoprostol in Alzheimer's disease. *Neurology.* 1999;**53**:197–201.

147. Rich JB, Rasmusson DX, Folstein MF, et al. Nonsteroidal anti-inflammatory drugs in Alzheimer's disease. *Neurology.* 1995;**45**:51–5.

148. Coker LH, Espeland MA, Hogan PE, et al. Change in brain and lesion after CEE therapies: the WHIMS-MRI studies. *Neurology.* 2014;**82**:427–34.

149. Coker LH, Espeland MA, Rapp SR, et al. Postmenopausal hormone therapy and cognitive outcomes: the Women's Health Initiative Memory Study (WHIMS). *J Steroid Biochem Mol Biol.* 2010;**118**:304–10.

150. Birks J, Grimley EV, Van Dongen M. Ginkgo biloba for cognitive impairment and dementia. *Cochrane Database Syst Rev.* 2002;CD003120.

151. Snitz BE, O'Meara ES, Carlson MC, et al. Ginkgo biloba for preventing cognitive decline in older adults: a randomized trial. *JAMA.* 2009;**302**:2663–70.

152. Angell M, Kassirer JP. Alternative medicine – the risks of untested and unregulated remedies. *NEJM.* 1998;**339**:839–41.

153. Briones TL, Darwish H. Decrease in age-related tau hyperphosphorylation and cognitive improvement following vitamin D supplementation are associated with modulation of brain energy metabolism and redox state. *Neuroscience.* 2014;**262**:143–55.

154. Briones TL, Darwish H. Vitamin D mitigates age-related cognitive decline through the modulation of pro-inflammatory state and decrease in amyloid burden. *J Neuroinflammation.* 2012;**9**:244.

155. Craft S, Baker LD, Montine TJ, et al. Intranasal insulin therapy for Alzheimer disease and amnestic mild cognitive impairment: a pilot clinical trial. *Arch Neurol.* 2012;**69**:29–38.

156. Newhouse P, Kellar K, Aisen P, et al. Nicotine treatment of mild cognitive impairment: A 6-month double-blind pilot clinical trial. *Neurology.* 2012;**78**:91–101.

157. Salloway S, Sperling R, Brashear HR. Phase 3 trials of solanezumab and bapineuzumab for Alzheimer's disease. *N Engl J Med.* 2014;**370**:1459–60.

158. Blennow K, Zetterberg H, Rinne JO, et al. AAB-001 201/202 Investigators: effect of immunotherapy with bapineuzumab on cerebrospinal fluid biomarker levels in patients with mild to moderate Alzheimer disease. *Arch Neurol.* 2012;**69**:1002–10.

159. Farlow M, Arnold SE, van Dyck CH, et al. Safety and biomarker effects of solanezumab in patients with Alzheimer's disease. *Alzheimer's & Dementia.* 2012;**8**: 261–71.

160. Dodel R, Rominger A, Bartenstein P, et al. Intravenous immunoglobulin for treatment of mild-to-moderate Alzheimer's disease: a phase 2, randomised, double-blind, placebo-controlled, dose-finding trial. *Lancet Neurology.* 2013;**12**:233–43.

161. Shah S, Federoff HJ. Therapeutic potential of vaccines for Alzheimer's disease. *Immunotherapy.* 2011;**3**: 287–98.

162. Wiessner C, Wiederhold KH, Tissot AC, et al. The second-generation active abeta immunotherapy CAD106 reduces amyloid accumulation in APP transgenic mice while minimizing potential side effects. *Journal of Neuroscience.* 2011;**31**:9323–31.

163. Winblad B, Andreasen N, Minthon L, et al. Safety, tolerability, and antibody response of active abeta

immunotherapy with CAD106 in patients with alzheimer's disease: Randomised, double-blind, placebo-controlled, first-in-human study. *Lancet Neurology.* 2012;**11**:597–604.

164. Wilson RS, Mendes De Leon CF, Barnes LL, et al. Participation in cognitively stimulating activities and risk of incident Alzheimer disease. *JAMA.* 2002;**287**: 742–8.

165. Wilson RS, Bennett DA, Bienias JL, et al. Cognitive activity and incident AD in a population-based sample of older persons. *Neurology.* 2002;**59**:1910–14.

166. Verghese J, Lipton RB, Katz MJ, et al. Leisure activities and the risk of dementia in the elderly. *NEJM.* 2003;**348**:2508–16.

167. Weuve J, Kang JH, Manson JE, et al. Physical activity, including walking, and cognitive function in older women. *JAMA.* 2004;**292**:1454–61.

168. Van Gelder BM, Tijhuis MAR, Kalmijn S, et al. Physical activity in relation to cognitive decline in elderly men; the FINE study. *Neurology.* 2004;**63**: 2316–21.

169. Teri L, Gibbons LE, McCurry SM, et al. Exercise plus behavioral management in patients with Alzheimer disease: a randomized controlled trial. *JAMA.* 2003;**290**:2015–22.

170. Rolland Y, Rival L, Pillard F, et al. Feasibility of regular physical exercise for patients with moderate to severe Alzheimer disease. *J Nutr Health Aging.* 2000;**4**: 109–13.

171. Dvorak RV, Poehlman ET. Appendicular skeletal muscle mass, physical activity, and cognitive status in patients with Alzheimer's disease. *Neurology.* 1998;**51**: 1386–90.

172. Lauque S, Arnaud-Battandier F, Gillette S, et al. Improvement of weight and fat-free mass with oral nutritional supplementation in patients with Alzheimer's disease at risk of malnutrition: a prospective randomized study. *J Am Geriatr Soc.* 2004;**52**:1702–7.

173. Scarmeas N, Luchsinger JA, Schupf N, et al. Physical activity, diet, and risk of Alzheimer disease. *JAMA.* 2009;**302**:627–37.

174. Ngandu T, Lehtisalo J, Solomon A, et al. A 2 year multidomain intervention of diet, exercise, cognitive training, and vascular risk monitoring versus control to prevent cognitive decline in at-risk elderly people (FINGER): a randomised controlled trial. *Lancet.* 2015;**385**(9984):2255–63.

175. Mohamed S, Rosenheck R, Lyketsos CG, et al. Caregiver burden in Alzheimer disease: cross-sectional and longitudinal patient correlates. *Am J Geriatr Psychiatry.* 2010;**18**: 917–27.

176. Okura T, Langa KM. Caregiver burden and neuropsychiatric symptoms in older adults with cognitive impairment: the aging, demographics, and memory study (ADAMS). *Alzheimer Dis Assoc Disord.* 2011;**25**: 116–21.

177. Okura T, Plassman BL, Steffens DC, et al. Prevalence of neuropsychiatric symptoms and their association with functional limitations in older adults in the United States: the aging, demographics, and memory study. *J Am Geriatr Soc.* 2010;**58**: 330–7.

178. Brodaty H, Arasaratnam C. Meta-analysis of nonpharmacological interventions for neuropsychiatric symptoms of dementia. *Am J Psychiatry.* 2012;**169**:946–53.

179. Teri L, Rabins P, Whitehourse P, et al. Management of behavior disturbance in Alzheimer disease: current knowledge and future directions. *Alzheimer Dis Assoc Disord.* 1992;**6**:77–88.

180. Roca RP. Managing the behavioral complications of dementia. In: Cobbs EL, Duthie EH, Murphy JB, eds. *Geriatric Review Syllabus: A Core Curriculum in Geriatric Medicine.* 4th ed., Iowa: Kendall/Hunt; 1999: 183–6.

181. Gitlin LN, Winter L, Dennis MP, Hodgson N, Hauck WW. Targeting and managing behavioral symptoms in individuals with dementia: a randomized trial of a nonpharmacological intervention. *J Am Geriatr Soc.* 2010;**58**:1465–74.

182. Lyketsos CG, Steinberg M, Tschanz JT, et al. Mental and behavioral disturbances in dementia. *Am J Psychiatry.* 2000;**157**:708–14.

183. Khachiyants N, Trinkle D, Son SJ, et al. Sundown syndrome in persons with dementia: an update. *Psychiatry Investig.* 2011;**4**:275–87.

184. Cohen-Mansfield J, Werner P. Management of verbally disruptive behaviors in nursing home residents. *J Gerontol Med Sci.* 1996;**52**:M369–77.

185. Sloane PD, Hoeffer B, Mitchell CM, et al. Effect of person-centered showering and the towel bath on bathing-associated aggression, agitation, and discomfort in nursing home residents with dementia: a randomized, controlled trial. *J Am Geriatr Soc.* 2004;**52**:1795–1804.

186. Porsteinsson AP, Drye LT, Pollock BG, et al. Effect of citalopram on agitation in Alzheimer disease: the CitAD randomized clinical trial. *JAMA.* 2014;**311**: 682–91.

187. Lonergan, E, Luxenberg, J, Colford, J. Haloperidol for agitation in dementia. *Cochrane Database Syst Rev.* 2002;CD003154.

188. Wilson MP, Pepper D, Currier GW, et al. The psychopharmacology of agitation: consensus statement of the American Association for Emergency Psychiatry Project Beta psychopharmacology workgroup. *West J Emerg Med.*2012;**13**:26–34.

189. Schneider LS, Tariot PN, Dagerman KS, et al. for the CATIE-AD Study Group. Effectiveness of atypical antipsychotic drugs in patients with Alzheimer's disease. *NEJM*. 2006;**355**:1525–1538.

190. Sink KM, Holden KF, Yaffe K. Pharmacological treatment of neuropsychiatric symptoms of dementia: a review of the evidence. *JAMA*. 2005;**293**:596–608.

191. Lee PE, Gill SS, Freedman M, et al. Atypical antipsychotic drugs in the treatment of behavioural and psychological symptoms of dementia: systematic review. *BMJ*. 2004;**329**:75.

192. Kuehn, BM. FDA warns antipsychotic drugs may be risky for elderly. *JAMA*. 2005;**293**:2462.

193. Schneider LS, Dagerman KS, Insel P. Risk of death with atypical antipsychotic drug treatment for dementia: meta-analysis of randomized placebo-controlled trials. *JAMA*. 2005;**294**:1934–42.

194. Wang PS, Schneeweiss S, Avorn J, et al. Risk of death in elderly users of conventional vs. atypical antipsychotic medications. *NEJM*. 2005;**353**:2335 41.

195. Nelson JC, Devanand DP. A systematic review and meta-analysis of placebo-controlled antidepressant studies in people with depression and dementia. *J Am Geriatr Soc*. 2011;**59**:577–85.

196. Weintraub D, Rosenberg PB, Drye LT, et al. Sertraline for the treatment of depression in Alzheimer disease: week-24 outcomes. *Am J Geriatr Psychiatry*. 2010;**18**:332–40.

197. Banerjee S, Hellier J, Dewey M et al. Sertraline or mirtazapine for depression in dementia (HTA-SADD): a randomised, multicentre, double-blind, placebo-controlled trial. *Lancet*. 2011 Jul 30;**378**(9789):403–11.

198. Banerjee S, Hellier J, Romeo R, et al. Study of the use of antidepressants for depression in dementia: the HTA-SADD trial – a multicentre, randomised, double-blind, placebo-controlled trial of the clinical effectiveness and cost-effectiveness of sertraline and mirtazapine. *Health Technol Assess*. 2013;**17**:1–166.

199. Coupland C, Dhiman P, Morriss R, et al. Antidepressant use and risk of adverse outcomes in older people: population based cohort study. *BMJ*. 2011;**343**:d4551.

200. Burrows G, Kremer C. Mirtazipine: clinical advantages in the treatment of depression. *Psychopharmacology*. 1997;**17**(Suppl): 34S–39S.

201. Camargos E, Louzado L, Quintas J. Trazodone improves sleep parameters in Alzheimer disease patients: a randomized, double-blind, and placebo-controlled study. *Am J Geriatr Psychiatry*. 2014 Dec;**22**(12):1565–74.

202. Drachman DA, Swearer JM. Driving and Alzheimer's disease: the risk of crashes [published erratum appears in *Neurology*. 1994;44:4]. *Neurology*. 1993;**43**:2448–56.

203. Iverson DJ, Gronseth GS, Reger MA, et al. Practice parameter update: evaluation and management of driving risk in dementia. Report of the quality standards subcommittee of the American Academy of Neurology. *Neurology*. 2010;**74**:1316–24.

204. American Geriatric Society Ethics Committee and Clinical Practice and Models of Care Committee. American Geriatrics Society feeding tubes in advance dementia position statement. *J Am Geriatr Soc*. 2014;**62**:1590–3.

205. Mitchell SL, Teno JM, Kiely DK, et al. The clinical course of advanced dementia. *N Engl J Med*. 2009;**361**: 1529–38.

206. Gillick MR. Rethinking the role of tube feeding in patients with advanced dementia. *NEJM*. 2000;**342**: 206–10.

207. Arai Y, Sugiura M, Washio M, Miura H, Kudo K. Caregiver depression predicts early discontinuation of care for disabled elderly at home. *Psychiatry Clin Neurosci*. 2001;**55**:379–82.

208. Belle SH, Burgio L, Burns R, et al. Enhancing the quality of life of dementia caregivers from different ethnic or racial groups. *Ann Intern Med*. 2006;**145**: 727–38.

209. Newcomer R, Yordi C, DuNah R, Fox P, Wilkinson A. Effects of the Medicare Alzheimer's Disease Demonstration on caregiver burden and depression. *Health Serv Res*. 1999;**34**:669–89.

210. Gaugler JE, Jarrott SE, Zarit SH, Stephens MA, Townsend A, Greene R. Respite for dementia caregivers: the effects of adult day service use on caregiving hours and care demands. *Int Psychogeriatr*. 2003;**15**:37–58.

211. Kennedy GJ. Dementia. In: Cassel CK, Leipzig R, Cohen HJ, Larson EB, Meier DE. eds. *Geriatric Medicine: An Evidence-Based Approach*. 4th ed. New York: Springer-Verlag; 2003:1074–93.

147

Recognition, management, and prevention of delirium

Lindsay A. Wilson, MD, MPH, and Margaret Drickamer, MD

Introduction

Delirium is a serious neuropsychiatric condition characterized by an acute change in cognition and attention that affects a significant proportion of hospitalized older adults. The prevalence of delirium (Table 11.1) varies depending on the care setting and patient population; in one large tertiary care teaching hospital, 34.8% of patients over the age of 80 met the diagnostic criteria for delirium.[1]

Delirium portends a poor prognosis; it is associated with an increased risk of death, a functional decline, and institutionalization.[2] The one-year mortality rate for delirium is high, found to be 39% in one study.[3] Institutionalization is more common among those who have been delirious, with one study determining an odds ratio of 4:53.[4] The association is not necessarily causal – delirium may initiate a decline in health, or patients who develop delirium may be more ill.

The economic costs of delirium are significant. In one study, delirium more than doubled a patient's average health care costs per day for the entire year. [5] Total costs per patient for the delirium alone ranged from $16,303 to $64,421, which translated to an overall burden to the US health-care system of $38 billion to $152 billion per year.[5] The study did not account for indirect costs, such as caregiver burden or decreased quality of life.

Despite its association with substantial adverse events and healthcare costs, delirium remains underdiagnosed.[1] Challenges to diagnosing delirium are often present but vary depending on the provider and the patient. One common challenge results from the difficulty in differentiating between delirium and dementia as providers might attribute the signs and symptoms of delirium to "dementia,"

assuming that the cognitive change is not new to the patient. Determining the acuity of onset of the cognitive change often requires some detective work such as calling a nursing facility or querying a caregiver. The physician must then trust this assessment of the patient's baseline mental status. Providers might also have difficulty determining if a somnolent or lethargic patient has delirium as this takes time and effort. The provider must attempt to arouse the patient to perform a cognitive assessment or initiate a conversation. Another challenge arises from the natural history of delirium. With delirium, cognition waxes and wanes, making brief assessments at discrete points in time sometimes inadequate. Providers again have to obtain collateral information from a caregiver to better determine whether the patient has displayed signs of delirium at other points in time. Finally, delirium can be called many names; examples include altered mental status, sundowning, agitation, and encephalopathy. Health care providers might not know if their patients have delirium due to the lack of consistent terminology used by caregivers and colleagues. Despite these challenges, delirium prevention, recognition, and management are key to the care of the older patient.

Definition

The American Psychiatric Association's *Diagnostic and Statistical Manual*, 5th edition (DSM-5), provides the following diagnostic criteria for delirium:

1. Inattention and reduced awareness
2. Change in cognition
3. Acute onset and fluctuating course
4. Presence of underlying medical cause based on evidence from the history and physical exam

---

Reichel's Care of the Elderly, 7th Edition, ed. Jan Busby-Whitehead *et al.* Published by Cambridge University Press.
© Cambridge University Press 2016.

Table 11.1 Prevalence and incidence of delirium in different care settings

Care setting	Prevalence (%)	Incidence
General medical ward	18–35	11–14
Medical ward, patients with dementia	18	56
Emergency department	8–17	
Nursing home	14	20–22
Intensive care	7–50	19–82

Source: Adapted from Inouye 2013.[6]

Table 11.2 Predisposing and precipitating factors for delirium

Predisposing	Precipitating
Cognitive impairment	Infection
Comorbidity	New medication
Polypharmacy	Surgery
Frailty	Restraint use
Malnutrition	Immobility
Dementia	New medication
Depression	Sleep deprivation
History of falls	Illness
Alcohol abuse	Dehydration
Vision Impairment	Fracture
Hearing Impairment	Neurologic disease
Age >65	Constipation
Male sex	Urinary retention
Neurologic disease	New environment or schedule
Low level of activity	Polypharmacy
Functional dependence	Pain

Source: Adapted from *NEJM* 2006.[9]

Pathophysiology

The pathophysiology of delirium remains incompletely understood and is likely diverse depending on the individual and the factors contributing to the delirium. Cerebral hypometabolism, cerebral hypoperfusion, deficiencies in glucose and oxygen at a cellular level, and an imbalance of cholinergic, serotonergic, dopaminergic, noradrenergic, and other neurotransmitter systems have all been implicated in the development of delirium in studies using techniques such as EEGs, proton emission computed tomography (PET), and measurement of serum biomarkers via immunocytochemistry.[7] Specific clinical scenarios may have other contributing factors. For example, in sepsis, circulating inflammatory cytokines may cause dysfunction in brain cells and blood vessels that alters permeability of the blood-brain barrier.[7] Further research is needed to elucidate a definitive pathway that may be targeted for prevention and treatment of delirium.

Etiology

Like many geriatric syndromes, the cause of delirium is usually multifactorial, and the multifactorial model of delirium is well described and widely accepted.[6] This model focuses on the interplay between predisposing factors and precipitating factors.[6] Predisposing factors, also termed intrinsic factors, are characteristics that patients have at baseline that increase their vulnerability to delirium.[6]

Precipitating factors, or extrinsic factors, are the additional insults that patients encounter that result in delirium when combined with the predisposing factors.[6] Patients with significant predisposing factors, such as cognitive impairment, high medical comorbidity, and polypharmacy, may only need a small precipitating factor, such as constipation or bed rest, to tip them into delirium.[6] Patients with either few or minor predisposing factors will need the addition of several significant precipitating factors, such as heart failure, pneumonia, and electrolyte abnormalities, to develop delirium.[6] The most common predisposing factor is cognitive impairment, but other examples of predisposing factors and precipitating factors are listed in Table 11.2.

> The cause of delirium is usually multifactorial resulting from a combination of predisposing and precipitating factors.

Table 11.3 Recommended strategies for using medications in patients at risk for delirium

Opioids	Utilize opioid-sparing techniques and medications such as routine administration of acetaminophen, heating pads, gentle massage, patches, or gels. Start with a low dose of opioids and frequently reassess, increasing dose as needed to achieve pain control. Use a bowel regimen to prevent constipation.
Benzodiazepines	Use the lowest dose possible for the shortest duration possible. Address anxiety and insomnia with nonpharmacological measures such as psychotherapy and sleep hygiene. Taper when discontinuing to avoid withdrawal as withdrawal can also precipitate delirium.
Diphenhydramine	Avoid; use second-generation antihistamines if possible. Use the lowest dose possible and for the shortest duration possible.

Certain medications, such as sedatives, opioids, and anticholinergics, are associated with the development of delirium.[6] These medications should be used cautiously in older adults at risk for delirium, and stopping or tapering these medications may be part of the management plan (refer to Table 11.3 and Management section). An important caveat is that uncontrolled pain can also precipitate delirium, so opioid pain medications should be used if necessary to alleviate discomfort.[8]

Prediction of delirium

The multifactorial model forms the basis for tools used to predict delirium in patient populations. For example, a prediction tool designed specifically for patients undergoing cardiac surgery gives points for prior stroke or transient ischemic attack, Mini-Mental Status Examination score, abnormal albumin, and Geriatric Depression Scale score. Higher scores are associated with higher rates of delirium.[10] Other tools have been developed for other specific patient populations, such as patients in the emergency department or at hospital discharge.[11, 12] While helpful for population use, these tools cannot accurately predict which individual will develop delirium.

Prevention

Inouye et al. reported important results of a multi-component intervention to prevent delirium in hospitalized older patients in the *New England Journal of Medicine* in 1999.[13] Hospitalized patients at risk for delirium were studied using a prospective matching strategy rather than a randomized controlled trial design, as this was the most cost-effective approach. Patients in the experimental arm received a multi-component, protocoled intervention addressing six risk factors for delirium: cognitive impairment, sleep deprivation, immobility, visual impairment, hearing impairment, and dehydration. The study found that the 15% of patients in the control arm developed delirium compared with 9% in the experimental arm.[13]

This pivotal study resulted in the development of the Hospital Elder Life Program, which has been implemented at more than 60 sites in five countries.[14] More information on the components of the Hospital Elder Life Program is provided in Table 11.4.

Geriatric consultation may have a role in the prevention of delirium in hip fracture patients, as demonstrated by a small randomized controlled trial.[15] Medications, including haloperidol, atypical antipsychotics, gabapentin, acetylcholinesterase inhibitors, and melatonin, have been studied, usually in the postoperative setting, but they were not efficacious in delirium prevention.[16]

> Up to one-third of delirium cases can be prevented with a multifactorial intervention (the Hospital Elder Life Program).

Diagnosis

The diagnosis of delirium is best made by using the Confusion Assessment Method, or CAM.[17] This algorithm, which was developed by an expert panel, utilizes four cardinal diagnostic criteria for delirium: acute onset and fluctuating course, inattention, disorganized thinking, and altered level of

Table 11.4 Components of the Hospital Elder Life Program

Daily visitor program: orientation, socialization

Therapeutic activities program: cognitive and social stimulation

Early mobilization program: daily exercise

Nonpharmacological sleep protocol: back rub, warm drink, relaxation tapes

Hearing and vision protocol: adaptations provided

Oral volume repletion and feeding assistance program: assistance with meals

Source: Adapted from the Hospital Elder Life Program.[13]

Confusion Assessment Method (CAM)(17)

- Does the patient have inattention?

- If yes, is it an acute onset and/or fluctuating?

- If yes, does the patient have either disorganized thinking OR altered level of consciousness?

- If yes, to all three *questions*--the patient is CAM positive.

Figure 11.1 Confusion Assessment Method (CAM).

consciousness. The patient must have the first two criteria and either the third or fourth to have a positive test. The test was validated against psychiatrists' diagnoses and was determined to have a sensitivity of 94%–100% and specificity of 90%–95%.[17]

An acute onset of cognitive change (criteria 1 of the CAM) is key to the diagnosis of delirium and helps differentiate delirium from dementia. The interviewer must question the caregiver regarding the patient's baseline mental status and rely on the history provided to determine the acuity of onset and fluctuating course.

Patients with inattention (criteria 2 of the CAM) have difficulty engaging in conversation, following commands, and performing simple repetitive tasks, such as subtracting serial sevens, tapping on the letter A in SAVEAHEART, or spelling "world" backward. They may attend to other stimuli, either internal such as their own thoughts, or external, such as their bed sheets, clothing, or IVs. A classic presentation of an inattentive delirious patient is the patient who is too busy picking at the bed sheets to focus on conversation.

Disorganized thinking (criteria 3 of the CAM) is not required for the diagnosis of delirium unless the patient has a normal level of consciousness (criteria 4 of the CAM).[17] Disorganized thinking is noted when a patient's speech is unpredictable, incoherent, paranoid, or illogical. A patient, for example, might refuse medications, believing that the drugs are poison.

The last diagnostic criteria is an altered level of consciousness. A patient with an altered level of consciousness is either more or less active than a person with normal alertness. A patient with delirium who is agitated, hyper vigilant, easily startled, and restless has hyperactive delirium. Alternatively, a patient who is difficult to arouse, lethargic, and sleepy has hypoactive delirium. Both of these variations can be alarming and difficult to manage.

> The Confusion Assessment Method is very sensitive and specific for the detection of delirium.

Evaluation

Once a patient has been diagnosed with delirium using the CAM, an evaluation to determine the possible underlying causes of the delirium starts with a full history, including a complete medication review, and thorough physical exam.[8] If the history is limited by the patient's mental state or ability to cooperate, an attempt should be made to question available caregivers about the patient's health and behavior in the days prior to the presentation.[8]

Possible underlying etiologies of delirium may be remembered using the mnemonic DELIRIUM (see Table 11.5), which can guide the history and physical.

Delirium can be the only manifestation of a severe illness, but it usually results from more than one factor.[8] The diagnostic workup should be guided by clinical suspicion coupled with findings on the history and physical exam.[8] Additionally, the patient's goals of care should be factored into the evaluation and treatment plan. Delirium is often present at the end of life when a palliative or comfort-oriented approach should be considered with the patient and his or her primary decision maker. Patients with delirium often lack capacity to make significant medical decisions so this role may be delegated to the designated decision maker: the person with health care power of attorney or next of kin.

151

Table 11.5 Delirium mnemonic to guide evaluation

Letter		Examples	Questions for caregiver	Examples of diagnostic studies
D	Drugs/lack of drugs	New or recent medications (e.g., benzodiazepines), alcohol intoxication/ withdrawal	Any new or recent medication changes? Any OTC medications? Illicit drugs? Alcohol use? When was his/her last drink of alcohol?	Urine drug screen, blood alcohol level
E	Electrolyte abnormalities	High or low glucose, sodium, calcium, urea nitrogen	Has the patient been eating and drinking well? How does s/he access food? Has s/he lost/ gained weight?	Chemistry panel, albumin, pre-albumin
L	Lack of sleep/ consistent routine	New home, new caregiver	Describe the patient's routine. Any changes recently?	
I	Infections	Pneumonia, UTI, acute cholecystitis, cellulitis, abscess, diverticulitis, appendicitis, gastroenteritis	Has the patient had a fever? Cough? Abdominal pain? Nausea or vomiting?	Lung, skin, and abdominal exams; CBC, urinalysis, urine culture, CT scan, *C. difficile* assay
R	Reduced sensory input	Vision or hearing loss	Does the patient wear eyeglasses or hearing aids?	Ear exam, eye exam, examination of hearing aids
I	Intracranial	Intracranial hemorrhage, stroke, seizure	Has the patient hit his/ her head? Is the patient on a blood thinner?	Neuro exam, head CT, EEG
U	Urinary retention, constipation	Fecal impaction, acute urinary retention	Has the patient had difficulty with urination, bowel movements? When was the last bowel movement?	Abdominal x-ray, bladder scan, rectal exam
M	Major organ dysfunction	Myocardial infarction, kidney failure, respiratory failure with CO_2 retention, mesenteric ischemia	Has the patient complained of chest pain, shortness of breath, abdominal pain, blood in the stools?	Cardiac exam, EKG, CBC, cardiac enzymes, chemistry panel, ABG, hemoccult

Although many additional studies may be part of the delirium evaluation, some tests to consider are listed in Table 11.6.

Management

The management of delirium requires multiple interventions targeting the precipitating and predisposing factors that contributed to the development of delirium.[8] Management should focus on treatments that enhance recovery, maximize function, and improve outcomes while minimizing the negative consequences of delirium.[8] These vary from patient to patient; therefore, certain aspects of the management approach are unique to each patient. For

Table 11.6 Examples of diagnostic studies in the evaluation of patients with delirium

Test	Diagnoses considered	Threshold for ordering	Comments
Chest x-ray	Pneumonia, pulmonary edema from congestive heart failure	Low	Chest x-ray can rarely be negative early in the course of pneumonia
EKG	Arrhythmia, ischemia	Low	Compare to baseline EKG, if available
Basic metabolic panel	Renal failure, electrolyte abnormalities	Low	Compare renal function to baseline renal function, if available
CBC	Leukocytosis, anemia	Low	Compare to baseline counts, if available
Cardiac enzymes	Ischemia	Low	
Urinalysis	Infection	Low	Older women may have abnormal findings that do not indicate infection unless signs and symptoms of infection are present
Urine culture	Infection	Low	Older women may have positive cultures that do not indicate infection unless signs and symptoms of infection are present
Liver function tests	Cholestasis, hepatitis	Intermediate	If fever is present, consider obtaining a right upper quadrant ultrasound to evaluate for acute cholecystitis, which can present atypically in older adults
Abdominal x-ray	Constipation, bowel obstruction	Intermediate	Consider CT if significant concern for intra-abdominal pathology (such as diverticulitis, appendicitis)
Head CT or MRI	Hemorrhage, stroke	Intermediate	Lower threshold in patients who have fallen or are on blood thinners, such as warfarin
EEG	Seizure	Very high	Can help differentiate delirium from other conditions, assess for occult seizures
Urine drug screen	Drug exposure	Low	
Blood alcohol level	Intoxication	Low	Only helpful in acute intoxication
Vitamin B12 level	Low B12	Intermediate	Rare to be the cause of acute delirium
Thyroid function tests	Hypothyroidism, hyperthyroidism	Low–intermediate	
Arterial blood gas	Hypercarbia, hypoxia	Intermediate	
Lumbar puncture	Meningitis	High	Consider in patients with fever and/or headache and/or nuchal rigidity

example, a palliative or comfort-oriented approach may be preferred by a patient who is at the end of life. Research on the effectiveness of these individualized management plans is difficult to perform and not available at this time; nonetheless, this approach is recommended until further research results are available.

Precipitating factors, such as infections, dehydration, and constipation, are often easier to address in the management plan than predisposing factors, such as cognitive impairment or hearing impairment, which may be longstanding issues. Nonetheless, even persistent conditions may be improved; for example, providers can address hearing impairment by removing cerumen impaction and providing noise amplifiers or hearing aids.

Pain can be difficult to assess in a patient with delirium since patients may have difficulty self-reporting, and agitation and somnolence from the delirium can mimic under- and over-treatment with opioids. Under-treatment of pain can lead to delirium; therefore, adequate pain control is essential in the management of delirium.[8] A combination of opioid-sparing agents, such as acetaminophen, lidocaine patches, and topical NSAID creams, and approaches, such as heating pads and gentle massage, in addition to opioids may ensure pain relief (see Table 11.3).

All patients with delirium would likely benefit from certain interventions, and this recommendation is extrapolated from the delirium prevention trials [13] and studies on the "delirium room" (DR), also called the "restraint-free room."[18] This room operates on the principle of "Tolerate, Anticipate, and Don't Agitate," and has special features (outlined in Table 11.5) that may lessen the negative outcomes associated with delirium.[18] For example, in the delirium room, physicians try to limit continuous intravenous infusions that tether the patient to an IV pole for prolonged periods, instead using boluses through IVs that are covered by soft gauze.

Physicians should try to untether patients as much as possible to allow for maximum mobility.[18] Restraints, ranging from soft wrist restraints to telemetry leads and intravenous infusions, should be minimized.[18] Bladder catheters should be removed as soon as possible, and patients should be encouraged and, if needed, assisted, to use the toilet.[18]

Another recommendation in the management of delirium is to encourage a normal sleep-wake cycle.

Table 11.7 Features and strategies of the delirium room

All patients can be seen by the nursing staff
The DR is near the nurses' station
Physical restraints are banned
Patients are screened for delirium every shift
Nurse and physician are involved in evaluation of delirium
Pharmacological interventions are a last resort
Physicians should evaluate an agitated patient at the bedside
If reorientation is not successful, do not continue to attempt reorientation
Hide necessary and remove unnecessary "attachments"
Encourage patients to be out of bed and assist or observe depending on patient safety

Source: Adapted from Flaherty 2011.[18]

[13] Allowing natural daylight and artificial light to keep a room well lit during the day and avoiding nighttime disruptions, such as lab draws and vital sign checks, help patients attend to their natural biological rhythm.

Family members or familiar caregivers should be encouraged to stay with a patient with delirium to provide reassurance and orientation.[13] Education on how to interact with the patient, particularly if the patient is agitated, may be needed, but families and caregivers are usually able to quickly learn this skill set (see Figure 11.2).

If these measures are not able to adequately address severe behavioral and emotional symptoms, most experts in the field concede that antipsychotics may be added to the non-pharmacological approach. Antipsychotics and their role in treating delirium are discussed further in the next section.

> The management of delirium first involves addressing predisposing and precipitating factors that contributed to its development.

Pharmacological treatment

Delirium can resolve and improve over time without pharmacological intervention, and studies do not

Recommendations of How to Interact with Patients with Delirium

Hyperactive

--Remain calm

--Approach the patient slowly

--Use a reassuring and calming tone

--Use gentle touch if patient appears receptive; if patient appears guarded, respect his/her

personal space as much as possible

--Ask easy-to-follow questions or speak using easy-to-follow statements

--Avoid restricting the patient's movements with tethers, such as oxygen tubing, telemetry,

catheters, and IVs

--Distract the patients from any distressing stimuli by providing alternative stimuli such as

a vest or apron that has strings, buttons, and other texture to provide tactile stimulation

(often called a busy-vest/apron)

Hypoactive

--Get close to the patient's face so that he can hear and see you as easily as possible

--Speak using easy-to-follow statements

--Touch the patient's arm or shoulder with increasing firmness to attempt to arouse

--Put glasses and hearing aids on the patient after ensuring that these assistive devices are

clean and functional

--Help the patient sit in an upright position, preferably in a chair

Figure 11.2 How to interact with patients with delirium

consistently show that any medication lessens the severity or reduces the duration of delirium.[19] The most commonly studied medications are in the class of antipsychotics, and most of the studies are small, with methodological challenges.[19] Additionally, these medications are associated with harms such as extrapyramidal symptoms, prolonged QT interval, and sedation.[19]

Antipsychotics should be reserved for patients who have severe distress from their delirium and cannot cooperate with essential medical care.[9] A recommended approach is to start with a very low dose of an antipsychotic, such as 0.5 mg of intravenous haloperidol or 0.25 mg of oral risperdone, and titrate the dose to a calming, but not sedating, effect on the patient.[9] The lowest dose possible should be used for the shortest duration possible. Given these medications have a black box warning for use in older adults, providers should attempt to communicate with families and caregivers about the risks and benefits. If time allows, a baseline EKG should be obtained to ensure that the patient does not have a prolonged QT interval, as almost all antipsychotics prolong the QT interval.

Conclusions

Delirium, a neurocognitive disorder characterized by an acute change in attention, usually results from a combination of precipitating and predisposing factors and can be the only manifestation of a severe underlying illness. The prevention, recognition, and management of delirium are essential to reducing the morbidity and mortality associated with this disorder. The components of the Hospital Elder Life Program should be part of the daily routine of our hospitalized older patients to reduce the incidence of delirium. Providers should regularly screen hospitalized older adults for delirium using the Confusion Assessment Method to improve detection. Once identified, a thorough history and physical should guide further evaluation and management, which involves addressing the precipitating and predisposing factors and providing support to the patient to maximize independence and functionality. Addressing delirium in these ways is a fundamental and critical part of geriatric patient care.

References

1. Ryan DJ, O'Regan NA, Caoimh RO, et al. Delirium in an adult acute hospital population: predictors, prevalence and detection. *BMJ Open* 2013 Jan 7;3(1):pii: e001772. DOI: 10.1136/bmjopen-2012-001772.

2. Dasgupta M. Prognosis of delirium in hospitalized elderly: worse than we thought. *Geriatric Psychiatry* 2013 May;29(5):497–505.

3. Kiely DK, Marcantonio ER, Inouye SK, et al. Persistent delirium predicts greater mortality. *J Am Geriatr Soc* 2009 Jan;57(1):55–61.

4. George J, Bleasdale S, Singleton S. Causes and prognosis of delirium in elderly patients admitted to a district general hospital. *Age Ageing* 1997 Nov 26(6):423–7.

5. Leslie DL, Inouye SK. The importance of delirium: economic and societal costs. *J Am Geriatr Soc* 2011 Nov;59(2):241–3.

6. Inouye SK, Westendorp RG, Saczynski JS. Delirium in elderly people. *Lancet* 2014 Mar 8;383(9920):911–22.

7. Williams ST. Pathophysiology of encephalopathy and delirium. *Journal of Clinical Neurophysiology* 2013;30(5):435–7.

8. Morrison RS1, Magaziner J, Gilbert M, et al. Relationship between pain and opioid analgesics on the development of delirium following hip fracture. *J Gerontol A Biol Sci Med Sci.* 2003 Jan;58(1):76–81.

9. Inouye SK. Delirium in older persons. *NEJM* 2006 Mar;354:1157–65.

10. Rudolph JL, Jones RN, Levkoff SE, et al. Derivation and validation of a preoperative prediction rule for delirium after cardiac surgery. *Circulation* 2009 Jan 20;119(2):229–36.

11. Kennedy M, Enander RA, Tadiri SP, Wolfe RE, Shapiro NI, Marcantonio ER. Delirium risk prediction, healthcare use and mortality of elderly adults in the emergency department. *J Am Geriatr Soc* 2014 Mar;62(3):462–69.

12. Inouye SK, Zhang Y, Jones RN, Kiely DK, Yang F, Marcantonio ER. Risk factors for delirium at discharge: development and validation of a predictive model. *Arch Intern Med* 2007 Jul 9;167(13):1406–13.

13. Inouye SK. A multicomponent intervention to prevent delirium in hospitalized older patients. *NEJM* 1999 Mar 4;340(9):669–76.

14. Inouye SK, Rubin FH, Wierman HR, Supiano MA, Fenlon K. No shortcuts for delirium prevention. *J Am Geriatr Soc* 2010 May;58(5):998–9.

15. Marcantonio ER. Reducing delirium after hip fracture: a randomized trial. *J Am Geriatr Soc* 2001 May;49(5):516–22.

16. Gorsch M, Nicholas JA. Pharmacologic prevention of postoperative delirium. *Z Gerontol Geriatri* 2014;47(2):105.

17. Inouye SK, van Dyck CH, Alessi CA, Balkin S, Siegal AP, Horwitz RI. Clarifying confusion: the confusion assessment method. A new method for detection of delirium. *Ann Intern Med* 1990 Dec 15;113 (12):941–8.

18. Flaherty JH, Little MO. Matching the environment to patients with delirium: lessons learned from the delirium room, a restraint-free environment for older hospitalized adults with delirium. *J Am Geriatr Soc* 2013;59:295–300.

19. Lonergan E, Britton AM, Luxenberg J, Wyller T. Antipsychotics for delirium. *Cochrane Database Syst Rev* 2007 Apr 18;2:CD005594.

Chapter 12

Diagnosis and management of heart disease in the elderly

Michael W. Rich, MD, and Joshua M. Stolker, MD

Global burden of heart disease in older adults

Cardiovascular disease is the leading cause of death and major disability in the United States and around the world, and the global burden of heart disease is increasing, in large part due to the aging of the population.[1, 2] In the United States, nearly two-thirds of all cardiovascular hospitalizations occur in patients aged 65 and older, more than 80% of cardiovascular deaths occur in geriatric individuals, and an estimated 70% of Americans over age 70 have clinically recognized cardiovascular diseases.[3] For these reasons, practitioners should become familiar with strategies for the prevention and management of cardiovascular disease in older adults.

Effects of aging on the cardiovascular system

Aging is associated with diverse alterations in cardiovascular structure and function (Table 12.1).[4] Some of the most clinically relevant changes include increasing vascular stiffness, impaired endothelial function, impaired left ventricular relaxation and compliance, diminished responsiveness to neurohormonal signals such as β-adrenergic stimulation, and degeneration of the sinus node and electrical conduction system. These factors contribute to the development of systolic hypertension, heart failure, coronary artery disease, aortic and mitral valve disease, and electrical disturbances including bradyarrhythmias and atrial fibrillation. In addition, the effects of aging modulate the clinical presentation and response to cardiovascular therapies in the geriatric population. Similarly, aging affects other organ systems (Table 12.2) that frequently interact with cardiovascular diseases and therapeutics.

Medical co-morbidities, altered pharmacokinetics and pharmacodynamics, behavioral and social factors, and financial concerns also impact prognosis and goals of care in older individuals with cardiovascular disease.[5]

Ischemic heart disease

Epidemiology and primary prevention

In 2010, approximately 7 million deaths worldwide were attributed to ischemic heart disease (IHD).[1] In men, the median age at death from IHD was about 70 years, while in women the median age at death was about 80 years (i.e., half of all IHD deaths in women occur in the small fraction of the population 80 years of age or older).[1]

Increasing age is the strongest predictor of coronary artery disease (CAD), as exemplified in risk assessment tools such as the Framingham Risk Score.[6] Age-related changes in the arterial wall and prolonged exposure to traditional atherosclerotic risk factors contribute to the paramount importance of advancing age as a predictor of CAD. Apart from age, major risk factors for CAD include hypertension, dyslipidemia, tobacco use, family history (via incompletely defined genetic factors), and behavioral and environmental factors such as atherogenic diet and sedentary lifestyle. Diabetes mellitus is considered a CAD risk-equivalent, since diabetics without known CAD experience seven-year rates of myocardial infarction (MI) that are similar to patients without diabetes who already have experienced an MI.[7] Importantly, the prevalence of hypertension, dyslipidemia, diabetes, and sedentary lifestyle all tend to increase with age, further predisposing older individuals to the development of CAD. In addition, subclinical cardiovascular disease is highly prevalent in the geriatric population and magnifies the risk of developing symptomatic CAD.[8]

Reichel's Care of the Elderly, 7th Edition, ed. Jan Busby-Whitehead *et al.* Published by Cambridge University Press.
© Cambridge University Press 2016.

Table 12.1 Effects of aging on the cardiovascular system

Gross anatomy
- Increased left ventricular wall thickness and decreased cavity size
- Endocardial thickening and sclerosis
- Increased left atrial size
- Valvular fibrosis and sclerosis
- Increased epicardial fat

Histology
- Increased lipid and amyloid deposition
- Increased collagen deposition and fibrosis
- Calcification of fibrous skeleton, valve rings, and coronary arteries
- Shrinkage of myocardial fibers with focal hypertrophy
- Decreased mitochondria, altered mitochondrial membranes
- Decreased nucleus: myofibril size ratio

Biochemical changes
- Decreased protein elasticity
- Numerous changes in enzyme content and activity affecting most metabolic pathways, but no change in myosin ATPase activity
- Decreased catecholamine synthesis, especially norepinephrine
- Decreased acetylcholine synthesis
- Decreased activity of nitric oxide synthase

Conduction system
- Degeneration of sinus node pacemaker and transition cells
- Decreased number of conducting cells in the AV-node and His-Purkinje system
- Increased connective tissue, fat, and amyloid
- Increased fibrosis in and around the atrial conduction system
- Increased calcification around conduction system

Vasculature
- Decreased distensibility of large and medium-sized arteries
- Impaired endothelial function
- Aorta and muscular arteries become dilated, elongated, and tortuous
- Increased wall thickness
- Increased connective tissue and calcification

Autonomic nervous system
- Decreased responsiveness to β-adrenergic stimulation
- Increased circulating catecholamines, decreased tissue catecholamines
- Decreased β-adrenergic receptors in cardiac myocytes
- Decreased cholinergic responsiveness
- Diminished response to valsalva and baroreceptor stimulation
- Decreased heart rate variability

Clinical presentation

Whereas substernal chest pain or pressure is considered the hallmark of obstructive CAD, geriatric individuals frequently present without classic angina. Elderly patients may experience dyspnea, nausea or gastrointestinal distress, presyncope or syncope, generalized malaise or fatigue, diaphoresis, altered mental status, or even no symptoms at all when experiencing acute coronary syndromes. Thus, the proportion of subjects with acute MI who present with chest pain decreases with age, although dyspnea remains a prominent presenting symptom. Exertional angina may not occur due to sedentary lifestyle or limited functional capacity in

Table 12.2 Effects of aging on other organ systems

Kidneys
- Gradual decline in glomerular filtration rate, ~8 mL/min/decade
- Impaired fluid and electrolyte homeostasis

Lungs
- Reduced ventilatory capacity
- Increased ventilation/perfusion mismatching

Neurohumoral system
- Reduced cerebral perfusion autoregulatory capacity
- Diminished reflex responsiveness
- Impaired thirst mechanism

Hemostatic system
- Increased levels of coagulation factors
- Increased platelet activity and aggregability
- Increased inflammatory cytokines and C-reactive protein
- Increased inhibitors of fibrinolysis and angiogenesis

Musculoskeletal system
- Decreased muscle mass (sarcopenia)
- Decreased bone mass (osteopenia), especially in women

frail individuals, so the diagnosis of CAD may be delayed.

Physical findings are variable, but subacute or late presentations in the geriatric population with MI may lead to more profound cardiovascular decompensation and associated signs of heart failure, hypotension, or shock. Other findings may include pallor, confusion, tachycardia, low-grade fever, leukocytosis, or elevated C-reactive protein. Individuals presenting with hemodynamic compromise, prolonged ischemia, or life-threatening arrhythmias have a markedly increased risk of death, and the mortality rate following acute MI increases exponentially with age (Figure 12.1).[9]

Diagnosis of myocardial infarction

In patients with acute myocardial ischemia, the electrocardiogram (ECG) often demonstrates ST-segment elevations and/or depressions, as well as T-wave abnormalities. However, older patients are less likely to exhibit diagnostic ECG changes due to preexisting conduction system disease (e.g., left bundle branch block), ventricular paced rhythm, left ventricular hypertrophy, prior MI, metabolic and electrolyte abnormalities, or medications such as digoxin or antiarrhythmic drugs.

The diagnosis of MI is confirmed when serum biomarkers of myocardial necrosis are elevated. Troponin-I and troponin-T have excellent sensitivity and specificity for diagnosing acute MI. Recently, the development of high sensitivity troponin assays has

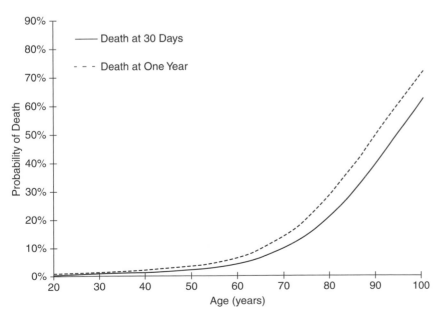

Figure 12.1 Probability of mortality at 30 days and 1 year as a function of age in the GUSTO-I trial ($N = 41,021$).

led to improved early detection of myocardial ischemia, but at the cost of a higher "false positive" rate.[10] This may lead to overdiagnosis of acute MI, especially in older adults who tend to have higher ambulatory troponin levels.[11] Additionally, troponin levels may be mildly elevated in the presence of renal insufficiency, which is highly prevalent in older patients.

The high prevalence of atypical presentations and nondiagnostic ECG findings in the geriatric population requires a higher index of suspicion for acute MI in elderly subjects. Delayed diagnosis is common in older patients, reducing the "window of opportunity" for implementing appropriate treatment and limiting the extent of ischemic damage. Treatment delays also increase the risk for complications, including heart failure, arrhythmias, hypotension, myocardial rupture, and shock.

Other cardiovascular and medical conditions with similar symptom complexes should be included in the differential diagnosis for MI, especially because many of these diseases also occur more frequently in elderly individuals. Chest pain without ECG changes could signify unstable angina, but other life-threatening conditions such as pulmonary embolus, aortic dissection, acute pericardial disease, pneumonia, severe peptic ulcer disease, cholecystitis, pancreatitis, or esophageal rupture must also be considered.

Pharmacologic management of myocardial infarction

Acute MI with ST-segment elevation usually involves atherosclerotic plaque rupture and associated thrombotic occlusion of an epicardial coronary artery. However, a large proportion of infarctions in the geriatric population occur without ST-segment elevation and arise because of a mismatch between oxygen supply and demand in the setting of fixed coronary obstruction. These infarcts are designated type II MIs in the universal classification of MI schema.[12] Thus, type II MI in the elderly often occurs in association with an infection (e.g., pneumonia or sepsis), significant hypertension or hypotension, anemia, perioperative volume shifts, or other systemic illness such as thyroid disease. Therapies are directed toward improving coronary blood flow, reducing myocardial oxygen demand, reducing the risk of coronary thrombosis, correcting the precipitating illness (e.g., infection), reducing sympathetic tone, and preventing adverse remodeling of hypoperfused myocardium.

The major therapeutic options for acute MI are listed in Table 12.3. Supplemental oxygen should be administered to maintain an arterial oxygen saturation $\geq 92\%$. Intravenous access and telemetry monitoring are imperative to identify and treat potential complications of MI. Morphine and nitroglycerin should be administered as needed to control pain and dyspnea.

Antiplatelet therapy Aspirin 160 mg–325 mg should be administered immediately and continued indefinitely at a dose of 75 mg–162 mg daily.[13, 14] Aspirin reduces mortality in patients with unstable angina or acute MI, and the benefit of aspirin therapy increases with age, from a 1% absolute mortality reduction below age 60 to a 4.7% absolute mortality reduction at age 70 and older.[15] Clopidogrel, a $P2Y_{12}$ receptor inhibitor, is a reasonable alternative (300 mg–600 mg loading dose followed by 75 mg daily) in subjects unable to take aspirin. Among patients with acute coronary syndromes, 12 months of aspirin plus clopidogrel reduces the risk of death or reinfarction by about 20% compared to aspirin alone.[16] Newer $P2Y_{12}$ receptor antagonists, such as prasugrel and ticagrelor, have been associated with improved outcomes relative to clopidogrel in younger patients, but prasugrel should be avoided in patients ≥ 75 years of age due to increased risk of bleeding.[17] In contrast, ticagrelor has demonstrated improved outcomes relative to clopidogrel, including lower rates of recurrent MI and cardiovascular death, and without higher bleeding rates in elderly subjects.[18, 19] The optimal duration of dual anti-platelet therapy remains controversial, with recent studies suggesting that treatment for up to 30 months is associated with a reduction in ischemic events at a cost of increased bleeding.[20] Thus, use of prolonged dual antiplatelet therapy in the geriatric population should be individualized. Whenever possible, all of the $P2Y_{12}$ agents should be withheld for five to seven days prior to elective coronary bypass or other surgery due to increased risk for perioperative bleeding. The recent U.S. approval of the intravenous P2Y12 agent cangrelor has provided an opportunity to bridge antiplatelet therapy for patients with recent MI or PCI who require urgent surgery, although its safety in older patients is not well established. An additional antiplatelet agent, vorapaxar, has been approved in the United States for add-on therapy for patients with prior MI or peripheral arterial disease, but the higher rates of bleeding and lesser benefit in elderly patients

Table 12.3 Management of acute myocardial infarction

General measures
- Oxygen to maintain arterial saturation ≥92%
- Telemetry monitoring
- Morphine for pain and dyspnea
- Nitroglycerin for ischemia and heart failure

Antiplatelet and antithrombotic therapy
- Aspirin
- Platelet $P2Y_{12}$ receptor inhibitors (clopidogrel, prasugrel,* ticagrelor, cangrelor)
- Glycoprotein IIb/IIIa inhibitors *(abciximab, eptifibatide, tirofiban)
- Systemic parenteral anticoagulants during MI (unfractionated heparin, enoxaparin, dalteparin, bivalirudin)

Oral beta-blockers
- (if heart rate and blood pressure are adequate)

Angiotensin-converting enzyme (ACE) inhibitors
- (or angiotensin receptor blockers if ACE inhibitors are contraindicated)

Other disease-modifying agents
- Eplerenone (if there is reduced left ventricular systolic function or diabetes at time of MI)
- High-potency statins

Other medications for compelling indications only
- Calcium channel blockers (if there is persistent hypertension; immediate-release nifedipine is contraindicated)
- Antiarrhythmic agents (if there are refractory ventricular arrhythmias after acute MI)
- Oral anticoagulation (select patients with anterior MI, atrial fibrillation, mechanical heart valves)

Reperfusion therapy
- Fibrinolysis (ST-elevation or new left bundle branch block only)
- Percutaneous coronary intervention (PCI)
- Urgent coronary bypass surgery in selected cases

Prior to hospital discharge
- Assessment of left ventricular systolic function (e.g., echocardiogram)
- Tobacco cessation counseling
- Nutritional evaluation
- Screening for depression
- Exercise counseling and cardiac rehabilitation referral

* Rarely indicated outside of the catheterization laboratory in patients >75 years of age

likely limit the use of this agent to very select older patients with low bleeding risk.[21]

Glycoprotein IIb/IIIa inhibitors (eptifibatide, tirofiban, abciximab) block the final common pathway of platelet aggregation and reduce infarct size in subjects with non-ST-elevation acute coronary syndromes. High-risk patients tend to gain the most benefit, particularly when undergoing percutaneous coronary intervention (PCI), but the risk of bleeding increases with age. Few studies have enrolled individuals over age 75, and one study demonstrated higher event rates in patients over age 80 receiving eptifibatide,[22] so the value of these agents in the elderly remains unclear. Due to a high risk of hemorrhage, glycoprotein IIb/IIIa inhibitors are contraindicated in patients over age 75 receiving thrombolytic therapy for ST-elevation MI,[13] and their incremental benefit in older patients receiving clopidogrel or other $P2Y_{12}$ inhibitors remains unclear.

Antithrombotic therapy In patients with acute MI, unfractionated or low-molecular-weight heparin should be administered immediately in addition to the antiplatelet agents already described – particularly in patients with high-risk features such as anterior MI, large MI, associated atrial fibrillation, or recurrent ischemia.[13, 14] Low-molecular-weight heparins (e.g., enoxaparin, dalteparin) offer more predictable anticoagulation than unfractionated heparin, but these agents are almost exclusively cleared through renal mechanisms. As a result, the low-molecular-weight heparins must be used with caution given the higher rates of hemorrhagic complications with the age-associated decline in renal function. Nevertheless, the combined endpoint of death, MI, and recurrent angina is reduced,[23] with significant benefits in older subjects.[24] Low-molecular-weight heparin must be used with caution, if at all, in patients with severe renal insufficiency (creatinine clearance <30 mL/min).

Patients with large anterior MI or evidence for left ventricular thrombus should be treated with warfarin for three months after MI to maintain an international normalized ratio (INR) of 2.0–3.0. Long-term therapy with warfarin is indicated in patients with atrial fibrillation, mechanical prosthetic heart valves, or other conditions requiring systemic anticoagulation. Older patients are at increased risk for warfarin-associated bleeding complications, especially when warfarin is used in combination with aspirin or other anti-platelet agents. The utility of newer oral anticoagulants, such as dabigatran, rivaroxaban, apixaban, and edoxaban, as alternatives to warfarin in patients with recent MI has not been assessed. Among patients with indications for chronic systemic anticoagulation undergoing PCI, one study demonstrated lower rates of bleeding and similar ischemic outcomes when withholding aspirin and treating patients with clopidogrel and warfarin alone. [25] However, the number of elderly subjects enrolled was small (maximum age was 80 years), and this approach has not yet been confirmed in larger trials.

Beta blockers Beta blockers reduce mortality, recurrent ischemia, and arrhythmias in patients with acute MI.[13, 14] Contraindications include bradyarrhythmias, hypotension, moderate or severe heart failure during MI, or active bronchospasm. A history of obstructive lung disease alone should not preclude beta-blocker therapy. In a pooled analysis of several clinical trials, early treatment with beta blockers reduced mortality by 23% in older patients with acute coronary syndromes, but had no effect in younger patients.[5] In addition, long-term beta-blocker treatment after MI is associated with 6 lives saved per 100 older patients treated, versus only 2.1 lives saved per 100 younger patients. However, older patients with acute MI are also at increased risk for serious adverse events associated with beta-blocker therapy, including heart failure, hypotension, shock, and death.[26] Current guidelines recommend institution of oral metoprolol or carvedilol within 24 to 48 hours only in hemodynamically stable patients.[13] Doses should be lower and titration slower in older adults. Following MI, metoprolol, propranolol, and timolol are approved for long-term use, while carvedilol and metoprolol succinate are approved for use after MI in patients with LV ejection fractions less than 40%.

Angiotensin and aldosterone inhibition Angiotensin converting enzyme inhibitors (ACEI) reduce mortality in MI, particularly in geriatric individuals aged 65–74, and in the setting of heart failure, left ventricular (LV) dysfunction, or anterior ST-elevation MI.[27] Following MI, ACEIs reduce mortality by 17%–34% in older patients, with an absolute benefit that is three times greater than in younger individuals. [28–30] Angiotensin receptor blockers (e.g., candesartan or valsartan) are suitable alternatives for ACEI-intolerant patients, but head-to-head trials have confirmed that ACEIs are the preferred medications in subjects with MI.[31] Serious potential adverse effects with both classes of drugs include hypotension, renal failure, and hyperkalemia – initiation and up-titration of these medications must be performed with caution in elderly patients with renal dysfunction or low blood pressure in the MI setting.

Eplerenone is a selective aldosterone antagonist that reduces mortality and cardiovascular hospitalizations in acute MI patients with LV systolic dysfunction (ejection fraction $\leq$40% at time of event) and either heart failure or diabetes.[32] Like spironolactone, eplerenone is a potassium-sparing diuretic that requires close monitoring of renal function and serum potassium levels during initiation and follow-up, particularly in the geriatric population.

Statins Statin therapy improves clinical outcomes after acute MI and should be initiated in all patients prior to hospital discharge.[6] The benefits of statin treatment have been verified in geriatric patients with known CAD or vascular disease,[33–36] with one study demonstrating a 15% reduction in recurrent MI, stroke, or cardiovascular death in subjects aged 70–82.[36] However, the utility of statins in patients over 80 years of age is controversial, as none of the clinical trials have enrolled patients in this age group. [37, 38] In addition, older patients may be at increased risk for statin-related myalgias,[39] and statins may be associated with fatigue, reduced physical activity levels, and cognitive impairment in susceptible older individuals.[40–42] Therefore, use of statins in patients of advanced age must be individualized, taking cardiovascular risk profile, life expectancy, prevalent comorbidities, and patient preferences into due consideration.

Other agents Nitrates and morphine are recommended for ongoing chest pain, but neither agent has been shown to reduce mortality or recurrent cardiovascular events. Calcium channel blockers have not been shown to improve outcomes in patients with acute MI, but may be useful in patients with ongoing ischemia, poorly controlled hypertension, or supraventricular tachyarrhythmias (diltiazem or verapamil). Empiric antiarrhythmic drugs (e.g., lidocaine or amiodarone), magnesium therapy, and glucose-insulin-potassium infusions are not recommended in acute MI in the absence of a specific indication. As noted earlier, systemic anticoagulation may be reasonable in select elderly patients with large anterior MI, even in the absence of other compelling indications (atrial fibrillation, mechanical valves, etc.).

Reperfusion in acute ST-segment elevation myocardial infarction (STEMI)

Acute MI associated with ST-segment elevation or new left bundle branch block is usually caused by thrombotic occlusion of the infarct-related coronary artery, and numerous large trials have confirmed that prompt pharmacological or mechanical reperfusion reduces mortality and morbidity.[13] Importantly, although the potential risks of pharmacological reperfusion with fibrinolytic therapy or mechanical reperfusion with percutaneous coronary intervention (PCI) are higher in older patients, the potential benefits are also higher, and the net benefit of reperfusion is at least as great in older as in younger patients. Therefore, older age per se is not a contraindication to thrombolytic therapy, but the benefits of reperfusion must be weighed against the risks of bleeding, which increase exponentially above 75 years of age. Primary PCI is the preferred reperfusion strategy in patients of all ages with STEMI if it can be performed within 90 minutes of presentation because it is associated with higher efficacy and lower risk of intracranial hemorrhage (ICH) relative to fibrinolytic therapy.[13, 43, 44] In situations where PCI cannot be performed within 90 minutes, fibrinolysis is considered a suitable alternative, provided that the risk of bleeding is

Table 12.4 Criteria for fibrinolytic therapy in older adults

Indications
- Symptoms of acute myocardial infarction within 6–12 hours of onset,* *and*
- ST-elevation ≥1 mm in two or more contiguous leads, or left bundle branch block not known to be present previously

Contraindications (absolute)
- Any prior intracranial hemorrhage or hemorrhagic stroke
- Ischemic stroke within the past three months (except if within the past three hours)
- Known malignant intracranial neoplasm or structural vascular lesion
- Active internal bleeding (excluding menses)
- Suspected aortic dissection
- Significant closed head or facial trauma within three months

Contraindications (relative)
- Blood pressure ≥180/110 mmHg on presentation, not readily controlled
- Prior ischemic stroke (>3 months ago)
- Advanced dementia, other intracranial pathology not described in contraindications
- Traumatic or prolonged cardiopulmonary resuscitation (>10 minutes)
- Recent major trauma, surgery, or internal bleeding (within two to four weeks)
- Noncompressible vascular puncture (e.g., subclavian intravenous line)
- Active peptic ulcer
- Pregnancy
- For streptokinase/anistreplase: prior exposure or allergic reaction to these agents
- Systemic anticoagulation with warfarin or heparin products at MI presentation (greater coagulopathy = greater hemorrhagic risk)

* Within six hours in patients ≥75 years of age.

acceptable (Table 12.4). In this regard, the risk of ICH is approximately twofold higher in patients ≥75 years of age treated with fibrinolysis compared to younger patients (1%–2% vs. 0.5%–1%).

Reperfusion in non-ST-elevation acute coronary syndromes (NSTEACS)

In elderly patients with acute coronary syndromes without ST-segment elevation, thrombolytic therapy

Table 12.5 TIMI Risk Score variables for predicting adverse clinical outcomes in NSTEACS*

- Aged 65 years or older
- Three or more risk factors for coronary artery disease
- Prior coronary stenosis of 50% or more
- ST-segment deviation on presenting electrocardiogram
- At least two anginal events in the prior 24 hours
- Use of aspirin in prior seven days
- Elevated serum cardiac markers (e.g., troponin)

*The combined endpoint of mortality, myocardial infarction, and urgent revascularization increases in linear fashion, with risk scores 0–1 associated with a 4.7% risk of events at two weeks, versus 8.3% for risk score 2, 13.2% for risk score 3, 19.9% for risk score 4, 26.2% for risk score 5, and 40.9% for risk scores 6–7.

is contraindicated and the role of PCI is less clear. Investigators from the thrombolysis in myocardial infarction (TIMI) group have identified seven variables that confer increased risk in individuals presenting with unstable angina or non-ST-elevation MI (Table 12.5).[45] This TIMI Risk Score may aid in triaging patients to an early invasive (i.e., coronary angiography) versus early conservative strategy (i.e., medical therapy, with invasive assessment only for subjects with recurrent ischemia or other clinical indications), and a similar approach is recommended by national guidelines for non-ST-elevation MI.[14] Several of the most important discriminators – including aged 65 and older, elevated cardiac biomarkers (i.e., troponin, creatine kinase-MB), and ST-segment deviation at presentation – have also been associated with higher rates of in-hospital mortality in large observational databases.[46] Since older age is associated with worse outcomes in acute MI, early coronary angiography is recommended in geriatric patients with MI complicated by recurrent ischemia, heart failure, or hemodynamic instability who are suitable candidates for percutaneous or surgical revascularization.[47] However, individualized decision making is required to carefully weigh the risks (e.g., contrast nephropathy, bleeding, potential for stroke or other embolic events) versus benefits related to invasive procedures.

Patients with acute MI at highest risk for death are those presenting with cardiac arrest, heart failure, hypotension, or significant tachycardia, and the in-hospital mortality rate approaches 50% for subjects with cardiogenic shock.[48] Although early coronary

revascularization is beneficial in patients up to age 75 presenting with acute MI complicated by cardiogenic shock, the value of this approach in patients over age 75 is less certain.[49, 50] Nevertheless, urgent revascularization is a reasonable option in selected elderly patients in the absence of other life-threatening conditions.

Complications of MI

Heart failure occurs in up to 50% of older patients with acute MI and is the most common cause of in-hospital death. Treatment includes diuretics and vasodilator therapy, especially nitroglycerin and ACE inhibitors. Beta blockers should be administered if blood pressure and heart rate are adequate, and if volume overload is manageable with diuretics. In more advanced heart failure, inotropic agents may be required transiently until the patient stabilizes (e.g., dopamine, dobutamine, milrinone – see the Heart Failure section in this chapter).

Clinically significant right ventricular (RV) ischemia or infarction occurs in 10%–20% of patients with acute inferior STEMI and portends an ominous prognosis in the elderly.[51] Manifestations of RV infarction include hypotension and signs of right-sided heart failure. Treatment involves intravenous fluid administration to maintain LV filling pressure and inotropic therapy if needed.

Life-threatening mechanical complications of MI occur in 1%–2% of all patients and appear to be decreasing in incidence since the advent of acute reperfusion therapy. Mechanical complications include LV free wall rupture with pericardial tamponade, papillary muscle dysfunction or rupture with severe acute mitral regurgitation, rupture of the interventricular septum, and aneurysm or pseudoaneurysm formation. Advanced age is a potent risk factor for each of these catastrophic consequences of acute MI.[52] Care should be individualized, but all forms of rupture require urgent attention and surgical repair, if at all possible. Management of ventricular aneurysm depends on size and degree of hemodynamic instability; in most cases, smaller aneurysms can be managed medically whereas surgical repair should be considered for large aneurysms associated with heart failure or thromboembolic complications. LV pseudoaneurysm refers to a situation in which a free wall rupture has been locally contained by adherent pericardium. Pseudoaneurysms are prone to expand, leading to pericardial tamponade, so surgical repair is recommended.

Sustained ventricular tachyarrhythmias are generally treated with direct-current cardioversion or defibrillation, beta-blocker therapy, and correction of electrolyte abnormalities and ischemia. Selected individuals may require anti-arrhythmic therapy or implantable defibrillators, particularly if new life-threatening ventricular arrhythmias occur more than 48 hours after MI, but these approaches are not indicated for routine management or for prophylactic purposes.[13] Supraventricular arrhythmias such as atrial fibrillation should be treated according to standard recommendations (see the Arrhythmias section in this chapter). Bradyarrhythmias frequently resolve spontaneously once ischemia has been treated, but patients may occasionally require temporary transvenous or transcutaneous pacing. Permanent pacing may be necessary in subjects with persistent high-grade heart block (e.g., Mobitz type II second-degree atrioventricular block or complete heart block in the setting of anterior MI).

Diagnosis and management of chronic coronary disease

After experiencing MI, all patients should be counseled in conjunction with their families or caregivers regarding the medication regimen, diet, and long-term recommendations for CAD management.[53] This is particularly important in elderly patients, for whom sensory or memory deficits combined with polypharmacy may adversely affect medication compliance. Assessment of risk factors should be targeted during the convalescent phase after MI, with nutritional counseling and tobacco cessation efforts addressed prior to discharge.[13, 14] Systolic blood pressure should be controlled in accordance with current guidelines,[54] lipid therapy should be initiated or titrated appropriately using higher potency statins,[55] diabetes management should be addressed,[56] and medical follow-up should be arranged. Cardiac rehabilitation reduces mortality and improves quality of life after MI, with similar benefits in younger and older patients. However, cardiac rehabilitation is significantly under-utilized in the geriatric population relative to younger patients.[57]

Chronic CAD, with or without prior MI, increases in prevalence with age – likely as a result of prolonged exposure to multiple cardiac risk factors in conjunction with structural and metabolic changes related to vascular aging. Atherosclerotic changes tend to be more diffuse in older adults, with a higher likelihood of left main and multivessel CAD. Compared to younger patients, geriatric patients tend to present with more advanced disease and fewer or no anginal symptoms due to comorbidities (e.g., diabetes), neuropsychiatric changes, and more sedentary lifestyles. Indications for stress testing are similar to those for younger individuals. However, clinicians should carefully screen geriatric patients prior to stress testing, taking into consideration whether the patient is a suitable candidate for coronary angiography and revascularization, in the event the stress test is abnormal and symptoms persist despite anti-anginal therapy. Often, elderly patients are unable to perform an exercise stress test; in such cases, a pharmacologic test such as a regadenoson nuclear scan or dobutamine echocardiogram is appropriate.[58]

Medical management of chronic stable angina includes aspirin, beta blockers, nitrates, calcium channel blockers, and ranolazine – with beta blockers being the anti-ischemic agents of first choice unless contraindicated.[53] Compared to medical management, coronary revascularization with PCI or coronary artery bypass graft (CABG) surgery reduces symptoms and improves quality of life; CABG also decreases mortality in certain high-risk subgroups (e.g., left main coronary disease, three-vessel disease with LV dysfunction). [59, 60] Coronary angiography, PCI, and CABG in the geriatric population are associated with higher complication rates than in younger patients. [61, 62] Higher mortality in the elderly is due in part to more advanced and diffuse CAD, worse LV function resulting from prior MI, and diminished cardiac reserve related to aging itself. Comorbidities play an important role as well, with vascular and renal disease contributing to procedural difficulty, bleeding complications, and contrast nephropathy. Stroke and other thromboembolic events, as well as heart failure, occur more commonly after either percutaneous or surgical revascularization in older patients. In addition, older patients undergoing CABG experience higher rates of arrhythmias (particularly atrial fibrillation), cognitive dysfunction, and pulmonary complications than younger patients, and these adverse events contribute to increased length of stay and mortality.[63] Despite the attendant risks, outcomes following PCI and CABG in older adults are generally favorable and over 50% of patients undergoing these procedures in the United States are over age 65.[3]

Heart failure and cardiomyopathy

Epidemiology and pathophysiology

More than 5 million Americans have heart failure (HF), and there are more than 1 million hospitalizations with HF as a primary diagnosis each year.[64] HF increases in both incidence and prevalence with increasing age, with up to 75% of HF hospitalizations occurring in patients aged 65 and older and approximately 50% occurring in patients over age 75. In addition, HF is the most costly Medicare diagnosis-related group (DRG), and mortality from HF rises exponentially with age. Age-related changes in cardiovascular structure and function – including increased arterial stiffness, impaired LV diastolic relaxation and compliance, diminished responsiveness to β-adrenergic stimulation, and dysfunction of the sinus node – all contribute to a marked reduction in cardiovascular reserve, predisposing older adults to the development of HF. In addition, increased vascular stiffness leads to a progressive rise in systolic blood pressure, which is a major risk factor for the development of HF in geriatric patients. Indeed, approximately 75% of HF cases have antecedent hypertension, although the increasing prevalence rates of CAD, diabetes, and valvular disease also contribute to the exponential rise in geriatric HF.

Etiology and prevention

Most HF in the geriatric population is related to hypertension and/or CAD. Other common causes include nonischemic dilated cardiomyopathy, valvular disease, and hypertrophic cardiomyopathy. Less common etiologies include myocarditis, constrictive pericarditis, thyroid disease, high-output states such as an arteriovenous fistula or anemia, and infiltrative diseases such as amyloid or hemochromatosis. Individuals with exposure to certain drugs, such as cocaine or chemotherapeutic agents (e.g., anthracyclines and trastuzumab), are also at risk for developing LV dysfunction.

Clinical guidelines emphasize prevention in high-risk populations – especially in subjects with multiple cardiovascular risk factors – and more aggressive titration of therapies in the presence of asymptomatic LV dysfunction, significant valvular disease, or symptomatic HF.[64] Large-scale clinical trials have verified that lowering blood pressure reduces the risk of developing HF,[65] and the greatest benefit is derived from control of systolic hypertension in subjects over age 80.[66] In patients with MI, the syndrome of HF may be delayed for months or years through implementation of the secondary prevention therapies described earlier. In the geriatric population, deconditioning and pulmonary disease may contribute to exercise intolerance, for which rehabilitation and lifestyle modifications are beneficial. Exercise training in particular is recommended in patients with asymptomatic LV dysfunction or chronic HF in the absence of severe symptoms.[64] Pharmacologic regression of LV hypertrophy in hypertensive subjects also reduces the incidence of HF and cardiovascular events.[67] Dietary counseling, including modest sodium restriction and avoidance of excessive fluid intake, may help reduce fluid retention and subsequent HF exacerbations. The importance of medication compliance should be discussed early after diagnosing HF, since medication nonadherence is a leading cause of rehospitalization for HF.

Clinical features and diagnosis

Classic symptoms of HF include shortness of breath (especially with exertion), exercise intolerance, orthopnea, paroxysmal nocturnal dyspnea, lower extremity edema, fatigue, and weakness. Elderly patients with HF also commonly experience anorexia, bloating, psychomotor slowing, lethargy, altered sensorium, and gastrointestinal disturbances. Because elderly persons are often sedentary, exertional symptoms may be less prominent than in younger patients. Conversely, "atypical" symptoms such as anorexia and altered cognition become increasingly prevalent.

Assessing symptom severity in patients with HF is useful for identifying therapeutic goals, monitoring disease progression, and determining prognosis. Although there are several metrics available, the New York Heart Association functional classification is most widely used (Table 12.6).[68] Nearly 70% of patients with HF are in class I or II, with mild limitations to routine physical activities. About 25% of patients experience more severe activity limitations (class III), whereas only 5% of patients are class IV, with symptoms during minimal exertion (e.g., going to the bathroom) or at rest. Patients with class IV HF have a one-year mortality rate of 25%–50% – worse than for many forms of metastatic cancer.

Table 12.6 New York Heart Association functional classification

Class	General characteristics
I	Cardiac disease does not limit physical activity. • Ordinary physical activity does not cause undue fatigue, palpitation, dyspnea, or anginal pain.
II	Cardiac disease results in slight limitation of physical activity. • Patients are comfortable at rest. • Ordinary physical activity results in fatigue, palpitation, dyspnea, or anginal pain.
III	Cardiac disease results in marked limitation of physical activity. • Patients are comfortable at rest. • Less than ordinary physical activity causes fatigue, palpitation, dyspnea, or anginal pain.
IV	Cardiac disease results in inability to carry on any physical activity without discomfort. • Symptoms of cardiac insufficiency or anginal syndrome may be present even at rest. • If any physical activity is undertaken, discomfort is increased.

Initial assessment should include a detailed history and physical examination. This is essential in the geriatric population, since patients may not present with typical symptoms or signs, and other medical conditions such as pulmonary disease or deconditioning may confound the clinical picture. Common precipitants of HF exacerbations in the elderly include medication or dietary noncompliance, ischemia, uncontrolled hypertension, new arrhythmias (especially atrial fibrillation), infection, volume overload (e.g., perioperatively or with blood transfusions), anemia, and drug interactions that adversely affect renal or cardiac function. Vital signs and volume status should be evaluated, and complete examination of the neck, chest, cardiovascular system, abdomen, and extremities should be performed. Routine laboratory studies include an assessment of electrolytes and renal function, and a complete blood count.[64] Select patients may require thyroid hormone assessment. An electrocardiogram is indicated, since HF is often precipitated by ischemia or arrhythmia. Chest radiography may be useful for diagnosing volume overload. Echocardiography should be performed at the time of initial diagnosis or when there is unexplained clinical deterioration in order to assess LV systolic and diastolic function, and to identify other structural abnormalities that may be contributing to the HF syndrome.

B-type natriuretic peptide (BNP) and its precursor N-terminal proBNP (NT-proBNP) are released by the myocardium when ventricular filling pressures are elevated, and these biomarkers are useful for both the diagnosis and management of HF.[69, 70] In one large trial, BNP was effective in distinguishing cardiac versus non-cardiac causes of dyspnea in the emergency department.[69] BNP levels increase with age and tend to be higher in women than in men.[71, 72] Other disorders in the geriatric population also contribute to higher BNP levels, including atrial fibrillation, renal dysfunction, and pulmonary hypertension. The predictive accuracy of BNP for diagnosing HF therefore declines with increasing age.[71] Nonetheless, BNP and NT-proBNP frequently add useful diagnostic and prognostic information to the evaluation of subjects with suspected HF. Thus, a normal BNP or NT-proBNP level makes acute HF unlikely, whereas a substantially elevated level of either biomarker greatly increases the likelihood of active HF. Similarly, persistently elevated biomarker levels despite aggressive treatment portend a less favorable prognosis.

Management

Initial goals of therapy for acute HF exacerbations include hemodynamic stabilization and correction of volume overload. Care for elderly patients must be individualized, with comorbid conditions, functional limitations, and personal preferences being taken into consideration in designing a therapeutic plan. In addition, since few clinical trials have enrolled substantial numbers of subjects over age 75, most HF therapies are of unproven benefit in older patients.[73] Multidisciplinary programs that provide individualized patient education and close follow-up have been shown to reduce hospitalizations and improve quality of life in elderly HF subjects.[74, 75] Furthermore, exercise training and cardiac rehabilitation have been associated with improved exercise tolerance in all age groups, leading to recent endorsement of cardiac rehabilitation for stable HF patients with LVEF ≤35% by the Centers for Medicare and Medicaid Services.[76]

Diuretics Loop diuretics are an essential component of the acute management of HF with volume overload. Administered intravenously, these agents promote rapid natriuresis and increased urine output. Older patients are more sensitive to diuretic-induced electrolyte disturbances and volume shifts than younger subjects, so close monitoring is imperative in conjunction with regular assessments of renal function and electrolytes. Although loop diuretics have not been shown to improve survival, and there are conflicting data concerning the short and long-term benefits of these agents,[77–79] relief of congestion is a primary goal of initial HF therapy.[80] In patients who do not respond adequately to loop diuretics, the addition of metolazone (usually administered 30–60 minutes before the loop diuretic) may facilitate diuresis, but renal and electrolyte disturbances are common. Dietary sodium restriction helps prevent fluid retention, and patients should be counseled to avoid salty foods and limit sodium intake to no more than 2 grams per day. Conversely, over-zealous sodium restriction has not been shown to improve outcomes and may be harmful.[81] Patients should also be instructed to monitor daily weights at home. A baseline "dry weight" should be defined, and subjects should be advised to adjust their diuretic dosage or contact their healthcare provider if their weight varies by more than two to three pounds from baseline over several days.

ACE inhibitors In patients with HF and reduced ejection fraction (HFrEF), angiotensin converting enzyme inhibitors (ACEI) reduce HF hospitalizations, improve quality of life, and decrease mortality by 25%–30% – with similar effects in older and younger subjects.[82, 83] Older patients experience higher rates of hypotension, hyperkalemia, and renal dysfunction during ACEI titration than younger individuals; close monitoring of these parameters is warranted. Up to 20% of patients may experience cough and a small percentage may experience angioedema from ACEI, but these side effects do not appear to increase in frequency with advancing age. In the absence of adverse effects, ACEI dosages should be titrated to those studied in clinical trials (e.g., captopril 50 mg tid, enalapril 10 mg bid, lisinopril 20 mg–40 mg q day, ramipril 10 mg q day). In addition, ACEI therapy in patients with asymptomatic LV dysfunction reduces progression to clinical HF,[84] so ACEI are indicated in patients with LV systolic dysfunction (LV ejection fraction

<40%–45%) regardless of New York Heart Association functional class.[64]

Angiotensin receptor blockers While ACEI are recommended as first line therapy for patients with HFrEF, angiotensin receptor blockers (ARBs) are suitable alternatives in individuals intolerant to ACEI due to cough or angioedema.[85,86] In a series of three trials involving patients with HF, the ARB candesartan reduced the composite endpoint of death or HF hospitalization by 13.8% among 1,736 subjects ≥ 75 years of age ($p = 0.007$), and the benefit was at least as great in this age group as in younger patients.[87] As with ACEI, older patients receiving ARBs are at increased risk for hypotension, renal dysfunction, and hyperkalemia. In addition, combination therapy with an ACEI and ARB is not recommended due to lack of proven benefit and increased risk for adverse effects.[88]

Hydralazine-nitrates The combination of hydralazine and nitrates improves clinical outcomes in HFrEF.[89] Although mortality reduction is less than with ACEI therapy, this combination is useful in subjects with renal dysfunction or hyperkalemia that precludes the use of ACEIs or ARBs.[90] Moreover, in the African-American Heart Failure Trial (A-HeFT), the combination of hydralazine and isosorbide dinitrate taken three times daily improved clinical outcomes in class III–IV HF subjects already treated with standard therapies including ACEIs and beta blockers.[91] All subjects in A-HeFT were African American, and the mean age was 57, so the role of these agents in older patients and in other racial/ethnic groups remains to be determined. Another important concern is the need for multiple daily doses of both agents, which may be problematic in elderly patients with polypharmacy and medication adherence difficulties.

Beta blockers Beta blockers improve LV function, decrease hospitalizations, and reduce mortality in a broad range of patients with HFrEF, and three beta blockers are indicated for management of HFrEF (metoprolol succinate, carvedilol, and bisoprolol).[92–94] However, geriatric patients are often sensitive to beta blockade, so initiation at a low dose with slow upward titration is imperative in order to avoid bradycardia, heart block, hypotension, or worsening HF. In particular, patients with class III–IV HF require meticulous and slow titration due to the potential for transient worsening of symptoms. Active bronchospasm is a contraindication to beta-blocker therapy, but chronic pulmonary disease does not preclude use of these drugs. Other contraindications include marked bradycardia, advanced heart block, hypotension, and severe decompensated HF.

Mineralocorticoid antagonists Spironolactone and eplerenone are mineralocorticoid antagonists (MRAs) with weak diuretic potency but with antifibrotic properties and other beneficial cardiovascular effects. When added to other therapies in class II–IV HFrEF, LVEF ≤35%, and class II–IV symptoms, these agents reduce mortality and hospitalizations by approximately 25%–30%.[95, 96] The benefits are similar in older and younger subjects, but older patients are more susceptible to worsening renal function and hyperkalemia.[97] Meticulous electrolyte and renal surveillance is therefore required in geriatric HF patients treated with MRA. Up to 10% of patients may develop gynecomastia and breast tenderness with spironolactone, but these side effects are rare with eplerenone.

Digoxin Digoxin reduces HF symptoms and hospitalizations but has no effect on mortality.[98] The benefits and adverse effects of digoxin are similar in older and younger patients – including those over age 80.[99] In addition, retrospective analysis of the Digitalis Investigation Group (DIG) trial suggests that digoxin may have a favorable effect on mortality when the serum digoxin level is maintained at <1.0 ng/mL.[100] In geriatric patients with persistent HF symptoms despite other therapeutic measures, digoxin should be initiated at a low dose (0.125 mg daily in the absence of renal dysfunction) with close monitoring for side effects such as bradycardia, heart block, arrhythmias, gastrointestinal symptoms, and mental status changes or visual disturbances. Digoxin toxicity occurs more frequently in the setting of hypokalemia, hypomagnesemia, hypercalcemia, and concurrent use of amiodarone, verapamil, and several other medications.

Anticoagulant and anti-inflammatory drugs Although the thromboembolic risk associated with HFrEF approaches that seen in atrial fibrillation, two large clinical trials failed to demonstrate a net clinical benefit from therapeutic anticoagulation with warfarin in HF patients.[101, 102] Warfarin or other anticoagulant treatment should therefore be reserved for patients with mechanical heart valves, atrial fibrillation, or other compelling indications.[64] Aspirin should be prescribed in patients with CAD, peripheral arterial disease, diabetes, or other indications for antiplatelet therapy. The value of aspirin in HF patients without clear indications for its use is uncertain. Nonsteroidal anti-inflammatory medications (other than aspirin) – commonly used to treat arthritis and chronic pain in older individuals – should be avoided in HF patients whenever possible because these agents promote sodium and water retention, antagonize ACEIs and other HF medications, and may worsen renal function.

Inotropic agents and intravenous vasodilators Intravenous inotropic agents, such as dobutamine and milrinone, have not been shown to improve clinical outcomes and have been associated with increased mortality rates in patients with advanced HF.[103, 104] Nevertheless, many clinicians utilize intravenous inotropes to alleviate symptoms in patients with severe intractable HF unresponsive to standard therapies. Intravenous nitroglycerin and nitroprusside have favorable hemodynamic effects in patients with severe HF, especially in those with poorly controlled hypertension or significant aortic or mitral regurgitation. Both agents may cause hypotension, and caution is advised in using nitroprusside in older patients, especially those with impaired renal function. Nesiritide, a recombinant form of BNP administered intravenously, has been shown to reduce LV filling pressures more effectively than intravenous nitrates or standard therapy (including diuretics), but nesiritide has not been shown to reduce morbidity or mortality.[105, 106] Routine use of nesiritide in patients with HF is not currently recommended.[64]

Heart transplantation and mechanical circulatory support

Although being 75 or more years of age is considered a contraindication to orthotopic heart transplantation (OHT) at most centers in the United States, a growing proportion of transplant recipients are 65–74 years of age, and outcomes are similar in this age group compared to younger patients.[107] However, the number of candidates for OHT greatly exceeds the number of donor hearts available, so only a small proportion of highly selected patients with advanced HF undergo the procedure. More recently, technological advances in mechanical circulatory support systems, particularly the development of continuous-flow left ventricular assist devices (LVADs), have led to more widespread use of LVADs as "destination therapy," rather than as a bridge to transplantation. To date, experience with LVADs in patients 70–74 years of age has been generally favorable with improved quality of life and functional status and an acceptable complication rate.[108] Data are limited in patients ≥80 years of age, but use of LVADs in this population is likely to increase as the technology continues to improve and complication rates decline. The most common complications associated with continuous-flow LVADs include bleeding (especially gastrointestinal bleeding), infections, and stroke. Outcomes following LVAD implantation are also dependent on comorbidity burden, baseline function status, and frailty, so careful patient selection is critical to the long-term success of mechanical circulatory support.

Heart failure with preserved ejection fraction

Approximately half of older adults with HF have a preserved LV ejection fraction (HFpEF).[109, 110] The impact of HFpEF on exercise tolerance, symptoms, and hospitalization rates is similar to that of HFrEF, although mortality rates tend to be somewhat lower.[111–113] In contrast to HFrEF, however, for which multiple pharmacological and device-based interventions have been associated with improved clinical outcomes, including mortality, to date no therapies have been shown to reduce mortality in patients with HFpEF.[114–123] As shown in Table 12.7, some studies have reported favorable effects on hospitalizations and/or exercise tolerance, but in general the magnitude of these effects has been modest. Thus, optimal management of HFpEF remains undefined.

Current recommendations for managing HFpEF focus on controlling heart rate, blood pressure, and volume status.[64] Hypertension should be treated in accordance with existing guidelines. Precipitating factors, such as ischemia or arrhythmia, should be managed appropriately, and judicious diuresis should be undertaken with close monitoring of blood pressure and renal function. Important differential diagnostic considerations in patients with HFpEF include valvular heart disease, pericardial constriction, restrictive cardiomyopathy (e.g., amyloidosis, hemochromatosis, sarcoidosis), and noncardiac etiologies such as pulmonary disease with right heart failure. Hypertrophic cardiomyopathy (HCM) may also mimic HFpEF and may be associated with exertional chest pain and syncope. Since the therapeutic armamentarium for HFpEF is limited, identification and treatment of potentially reversible causes of the patient's symptoms is essential.

Device therapy in advanced heart failure

Implantable devices Although pharmacological and behavioral therapies are the cornerstones of HF management, implantable devices are playing an increasingly important role in the treatment of HF patients. Advanced HF frequently is associated with dyssynchronous LV contraction related to abnormalities of electrical conduction, and cardiac resynchronization therapy (CRT) improves symptoms and clinical outcomes in patients with NYHA class II–IV HF, LVEF ≤35%, and a QRS duration ≥150 msec on the electrocardiogram, especially with left bundle branch block morphology.[124–126] Interestingly, the benefits of CRT appear to be greater in women than in men, and recent data suggest that some women with QRS duration ≥130 msec but <150 msec may also benefit.[127, 128] Although none of the CRT trials enrolled patients over 80 years of age, observational studies indicate that selected octogenarians may derive significant quality of life benefit from CRT.[129] Thus, CRT should be considered in elderly patients with persistent advanced HF symptoms who otherwise meet criteria for the device.

Implantable cardioverter-defibrillators (ICDs) reduce the risk for sudden cardiac death (SCD) in selected patients at increased risk for such events.[130, 131] Current criteria for ICD implantation include an LVEF ≤35%, NYHA class II–III symptoms, and a life-expectancy of at least 1 year with good functional status.[126] However, few patients over 80 years of age were enrolled in the major ICD trials, and there is evidence that the life-saving benefits of ICDs decline with age, most likely due to competing morbidities.[132] Thus, although age is not a contraindication to an ICD, device implantation should be undertaken only after careful consideration of the potential benefits and risks through a process of shared decision making. In addition, a discussion of circumstances under which the patient would want to disable the ICD to avoid painful shocks (e.g., in the event of terminal illness) should occur prior to device implantation in all patients, regardless of age.[133]

Table 12.7 Pharmacotherapy trials for heart failure with preserved ejection fraction

Trial*	Patients	Treatment	LVEF	Age	Outcomes compared to placebo**
PEP-CHF	850	Perindopril	65 (56–66)	75 (72–79)	Death/hospitalization by 1 year – HR 0.69 (0.47–1.01, $p = 0.055$); HF hospitalization by 1 year – HR 0.63 (0.41–0.97, $p = 0.033$)
CHARM-Preserved	3,023	Candesartan	54 ± 9	67 ± 11	CV death/HF admission – HR 0.89 (0.77–1.03, $p = 0.118$); HF admission – HR 0.85 (0.72–1.01, $p = 0.072$)
I-PRESERVE	4,128	Irbesartan	50 ± 9	72 ± 7	Death/hospitalization – HR 0.95 (0.86–1.05, $p = 0.35$)
SENIORS (EF >35% subgroup)	643	Nebivolol	49 ± 10	76 ± 5	All cause death/CV hospitalization – HR 0.81 (0.63–1.04)
TOPCAT	3,445	Spironolactone	56 (51–62)	69 (61–76)	CV death/HF hospitalization/aborted SCD – HR 0.89 (0.77–1.04, $p = 0.14$); HF hospitalization – HR 0.83 (0.69–0.99, $p = 0.04$)
Aldo-DHF	422	Spironolactone	67 ± 8	67 ± 8	Reduced E/e' avg 1.5 ($p < 0.001$)
RELAX	216	Sildenafil	60 (56–65)	69 (62–77)	No difference Δ VO2 peak at 24 weeks
ESS-DHF	192	Sitaxsentan	51 ± 12	65 ± 10	Median 43 second relative increase in Naughton treadmill time ($p = 0.03$)
DIG Ancillary	988	Digoxin	55 ± 8	67 ± 10	HF hospitalization – HR 0.79 (0.59 – 1.04, $p = 0.09$; hospitalization for unstable angina – HR 1.37 (0.99–1.91, $p = 0.06$)

Abbreviations: LVEF = left ventricular ejection fraction; E/e' avg = echocardiographic mitral inflow velocity/tissue Doppler velocity ratio; CV = cardiovascular; VO2 = oxygen consumption; SCD = sudden cardiac death; HR = hazard ratio (with 95% confidence interval)

Age (in years) and LVEF (%) presented as mean ± Standard Deviation (SD), or Interquartile Range (IQR).

* Trial acronyms: PEP-CHF = Perindopril in Elderly People with Chronic Heart Failure; CHARM-Preserved = Candesartan in Heart failure: Assessment of Reduction in Mortality and morbidity – Preserved LVEF; I-PRESERVE = Irbesartan in heart failure with Preserved ejection fraction study; SENIORS = Study of the Effects of Nebivolol Intervention on Outcomes and Rehospitalisation in seniors with heart failure; TOPCAT = Treatment Of Preserved Cardiac function heart failure with an Aldosterone antagonist; Aldo-DHF = Aldosterone receptor blockade in Diastolic Heart Failure; RELAX = Phosphodiesterase-5 inhibition to improve clinical status and exercise capacity in heart failure with preserved ejection fraction; ESS-DHF = Effectiveness of Sitaxsentan Sodium in patients with Diastolic Heart Failure; DIG Ancillary = Digitalis Investigation Group Ancillary trial

** All-cause mortality was not significantly reduced in *any* trial.

Rehospitalizations and prognosis

Approximately 20%–25% of patients discharged from the hospital with a primary diagnosis of HF are readmitted within 30 days, and up to 50% are readmitted within six months. These readmissions contribute substantially to the total cost of caring for HF patients, and hospitals with excess risk-adjusted 30-day readmission rates are subject to financial penalties under the Affordable Care Act's Hospital Readmission Reduction Program. In addition, 30-day readmission rates are widely used as quality metrics to assess performance of both hospitals and physicians. Over the past two decades, numerous studies have tested various interventions designed to reduce readmissions in selected patients with HF. These interventions generally include individualized patient and family education aimed at enhancing HF self-care in conjunction with close follow-up in the days and weeks immediately following discharge. Although randomized trials and meta-analyses have shown that such interventions reduce all-cause readmissions by 20%–25%, the effectiveness of "disease management" programs in improving outcomes on a population-wide basis has not been established.[134] Furthermore, since approximately two-thirds of early readmissions are for reasons other than HF, additional research is needed to develop and test novel interventions designed to manage HF in the context of multiple chronic conditions.

The overall prognosis for elderly patients with HF remains poor, with one-year mortality rates of up to 25% and five-year mortality rates of 75%–80%. Factors associated with worse prognosis include older age, more severe symptoms (New York Heart Association functional class III–IV), ischemic etiology, renal insufficiency, hyponatremia, peripheral arterial disease, and dementia.[135] Patients with HFpEF have a somewhat more favorable short-term prognosis than subjects with HFrEF, but long-term prognosis is similar. In light of the high mortality associated with HF, which is equivalent or worse than many forms of cancer, it is appropriate to begin to address goals of care and end-of-life issues early in the course of illness.[136] HF patients should be advised to develop a living will or advance directive and to designate durable power of attorney for health care in the event that decision-making capacity is lost, either temporarily or permanently. In patients with advanced HF and NYHA class IV symptoms despite optimal therapy, life expectancy is less than six months. In such cases, transition to palliative care or hospice should be considered.

Valvular heart disease

Aortic stenosis

The prevalence of aortic stenosis (AS) increases with age, from 0.2% in persons 50–59 years of age to 9.8% in octogenarians.[137] AS is the most common valvular abnormality requiring intervention in older adults, and more than 70% of aortic valve procedures are performed in patients over 65 years of age.[137] In the geriatric population, most AS is related to progressive calcific and fibrotic changes of the valve leaflets. Classic symptoms of AS include chest pain, shortness of breath, and light-headedness or syncope. Physical examination findings include a harsh systolic ejection murmur that tends to peak later in systole as the degree of stenosis worsens, and delayed and low-amplitude carotid arterial pulses. Once symptoms attributable to AS develop, the prognosis is poor, with an average survival of two to three years without intervention.[138] As with CAD and HF, the presentation of severe AS may be delayed in the geriatric population due to reduced physical activity levels. Symptoms may not be evident until another medical illness or need for surgery arises, at which time stenosis may be more advanced than in younger patients at the time of diagnosis.

An aortic valve (AV) area of 1.0 cm^2 or less is generally considered severe stenosis, whereas a valve area of 1.0 cm^2–1.5 cm^2 defines moderate stenosis and a valve area of 1.5 cm^2–2.0 cm^2 is considered mild stenosis.[138] LV hypertrophy commonly results from chronic LV pressure overload, and conduction system disease may be present as a result of concurrent calcium deposition. CAD frequently coexists in calcific AS due to the overlap in underlying pathophysiology and the age of the affected population.

Traditionally, the treatment of AS has required surgical aortic valve replacement, as medical therapy has not been shown to delay disease progression or improve outcomes. In addition, percutaneous balloon aortic valvuloplasty is ineffective for long-term management. More recently, however, the availability of transcatheter aortic valve implantation (TAVI) has revolutionized the treatment of severe AS in elderly patients at high or prohibitive risk for surgical aortic valve replacement.[138] Most commonly, TAVI is performed via the femoral artery in a manner analogous to PCI. After dilating the native valve with a balloon catheter, a bioprosthetic valve is inserted in the aortic valve position and expanded. In a series of prospective randomized trials, TAVI was shown to be superior to medical therapy with respect to survival and quality of life in patients deemed "inoperable" by cardiac surgeons, and to be equivalent to surgical AVR in high-risk patients.[139–142] Importantly, the average age of patients enrolled in these trials was 83–84 years, many patients were over 90 years of age, and the majority had significant comorbidities. A limitation of TAVI is that in some older patients the femoral artery is too small to allow introduction of the catheter, thus necessitating the use of an alternate approach (e.g., transapical or transaortic). Complication rates are generally acceptable, although the risk of stroke is somewhat higher with TAVI than with surgical valve replacement. Conversely, hospital length of stay and especially post-procedural recovery times are substantially shorter with TAVI. However, despite the fact that TAVI is associated with excellent outcomes in the majority of patients, not all patients derive benefit. Indeed, up to 25% of TAVI patients die within one year of the procedure or survive but without improvement in exercise tolerance or quality of life. Several factors, including frailty, help identify older patients less likely to benefit from TAVI, and ongoing research is aimed at better clarifying situations in which TAVI (and other aggressive interventions) are likely to be futile.[143]

Prior to valve replacement by either the surgical or transcatheter approach, coronary angiography is warranted in most older individuals to assess for CAD and the potential need for concomitant coronary revascularization. In geriatric patients referred for surgical valve replacement, bioprosthetic valves are preferred over mechanical valves because they offer satisfactory durability while avoiding the need for long-term systemic anticoagulation. Procedural mortality is less than 5% for both isolated surgical AV replacement and TAVI. Post-procedural quality of life is substantially improved among patients with uncomplicated recovery from valve intervention, and long-term survival is excellent – even in octogenarians. Lifelong endocarditis prophylaxis is indicated for dental or surgical procedures in all patients with prosthetic heart valves.

Aortic insufficiency

Chronic regurgitation at the AV is often well tolerated for many years, as the LV can effectively compensate for chronic volume overload. Common geriatric causes of chronic AV insufficiency include long-standing hypertension, myxomatous degeneration of the AV leaflets, and disorders of the ascending aorta (e.g., aneurysmal dilation). Other causes include rheumatic valve disease, other autoimmune conditions, prior endocarditis, and tumors. Many patients are asymptomatic but may exhibit findings of elevated stroke volume such as increased pulse pressure or prominent arterial pulsations ("bounding pulses"). A decrescendo diastolic murmur is usually heard along the left sternal border. LV hypertrophy is often present on the electrocardiogram.

Optimal medical therapy for severe chronic AV regurgitation is undefined. Vasodilators such as ACEIs or nifedipine are often prescribed, but the value of such treatment in delaying surgery and improving clinical outcomes remains controversial.[144, 145] Progressive exertional dyspnea or HF signifies a failing LV and necessitates AV replacement.[138] Other indications for surgery include increasing LV dilation or a reduction in LV systolic function with exercise. Operative mortality in geriatric patients undergoing AV replacement is acceptable, and long-term outcomes are generally favorable.

Mitral stenosis

In younger patients, stenosis of the mitral valve (MV) is almost always rheumatic in origin, although rare inflammatory or infectious processes may result in MV scarring and narrowing. In older individuals, calcification of the MV annulus with impingement into the valve orifice is the most common cause of MV stenosis, although it is rarely severe enough to warrant surgery. Mitral stenosis in older patients usually runs an indolent course, with gradual progression over several decades. Common symptoms include exertional dyspnea and fatigue. In advanced cases, signs of biventricular failure and pulmonary hypertension are evident. The left atrium is often markedly enlarged, increasing the risk for atrial fibrillation and systemic thromboembolism. Pulmonary hypertension is also common, which contributes to the development of right-sided HF. Classic physical findings include an early diastolic opening snap and a mid-diastolic low-pitched rumbling murmur best heard at the cardiac apex, often with pre-systolic accentuation. A MV area less than 1.0 cm^2 indicates severe stenosis, whereas valve areas of 1.0 cm^2–1.5 cm^2 and 1.6 cm^2–2.0 cm^2 indicate moderate and mild stenosis, respectively.

Diuretics and sodium restriction are recommended to maintain euvolemia in patients with MV stenosis. If atrial fibrillation is present, anticoagulation with warfarin should be initiated to maintain an international normalized ratio (INR) of 2.0–3.0.[138] Importantly, the new oral anticoagulants (dabigatran, rivaroxaban, apixaban, edoxaban) have not been studied and are not approved for use in patients with atrial fibrillation attributable to valvular heart disease. Unlike AV stenosis, the MV can be dilated via percutaneous valvuloplasty with good intermediate-to-long-term success, provided there is no significant MV regurgitation or other technical factors such as heavy valvular calcification. As these contraindications to valvuloplasty are more common in older than in younger patients, most elderly patients with severe symptomatic MV stenosis will require MV replacement. As with AV surgery, bioprosthetic valves are generally recommended in geriatric patients, although many older patients will still require anticoagulation for atrial fibrillation. Operative mortality is generally higher with MV replacement than with AV replacement, ranging from 5% to 15% depending on age, functional status, prevalent comorbidities, and the experience of the surgical team. The risk of developing atrial fibrillation after surgery increases with age, and is particularly high after MV surgery.[146] Preoperative beta-blocker or amiodarone therapy reduces postoperative morbidity from atrial fibrillation.[147, 148] Recovery following MV surgery may be slow, often requiring prolonged rehabilitation.

Mitral regurgitation

MV regurgitation can occur as a result of CAD, myxomatous degeneration, rheumatic MV disease, or stretching of the MV annulus from progressive LV dilatation and HF. All of these processes occur more commonly in the elderly, and the majority of MV surgeries are performed in the Medicare population. Severe chronic MV regurgitation may be asymptomatic until the LV begins to fail, particularly in older patients with reduced activity levels, at which point symptoms typical of HF may ensue. An apical

holosystolic murmur with radiation to the axilla is usually present, occasionally accompanied by an S3 gallop. Echocardiography – especially transesophageal echocardiography – is useful for defining the severity of MV regurgitation and identifying other structural abnormalities.

Medical therapy has not been shown to reduce progression of MV regurgitation, although many physicians recommend empiric afterload reduction with ACEIs or other vasodilators. Symptomatic patients with severe MV regurgitation and an LV ejection fraction of 30% or higher should be evaluated for MV surgery. Surgery should also be considered in asymptomatic individuals with LV dilatation and/or mild to moderate LV dysfunction, as early intervention has been associated with improved long-term outcomes in these patients.[149] MV repair, when feasible, is preferable to MV replacement.[138] Operative mortality and long-term outcomes following MV repair for nonischemic regurgitation are generally good in patients with preserved LV systolic function, but are less favorable in subjects with an ischemic etiology or with impaired LV systolic function.[136] More recently, transcatheter MV repair has been shown to be an effective alternative to surgery in selected patients, including older adults.[150, 151] Since elderly patients often have other comorbid conditions that may affect post-procedural outcomes and long-term prognosis, the decision to proceed with a MV intervention must be individualized.

Tricuspid and pulmonic valve disease

In geriatric patients, the right-sided heart valves generally become dysfunctional as a consequence of left heart problems or *cor pulmonale* from acute or chronic lung disease. Tricuspid regurgitation often results from right ventricular dilatation in the setting of pulmonary hypertension or HF. Symptoms and signs reflect right-sided HF and may include dyspnea, elevated jugular venous pressure, a murmur of tricuspid regurgitation, hepatic congestion, and lower extremity edema. Tricuspid valve repair (i.e., annuloplasty) is occasionally performed at the time of cardiac surgery for other reasons, but tricuspid regurgitation is rarely the primary indication for heart surgery. Similarly, pulmonic insufficiency may result from left-sided HF or pulmonary hypertension but usually does not require surgical intervention.

Endocarditis

Age-associated valvular degeneration and stenosis increase the risk for infective endocarditis in older adults. The risk is further compounded by higher rates of blood-borne infection in older patients, as conditions such as cancer, hemodialysis, dental disease, pneumonia, indwelling catheters, and non-cardiac surgery are common sources of bacteremia. Management of endocarditis includes intravenous antibiotic therapy and consideration of valve repair or replacement in patients with high-risk features such as embolic phenomena, large vegetations (>1 cm), perivalvular abscess, heart failure, hemodynamic instability, or failure to respond to antibiotics.[138]

Pericardial diseases

Pericarditis

Acute pericarditis usually presents as pleuritic chest pain that is often worse in the supine position and improved with sitting. Fever and leukocytosis are common with infectious etiologies, which represent the majority of cases worldwide. Additional etiologies in the geriatric population include recent MI, hypothyroidism, uremia, recent cardiac or thoracic surgery, malignancy, and prior radiation therapy to the chest. The ECG may show diffuse ST-segment elevation with PR-segment depression. Sinus tachycardia is common, but new pathologic Q waves are absent. The cardinal sign is a pericardial friction rub, although this may be transient or absent. Serum troponin levels may be slightly elevated, indicating myocardial involvement. Echocardiography may demonstrate a pericardial effusion, but the absence of an effusion does not preclude the diagnosis of pericarditis. Most cases of acute pericarditis respond to a nonsteroidal anti-inflammatory drug, alone or in combination with colchicine, which has been shown to reduce recurrences. Corticosteroids should be reserved for refractory cases. Anticoagulation should be avoided due to the risk of hemorrhagic transformation.

Pericardial effusion and tamponade

Common etiologies of pericardial effusion are similar to those for pericarditis but also include HF, hypoalbuminemia, rheumatologic disorders, chest wall trauma, hemorrhage, and certain medications (e.g.,

minoxidil). Although most pericardial effusions do not progress to tamponade, patients with malignant, traumatic, or infectious etiologies are at increased risk. Clinical manifestations of pericardial tamponade include dyspnea, tachycardia, hypotension, jugular venous distension, and pulsus paradoxus (although the latter is not always present). In addition to a moderate or large pericardial effusion, echocardiographic features of tamponade include respiratory variability in flow velocities, right atrial or ventricular compression by the effusion, and a dilated inferior vena cava. Treatment of tamponade involves percutaneous pericardiocentesis (preferably with echocardiographic, hemodynamic, and/or fluoroscopic guidance) or surgical drainage with creation of a pericardial "window" – the therapy of choice when the effusion is likely to recur (e.g., with malignancy).

Pericardial constriction

Pericardial constriction is a late complication of an inflammatory or infectious pericarditis. The pericardium becomes thickened and scarred, inhibiting ventricular filling. In the past, tuberculous pericarditis was the most commonly identified cause of constriction. Currently, most cases occur following one or more episodes of acute pericarditis, radiation therapy for thoracic cancer, or after open heart surgery; as a result, the diagnosis is becoming more common in the geriatric population. The clinical course is usually characterized by exertional dyspnea and fatigue, lower extremity edema, ascites, hepatic congestion, and bowel edema leading to bloating and anorexia. Cirrhosis of the liver may occur in long-standing cases. Inspiratory expansion of the jugular veins (Kussmaul's sign) is a hallmark of pericardial constriction but may also occur in other disease states (e.g., pulmonary hypertension). Echocardiographic findings include small ventricular cavities with normal systolic function but restrictive filling, a thickened pericardium, and a characteristic pattern of respiratory variation in hepatic vein blood flow. Chest imaging may reveal pericardial thickening or calcification. Simultaneous right and left heart catheterization demonstrates equalization of diastolic pressures throughout all chambers with an early plateau in the right and left ventricular diastolic wave form ("square root sign") and discordant respiratory variation of right and left ventricular systolic pressures. The only effective treatment is surgical pericardiectomy, which is associated with substantial morbidity and mortality and may not be feasible for elderly patients with advanced comorbidities. Constriction must be differentiated from restrictive cardiomyopathy, which presents a similar clinical and hemodynamic picture, but which cannot be treated by surgical pericardial removal.

Arrhythmias and conduction disturbances

Most forms of arrhythmia and conduction system disease increase with age, and over 75% of pacemakers and more than half of ICDs are placed in patients 65 years of age or older.[3] Aging is associated with fibrosis and calcification throughout the cardiac skeleton, leading to slower impulse generation and conduction and an increased frequency of atrial and ventricular premature depolarizations. In the absence of symptoms, most age-associated bradyarrhythmias, conduction abnormalities, and nonsustained tachyarrhythmias do not require treatment.

Bradycardia

Sinoatrial dysfunction, often referred to as "sick sinus syndrome," refers to various disorders related to impaired function of the sinus node and supraventricular conduction system. Sinus node pacemaker cells degenerate with age, and only around 10% of these cells continue to function normally by age 75. Similarly, conduction of the sinus impulse to atrial tissue or to the ventricles may become impaired, causing sinus node exit block or atrioventricular nodal block, respectively. Age-related stiffening of the carotid arteries also predisposes elderly individuals to carotid sinus hypersensitivity and associated vagally mediated bradyarrhythmias. Symptoms attributable to bradycardia may include dizziness and lightheadedness, angina, dyspnea, exercise intolerance, impaired mental function, fatigue, and syncope. Symptoms may occur at rest, upon standing, with positional changes of the head or neck (e.g., in patients with carotid sinus hypersensitivity), or during exertion (e.g., chronotropic incompetence, the inability to increase heart rate commensurate with increased metabolic demands). Often, 24-hour or 30-day ambulatory monitoring is required to correctly diagnose symptomatic bradycardia. A treadmill exercise test may facilitate the diagnosis of chronotropic incompetence.

Acute bradycardia is treated with atropine but the effect is short-lived. Reversible causes such as CAD (especially inferior ischemia), autonomic dysfunction, hypothyroidism, and electrolyte abnormalities should be treated if possible. Beta blockers, certain calcium channel blockers (diltiazem, verapamil), digoxin, clonidine, and many antiarrhythmic drugs may also precipitate symptomatic bradycardia, and a reduction in dosage or discontinuation of these agents may be required. Cholinesterase inhibitors, such as donepezil, can also cause bradycardia. Pacemaker implantation is indicated for non-reversible symptomatic bradycardia.[126] A prophylactic pacemaker is occasionally recommended in asymptomatic patients with severe bradycardia (heart rate less than 35–40 beats per minute) or high-degree atrioventricular block. In sick sinus syndrome, dual-chamber pacing is associated with lower risks of developing atrial fibrillation or requiring hospitalization compared to single-chamber pacing, but dual-chamber pacing does not reduce mortality.[152]

Supraventricular tachycardias

Supraventricular tachycardias (SVTs) increase in prevalence with advancing age. In many cases, brief episodes of SVT respond to beta blockers or calcium channel blockers. Some individuals may require the addition of digoxin or treatment with an antiarrhythmic drug. Radiofrequency ablation is also effective in selected cases. Of note, termination of SVT may be associated with prolonged sinus pauses and syncope in elderly patients ("tachy-brady syndrome"), occasionally requiring pacemaker placement to enable suppression of the tachyarrhythmias with medications. Multifocal atrial tachycardia (MAT) is an irregular SVT characterized by three or more P-wave morphologies on the electrocardiogram. MAT is most commonly seen in subjects with severe chronic lung disease, and often responds to treatment of the underlying lung disorder in conjunction with diltiazem, verapamil, or a beta blocker (if tolerated).

The most common sustained tachyarrhythmia in the geriatric population is atrial fibrillation (AF). Nearly 20%–25% of individuals will develop AF or atrial flutter during their lifetime,[3] but the prevalence increases from <1% before age 40 to approximately 10% after age 80 (Figure 12.2).[153] In older adults, most AF arises in the context of age-related atrial fibrosis leading to adverse remodeling and intra-atrial electrical abnormalities. AF may be

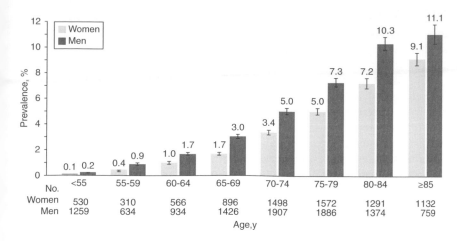

Figure 12.2 Prevalence of atrial fibrillation by age and gender in a large health maintenance organization in 1996–1997.

precipitated by uncontrolled hypertension, ischemia or acute MI, hyperthyroidism, alcohol excess or illicit drug use, HF, progressive valvular disease, acute or chronic lung conditions (e.g., pulmonary embolus or pneumonia), hypokalemia, cardiac or noncardiac surgery, stimulant medications (caffeine, pseudoephedrine), and chemotherapy for cancer.

Echocardiography is indicated in patients with new AF to evaluate for structural heart disease or pulmonary hypertension.[154] Electrolyte and thyroid hormone levels should be assessed as well. Patients with acute or chronic AF may be asymptomatic or experience palpitations, chest discomfort, effort intolerance, lightheadedness, syncope, or symptoms of HF. Occasionally elderly patients with acute-onset AF present with pulmonary edema due to the sudden loss of the atrial contribution to LV filling (the "atrial kick") and associated fall in cardiac output. Some elderly subjects present with bradycardia in the setting of AF due to underlying conduction system disease or therapy with AV nodal blocking agents. Unfortunately, in some cases AF is first diagnosed after a thromboembolic event such as a stroke.

Postoperative AF occurs in up to 50% of older patients undergoing major cardiac or thoracic surgery. Beta blockers, sotalol, and amiodarone reduce the risk of AF after cardiac surgery in the geriatric population.[155, 156] Although no mortality benefit has been demonstrated with these perioperative interventions, length of stay is reduced relative to subjects experiencing postoperative AF.

Management of acute AF focuses on rate control and prevention of thromboembolism. The majority of patients presenting with AF have a rapid heart rate that is irregularly irregular, so therapy is directed at slowing the ventricular rate with a beta blocker or calcium channel blocker (diltiazem or verapamil). Digoxin is less effective than other agents but may be used as adjunctive therapy or when beta blockers and calcium channel blockers are contraindicated (e.g., due to hypotension). Concurrent HF should be treated with diuretics, and hemodynamically unstable patients should undergo immediate electrical cardioversion. In hemodynamically stable patients, the need for and timing of pharmacologic or electrical cardioversion is unclear, since clinical trials indicate that cardioversion of asymptomatic or mildly symptomatic patients with AF does not improve quality of life or reduce mortality or stroke risk compared with a strategy of rate control and long-term anticoagulation.[157, 158] Nonetheless, these studies suggest that individuals maintaining sinus rhythm have better quality of life than those with persistent AF (irrespective of treatment strategy), so many clinicians recommend at least one attempt to restore sinus rhythm for recent-onset AF. In cases where AF has clearly been present for less than 48 hours (e.g., in the postoperative setting), the risk of thromboembolism is low, so pharmacologic or electrical cardioversion (if necessary) can be undertaken with relative safely. In patients with AF of longer or unknown duration, elective cardioversion should be preceded by a period of three to four weeks of systemic anticoagulation. Alternatively, transesophageal echocardiography may be performed, and if no atrial thrombus is demonstrated, electrical or pharmacologic cardioversion can then be undertaken. In either case, systemic anticoagulation is essential for a minimum of four weeks following cardioversion due to transient atrial stunning and significantly higher thromboembolic risk during the first several weeks after cardioversion. Furthermore, long-term anticoagulation is warranted for most older patients with AF.[154] In subjects who remain highly symptomatic despite efforts to control rate and/or maintain sinus rhythm with antiarrhythmic drug therapy, additional therapeutic options include catheter-based pulmonary vein isolation, ablation of the atrioventricular node with pacemaker implantation, and the surgical "Maze" procedure.

Systemic thromboembolism, most commonly an acute stroke, is the most devastating complication of AF, and results from thrombus arising in the left atrial appendage. In addition to being a risk factor for the development of AF, increasing age is a potent risk factor for stroke in patients with either paroxysmal or persistent AF. In the Framingham Heart Study, prior to the use of contemporary anticoagulation therapies, the proportion of strokes related to AF increased from 1.5% for patients in their fifties to 23.5% for patients over 80 years old.[159]

In clinical practice, the $CHADS_2$ and CHA_2DS_2-VASc scores are often used to estimate stroke risk in patients with AF and to identify patients who may benefit from long-term anticoagulation.[160, 161] $CHADS_2$ assigns one point each for congestive heart failure, hypertension, age of ≥ 75 years, and diabetes, and two points for prior stroke or transient ischemic attack (maximum score = 6). CHA_2DS_2-VASc is similar, but assigns two points for age of ≥ 75 years, and one point each for vascular disease (coronary artery disease, peripheral arterial disease, or abdominal aortic aneurysm), age of 65–74 years, and sex category female (maximum score = 9). Patients with AF and a $CHADS_2$ or CHA_2DS_2-VASc score ≥ 2 have an annual stroke risk of at least 4%, and systemic anticoagulation is recommended in the absence of major contraindications. In patients with a score of 1 using either instrument, anticoagulation is the preferred treatment, but antiplatelet therapy with aspirin and/or clopidogrel may be considered based on individual circumstances (e.g., moderate or high risk of bleeding) or patient preferences. Patients with a score of 0 (especially a CHA_2DS_2-VASc score of 0) are at relatively low risk and may be managed with antiplatelet therapy or no antithrombotic treatment. Note that all men ≥ 75 years of age and all women ≥ 65 years of age have a CHA_2DS_2-VASc score of at least 2 and are therefore candidates for anticoagulation.

Until recently, vitamin K antagonists such as warfarin were the only effective orally administered agents for long-term anticoagulation. In the past few years, several new antithrombotic agents (dabigatran, rivaroxaban, apixaban, edoxaban) have been approved for use in the United States, and additional alternatives may soon become available. Warfarin, at a dose adjusted to maintain the international normalized ratio (INR) in the range of 2.0–3.0, reduces the risk of stroke by 60%–70% in patients with AF, including patients over age 75.[154] Each of the newer agents has been shown to be at least as effective as warfarin in reducing the risk of ischemic stroke with lower risk of hemorrhagic stroke and equivalent or lower risk of major bleeding.[162–164] Principal advantages of the newer agents include fixed dosing, lack of need for monitoring INR or other blood tests, and markedly fewer drug–drug and drug–food interactions relative to warfarin. Disadvantages include contraindication in patients with severe renal impairment, lack of an effective antidote in the event of bleeding (except for dabigatran), higher cost, and uncertain safety and efficacy in patients over age 75 with multiple comorbidities due to limited enrollment of such patients in the pivotal clinical trials. In light of these advantages and disadvantages, selection of an anticoagulant agent is best accomplished through shared decision making on an individualized basis.

The most important and serious adverse event associated with the use of anticoagulants is bleeding, and older patients are at increased risk for this complication. Although several bleeding risk scores have been developed, the HAS-BLED score is most widely used. HAS-BLED assigns one point for hypertension (systolic blood pressure ≥ 160 mmHg), abnormal renal function, abnormal hepatic function, prior stroke, prior major bleeding or bleeding disorder, labile INR (<60% of time in therapeutic range), age >65 years ("elderly"), drugs predisposing to bleeding (antiplatelet agents, nonsteroidal anti-inflammatory drugs), and alcohol use (maximum score = 9).[165] Patients with a HAS-BLED score ≥ 3 are at increased risk for bleeding and warrant close follow-up. Utilizing the HAS-BLED score in combination with either the $CHADS_2$ or CHA_2DS_2-VASc score may be useful for evaluating the risks and benefits of anticoagulation in individual patients.[166] For example, a patient with a CHA_2DS_2-VASc score of 1 and HAS-BLED score of 4 may not be a good candidate for anticoagulation, whereas a similar patient with a HAS-BLED score of 1 may benefit from treatment.

A common conundrum in older patients with AF is an increased risk for falls, and concern about fall-related bleeding is the most common reason for withholding anticoagulants in older patients. However, several studies have shown that in the majority of patients, the risk of serious bleeding related to a fall is greatly outweighed by the beneficial effects of anticoagulation in reducing the risk of stroke and other embolic events in AF.[167, 168] Therefore, in most cases a perceived high risk of falls should not be considered a contraindication to anticoagulation. Of note, a meta-analysis of patients aged 75 and older enrolled in 10 randomized trials of dabigatran, rivaroxaban, and apixaban demonstrated no significant increase in bleeding with these drugs when compared with warfarin, and either equal or greater efficacy than warfarin with respect to the risk of stroke.[169]

Since AF and atrial flutter frequently coexist in the same patient, atrial flutter is managed using the same approach as for AF. In an occasional patient with isolated atrial flutter, radiofrequency ablation of the re-entrant pathway may be curative, and success rates in this setting are higher than for ablation of AF.

Ventricular arrhythmias

Ventricular arrhythmias, both isolated ventricular premature depolarizations (VPDs) and ventricular tachycardia (VT), increase in frequency with age – in part due to age-related changes in the cardiac conduction system, and in part related to the higher prevalence of cardiac disease at older age (especially CAD, cardiomyopathy, and hypertensive heart disease). In general, management of ventricular arrhythmias is similar in older and younger individuals and is dependent on symptoms, hemodynamic impact, and the severity of underlying heart disease. CAD, hypertension, and valvular heart disease should be treated as previously discussed. Electrolyte abnormalities, including hypokalemia, hyperkalemia, and hypomagnesemia, should be corrected. Isolated VPDs require no specific therapy unless the patient experiences disabling symptoms, in which case beta blockers are first-line treatment, followed by antiarrhythmic drugs if needed.

In the absence of HF or LV systolic dysfunction, asymptomatic nonsustained VT also requires no treatment, and symptomatic patients should be

managed in the same manner as for symptomatic VPDs. Sustained VT in geriatric patients almost always occurs in the context of advanced structural heart disease and portends an increased risk for sudden death. Acute sustained VT with hypotension or hypoperfusion should be treated with immediate electrical cardioversion, followed by an evaluation for precipitating causes. Recurrent sustained VT, whether symptomatic or asymptomatic, may warrant antiarrhythmic drug therapy and/or implantation of an ICD.[126, 170] Finally, as noted previously, patients with New York Heart Association class II–III HF and an LV ejection fraction of 35% or lower should be considered for an ICD on an individual basis in the absence of very advanced age, frailty, or other major life-limiting comorbidities.[126] In this context, subjects with CAD and documented VT (sustained or nonsustained) are at greatest risk for sudden cardiac death – a factor that should be taken into account in the decision-making process. Ventricular fibrillation is immediately life threatening and requires emergent defibrillation. Since primary ventricular fibrillation is almost always caused by ischemia, urgent coronary angiography is usually warranted in survivors of this arrhythmia.

Summary

Aging is associated with diffuse changes throughout the cardiovascular system as well as increasing prevalence of most forms of cardiovascular disease. As a result, the majority of men and women over the age of 65 have clinically manifest cardiovascular disorders, and such disorders are the leading cause of death, as well as a major source of disability and impaired quality of life in older adults. In general, the diagnosis and treatment of cardiovascular diseases are similar in older and younger patients. However, most cardiovascular therapies have been less well studied in elderly subjects, especially women, patients with more advanced age (e.g., over age 80), and individuals with multiple comorbid conditions. As a result, treatment of the older patient with cardiac disease must be individualized, taking into consideration each patient's unique set of circumstances, needs, and personal preferences. Finally, as the population ages, there is a clear need for additional research focusing specifically on the prevention and management of cardiovascular diseases in the geriatric age group.

References

1. Moran AE, Forouzanfar MH, Roth GA, et al. Temporal trends in ischemic heart disease mortality in 21 world regions, 1980–2010: the Global Burden of Disease 2010 Study. *Circulation* 2014;**129**:1483–1492.

2. Lozano R, Naghavi M, Foreman K, et al. Global and regional mortality from 235 causes of death for 20 age groups in 1990 and 2010: a systematic analysis for the Global Burden of Disease Study 2010. *Lancet* 2012;**380**:2095–2128.

3. Go AS, Mozaffarian D, Roger VL, et al. Heart disease and stroke statistics – 2014 update: a report from the American Heart Association. *Circulation* 2014;**129** (3):399–410.

4. Lakatta EG. Age-associated cardiovascular changes in health: impact on cardiovascular disease in older persons. *Heart Failure Reviews* 2002;7:29–49.

5. Rich MW. Heart disease in the elderly. In: Rosendorff C, ed. *Essential Cardiology: Principles and Practice*, Third Edition. New York: Springer, 2013:669–686.

6. D'Agostino RB, Vasan RS, Pencina MJ, et al. General cardiovascular risk profile for use in primary care: the Framingham Heart Study. *Circulation* 2008;**117**:743–753.

7. Haffner SM, Lehto S, Ronnemaa T, et al. Mortality from coronary heart disease in subjects with type 2 diabetes and in nondiabetic subjects with and without prior myocardial infarction. *New Engl J Med* 1998;**339**:229–234.

8. Kuller LH, Arnold AM, Psaty BM, et al. Ten-year follow-up of subclinical cardiovascular disease and risk of coronary heart disease in the Cardiovascular Health Study. *Arch Int Med* 2006;**166**:71–78.

9. White HD, Barbash GI, Califf RM, et al. Age and outcome with contemporary thrombolytic therapy: results from the GUSTO-I trial. *Circulation* 1996;**94**:1826–1833.

10. Scirica BM. Acute coronary syndrome: emerging tools for diagnosis and risk assessment. *J Am Coll Cardiol* 2010;**55**:1403–1415.

11. Eggers KM, Venge P, Lindahl B, Lind L. Cardiac troponin I levels measured with a high-sensitivity assay increase over time and are strong predictors of mortality in an elderly population. *J Am Coll Cardiol* 2013;**61**:1906–1913.

12. Thygesen K, Alpert JS, Jaffe AS, et al. Third universal definition of myocardial infarction. *J Am Coll Cardiol* 2012;**60**:1581–1598.

13. O'Gara PT, Kushner FG, Ascheim DD, et al. 2013 ACCF/AHA guideline for the management of ST-elevation myocardial infarction. *J Am Coll Cardiol* 2013;**61**:e78–140.

14. Amsterdam EA, Wenger NK, Brindis RG, et al. 2014 AHA/ACC Guideline for the Management of Patients with Non-ST-Elevation Acute Coronary Syndromes. *J Am Coll Cardiol* 2014;**64**(24):e139–e228.

15. ISIS-2 (Second International Study of Infarct Survival) Collaborative Group. Randomised trial of intravenous streptokinase, oral aspirin, both, or neither among 17,187 cases of suspected acute myocardial infarction: ISIS-2. *Lancet* 1988;**332**: 349–360.

16. The Clopidogrel in Unstable Angina to Prevent Recurrent Events Trial Investigators. Effects of clopidogrel in addition to aspirin in patients with acute coronary syndromes without ST-segment elevation. *N Engl J Med* 2001;**345**: 494–502.

17. Wiviott SD, Braunwald E, McCabe CH, et al. Prasugrel versus clopidogrel in patients with acute coronary syndromes. *N Engl J Med* 2007;**357**:2001–2015.

18. Wallentin L, Becker RC, Budaj A, et al. Ticagrelor versus clopidogrel in patients with acute coronary syndromes. *N Engl J Med* 2009;**361**:1045–1057.

19. Steen H, James S, Becker RC, et al. Ticagrelor versus clopidogrel in elderly patients with acute coronary syndromes: a substudy from the Prospective Randomized PLATelet Inhibition and Patient Outcomes (PLATO) trial. *Circ Cardiovasc Qual Outcomes* 2012;680–688.

20. Mauri L, Kereiakes DJ, Yeh RW, et al. Twelve or 30 months of dual antiplatelet therapy after drug-eluting stents. *N Engl J Med* 2014;**371**:2155–2166.

21. Morrow DA, Braunwald E, Bonaca MP, et al. Vorapaxar in the secondary prevention of atherothrombotic events. *N Engl J Med* 2012;**366**:1404–1413.

22. The PURSUIT Trial Investigators. Inhibition of platelet glycoprotein IIb/IIIa with eptifibatide in patients with acute coronary syndromes. *N Engl J Med* 1998;**339**: 436–443.

23. Antman EM, Cohen M, Radley D, et al. Assessment of the treatment effect of enoxaparin for unstable angina/non-Q-wave myocardial infarction: TIMI 11B-ESSENCE meta-analysis. *Circulation* 1999;**100**:1602–1608.

24. FRagmin and Fast Revascularization during InStability in Coronary artery disease (FRISC II) Investigators. Long-term low-molecular-mass heparin in unstable coronary-artery disease: FRISC II prospective randomised multicentre study. *Lancet* 1999;**354**: 701–707.

25. Dewilde WJ, Oirbans T, Verheugt FW, et al. Use of clopidogrel with or without aspirin in patients taking oral anticoagulant therapy and undergoing percutaneous coronary intervention: an open-label, randomized, controlled trial. *Lancet* 2013;**381**:1107–1115.

26. COMMIT Collaborative Group. Early intravenous then oral metoprolol in 45,852 patients with acute

myocardial infarction: randomised placebo-controlled trial. *Lancet* 2005;**366**:1622–1632.

27. ACE Inhibitor Myocardial Infarction Collaborative Group. Indications for ACE inhibitors in the early treatment of acute myocardial infarction: systematic overview of individual data from 100,000 patients in randomized trials. *Circulation* 1998;**97**:2202–2212.

28. Gruppo Italiano per lo Studio della Sopravvivenza nell'Infarto Miocardico. GISSI-3: effects of lisinopril and transdermal glyceryl trinitrate singly and together on 6-week mortality and ventricular function after acute myocardial infarction. *Lancet* 1994;**343**:1115–1122.

29. Ambrosioni E, Borghi C, Magnani B, for the Survival of Myocardial Infarction Long-Term Evaluation (SMILE) Study Investigators. The effect of the angiotensin-converting-enzyme inhibitor zofenopril on mortality and morbidity after anterior myocardial infarction. *N Engl J Med* 1995;**332**:80–85.

30. The Acute Infarction Ramipril Efficacy (AIRE) Study Investigators. Effect of ramipril on mortality and morbidity of survivors of acute myocardial infarction with clinical evidence of heart failure. *Lancet* 1993;**342**:821–828.

31. Dickstein K, Kjekshus J. Effects of losartan and captopril on mortality and morbidity in high-risk patients after acute myocardial infarction: the OPTIMAAL randomised trial. *Lancet* 2002;**360**:752–760.

32. Pitt B, Remme W, Zannad F, et al. Eplerenone, a selective aldosterone blocker, in patients with left ventricular dysfunction after myocardial infarction. *N Engl J Med* 2003;**348**:1309–1321.

33. Miettinen TA, Pyorala K, Olsson AG, et al. Cholesterol-lowering therapy in women and elderly patients with myocardial infarction or angina pectoris: findings from the Scandinavian Simvastatin Survival Study (4S). *Circulation* 1997;**96**:4211–4218.

34. Lewis SJ, Moye LA, Sacks FM, et al. Effect of pravastatin on cardiovascular events in older patients with myocardial infarction and cholesterol levels in the average range: results of the Cholesterol and Recurrent Events (CARE) trial. *Ann Intern Med* 1998;**129**:681–689.

35. The Long-Term Intervention with Pravastatin in Ischaemic Disease (LIPID) Study Group. Prevention of cardiovascular events and death with pravastatin in patients with coronary heart disease and a broad range of initial cholesterol levels. *N Engl J Med* 1998;**339**:1349–1357.

36. Shepherd J, Blauw GJ, Murphy MB, et al. Pravastatin in elderly individuals at risk of vascular disease (PROSPER): a randomised controlled trial. *Lancet* 2002;**360**:1623–1630.

37. Stone NJ, Intwala S, Katz D. Statins in very elderly adults. *J Am Geriatr Soc* 2014;**62**:943–945.

38. Rich MW. Aggressive lipid management in very elderly adults: less is more. *J Am Geriatr Soc* 2014;**62**:945–947.

39. Sathasivam S. Statin induced myopathy. *BMJ* 2008;**337**:a2286.

40. Lee DS, Markwardt S, Goeres L, et al. Statins and physical activity in older men: the osteoporotic fractures in men study. *JAMA Intern Med* 2014;**174**:1263–1270.

41. Golomb BA, Evans MA, Dimsdale JE, et al. Effects of statins on energy and fatigue with exertion: Results from a randomized controlled trial. *Arch Intern Med* 2012;**172**:1180–1182.

42. Evans MA, Golomb BA. Statin-associated adverse cognitive effects: survey results from 171 patients. *Pharmacotherapy* 2009;**29**:800–811.

43. The Global Use of Strategies to Open Occluded Coronary Arteries in Acute Coronary Syndromes (GUSTO IIb) Angioplasty Substudy Investigators. A clinical trial comparing primary coronary angioplasty with tissue plasminogen activator for acute myocardial infarction. *N Engl J Med* 1997;**336**:1621–1628.

44. De Boer MJ, Ottervanger JP, van't Hof AW, et al. Reperfusion therapy in elderly patients with acute myocardial infarction: a randomized comparison of primary angioplasty and thrombolytic therapy. *J Am Coll Cardiol* 2002;**39**:1723–1728.

45. Antman EM, Cohen M, Bernink PJLM, et al. The TIMI Risk Score for unstable angina/non-ST elevation MI: a method for prognostication and therapeutic decision making. *JAMA* 2000;**284**:835–842.

46. Granger CB, Goldberg RJ, Dabbous O, et al. Predictors of hospital mortality in the Global Registry of Acute Coronary Events (GRACE). *Arch Intern Med* 2003;**163**:2345–2353.

47. FRagmin and Fast Revascularization during InStability in Coronary artery disease (FRISC II) Investigators. Invasive compared with non-invasive treatment in unstable coronary-artery disease: FRISC II prospective randomised multicentre study. *Lancet* 1999;**354**: 708–715.

48. Hochman JS. Cardiogenic shock complicating acute myocardial infarction: expanding the paradigm. *Circulation* 2003;**107**:2998–3002.

49. Hochman JS, Sleeper LA, White HD, et al. for the SHOCK Investigators. One-year survival following early revascularization for cardiogenic shock. *JAMA* 2001;**285**:190–192.

50. Dzavik V, Sleeper LA, Cocke TP, et al. for the SHOCK Investigators. Early revascularization is associated with improved survival in elderly patients with acute myocardial infarction complicated by cardiogenic

shock: a report from the SHOCK Trial Registry. *Eur Heart J* 2003;**24**:828–837.

51. Bueno H, Lopez-Palop R, Perez-David E, et al. Combined effect of age and right ventricular involvement on acute inferior myocardial infarction prognosis. *Circulation* 1998;**98**:1714–1720.

52. Hasdai D, Topol EJ, Califf RM, et al. Cardiogenic shock complicating acute coronary syndromes. *Lancet* 2000;**356**:749–756.

53. Fihn SD, Gardin JM, Abrams J, et al. 2012 ACCF/AHA/ACP/AATS/PCNA/SCAI/STS guideline for the diagnosis and management of patients with stable ischemic heart disease. *J Am Coll Cardiol* 2012;**60**:e44–e164.

54. James PA, Oparil S, Carter BL, et al. 2014 evidence-based guideline for the management of high blood pressure in adults. *JAMA* 2014;**311**:507–520.

55. Stone NJ, Robinson JG, Lichtenstein AH, et al. 2013 ACC/AHA guideline on the treatment of blood cholesterol to reduce atherosclerotic cardiovascular risk in adults. *J Am Coll Cardiol* 2014;**63**:2889–2934.

56. American Geriatrics Society Expert Panel on the Care of Older Adults with Diabetes Mellitus. Guidelines abstracted from the American Geriatrics Society guidelines for improving the care of older adults with diabetes mellitus: 2013 update. *J Am Geriatrc Soc* 2013;**61**:2020–2026.

57. Witt BJ, Jacobsen SJ, Weston SA, et al. Cardiac rehabilitation after myocardial infarction in the community. *J Am Coll Cardiol* 2004;**44**:988–996.

58. American College of Cardiology/American Heart Association Task Force on Practice Guidelines (Committee to Update the 1997 Exercise Testing Guidelines). ACC/AHA 2002 guidelines update for exercise testing. *Circulation* 2002;**106**:1883–1892.

59. The TIME Investigators. Trial of invasive versus medical therapy in elderly patients with chronic symptomatic coronary-artery disease (TIME): a randomised trial. *Lancet* 2001;**358**:951–957.

60. Boden WE, O'Rourke RA, Teo KK, et al. Optimal medical therapy with or without PCI for stable coronary disease. *N Engl J Med* 2007;**356**:1503–1516.

61. Weintraub WS, Veledar E, Thompson T, Burnette J, Jurkovitz C, Mahoney E. Percutaneous coronary intervention outcomes in octogenarians during the stent era (National Cardiovascular Network). *Am J Cardiol* 2001;**88**:1407–1410.

62. Alexander KP, Anstrom KJ, Muhlbaier LH, et al. Outcomes of cardiac surgery in patients ≥80 years: results from the National Cardiovascular Network. *J Am Coll Cardiol* 2000;**35**:731–738.

63. Newman MF, Kirchner JL, Phillips-Bute B, et al. for the Neurological Outcome Research Groups and the Cardiothoracic Anesthesiology Research Endeavors Investigators. Longitudinal assessment of neurocognitive function after coronary-artery bypass surgery. *N Engl J Med* 2001;**344**:395–402.

64. Yancy CW, Jessup M, Bozkurt B, et al. 2013 ACCF/AHA guideline for the management of heart failure. *Circulation* 2013;**128**:e240–e327.

65. The ALLHAT Collaborative Research Group. Major outcomes in high-risk hypertensive patients randomized to angiotensin-converting enzyme inhibitor or calcium channel blocker versus diuretic: the Antihypertensive and Lipid-Lowering Treatment to Prevent Heart Attack Trial (ALLHAT). *JAMA* 2002;**288**:2981–2997.

66. Moser M, Hebert PR. Prevention of disease progression, left ventricular hypertrophy and congestive heart failure in hypertension treatment trials. *J Am Coll Cardiol* 1996;**27**:1214–1218.

67. Okin PM, Devereux RB, Jern S, et al. Regression of electrocardiographic left ventricular hypertrophy during antihypertensive treatment and the prediction of major cardiovascular events. *JAMA* 2004;**292**:2343–2349.

68. Goldman L, Hashimoto B, Cook EF, Loscalzo A. Comparative reproducibility and validity of systems for assessing cardiovascular functional class: advantages of a new specific activity scale. *Circulation* 1981;**64**:1227–1234.

69. Maisel AS, Krishnaswamy P, Nowak RM, et al. for the Breathing Not Properly Multinational Study Investigators. Rapid measurement of B-type natriuretic peptide in the emergency diagnosis of heart failure. *N Engl J Med* 2002;**347**:161–167.

70. Gaggin HK, Mohammed AA, Bhardwaj A, et al. Heart failure outcomes and benefits of NT-proBNP-guided management in the elderly: Results from the Prospective, Randomized ProBNP Outpatient Tailored Chronic Heart Failure Therapy (PROTECT Study). *J Cardiac Fail* 2012;**18**:626–634.

71. Redfield MM, Rodeheffer RJ, Jacobsen SJ, et al. Plasma brain natriuretic peptide concentration: impact of age and gender. *J Am Coll Cardiol* 2002;**40**:976–982.

72. Wang TJ, Larson MG, Levy D, et al. Impact of age and sex on plasma natriuretic peptide levels in healthy adults. *Am J Cardiol* 2002;**90**:254–258.

73. Heiat A, Gross CP, Krumholz HM. Representation of the elderly, women, and minorities in heart failure clinical trials. *Arch Intern Med* 2002;**162**:1682–1688.

74. Rich MW, Beckham V, Wittenberg C, et al. A multidisciplinary intervention to prevent the readmission of elderly patients with congestive heart failure. *N Engl J Med* 1995;**333**:1190–1195.

75. Whellan DJ, Hasselblad V, Peterson E, O'Connor CM, Schulman KA. Meta-analysis and review of heart failure disease management randomized controlled clinical trials. *Am Heart J* 2005;**149**:722–729.

76. Ades PA, Keteyian SJ, Balady GJ, et al. Cardiac rehabilitation exercise and self-care for chronic heart failure. *J Am Coll Cardiol HF* 2013;**1**(6):540–547.

77. Faris R, Flather M, Purcell H, et al. Current evidence supporting the role of diuretics in heart failure: a meta analysis of randomised controlled trials. *Int J Cardiol* 2002;**82**:149–158.

78. Domanski M, Norman J, Pitt B, et al. Diuretic use, progressive heart failure, and death in patients in the Studies of Left Ventricular Dysfunction (SOLVD). *J Am Coll Cardiol* 2003;**42**:705–708.

79. Neuberg GW, Miller AB, O'Connor CM, et al. Diuretic resistance predicts mortality in patients with advanced heart failure. *Am Heart J* 2002;**144**:31–38.

80. Gheorghiade M, Zannad F, Sopko G, et al. Acute heart failure syndromes: current state and framework for future research. *Circulation* 2005;**112**:3958–3968.

81. Gupta D, Georgiopoulou VV, Kalogeropoulos AP, et al. Dietary sodium intake in heart failure. *Circulation* 2012;**126**:479–485.

82. Flather MD, Yusuf S, Kober L, et al. for the ACEI-Inhibitor Myocardial Infarction Collaborative Group. Long-term ACEI-inhibitor therapy in patients with heart failure or left-ventricular dysfunction: a systematic overview of data from individual patients. *Lancet* 2000;**355**:1575–1581.

83. Garg R, Yusuf S for the Collaborative Group on ACE Inhibitor Trials. Overview of randomized trials of angiotensin-converting enzyme inhibitors on mortality and morbidity in patients with heart failure. *JAMA* 1995;**273**:1450–1456.

84. The SOLVD Investigators. Effect of enalapril on mortality and the development of heart failure in asymptomatic patients with reduced left ventricular ejection fraction. *N Engl J Med* 1992;**327**:685–691.

85. Maggioni AP, Anand I, Gottlieb SO, et al. Effects of valsartan on morbidity and mortality in patients with heart failure not receiving angiotensin-converting enzyme inhibitors. *J Am Coll Cardiol* 2002;**40**:1414–1421.

86. Granger CB, McMurray JJV, Yusuf S, et al. Effects of candesartan in patients with chronic heart failure and reduced left-ventricular systolic function intolerant to angiotensin-converting-enzyme inhibitors: the CHARM-Alternative trial. *Lancet* 2003;**362**:772–776.

87. Pfeffer MA, Swedberg K, Granger CB, et al. Effects of candesartan on mortality and morbidity in patients with chronic heart failure: the CHARM-Overall programme. *Lancet* 2003;**362**:759–766.

88. Kuenzli A, Bucher HC, Anand I, et al. Meta-analysis of combined therapy with angiotensin receptor antagonists versus ACE inhibitors alone in patients with heart failure. *PloS One* 2010;**5**:e9946.

89. Cohn JN, Archibald DG, Ziesche S, et al. Effect of vasodilator therapy on mortality in chronic congestive heart failure: results of a Veterans Administration Cooperative Study. *N Engl J Med* 1986;**314**:1547–1552.

90. Cohn JN, Johnson G, Ziesche S, et al. A comparison of enalapril with hydralazine-isosorbide dinitrate in the treatment of chronic congestive heart failure. *N Engl J Med* 1991;**325**:303–310.

91. Taylor AL, Ziesche S, Yancy C, et al. for the African-American Heart Failure Trial Investigators. Combination of isosorbide dinitrate and hydralazine in blacks with heart failure. *N Engl J Med* 2004;**351**:2049–2057.

92. MERIT-HF Study Group. Effect of metoprolol CR/XL in chronic heart failure: Metoprolol CR/XL Randomised Intervention Trial in Congestive Heart Failure (MERIT-HF). *Lancet* 1999;**353**:2001–2007.

93. Packer M, Coats AJS, Fowler MB, et al. for the Carvedilol Prospective Randomized Cumulative Survival Study Group. Effect of carvedilol on survival in severe chronic heart failure. *N Engl J Med* 2001;**344**:1651–1658.

94. Deedwania PC, Gottlieb S, Ghali JK, et al. Efficacy, safety and tolerability of beta-adrenergic blockade with metoprolol CR/XL in elderly patients with heart failure. *Eur Heart J* 2004;**25**:1300–1309.

95. Pitt B, Zannad F, Remme WJ, et al. for the Randomized Aldactone Evaluation Study Investigators. The effect of spironolactone on morbidity and mortality in patients with severe heart failure. *N Engl J Med* 1999;**341**:709–717.

96. Zannad F, McMurray JJV, Krum H, et al. Eplerenone in patients with systolic heart failure and mild symptoms. *N Engl J Med* 2011;**364**:11–21.

97. Juurlink DN, Mamdani MM, Lee DS, et al. Rates of hyperkalemia after publication of the Randomized Aldactone Evaluation Study. *N Engl J Med* 2004;**351**:543–551.

98. The Digitalis Investigation Group. The effect of digoxin on mortality and morbidity in patients with heart failure. *N Engl J Med* 1997;**336**:525–533.

99. Rich MW, McSherry F, Williford WO, Yusuf S, for the Digitalis Investigation Group. Effect of age on mortality, hospitalizations and response to digoxin in patients with heart failure: the DIG study. *J Am Coll Cardiol* 2001;**38**:806–813.

100. Ahmed A, Rich MW, Love TE, et al. Digoxin and reduction in mortality and hospitalization in heart failure: a comprehensive post hoc analysis of the DIG trial. *Eur Heart J* 2006;**27**:178–186.

101. Massie BN, Collins JF, Ammon SE, et al. Randomized trial of warfarin, aspirin, and clopidogrel in patients with chronic heart failure: the Warfarin and

Antiplatelet Therapy in Chronic Heart Failure (WATCH) Trial. *Circulation* 2009;**119**:1616–1624.

102. Homma S, Thompson JLP, Pullicino PM, et al. Warfarin and aspirin in patients with heart failure and sinus rhythm. *N Engl J Med* 2012;**366**:1859–1869.

103. O'Connor CM, Gattis WA, Uretsky BF, et al. Continuous intravenous dobutamine is associated with an increased risk of death in patients with advanced heart failure: Insights from the Flolan International Randomized Survival Trial (FIRST). *Am Heart J* 1999;**138**:78–86.

104. Cuffe MS, Califf RM, Adams KFJ, et al. Short-term intravenous milrinone for acute exacerbation of chronic heart failure: a randomized controlled trial. *JAMA* 2002;**287**:1541–1547.

105. Publication Committee for the VMAC Investigators (Vasodilation in the Management of Acute CHF). Intravenous nesiritide vs nitroglycerin for treatment of decompensated congestive heart failure: a randomized controlled trial. *JAMA* 2002;**287**:1531–1540.

106. O'Connor CM, Starling RC, Hernandez AF, et al. Effect of nesiritide in patients with acute decompensated heart failure. *N Engl J Med* 2011;**365**:32–43.

107. Daneshvar DA, Czer LS, Phan A, Trento A, Schwarz ER. Heart transplantation in the elderly: why cardiac transplantation does not need to be limited to younger patients but can be safely performed in patients above 65 years of age. *Ann Transplant* 2010;**15**:110–119.

108. Atluri P, Goldstone AB, Kobrin DM, et al. Ventricular assist device implant in the elderly is associated with increased, but respectable risk: A multi-institutional study. *Ann Thorac Surg* 2013;**96**:141–147.

109. Kitzman DW, Gardin JM, Gottdiener JS, et al. for the Cardiovascular Health Study Research Group. Importance of heart failure with preserved systolic function in patients > or = 65 years of age. *Am J Cardiol* 2001;**87**:413–419.

110. Owan TE, Hodge DO, Herges RM, Jacobsen SJ, Roger VL, Redfield MM. Trends in prevalence and outcome of heart failure with preserved ejection fraction. *N Engl J Med* 2006;**355**:251–259.

111. Bhatia RS, Tu JV, Lee DS, et al. Outcome of heart failure with preserved ejection fraction in a population-based study. *New Engl J Med* 2006;**355**:260–269.

112. Owan TE, Hodge DO, Herges RM, et al. Trends in prevalence and outcome of heart failure with preserved ejection fraction. *New Engl J Med* 2006;**355**:251–259.

113. Meta-analysis Global Group in Chronic Heart Failure (MAGGIC). The survival of patients with heart failure with preserved or reduced left ventricular ejection fraction: an individual patient data meta-analysis. *Eur Heart J* 2011; doi:10.1093/eurheartj/ehr254.

114. Yusuf S, Pfeffer MA, Swedberg K, et al. for the CHARM investigators and Committees. Effects of candesartan in patients with chronic heart failure and preserved left-ventricular ejection fraction: the CHARM-Preserved Trial. *Lancet* 2003;**362**:777–781.

115. Ahmed A, Rich MW, Fleg JL, et al. Effects of digoxin on morbidity and mortality in diastolic heart failure: the Ancillary Digitalis Investigation Group Trial. *Circulation* 2006;**114**:397–403.

116. Cleland JGF, Tendera M, Adamus J, et al. The perindopril in elderly people with chronic heart failure (PEP-CHF) study. *Eur Heart J* 2006;**27**:2338–2345.

117. Massie BM, Carson PE, McMurray JJ, et al. Irbesartan in patients with heart failure and preserved ejection fraction. *N Engl J Med* 2008;**359**:2456–2467.

118. Van Veldhuisen DJ, Cohen-Solal A, Bohm M, et al. Beta-blockade with nebivolol in elderly heart failure patients with impaired and preserved left ventricular ejection fraction. *J Am Coll Cardiol* 2009;**53**:2150–2158.

119. Pitt B, Pfeffer MA, Assmann SF, et al. Spironolactone for heart failure with preserved ejection fraction. *N Engl J Med* 2014;**370**:1383–1392.

120. Edelmann F, Wachter R, Schmidt AG, et al. Effect of spironolactone on diastolic function and exercise capacity in patients with heart failure with preserved ejection fraction: the Aldo-DHF randomized controlled trial. *JAMA* 2013;**309**:781–791.

121. Redfield MM, Chen HH, Borlaug BA, et al. Effect of phosphodiesterase-5 inhibition on exercise capacity and clinical status in heart failure with preserved ejection fraction: a randomized clinical trial. *JAMA* 2013;**309**:1268–1277.

122. Zile MR, Bourge RC, Redfield MM, Zhou D, Baicu CF, Little WC. Randomized, double-blind, placebo-controlled study of sitaxsentan to improve impaired exercise tolerance in patients with heart failure and a preserved ejection fraction. *J Am Coll Cardiol HF* 2014;**2**:123–130.

123. Conraads VM, Metra M, Kamp O, et al. Effects of long-term administration of nebivolol on the clinical symptoms, exercise capacity, and left ventricular function of patients with diastolic dysfunction: results of the ELANDD study. *Eur J Heart Fail* 2012;**14**:219–225.

124. Bristow MR, Saxon LA, Boehmer J, et al. for the Comparison of Medical Therapy, Pacing, and Defibrillation in Heart Failure (COMPANION) Investigators. Cardiac-resynchronization therapy

with or without an implantable defibrillator in advanced chronic heart failure. *N Engl J Med* 2004;**350**:2140–2150.

125. Cleland JGF, Daubert JC, Erdmann E, et al. for the Cardiac Resynchronization-Heart Failure (CARE-HF) Study Investigators. The effect of cardiac resynchronization on morbidity and mortality in heart failure. *New Engl J Med* 2005;**352**:1539–1549.

126. Tracy CM, Epstein AE, Darbar D, et al. 2012 ACCF/ AHA/HRS Focused update incorporated into the ACCF/AHA/HRS 2008 Guidelines for Device-Based Therapy of Cardiac Rhythm Abnormalities. *Circulation* 2013;**127**:e283–e352.

127. Cheng YJ, Zhang J, Li WJ, et al. More favorable response to cardiac resynchronization therapy in women than in men. *Circ Arrhythm Electrophysiol* 2014;**7**(5):807–815.

128. Zusterzeel R, Selzman KA, Sanders WE, et al. Cardiac resynchronization therapy in women: US Food and Drug Administration meta-analysis of patient-level data. *JAMA Intern Med* 2014;**174**:1340–1348.

129. Verbrugge FH, Dupont M, De Vusser P, et al. Response to cardiac resynchronization therapy in elderly patients (≥70 years) and octogenarians. *Eur J Heart Fail* 2013;**15**:203–210.

130. Moss AJ, Zareba W, Hall WJ, et al. for the Multicenter Automatic Defibrillator Implantation Trial II Investigators. Prophylactic implantation of a defibrillator in patients with myocardial infarction and reduced ejection fraction. *N Engl J Med* 2002;**346**:877–883.

131. Bardy GH, Lee KL, Mark DB, et al. for the Sudden Cardiac Death in Heart Failure Trial (SCD-HeFT) Investigators. Amiodarone or an implantable cardioverter-defibrillator for congestive heart failure. *N Engl J Med* 2005;**352**:225–237.

132. Santangeli P, Di Biase L, Dello Russo A, et al. Meta-analysis: age and effectiveness of prophylactic implantable cardioverter-defibrillators. *Ann Intern Med* 2010;**153**:592–599.

133. Lampert R, Hayes DL, Annas GJ, et al. HRS Expert Consensus Statement on the Management of Cardiovascular Implantable Electronic Devices (CIEDs) in patients nearing end of life or requesting withdrawal of therapy. *Heart Rhythm* 2010;**7**:1008–1026.

134. Feltner C, Jones CD, Cene CW, et al. Transitional care interventions to reduce readmissions for persons with heart failure: a systematic review and meta-analysis. *Ann Intern Med* 2014;**160**:774–784.

135. Huynh BC, Rovner A, Rich MW. Long-term survival in elderly patients hospitalized for heart failure: 14 year follow-up from a prospective randomized trial. *Arch Intern Med* 2006;**166**:1892–1898.

136. Whellan DJ, Goodlin SJ, Dickinson MG, et al. End-of-life care in patients with heart failure. *J Cardiac Failure* 2014;**20**:121–134.

137. Otto CM, Prendergast B. Aortic-valve stenosis – from patients at risk to severe valve obstruction. *N Engl J Med* 2014;**371**:744–756.

138. Nishimura RA, Otto CM, Bonow RO, et al. 2014 AHA/ACC guideline for the management of patients with valvular heart disease. *J Am Coll Cardiol* 2014;**63**: e57–e185.

139. Leon MB, Smith CR, Mack M, et al. Transcatheter aortic-valve implantation for aortic stenosis in patients who cannot undergo surgery. *N Engl J Med* 2010;**363**:1597–1607.

140. Smith CR, Leon MB, Mack MJ, et al. Transcatheter versus surgical aortic-valve replacement in high-risk patients. *N Engl J Med* 2011;**364**:2187–2198.

141. Kodali SK, Williams MR, Smith CR, et al. Two-year outcomes after transcatheter or surgical aortic-valve replacement. *N Engl J Med* 2012;**366**:1686–1695.

142. Reynolds MR, Magnuson EA, Lei Y, et al. Health-related quality of life after transcatheter aortic valve replacement in inoperable patients with severe aortic stenosis. *Circulation* 2011;**124**:1964–1972.

143. Lindman BR, Alexander KP, O'Gara PT, Afilalo J. Futility, benefit, and transcatheter aortic valve replacement. *J Am Coll Cardiol Cardiovasc Intervent*; 2014;**7**:707–716.

144. Scognamiglio R, Rahimtoola SH, Fasoli G, et al. Nifedipine in asymptomatic patients with severe aortic regurgitation and normal left ventricular function. *N Engl J Med* 1994;**331**:689–694.

145. Evangelista A, Tornos P, Sambola A, et al. Long-term vasodilator therapy in patients with severe aortic regurgitation. *N Engl J Med* 2005;**353**:1342–1349.

146. Mathew JP, Fontes ML, Tudor IC, et al. A multicenter risk index for atrial fibrillation after cardiac surgery. *JAMA* 2004;**291**:1720–1729.

147. Crystal E, Connolly SJ, Sleik K, et al. Interventions on prevention of postoperative atrial fibrillation in patients undergoing heart surgery: a meta-analysis. *Circulation* 2002;**106**:75–80.

148. Mitchell LB, Exner DV, Wyse DG, et al. Prophylactic oral amiodarone for the prevention of arrhythmias that begin early after revascularization, valve replacement, or repair – PAPABEAR: a randomized controlled trial. *JAMA* 2005;**294**:3093–3100.

149. Enriquez-Sarano M, Avierinos JF, Messika-Zeitoun D, et al. Quantitative determinants of the outcome of asymptomatic mitral regurgitation. *N Engl J Med* 2005;**352**:875–883.

150. Feldman T, Foster E, Glower DD, et al. Percutaneous repair or surgery for mitral regurgitation. *N Engl J Med* 2011;**364**:1395–1406.

151. Wan B, Rahnvavardi M, Tian DH, et al. A meta-analysis of MitraClip system versus surgery for treatment of severe mitral regurgitation. *Ann Cardiothorac Surg* 2013;**2**:683–692.

152. Lamas GA, Lee KL, Silverman R, et al. Ventricular pacing or dual-chamber pacing for sinus-node dysfunction. *N Engl J Med* 2002;**346**:1854–1862.

153. Go AS, Hylek EM, Phillips KA, et al. Prevalence of diagnosed atrial fibrillation in adults: national implications for rhythm management and stroke prevention: the AnTicoagulation and Risk factors In Atrial fibrillation (ATRIA) study. *JAMA* 2001;**285**:2370–2375.

154. January CT, Wann LS, Alpert JS, et al. 2014 AHA/ACC/HRS guideline for the management of patients with atrial fibrillation. *J Am Coll Cardiol* 2014;**64**(21):e1–e76.

155. Coleman CI, Perkerson KA, Gillespie EL, et al. Impact of prophylactic beta blockade on post-cardiothoracic surgery length of stay and atrial fibrillation. *Ann Phamacother* 2004;**38**:2012–2016.

156. Kluger J, White CM. Amiodarone prevents symptomatic atrial fibrillation and reduces the risk of cerebrovascular events and ventricular tachycardia after open heart surgery: results of the Atrial Fibrillation Suppression Trial (AFIST). *Card Electrophysiol Rev* 2003;**7**:165–167.

157. Wyse DG, Waldo AL, DiMarco JP, et al. A comparison of rate control and rhythm control in patients with atrial fibrillation. *N Engl J Med* 2002;**347**:1825–1833.

158. The AFFIRM Investigators. Quality of life in atrial fibrillation: the Atrial Fibrillation Follow-up Investigation of Rhythm Management (AFFIRM) study. *Am Heart J* 2005;**149**:112–120.

159. Wolf PA, Abbott RD, Kannel WB. Atrial fibrillation as an independent risk factor for stroke: the Framingham Study. *Stroke* 1991;**22**:983–988.

160. Gage BF, Waterman AD, Shannon W, et al. Validation of clinical classification schemes for predicting stroke: results from the National Registry of Atrial Fibrillation. *JAMA* 2001;**285**:2864–2870.

161. Lip GY, Nieuwlaat R, Pisters R, Lane DA, Crijns HJ. Refining clinical risk stratification for predicting stroke and thromboembolism in atrial fibrillation using a novel risk factor-based approach: the Euro Heart Survey on Atrial Fibrillation. *Chest.* 2010;**137**:263–72.

162. Connolly SJ, Ezekowitz MD, Yusuf S, et al. Dabigatran versus warfarin in patients with atrial fibrillation. *N Engl J Med* 2009;**361**:1139–1151.

163. Patel MR, Mahaffey KW, Garg J, et al. Rivaroxaban versus warfarin in nonvalvular atrial fibrillation. *N Engl J Med* 2011;**365**:883–891.

164. Granger CB, Alexander JH, McMurray JJV, et al. Apixaban versus warfarin in patients with atrial fibrillation. *N Engl J Med* 2011;**365**:981–992.

165. Pisters R, Lane DA, Nieuwlaat R, Vos CB, Crijns HJ, Lip GY. A novel user-friendly score (HAS-BLED) to assess 1-year risk of major bleeding in patients with atrial fibrillation: the Euro Heart Survey. *Chest* 2010;**138**:1093–1100.

166. Lane DA, Lip GYH. Clinician update: use of the CHA_2DS_2-VASc and HAS-BLED scores to aid decision making for thromboprophylaxis in nonvalvular atrial fibrillation. *Circulation* 2012;**126**:860–865.

167. Gage BF, Birman-Deych E, Kerzner R, Radford MJ, Nilasena DS, Rich MW. Incidence of intracranial hemorrhage in patients with atrial fibrillation who are prone to fall. *Am J Med* 2005;**118**:612–617.

168. Donze J, Clair C, Hug B, et al. Risk of falls and major bleeds in patients on oral anticoagulation therapy. *Am J Med* 2012;**125**:773–778.

169. Sardar P, Chatterjee S, Chaudhari S, Lip GY. New oral anticoagulants in elderly adults: evidence from a meta-analysis of randomized trials. *J Am Geriatr Soc* 2014;**62**:857–864.

170. Buxton AE, Lee KL, Fisher JD, et al. for the Multicenter Unsustained Tachycardia Trial Investigators. A randomized study of the prevention of sudden death in patients with coronary artery disease. *N Engl J Med* 1999;**341**:1882–1890.

Chapter 13

Hypertension in the elderly

Sonia Sehgal, MD, Neetu Bhola, MD, and Jung Hee Han, DO

Introduction

The number of older adults is growing, and the majority of this population has hypertension. Essential hypertension is the leading diagnosis in outpatient visits in the United States in the geriatric population. [1] It is brought on in part due to the physiologic changes of aging, but for some it occurs earlier due to lifestyle or other risk factors. Hypertension increases the risk for multiple medical conditions which can lead to decreased health status, functional ability and survival. Adequately treating hypertension in the elderly is beneficial and can reduce the risk of stroke, heart failure, and death due to cardiovascular disease. Owing to the unique characteristics of this special population, treatment recommendations require special consideration. This chapter will review both the evaluation and management of hypertension in elderly persons.

Epidemiology

Hypertension remains a chronic and prominent health condition affecting the morbidity and mortality of a great proportion of the elderly population. According to the National Health and Nutrition Examination Survey (NHANES) 2007 to 2010, age-adjusted prevalence of hypertension among people 18 years of age and older was 29.6%. The prevalence sharply increases to 71.6% in those 65 years of age and over.[2] In the Framingham Heart Study, 90% of those 55 years of age and older who were not diagnosed with hypertension went on to develop the condition.[3] Although increasing awareness has improved control rates among all age groups, the rates are unacceptably high in older adults with only 48.6% of this population having controlled hypertension, with highest rates in certain minority populations. Despite improved control, hypertension remains an important risk factor for cardiovascular disease, congestive heart failure and stroke.

Pathophysiology

Age related changes in arterial structure and function predispose older individuals to hypertension. Large vessels stiffen due to impaired function of elastin protein, increased collagen and loss of smooth muscle cells. Also contributing to this vascular dysfunction is atherosclerosis and calcium deposition within the vessel wall. This increased arterial stiffness leads to increased peripheral vascular resistance and decreased vascular compliance. Increased afterload and left ventricular hypertrophy follow.

Progressive renal dysfunction with a decrease in glomerular filtration rate and changes in the kidneys' ability to manage sodium regulation result in heightened sensitivity to dietary sodium intake and elevated blood pressures. Two-thirds of older adults have salt-sensitive hypertension.

Age associated changes in the sympathetic nervous system also contributes to impaired blood pressure regulation. Decreased baroreflex sensitivity leads to increased blood pressure variability – most noticeably a delayed response in heart rate to decreased blood pressure.

Additional factors contributing to blood pressure dysfunction in the elderly include increased risk of orthostatic and postprandial hypotension – often complicating management strategies. Also, circadian variability in blood pressure leads to relatively higher nighttime and early morning blood pressures increasing an older adult's risk of myocardial infarction and stroke.

Lifestyle, tobacco, alcohol, caffeine, and certain medications such as nonsteroidal anti-inflammatory

Reichel's Care of the Elderly, 7th Edition, ed. Jan Busby-Whitehead *et al.* Published by Cambridge University Press.
© Cambridge University Press 2016.

Table 13.1 Classification of blood pressure levels

Category	Systolic (mmHg)		Diastolic (mmHg)
Normal	<120	*and*	<80
Prehypertension	120–139	*or*	80–89
Hypertension:			
Stage 1	140–159	*or*	90–99
Stage 2	>160	*or*	>100

drugs (NSAIDs), steroids, antidepressants, decongestants, and migraine medications also negatively impact blood pressure control in the elderly patient.

Diagnosis and evaluation

Blood pressure levels as defined by the JNC7 (the Seventh Report of the Joint National Committee on Prevention, Detection, Evaluation, and Treatment of High Blood Pressure) are noted in Table 13.1. Although the most recent evaluation of available literature conducted by the Eighth Joint National Committee (JNC8) did not redefine blood pressure levels, it did recommend treating hypertensive patients older than 60 years of age to a blood pressure goal of less than 150/90 mmHg.[4]

To diagnose hypertension in the elderly, at least three separate blood pressure measurements obtained on two different office visits are needed. Additional measurements as well as orthostatic readings may be required due to increased variability in blood pressure in older adults. Particular attention should be given to using the appropriate cuff size, placing the arm at the level of the heart, and obtaining the readings in a relaxed setting – preferably with the patient seated comfortably for five minutes.

Ambulatory (home) blood pressure monitoring is useful for the evaluation of "white coat" hypertension or patients with a great deal of variability between readings. Increased rigidity of the peripheral arteries due to calcification and atherosclerosis in the rare patient can lead to pseudohypertension. Due to the incomplete compression of the brachial artery when the blood pressure cuff is inflated, falsely elevated systolic readings are obtained. Pseudohypertension should be suspected in patients with refractory hypertension without expected end organ damage or when hypotension results unexpectedly after starting antihypertensive medications. When measuring blood

pressures the auscultatory gap (an indication of arterial stiffness) can lead to artificially low readings. To avoid such inaccuracies, inflate the blood pressure cuff 40 mmHg higher than the pressure needed to occlude the brachial pulse.

Initial history should include a review of personal cardiac risk factors, family history as it relates to cardiac disease, evaluation of medications (including prescribed and over-the-counter), herbal remedies, and other supplements. In addition, discussing lifestyle choices (tobacco, alcohol and substance, exercise history, and dietary preferences) is useful. Compliance with sodium restriction and antihypertensive medications may be useful for those patients diagnosed with hypertension who have poor control. High-risk comorbid conditions such as diabetes mellitus, congestive heart failure, stroke, and hyperlipidemia should also be assessed.

Physical exam maneuvers should focus on the cardiovascular system and potential sites of end organ damage from uncontrolled blood pressure. Funduscopic examination to identify papilledema or retinopathy, carotid examination to evaluate bruits, heart examination with particular focus on murmurs, cardiac rhythm, and heart size as well as peripheral pulses and abdominal bruits are cardinal elements of the physical exam needed to evaluate a patient with hypertension. Laboratory and investigative studies should include an electrocardiogram, basic metabolic panel to examine electrolytes, kidney function and glucose, a fasting lipid panel, and urinalysis.

As in younger patients, secondary causes of hypertension such as renal artery stenosis, renal failure, hyperaldosteronism, Cushing's syndrome, pheochromocytoma, obstructive sleep apnea, and hyperthyroidism should be evaluated in those with refractory hypertension.

Comorbidities and end-organ effects

Uncontrolled hypertension affects multiple organ systems and can exacerbate other chronic conditions. Most commonly, effects are seen in the cardiovascular, cerebrovascular, and renal systems. Coronary artery disease, including myocardial infarction and angina as well as left ventricular dysfunction, are prevalent among people with hypertension. Arrhythmias, such as atrial fibrillation may also be related. Uncontrolled blood pressures can also increase the risk of aortic or peripheral arterial disease, such as abdominal or thoracic aortic aneurysms and dissection. Hypertension is linked to cerebrovascular disease, in particular ischemic stroke and cerebral hemorrhage. Studies are evaluating a possible link between cognitive impairment (vascular dementia and Alzheimer's disease) and uncontrolled blood pressure. Although renal function declines with age, hypertension is an independent risk factor for further kidney disease. Retinopathy can also result from uncontrolled blood pressure, with increased risk for retinal artery occlusion and ischemic optic neuropathy.

Diabetes mellitus and hypertension affect many of the same end organs and an additive effect is seen in the risk of complications. The combined presence of both conditions accelerates the risk of cardiovascular disease, retinopathy, nephropathy, and cerebral disease.

Benefits of treatment

Despite the benefits of treating hypertension in elderly patients, medical providers remain reluctant to treat moderately elevated blood pressures in older adults. Appropriate treatment of hypertension reduces the risk of cerebrovascular disease, congestive heart failure, and cardiovascular disease, regardless of age. Multiple studies have shown significant reduction in morbidity and mortality when elevated blood pressures are appropriately treated to goal. In the Systolic Hypertension in the Elderly Program (SHEP) trial, hypertension management led to a 36% reduction in strokes, 27% reduction in myocardial infarctions, 27% reduction in coronary artery disease, 32% reduction in cardiovascular disease, and a 13% reduction in mortality. A further analysis of the data obtained in this study revealed a reduction of all stroke types, including subtypes of both ischemic and hemorrhagic strokes.[5] Similar benefits were seen in the HYpertension in the Very Elderly Trial (HYVET) study, which included individuals aged 80–105 years. [6] This study showed reduction in strokes by 34%, heart failure by 72%, cardiovascular mortality by 27%, and all-cause mortality by 28%.

Treatment

Treating hypertension in the elderly can be a challenging task given the limited information for evidence-based guidelines for the management of elevated blood pressure in older adults. Current recommendations developed by national working groups provide recommendations based on expert opinion. Individualized treatment plans should be created for each patient, paying particular attention to concurrent medical conditions, current life expectancy, and social situation (such as whom they are living with and where). Geriatric patients are more prone to adverse drug events, and the "start low, go slow" adage should dictate medication management. If appropriate, family members and caregivers should be included in the discussion to determine treatment goals.

The JNC8 recommends a blood pressure target of less than 150/90 mmHg for patients aged 60 years and older. However, patients who are already receiving treatment and are stable with a systolic blood pressure of less than 140 mm Hg do not require alterations to the current medication regimen if no adverse effects are experienced with the lower blood pressure (orthostatic hypotension, dizziness, etc.).[4]

Earlier guidelines emphasized the importance of controlling diastolic blood pressure. At one time, systolic blood pressure elevation was attributed to the physiologic changes associated with aging. However, newer recommendations focus on the management of systolic blood pressure values known to increase cardiovascular risk.

Nonpharmacologic treatment

For patients with mild hypertension, lifestyle modification may be the only adjustment required to manage elevated blood pressure. For those with moderate to severe hypertension, nonpharmacologic therapies will augment medication management and likely result in lower doses of medications needed to adequately control the disease. A detailed social history including elements of tobacco and alcohol use as well as a formal dietary history, including how meals are prepared (e.g., premade meals may be salt rich), help to determine modifiable risk factors.[7] Additionally, stress reduction and maintaining a healthy body weight may help control elevated blood pressure levels. Moderate exercise and a diet rich in fruits and vegetables also help to control mild hypertension. The dietary approaches to stop hypertension (DASH) diet incorporates foods high in fiber, calcium, potassium, and magnesium and low in cholesterol, and it has been shown to reduce blood pressure. Consultation with a dietitian may be beneficial for some patients. Weight loss can be considered in an elderly patient with a body mass index (BMI) greater than 26. Patients that are able to ambulate on their own and that are not wheelchair bound should be encouraged to participate in exercise and walk at least 30 minutes per day for the majority of the week.[7]

Considerations in treatment

Nonpharmacologic therapies should be attempted prior to medication management in stable patients. Individual drugs can be selected based on patient comorbidities and side effect profiles. The risks and benefits of medication management of hypertension should be discussed with each patient. The side effect profile of medications, such as electrolyte disturbances, edema, or cough, should be considered in regard to the patient's current medical conditions and/or comorbidities. Certain patients that are more prone to dehydration may have worsening of orthostatic hypotension. Elderly patients can have drug accumulation due to renal dysfunction; therefore, doses need to be managed accordingly. Antihypertensive medications should be initiated at the lowest possible dose and slowly increased if needed. If after one month of treatment, the blood pressure is not at goal, this medication dose should be slowly increased.[4] A second agent from another class can be added if further blood pressure control is needed after reaching the full dose of the first drug – again starting at the lowest possible dose. Nonadherence, drug interactions, and polypharmacy should be considered with each dose escalation and addition of new drugs.

Classes of antihypertensive medications

Thiazide-type diuretics, angiotensin converting enzyme inhibitors, angiotensin receptor blockers, and calcium channel blockers are appropriate first-line antihypertensive medications to consider when managing elevated blood pressure in the geriatric population.[4]

Thiazide-type diuretics

Randomized controlled trials have shown significant benefit in the prevention of stroke, cardiovascular events, and mortality when low-dose thiazide diuretics are used for the management of hypertension in the elderly. Side effects to be noted with this class of medication include hypokalemia, hyponatremia, hypomagnesemia, and glucose intolerance. Caution should be exercised when using this medication in a patient known to have gout, as uric acid levels can rise with the drug. Side effects can be minimized when using these drugs at a lower dose. Potassium replacement may be needed and can decrease the risk of arrhythmias. Loop diuretics can be used in the management of hypertension but are generally reserved for patients with congestive heart failure.

Calcium channel blockers

Dihydropyridine calcium channel blockers are effective in decreasing stroke risk in older patients with elevated blood pressure. Calcium channel blockers act by causing vasodilation, increasing vascular permeability, or by affecting cardiac contractility. Common side effects include peripheral edema, constipation, and gastro-esophageal disease. Headaches and postural hypotension may occur. Non-dihydropyridine and short-acting calcium channel blockers should be avoided as first-line agents for the management of hypertension. Non-dihydropyridine drugs can induce heart block and should be avoided in patients with conduction defects.

Angiotensin-converting enzyme inhibitors

Angiotensin-converting enzyme (ACE) inhibitors can also be used as monotherapy for the management of hypertension. Clinicians may prefer this class of medication in the elderly due to their end-organ protective features for patients with either cardiac or renal disease, such as congestive heart failure and diabetic nephropathy, respectively.[8] In addition, a protective effect is seen in patients with hypertensive nephrosclerosis. Side effects related to these drugs include: hyperkalemia, elevated creatinine (in those with renal artery stenosis), dry cough, angioedema, neutropenia, and agranulocytosis.

Angiotensin receptor blockers

Angiotensin receptor blockers can be considered first-line therapy for elevated blood pressures, particularly in patients with diabetic nephropathy and congestive heart failure. The side-effect profile is similar to ACE inhibitors, except for much decreased risk of cough. These medications may be considered for those who are not able to tolerate ACE inhibitors.

Other classes

Beta blockers are not a preferred first-line therapy for the management of uncomplicated hypertension. Beta blockers, as compared to placebo, provided no reduction in all-cause mortality and myocardial infarction. Risk reduction for stroke was much less in beta blockers as compared to other medications.[9] Adults with coronary artery disease, congestive heart failure, prior myocardial infarction, angin, or hypertrophic cardiomyopathy may benefit from these medications owing to effectiveness in secondary prevention of cardiac events, and they may be considered first-line therapy for patients with these issues. Alpha receptor antagonists should not be used as first-line therapy for the management of elevated blood pressure due to potential orthostatic hypotension and congestive heart failure exacerbation.

Summary

Evidence and expert opinion support treating hypertensive persons aged 60 years or older to a blood pressure goal of less than 150/90 mmHg.[4] When considering treatment options, both nonpharmacologic and pharmacologic treatments must be considered in the context of an individual treatment plan keeping in mind quality of life, comorbid conditions, and patient goals. The possible risks and benefits of antihypertensive medications should be discussed with the patient and/or caregivers. Several medications are available for treatment, and the "start low, go slow" adage should dictate management strategies.

References

1. US Census Bureau, Statistical Abstract of the United States: 2012. Table 169. Visits to Office-Based Physicians and Hospital Outpatient Departments by Diagnosis: 2003 and 2008. Health and Nutrition, page 117. Available at: www.census.gov/prod/2011pubs/12statab/health.pdf (accessed August 15, 2014).

2. Gillespie CD, Hurvitz KA, National Center for Chronic Disease Prevention and Health Promotion, National Center for Health Statistics. Prevalence of hypertension and controlled hypertension – United States, 2007–2010. CDC Health Disparities and Inequalities Report – United States, 2013. *MMWR* Supplement. 2013;62(3):144–8.

3. Vasan RS, Larson MG, Leip EP, et al. Impact of high-normal blood pressure on the risk of cardiovascular disease. *N Engl J Med.* 2001;345:1291–7.

4. James PA, Oparil S, Carter BL, et al. 2014 evidence-based guideline for the management of high blood pressure in adults: report from the panel members appointed to the eighth joint national committee (JNC 8). *JAMA.* 2014;311(5):507–20.

5. Perry HM Jr, Davis BR, Price TR, et al. Effect of treating isolated systolic hypertension on the risk of developing various types and subtypes of stroke: the systolic hypertension in the elderly program (SHEP). *JAMA.* 2000;824:465–71.

6. Beckett NS, Peters R, Fletcher AE, et al. Treatment of hypertension in patients 80 years of age or older. *N Engl J Med.* 2008;358:1887–98.

7. Laubscher T, Regier L, Stone S. Hypertension in the elderly: new blood pressure targets and prescribing tips. *Canadian Family Physician.* 2014;60(5):453–6.

8. Sica D. Assessment of the role of ACE inhibitors in the elderly. In: Prisant LM, ed. *Hypertension in the Elderly.* Totowa, NJ: Humana Press, 2005: 321–48.

9. *JNC7 Express: The Seventh Report of the Joint National Committee on Prevention, Detection, Evaluation, and Treatment of High Blood Pressure.* Bethesda, MD: National High Blood Pressure Education Program, Department of Health and Human Services, 2003:3 (table 1).

Peripheral artery disease in the elderly

Belinda J. Parmenter, PhD, AEP, Christopher D. Askew, PhD, and
Jonathan Golledge, MChir, FRACS

Introduction

"Peripheral arterial disease" (PAD) is a term that encompasses atherosclerotic, aneurysmal and thromboembolic diseases of the peripheral arteries. As the term generally refers to a range of arterial disorders, for the purpose of this chapter, the authors have chosen to focus on atherosclerotic diseases of the abdominal aorta, trunk, and lower extremity arteries. Lower extremity PAD is caused by atherosclerosis of the underlying arteries (excluding coronary and cerebral), resulting in a narrowing or complete occlusion of these vessels and consequent reduction in blood flow to the extremities. In most people PAD is asymptomatic, and thus commonly remains undetected; however, others may experience pain with activity (known as intermittent claudication), thereby limiting walking ability and physical activity levels. Therefore, the clinical sequelae of symptomatic disease can be devastating. PAD is associated with reduced cardiorespiratory fitness, sarcopenia,[1, 2] impaired lower extremity functioning,[2, 4] and reduced quality of life (QOL),[5] as well as increased risk of morbidity and mortality.[6] In addition to the morbidity directly associated with PAD, persons with PAD have an increased risk of coexisting coronary and cerebrovascular disease due to reduced activity levels. In fact, a diagnosis of PAD is critical evidence of more widespread cardiovascular disease (CVD) with substantially increased risk of subsequent CVD events and mortality.[6]

Being an atherosclerotic disease, PAD shares similar risk factors to cerebrovascular and coronary artery disease. Traditional risk factors include increasing age, cigarette smoking,[7, 8] hypertension,[9] dyslipidaemia,[9] diabetes,[9] and physical inactivity,[10] with emerging risk factors including elevated homocysteine, lipoprotein A, fibrinogen, and c-reactive protein levels.[11] Cigarette smoking, however, is still one of the strongest contributing risk factors with some epidemiological studies reporting that smoking increases the risk of developing PAD up to six times.[12] Recent research has shown that both men and women with PAD have greater long-term risks of cardiovascular and all-cause mortality when compared to those with a history of myocardial infarction alone, with recommendations that PAD should be considered a coronary artery disease equivalent.[13] However, even though the incidence and prevalence of PAD is rising, it largely remains underdiagnosed and undertreated.[14] With its presence being linked to a number of other significant health conditions and due to the asymptomatic nature of the disease, recent recommendations have been made of screening for and early detection of PAD in adults with the use of the ankle brachial pressure index (ABI).[15] The ABI is a PAD specific diagnostic tool that compares ankle pressures to brachial pressures and is explained in more detail later in this chapter. It has been recently recommended to be used as a screening tool in patients at increased risk of the disease, which includes all adults over the age of 65 years.[16] For prevention of disease progression, early identification is vital and may in fact improve the health, quality of life, morbidity, and mortality of elderly populations.

Epidemiology

Atherosclerotic PAD affects up to 8.5 million (one in sixteen, or 7.2%) Americans aged ≥ 40 years.[17] Prevalence increases exponentially across age groups,[17] with approximately 12%–20% of individuals older than 60 years having PAD.[18] PAD is associated with significant morbidity and mortality, with prevalence higher in older individuals and black

---

Reichel's Care of the Elderly, 7th Edition, ed. Jan Busby-Whitehead *et al.* Published by Cambridge University Press.
© Cambridge University Press 2016.

race/ethnicity.[17] Historically, PAD has been known to affect men, more so than women. However, while most studies suggest that the prevalence of PAD is now similar in men and women,[19, 20] a recent epidemiological study reported a higher prevalence of PAD among women.[20] Non-Hispanic whites contributed the most individuals to the total prevalence, however, among older ages, the prevalence rate for African Americans was two to three times higher.[17] This same study concluded that people of Hispanic origin may have similar to slightly higher rates of PAD compared to non-Hispanic whites.[17]

Among the general population, approximately 10% of people with PAD have the classic symptom of intermittent claudication. Approximately 40% are asymptomatic, and the remaining 50% experience a variety of leg symptoms different from the classic intermittent claudication.[4, 21] Data from NHANES 1999–2002 suggests that up to one-quarter of adults have severe PAD (ABI ≤ 0.7).[22] Data from a 2006 systematic review found that PAD (defined by ABI ≤ 0.9) is a marker for systemic atherosclerosis,[23] further supporting the notion that a diagnosis of PAD is critical evidence of more widespread cardiovascular disease (CVD) with substantially increased risk of subsequent CVD events and mortality.[6] A further meta-analysis conducted in 2008 on up to 49,000 people reported an association between ABI and mortality where persons with an ABI of between 1.11 and 1.40 are at lowest risk of mortality. A low ABI of ≤ 0.9 carried a threefold risk of all-cause death compared to persons with a normal ABI of between 1.11 and 1.40.[24]

In addition, further studies identified that a decline in ABI of >0.15 within a 10-year period was associated with a subsequent 2.4-fold increased risk in all-cause mortality and 2.8-fold increased risk of CVD mortality.[25]

Lower limb atherosclerosis usually manifests at different levels, however, may also be restricted to a particular region. Typically it is classified as either "proximal" or "distal." Proximal usually refers to the aortoiliac arteries,[26] with distal involving only the femoropopliteal and/or tibial vessels.[27] One further classification known as multilevel disease includes atherosclerotic lesions of both proximal and distal arteries.[27] One study found that among 440 patients with PAD, male sex and smoking were associated more with proximal rather than distal disease and proximal disease was associated with a threefold increased risk of mortality.[28]

Pathophysiology

PAD is characterized by stenosis or occlusion of the lower limb arteries, leading to a reduction in blood flow capacity. Although arterial obstruction may occasionally result from conditions such as fibromuscular dysplasia, Buerger's disease, or arteritis, PAD is most commonly a manifestation of atherosclerosis – the same underlying disease process that is responsible for coronary and cerebrovascular disease. Atherosclerosis is initiated by injury or irritation of the vessel walls, which results in a chronic, systemic inflammatory process leading to the development of arterial wall lesions, the accumulation of lipid deposits and the gradual formation of fibrous atherosclerotic plaques.[29] These plaques protrude into the lumen of the vessel causing a chronic impairment in blood flow capacity. Furthermore, unstable plaques may ulcerate and cause thrombotic occlusion or embolization.[30] Arterial lesions most commonly develop in regions of low shear stress and turbulent flow, including the proximal regions of the aorto-iliac and femoro-popliteal segments, and there is some evidence that distal lesions are more common in older patients.[31] Atherosclerosis and the presence of PAD is associated with vascular endothelial dysfunction and a limited capacity for arterial vasodilation, which may further exacerbate the blood flow impairment to the lower limbs and contribute to the elevated cardiovascular risk of PAD patients.[32]

Risk factors

PAD has a risk factor profile similar to those associated with coronary artery disease. Traditional risk factors include age, diabetes, smoking, hypertension, and hyperlipidemia.[19] Past studies have shown chronic kidney disease,[33] hyperhomocystinemia, [34] elevated fibrinogen concentration,[35] and certain ethnic backgrounds [17] as also contributing to the development of PAD. A more recent study has highlighted more nontraditional biomarkers of elevated risk including soluble intercellular adhesion molecule-1, high sensitivity C-reactive protein, high-density lipoprotein cholesterol (HDL-C) and the ratio of total cholesterol to HDL-C being significantly associated with incident symptomatic PAD in women. [11] Cigarette smoking, both tobacco and marijuana, is the most modifiable risk factor for the development of PAD, whereas age is the most significant nonmodifiable risk factor, with prevalence increasing exponentially across the age groups reaching approximately 20% of persons older than 60 years.[18] Many studies have shown that the distribution, extent and progression of PAD are influenced by CVD risk factors but the findings are inconsistent among certain risk factors.[31] However, most studies tend to suggest that smoking related PAD predominantly affects the proximal arteries, with diabetes predominantly affecting the distal arteries.[31] A recent "call to action" from the AHA association highlighted the increasing prevalence of PAD among women, with data from the 2010 US census showing that there were more women than men with PAD among US adults ≥40 years of age.[36]

Clinical presentation

PAD is associated with a wide range of symptoms and presentations. Symptoms will depend on the size and location of the affected artery (Table 14.1). PAD is typically asymptomatic in its early stages; however, as the disease develops the most commonly recognized/reported symptom is intermittent claudication, meaning "to limp," which has historically been described as a cramplike pain in the muscles of the calf. This pain is "intermittent" in nature in that it reproducibly appears with exertion (e.g., during walking), dissipates quickly with rest, and does not dissipate if exertion continues.[37] It is now recognized that exertional symptoms may be more varied and include tingling, numbness, burning, throbbing or shooting-pain; and symptoms may present in other regions of the limb such as the buttocks, thighs, and feet.[38]

Table 14.1 Location of lesion and corresponding location of intermittent claudication

Location of lesion	Frequency of involvement	Common location of symptoms
Aortoiliac arteries	25%–30%	Hips and buttocks, thigh, calf
Superficial femoral artery, deep femoral artery, popliteal artery	80%–90%	Thigh, calf
Tibial artery, peroneal artery	40%–50%	Calf, shin, ankle/foot

With proximal aortoiliac disease, thigh, hip, or buttock claudication may develop with activity and will usually precede calf pain. More distal disease may cause calf, ankle or foot pain while walking. Intermittent claudication tends to be more frequently reported in those with distal lesions.[28] Buttock and thigh pain seem to be more commonly present with proximal lesions, whereas calf pain is more common with distal lesions; however, patients may still report pain at a variety of levels throughout their legs, regardless of the location of the lesion.[28] Many older patients with PAD may present as being asymptomatic because their lower physical activity levels are below the threshold that induces symptoms.[39]

More severe disease with greater hemodynamic impairment is associated with critical limb ischemia (CLI), which manifests as rest pain, or tissue loss through ulceration or gangrene (tissue necrosis). Rest pain commonly affects the feet or toes, usually when the patient is lying down, and patients may find relief by placing the limb in a dependent position. The term "CLI" is used to describe chronic symptoms that have been present for more than two weeks,[19] which distinguishes it from acute limb ischemia where there is a sudden reduction in limb perfusion. The symptoms of PAD, from asymptomatic through to major tissue loss as a result of gangrene, may be classified according to Fontaine or Rutherford categorization systems.[19]

Screening, diagnosis, and investigation

A number of methods are available to investigate PAD and determining which methods are most appropriate depends on a number of factors including the setting the test is being applied in (screening, diagnosis or investigation), the intention of the investigating physician (medical or interventional management) and the comorbidities of the patients (e.g., renal impairment increases the risk of contrast requiring imaging).[40–42] In elderly subjects comorbidities are common, which may impact in a number of ways. Firstly, the concurrent presence of respiratory, cardiac, joint, or other musculoskeletal problems, common in elderly patients, may complicate the diagnosis since patients may not be able to ambulate adequately to appreciate classical symptoms of PAD. Secondly, patients may be unable to complete or are at increased risk with some investigations, such as

Table 14.2 Classification of Ankle Brachial Index according to American Heart Association guidelines

Ankle Brachial Index	Classification
>1.40	Noncompressible arteries
1.00–1.40	Normal range
0.91–0.99	Borderline PAD
0.71–0.90	Mild PAD
0.41–0.70	Moderate PAD
<0.41	Severe PAD

treadmill tests or imaging tests requiring contrast. Thirdly, the interpretation of investigations maybe more complex, for example peripheral artery calcification may obscure imaging or provide falsely elevated ankle pressures. The following section describes the more commonly employed investigations in clinical practice although others such as questionnaires (e.g., the Edinburgh Claudication Questionnaire) were previously used in diagnosis or screening but are now thought to be too inaccurate due to the realization that many patients with PAD are asymptomatic or have atypical symptoms.[43]

The main objective diagnostic criteria used for PAD is based on the measurement of ankle brachial pressure index (ABI),[40–43] with cut-offs and classifications presented in Table 14.2. ABI assessment involves insonating the Doppler signals in the dorsalis pedis and posterior tibial arteries in both feet and assessing the calf cuff pressure required to obliterate these signals. The higher of the two pedal pressures in each foot is divided by the similarly measured highest brachial pressure and reported as the ABI separately for each foot.

Updates to the diagnosis criteria used is a resting ABI between 1.00 to 1.40 as normal range;[40–43] with abnormal values defined as those ≤0.90. ABI values of 0.91 to 0.99 are considered "borderline" and values ≥1.40 indicate non compressible arteries. [10,16] Some patients with PAD may have resting ABI of 0.9 or greater either because the lower limb atherothrombosis is not hemodynamically significant or because it only becomes relevant during exercise. In the later instance assessment of ABI after a treadmill test may identify an appreciable (≈15%) fall in ankle pressure. ABI readings can be falsely elevated, typically >1.4 or incompressible, in patients with very

calcified tibial arteries, sometimes found in subjects with renal failure or diabetes which are common comorbidities in the elderly. ABI readings have values beyond simple diagnosis of PAD since they provide a guide to the severity of the lower limb ischemia and also are independently associated with mortality and cardiovascular events in PAD patients.[44, 45] ABI should be routinely measured in patients suspected of having PAD; however, there is acknowledged reluctance by physicians in assessing ABI, mainly due to time and equipment limitations.[46] Physicians typically prefer to order anatomical imaging tests such as lower limb arterial duplex imaging, computed tomographic angiography (CTA) or magnetic resonance angiography (MRA) which are readily available from radiology providers in most Western countries, although these investigators are best reserved for patients being considered for interventions in whom the information provided is useful for planning the management. Duplex imaging utilizes B mode ultrasound and Doppler to provide anatomical and hemodynamic information. Typically the peak systolic velocity of the Doppler wave form is elevated at the site of a stenosis, with a twofold elevation being commonly used to define a 50% stenosis and a three- or fourfold elevation being used to define a 75% stenosis. [40, 42] The advantages of duplex imaging include its noninvasive nature and absence of established complications, however, detailed and accurate imaging requires a highly trained and experienced sonographer which are not available at every facility. Both CTA and MRA provide detailed mapping of the lower limb arteries with sufficient detail to plan interventional management.[47] CTA does involve ionising radiation and the injection of intravenous contrast with the associated rare but serious risks, such as renal failure (primarily in patients with pre-existing renal impairment), contrast allergy and lactic acidosis (a rare metabolic complication to contrast which may be seen in patients receiving metformin). CTA is also less accurate in patients with marked vascular calcification. MRA is frequently less available than CTA due to the longer time needed to acquire images, the lower number of MR machines established in many cities and the more complex processing needed to reconstruct images. Both CTA and MRA can provide similar accuracy to diagnostic conventional angiography, although typically they are less accurate at assessing tibial arteries than selective angiography.[47] Formal digital subtraction angiography (DSA) typically involves percutaneous placement of a femoral or brachial sheath and selective catheterization of lower limb arteries to provide detailed and high quality assessment of the lumen of the lower limb arteries. It is now unusual to undertake formal angiography for diagnostic purposes alone in patients with PAD, despite the fact that this imaging is still considered the gold standard, owing to its interventional nature and associated but rare risks of serious bleeding, atherothrombotic embolization, renal impairment, and contrast allergy. DSA is usually undertaken as part of directing and quality assessing therapeutic revascularization by angioplasty, stenting, or atherectomy. DSA also does not provide any information about the arterial wall, unlike CTA or MRA, which can limit its ability to identify and assess pathologies such as aneurysms.

Differential diagnosis

Important differential diagnoses to consider in patients presenting with symptoms of intermittent claudication include cauda equina syndrome or spinal claudication, nerve root pathologies such as degenerative lumbo-sacral disc disease, peripheral neuropathy and venous claudication. In patients with classical symptoms and signs, differentiating these diagnoses can be straightforward. Patients with spinal claudication, for example, typically find their symptoms of leg pain are improved on walking up hill whereas those with PAD typically have worse symptoms in this situation. Patients with obstructive venous disease and peripheral neuropathy would typically have signs of leg swelling and sensory loss, respectively. In many elderly patients a number of pathologies coexist. Patients with PAD commonly also have lumbo-sacral disc degeneration, for example. Approximately 30% of patients with PAD have atypical symptoms that can also contribute to difficulty in differentiating diagnoses.[43]

Management

Optimal treatment for the management of PAD is outlined in Table 14.3.

Smoking cessation

The recently updated American Heart Association (AHA) guidelines recommend the following regarding smoking cessation:[10, 16]

Table 14.3 Optimal medical management of PAD

1. Smoking cessation
2. Treatment of hypercholesterolemia (statin)
3. Treatment of hypertension (beta blocker or angiotensin-converting enzyme inhibitors)
4. Treatment of diabetes mellitus (foot care and blood glucose control)
5. Use of antiplatelet drugs (clopidogrel or aspirin)
6. Treatment of symptoms of claudication with use of vasodilator (pentoxyfilline or cilostazol)
7. Exercise rehabilitation

1. Patients who are smokers or former smokers should be asked about status of tobacco use at every visit.
2. Patients should be assisted with counseling and developing a plan for quitting that may include pharmacotherapy and/or referral to a smoking cessation program.
3. Individuals with lower extremity PAD who smoke cigarettes or use other forms of tobacco should be advised by each of their clinicians to stop smoking and offered behavioral and pharmacological treatment.
4. In the absence of contraindication or other compelling clinical indication, one or more of the following pharmacological therapies should be offered: varenicline, bupropion, and nicotine replacement therapy.

Hypercholesterolemia management

The American Heart Association (AHA) guidelines recommend the following for cardiovascular risk factor reduction in the form of lipid lowering drugs for persons with PAD:[45]

1. Treatment with a statin medication is indicated for all patients with PAD to achieve a target LDL cholesterol level of less than 100 mg/dL or 2.6 mmol/L.
2. Treatment with a statin medication is indicated for patients with PAD at high risk of cardiovascular events to achieve a target LDL cholesterol level of less than 70 mg/dL or 1.8 mmol/L.

Furthermore, Gardner et al. recommend that statins should be prescribed to all patients with PAD irrespective of the presence of coronary artery disease, with several studies reporting improvements in walking ability, ABI and symptoms of claudication after treatment with a statin.[48]

Hypertension management

The American Heart Association (AHA) guidelines recommend the following for cardiovascular risk factor reduction in the form of antihypertensive drugs for persons with PAD:[45]

1. Antihypertensive therapy should be administered to hypertensive patients with lower extremity PAD to achieve a goal of less than 140 mmHg systolic over 90 mmHg diastolic in nondiabetics.
2. In persons with diabetes and/or chronic renal disease therapy should aim to reduce blood pressure to less than 130 mmHg systolic over 80 mmHg diastolic to reduce the risk of myocardial infarction, stroke, congestive heart failure, and cardiovascular death.
3. Beta adrenergic antagonist drugs are effective antihypertensive agents and are not contraindicated in patients with PAD.
4. Level B evidence supports the use of angiotensin-converting enzyme inhibitors for symptomatic patients with lower extremity PAD to reduce the risk of adverse cardiovascular events.

Control of hypertension is critical to prevent adverse cardiovascular events; however, practitioners should be aware that although not common, antihypertensive therapy may decrease limb perfusion pressure potentially increasing symptoms of claudication and critical limb ischemia.

Diabetes management

Due to poor peripheral blood flow, persons with diabetes and lower extremity PAD are susceptible to increased risk of skin ulceration, necrosis, and subsequent amputation. Diabetes itself is a leading cause of nontraumatic lower extremity amputation (NLEA), and although rates of amputation are declining, NLEA continues to be substantially higher in the diabetic populations when compared to nondiabetics.[49] Therefore, to decrease the risk of NLEA in diabetics, the AHA guidelines recommend the following for management of diabetes in persons with PAD:[45]

1. Proper foot care, including use of appropriate footwear, podiatric medicine, daily foot inspection, skin cleansing and use of topical moisturizing creams should be encouraged and skin lesions and ulcerations should be addressed

urgently in all diabetic patients with lower extremity PAD.
2. Treatment of diabetes in individuals with lower extremity PAD should also include aiming to reduce hemoglobin A1c to at least less than 6.5% or 48 mmol/mol or 140 mg/dL. In fact, studies have shown that for every 1% reduction in HbA1c there is a corresponding 37% reduction in microvascular complication, with potentially improved cardiovascular outcomes, suggesting that ongoing reduction of HbA1c to normal values of less than 6% is optimal.[50]

Antiplatelet and antithrombotic drugs

The recently updated AHA guidelines recommend the following regarding the use of antiplatelet and antithrombotic drugs:[10, 16]

1. Antiplatelet therapy is indicated to reduce the risk of myocardial infarction, stroke, and vascular death in individuals with symptomatic atherosclerotic lower extremity PAD, including those with intermittent claudication or critical limb ischemia, prior lower extremity revascularization, or prior amputation for lower extremity ischemia.
2. Aspirin, typically ranging in doses of 75 mg–325 mg per day is recommended as safe and effective antiplatelet therapy to reduce the risk of stroke, myocardial infarction or vascular death in individuals with lower extremity PAD.
3. Clopidogrel, at a dose of 75 mg per day, is recommended as a safe and effective alternative antiplatelet therapy to aspirin to reduce the risk of stroke, myocardial infarction or vascular death in individuals with lower extremity PAD.

Vasodilators

Pharmacological therapy for the treatment of the symptom of intermittent claudication itself is limited and can be expensive. Studies have found that the use of pentoxyfilline or the cilostazol can significantly improve walking ability in persons with PAD, however exercise therapy has been shown to produce greater improvements in walking ability in persons who are able to complete exercise regimes.[48]

Exercise rehabilitation

Supervised exercise rehabilitation remains the gold standard medical treatment for PAD with multiple systematic reviews and meta-analyses showing that various modes of exercise improve walking ability, fitness and quality of life in persons with PAD.[3, 48, 51–53] Although the gold standard has traditionally been supervised intermittent walking therapy to moderate claudication pain, two recent reviews have shown that there is no clear evidence of differences between supervised walking exercise and alternative exercise modes in improving the maximum and pain-free walking distance of patients with intermittent claudication.[52, 53]

People with PAD have impaired function and quality of life.[3, 54] Furthermore, patients with PAD, including those who are asymptomatic, experience a significant decline in lower-extremity functioning over time.[1, 55–57] Among patients with established PAD, higher PA levels during daily life are associated with better overall survival rate, a lower risk of death because of CVD, and slower rates of functional decline.[58, 59] In addition, better six-minute walk performance and faster walking speed are associated with lower rates of all-cause mortality, cardiovascular mortality, and mobility loss,[9, 25, 58, 60] with exercise or peak aerobic capacity being the strongest predictor of mortality in patients with PAD.[60] Consequently, patients with intermittent claudication experience difficulty in performing activities of daily living and are at increased risk of becoming more sedentary and becoming dependent on other people. This increased sedentariness and reduced physical activity leads to increased cardiovascular risk and worsening of comorbid conditions such as hypertension, obesity, hypercholesterolemia, and diabetes. Each of these risk factors and conditions can all be treated with a specific exercise program.

Current AHA recommendations for exercise and lower extremity PAD rehabilitation include:[45]

1. A program of supervised exercise training as an initial treatment modality for patients with intermittent claudication (level of evidence: A).

2. Supervised exercise training should be performed for a minimum of 30–45 minutes, in sessions performed at least three times per week for a minimum of 12 weeks, with optimal improvements occurring at 24 weeks (level of evidence A).

3. Types of exercise that have been shown in randomized controlled trials (RCTs) to improve walking ability in persons with PAD include supervised intermittent walking, pole striding, and lower extremity aerobic exercise (level of evidence A). Arm cranking and progressive resistance training have also been shown in RCTs to be promising; however, fewer trials have been published on these modes (level of evidence B).[3, 52] Treadmill and track walking seems to be the most effective exercise mode for claudication; however, if patients are unable to tolerate walking due to comorbidities precluding them from participating, other modes may also be beneficial (level of evidence A).[3, 52, 53]

4. Direct supervision is recommended for patients undertaking an exercise program because as patients improve their walking ability, the exercise workload should be increased to ensure there is always the stimulus of claudication pain during the workout. In addition, with an increase in walking tolerance there is a possibility that cardiac signs and symptoms may appear. If these events do occur, a thorough medical re-evaluation should be completed.

The aim of an exercise program should therefore be to improve walking ability, exercise/aerobic capacity (cardiorespiratory fitness), lower extremity function, and general daily physical activity levels, with the overall aim of reducing the risk of cardiovascular events.

Recommendations for CLI endovascular and open surgical treatment for limb salvage

Patients with lifestyle limiting intermittent claudication resultant in rest pain can be considered for revascularization therapy, which includes endovascular or surgical therapy. The AHA guidelines recommend the following for persons with critical limb ischemia, including endovascular and open surgical treatment for limb salvage:[16, 45]

1. For individuals with combined inflow (aortoiliac) and outflow (typically superficial femoral) disease with critical limb ischemia, inflow lesions should be addressed first.

2. For individuals with combined inflow and outflow disease in whom symptoms of critical limb ischemia or infection persist after inflow revascularization, an outflow revascularization procedure should be performed.

3. If it is unclear whether hemodynamically significant inflow disease exists, intra-arterial

pressure measurements across suprainguinal lesions should be measured before and after the administration of a vasodilator.

4. For patients with limb-threatening lower extremity ischemia and an estimated life expectancy of two years or less or in patients in whom an autogenous vein conduit is not available, balloon angioplasty is reasonable to perform when possible as the initial procedure to improve distal blood flow.

5. For patients with limb-threatening ischemia and an estimated life expectancy of more than two years and when an autogenous vein conduit is available, bypass surgery is reasonable to perform as the initial treatment to improve distal blood flow.

Choosing between endovascular versus open surgery depends on a number of factors including a patient's age, comorbidities, and type of lesion. Surgery is normally reserved for those patients with whom the cardiovascular risk of surgery is low.[48]

Complications

Being an atherosclerotic disease, patients with PAD generally have coexisting coronary artery disease, cerebrovascular disease, or renal disease. Even in patients with asymptomatic PAD, the risk of coexisting coronary or cerebrovascular disease is elevated; therefore, patients may present with a history of myocardial infarction, angina, atrial fibrillation, transient ischemic attack, or stroke. Individuals with PAD have severely reduced physical fitness and functional capacities.[3] The maximal walking capacity of PAD patients is less than half that observed in healthy older adults,[61] and their cardiorespiratory fitness, measured as maximal oxygen consumption during exercise, is similar to that observed in patients with class III heart failure.[62] Patients may avoid physical activity because of the pain associated with activity and their poor exercise tolerance, and this physical inactivity exacerbates their limited functional capacity, increases their cardiovascular risk and is associated with elevated mortality.[58, 63, 64]

As patients with PAD are at high risk of other CVD, improvements in their walking ability may unmask signs and symptoms (e.g., angina, unusual shortness of breath, adverse blood pressure responses, ST-segment depression, other arrhythmias) of cardiac ischemia.[4] Care should be taken to establish and monitor closely those at risk of a cardiovascular event, especially as walking ability improves. If signs and symptoms appear, prompt re-evaluation from the patient's medical practitioners should occur. Peripheral neuropathy affects some patients with PAD, particularly those with concomitant diabetes, and this may in turn lead to poor balance and increase the risk of lower limb wounds or lesions. Patients with PAD have poor wound healing on the lower limb, and some patients may be prescribed antiplatelet agents (e.g., aspirin) or antiocoagulants (e.g., warfarin), which may further increase the risk of bleeding. Appropriate and proper fitting footwear should be worn by patients during exercise, and care should be taken with balance and transfers from exercise equipment.[1] Patients with PAD and systemic atherosclerosis have an elevated risk of abdominal aortic aneurysm (AAA), which is characterized by dilatation of the aorta beyond its normal size.[65] There is evidence that enhanced cardiorespiratory fitness improves surgical outcomes for patients who require AAA repair;[54] therefore, such exercise and physical activity should not be avoided by these patients.[4] However, further research is needed to help identify safe and effective exercise prescription guidelines for this cohort.

Many patients with PAD will have an array of other comorbidities including musculoskeletal conditions, diabetes, hypertension, and obesity that will affect their exercise tolerance and ability to complete an exercise program.[58, 59] Some patients may also have contra-indications to exercise such as unstable coronary artery disease, neurological impairments or musculoskeletal limitations. These patients should be stabilized and, if warranted, evaluated by their general practitioner or medical specialist prior to commencing any form of exercise therapy.

References

1. McDermott M, Hoff F, Ferrucci L, et al. Lower extremity ischemia, calf skeletal muscle characteristics, and functional impairment in peripheral arterial disease. *J Am Ger Soc.* 2007;**55**(3):400–406.

2. Parmenter B, Baker M, Barry B, et al. Muscle strength is impaired in peripheral arterial disease and predicts over ground walking ability. Submitted to *J Gerontol.* 30 Jun 2014.

3. Parmenter BJ, Raymond J, Fiatarone Singh M. The effect of exercise on fitness and functional outcomes in intermittent claudication: a systematic review of randomized controlled trials. *Sports Med.* 2013;**43**(6):513–552.

4. McDermott M, Greenland P, Liu K, et al. Leg symptoms in peripheral arterial disease. Associated clinical

characteristics and functional impairment. *JAMA*. 2001;**286**(13):1599.

5. Long J, Modrall J, Parker B, Swann A, Welborn III M, Anthony T. Correlation between ankle-brachial index, symptoms, and health-related quality of life in patients with peripheral vascular disease. *J Vasc Surg*. 2004;**39**:723–727.

6. Caro J, Migliaccio-Walle K, Ishak K, Proskorovsky I. The morbidity and mortality following a diagnosis of peripheral arterial disease: long-term follow-up of a large database. *BMC Cardiovascular Disorders*. 2005;**5**(14):1–8.

7. Criqui M, Deneberg J, Langer R, Fronek A. The epidemiology of peripheral arterial disease: importance of identifying the population at risk. *Vasc Med*. 1997;**2**(3):221–226.

8. Kannel W, Shurtleff D. The Framingham Study: cigarettes and the development of intermittent claudication. *Geriatrics*. 1973;**28**(2):61–68.

9. Smith G, Shipley M, Rose G. Intermittent claudication, heart disease risk factors, and mortality: the Whitehall Study. *Circulation*. 1990;**82**(6):1925–1931.

10. Anderson J, Halperin J, Albert N, et al. Management of patients with peripheral artery disease ACC/AHA 2005 and 2011 guidelines. *Circulation*. 2013;**127**. doi: 10.1161/CIR.1160b1013e31828b31882aa.

11. Pradhan A, Shrivastava S, Cook N, Rifai N, Creager M, Ridker P. Symptomatic peripheral arterial disease in women: nontraditional biomarkers of elevated risk. *Circulation*. 2008;**117**:823–831.

12. Fowkes F, Housley E, Riemersma R, et al. Smoking, lipids, glucose intolerance, and blood pressure as risk factors for peripheral atherosclerosis compared with ischemic heart disease in the Edinburgh Artery Study. *Am J Epidemiol*. 1992;**135**:331–340.

13. Subherwal S, Patel M, Kober L, et al. Peripheral artery disease is a coronary heart disease risk equivalent among both men and women: results from a nationwide study. *Eur J Prev Cardiol*. 2014;**22**(3). doi: 10.1177/2047487313519344.

14. McDermott M, Mehta S, Ahn H, Greenland P. Atherosclerotic risk factors are less intensively treated in patients with peripheral arterial disease than in patients with coronary artery disease. *J Gen Intern Med*. 1997;**12**(4):209–215.

15. Criqui M, Langer R, Fronek A, et al. Mortality over a period of 10 years in patients with peripheral arterial disease. *N Engl J Med*. 1992;**326**:381–386.

16. Rooke T, Hirsch A, Misra S, et al. ACCF/AHA focused update of the Guideline for the Management of Patients with Peripheral Artery Disease (updating the 2005 guideline). *J Am Coll Cardiol*. 2011;**58**(19):2020–2045.

17. Allison M, Ho E, Denenberg J, et al. Ethnic-specific prevalence of peripheral arterial disease in the United States. *Am J Prev Med*. 2007;**32**:328–333.

18. Go A, Mozaffarian D, Roger V, et al. Heart Disease and Stroke Statistics 2013 Update: a report from the American Heart Association. *Circulation*. 2013;**127**(2): e6–e245.

19. Norgren L, Hiatt WR, Dormandy JA, Nehler MR, Harris KA, Fowkes FGR. Inter-society consensus for the management of peripheral arterial disease. *J Vasc Surg*. 2007;**45**(1):S5–S67.

20. Eraso L, Fukaya E, Mohler E, Xie D, Sha D, Berger J. Peripheral arterial disease, prevalence and cumulative risk factor profile analysis. *Eur J Prev Cardiol*. 2014;**21**:704–711.

21. Hirsch AT, Criqui MH, Treat-Jacobson D. Peripheral arterial disease detection, awareness, and treatment in primary care. *JAMA*. 2001;**286**(11):1317–1324.

22. Centers for Disease Control and Prevention (CDC). Lower extremity disease among persons aged > or =40 years with and without diabetes: United States, 1999–2002. *MMWR*. 2005;**54**:1158–1160.

23. Heald C, Fowkes F, Murray G, Price J, Ankle Brachial Index Collaboration. Risk of mortality and cardiovascular disease associated with the ankle-brachial index: systematic review. *Atherosclerosis*. 2006;**189**:61–69.

24. Ankle Brachial Index Collaboration, Fowkes FG, Murray GD, et al. Ankle brachial index combined with Framingham Risk Score to predict cardiovascular events and mortality: a meta-analysis. *JAMA*. 2008;**300**(2):197–208.

25. Criqui M, Ninomiya J, Fronek A. Progression of peripheral arterial disease predicts cardiovascular disease morbidity and mortality. *J Am Coll Cardiol*. 2008;**52**(21):1736–1742.

26. Garcia L. Epidemiology and pathophysiology of lower extremity peripheral arterial disease. *J Endovasc Surg*. 2006;**13**(S2):113–119.

27. Kroger K, Buss C, Renzing-Kohler K, Santosa F, Rudofsky G. Segmental manifestation of peripheral atherosclerosis and its association to risk factors. *VASA*. 2000;**29**(3):199–203.

28. Van Zitteren M, Vriens P, Heyligers J, et al. Self-reported symptoms on questionnaires and anatomic lesions on duplex ultrasound examinations in patients with peripheral arterial disease. *J Vasc Surg*. 2012;**55**:1025–1034.

29. Gutstein D, Fuster V. Pathophysiology and clinical significance of atherosclerotic plaque rupture. *Cardiovasc Res*. 1999;**41**:323–333.

30. Okura H, Asawa K, Kubo T, et al. Incidence and predictors of plaque rupture in the peripheral arteries. *Circ Cardiovasc Interv*. 2010;**3**:63–70.

31. Chen Q, Shi Y, Wang Y, Li X. Patterns of disease distribution of lower extremity peripheral arterial disease. *Angiology*. 2015 Mar 19;**66**(3):211–218.

32. Brevetti G, Schiano V, Chiariello M. Endothelial dysfunction: a key to the pathophysiology and natural history of peripheral arterial disease? *Atherosclerosis.* 2008;**197**:1–11.

33. O'hare A. Management of peripheral arterial disease in chronic kidney disease. *Cardiol Clin.* 2005;**23**(3):225–236.

34. Graham I, Daly L, Refsum H, et al. Plasma homocysteine as a risk factor for vascular disease: the European Concerted Action Project. *JAMA.* 1997;**277**(22):1775–1781.

35. McDermott M, Greenland P, Guralnik J, et al. Inflammatory markers, D-dimer, pro-thrombotic factors, and physical activity levels in patients with peripheral arterial disease. *Vascular Medicine.* 2004;**9**(2):107–115.

36. Hirsch A, Allison M, Gomes A, et al. A call to action: women and peripheral artery disease: a scientific statement from the American Heart Association. *Circulation.* 2012;**125**:1449–1472.

37. Rose G. The diagnosis of ischaemic heart pain and intermittent claudication in field surveys. *Bulletin of the World Health Organisation.* 1962;**27**:645–658.

38. Schorr E, Treat-Jacobson D. Methods of symptom evaluation and their impact on peripheral artery disease (PAD) symptom prevalence: a review. *Vasc Med.* 2013;**18**:95–111.

39. McDermott M, Mehta S, Greenland P. Exertional leg symptoms other than intermittent claudication are common in peripheral arterial disease. *Arch Intern Med.* 1999;**159**:387–392.

40. Au T, Golledge J, Walker P, Haigh K, Nelson M. Peripheral arterial disease – diagnosis and management in general practice. *Aust Fam Physician.* 2013;**42**(6):397–400.

41. Haigh K, Bingley J, Golledge J, Walker P. Peripheral arterial disease – screening in general practice. *Aust Fam Physician.* 2013;**42**(6):391–395.

42. Golledge J. Lower-limb arterial disease. *Lancet.* 1997;**350**(9089):1459–1465.

43. McDermott M, Applegate W, Bonds D, et al. Ankle brachial index values, leg symptoms, and functional performance among community-dwelling older men and women in the lifestyle interventions and independence for elders study. *J Am Heart Assoc.* 2013;**2**(6):e0000257.

44. Fowkes F, Murray G, Butcher I, et al. Development and validation of an ankle brachial index risk model for the prediction of cardiovascular events. *Eur J Prev Cardiol.* 2014;**21**(3):310–320.

45. Hirsch A, Haskal Z, Hertzer N, et al. ACC/AHA 2005 guidelines for the management of patients with peripheral arterial disease (lower extremity, renal, mesenteric, and abdominal aortic): executive summary a collaborative report. *J Am Coll Cardiol.* 2006;**47**(6):1239–1312.

46. Haigh K, Bingley J, Golledge J, Walker P. Barriers to screening and diagnosis of peripheral artery disease by general practitioners. *Vasc Med.* 2013;**18**(6):325–330.

47. Jens S, Koelemay M, Reekers J, Bipat S. Diagnostic performance of computed tomography angiography and contrast-enhanced magnetic resonance angiography in patients with critical limb ischaemia and intermittent claudication: systematic review and meta-analysis. *Eur Radiol.* 2013;**23**(11):3104–3114.

48. Gardner A, Afaq A. Management of lower extremity peripheral arterial disease. *J Cardiopulm Rehabil Prev.* 2008;**28**(6):349–357.

49. Li Y, Burrows N, Gregg E, Albright A, Geiss L. Declining rates of hospitalization for nontraumatic lower-extremity amputation in the diabetic population aged 40 years or older: US, 1988–2008. *Diabetes Care.* 2012;**35**(2):273–277.

50. Stratton I, AI A, Neil H, et al. Association of glycaemia with macrovascular and microvascular complications of type 2 diabetes (UKPDS 35): prospective observational study. *BMJ.* 2000;**321**(7258):405–412.

51. Askew CD, Parmenter BJ, Leight AS, Walker PJ, Golledge J. Exercise prescription for patients with peripheral arterial disease and intermittent claudication: a position statement from Exercise and Sports Science Australia. *Journal of Science and Medicine in Sport.* 2013; http://dx.doi.org/10.1016/j.jsams.2013.10.251.

52. Parmenter BJ, Raymond J, Dinnen PJ, Fiatarone Singh MA. A Systematic Review of randomized controlled trials: walking versus alternative exercise prescription as treatment for intermittent claudication. *Atherosclerosis* 2011;**218**(1):1–12.

53. Lauret G, Fakhry F, Fokkenrood H, Hunink M, Teijink J, Spronk S. Modes of exercise training for intermittent claudication. *Cochrane Database Syst Rev.* 2014;7; CD009638.

54. Parmenter B, Dieberg G, Smart N. A Meta Analysis of exercise training to improve health related quality of life in peripheral arterial disease. Accepted for publication in *Vascular Medicine* 18 Oct 2014.

55. McDermott M, Criqui M, Greenland P, et al. Leg strength in peripheral arterial disease: associations with disease severity and lower-extremity performance. *J Vasc Surg.* 2004;**39**(3):523–530.

56. McDermott M, Greenland P, Liu K, et al. The ankle brachial index is associated with leg function and physical activity: the Walking and Leg Circulation Study. *Ann Intern Med.* 2002;**136**(12):873–883.

57. McDermott M, Guralnik J, Albay M, Bandinelli S, Miniati B, Ferrucci L. Impairments of muscles and nerves associated with peripheral arterial disease and

their relationship with lower extremity functioning: the InCHIANTI Study. *J Am Ger Soc.* 2004;**52**(3):405–410.

58. Gardner A, Montgomery P, Parker D. Physical activity is a predictor of all-cause mortality in patients with intermittent claudication. *J Vasc Surg.* 2008;**47**(1):117–122.

59. Gardner AW, Katzel LI, Sorkin JD, et al. Exercise rehabilitation improves functional outcomes and peripheral circulation in patients with intermittent claudication: a randomized controlled trial. *J Americ Geriatrics Soc.* 2001;**49**(6):755–762.

60. Leeper N, Myers J, Zhou M, et al. Exercise capacity is the strongest predictor of mortality in patients with peripheral arterial disease. *J Vasc Surg.* 2013;**57**(3):728–733.

61. Askew C, Green S, Walker P, et al. Skeletal muscle phenotype is associated with exercise tolerance in patients with peripheral arterial disease. *J Vasc Surg.* 2005;**41**:802–807.

62. Hiatt W. Medical treatment of peripheral arterial disease and claudication. *N Engl J Med.* 2001;**344**:1608–1621.

63. Garg P, Liu K, Tian L, et al. Physical activity during daily life and functional decline in peripheral arterial disease. *Circulation.* 2009;**119**:251–260.

64. Garg P, Tian L, Criqui M, et al. Physical activity during daily life and mortality in patients with peripheral arterial disease. *Circulation.* 2006;**114**:242–248.

65. Kurvers H, van der Graaf Y, Blankensteijn J, Visseren F, Eikelboom B, SMART Study Group. Screening for asymptomatic internal carotid artery stenosis and aneurysm of the abdominal aorta: comparing the yield between patients with manifest atherosclerosis and patients with risk factors for atherosclerosis only. *J Vasc Surg.* 2003;**37**(6):1226–1233.

Chapter 15

Neurologic problems in the elderly

Steven Tam, MD

Introduction

Neurological problems are common reasons for clinician visits among elderly patients. With the expected rise in this portion of the population, it is important for the clinician caring for the elderly to become familiar with various neurological conditions. The symptoms of neurological conditions affect physical health, as well as the social and psychological well-being of the older adult. Management of neurological complaints in this population can be challenging, however, due to the myriad of overlapping conditions with similar presentations, presence of comorbid conditions, and complex pharmacology that may be present in this age group. Nevertheless, familiarity with presentations, diagnostic workup and treatment options for these conditions helps to ensure quick and accurate care for the older patient.

In this chapter, several common neurological complaints of older people, their impact, as well as their evaluation and available treatment options will be reviewed. Other conditions including gait and movement disorders, dizziness, delirium, dementia, and cerebrovascular disease in the elderly will be discussed extensively in other chapters.

Important considerations

When evaluating the older adult for neurological complaints, there are some considerations to take into account while performing the history and physical exam. The clinician taking a history should be aware that the older adult may have comorbid conditions which may impair the patient's ability to accurately recount the history. Gathering information from collateral sources may become necessary in conditions that cause further alterations in cognition such as with syncope or seizures. Additional information may be limited, however, if the family member or friend is not in contact with the patient on a regular basis. Further, when assessing a patient's functional ability to perform activities of daily living, family members may under- or overestimate the elderly patient's abilities when it comes to performance of various activities such as driving, managing finances, and participating in household activities.

With neurological complaints, additional detail should be paid to the impact the symptom has on quality of life and any resulting disability. Assessment should be done for declines in the patient's performance of basic and instrumental activities of daily living, such as toileting, bathing, cooking, and managing medications. Treatment and care plans should be developed for the underlying etiology as well as address the impact on daily function and quality of life.

On physical examination, changes on the neurological exam can be seen with "normal aging" and should be distinguished from disease-related causes. Common findings on cranial nerve assessment include changes in visual accommodation and vision distance, as well as diminished pupillary responses. Decrease in pupil size and upward gaze impairment are other "normal findings" while examining the eye. [1] Hearing may decrease slowly with age, but this is a concern in the older patient who recognizes a deficit acutely or if there are other symptoms such as vertigo or headache. Memory assessment will be discussed separately in the chapters discussing delirium and dementia, but normal cognitive changes typically involve decreases in processing speed and efficiency.

Abnormal gait and falls are frequent complaints of the elderly patient in multiple health-care settings. Although gait and movement disorders will be discussed elsewhere, there are some changes that occur as part of the normal aging process. Measurable changes include shortened stride, stooped posture, slower cadence, decreases in arm swing, and decreased clearance with each stride.[1]

Reichel's Care of the Elderly, 7th Edition, ed. Jan Busby-Whitehead *et al.* Published by Cambridge University Press.
© Cambridge University Press 2016.

Slight increases in motor tone as well as axial and limb rigidity may also be seen in normal older patients. Decreases in muscle mass can lead to decreased power and weakness. Other observations include decreased myelinated fiber length, neuronal atrophy, changes in neuronal signaling, reduction in motor cortex plasticity, and motor unit changes with morphological, physiological, and behavior changes.[1] The most common reflex lost in the elderly is a decrease in the ankle reflex. Although the exact cause is unknown, its believed to be related to degenerative changes, tightening of the Achilles, and decreases in sensory pathways.[2] Reflex changes can also involve the presence of "frontal release reflexes" in the form of grasp, snout, and suck reflexes that may occur in many elderly patients, but may also be signs of frontal cerebral lobe damage.

Changes in the peripheral sensory system also occur with advancing age. Diminished vibratory, pinprick, and touch sensation can occur in 33%–50% of individuals over the age of 75, but may not be detected in normal clinical settings.[1, 2] While the exact etiology of what causes these normal changes is unknown, likely contributing factors include reduced sensory fibers, decreased amplitude of sensory actions potentials, and changes in connective tissue and the dorsal root ganglia.

Muscle weakness

Muscle weakness is one of the most common complaints for the older patient and impacts social and physical activities of the elderly patient. Acute muscle weakness can be due to a broad range of causes, with some etiologies that can be life threatening and increase disability. Unfortunately, symptoms of weakness in elderly people may be vague on presentation, making it difficult to diagnose the etiology and provide the appropriate treatment.

Fatigue occurs when a patient is unable to complete a task involving the muscles after several repetitions. *Intrinsic* (primary) muscle weakness indicates the inability to do a task altogether. *Asthenia* occurs when the patient complains of weakness when there is no true muscle weakness. Additional terminology includes *plegia*, referring to paralysis, and *paresis*, indicating partial loss of voluntary movement in a limb.

Causes of neurological weakness

As previously noted, changes in muscle strength occur in the aging adult and can add challenge to making the diagnosis in the patient complaining of weakness.

Table 15.1 Upper vs. lower motor neuron patterns of weakness

	Findings	Examples
Upper motor neuron	Increased motor tone, reflexes, presence of Babinski sign	CNS lesion/mass or stroke, CNS injury such as a spinal cord transection. ALS
Lower motor neuron	Decreased motor tone, reflexes, absence of Babinski sign	Neuropathies, ALS neuromuscular junction disorders.

With aging, sarcopenia occurs in the form of decreased muscle mass and strength. Between the ages of 70 and 79, it has been estimated that muscle strength decreases at a rate of up to 3% per year.[3] The clinician should be aware of this combination of factors to account for normal muscle weakness in the older adult when evaluating complaints of weakness.

The list of causes of muscle weakness is extensive and includes neurological and non-neurological etiologies. Neurological causes of muscle weakness can fit patterns of upper motor neuron or lower motor neuron weakness, and sometimes both (Tables 15.1 and 15.2). Other neurological etiologies can be located in the neuromuscular junction.

Multiple sclerosis

Multiple sclerosis is an idiopathic inflammatory disease that causes demyelination and axonal degeneration in the central nervous system. Classically, multiple sclerosis is described as lesions separated by time and space. Depending on location of the presenting area of inflammation, muscle weakness may be associated with upper or lower motor neuron findings or both. Multiple sclerosis can have a wide array of presentations and can include other symptoms of neuropathies, neuralgias such as trigeminal neuralgia, diplopia, urinary problems, and gait disturbances. The course of the disease can vary in presentation and can range from a relapsing–remitting course to one that is progressive. A secondary form following a relapsing–remitting course of disease is typically more common than a primary progressive course from onset. Typically the disease has a lower incidence in the elderly as it more commonly affects the younger female adult. However, late onset multiple sclerosis can occur in the elderly more frequently in a primary progressive form.[4] Also, long-term disability from

Table 15.2 Neurological causes of weakness and presentation

Neurological causes	Location/etiology	Presentation of symptoms	Additional workup
Guillain-Barré syndrome	Autoimmune disease with antibodies directed at myelin and/or the Schwann cells	Flaccid paralysis	CSF studies
Multiple sclerosis	Demyelination and axonal degeneration, lesions separated in space and time	Variable depending on location of the lesion	Neuroimaging and CSF studies
Amyotrophic lateral sclerosis	Degeneration involving the upper and/or lower motor neurons or both.	Weakness in any body part, hyperreflexia, spasticity, atrophy, fasciculation; bulbar and ocular symptoms	EMG/NCV
Myasthenia gravis	Neuromuscular junction, antibody response at the acetylcholine receptor	Fatigable weakness of the skeletal muscles	Edrophonium (tensilon) test, acetylcholine receptor antibody (AChR-Ab), muscle specific tyrosine kinase antibody (MuSK-Ab), electrophysiology
Spinal cord pathology, radiculopathies	Spinal cord, nerve roots	Radicular symptoms (weakness, with pain and sensory deficits)	Imaging, electrophysiology studies
Cerebrovascular disease	Cortical, intraparenchymal; ischemic, hemorrhagic etiologies	Weakness, sensory loss, cortical dysfunction in the distribution of the affected area	Neuroimaging studies

the disease may persist into late life if the onset occurs early on; the disease carries a higher mortality rate as well.[5]

Treatment consists of glucocorticoid therapy and other immunosuppressive agents such as methotrexate in progressive disease, while other medications continue to be evaluated as therapeutic options. In multiple sclerosis presenting with a relapsing–remitting course, treatment typically involves interferon therapy or other disease modifying agents. Acute exacerbations are treated with glucocorticoid therapy.

Guillain-Barré syndrome

Guillain-Barré syndrome (GBS) is a polyneuropathy caused by an autoimmune response directed against the myelin or Schwann cells causing diffuse demyelination. The neuropathy can involve the motor, sensory, as well as autonomic systems. Weakness traditionally has been described as an ascending paralysis with acute onset over a period of four weeks. Annual incidence has varied from 0.4 to 4 cases/100,000 per year affecting every age group with increasing incidence with age.[6, 7] Although uncommon, the disease can be life threatening and cause significant disability. It is often preceded by a respiratory or gastrointestinal illness, with the most common microorganism being *Campylobacter jejuni* and cytomegalovirus. There have also been some concerns of the development of post-vaccination GBS, although the true risk of vaccine-associated GBS is uncertain. Caution should be taken with certain vaccines including influenza and tetanus diphtheria if there has been prior GBS.

Findings usually consist of a flaccid paralysis of the legs with areflexia ascending into the arms. Variations of the syndrome include the acute inflammatory demyelinating polyneuropathy, acute motor axonal neuropathy, and the Miller Fisher Syndrome, in which ophthalmoplegia and other cranial nerve involvement is present along with ataxia and areflexia. Additionally, because of autonomic system involvement, respiratory muscle failure, and autonomic instability can occur. Patients may need to be hospitalized to monitor for development of respiratory muscle failure and require other supportive care. Cerebrospinal fluid (CSF) examination classically shows albuminocytologic dissociation with an elevated CSF protein level with a normal white blood cell count. Diagnosis may be confirmed with electromyography/nerve conducting velocity (EMG/NCV) studies, but demyelination may not be seen at first presentation. Onset in the older patient is associated with a poorer prognosis for recovery, so the clinician should have a high index of suspicion when the patient presents with acute weakness. Treatment usually involves providing supportive care and either plasma exchange or intravenous immunoglobulin (IVIG).

Motor neuron disease

Motor neuron disease causes degeneration of the upper or lower motor neurons or both and can lead to significant disability and increased mortality. Amyotrophic lateral sclerosis (ALS, Lou Gehrig's disease) is the most common of these diseases affecting both the upper and lower motor neuron. ALS can affect young adults, but increases in incidence with age, with higher numbers in those over the age of 75. [8] While affecting more males at earlier ages, the ratio shifts to more females during the later years. On history and examination, patients may present with weakness in any body part. Exam findings can include hyperreflexia and spasticity (upper motor neuron) along with atrophy and fasciculation (lower motor neuron). Dysphagia, facial weakness, and ocular symptoms can be seen when the cranial nerves are involved. Diagnosis is made based on clinical criteria showing progressive upper and lower motor neuron symptoms. Electromyography and nerve conduction studies can be helpful in providing supportive evidence for the diagnosis of ALS, or if there are conflicting findings. Treatment primarily consists of supportive care including ventilatory and nutritional

assistance. Currently the glutamate antagonist, riluzole, is approved in the treatment of ALS, which has been shown to prolong survival by three to six months.[9]

Additional forms of motor neuron diseases including spinal muscular atrophies (pure lower motor neuron disorders), primary lateral sclerosis (pure upper motor neuron disorders), and progressive bulbar palsy (upper and lower motor neuron disorder of the cranial muscles).[10] Symptoms typically arise from the neuronal location affected by neuron degeneration.

Myasthenia gravis

Myasthenia gravis is a clinical diagnosis involving fluctuating and fatigable weakness involving the skeletal muscle groups. It is caused by an antibody response directed at the acetylcholine receptor of the neuromuscular junction. It can occur at any age group, and there is a bimodal distribution to the incidence of disease. The incidence in those over the age of 65 is 52.9 cases a year per million with a predilection for men in the sixth and seventh decades of life, while women are typically affected at younger ages.[11, 12]

Presenting symptoms can include any skeletal muscle group with often-times transient symptoms at the beginning of the disease with progressive worsening (Table 15.3). Diagnosis is made on a clinical basis, while the bedside ice pack test (improvement in eyelid ptosis with application of the ice pack) and the edrophonium test (improvement in muscle strength with injection of edrophonium) can be used to support the diagnosis. Further confirmation of the diagnosis can be made with acetylcholine receptor antibody (AChR-Ab) and muscle specific tyrosine kinase antibody (MuSK-Ab) testing, along with electrophysiologic analysis showing decreased muscle action potential.[11, 12] Additional evaluation for

Table 15.3 Skeletal manifestations of myasthenia gravis

Ocular weakness (ptosis, diplopia)

Bulbar weakness (dysarthria, dysphagia, weakness with chewing)

Neck extensor weakness

Limb weakness (proximal greater than distal)

Respiratory weakness (can lead to myasthenia crisis)

comorbid conditions causing or contributing to the myasthenia gravis includes evaluation for malignancy, thymoma, and autoimmune diseases. Treatment generally consists of acetylcholinesterase inhibition (pyridostigmine), and the use of plasmapheresis and IVIG during acute exacerbations. Chronic treatment with immunosuppression therapy can be done with various agents including corticosteroids, azathioprine, cyclosporine, and mycophenolate. The role of surgical thymectomy in the elderly population is still unclear, especially given the likelihood of thymic involution. Patients and their care providers should be careful to avoid medications that increase muscle weakness in myasthenia gravis.

Additional neurological causes of weakness

The presence of structural central nervous system (CNS) lesions can cause weakness with variable presentation depending on location of the lesion. Lesions due to stroke and CNS masses may be associated with other systemic and neurologic complaints. Spinal pathology from chronic progressive etiologies such as degenerative disc disease, spinal stenosis or acute disc herniation, and spinal cord injury can lead to radicular symptoms involving the affected nerve roots. Often this form of weakness may be accompanied by complaints of pain and sensory loss. The clinician should be aware of warning signs such as bowel or bladder dysfunction that may suggest myelopathy, and other systemic symptoms that may point to an infectious (abscess) or malignant etiology in the older adult. Further workup if indicated can include imaging and electrophysiologic studies, while management will depend on the acuity and resulting disability of the lesion and can range from conservative management with physical therapy and symptomatic treatment to surgical intervention.

Non-neurological causes of muscle weakness in the elderly

The list of non-neurological causes of muscle weakness complaints in the elderly is extensive (Table 15.4). Further workup based on a thorough history and physical examination will help to narrow down possible contributing etiologies and to help guide further workup.

As older patients may take multiple medications due to comorbid medical problems, medication history should be reviewed with the elderly patient thoroughly for medications and drug interaction that

Table 15.4 Non-neurological causes of weakness

Cause	Example
Cardiogenic	Congestive heart failure, cardiomyopathy, ischemic heart disease, arrhythmia
Pulmonary	Chronic obstructive pulmonary disease, emphysema, chronic asthma, pulmonary fibrosis
Myopathy/ rheumatologic	Polymyositis, dermatomyositis, inclusion body myositis, vasculitis, arthritic conditions, connective tissue diseases
Endocrine	Thyroid disease, adrenal disease, parathyroid disorder
Infection	Influenza, HIV, bacterial, viral, parasitic, facial weakness (Bell's palsy)
Renal	Renal failure, dehydration, infectious etiologies
Electrolyte	Potassium, sodium, calcium, magnesium disturbances
Medications	Glucocorticoids, antibiotics, statins, chemotherapeutic agents, immunosuppressive therapy
Psychiatric	Depression, mood disorders, psychogenic etiologies.

cause muscle weakness. For example, corticosteroids are used to treat a variety of conditions including inflammatory muscle and rheumatologic diseases, and may worsen any disease-associated weakness. The clinician should caution the patient regarding their usage, and should periodically review the necessity of continuing it. When the decision is made to discontinue corticosteroids, care should be taken to taper off to reduce the risk for adrenal insufficiency with rapid discontinuation of corticosteroids.

Statin use may be commonly seen in the elderly patient with treatment of hyperlipidemia, coronary artery disease, and vascular disease. Adverse effects affecting the muscles can range from myalgias to muscle injury to severe myopathy. Overall incidence appears to be low, but it is difficult to quantify.[13, 14] Genetics, drug interactions and metabolism have contributing components to muscle toxicity from statins, along with the presence of other conditions such as thyroid disease which can cause its own myopathy. Establishing a creatinine kinase level at baseline when starting therapy and monitoring for adverse muscle effects routinely at follow up visits may help to delineate if muscle complaints are related to the lipid-lowering agents from other causes. If lipid-lowering therapy is still indicated, the clinician can consider switching to a statin associated with lower risk of muscle toxicity.[13]

Evaluation

Muscle weakness in the elderly patient is often a vague complaint and should be clarified on history taking to help initiate the appropriate workup. Asthenia is typically accompanied by complaints of feeling weak, while patients that have primary muscle weakness will have difficulty performing the first repetition of the task. History taking should review onset, duration, and distribution along with associated symptoms and possible triggering etiologies. The presence of symptoms for a longer duration may indicate a more chronic etiology such as a systemic illness or the chronic use of a medication, whereas acute onset of symptoms might prompt an urgent workup for cerebrovascular disease, infection, or acute metabolic or other medical changes.

A thorough review of medications and supplements as well as social and family history intake is necessary to identify potential triggers and hereditary risk factors. Special attention should also be paid to any symptoms that indicate so-called red flags, thus prompting urgent evaluation (Table 15.5).

The pattern of muscle weakness helps to identify the etiology. Focal weakness is usually indicative of

Table 15.5 Potential red flags related to muscle weakness

Aphasia
Dysphagia and changes in voice
Vision changes
Respiratory difficulties
Falls
Presence of pain
Alterations in bowel and bladder function
Altered mental status

involvement of a peripheral nerve or a focal lesion in the cerebral cortex, whereas diffuse weakness may be more likely due to a widespread neurologic, metabolic, infectious, or other systemic etiology. Proximal weakness is suggested with difficulty getting out of a chair or walking up stairs, and can be caused by a myopathy or neuromuscular junction disorder. Distal weakness usually involving complaints of difficulties with grip strength, writing, and weakness of the feet may be seen in motor neuron disease and demyelinating conditions.

Physical examination helps determine if there is an underlying neurological cause or other etiology for the weakness. Some important observations include tenderness in the muscles, possibly indicating an inflammatory myopathy and the presence of atrophy, which can suggest a motor neuron etiology. Examining the cranial nerves identifies ocular muscle involvement and bulbar pathology; the motor examination should evaluate muscle tone, strength, and reflexes for upper and lower motor neuron and neuromuscular junction pathology. Sensory examination should be performed to detect associated deficits present in conditions, such as in Guillain-Barré syndrome.

Additional testing is guided by the history and physical examination for the appropriate workup. Laboratory testing typically includes a metabolic panel, with liver and kidney functions, along with creatinine kinase. Rheumatologic lab tests with sedimentation rates, C-reactive protein, and markers for lupus and other connective tissue and vasculitis diseases should be checked when indicated by the history and examination. Lumbar puncture may be indicated if there is a pertinent infectious, inflammatory, metabolic, or cerebrovascular etiology suspected, such as GBS. Radiographs of the spine are pertinent when there is concern for a radiculopathy (such as with sciatica or cervical radiculopathy). Neuroimaging with computed tomography (CT) or magnetic resonance imaging (MRI) is indicated where there is suspicion for CNS pathology, such as with a mass, cerebrovascular disease, intracranial hemorrhage, infection, or multiple sclerosis.

Nerve conduction and electromyography studies help clarify the affected site, confirm the diagnosis, and guide a muscle biopsy if indicated. Muscle biopsy is useful when a myositis is suspected or if the diagnosis remains uncertain. Further histologic and microscopic analysis can distinguish different myopathies, vasculitis, and metabolic and granulomatous diseases.

Treatment is dependent on determining the correct etiology of the muscle weakness, removing any triggering factors and providing appropriate available treatment options. Providing comprehensive care for affected aspects of daily function and supportive measures, such as ventilator support for respiratory dysfunction in ALS, should also be reviewed with the patient, especially if quality of life is significantly affected.

Sensory disorders/neuropathies

Changes in sensation are a common presenting symptom in the elderly, and frequency increases with age. Manifestations, including dysesthesias and neuralgias, have been shown to impact gait, restrict daily functioning, and decrease quality of life.[15] As previously noted, some sensory losses may be commonly found in the aging patient, including decreased vibratory and proprioception. Due to the often vague presentations in the elderly and complex sensory pathways involved, evaluation of neuropathic complaints can be a diagnostic challenge. Familiarity with some of the common presenting patterns and potential etiologies can help to alleviate some of the clinician's frustrations and guide the workup.

Pathology of sensory loss stems from processes that interrupt the normal flow of sensory input (Table 15.6). Pain, temperature, and touch stimuli are carried by small poorly myelinated fibers into the spinal cord via the dorsal nerve root, synapsing in the dorsal horns, and crossing the midline before ascending in the spinothalamic tract to synapse in the thalamus. On the other hand, large myelinated fibers carrying proprioceptive and vibratory stimuli enter via the dorsal roots into the dorsal columns and ascend ipsilaterally to synapse with the cuneate and gracile nuclei of the medulla. Second order neurons then cross the medulla and ascend to synapse in the thalamus. After synapsing in the thalamus, neurons carrying information from all of the different modalities finally terminate in the primary sensor cortex of the parietal lobe, which is arranged somatographically with the face laterally placed near the Sylvian fissure and the leg medially positioned similar to the layout for the motor homunculus. Brown-Séquard syndrome occurs when there is a lesion affecting one side of the spinal cord, resulting in ipsilateral impaired proprioception and vibration combined with decreased contralateral pain and temperature sensations due to crossing of the respective sensory fibers.[16]

Causes of sensory loss

Common changes in peripheral neurons with aging result in decrease fibers, declines in nerve conduction, and a decreased capacity for axonal reinnervation following injury.[17] Although common in the older adult, the resulting manifestations may be above the thresholds of detection on standard clinical exams in the office. The presence of signs and symptoms affecting daily quality of life and functional status in the elderly patient is usually indicative of pathology in excess of normal aging. Exact mechanisms of neuropathic damage are unknown though the common mechanistic pathways of nerve damage result in Wallerian degeneration of the axon, myelin sheath, and "dying back" of the nerve cell. In elderly patients, the causes of sensory loss are extensive, and it is useful to separate the etiologies into central and peripheral etiologies. CNS causes of sensory loss usually stem from structural and anatomical lesions, cerebrovascular disease, or demyelination. Various distribution

Table 15.6 Normal sensory pathways

Sensation	Nerve fibers	Crossover	Site of ascension
Pain, temperature, and touch	Small poorly myelinated fibers	Midline of the spinal cord in the anterior commissure	Contralateral anterior spinothalamic tract (touch) Lateral spinothalamic tract (pain and temperature)
Proprioception, vibratory pressure, and touch	Large myelinated fibers	Medulla (medial lemniscus)	Ipsilateral medial gracile column (lumbothoracic) Lateral cuneate column (cervical)

Table 15.7 Sensory patterns due to central nervous system pathology

Pattern	Site, laterality	Symptoms/findings	Cause	Examples
Cape distribution	Central cervical cord lesion, spinothalamic tract, bilateral	Decreased pinprick and temperature sensation (due to spinothalamic tract involvement)	Cord compression, demyelination	Tumor, syrinx, demyelinating diseases
Brown-Séquard	One side of spinal cord, ipsilateral and contralateral symptoms	Decreased proprioception, vibration, weakness (ipsilateral), decreased pinprick, temperature (contralateral)	Damage to unilateral aspect of spinal cord, hemisection of the spinal cord	Tumor, trauma
Brainstem	Brainstem, most well known is Wallenburg syndrome involving the lateral medulla, ipsilateral, and contralateral involvement	Brainstem location dependent, Wallenburg = decreased pain and temperature in the ipsilateral face and contralateral limb and trunk, Horner's syndrome, vestibular and cerebella symptoms can be associated	Damage to the brain stem, cerebrovascular disease	Vertebral artery disease, dissection, stroke
Thalamic	Thalamus, unilateral	Contralateral sensory loss in all modalities	Damage to the thalamus	Tumor, abscess, lacunar infarct
Cortical	Sensory cortex	Cortical symptoms, associated symptoms, aphasia, neglect	Damage to the cerebrum	Tumor, demyelination

Source: Adapted from Zawora et al.[18]

and presentations of CNS sensory loss symptoms are presented in Table 15.7, whereas peripheral etiologies are listed in Table 15.8. Common causes of peripheral neuropathy in the elderly include diabetes, infection, malignancy, autoimmune disease, and nutritional and vitamin deficiencies.

Diabetic neuropathy

Diabetes is the most common cause of neuropathy in the elderly and has a variety of presentations (Table 15.9). About 60%–70% of people with diabetes have mild to severe forms of nervous system damage, with approximately 20%–30% complaining of decreased sensation in the lower extremities and up to 26% of undiagnosed diabetics found to have peripheral neuropathy in one study.[19–21]

The most common presentation is a long axon distal sensory polyneuropathy. Symptoms most commonly consist of sensory loss and pain described as sharp, burning, or aching beginning in the distal extremities with proximal progression of symptoms forming the "stocking and glove" distribution. On examination, sensory loss can encompass large fiber function involving vibration and proprioception or small fiber involvement with pain, impaired temperature sensation, reduced distal reflexes, and distal muscle weakness. Consequences of progressive neuropathy include risk for infections, limb injury, and impairment of other major organ systems. Neuropathic symptoms also reduce participation in physical and social activities and lead to sleep impairment and difficult to control chronic pain syndromes.

Diabetes is also the most common form of small fiber neuropathy, which typically presents with painful dysesthesias and sensory loss involving thermal and pain perception. Small fibers are implicated

Table 15.8 Sensory patterns due to peripheral nervous system pathology

Pattern	Site, laterality	Symptoms/findings	Cause	Examples
Mononeuropathy	Individual nerve, unilateral	Sensory loss, paresthesias in distribution of nerve	Damage to the nerve, e.g., entrapment, trauma	Carpal and tarsal tunnel syndrome, ulnar nerve entrapment, meralgia paresthetica. Diabetic neuropathy
Radiculopathy	Nerve root, and corresponding dermatome and myotome, unilateral	Sensory loss, "lancinating pain" exacerbated by cough, sneezing, or straining	Damage to the nerve root, can also be caused by compression, trauma	Disc herniation, spinal stenosis, trauma, infection, malignancy
Axonal neuropathy (stocking-glove distribution)	Long nerve axons (small and large fiber), bilateral	Stocking, glove distribution of symptoms, starts distally and progresses proximally. More severe disease involving the hands (gloves). Can be loss of pinprick and temperature sensation, proprioception, vibratory sense.	Damage to long axon sensory nerves, starting distally; demyelination, inflammatory, vascular etiologies	Diabetes, vitamin B12 deficiency, alcohol, paraneoplastic syndrome, demyelinating neuropathy (GBS), central cervical cord lesions such as tumor, cervical spondylosis, infectious (HIV, syphilis)
Sensory neuropathy	Dorsal root ganglion, can be asymmetric	Numbness, paresthesias, lack motor involvement, but can be disabling. Rare	Degeneration, toxic metabolic, autoimmune	Paraneoplastic disease (small cell lung cancer and anti-Hu antibodies), GBS, Sjögren's, chemotherapy

Source. Adapted from Zawora et al.[10]

when diabetic neuropathy presents with painful paresthesias. Confirmatory exams with routine nerve conduction studies typically assessing for large nerve fiber function may be of limited utility and additional examination with newer diagnostic tools such as quantitative sensory testing may be needed when the diagnosis is in question.[22] Other causes of small fiber polyneuropathy include other endocrine diseases (hypothyroidism), amyloidosis, toxin exposure including alcohol, vitamin B12 deficiency, Sjögren's syndrome, medications (metronidazole), monoclonal gammopathy, and HIV infection; the remainder of cases have no clear identifiable etiology. [22, 23] Treatment usually consists of symptomatic treatment with anticonvulsants, antidepressants, and opioids.

Post-herpetic neuralgia

A common cause of a painful neuropathy in the elderly is post-herpetic neuralgia following a case of shingles. Estimated cases of shingles are between 600,000–800,000 cases per year in the United States, with higher incidences in the elderly population. Studies have reported 8%–24% of all age groups developing some degree of neuralgia, with higher occurrences in those over 50 years of age.[21] Presentation usually consists of a dermatomal vesicular rash, prodromal headache, malaise, paresthesias and initial pain due to the attack. Post-herpetic neuralgia occurs when the lesions resolve and there is persistent pain. Although pain typically decreases within months of onset, some elderly patients may have persistent and progressive pain despite multiple treatment attempts.

211

Table 15.9 Different forms of neuropathy due to diabetes [20]

Type of diabetic neuropathy	Presenting symptoms
Sensory long axon peripheral neuropathy	Varying degrees of sensory loss, paresthesias, allodynia, pain, stocking and glove distribution
Small fiber neuropathy	Pain, diminished temperature sensations
Autonomic neuropathy	Affects various organ systems: *Gastrointestinal*: esophageal dysmotility, gastroparesis, constipation or diarrhea, fecal incontinence *Genitourinary*: neurogenic bladder, sexual dysfunction *Cardiovascular*: tachycardia, orthostatic hypotension Anhidrosis, heat intolerance,
Cranial neuropathy	3rd cranial nerve palsy, double vision, eyelid droop, dysconjugate gaze Facial nerve palsy
Compression and entrapment neuropathy	Carpal tunnel syndrome (median nerve), radial, ulnar, and peroneal neuropathies
Trunk mononeuropathy	Dysesthesias of the thoracic dermatomes or radicular thoracic pain
Amyotrophy	Lumbosacral plexus neuropathy, asymmetric, lower limb atrophy and weakness, loss of reflexes. Sudden onset of sharp pain.
Mononeuropathy multiplex	Multiple mononeuropathies occurring in the same patient.

If the cranial nerves are affected, additional complications may arise, most notable if the first division of the trigeminal branch is involved causing herpes zoster ophthalmicus. An attack in this distribution can cause pain and ocular complications threatening vision.[24, 25]

Diagnosis is usually clinical, but sometimes sampling of the fluid from the lesions with viral culture or PCR analysis is necessary to provide confirmation if the presentation is atypical. Treatment usually consists of antiviral medications (acyclovir, valcyclovir) for the initial attack, with symptomatic treatment for the post herpetic neuralgia. A vaccine is available for herpes zoster that has shown efficacy in reducing the incidence of herpes zoster cases along with reducing the resultant complications of the disease.[24] Post-herpetic neuralgia, like diabetic neuropathy in the elderly, can lead to decreased social interactions, compromise of physical conditioning, problems with sleep, depression, and fatigue.

Demyelinating neuropathies

Demyelinating neuropathies include GBS, chronic inflammatory demyelinating polyneuropathy (CIDP), and multiple sclerosis. Guillain-Barré syndrome and multiple sclerosis as noted in our discussion of muscle weakness are demyelinating neuropathies that can affect the motor and sensory nerves. In GBS, sensory symptoms typically involve paresthesias of the distal extremities marching proximally, while in multiple sclerosis the presentation is varied depending on the location of the lesion.

CIDP is a heterogeneous sensorimotor neuropathy with different variations of proximal and distal muscle weakness along with sensory loss and different paresthesias.[26] The condition has a higher incidence and prevalence in the elderly population and is thought to be autoimmune driven though the antigenic cause remains unknown.[27, 28] The clinical course is variable with relapsing–recurring and chronic progressive courses. Treatment is directed at blocking the immune response and immunotherapy includes corticosteroid, IVIG, plasma exchange, and other corticosteroid sparing therapy.[26]

Others causes of neuropathy

Toxic metabolic etiologies are also common causes of neuropathy in the elderly. Alcohol as a toxin is a common cause of neuropathy in the elderly. Alcohol use is still common among the older population with heavy usage seen in up to 6% of old adults.[29] The cause of alcohol-related neuropathy is unknown, but previous theories include alcohol as a direct toxin versus indirectly leading to deficiency of vitamins and other nutrition elements.[30] Neuropathy related to alcohol usually presents with a distal sensory neuropathy but can have a variety of presentations, including painful paresthesias. Treatment is aimed at halting progression of the neuropathic symptoms with reduction or cessation of alcohol and symptomatic treatment when the neuropathic symptoms impair function and quality of life.

Vitamin B12 deficiency occurs in elderly patients due to dietary deficiency or malabsorption from atrophic gastritis, the chronic use of acid blocking medications, or *Helicobacter pylori* infection. Vitamin B12 is necessary for optimal nerve functioning and deficiency can lead to sub-acute combined degeneration of the dorsal and lateral spinal columns. The sensory findings of the polyneuropathy include decreased proprioception and vibratory sensation. Myelopathy, spastic paresis and the presence of an extensor plantar response (Babinski sign) are also associated findings. Laboratory findings, in addition to decreased vitamin B12 levels, can include elevated methylmalonic acid levels and homocysteine levels. If severe neurological dysfunction is present, parenteral therapy is usually required.[31]

Monoclonal gammopathy and other plasma cell disorders have a higher incidence in the elderly population and can present with peripheral neuropathy. Monoclonal protein are suspected to be involved in about 10% of unknown causes of peripheral neuropathy, with a higher association with peripheral neuropathy when an IgM monoclonal gammopathy is present.[32] Presentations include long axonal sensory neuropathies with variable paresthesias, pain, and sensory loss in stocking and glove distribution, along with an amyotrophy beginning in the lower extremities and progressing to the hands and upper extremities. Treatment is aimed at the monoclonal gammopathy with immune suppression and chemotherapeutic agents, along with therapy to treat symptoms.

Of note, in elderly patients (as in any age group) who present with an inconsistent sensory exam, a functional or psychogenic cause may be considered. History should assess for psychological and social stressors, whereas laboratory, imaging, and electrophysiological evaluations are likely to be normal in these circumstances. As in other age groups, this should be a diagnosis of exclusion.

Table 15.10 Sensory terms

Sensory term	Definition
Hypesthesia/hypoesthesia	Decreased ability to perceive pain, temperature, touch, or vibration
Anesthesia	Inability to perceive pain, temperature, touch, or vibration
Hypalgesia	Decreased sensitivity to pain, whereas analgesia is the complete insensitivity to pain
Hyperesthesia	Increased sensitivity to pain
Allodynia	Pain due to a stimulus that is not normally painful
Dysesthesia	Altered sensation
Mononeuropathy	Single peripheral nerve being affected (Example: compression, trauma)
Mononeuritis or mononeuropathy multiplex	Multiple single peripheral nerve lesions affected simultaneously due to the same disease process (Example: diabetes, cryoglobulinemia)
Polyneuropathy	Multiple peripheral nerves affected, with similar distribution on both sides (Example: diabetes)

Evaluation

Similar to complaints of muscle weakness in elderly patients, understanding the exact complaint of sensory loss can be challenging because the presenting complaint may be vague. Different terminology exists for alterations in sensation and efforts should be made to accurately describe the sensory symptom and the sites involved (Table 15.10). The time course of symptoms and progression of symptoms can provide valuable information as to possible underlying etiologies for the symptoms. Acute and subacute presentations may be seen with trauma, demyelination, CNS lesions, or vascular disease, whereas chronic symptoms can be seen with systemic metabolic or toxic etiologies such as alcoholism, diabetes, hypothyroidism, and autoimmune disease. A thorough review of medical problems, medication lists, and psychosocial history should be performed with the patient to identify any triggers or risk factors. Toxic exposures, travel history, and HIV risk factors should also be reviewed with the patient.

Sensory examinations in general are challenging in the primary care office given its extensive nature and the time constraints of most office visits. A thorough history and completed portions of the examination can help identify where to begin with the sensory examination. Key parts to identify include involvement of the extremity versus the trunk and head and if the symptoms lateralize or not. Further characterization of the paresthesias can help to localize to small fiber (burning, stinging) versus large fiber involvement (tingling, pins and needles). Associated abnormalities in muscle strength and gait may give additional clues to systemic etiologies.

Table 15.11 lists techniques to examine the different sensory modalities in the office. Since common neuropathic complaints involve the long axonal nerves, one can start the sensory exam distally and then march proximally to detect the level of the sensory deficit, with attention paid to the opposing

Table 15.11 Office sensory examination

Sensory modality	Technique
Pain	Safety pin, sharp end of cotton swab broken in half
Temperature	Temperature can be checked with small plastic bottles of hot or cold water, cool tuning fork, or metal handle of reflex hammer
Vibratory sense	128-Hz tuning fork to bony prominence in lower extremities
Proprioception	Ask the patient to identify movement of the great toe, in various directions. Romberg test integrates proprioception and postural stability (positive, if by closing eyes the patient loses balance – suggests that proprioception is impaired as stability is dependent on the visual system).

extremity to check for lateralization of the deficit. The Romberg test can be done to check for proprioception, but in the elderly patient, special care should be made to support the patient when there is a concern for falls.

Laboratory evaluation includes a comprehensive metabolic panel with electrolytes, kidney and liver function, and fasting glucose along with a complete blood count, sedimentation rate, B12 and folate levels, and thyroid function studies. A glucose tolerance test and hemoglobin A1c can be done to further evaluate for diabetes. Urine should be checked to evaluate for glucose and proteinuria, which can be seen in certain neuropathies related to multiple myeloma, amyloidosis, and monoclonal immunoglobulin disease. Rheumatologic workup when indicated involves additional testing encompassing antinuclear antibodies, angiotensin converting enzyme, anti-neutrophil cytoplasmic antibodies (ANCA), Sjögren antibodies, and anti-Hu antibody to evaluate for vasculitis and connective tissue disease.

Electromyography and nerve conduction studies (EMG and NCV) help distinguish sensory loss disorders from other myopathies and neuromuscular junction conditions. Obtaining cerebral spinal fluid with a lumbar puncture may be required if there is a high index of suspicion for infectious etiologies, or a demyelinating disorder such as GBS.

Treatment

Treatment for sensory neuropathies in the elderly patient involves treating the underlying condition, and providing symptomatic relief. Care should be taken to review the impact of the sensory loss and paresthesias on the patient. Counseling on reducing fall risks with an assistive device during ambulation and instructions on reducing safety risks in the home and during the performance of activities of daily living should be given to the elderly patient and family members. Although pain caused by the neuropathies can be debilitating, further treatment with medications is often limited by side effects, drug interactions, and pharmacokinetics.

First line medications for neuropathic pain generally include tricyclic antidepressants (TCAs), gabapentin, and topical lidocaine (Table 15.12). TCAs, however, generally have limited use in the geriatric patient due to their anticholinergic effects, whereas gabapentin and pregabalin can cause fatigue and sedation. Additionally their use may be further

Table 15.12 Neuropathic pain medications[20, 34]

Medications used for neuropathic pain	Advantages	Limiting factors in the elderly Patients
Tricyclic antidepressants (secondary amine nortriptyline, desipramine, tertiary amine amitriptyline)	Low cost, easy dosing, anti-depressant, works on sleep	Risk for anticholinergic side effects (dry mouth, constipation, orthostatic hypotension, cardiac toxicity)
Serotonin norepinephrine reuptake inhibitors (duloxetine, venlafaxine)	Duloxetine efficacy in painful diabetic peripheral neuropathy, treats depression, less cardiac effects Venlafaxine, effective in painful polyneuropathies	Duloxetine – nausea Venlafaxine – cardiac toxicity
Anticonvulsants: calcium channel alpha2-sigma ligands (gabapentin, pregabalin)	Efficacy in neuropathic pain, less drug interactions	Dizziness, sedation; limited use with renal insufficiency
Other anticonvulsants: carbamazepine	Carbamazepine – efficacy in trigeminal neuralgia	Mixed efficacy with other agents, oxcarbazepine, valproic acid. Side effects related to anticonvulsants
Tramadol	Efficacy in neuropathic pain	Lower seizure threshold, similar side effects to opioids, serotonin syndrome, abuse risk
Opioids	Efficacy in neuropathic pain	GI side effects, nausea, sedation, risk for confusion, risk for abuse
Topical lidocaine	Local efficacy for neuropathic pain	Rash, skin irritant

restricted with renal disease. Topical therapy with lidocaine is generally limited by local epidermal reactions and its cost, but can be effective with minimal systemic absorption. Due to potentially limiting side effects, opioids and tramadol are analgesics with limited use in neuropathic pain.[33, 34] If opioids and tramadol are used, consideration should be given to convert to long acting formulations to help with medication compliance. Antidepressant medications with serotonin-norepinephrine reuptake inhibitors such as Duloxetine and Venlafaxine appear to show some efficacy in the treatment of neuropathic pain, whereas serotonin reuptake inhibitors haven't shown significant improvement from placebo.[33]

Seizure disorders

Seizures can have a devastating impact on the elderly patient. Not only does this disorder cause physical injury and medical instability, it can adversely affect quality of life especially in an elderly patient with concerns of losing independence and a decreasing social sphere.[35] Seizures have the highest prevalence among children and the elderly, but they are still difficult to recognize in the older patient.[36] One of the challenges of recognition of seizures in the elderly is the myriad of conditions with overlapping symptoms and presentations, such as with transient ischemic attacks, cerebrovascular disease, delirium, and syncope.

A thorough workup to identify any provoking etiologies of seizure should be done along with assessing the risk for recurrence of seizures. Early neurology referral should be requested to aid in diagnosis and management when the diagnosis is suspected, especially in the presence of other comorbid medical conditions that are common in the elderly. Establishing follow up also needs to be ensured to evaluate for recurrence of seizures and tolerance of medications.

Background

At least 25% of all new onset seizures occur in the elderly, whereas the prevalence rate in the community elderly population is approximately 1.5% in the United States as compared to 0.5% in younger adults.[36–38] Those living in nursing facilities have seizure and epilepsy rates as high as 9% and possibly higher.[37, 39, 40] For epilepsy, defined as recurrent unprovoked seizures without treatment, annual incidence increases with age as well.[41, 42] Actual incidences may in fact be higher due to difficulties recognizing seizures.

The most common cause of seizures in the elderly is cerebrovascular disease; 30%–40% of epileptic seizures in the elderly occur in those who have had a stroke, and up to 9% of patients who have had a stroke will suffer a seizure.[37, 43] Further, the risk for epilepsy is increased up to twentyfold after a stroke.[44] Seizures are more likely to occur with hemorrhagic stroke, larger infarct size, and cortical rather than subcortical involvement.[36, 44]

Alzheimer's disease and other neurodegenerative dementias have a high prevalence in the elderly population and are a risk factor for the development of seizures.[45, 46] Up to 10%–20% of cases of epilepsies are thought to be due to underlying Alzheimer's disease and other neurodegenerative dementias found in elders, although the exact cause is still not understood. [44] Possible etiologies include neurotoxicity from beta amyloid protein, neurotransmitter disruption, and mutations of the gamma secretase, and amyloid precursor protein genes, which are associated with earlier onset familial dementias and the presence of seizures.[47] Younger age of onset of dementia, more advanced disease, and history of antipsychotic use are also characteristics that appear to be associated with greater incidence of seizures in elderly patients with dementia.[44, 45, 48, 47]

Additional causes include intracranial tumors, head trauma, and a variety of acute medical illnesses and medications that may cause an acute seizure. Up to 20% of cases of epilepsy in the elderly are associated with trauma, and 8%–45% of seizures are attributable to tumors.[36, 44] Subdural hematoma and skull fractures following trauma have greater association with seizures in cases of head injury, while primary and low grade brain tumors are also more commonly associated with seizures. Other common provoking causes include heavy alcohol use and withdrawal, metabolic disturbances, drugs/medications, and infectious etiologies that can cause an acute seizure or lower the seizure threshold in patients with epilepsy.

Seizure presentation in the elderly

Seizure presentation in the elderly is variable and may not always consist of convulsions. Often symptoms are vague and include confusion, dizziness, weakness, and/or paresthesias (Table 15.13). The older adult may have a seizure more typically originating in the frontal lobe with secondary generalization, while generalized seizures from primary disorders are more common in the younger patient. Longer periods of postictal weakness and confusion are also commonly found with elderly patients.

Status epilepticus is a presentation of seizures of which the clinician caring for the elderly should be aware. Although there are varying definitions, it is the ongoing occurrence of a seizure or frequent seizure episodes without a postictal return to baseline. Both convulsive and nonconvulsive forms of status epilepticus can happen with a higher frequency in the elderly.[36, 49] Convulsive status epilepticus is easier to recognize because of the presence of motor symptoms. With nonconvulsive status epilepticus, however, it is more difficult to detect because of indistinct presentations that can delay diagnosis. Often, findings in nonconvulsive status epilepticus include altered mental status, confusion, and lethargy in the ambulatory setting.

Table 15.13 Differences in seizures between the elderly and the young patient

	Younger patient	Elderly patient
Type of seizure	Generalized	Focal, partial with secondary generalization
Origin of seizure	Temporal lobe epilepsy is a common location	Focal areas due to previous stroke, tumors, head injury. Neurodegenerative dementia.
Symptoms	Prodromal symptoms including déjà vu or olfactory hallucinations, may include facial and motor automatisms	May include nonspecific symptoms, dizziness, paresthesias, confusion Longer periods of postictal confusion and weakness

Table 15.14 Common conditions with similar presentations to seizures

Condition	Additional workup
Altered mental status/delirium	Toxic, metabolic and infectious studies, medication and drug review
Syncope/dizziness	Toxic, metabolic and infectious workup, medication and drug review; cardiac and neurologic workup
Memory loss, transient global amnesia, dementia	Toxic, metabolic and infectious workup, medication and drug review; neurocognitive testing, neuroimaging, consideration for CSF studies
TIAs	Neuroimaging with CT/MRI, carotid evaluation, ECG, and telemetry monitoring
Sleep disorders	Sleep testing, polysomnography

Table 15.15 Risk factors for seizures to assess for on history taking

Cerebrovascular disease history
Previous seizure episodes and provoking factors if known
History of and risk factors for malignancy
Previous infections, especially intracranial/CNS infections
Head trauma, brain injury
Alcohol and drug use/abuse

Exacerbations of an existing epilepsy condition or the presence of toxic metabolic disturbances, including alcohol, drug, and medication withdrawal, are the most common causes of nonconvulsive status in the elderly population.[49] Intracranial pathologies including tumor, trauma, and hemorrhage are other etiologies.[50] In certain clinical scenarios such as unexplained coma, the presence of nonconvulsive status epilepticus should be considered as a possible diagnosis. EEG findings can be variable, but include detecting generalized spike and slow wave discharges or focal spikes stemming from frontal and/or temporal regions.[49]

Differential diagnosis

Recognizing a seizure in the elderly can be difficult because of the wide array of presentations with similar overlapping and often vague symptoms. Various common conditions in the elderly patient with similar symptoms are listed in Table 15.14.

Evaluation

History taking in the elderly patient presenting with a seizure should obtain information on the presentation and time course of the episode, provoking factors, and assessment for sustained injuries and loss of consciousness. Associated symptoms, concurrent medical illnesses, and an accurate medication review should be ascertained. Prior medical, social and family history should assess for risk factors for seizure (Table 15.15). Postictal confusion or an underlying cognitive condition can limit obtaining an accurate history from the older patient. Seeking out witnesses when available for collateral information is often necessary to provide additional details.

A thorough physical and neurological exam should evaluate for possible contributing conditions and assess for injuries and any residual deficits. Laboratory workup includes evaluation for metabolic disturbances, hepatic and renal function, a complete blood count, and thyroid function tests. Urine tests, cultures, toxicology and alcohol screening, along with a syphilis test and other infectious screens may be indicated by the history. Further concerns for CNS infection and hemorrhage may prompt lumbar puncture and further cerebrospinal fluid analysis. Neuroimaging should be checked in the elderly patient with new onset seizures to exclude ischemia, space occupying lesions, or inflammatory conditions due to their higher prevalence in this population.

Use of EEG in the elderly can provide additional information in the diagnosis of seizures and epilepsy. EEG can identify an epileptogenic focus, as well as periodic lateralizing epileptiform discharges (PLEDS) which suggests increased risk for the development of seizures.[37] If there is concern for status epilepticus, especially nonconvulsive seizures, EEG is useful for confirming the diagnosis. A limitation of EEG use, however, is that seizure activity may not always be present during interictal periods and a normal EEG may not exclude epilepsy. Conversely, other nonspecific findings in the elderly patient such as generalized slowing can occur in a variety of medical conditions, and may be present in the absence of seizures. Video and ambulatory EEG may have additional value in the elderly, and may also assist in the diagnosis of other etiologies when evaluating for seizures.[51]

Management of seizures

Initial management of an active seizure episode in the elderly is like that of any age group. The patient needs to be triaged and stabilized with attention to prevention of injury. Basic life support is initiated, followed by administering diazepam or lorazepam, and then phenytoin or fosphenytoin to abort the seizure activity. Identification of any provoking causes is important to help understand the risk for recurrence of seizures and assess the need for further maintenance anti-epileptic therapy. A seizure caused by an acute metabolic disturbance, medication, or medication withdrawal will generally not require ongoing anti-epileptic therapy. Seizures due to certain intracranial events, such as a hemorrhagic stroke or head trauma, may warrant treatment for a limited defined period of time. A neurologist should be consulted to help assist in the diagnosis and management of seizures.

Initiation of treatment in recurrent unprovoked seizures in the elderly, however, can sometimes be a difficult decision, and is further limited by sparse randomized trial data involving the elderly. Typically anti-epileptic therapy is started after a second seizure. However, given the presence of risk factors in the older patient that can increase the risk for recurrence such as stroke, consideration is often given to initiate anti-epileptic therapy after the first seizure. [44] Discussion should be had with the patient regarding risks and benefits of initiation of anti-epileptic (AED) therapy versus no maintenance therapy prior to starting treatment.

Aging related changes in pharmacokinetics, renal and hepatic function, possible drug interactions, and side effects should all be considered when choosing a seizure medication. Once started, close monitoring of levels with certain AEDs and follow-up to review for adverse effects should be done routinely to ensure tolerability and adherence to the medication. General complaints after starting AEDs include sedation and fatigue, lightheadedness, changes in balance, and cognitive complaints. Other factors, including dosing schedule and cost, may influence the choice of medication.

Although choosing an AED medication should be individualized, many clinicians have preferred newer agents due to simpler pharmacokinetics, decreased side effects, and decreased drug interactions compared to older antiepileptic medications (Table 15.16).[44, 52, 53] Few data is available however, to suggest that the effectiveness between newer and older agents are significantly different, especially in the elderly population.[41] Previously published guidelines have stated that gabapentin, lamotrigine, and possibly carbamazepine are effective as initial monotherapy agents for partial onset seizures in the elderly population, whereas other AED agents are lacking in data in the elderly but generally are effective in adults.[54, 55] Gabapentin and lamotrigine in comparison to carbamazepine have shown similar efficacy, but decreased tolerability was generally found in those receiving carbamazepine. Levetiracetam is also a newer agent showing better tolerability and similar efficacy in the elderly population.[41, 53] Lastly, while some benzodiazepines and barbiturates may be indicated during an acute seizure, these classes have a higher risk for side effects and toxicity and should be avoided in maintenance therapy in the treatment of epilepsy.

The clinician should be aware of additional serious though rare adverse effects and conditions to monitor for after initiating anti-epileptic therapy. Agranulocytosis, aplastic anemia, Stevens Johnson syndrome, hepatic failure, and cardiac arrhythmias can be seen with carbamazepine, phenytoin, and valproic acid along with other anti-epileptic medications. Osteomalacia and osteoporosis are also bone disorders at a greater risk of occurring with long term use of certain anti-epileptic therapies. Osteoporosis is common in elderly patients, especially amongst post-menopausal women. Bone density monitoring and therapy with calcium, vitamin D, and bisphosphonates should be considered when anti-epileptics are used long term.

Duration of AED therapy is controversial. In elderly patients, the risk for recurrence of seizures is high due to the previously mentioned risk factors that often persist. With appropriate treatment, however, control of seizures is attained in 70% or more of elderly patients.[36] In general, treatment is usually life long as many of the risk factors for recurrence in the elderly are not likely to resolve during the period of seizure freedom. For those patients looking to

Table 15.16 Seizure medications used in the elderly population

Medication	Adverse effects	Pharmacological considerations	Special considerations in the elderly
Carbamazepine	Many drug interactions; can cause aplastic anemia, agranulocytosis, SIADH, rash; can cause CNS depression	High protein binding, enzymatic inducer; hepatic metabolism, urine and feces excretion	Partial seizure use; can cause cardiac conduction abnormalities, bone marrow disorders. Contraindicated if using MAOIs. Can cause bone loss, SIADH. Relatively cheap.
Eslicarbazepine	Dizziness, somnolence, headache, fatigue, hepatotoxicity	Caution in renal and hepatic impairment	Adjunctive use in partial seizures, hyponatremia, multiorgan hypersensitivity reactions, enzyme induction, drug interactions.
Gabapentin	Somnolence and fatigue, weight gain, dizziness, ataxia	Caution in renal insufficiency	Well tolerated, for partial seizures. Renal adjust dosing. Limited by multiple dosing, dizziness. Few interactions.
Lamotrigine	Aseptic meningitis reported, skin reactions, multiorgan hypersensitivity, sleep complaints	Hepatic and renal, glucuronic acid conjugation	Partial, tonic-clonic seizures, not altered by renal impairment,[36] good tolerability in the elderly.[52]
Levetiracetam	Behavior problems, sedation	Enzymatic hydrolysis, excreted in urine. Dosage adjustment with renal impairment.	Fewer drug interactions. Partial, tonic-clonic seizures. Cognitively benign profile, may be better tolerated in dementia patients.[53]
Oxcarbazepine	Better tolerability, allergic rash, hyponatremia, ataxia, tremor, fatigue; dizziness a big side effect	Selective enzymatic induction, still with drug interactions. Glucuronidation, excreted in urine	Partial seizures; better tolerance than carbamazepine. Can cause hyponatremia, neurotoxicity, cardiac toxicity. Contributes to vertigo, dizziness, tremor. Potential hematologic adverse effects.
Phenytoin/ fosphenytoin	Neuropathy, osteomalacia, gingival hypertrophy, pancytopenia, hepatotoxicity, cardiac arrhythmias, dizziness, psych changes	Heavy protein binding, urine exertion, saturation metabolism, nonlinear kinetics, enzyme induction	Partial, tonic-clonic seizures including status epilepticus, cheap, cognitive effects, osteomalacia, and osteoporosis. Many drug interactions (warfarin, TCAs, diabetes, chemotherapeutics).
Pregabalin	Dizziness, somnolence, CNS effects	Urine excretion, caution in renal insufficiency	Lower doses needed for therapeutic benefit, adjunctive therapy for partial seizures, useful in other conditions, (neuropathic pain). Renal dosing.
Tiagabine	Sedation, dizziness, CNS effects	Hepatic metabolism	Adjunctive use in partial seizures, drug interactions

Table 15.16 (cont.)

Medication	Adverse effects	Pharmacological considerations	Special considerations in the elderly
Topiramate	CNS effects, anorexia, weight loss, weakness	Urine excretion, renal adjustments, some liver metabolism, possible decreased clearance with age	Partial and tonic-clonic seizures, can cause cognitive impairment, renal stones. Can cause weight loss.
Valproic acid	Weight gain, GI upset, hair loss, bruising, tremor dizziness, changes in mood, parkinsonism, osteoporosis, ataxia, hepatotoxicity	High protein binding, longer half life, drug interactions, hepatic metabolism, not recommended in hepatic impairment, and urine clearance, caution in renal impairment	Partial and complex seizures, broad spectrum, drug interactions, enzymatic induction, drug interactions, can be useful in other conditions (bipolar disorder, migraine prophylaxis)
Zonisamide	Somnolence, dizziness, weight loss	Use with caution in renal and hepatic impairment. Not recommended in more severe renal impairment. Hepatic metabolism	Adjunctive use in partial seizures, limited data for use in the elderly, can cause kidney stones. Drug interactions

Source: Adapted from Zawora et al.[18]

discontinue anti-epileptic therapy, recommendations on when to start a weaning trial vary from six months to three years after a seizure free period.[56] The patient needs to be counseled on the risk for recurrence and possible consequences of having seizures. Discontinuing the anti-epileptic therapy should be done slowly to titrate off the medication.

Resection of an epileptic focus and vagal nerve stimulation are additional treatment options in epilepsy treatment for refractory cases. However, due to the lack of more generalizable data and the invasive nature of these treatment options, consideration for these interventions should be on an individualized basis. Other long-term management issues to discuss with elderly patients surround life style and safety issues. Individual states have safety laws regarding driving safety and elderly patients with seizures need to be counseled regarding the safety risks, especially when other comorbidities that compromise safety are present. Additional discussions over safety, such as regarding taking baths and swimming should also be had with the patient.

Headaches

Headaches are a common complaint in the physician's office and should be evaluated carefully in the elderly patient due to serious underlying causes that may be present in this population. Primary headaches are defined as headache condition (such as migraines, tension, and cluster) without clear anatomical reasons whereas secondary headaches are due to an underlying condition. In general, new onset of primary headaches decreases with age but still make up a large portion of headaches in older people.[57] In one study, the prevalence of primary headaches was found to decrease from 35.4% in men and 53.2% in women between ages of 55 and 64 years to 22.5% and 38.3% respectively in men and women greater than 85 years of age.[58]

Often, primary headache symptoms from a younger age will carry over to the older population as well. With new headaches, however, the history and examination should carefully search for secondary causes. Although the incidence of primary headaches decreases with age, secondary headaches due to serious and potentially life-threatening intracranial pathology or other systemic etiologies increase with age, found in about 15%.[59, 60]

Primary headaches

Tension type headache

Tension type headaches decline with age but still are the most common headache in the elderly, with prevalence ranging between 35.8% and 44.5%.[57, 59] Often described as a bilateral headache with noncharacteristic tightness or pressing pain, it is usually less disabling and doesn't prevent participation in daily activities. Usually lasting minutes to days, common precipitating factors include stress and sleep disruptions. Chronic tension type headaches also are often associated with stress and mood disorders. Features such as nausea, vomiting, and photophobia are typically absent, and examination may reveal tenderness of the head, neck or shoulder muscles. The diagnosis is a clinical one as there are no specific diagnostic tests.

Simple analgesics such as aspirin, NSAIDs, and acetaminophen generally have good efficacy in treating acute tension type headaches and are reasonable initial therapies for tension type headache (Table 15.17). NSAID use should be cautioned in elderly people, especially if concurrent gastrointestinal or renal disease is present or if other anticoagulant therapy is being used. Combinations of simple analgesics with caffeine are also effective but are also associated with increased adverse effects.[57] Opioids and butalbital should be avoided in the treatment of tension type headaches due to the risk of dependency, adverse effects, and a higher risk of transformation into chronic daily headaches. Of note, patients with this type of headache frequently self-diagnose and self-treat the headache. It is important to review and counsel with patients that frequent use of analgesics can transform tension type headaches and other primary headache syndromes into medication overuse headache and chronic daily headaches. Additional nonpharmacological treatment with biofeedback, massage, heat, and ice may also be used as treatment options.

Table 15.17 Acute primary headache treatments

Medication	Indications	Considerations for use in the elderly
Oxygen, high flow	Acute cluster headache	Relatively safe in the elderly; caution in chronic obstructive pulmonary disease
Caffeine	Migraines, tension-type headaches	Risk for developing chronic daily headache, GI upset, palpitations, and tachyarrhythmia
Acetaminophen	Migraine, tension-type headaches	Caution in liver dysfunction; risk for chronic daily headache
NSAIDs	Migraines, tension-type headaches	Risk for GI side effects, bleeding. Caution with renal dysfunction
Opioids and barbiturates	Broad range of acute headache	Risk for abuse and dependency; overuse can lead to chronic daily headaches
Antiemetics (metoclopramide, chlorpromazine)	Migraines with nausea and vomiting	Extrapyramidal side effects, parkinsonism, QT prolongation, sedation, orthostatic hypotension
Triptans	Moderate to severe migraines, tension headaches in conjunction with migraines	Comes in oral, nasal, and parenteral preparations; limited use in patients with vascular disease
Ergotamines	Migraines	Also available in oral, nasal, and parenteral preparations; limited use in patients with vascular disease

Table 15.18 Prophylactic treatment for primary headaches

Medication	Indications	Considerations for use in the elderly
Tricyclic antidepressants (amitriptyline, nortriptyline, doxepin)	Migraines, tension-type headaches	Anticholinergic adverse effects, sedation, hypotension, QT prolongation, urinary retention, confusion
Venlafaxine	Migraines[61]	Useful for coexisting mood disorder or anxiety
Valproate	Migraines, cluster headache	Adverse effects include GI symptoms, liver dysfunction, tremor, weight gain, sedation
Topiramate	Migraines, cluster headache	CNS effects, cognitive side effects, dizziness, sedation, nausea, anorexia; avoid/contraindicated if nephrolithiasis is present
Beta blockers	Migraines	May have benefits if other co-existing conditions (tremor, CHF). Caution in elderly patients with diabetes, COPD, asthma, depression. Adverse effects include hypotension, bradycardia, lethargy, and sedation.
Calcium channel blockers	Migraines (weaker data), cluster headaches (verapamil)	High doses may be required, arrhythmia, hypotension, edema, constipation. Drug interactions; dizziness.
Lithium	Cluster, hypnic headaches[57]	Many side effects including tremor, cognitive impairment, weakness, nausea

When frequent use of analgesics is required, a prophylactic medication can be considered (Table 15.18). Tricyclic antidepressants are an effective prophylactic medication for reducing the severity and frequency of daily tension headaches, but they are limited by their anticholinergic adverse effects and potential cardiac toxicity in the elderly. If a prophylactic medication is initiated, considerations in the elderly include starting at a low dose and titrating to the lowest effective dose or when adverse effects develop. Also of importance is giving the prophylactic medication an adequate duration of time, measuring the effectiveness by tracking reductions in headache frequency, and avoiding analgesic use. Other agents including SSRIs, SNRIs, and anticonvulsants such as gabapentin and topiramate may have some benefits, but do not have a proven efficacy.[57]

Migraines

Migraines are the second most common primary headache syndrome in the elderly and can cause significant disability. New onset migraines in the elderly, however, are unusual and have an annual incidence of only 2% in this age group. Other older patients have a preexisting diagnosis with continued symptoms as they age.[59] The pathophysiology is complex and incompletely understood, although proposed mechanisms include vasospasms and trigeminovascular system activation.

Migraines may evolve through four phases: the premonitory phase, aura, headache, and the postdromal phase. The premonitory phase can occur hours to days before the aura or headache and commonly consists of fatigue, irritability, poor concentration, mood changes, and other systemic complaints.[62] An aura may follow the premonitory phase, where visual disturbances (including visual scotoma and flashes) are most common, but can consist of almost any neurological symptom. The aura typically develops over five minutes or more and may precede the actual headache, which can last up to several days with variable intensity and worsens with physical activity. In the early stages, migraines are commonly described as being achy with later progression to throbbing pain that is usually unilateral. Additional features may include photophobia, phonophobia, vegetative symptoms, and involvement of both sides of the head.[57] Finally a prodromal phase can be present and typically consists of fatigue, lethargy, and mood changes.

It is important to remember that patients may not experience all four phases of migraines, and as patients age, there can experience different presentations. For example, many older adults can experience aura without the migraine headache, which may present similar to transient ischemic attacks, cerebrovascular disease, or partial. The resulting heterogeneity may lead to diagnostic confusion and migraine attacks can be a consideration when the older patient presents with neurological symptoms without a clear identifiable cause.

Treatment typically involves attempts to abort the acute headache and initiation of a preventative medication if the attacks are frequent (Tables 15.17 and 15.18). Nonspecific analgesics such as NSAIDs and acetaminophen are effective for treatment of migraine headaches, but are limited by the same side effects when used for treatment of other conditions. Antiemetic therapy with metoclopramide or chlorpromazine is useful for reducing the headache pain and also treating associated nausea and vomiting. Intravenous and intramuscular forms are also available when there is significant nausea and vomiting present; however, their use may be limited by extrapyramidal symptoms, medication induced parkinsonism and cardiac toxicity (QT prolongation) in the elderly. Anti emetics can also be used in combination with simple analgesics when the migraine is mild to moderate. Opioids and butalbital containing compounds are used to treat acute headaches, but they carry the same risks with treating other headaches.

Serotonin 5-HT 1b/1d receptor agonist (triptans) and ergotamines are migraine specific medications that are effective in aborting acute migraines. Triptans come in oral, nasal, and parenteral forms which allow for alternative treatment delivery options when there is severe nausea or vomiting. Triptans affect the meningeal blood vessels, the trigeminal nerve endings, and second order neuron synapses in the trigeminocervical complex.[57] Use of triptans in the elderly and adults is recommended against when there is a history of ischemic heart disease and stroke due to the potential vasoconstriction activity of these medications. Ergotamines are alkaloids that also bind to serotonin receptors as well as dopamine and noradrenergic receptors. Although effective at treating

migraines, their use is limited by nausea and should also not be used in patients with coronary artery disease, peripheral vascular disease, or a history of ischemic stroke due to their ability to vasoconstrict cerebral, coronary, and peripheral blood vessels. Dihydroergotamine is available in nasal and intramuscular forms.

Preventive medications may be considered in the elderly if the migraines occur with increased frequency, interfere with daily activities, or based on patient preference. Prophylactics should also be considered if acute treatments are unable to be used, or if there are associated neurological complications to the migraine such as in hemiplegia or infarct.[57] Various treatment options can be chosen based on tolerability to side effects and coexisting medical conditions.

Cluster headache

Cluster headaches are the most common form of trigeminal autonomic cephalalgias (TACs), and classically described as unilateral sharp stabbing headaches in the temporal and orbital regions that are more common in middle-aged than older men.[63] Cluster headaches are associated with ipsilateral autonomic features of nasal congestion, ptosis, and rhinorrhea, and can occur in short-lived episodes throughout the day and are not relieved with sleep or rest.

First-line therapy for treatment of acute attacks includes oxygen at a flow rate of 7 liters per minute or greater and triptans. Oxygen has been shown to be safe and effective when available but should be used with caution in those with concomitant COPD. Sumatriptan is effective for cluster headaches and comes in subcutaneous (6 mg) and intranasal formulations (20 mg). The intranasal formulation, while more convenient, is slower acting and may not be as effective since the onset of cluster headaches tends to be very quick. Triptans are limited by the same adverse effect profile as in their use for migraines. Preventive treatment with the goal of suppressing recurrent attacks and minimizing adverse effects of frequent treatments can also be used for cluster headaches. Lithium and high dose verapamil are effective in prophylaxis of cluster headaches, but they are limited by their adverse effects. Topiramate may be an effective add-on, so high doses of verapamil monotherapy can be avoided, but it is also limited by tolerability.

Table 15.19 Other primary headache types [57, 63, 64]

Primary headache types	Characteristics	Treatment considerations in the elderly
Hypnic	"Alarm clock headache"; low prevalence, but affecting the elderly primarily. Nocturnal onset; lacks migrainous/autonomic features. Generally described as diffuse, nonthrobbing moderate severity, can be frontotemporal in location. More common in women.	Reported relief with sitting up and pacing. Prophylaxis with lithium or indomethacin, but may be limited due to their associated side effects. Nighttime caffeine or melatonin may also be effective.
Exploding headache syndrome	Rare, usually encountered in the elderly; awakes them from sleep with the sense of a loud, painless, explosive noise has occurred in the head. Usually upon awakening, or while falling asleep; some patients also note flashing lights. Triggers include sleep deprivation and stress.	Benign condition; avoid triggers. Tricyclic antidepressants and topiramate may be useful for treatment of recurrent attacks.
Uncommon trigeminal autonomic cephalalgias (TACs)	(SUNCT) (SUNA). Unilateral, sharp, stabbing, severe pain, usually in the orbital or temporal areas. Usually involves V1 distribution of trigeminal nerve. Associated with conjunctival injection and tearing (SUNCT) or cranial autonomic features (SUNA) including nasal stuffiness, rhinorrhea, ptosis. Duration lasting minutes, with high frequency of attacks (separates from trigeminal neuralgia)	Evaluate for secondary causes, including tumors, meningioma, cerebellar pontine angle tumors, brainstem infarcts, intraorbital lesions. Oxygen, sumatriptan, verapamil not effective as in cluster headaches; can do trial with anticonvulsants (lamotrigine, topiramate, gabapentin).
Primary cough headaches	Paroxysmal pain, occurring during cough, Valsalva maneuver, usually following upper respiratory illness. May be due to temporary sensitivity of the carotid baroreceptors to increased intrathoracic pressure. More common in older patients. Secondary causes occur 40% of the time, but are more common in younger patients.	Generally a condition that remits following the resolution the preceding illness. Effective treatments include indomethacin and lumbar puncture to lower intracranial pressures and reset receptors.

Additional primary headache types

Additional primary headache types that are rare but more common to the elderly patient are listed in Table 15.19. Although occurring less frequently, they are important for the clinician to recognize to ensure proper diagnosis and evaluation.

Secondary headache syndromes

New onset headaches, headaches with warning flags, and conversion of preexisting headache conditions should prompt urgent evaluation in the elderly patient as up to 15% of headaches in the elderly can be caused by potentially life-threatening conditions

(Table 15.20).[59] Early recognition of potentially life-threatening neurological conditions causing headaches such as with subarachnoid hemorrhage, subdural hematoma, and stroke can help with treatment outcomes in this patient population.

Headache induced by neuralgias

Secondary headaches in the elderly can include neurologic etiologies and a broad range of non-neurologic causes. Neuralgias that cause headaches with higher incidences in the elderly include post-herpetic neuralgia and trigeminal neuralgia. Headache with herpes zoster can occur in the form of a generalized prodromal headache or a more focal craniofacial pain

Table 15.20 Secondary headaches[59, 63]

Secondary headache types	Presenting features	Diagnostics and treatment considerations in the elderly
Subarachnoid hemorrhage	Sudden onset of "thunderclap" headache; "worst headache" of life; can be associated with nausea, vomiting, hypertension syncope, neck pain, coma, confusion. Sometimes a sentinel headache in the days prior to the SAH is reported. May present subtly and with a normal neuro examination.	Noncontrast CT scan of the head. Lumbar puncture may have more diagnostic utility if further out from onset of symptoms (looking for xanthochromia). Prognosis is worse in older patients (15% of patients >75 returning to independent living at discharge). Early surgical consultation and treatment if possible.
Subdural hematoma	Complaints of mild headache (up to 90% of patients with chronic subdural hematoma). Peak incidence in sixth and seventh decades of life for chronic subdural hematomas (greater than 20 days); 80% occurring in elderly men.	Noncontrast enhanced CT scan of the head. Early surgical consultation recommended
Stroke (cerebral vascular accident)	Headache, relatively uncommon feature, but can occur in up to 17% of patients. Described as dull/throbbing, mild to severe. Can be associated with nausea and vomiting; may have a preceding premonitory headache.	Noncontrast enhanced CT/MRI. Early neurology evaluation; TPA and antiplatelet therapy.
Neoplasm/mass	Incidence of primary and metastatic tumors increases with age. Typically described as morning headache that worsens with positional change; associated with nausea and vomiting. Sometimes bifrontal, resembling tension-type headache. Worsens with bending over. May have other neurological deficits.	CT/MRI. Metastatic disease increases with age.
Meningitis/ encephalitis	Initial symptoms include headache, fever, altered mental status. Associated symptoms can include nuchal rigidity. All symptoms may not be present in elderly patients. Additional symptoms can include confusion, nausea, vomiting, altered mental status, photophobia, malaise.	Meningitis: Lumbar puncture, with gram stain and culture; 18% mortality in meningitis in all age groups, but increases with age. Start empiric antibiotics on suspicion of bacterial meningitis, based on age and health status. Aseptic meningitis usually requires supportive care. Encephalitis: Lumbar puncture may show lymphocytic pleocytosis in the CSF. High mortality, up to 10%. Can result in neurologic damage, herpes is most common (HSV-1). Treat with acyclovir. Intensive monitoring required.
Giant cell arteritis	Classic symptoms are temporal orbital headache, jaw/tongue claudication and visual changes. Headache occurs in approximately two-thirds of patients. Can be a continuous or intermittent headache, typically throbbing. Approximately 50% of patients with painful chewing. Permanent loss of vision in up to 20% of patients.	Examination may reveal temporal artery tenderness or nodularity, possible erythema. Absence does not exclude the diagnosis. Check erythrocyte sedimentation rate, C-reactive protein. Temporal artery biopsy may be required. High dose corticosteroids should be started on suspicion; temporary artery biopsy can still be performed up to 7 days after initiation of corticosteroids

Table 15.20 (cont.)

Secondary headache types	Presenting features	Diagnostics and treatment considerations in the elderly
Acute-angle closure glaucoma	Prevalence increases with age, more common in elderly women. Usually sudden onset of severe pain, with unilateral headache, may also have blurred vision, nausea, and vomiting. Exam with fixed mid position pupil, hazy cornea, "rock hard" globe on palpation of the eye.	Examination of the eye, referral to ophthalmology to measure the intraocular pressure (normal <20 mmHG). Early recognition/referral to ophthalmology, treatment to lower pressures – beta blockers, acetazolamide, topical parasympathomimetic agents, mannitol, definitive treatment with laser iridectomy.
Hypoxia/carbon monoxide	No characteristic pattern to headache or location. Associated symptoms: altered mental status, blurred vision, weakness, lethargy. Look for multiple members with similar symptoms. Ask about living situation, furnace, indoor use of grills/gas stoves for heating (may be seen in dementia patients).	Elevated carboxyhemoglobin level on ABG. Requires high index of suspicion Treatment with oxygen, treat underlying cause
Headache from post-herpetic neuralgia	Following shingles episode, can involve craniofacial dermatome. Burning/lancinating pain; can affect vision if eyes involved.	Shingles vaccination, treatment with antiviral medications during the acute episode, symptomatic relief
Trigeminal neuralgia headache	Paroxysmal, unilateral headache, sharp, electrical pains, usually V2/V3 of the trigeminal nerve related. Short pains, recurrent.	Carbamazepine effective; may be limited by side effects. Other agents include lamotrigine, gabapentin
Medication-induced headaches	Adverse effects of medication, or from rebound headaches that occur with chronic analgesic use for chronic headache disorder.	Discontinue drugs that trigger the headaches. For medication withdrawal headaches, discontinue the offending agent and use different agent for symptomatic relief.

if the trigeminal nerve is involved. As in any other dermatome, persistence of the often burning and lancinating pain can lead to a debilitating post-herpetic neuralgia. Antiviral medications to reduce the severity and duration of the acute attack and neuropathic pain relief with tricyclic antidepressant agents and anti-epileptic medications have been the mainstay of treatment options. Vaccination with the herpes zoster vaccine has been effective in reducing cases of herpes zoster and complications of the attacks.

Trigeminal neuralgia is the most common neuralgia in the elderly and causes a paroxysmal unilateral headache characterized by sharp or electrical pains occurring in the V2 or V3 divisions of the trigeminal nerve with less frequent involvement of the V1 (ophthalmic) branch. The pain is usually short lived but can be recurrent.[59] Triggers include cold air, speaking, chewing, grimacing, or light touch along the distribution of the affected nerve. The pain can be so severe that chewing and speaking are difficult during an attack. Etiologies include compression of the trigeminal nerve from a structural lesion including tortuous blood vessels, arteriovenous malformations, and tumors such as acoustic neuroma and meningioma. Demyelination of the trigeminal nerve in multiple sclerosis can also cause trigeminal neuralgia symptoms. Further evaluation with neuroimaging may be required if there are other focal findings on neurologic examination.

Pharmacological treatment has generally involved anti-epileptic therapy, with carbamazepine the best studied. Doses range from 400 mg–800 mg/day in divided doses, with side effects more manageable starting at lower doses and titrating up slowly. Additional agents include lamotrigine, gabapentin, phenytoin, and baclofen, which have vary degrees of efficacy. Lamotrigine and gabapentin are generally better tolerated. When tolerated, medical treatment is effective in about 70% of patients. Cases of trigeminal neuralgia that are refractory to medical treatment may be candidates for surgical treatment with microvascular decompression, rhizotomy, or radiosurgery.

Giant cell arteritis

A common non-neurological cause of secondary headaches in the elderly is giant cell arteritis (GCA). GCA or temporal arteritis is a medium to large vessel vasculitis that typically affects the vessels in the head and neck including the temporal arteries with peak incidences in the elderly population between the ages of 70 and 80. The thoracic aorta, axillary, and vertebral arteries may be involved as well. Ophthalmic artery involvement can lead to permanent loss of vision in up to 15% of patients.[65] The most common symptom, however, is a headache located over the temporal artery and the temporal and orbital regions. Pain in the jaw with chewing and myalgias from polymyalgia rheumatica are also associated findings. Symptoms often escalate over days to weeks. Examination may reveal a tender or pulseless temporal artery while the sedimentation rate and C-reactive protein level are usually elevated, although 4% of cases will present with normal levels.[66]

Definitive diagnosis requires a temporal artery biopsy, although a negative biopsy does not rule out giant cell arteritis. If the diagnosis is suspected high dose oral corticosteroids should be initiated while waiting for the biopsy to be done. Effective treatment recommendations for corticosteroid doses range from 1 mg/kg daily to higher IV pulse doses (1,000 mg), although dosing is largely based on clinical experience. Once symptoms are improved and laboratory values have normalized, slow tapering of glucocorticoids can be attempted. Flare-ups can occur during a taper and are generally responsive to raising the dose of glucocorticoids.[65]

Medication-related headaches

Medications are also associated with headaches. Some common medications that can cause headaches include antibiotics (trimethoprim-sulfamethoxazole, tetracycline), beta blockers, calcium channel blockers, hormonal therapies, H-2 blockers, NSAIDs, sedatives, and stimulants including caffeine.[59, 63] Chronic or overuse of analgesics can also transform previous episodic primary headache conditions into chronic daily headaches. While peak prevalence occurs in the late forties and declines with age, clinicians should be aware that medication overuse headaches can still occur in those over the age of 65.[67] Withdrawal or rebound headaches are most common with opioids and analgesics in combination with barbiturates and caffeine, but can also be seen with triptans and NSAIDs.[59] Treatment usually requires discontinuation of the offending agent, or analgesic. Withdrawal symptoms after discontinuation include worsening headache, nausea, vomiting, anxiety, and sleep disturbances. Rescue treatments for withdrawal symptoms include anti-emetics, alternate analgesics, intravenous hydration, and other nonpharmacologic approaches.[67] If the patient is able to revert back to baseline and persistent episodic headaches still occur, a prophylactic headache medication can be tried to reduce the frequency of episodes.

Intracranial mass

The incidence of tumors increase with age and presence of an intracranial neoplasm should be excluded in the workup of new or different headache symptoms in the elderly patient. Due to the higher incidence of malignancies in this age group, intracranial neoplasms can be from primary or metastatic disease. [59] Classic presentations of headaches related to neoplasm usually are described as a severe morning headache that changes in intensity with positional change and associated nausea and vomiting. However, in elderly people these headaches may be milder and have more of a resemblance to a tension-type headache that may confound the history. Additional supportive findings for the clinician examining the older patient to be aware include focal deficits, mental status changes, papilledema, or other neurological symptoms.

Cerebrovascular disease

Headache in the older patient can also be a symptom of cerebrovascular disease. With ischemic stroke, headache is somewhat uncommon, occurring in up to 17%–25% of cases.[59, 68] When present, it can be ipsilateral or generalized, and it is often described as a dull or throbbing headache with varying intensity level. It may manifest as a "premonitory headache" and can precede the cerebrovascular event by days to weeks.

Hemorrhagic stroke from an intracerebral or subarachnoid hemorrhage, caused by a ruptured aneurysm, bleeding from an arteriovenous malformation, trauma, high blood pressure, or other condition affecting the cerebral vasculature can be associated with headache as well. Headaches associated with hemorrhage stroke occur in about 40%–60% of cases and may also occur as a sentinel event preceding the hemorrhage for days to weeks prior to the actual bleed.[59, 68] In subarachnoid hemorrhage, the headache is classically described as the worse headache of the patient's life, with sudden onset and association with nausea, vomiting, confusion, lethargy, nuchal rigidity, and neck pain. Not all associated symptoms will be present, however. In the case of a sentinel headache, there may be a normal physical exam. Noncontrast CT scanning is used initially for the confirmation of SAH, but may have a lower sensitivity further away from the onset of symptoms. A lumbar puncture can be performed, with xanthochromia being the pathognomonic finding. Treatment involves medical management with early neurosurgical consultation.

Subdural hematomas occur as a result of trauma including falls and the resulting headache varies in presentation but may be mild and generalized. Elderly patients on blood thinners presenting with generalized headaches and altered mental status after trauma should trigger an evaluation for subdural hematomas. Treatment is medical support, with discontinuation of the blood thinning agent and possible surgical intervention.

Other secondary causes of headaches

More than 50% of cases of community acquired cases of meningitis occur in patients over the age of 50, with higher mortality rates with increasing age.[59] The classic presentation of meningitis is headache, fever, and nuchal rigidity, but all features may not be present in elderly patients. Additional symptoms include photophobia, nausea, vomiting, and altered level of consciousness. When meningitis is suspected, workup requires a lumbar puncture for confirmation of the disease, antibiotic therapy for bacterial meningitis, and supportive therapy for aseptic meningitis.

Headaches related to other infectious, metabolic, or other organ system disease can be of variable presentation and intensity. Acute angle closure glaucoma is an ophthalmologic emergency, and is more common in elderly women.[59] It is often mistaken for other primary and secondary causes of headaches. Distinguishing features include a unilateral headache with acute onset, clouded cornea, a fixed pupil, a painful hard globe of the eye, blurred vision, nausea,

and vomiting. Early recognition, measurement of intraocular pressures, and emergent ophthalmologic consultation should be obtained to help with preservation of vision. Additional ocular etiologies of headache include optic neuritis and scleritis.

Carbon dioxide retention headaches, and headaches with hypoxia, such as in patients with COPD and sleep apnea, usually consist of pain in the frontal or occipital regions. With sleep apnea, the headache is described as being more intense upon waking, with resolution during the course of the day.[68] Improvement in headaches can be seen with treating the underlying condition.

Headaches related to neck disease usually involve cervical/occipital pain and limited range of motion of the neck. If significant structural disease is present, the patient may also have radicular symptoms. Treatment is aimed at symptomatic relief with analgesics and physiotherapy, while the presence of neurological deficits and functional impairment may necessitate further surgical intervention.

Headache evaluation

Due to the higher prevalence of headaches in the elderly caused by secondary conditions, evaluation in this age group should carefully assess for underlying causes. History taking should evaluate for "red flag" complaints, which includes a history of "the worst headache of my life," signs of meningismus, or the presence of focal neurological deficits. Additional assessment for sequelae of falls, head trauma, and uncontrolled medical conditions such as diabetes, hypertension, and pain should also be performed when suggested by the history. Past medical and social history reviewing for a history of malignancy as well as alcohol and drug use provides useful information in guiding further workup. A detailed medication history to search for analgesic use and medications that can cause headaches should be reviewed with the patient.

Associated symptoms often help to distinguish between different types of headaches. Among primary headache syndromes, the presence of photophobia and aura are more suggestive of migraines, whereas unilateral head pain, rhinorrhea, ptosis, and nasal congestions (autonomic symptoms) with repeated attacks can indicate a cluster headache. Tension type headache will be a more nondescript bilateral non-throbbing headache, without other associated features (Figure 15.1).

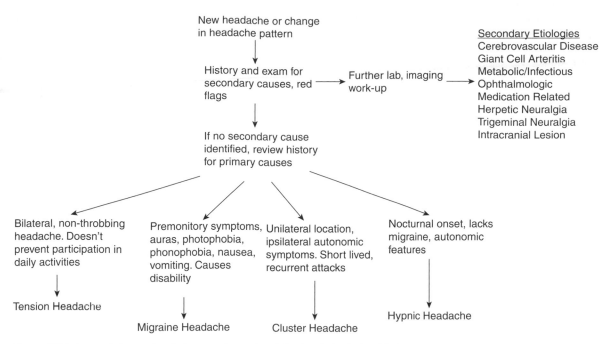

Figure 15.1 Approach to new headaches or a change in existing headache in the elderly.

Neurological examination of the elderly patient with complaints of headache assesses for neurological deficits while examining cranial nerves, motor and sensory function. Mental status and altered level of consciousness are generally associated with more systemic or intracranial processes. Abnormalities of balance, coordination, and reflexes may be seen in intracranial or spinal pathology. General physical examination should include assessments of vital signs and searching for any ocular and cardiopulmonary abnormalities suggesting of headaches from ophthalmologic and cardiogenic causes. If there is a history concerning for trauma or falls, examination of the head and scalp along with the skin and musculoskeletal system to assess for injuries is necessary.

Additional laboratory workup is guided by the history and exam to identify secondary causes. Laboratory studies may include checking for infectious etiologies, hormone distortions, toxicology studies, and comprehensive metabolic panels may be indicated depending on the history. Neuroimaging is indicated when there are red flag symptoms reported. Although there is yet to be consensus guidelines on imaging with CT or MRI of the brain, imaging should also be considered with new onset headache in the elderly. CT/MRI should also be done if mental status changes, focal neurologic deficits, seizures, post-trauma headaches, or papilledema are present, with the goal of evaluating for any intracranial lesion.

Conclusion

Neurological problems are common in elderly patients. Weakness, sensory complaints and headaches are very common complaints in any medical setting and seizures are becoming increasingly prevalent with advancing age. Significant disability can occur if neurological issues are not addressed in the elderly patient. It is important for the primary care clinician to become familiar with these disorders in order to promptly recognize and manage the underlying cause to help alleviate unnecessary decreases in the quality of life of older patients.

References

1. D.A. Drachman, J.M. Swearer. Neurological Evaluation of the Elderly Patient. In: Albert M.L., Knoefel J.E., eds. *Clinical Neurology of Aging.* 3rd Edition. New York, Oxford University Press, 2011; 41–53.

2. J.I. Sirven, E.L. Mancall. Neurological Examination of the Older Adult. In: Sirven J.I., Malamut B.L., eds. *Clinical Neurology of the Older Adult.* 2nd Edition. Philadelphia, Lippincott Williams and Wilkins, 2008; 5–7.

3. T.M. Manini, S.L. Hong, B.C. Clark. Aging and muscle: a neuron's perspective. *Curr Opin Clini Nutr Metab Care* 2013; **16(1)**: 1–10.

4. T. Chitnus, H.L. Weiner. Multiple Sclerosis in the Elderly. In: Albert M.L., Knoefel J.E., eds. *Clinical Neurology of Aging.* 3rd Edition. New York, Oxford University Press, 2011; 536–543.

5. A. Scalfari, V. Knappertz, G. Cutter, et al. Mortality in patients with multiple sclerosis. *Neurology* 2013; **81**: 184–192.

6. R.A. Hughes, J.H. Rees. Clinical and epidemiologic features of Guillain-Barré syndrome. *The Journal of Infectious Diseases* 1997; **176**: S92–8.

7. N. Yuki, H.P. Hartung. Guillain-Barré syndrome. *N Engl J Med* 2012; **366**: 2294–2304.

8. P.M. Worms. The epidemiology of motor neuron disease: a review of recent studies. *Journal of the Neurological Sciences* 2001; **191**: 3–9.

9. L.P. Rowland, N.A. Shneider. Amyotrophic lateral sclerosis. *N Engl J Med* 2001; **344**: 1688–1700.

10. M. Donaghy. Classification and clinical features of motor neurone diseases and motor neuropathies in adults. *J. Neurol* 1999; **246**: 331–333

11. J.P. Sieb. Myasthenia gravis: an update for the clinician. *Clinical and Experimental Immunology* 2013; **175**: 408–418.

12. D.B. Drachman. Myasthenia gravis. *N Engl J Med* 1994; **330**: 1797–1810.

13. R. Bitzur, H. Cohen, Y. Kamai, D. Harats. Intolerance to statins: mechanisms and management. *Diabetes Care* 2013; **36**: S325–S330.

14. A.F. Macedo, F.C. Taylor, J.P. Casas, et al. Unintended effects of statins from observational studies in the general population: systematic review and meta-analysis. *BMC Medicine* 2014; **12**: 51–64.

15. J.W. Mold, S.K. Vesely, B.A. Keyl. The prevalence, predictors, and consequences of peripheral sensory neuropathy in older patients. *J Am Board Fam Pract* 2004; **17**: 309–318.

16. K.K. Hreib, H.R. Jones. Clinical Neurologic Evaluation. In: Jones H.R., ed. *Netter's Neurology.* New Jersey, Icon Learning Systems, 2005; 2–39.

17. C.R. Hoffman Snyder, B.E. Smith. Common Peripheral Neuropathies in the Older Adult. In: Sirven J.I., Malamut B.L., eds. *Clinical Neurology of the Older Adult.* 2nd Edition. Philadelphia, Lippincott Williams and Wilkins, 2008; 402–419.

18. M. Zawora, T.W. Liang, H. Jarra. Neurological Problems in the Elderly. In: Arenson S., Busby-Whitehead J., Brummel-Smith K., et al., eds. *Reichel's Care of the Elderly: Clinical Aspects of Aging.* 6th Edition. New York, Cambridge University Press, 2009; 140–170.

19. Centers for Disease Control and Prevention. *National Diabetes Statistics Report: Estimates of Diabetes and Its Burden in the United States, 2014.* Atlanta, GA: US Department of Health and Human Services; 2014. Available at: www.cdc.gov/diabetes/pubs/statsre port14/national-diabetes-report-web.pdf (accessed August 3, 2014).

20. G. Charnogursky, H. Lee, N. Lopez. Diabetic neuropathy. *Handbook of Clinical Neurology* 2014; **120**: 773–785.

21. K.E. Schmader. Epidemiology and impact on quality of life of postherpetic neuralgia and painful diabetic neuropathy. *Clinical Journal of Pain* 2002; **18**: 350–354.

22. D. Lacomis. Small-fiber neuropathy. *Muscle and Nerve* 2002; **26**: 173–188.

23. T.H. Brannagan, L.H. Weimer, N. Latov. Acquired Neuropathies. In: Rowland L.P., ed. *Merritt's Neurology.* 11th Edition. Philadelphia, Lippincott Williams and Wilkins, 2005; 748–767.

24. N. Ghaznawi, A. Virdi, A. Dayan, et al. Herpes zoster ophthalmicus: comparison of disease in patients 60 years and older versus younger than 60 years. *Ophthalmology* 2011; **118**: 2242–2250.

25. J.W. Gnann, R.J. Whitley. Herpes zoster. *N Engl J Med* 2002; **347**: 340–346.

26. A.H. Eldar, J. Chapman. Guillain-Barré syndrome and other immune mediated neuropathies: diagnosis and classification. *Autoimmunity Reviews* 2014; **13**: 525–530.

27. M. Mahdi-Rogers, R.A. Hughes. Epidemiology of chronic inflammatory neuropathies in southeast England. *European Journal of Neurology* 2014; **21**: 28–33.

28. M. Lijima, H. Koike, N. Nattori, et al. Prevalence and incidence rates of chronic inflammatory demyelinating polyneuropathy in the Japanese population. *J Neurol Neurosurgery Psychiatry* 2008; **79(9)**: 1040–1043.

29. S.K. Rigler. Alcoholism in the elderly. *American Family Physician* 2000; **61**: 1710–1716.

30. M. Mellion, J.M. Gilchrist, S. De La Monte. Alcohol-related peripheral neuropathy: nutritional, toxic, or both? *Muscle and Nerve* 2011; **43**: 309–316.

31. N. Kumar. Neurologic aspects of cobalamin (B12) deficiency. *Handbook of Clinical Neurology* 2014; **120**: 915–926.

32. R. Nemni, E. Gerosa, G. Piccolo, G. Merlinii. Neuropathies associated with monoclonal Gammopathies. *Haematologica* 1994; **79**: 557–566.

33. R. Pop-Busui, L. Roberts, S. Pennathur, et al. The management of diabetic neuropathy in CKD. *Am J Kidney Dis* 2010; **55**: 365–385

34. R.H. Dworkin, A.B. O'Connor, M. Backonja, et al. Pharmacologic management of neuropathic pain:

evidence-based recommendations. *Pain* 2007; **132**: 237–251.

35. I. Laccheo, E. Ablah, R. Heinrichs, et al. Assessment of quality of life among the elderly with epilepsy. *Epilepsy Behav* 2008; **12**: 257–261.

36. L.J. Stephen, M.J. Brodie. Epilepsy in elderly people. *Lancet* 2000; **355**: 1441–1446.

37. I.E. Leppik, A.K. Birnbaum. Epilepsy in the elderly. *Annals of the New York Academy of Sciences* 2010; **1184**: 208–224.

38. R.E. Ramsay, A.J. Rowan, F.M. Pryor. Special considerations in treating the elderly patient with epilepsy. *Neurology* 2004; **62**: S24–9.

39. F. Huying, S. Limpe, K.J. Werhahn. Antiepileptic drug use in nursing home residents: a cross-sectional, regional study. *Seizure* 2006; **15**: 194–197

40. N.A. Hardie, J. Garrard, C.R. Gross, et al. The validity of epilepsy or seizure documentation in nursing homes. *Epilepsy Research* 2007; **74**: 171–175.

41. M.J. Brodie, K. Kelly, L.J. Stephen. Prospective adults with new antiepileptic drugs in focal epilepsy: insights into population responses? *Epilepsy and Behavior* 2014; **31**: 73–76.

42. H. Wallace, S. Shorwon, R. Tallis. Age-specific incidence and prevalence rates of treated epilepsy in an unselected population of 2,052,922 and age-specific fertility rates of women with epilepsy. *Lancet* 1998; **352**: 1970–73.

43. C.F. Bladin, A.V. Alexandrov, A. Bellavance, et al. Seizures after stroke: a prospective multicenter study. *Arch Neurol* 2000; **57**: 1617–1622.

44. M.J. Brodie, A.T. Elder, P. Kwan. Epilepsy in later life. *Lancet Neurol* 2009; **8**: 1019–30.

45. P. Imfeld, M. Bodmer, M. Schuerch, et al. Seizures in patients with Alzheimer's disease or vascular dementia: a population-based nested case control analysis. *Epilepsia* 2013; **54**: 700–707.

46. M.C. Irizarry, S. Jin, F. He, et al. Incidence of new-onset seizures in mild to moderate Alzheimer disease. *Arch Neurol* 2012; **69**: 368–372.

47. D. Sherzai, T. Losey, S. Vega, A. Sherzai. Seizures and dementia in the elderly: nationwide inpatient sample 1999–2008. *Epilepsy and Behavior* 2014; **36**: 53–56.

48. K.A. Vossel, A.J. Beagle, G.D. Rabinovici, et al. Seizures and epileptiform activity in the early stages of Alzheimer disease. *JAMA Neurol* 2013; **70**: 1158–1166.

49. H. Meierkord, M. Holtkamp. Non-convulsive status epilepticus in adults: clinical forms and treatment. *Lancet Neurol* 2007; **6**: 329–339.

50. J. Jirsch, L.J. Hirsch. Nonconvulsive seizures: developing a rational approach to the diagnosis and management in the critically ill population. *Clinical Neurophysiology* 2007; **118**: 1660–1670.

51. A.E. McBride, T.T. Shih, L.J. Hirsch. Video-EEG monitoring in the elderly: a review of 94 patients. *Epilepsia* 2002; **43**: 165.

52. A.J. Rowan, R.E. Ramsay, J.F. Collins, et al. New onset geriatric epilepsy: a randomized study of gabapentin, lamotrigine, and carbamazepine. *Neurology* 2005; **64**: 1868–1873.

53. E. Cumbo, L.D. Ligori. Levitiracetam, lamotrigine, and phenobarbital in patients with epileptic seizures and Alzheimer's disease. *Epilepsy Behavior* 2010; **17**: 461.

54. T. Glauser, E. Ben-Menachem, B. Bourgeois, et al. ILAE treatment guidelines: evidence-based analysis of antiepileptic drug efficacy and effectiveness as initial monotherapy for epileptic seizures and syndromes. *Epilepsia* 2006; **47**: 1094–1120.

55. T. Glauser, E. Ben-Menachem, B. Bourgeois, et al. Updated ILAE evidence review of antiepileptic drug efficacy and effectiveness as initial monotherapy for epileptic seizures and syndromes. *Epilepsia* 2013; **54**: 551–563.

56. L.M. Speechio, L. Tramacere, A. La Neve, E. Beghi. Discontinuing antiepileptic drugs in patients who are seizure free on monotherapy. *J Neurol, Neurosurg Psychiatry* 2002; **72**: 22–25.

57. M.S. Robbins, R.B. Lipton. Management of headache in the elderly. *Drugs Aging* 2010; **27**: 377–398.

58. J. Schwaiger, S. Kiechl, K. Seppi, et al. Prevalence of primary headaches and cranial neuralgias in men and women aged 55–94 years (Bruneck Study). *Cephalagia* 2009; **29**: 179–187.

59. R.A. Walker, M.C. Wadman. Headache in the elderly. *Clin Geriatr Med* 2007; **23**: 291–305.

60. M. Prencipe, A. Casini, C. Ferretti, et al. Prevalence of headache in an elderly population: attack frequency, disability and use of medication. *J Neurol Neurosurg Psychiatry* 2001; **70**: 377–81.

61. T. Pringsheim, J. Davenport, W. Becker. Prophylaxis of migraine headache. *CMAJ* 2010; **182**: E269–276.

62. A. Charles. The evolution of a migraine attack – a review of recent evidence. *Headache* 2013; **53**: 413–419.

63. C.C. Bamford, M. Mays, S.J. Tepper. Unusual headaches in the elderly. *Curr Pain Headache Rep* 2011; **15**: 295–301.

64. A. Özge. Chronic daily headache in the elderly. *Curr Pain Headache Rep* 2013; **17**: 382–389.

65. C.M. Weyand, J.J. Goronzy. Giant-cell arteritis and polymalgia rheumatica. *N Engl J Med* 2014; **371**: 50–57

66. T.A. Kermani, J.S. Schmidt, C.S. Crowson, et al. Utility of erythrocyte sedimentation rate and C-reactive protein for the diagnosis of giant cell arteritis. *Semin Arthritis Rheum* 2012; **41**: 866–871.

67. E.S. Kristoffersen, C. Lundqvist. Medication-overuse headache: epidemiology, diagnosis and treatment. *TherAdv Drug Saf.* 2014; **5**: 87–99.

68. D.W. Dodick, D.J. Capobianco. Headaches. In: Sirven J.I., Malamut B.L., eds. *Clinical Neurology of the Older Adult.* 2nd Edition. Philadelphia, Lippincott Williams and Wilkins, 2008; 197–212.

Chapter 16

Prevention, diagnosis, and management of stroke and TIA in the elderly

Ana C. G. Felix, MBBCh

Introduction

Stroke is the leading cause of physical and cognitive disability in the United States and the fourth leading cause of death.[1–3] Strokes occur across all continents, age groups, and socioeconomic groups, but are much more common in those over age 65.[4]

Although the term "stroke" is generally understood to reflect a sudden and abrupt onset of neurological symptoms and signs that correspond to an underlying vascular etiology, only in recent years has the definition been updated to reflect trends in neuroimaging and histopathology. Stroke is defined as an episode of loss of neurological function due to a *focal infarction* of the brain, spinal cord, or retina. [5] This term includes ischemic stroke and all types of intracerebral hemorrhage (ICH), including subdural hemorrhage (SDH) and subarachnoid hemorrhage (SAH).

In the 1960s, the term "transient ischemic attack" (TIA) came into use, to separate patients who had brief and self-limited neurological symptoms from those who had more prolonged neurological deficits. The definition of TIA was updated in 2009 to reflect that TIA is a transient episode of neurological dysfunction caused by focal ischemia of the brain, spinal cord, or retina *without acute infarction*.[6] These updated definitions highlight the importance of a tissue-based diagnosis of infarction, rather than a purely clinical diagnosis, for both stroke and TIA.

Epidemiology

There are approximately 800,000 strokes annually in the United States. Half of these occur in people who are 75 or older,[2] while only 34% of hospitalized patients with stroke are under age 65.[6] In the United States alone, there are approximately 7 million stroke survivors, and this number is likely to increase

due to a combination of an increasingly aging population and declining stroke mortality.[7] The cost of caring for stroke patients in the United States alone is estimated at $38.6 billion annually.[1]

There has been a decrease in the incidence of stroke since 1987, with the biggest decline occurring in patients above age 65.[2] Between 2000 and 2010, the relative rates of stroke death fell by 35.8%, while the actual number of stroke deaths fell by almost 23%. [2] While there are likely many reasons for this change, one factor is the improved management of modifiable vascular risk factors. However, despite the improvement in overall stroke incidence, mortality continues unchanged in the older population. The higher mortality in the elderly may be driven partly by early withdrawal of care,[8] as well as the increased use of advance directives in hospitalized patients over the last decade.[8–10]

Stroke types

Stroke is a heterogeneous disorder with many causes. [5] Management of the stroke itself and prevention of future strokes relies on establishing the mechanism of the stroke and reducing triggers for stroke recurrence.

Approximately 85% of all strokes are ischemic strokes, and 15% of all strokes are hemorrhagic strokes (including intracerebral, subarachnoid, and subdural hemorrhages). Hemorrhagic strokes are more likely to be fatal than ischemic strokes.[11]

Efforts to understand causes of stroke have led to two major classification systems for ischemic stroke. Although not interchangeable, both classification systems have been validated, particularly in categorizing stroke into large vessel, small vessel, and cardioembolic.[12] The Trial of Org 10172 in Acute Stroke Treatment (TOAST) classification is outlined in Table 16.1.[13] The Causative Classification of

Reichel's Care of the Elderly, 7th Edition, ed. Jan Busby-Whitehead *et al.* Published by Cambridge University Press.
© Cambridge University Press 2016.

Table 16.1 TOAST classification of subtypes of acute ischemic stroke

Large artery atherosclerosis

Cardioembolism

Small vessel occlusion

Stroke of other determined etiology

Stroke of undetermined etiology:
- Two or more causes identified
- Negative evaluation
- Incomplete evaluation

Table 16.2 ABCD2 criteria for TIA risk stratification

Criteria	Details	Points
Age	More than 60 years	1
Blood pressure	More than 140/90 at initial presentation	1
Clinical features	Weakness Aphasia/speech disruption	21
Duration of episode	10–59 minutes 60 minutes or more	12
Diabetes	History of diabetes	1

Stroke System (CSS) is an online database that uses an evidence-based algorithm that provides both causative and phenotypic stroke subtypes (css.mgh.harvard.edu).[14]

Transient ischemic attack

Approximately 240,000 adults experience a TIA in the United States every year, and evidence suggests a very high risk for adverse events afterward. TIAs are stroke-events that resolve spontaneously, without persistent neurological dysfunction or magnetic resonance imaging (MRI) evidence for infarction.[15,16]

The diagnosis of stroke and TIA has shifted from a time-based to a tissue-based diagnosis, requiring imaging for confirmation. Early on after the symptom onset, computerized tomography (CT) scanning does not usually reveal ischemic changes, but is very sensitive to identification of hemorrhagic stroke. CT scan is still recommended as the first imaging modality in the acute presentation of symptoms suggestive of stroke and TIA. MRI is more sensitive to identification of ischemic brain tissue,[17] but it is not always feasible, particularly in the elderly population, due to unstable clinical symptoms, claustrophobia, or presence of pacemakers or other devices, among other factors.

In one population-based study, the risk for ischemic stroke during the six months following a TIA was 17%,[18] with the highest risk of recurrent TIA or stroke occurring in the first two days (6%). These data have been reproduced in several studies, suggesting the TIA be considered the "unstable angina" of the brain. TIA events represent an opportunity to identify risk factors, such as intermittent atrial fibrillation. Modification of risk factors will reduce future risk for recurrent TIA or stroke.

Risk stratification for TIA

After the initial presentation with TIA symptoms, the ABCD2 criteria (Table 16.2) can be used in the clinical setting to identify patients at high risk for stroke, using clinical data obtained at the time of the initial clinical assessment.[15, 17, 19] The ABCD2 criteria can also be useful in identifying patients likely to require hospitalization rather than an expedited outpatient evaluation, due to elevated risk for stroke in the near future. For example, a total ABCD2 score of 6–7 is associated with an 8% risk for stroke in the 48 hours after the TIA.

It is reasonable to hospitalize patients who present with symptoms suggestive of TIA, if they present within 72 hours of the TIA event *and* any of the following criteria are present:

1. ABCD2 score of 3 or higher
2. ABCD2 score of 0–2 and uncertainty that diagnostic workup can be completed within two days as an outpatient
3. ABCD2 score of 0–2 and other evidence that indicates the patient's event was caused by focal ischemia

Risk factors for stroke and TIA

Stroke and TIA are known to be associated with risk factors that often overlap for atherosclerosis and heart disease and are typically described in two categories: "modifiable" risk factors (those risk factors that may be altered with some intervention) and "nonmodifiable" risk factors (those risk factors which cannot be altered with medication or simple intervention) (see Table 16.3). Since 25% of all strokes are recurrent, identifying the underlying cause for the stroke, and

Table 16.3 Risk factors for ischemic stroke

Modifiable	Nonmodifiable
Atrial fibrillation	Older age
Hypertension	Gender
Heart disease	Genetics (e.g., ethnicity, sickle cell disease)
Hyperlipidemia	
Diabetes	
Obesity	
Tobacco use	
Alcohol abuse	
Less well identified: • Hyperhomocysteinemia • Stress • Sleep apnea	

associated modifiable risk factors, may provide opportunities to reduce the risk for future stroke events.

Identification and management of modifiable risk factors is a key factor in stroke prevention and is discussed in detail later in this chapter.

Of the nonmodifiable risk factors, age is the most important. Stroke affects people over the age of 65 more so than any other group.[20] Gender and genetics are the other two significant nonmodifiable risk factors, with notable racial and ethnic disparities in stroke incidence and outcome. Socioeconomic factors also affect stroke risk and are not easily modifiable.

There is a higher incidence of stroke in African-American men in the United States; they also have poorer outcomes after stroke.[7] Similar disparities have been found in ethnic minorities in Europe.[21] There is a higher rate of major cardiovascular events in low-income countries and rural communities despite the fact that these countries have a lower risk-factor burden. Additionally, case fatality rates after major cardiovascular events are highest in low-income countries and rural areas, although the risk-factor burden is higher in urban communities than in the rural communities.[4]

Sickle cell disease (SCD) is associated with increased ischemic stroke risk in children and young adults. As longevity increases for those who have sickle cell disease, the risk for stroke increases again after age 29; however, there is very little data on the treatment of older adults with SCD, with most data extrapolated from the pediatric experience.[22, 23]

Hemorrhagic stroke

Hemorrhagic strokes represent a heterogeneous group of conditions, including intracerebral, subarachnoid, subdural, epidural, and intraventricular hemorrhage.

Risk factors for hemorrhagic stroke

Trauma is a major risk factor for hemorrhagic strokes of all types, more so in elderly and frail patients because of their high rate of falls.

Hypertension increases the risk for spontaneous intracerebral hemorrhage. However, hypertension treatment itself presents a challenge in the elderly patient and requires careful weighing of risk and benefit, as antihypertensive medications increase the risk of falls in elderly patients.[24, 25]

In contrast to these long-term data regarding stroke risk, reducing blood pressure aggressively in the setting of acute intracerebral hemorrhage has been considered an opportunity to reduce hematoma size, but there remains no clear association with improved neurological function or outcomes.[11]

Another risk factor for hemorrhagic stroke in the elderly is medications, particularly anticoagulants and antiplatelet drugs.

Stroke prevention

Prevention of stroke is the key element in preventing stroke-related disability and should focus on the modifiable risk factors, previously discussed and outlined in Table 16.3. Almost a quarter of all strokes are recurrent strokes and are associated with twice the probability of death as well as increased cardiovascular complications compared to first-ever stroke.[26]

A reasonable strategy for the clinical management of patients presenting with TIA or stroke is to try to identify the stroke type and subtype, followed by a careful analysis of their individual risk factors, a process referred to as risk stratification (as described in the section on TIA). This allows for targeted opportunities to reduce modifiable risk factors.[27] (See Table 16.3.)

In addition to obtaining a detailed clinical history, a baseline assessment of blood pressure (BP) at the time of hospital discharge is important, since BP is elevated initially after stroke and may return to normal within a few days of the stroke. Screening fasting lipid profile and glucose at the time of the event is also reasonable. A drug history is also important since anticoagulants and antiplatelet drugs are associated with elevated risk for hemorrhagic stroke, and atypical antipsychotics are associated with increased ischemic stroke risk.[28]

For some risk factors, such as hyperhomocysteneimia, which may be associated with increased risk for ischemic stroke, there is no recommendation for routine screening. Furthermore, it remains unclear whether reducing the levels of homocysteine with supplementation of folate, vitamin B6, and vitamin B12 reduces future stroke risk.[27]

High levels of chronic stress, depressive symptoms, and higher levels of hostility are associated with higher stroke and TIA risk, independent of other risk factors. Assessing for depression and stress in elderly patients may provide additional opportunities for reducing risk factor burden.[29, 30]

Atrial fibrillation

Atrial fibrillation (AF) is the most common sustained cardiac arrhythmia, occurring in 1%–2% of the general population, with an increased prevalence with age. The prevalence of atrial fibrillation in those over age 65 is 5%, and 10% in people over 80 years of age.[31–33] Factors associated with atrial fibrillation include age, hypertension, diabetes, cardiomyopathy, chronic obstructive pulmonary disease, obesity, and sleep apnea, most of which overlap with other vascular and stroke risk factors, as outlined in Table 16.3.

Cryptogenic stroke is defined as ischemic stroke of undetermined cause and accounts for approximately 20%–40% of ischemic strokes. Atrial fibrillation can be intermittent and asymptomatic, thus creating a challenge for diagnosis. Although AF is identified in about 15% of strokes,[31] it is suspected in older patients with cryptogenic stroke. The importance of identifying the presence of AF in cryptogenic stroke is self-evident, given the risk associated with anticoagulation therapy. Particularly in elderly patients, anticoagulation is not indicated for secondary stroke prevention unless there is clear evidence for AF. In addition, strokes in patients with AF are associated with higher morbidity and mortality than those without AF.[32, 33]

The use of prolonged cardiac monitoring increases the likelihood of finding AF and should be considered within six months of a cryptogenic stroke or TIA in patients over age 65.[27, 34, 35] There are many strategies and devices to detect paroxysmal AF. Although the mode and duration of enhanced electrocardiogram (ECG) monitoring remains under investigation, noninvasive ambulatory ECG monitoring for 30 days increases the detection of paroxysmal atrial fibrillation by a factor of 5, as compared to standard 24-hour ECG monitoring.[36, 37]

The risk for stroke related to paroxysmal AF appears to be similar to the risk with chronic AF and atrial flutter. Nonvalvular AF confers an increased stroke risk of two to seven times that of patients without AF, whereas rheumatic AF confers a risk up to 17 times higher than in those without the disease and five times higher than nonvalvular AF.

The decision to consider anticoagulant or antithrombotic treatment to reduce stroke risk should be balanced against the risk of bleeding, cost of monitoring, and difficulty of monitoring therapy.

Risk stratification provides an estimate of stroke risk without anticoagulants. The CHADS2 score is an acronym for five clinical factors (congestive heart failure, hypertension, age 75 or older, diabetes, and prior stroke or TIA), the presence of which counts as one point, except for stroke or TIA, that count as two points. Patients with a CHADS2 score of 0 are considered low risk for recurrent stroke, and those with scores of 2 or higher are considered high risk for stroke.

The CHA2DS2-VASc score adds female gender, additional age strata, and vascular disease. This enhanced score performs similarly to the CHADS2 score, but considers all women and people aged 65–74 at intermediate risk for stroke, and therefore leads to a larger percentage of patients being considered for anticoagulation therapy.[33]

Antincoagulants

Timing of anticoagulation initiation

Timing of anticoagulation is another important clinical consideration. Although anticoagulants are usually initiated within 14 days after the onset of the neurological symptoms, this may be delayed if there is a concern for hemorrhagic transformation of the ischemic infarct (such as with large infarct size, hemorrhagic transformation on imaging, uncontrolled hypertension, or tendency to hemorrhage).

Selection of an anticoagulant

The selection of an anticoagulant is very individualized, with recent data suggesting that newer anticoagulants are probably as safe as warfarin in the elderly.[38] Combining oral anticoagulation with antiplatelet therapy is not recommended for stroke or TIA prevention, although this combination may be appropriate for other cardiovascular indications.[27] A more detailed discussion of anticoagulants follows later in this chapter. For those patients unable to take oral anticoagulants, aspirin alone is recommended, with the addition of clopidogrel in some patients.[27]

Use of anticoagulants

Overall, the newer anticoagulants appear to be equal in efficacy to conventional therapy and do not cause excess bleeding.[32,39] In particular, the risk for intracranial hemorrhage, which is related to age, is reduced by the new anticoagulants relative to warfarin, making newer agents particularly attractive for older patients. In addition, warfarin remains the only oral anticoagulant that can be reversed, if necessary.

Vitamin K antagonists: warfarin

Vitamin K antagonists, such as warfarin, have been used for many years and reduce stroke risk by 68% and overall mortality by 33%, with the recommended target international normalized ratio (INR) of 2.0–3.0. [33] However, warfarin carries significant potential for drug–drug interactions, and dietary interactions create a significant burden for monitoring and dose adjustment. However, a major advantage of warfarin is in the potential for reversibility using fresh frozen plasma (FFP), Vitamin K and, more recently prothrombin complex concentrates (PCCs). This is particularly important in the setting of emergency management of patients with bleeding complications or the need for intervention that may require reversing anticoagulation effects.[40] RFVIIa is not recommended as a solo agent to reverse anticoagulation, although it can shorten the measured INR.[40]

Direct thrombin inhibitors: dabigatran

Dabigatran is the only oral direct thrombin inhibitor available since ximelagatran was withdrawn from the market due to hepatotoxicity. It features twice daily dosing that does not require coagulation monitoring, lower rates of ischemic stroke, and a lower intracranial hemorrhage risk.[33] Issues that remain under review are overall cost and risk for use in those with renal insufficiency (a major factor in the older adult population), who require lower-dose therapy. Furthermore, as previously outlined, there is no known agent that allows reversibility of anticoagulation effects, particularly in the emergency management of older adults.

Oral factor Xa agents

Rivaroxaban and apixaban directly inhibit factor Xa, which is the enzyme that converts prothrombin to active thrombin (similar to low-molecular-weight heparin). There are other agents under development, including edoxaban and betrixaban, with pending efficacy data at the time of writing. These drugs do not require monitoring, but require lower dosing in patients with renal insufficiency. Unlike warfarin, this drug does not have a known antidote or agent for reversibility of anticoagulation effects.

Antiplatelet therapy

Antiplatelet agents are effective in stroke risk reduction, with aspirin conferring approximately 20% reduction in stroke risk but associated with slightly increased bleeding risk. There is debate regarding the optimal dosing of aspirin, but it generally ranges between 81 mg and 325 mg. There is a lack of evidence indicating superior efficacy with higher doses.

As described earlier in the chapter, there may be a role for using aspirin or other antiplatelet agents along with full-dose warfarin in some patients with indications such as atrial fibrillation and coronary artery disease or coronary stenting. However, antiplatelet and anticoagulant agents are among the most frequent cause of adverse drug-event-related hospitalizations.[41] Dual antiplatelet therapy combining the use of aspirin and clopidogrel has been associated with slightly increased risk for hemorrhagic complications, although there appears to be benefit to the early use of this combination after an ischemic stroke or TIA, particularly in patients with carotid disease TIA.[42–44]

Blood pressure for risk modification

Normalizing blood pressure (BP) is an important factor in long-term risk reduction for stroke and other vascular diseases. However, following an acute ischemic stroke, 80% of patients will have elevated BP with a spontaneous return to baseline within days, and the timing and degree of BP lowering after acute stroke, particularly hemorrhagic stroke, remains under investigation.[45] The benefit must be weighed against the risk of recurrent falls in those over the age of 70 associated with antihypertensive medications in all classes.[24, 25]

Current guidelines recommend the initiation of BP therapy for previously untreated patients with ischemic stroke or TIA who, after the first several days, have an established systolic blood pressure of 140 mmHg or higher or diastolic blood pressure of 90 or higher. The benefit of reducing BP lower than that is of unclear benefit and may be risky in older adults. In patients with an established diagnosis of hypertension, BP therapy should be re-initiated after the first few days, although the BP target is not clear. The routine use of beta blockers to lower stroke recurrence for secondary prevention has not been demonstrated to be effective.[46]

Myocardial infarction and cardiomyopathy in stroke

Stroke following acute anterior myocardial infarction is more frequently associated with anterior apical akinesis or dyskinesia on echocardiography, left ventricular mural thrombus, or anterior or apical wall-motion abnormalities with a left ventricular ejection fraction of less than 40%. In these patients, anticoagulation (or low-molecular-weight heparin) for three months may be reasonable to prevent recurrence of ischemic stroke or TIA.

Valvular heart disease

In patients with rheumatic mitral valve disease and AF who present with stroke or TIA, long-term anticoagulation is indicated, with INR target 2.5. In the absence of AF but with no evidence for another cause of symptoms such as carotid disease, long-term use of anticoagulation is reasonable rather than antiplatelet therapy. If the ischemic stroke or TIA occurs in the setting of appropriate anticoagulation, adding aspirin is reasonable. Antiplatelets are also recommended for those who do not have an indication for anticoagulation, including mitral valve prolapse.

Patent foramen ovale

The presence of patent foramen ovale (PFO) is associated with higher risk for stroke, although closure of PFO in young (less than 65 years of age) patients with

stroke or TIA has not been associated with improved outcomes. The use of antiplatelets is reasonable unless there is evidence for venous thromboembolism, in which case either anticoagulation or an inferior vena cava filter may be reasonable. In patients with PFO and deep venous thrombosis (DVT), closure may be considered, depending on risk for recurrent DVT.[47]

Mechanical closure

Embolization from the left atrial appendage remains a concern, although closure of the appendage using devices remains under investigation.

Lipid lowering

Current American Heart Association (AHA) guidelines recommend the initiation of statin therapy for patients with recent stroke or TIA whose LCL-C is greater than 100 mg/dL. However, most studies of lipid lowering have either not been validated in the elderly, or their use is predicated upon long-term use with questionable translation of benefit to an elderly population.[48, 49] The use of statins in elderly people, in particular, presents a significantly increased burden of liver enzyme abnormalities,[50] myalgias, and concerns about adverse cognitive effects.[51, 52]

Glycemic control and stroke

All patients who present with TIA or stroke should be screened for diabetes.[27] Increased glucose levels within 24 hours of hypertensive spontaneous intracerebral hemorrhage correlate with poorer outcomes.[53] Diagnosis of diabetes or pre-diabetes following acute ischemic stroke is associated with poor long-term outcomes and a higher risk for recurrent stroke.[54, 55]

Obesity and physical inactivity

All patients with stroke or TIA should have a body mass index (BMI) calculation. Obesity is an increasing problem across all age groups, although weight fluctuations appear to be greater in the older adult.[56] Physical inactivity and poor nutrition remain a major concern in older people, often compounded by comorbid and social conditions, and may impact recovery after stroke.

Carotid disease

Carotid revascularization in symptomatic carotid stenosis should be considered for all patients to reduce stroke risk. Carotid endarterectomy (CEA) and carotid artery stenting (CAS) have been found equally effective carotid revascularization procedures.

Although there are several factors when selecting a procedure, it is clear that only operators with established periprocedural stroke and mortality rates of less than 6% should perform the procedures for symptomatic patients. Both surgeons and interventionalists need to be rigorously trained to minimize the pitfalls of learning curve on outcomes of patients undergoing either procedure.

The North American Symptomatic Carotid Endarterectomy Trial (NASCET) demonstrated that patients older than 75 years of age benefited more from CEA than younger patients, due to high risk for ipsilateral stroke in the medical therapy arm. [57] However, medical therapy has changed outcomes in the intervening time since the NASCET publication in 2001.

The Carotid Revascularization Stenting versus Endarterectomy for Treatment of Carotid-Artery Stenosis (CREST) trial discontinued enrollment of patients over the age of 80 due to the higher rate of complications associated with this age group.[58] A recent meta-analysis suggests that carotid artery stenting carries an increased risk for stroke in older adults, while mortality (at least in the short term) is equivalent to younger patients. CAS should only be considered in older adults if the risk for surgery is very high or unacceptable.[59, 60] Carotid endarterectomy is associated with increased mortality but similar stroke outcomes when compared to younger patients.[61]

Routine long-term follow-up imaging of the extracranial carotid circulation with carotid duplex ultrasonography is *not recommended*.

Intracranial stenosis

For patients with recent TIA or stroke attributable to severe stenosis (70%–99%) of a major intracranial artery, the addition of clopidogrel 75 mg/d to aspirin for 90 days may be reasonable. In addition, maintaining systolic BP below 140 mmHg and initiating high-intensity statin therapy may reduce stroke recurrence risk. Endovascular intervention of intracranial vessels, particularly for patients failing medical therapy, remains under investigation, and the use of warfarin offers no benefit over antiplatelet therapy.[27, 62]

Sleep apnea

Sleep disordered breathing and sleep apnea are emerging risk factors for stroke, associated with two to three times higher risk for stroke, poorer outcome after stroke, higher rate of stroke recurrence, and overall higher health care utilization in elderly patients.[63] The use of over-the-counter and prescription sleep medications is also associated with higher risk for stroke and mortality in older adults, although the mechanisms are unclear.[64] Screening for and treatment of sleep-disordered breathing in elderly patients may help reduce risk and cost of care; however, there are no data regarding outcomes in treatment of sleep apnea in older adults.[65, 66]

Aortic arch atheroma

The use of antiplatelet therapy and statin therapy is recommended in patients with aortic arch atheroma who present with stroke or TIA.

Treatment of ischemic stroke

Treatment of ischemic stroke currently revolves around defining the time of onset of stroke symptoms. Onset of symptoms is defined as the time the patient was last known to be normal. In situations where the patient wakes up with symptoms, the time the patient was last normal will be the time he or she went to sleep, feeling normal. In patients with symptoms of longer than three hours in duration prior to presentation, standard treatment consists of supportive care, prevention of complications, rehabilitation, and secondary prevention of future events. If symptoms began within three hours of arrival to medical evaluation, consideration should be given to intravenous thrombolytic therapy (Alteplase, recombinant tPA, or rtPA).[67]

Role of thrombolytics in older adults with acute ischemic stroke

The original study that led to FDA approval of intravenous thrombolytic therapy in acute ischemic stroke excluded patients over the age of 80. Since then, data has shown that rtPA can be administered safely in patients who are over the age of 80, and there is no difference in the rates of neurological improvement in elderly and nonelderly patients or males and females. This would suggest that all patients representing with ischemic stroke symptoms within three hours of onset should receive thrombolysis.[68–70]

Stroke rehabilitation and recovery

The treatment of stroke must focus on both recovery and rehabilitation of neurological function as well as prevention of complications, including immobility, swallowing difficulties, and medication side effects. Stroke recovery is challenging, more so in the elderly patient who may have preexisting mobility or cognitive impairments and a higher rate of comorbid medical conditions. There are estimated to be over seven million stroke survivors in the United States alone.[7] Addressing the impact of stroke-related disability, particularly in the elderly, is an increasingly complex challenge, particularly given the increasing aging population coupled with reduced stroke mortality.[2]

A single study describes outcome 10 years after first-ever stroke. In this study, more than half the patients were older than 75. Of the 35% ischemic stroke survivors who survived for 10 years, 68% lived independently and 14% had major dependence for all activities of daily living (ADL). This suggests that elderly patients have the potential for recovery and long-term survival after stroke.[71]

Non-Hispanic black people have twice the number of strokes as non-Hispanic white people. However, it appears that in the United States, older black people also have greater disability related to their strokes than white people, including difficulties with self-care, mobility, and household activities.[7]

Gastrointestinal complications after stroke

Gastrointestinal complications after stroke are common and contribute significantly to morbidity and mortality.[72] Dysphagia is the most common gastrointestinal complication following stroke (particularly ischemic stroke) and is associated with post-stroke malnutrition and pneumonia, a major cause of post-stroke mortality.[73] Aggressive screening for dysphagia is warranted to minimize the risk for associated complications, with clear guidelines established by both the American Heart Association and the Joint Commission to ensure that all stroke and TIA patients are screened appropriately.

Impaired gastrointestinal motility is another common complication following ischemic stroke, which increases risk for aspiration, vomiting, and feeding tube failure as well as reduced drug absorption.[72]

Other complications include constipation and fecal incontinence, which impact quality of life after stroke. Up to 80% of post-stroke survivors who live in skilled nursing facilities have constipation, and screening for fecal incontinence should be considered.[74] Treatment should include common-sense conservative measures and reducing anticholinergic and other drugs

Gastrointestinal bleeding is associated with poor outcome after stroke and is present in up to 8% of stroke patients. Although the cause remains unclear, factors such as stress, prior history of peptic ulcer disease, *H. pylori* infection, cancer, stroke severity, and aspirin use have been implicated.[72]

Venous thromboembolism

Venous thromboembolism (VTE) includes both deep venous thrombosis (DVT) and pulmonary embolus (PE), occurring in approximately 3% of hospitalized patients with stroke.[75] The use of low-molecular-weight heparin (LMWH) or unfractionated heparin (UFH) is more effective than aspirin and/or intermittent pneumatic compression in preventing VTE.[76]

Fever

Fever occurs in up to half of patients after stroke and is associated with an increased morbidity and mortality.[77]

Long-term complications of stroke

Depression

Depression is very common in elderly people, estimated to range from 25% to 37%.[78] The geriatric depression score (GDS) appears to yield reliable and reproducible results in this population. A score of 5 or more supports a diagnosis of depression. Suicidal ideation has been reported in 7%–15% of stroke patients and is associated with depression and post-stroke apathy.[79–81] Up to 50% of people who survive a stroke will become depressed. Depression impacts recovery, severity of impairment, and disability. Depression post-stroke also contributes to lower quality of life and increased use of health care resources. Treatment appears to be more effective when multifaceted, including counselling of patient and caregivers as well as providing both psychosocial and physiological support, including antidepressants.[79–81]

Urinary incontinence

Forty to sixty percent of patients admitted to a hospital after strokes have some form of urinary incontinence (UI). Although this improves over time, up to 37% continue to have symptoms at one year, with the associated increased risk for skin breakdown and urinary tract infection (UTI).[82] This leads to a higher physical, emotional, and economic burden for stroke survivors and their caregivers. There appear to be several contributing mechanisms to post-stroke UI, including disruption of the neuromicturition pathways, cognitive or language deficits, and medication side effects.

Caregiving for stroke

Whereas caregiving of elderly people is a common element in society, the unique nature of stroke is such that the caregiving role is thrust upon loved ones and close relatives very suddenly. Caregivers of older adults with stroke carry a greater burden, regardless of socioeconomic status, due to factors that may include differences in acute medical care and rehabilitation care, as well as preferences for care on the part of patients and their families.[83]

End-of-life decision making

Understanding the outcomes of stroke may be helpful when guiding patients and caregivers in the process of decision making after a stroke event. Living with multiple chronic conditions, including stroke, has a negative impact on life expectancy. Life expectancy is reduced by an average of 1.8 years with each additional chronic condition. This appears consistent across age and gender, but not across ethnicity.[84]

In general, very large intracerebral hemorrhages (ICH) and subarachnoid hemorrhages have a very poor prognosis for meaningful neurological recovery, particularly in older persons or patients with prior neurological or comorbid conditions.[85] Up to 50% of patients die in the first month, with only 20% independent at six months.[86] Factors that impact outcomes negatively include advanced age, impaired neurological examination or impaired level of consciousness at presentation, and large hemorrhage size.[85–87]

However, with ischemic stroke, recovery depends on many variables and is largely unpredictable. Consideration should be given to rates of complications; for example, if a patient develops aspiration pneumonia, the likelihood of returning home is very low.[73]

One area of debate is whether patients with aphasia are less likely to benefit from rehabilitation than those with non-dominant hemispheric strokes. Patients with severe hemi-neglect may recover very poorly and at rates similar to those with severe or global aphasia. This should be taken into account when making decisions about end-of-life care. Another factor to consider is that older patients usually have some degree of global cerebral atrophy and may not succumb to the effects of the stroke in the short term, such as raised intracranial pressure or cerebral edema.

Active decision making rather than passive expectation of death by families and caregivers is important when considering quality of life and end-of-life care.

References

1. Feigin VL, Lawes CM, Bennett DA, Anderson CS. Stroke epidemiology: a review of population-based studies of incidence, prevalence, and case-fatality in the late 20th century. *Lancet Neurol* 2003 Jan;**2**(1):43–53.

2. Koton S, Schneider AL, Rosamond WD, et al. Stroke incidence and mortality trends in US communities, 1987 to 2011. *JAMA* 2014 Jul 16;**312**(3):259–268.

3. Go AS, Mozaffarian D, Roger VL, et al. Executive summary: heart disease and stroke statistics–2014 update: a report from the American Heart Association. *Circulation* 2014 Jan 21;**129**(3):399–410.

4. Yusuf S, Rangarajan S, Teo K, et al. Cardiovascular risk and events in 17 low-, middle-, and high-income countries. *N Engl J Med* 2014 Aug 28;**371**(9):818–827.

5. Sacco RL, Kasner SE, Broderick JP, et al. An updated definition of stroke for the 21st century: a statement for healthcare professionals from the American Heart Association/American Stroke Association. *Stroke* 2013 Jul;**44**(7):2064–2089.

6. Marini C, Baldassarre M, Russo T, et al. Burden of first-ever ischemic stroke in the oldest old: evidence from a population-based study. *Neurology* 2004 Jan 13;**62**(1):77–81.

7. Burke JF, Freedman VA, Lisabeth LD, et al. Racial differences in disability after stroke: results from a nationwide study. *Neurology* 2014 Jul 29;**83**(5):390–397.

8. Kelly AG, Hoskins KD, Holloway RG. Early stroke mortality, patient preferences, and the withdrawal of care bias. *Neurology* 2012 Aug 28;**79**(9):941–944.

9. Qureshi AI, Chaudhry SA, Connelly B, et al. Impact of advanced healthcare directives on treatment decisions by physicians in patients with acute stroke. *Crit Care Med* 2013 Jun;**41**(6):1468–1475.

10. Silveira MJ, Wiitala W, Piette J. Advance directive completion by elderly Americans: a decade of change. *J Am Geriatr Soc* 2014 Apr;**62**(4):706–710.

11. Barber PA, Kleinig TJ. INTERACT2: a reason for optimism with spontaneous intracerebral hemorrhage? *Int J Stroke* 2014 Jan;**9**(1):59–60.

12. McArdle PF, Kittner SJ, Ay H, et al. Agreement between TOAST and CCS ischemic stroke classification: The NINDS SIGN Study. *Neurology* 2014 Oct 28;**83**(18):1653–1660. Epub 2014 Sep 26.

13. Adams HP Jr, Bendixen BH, Kappelle LJ, et al. Classification of subtype of acute ischemic stroke. Definitions for use in a multicenter clinical trial. TOAST. Trial of Org 10172 in Acute Stroke Treatment. *Stroke* 1993 Jan;**24**(1):35–41.

14. Arsava EM, Ballabio E, Benner T, et al. The Causative Classification of Stroke system: an international reliability and optimization study. *Neurology* 2010 Oct 5;**75**(14):1277–1284.

15. Asimos AW, Johnson AM, Rosamond WD, et al. A multicenter evaluation of the ABCD2 score's accuracy for predicting early ischemic stroke in admitted patients with transient ischemic attack. *Ann Emerg Med* 2010 Feb;**55**(2):201–210.e5.

16. Easton JD, Saver JL, Albers GW, et al. Definition and evaluation of transient ischemic attack: a scientific statement for healthcare professionals from the American Heart Association/American Stroke Association Stroke Council; Council on Cardiovascular Surgery and Anesthesia; Council on Cardiovascular Radiology and Intervention; Council on Cardiovascular Nursing; and the Interdisciplinary Council on Peripheral Vascular Disease. The American Academy of Neurology affirms the value of this statement as an educational tool for neurologists. *Stroke* 2009 Jun;**40**(6):2276–2293.

17. Giles MF, Albers GW, Amarenco P, et al. Early stroke risk and ABCD2 score performance in tissue- vs time-defined TIA: a multicenter study. *Neurology* 2011 Sep 27;**77**(13):1222–1228.

18. Kleindorfer D, Panagos P, Pancioli A, et al. Incidence and short-term prognosis of transient ischemic attack in a population-based study. *Stroke* 2005 Apr;**36**(4):720–723.

19. Johnston SC, Gress DR, Browner WS, Sidney S. Short-term prognosis after emergency department diagnosis of TIA. *JAMA* 2000 Dec 13;**284**(22):2901–2906.

20. Rojas JI, Zurru MC, Romano M, et al. Acute ischemic stroke in patients aged 80 or older. *Medicina (B Aires)* 2007;**67**(6 Pt 2):701–704.

21. Agyemang C, van Oeffelen AA, Norredam M, et al. Ethnic disparities in ischemic stroke, intracerebral hemorrhage, and subarachnoid hemorrhage incidence in the Netherlands. *Stroke* 2014 Sep 30;**45**(11):3236–3242.

22. Talahma M, Strbian D, Sundararajan S. Sickle cell disease and stroke. *Stroke* 2014 Jun;**45**(6):e98–e100.

23. Gueguen A, Mahevas M, Nzouakou R, et al. Sickle-cell disease stroke throughout life: a retrospective study in an adult referral center. *Am J Hematol* 2014 Mar;**89**(3):267–272.

24. Tinetti ME, Han L, Lee DS, et al. Antihypertensive medications and serious fall injuries in a nationally representative sample of older adults. *JAMA Intern Med* 2014 Apr;**174**(4):588–595.

25. Aronow WS, Fleg JL, Pepine CJ, et al. ACCF/AHA 2011 expert consensus document on hypertension in the elderly: a report of the American College of Cardiology Foundation Task Force on Clinical Expert Consensus Documents developed in collaboration with the American Academy of Neurology, American Geriatrics Society, American Society for Preventive Cardiology, American Society of Hypertension, American Society of Nephrology, Association of Black Cardiologists, and European Society of Hypertension. *J Am Soc Hypertens* 2011 Jul–Aug;**5**(4):259–352.

26. Gouya G, Arrich J, Wolzt M, et al. Antiplatelet treatment for prevention of cerebrovascular events in patients with vascular diseases: a systematic review and meta-analysis. *Stroke* 2014 Feb;**45**(2):492–503.

27. Kernan WN, Ovbiagele B, Black HR, et al. Guidelines for the prevention of stroke in patients with stroke and transient ischemic attack: a guideline for healthcare professionals from the American Heart Association/American Stroke Association. *Stroke* 2014 Jul;**45**(7):2160–2236.

28. Shin JY, Choi NK, Jung SY, et al. Risk of ischemic stroke with the use of risperidone, quetiapine and olanzapine in elderly patients: a population-based, case-crossover study. *J Psychopharmacol* 2013 Jul;**27**(7):638–644.

29. Everson-Rose SA, Roetker NS, Lutsey PL, et al. Chronic stress, depressive symptoms, anger, hostility, and risk of stroke and transient ischemic attack in the multi-ethnic study of atherosclerosis. *Stroke* 2014 Aug;**45**(8):2318–2323.

30. Lambiase MJ, Kubzansky LD, Thurston RC. Prospective study of anxiety and incident stroke. *Stroke* 2014 Feb;**45**(2):438–443.

31. Helms TM, Duong G, Zippel-Schultz B, et al. Prediction and personalised treatment of atrial fibrillation-stroke prevention: consolidated position paper of CVD professionals. *EPMA J* 2014 Sep 2;**5**(1):15.

32. Coppens M, Hart RG, Eikelboom JW. Stroke prevention in older adults with atrial fibrillation. *CMAJ* 2013 Nov 19;**185**(17):1479–1480.

33. Quinn GR, Fang MC. Atrial fibrillation: stroke prevention in older adults. *Clin Geriatr Med* 2012 Nov;**28**(4):617–634.

34. Moran PS, Flattery MJ, Teljeur C, et al. Effectiveness of systematic screening for the detection of atrial fibrillation. *Cochrane Database Syst Rev* 2013 Apr 30;**4**: CD009586.

35. Sanna T, Diener HC, Passman RS, et al. Cryptogenic stroke and underlying atrial fibrillation. *N Engl J Med* 2014 Jun 26;**370**(26):2478–2486.

36. Gladstone DJ, Spring M, Dorian P, et al. Atrial fibrillation in patients with cryptogenic stroke. *N Engl J Med* 2014 Jun 26;**370**(26):2467–2477.

37. Weber-Kruger M, Gelbrich G, Stahrenberg R, et al. Finding atrial fibrillation in stroke patients: randomized evaluation of enhanced and prolonged Holter monitoring – Find-AF$_{RANDOMISED}$ – rationale and design. *Am Heart J* 2014 Oct;**168**(4):438–445.e1.

38. Halperin JL, Hankey GJ, Wojdyla DM, et al. Efficacy and safety of rivaroxaban compared with warfarin among elderly patients with nonvalvular atrial fibrillation in the Rivaroxaban Once Daily, Oral, Direct Factor Xa Inhibition Compared With Vitamin K Antagonism for Prevention of Stroke and Embolism Trial in Atrial Fibrillation (ROCKET AF). *Circulation* 2014 Jul 8;**130**(2):138–146.

39. Sardar P, Chatterjee S, Chaudhari S, Lip GY. New oral anticoagulants in elderly adults: evidence from a meta-analysis of randomized trials. *J Am Geriatr Soc* 2014 May;**62**(5):857–864.

40. Dzik WS. Reversal of drug-induced anticoagulation: old solutions and new problems. *Transfusion* 2012 May;**52** Suppl 1:45S–55S.

41. Salvi F, Marchetti A, D'Angelo F, et al. Adverse drug events as a cause of hospitalization in older adults. *Drug Saf* 2012 Jan;**35** Suppl 1:29–45.

42. Wang C, Yi X, Zhang B, et al. Clopidogrel plus aspirin prevents early neurologic deterioration and improves 6-month outcome in patients with acute large artery atherosclerosis stroke. *Clin Appl Thromb Hemost* 2015 Jul;**21**(5):453–461. Epub 2014 Sep 23.

43. Wong KS, Chen C, Fu J, et al. Clopidogrel plus aspirin versus aspirin alone for reducing embolisation in patients with acute symptomatic cerebral or carotid artery stenosis (CLAIR study): a randomised, open-label, blinded-endpoint trial. *Lancet Neurol* 2010 May;**9**(5):489–497.

44. Markus HS, Droste DW, Kaps M, et al. Dual antiplatelet therapy with clopidogrel and aspirin in symptomatic carotid stenosis evaluated using doppler embolic signal detection: the clopidogrel and aspirin for reduction of emboli in symptomatic carotid stenosis (CARESS) trial. *Circulation* 2005 May 3;**111**(17):2233–2240.

45. Boan AD, Lackland DT, Ovbiagele B. Lowering of blood pressure for recurrent stroke prevention. *Stroke* 2014 Aug;**45**(8):2506–2513.

46. De Lima LG, Saconato H, Atallah AN, da Silva EM. Beta-blockers for preventing stroke recurrence. *Cochrane Database Syst Rev* 2014 Oct 15;**10**:CD007890.

47. Udell JA, Opotowsky AR, Khairy P, et al. Patent foramen ovale closure vs medical therapy for stroke prevention: meta-analysis of randomized trials and review of heterogeneity in meta-analyses. *Can J Cardiol* 2014 Oct;**30**(10):1216–1224.

48. Kmietowicz Z. Geriatrician questions prescribing for stroke prevention in people over 80. *BMJ* 2014 Feb 26;**348**:g1788.

49. Byatt K. Overenthusiastic stroke risk factor modification in the over-80s: are we being disingenuous to ourselves, and to our oldest patients? *Evid Based Med* 2014 Aug;**19**(4):121–122.

50. Manocha D, Bansal N, Gumaste P, Brangman S. Safety profile of high-dose statin therapy in geriatric patients with stroke. *South Med J* 2013 Dec;**106**(12):658–664.

51. Raley KA, Hutchison AM. Statin use and cognitive changes in elderly patients with dementia. *Consult Pharm* 2014;**29**(7):487–489.

52. Mandas A, Congiu MG, Abete C, et al. Cognitive decline and depressive symptoms in late-life are associated with statin use: evidence from a population-based study of Sardinian old people living in their own home. *Neurol Res* 2014 Mar;**36**(3):247–254.

53. Tapia-Perez JH, Gehring S, Zilke R, Schneider T. Effect of increased glucose levels on short-term outcome in hypertensive spontaneous intracerebral hemorrhage. *Clin Neurol Neurosurg* 2014 Mar;**118**:37–43.

54. Tanaka R, Ueno Y, Miyamoto N, et al. Impact of diabetes and prediabetes on the short-term prognosis in patients with acute ischemic stroke. *J Neurol Sci* 2013 Sep 15;**332**(1–2):45–50.

55. Nardi K, Milia P, Eusebi P, et al. Predictive value of admission blood glucose level on short-term mortality in acute cerebral ischemia. *J Diabetes Complications* 2012 Mar–Apr;**26**(2):70–76.

56. Murphy RA, Patel KV, Kritchevsky SB, et al. Weight change, body composition, and risk of mobility disability and mortality in older adults: a population-based cohort study. *J Am Geriatr Soc* 2014 Aug;**62**(8):1476–1483.

57. Alamowitch S, Eliasziw M, Algra A, et al. Risk, causes, and prevention of ischaemic stroke in elderly patients with symptomatic internal-carotid-artery stenosis. *Lancet* 2001 Apr 14;**357**(9263):1154–1160.

58. Brott TG, Hobson RW 2nd, Howard G, et al. Stenting versus endarterectomy for treatment of carotid-artery stenosis. *N Engl J Med* 2010 Jul 1;**363**(1):11–23.

59. Gonzales NR, Demaerschalk BM, Voeks JH, et al. Complication rates and center enrollment volume in the carotid revascularization endarterectomy versus stenting trial. *Stroke* 2014 Sep 25.

60. Rerkasem K, Rothwell PM. Carotid endarterectomy for symptomatic carotid stenosis. *Cochrane Database Syst Rev* 2011 Apr 13;(4):CD001081.

61. Antoniou GA, Georgiadis GS, Georgakarakos EI, et al. Meta-analysis and meta-regression analysis of outcomes of carotid endarterectomy and stenting in the elderly. *JAMA Surg* 2013 Dec;**148**(12):1140–1152.

62. Kasner SE, Lynn MJ, Chimowitz MI, et al. Warfarin vs aspirin for symptomatic intracranial stenosis: subgroup analyses from WASID. *Neurology* 2006 Oct 10;**67**(7):1275–1278.

63. Birkbak J, Clark AJ, Rod NH. The effect of sleep disordered breathing on the outcome of stroke and transient ischemic attack: a systematic review. *J Clin Sleep Med* 2014 Jan 15;**10**(1):103–108.

64. Petrov ME, Howard VJ, Kleindorfer D, et al. Over-the-counter and Prescription Sleep Medication and Incident Stroke: The REasons for Geographic And Racial Differences in Stroke Study. *J Stroke Cerebrovasc Dis* 2014 Sep;**23**(8):2110–2116.

65. Birkbak J, Clark AJ, Rod NH. The effect of sleep disordered breathing on the outcome of stroke and transient ischemic attack: a systematic review. *J Clin Sleep Med* 2014 Jan 15;**10**(1):103–108.

66. Diaz KM, Booth 3rd JN, Calhoun DA, et al. Healthy lifestyle factors and risk of cardiovascular events and mortality in treatment-resistant hypertension: the reasons for geographic and racial differences in stroke study. *Hypertension* 2014 Sep;**64**(3):465–471.

67. Marler JR. Tissue plasminogen activator for acute ischemic stroke. *N Engl J Med* 1995 Dec 14;**333**(24):1581–1588.

68. Yayan J. Effectiveness of alteplase in the very elderly after acute ischemic stroke. *Clin Interv Aging* 2013;**8**:963–974.

69. Gomez-Choco M, Obach V, Urra X, et al. The response to IV rt-PA in very old stroke patients. *Eur J Neurol* 2008 Mar;**15**(3):253–256.

70. Engelter ST, Bonati LH, Lyrer PA. Intravenous thrombolysis in stroke patients of > or = 80 versus < 80 years of age – a systematic review across cohort studies. *Age Ageing* 2006 Nov;**35**(6):572–580.

71. Jonsson AC, Delavaran H, Iwarsson S, et al. Functional status and patient-reported outcome 10 years after stroke: the Lund Stroke Register. *Stroke* 2014 Jun;**45**(6):1784–1790.

72. Camara-Lemarroy CR, Ibarra-Yruegas BE, Gongora-Rivera F. Gastrointestinal complications after ischemic stroke. *J Neurol Sci* 2014 Aug 28.

73. Martino R, Foley N, Bhogal S, et al. Dysphagia after stroke: incidence, diagnosis, and pulmonary complications. *Stroke* 2005 Dec;**36**(12):2756–2763.

74. Lin CJ, Hung JW, Cho CY, et al. Poststroke constipation in the rehabilitation ward: incidence, clinical course and associated factors. *Singapore Med J* 2013 Nov;**54**(11):624–629.

75. Douds GL, Hellkamp AS, Olson DM, et al. Venous thromboembolism in the Get with the Guidelines-Stroke acute ischemic stroke population: incidence and patterns of prophylaxis. *J Stroke Cerebrovasc Dis* 2014 Jan;**23**(1):123–129.

76. Naccarato M, Chiodo Grandi F, Dennis M, Sandercock PA. Physical methods for preventing deep vein thrombosis in stroke. *Cochrane Database Syst Rev* 2010 Aug 4;**8**:CD001922.

77. Drury P, Levi C, McInnes E, et al. Management of fever, hyperglycemia, and swallowing dysfunction following hospital admission for acute stroke in New South Wales, Australia. *Int J Stroke* 2014 Jan;**9**(1):23–31.

78. Allan LM, Rowan EN, Thomas AJ, et al. Long-term incidence of depression and predictors of depressive symptoms in older stroke survivors. *Br J Psychiatry* 2013 Dec;**203**(6):453–460.

79. Tang WK, Caeiro L, Lau CG, et al. Apathy and suicide-related ideation 3 months after stroke: a cross-sectional study. *BMC Neurol* 2015 Apr 23;**15**(1):60.

80. Santos CO, Caeiro L, Ferro JM, Figueira ML. A study of suicidal thoughts in acute stroke patients. *J Stroke Cerebrovasc Dis* 2012 Nov;**21**(8):749–754.

81. Vallury KD, Jones M, Gray R. Do family-oriented interventions reduce poststroke depression? A systematic review and recommendations for practice. *Top Stroke Rehabil* 2015 Dec;**22**(6):459–465. doi: 10/1179/1074935715Z00000000061. Epub 2015 Mar 28.

82. Cai W, Wang J, Wang L, et al. Prevalence and risk factors of urinary incontinence for post-stroke inpatients in Southern China. *Neurourol Urodyn* 2015;**34**(3):231–235.

83. Gregory P, Edwards L, Faurot K, et al. Patient preferences for stroke rehabilitation. *Top Stroke Rehabil* 2010 Sep–Oct;**17**(5):394–400.

84. DuGoff EH, Canudas-Romo V, Buttorff C, et al. Multiple chronic conditions and life expectancy: a life table analysis. *Med Care* 2014 Aug;**52**(8):688–694.

85. Bilbao G, Garibi J, Pomposo I, et al. A prospective study of a series of 356 patients with supratentorial spontaneous intracerebral haematomas treated in a neurosurgical department. *Acta Neurochir (Wien)* 2005 Aug;**147**(8):823–829.

86. Bhatia R, Singh H, Singh S, et al. A prospective study of in-hospital mortality and discharge outcome in spontaneous intracerebral hemorrhage. *Neurol India* 2013 May–Jun;**61**(3):244–248.

87. Flemming KD, Wijdicks EF, Li H. Can we predict poor outcome at presentation in patients with lobar hemorrhage? *Cerebrovasc Dis* 2001;**11**(3):183–189.

Movement disorders in the elderly

Laura Scorr, MD, Mihai Cosmin Sandulescu, MD, and Tsao-Wei Liang, MD

Tremor

Tremors are the most common movement disorder and occur as a result of dysfunction of the basal ganglia, cerebellum, or the brainstem connections between these systems. Tremors are defined as involuntary, rhythmic, oscillatory movements that can affect any part of the body. Furthermore, they are categorized based upon the type of activity that maximizes the tremor.

Action tremors appear when holding a certain posture (e.g., arms outstretched) or during deliberate targeted movement (e.g., writing, holding a fork) and disappear when the affected body part is relaxed or at rest. A *rest tremor* is observed when the affected body part is supported and completely at rest; for example, when the hands are supported in one's lap or hanging at the side. Voluntary action typically suppresses this tremor temporarily, but it may reemerge with a sustained posture. The primary question that a geriatrician will likely face regarding tremor is to differentiate between the tremor of Parkinson's disease or essential tremor (see Table 17.1). In general, a rest tremor is a parkinsonian tremor until proven otherwise. Rarely, a parkinsonian tremor can occur as a result of cerebellar or brainstem lesions. The characteristics of the parkinsonian tremor will be discussed in detail in the subsequent section on parkinsonism. Dopaminergic agents such as levodopa and anticholinergic agents such as trihexyphenidyl are often highly effective for this type of tremor.

Essential tremor (ET) is the prototypical action tremor, and the most common adult-onset movement disorder with a prevalence of 0.9% in persons over the age of 65.[1] The term "benign" refers to the fact that the majority of persons with ET have mild, minimally progressive symptoms at onset and do not seek medical attention for years. However, the condition has a

Table 17.1 Comparison of essential tremor and parkinsonian tremor

	Essential tremor	Parkinsonian tremor
Body regions affected	Head, vocal tremor, hands	Jaw/chin, hands, legs
	Often bilateral, symmetric	Often unilateral onset
Associated neurological symptoms	None	Cardinal symptoms of Parkinson's disease
Typical treatment	Primidone or beta blockers	Dopaminergic and anticholinergic agents
Typical deep brain stimulation target	Thalamus	Subthalamic nucleus or globus pallidus interna

tendency to progress with age and can lead to significant disability. Because of the hereditary nature of the condition, a family history of similar tremor may be present. ET most commonly affects the arms and hands, but may also involve the head or voice, either in combination or in isolation. The chief complaints of patients with ET are difficulties writing, holding utensils, or drinks. Tremulous handwriting can be demonstrated in the office and used to document responses to therapy. When the head and neck are involved, the tremor can result in horizontal ("no-no") or vertical ("yes-yes") bobbing.

The main indicators for treatment are social, occupational, or functional disability. Beta blockers (e.g., propanolol and atenolol) and primidone are considered first-line agents for the treatment of ET

Reichel's Care of the Elderly, 7th Edition, ed. Jan Busby-Whitehead *et al.* Published by Cambridge University Press.
© Cambridge University Press 2016.

Table 17.2 First-line agents for treatment of essential tremor

	Propranolol (Inderal, Inderal LA)	Primidone (Mysoline)
Mechanism of action	Nonspecific adrenergic blockade	Phenobarbital
Daily dose range	60 mg–240 mg	50 mg–1,000 mg
Side effects	Fatigue, impotence, bradycardia, dizziness, depression	Sedation, confusion, dizziness, ataxia, vertigo
Relative contraindications	AV block, diabetes, heart failure, asthma/emphysema	Hepatic or renal failure, benzodiazepine/barbiturate use

(see Table 17.2).[2] Both agents decrease tremor amplitude, but generally do not abolish the tremor. Second-line agents such as topiramate, gabapentin, benzodiazepines, and phenobarbital should be tried in individuals who are intolerant of or refractory to first-line agents. Occasionally, medications may be more effective in combination, but the authors caution against polypharmacy in this population.

Both stereotactic thalamotomy and high frequency thalamic deep brain stimulation (DBS) can be dramatically effective for medically refractory ET.[3] The obvious limitations of the procedure are the invasive nature of a brain procedure, with a very low rate of serious complications (<1%–5%). The primary advantage of stimulation compared to thalamotomy is the ability to reverse and optimize response by adjusting electrical stimulation.[4]

An *intention tremor* is a specific type of action tremor in which the amplitude increases as the affected limb approaches a goal. A true intention tremor results from dysfunction of the tracts exiting the cerebellum, leading to the term "cerebellar outflow tremor." The term "rubral tremor" may also be used to describe an intention tremor and implies dysfunction of the midbrain red (rubral) nucleus, although intention tremors may arise from lesions outside the midbrain. Multiple sclerosis, head trauma, stroke, and degenerative diseases of the brainstem and cerebellum may produce a rubral tremor.[5] The full spectrum of a rubral tremor may include a rest component, titubation (head and trunk oscillation when the trunk is unsupported), gait ataxia, and a coarse "flapping" quality due to involvement of proximal muscle groups. Rubral tremors are very disabling as they can severely impair basic activities such as feeding, dressing, and hygiene. They are notoriously difficult to treat, and surgical therapies have been attempted with limited success.

Obtaining a thorough medication history in the geriatric population is imperative since polypharmacy is common and drug-induced tremors are often reversible and avoidable. The diagnosis of drug-induced tremor is made by exclusion of other causes of tremor, establishing a temporal relation with exposure to a tremorigenic drug, and a identifying a dose-response relationship. Table 17.3 provides a list of medications commonly associated with tremor. Antipsychotics and other psychotropic medications are often culprits, but other drugs associated with tremor include albuterol, amiodarone, prednisone, and theophylline. Chronic treatment with lithium carbonate causes a fine postural or kinetic tremor. In overdose or toxicity, lithium can also be associated with a cerebellar or parkinsonian syndrome.[6, 7] Withdrawal from benzodiazepines, alcohol, or other central nervous system depressants often results in tremor. If the causative medication cannot be discontinued, treatment with propranolol or primidone can be considered.

Parkinsonism and Parkinson's disease

General concepts

"Parkinsonism" is a general term used to describe a clinical syndrome characterized by rest tremor, bradykinesia, rigidity, and postural instability. Although most cases of parkinsonism are sporadic, idiopathic, and neurodegenerative, parkinsonism may also occur as a result of a structural lesion, drugs, or toxin affecting basal ganglia function. Common secondary causes of parkinsonism include vascular parkinsonism, drug-induced parkinsonism, and normal pressure hydrocephalus (NPH) and will be discussed individually in the following section.

Table 17.3 Medications and toxins that induce or exacerbate tremor

Beta adrenergic agonists
  Epinephrine
  Isoproterenol
  Albuterol

Theophylline

Amphetamines

Lithium

Phenothiazines, butyrophenones

Tricyclic antidepressants

Anti-arrhythmics
  Amiodarone
  Procainamide
  Mexiletine

Antimicrobials
  Trimethoprim-sulfamethoxazole
  Acyclovir

Antiepileptics
  Valproic acid
  Carbamazepine
  Lamotrigine

Immunosuppressants
  Prednisone
  Cyclosporine
  Tacrolimus

Xanthines (in coffee and tea)

Heavy metals
  Mercury
  Lead
  Arsenic
  Bismuth

The most common neurodegenerative form of parkinsonism is *Parkinson's disease* (PD). The prevalence of PD is estimated between 100 and 300 per 100,000.[8] Although PD can occur on a familial basis, the vast majority of cases are sporadic suggesting an unknown environmental risk factor. The hallmark of the condition is the selective degeneration of midbrain dopaminergic neurons, which leads to the cardinal features of the disorder and the characteristic response to levodopa.

Finally, several related degenerative disorders known as *Parkinson's plus or atypical parkinsonian*

syndromes are a part of the larger complex of parkinsonism and may be mistaken for Parkinson's disease. Features common to this group of disorders include poor response to levodopa, more rapid progression to severe disability compared to idiopathic PD, and additional neurological features that make them atypical for PD.

Clinical features of parkinsonism

"Bradykinesia," the hallmark of Parkinson's disease, refers to slowing of movements, hesitancy, arrests, decreased amplitude, or poverty of movements. Passively manipulating joints such as the wrist, elbow, or knee will reveal either a constant increase in tone (lead-pipe rigidity) or a ratchety increase in tone (cogwheel rigidity).

Tremor is the most recognizable aspect of parkinsonism, but may not be present in up to 40% of patients with parkinsonism. The typical parkinsonian tremor presents unilaterally at rest, may affect the hands, legs, jaw, or tongue, and remains asymmetric throughout the course of the disease. Mental concentration (e.g., counting backwards) and walking enhance a parkinsonian tremor. Furthermore, lifting the arms to sustain a posture will dampen the tremor temporarily, but the original amplitude and frequency will return after a delay of two to three seconds. This so-called *re-emergent tremor* is a pathognomonic clue to a parkinsonian tremor.

In early disease, the examination may reveal a subtle unilateral tremor, decreased arm swing or dragging of one leg. Patients often report that walking feels unnatural. Impaired finger dexterity, loss of facial expression (hypomimia), and small handwriting (micrographia) are often the earliest signs of bradykinesia and parkinsonism. The voice can be hypophonic and monotone with a loss of diction. The combination of rigidity and bradykinesia leads to difficulty with ordinary tasks such as turning in bed, rising from a chair, or getting in and out of a car. Because of the loss of dexterity and range of motion, dressing and routine hygiene can become laborious.

A characteristic stooped posture develops with forward flexion of the trunk, neck, elbows, shoulders, and knees. Stride height and length are reduced leading to a shuffling gait. The stooped posture and shift in the center of gravity contributes to a tendency to fall forward (propulsion) and an inability to stop (festination). Turning occurs "en-bloc," as the head, neck, torso, and extremities no longer rotate independently due to rigidity and bradykinesia. Start hesitation causes difficulty rising from a chair or initiating walking. Patients may describe freezing as though the feet are transiently stuck or "glued" to the ground. The phenomenon typically occurs in doorways, narrow hallways, or near obstacles. Patients often find that visual cues such as floor or sidewalk markings will release them from freezing. Freezing of gait (FOG) is one of the more debilitating symptoms encountered in parkinsonian states and often leads to falls and subsequent injury. Unfortunately, freezing can be refractory to dopaminergic therapy.

Postural stability is tested using the pull test in which the examiner firmly tugs the patient from behind and assesses the ability to maintain an upright stance. Retropulsion or toppling backward occurs when the ability to adjust or maintain the center of gravity is lost. Due to the combination of flexed posture and postural instability, forward falls are typical of moderate to advanced stages of PD.

Secondary or nonmotor features of parkinsonism include dysphagia, excess saliva or drooling (sialorrhea), constipation, overactive bladder, erectile dysfunction, seborrheic dermatitis, orthostatic hypotension, pain, paresthesias, and sleep disturbances including REM sleep behavior disorder (RBD), periodic limb movements of sleep (PLMS), restless legs syndrome (RLS), insomnia, and obstructive sleep apnea. Numbness, tingling, aching pains, fatigue, and weakness are common complaints of PD that may be dismissed early in the diagnosis or mistaken for other neurological or medical conditions.

Neuropsychiatric symptoms that may occur in a parkinsonian disorder include subcortical dementia, depression, apathy, anxiety, hallucinations, or delusions (see Table 17.4).

Differential diagnosis

The diagnosis of PD or an atypical parkinsonian disorder is made by a clinical exam. When all cardinal symptoms are present, the diagnosis is fairly obvious. Diagnostic difficulty usually arises in early stages of the disease when the predominant symptoms are subtle secondary symptoms. In the hands of experienced neurologists, up to 20% of patients have an alternate diagnosis at autopsy while cases with atypical features may prove to have PD.[9] Since 2011, the Dopamine Transporter SPECT scan (DaT)© has been available in the United States and can aid in the early

Table 17.4 Neuropsychiatric manifestations of parkinsonism

Cognitive and intellectual impairment and dementia
Visual hallucinations
Delusions
Depression, anhedonia, dysphoria
Anxiety
Akathisia
Apathy or amotivation
Sleep disorders such as insomnia, sleep fragmentation, excessive daytime somnolence, sleep attacks, REM behavior disorder, periodic leg movements of sleep
Impulse control behaviors

diagnosis of Parkinsonism. The radiotracer *ioflupane* labels the dopamine transporter found in nigrostriatal neurons. Therefore, it can distinguish parkinsonism from essential tremor, but it does not distinguish between parkinsonian disorders.

The single most important feature distinguishing idiopathic PD from secondary and atypical forms of parkinsonism is the response to levodopa. Patients with idiopathic PD display a robust response to levodopa that lasts for many years because PD primarily affects midbrain dopaminergic neurons in the substantia nigra (SN). The lack of response characteristic of other forms of parkinsonism is due to degeneration of post-synaptic receptors and non-dopaminergic systems (see Table 17.5).

Red flags suggesting an atypical or secondary form of parkinsonism include ocular motor palsy, cerebellar signs, early, prominent falls, gait, cognitive, or cranial nerve dysfunction, autonomic failure, or pyramidal signs. These conditions tend to be more rapidly progressive than PD due to the lack of disease specific treatment options.

Progressive supranuclear palsy (PSP) refers to the characteristic eye movement abnormality associated with the condition. The hallmarks of the condition are an akinetic-rigid parkinsonism with early imbalance leading to falls. Postural instability leading to falls is often a later manifestation of PD and should alert the physician to alternate forms of parkinsonism. The characteristic vertical gaze palsy is not always a presenting feature, but invariably develops over time. Other characteristic features include a prominent stare with a worried or

Table 17.5 Parkinson's plus syndromes

	First description	MRI findings	Primary pathology
Parkinson's disease	1817, James Parkinson	Normal	Nigrostriatal degeneration, Lewy bodies (LB)
Progresssive supranuclear palsy	1964, Steele, Richardson, Olszewski	Midbrain atrophy, "hummingbird sign"	Midbrain degeneration, frontal lobe degeneration, tau-positive neurofibrillary tangles
Multiple system atrophy	1900, Dejerine and Thomas 1960, Shy and Drager 1960, van der Eecken, Adams, van Bogaert 1969, Graham and Oppenheimer	Lower brainstem and cerebellar atrophy, "hot-cross bun sign," linear putaminal hyperintensity	Striatonigral, olivopontocerebellar, intermediolateral cell column degeneration, synuclein positive Glial cytoplasmic inclusions (GCI)
Dementia with Lewy bodies	1996, McKeith, Galasko, Kosaka, et al.	Global atrophy	Diffuse cortical and subcortical LB and synuclein positive dystrophic neurites
Corticobasal ganglionic degeneration	1968, Rebeiz, Kolodny, Richardson	Asymmetric frontoparietal atrophy	Ballooned neurons, Tau positive glial inclusions, plaques, and coiled bodies

astonished facial expression and dysarthria. Patients with PSP often develop personality changes and cognitive impairment due to concomitant frontal lobe degeneration. The combination of cognitive impairment and lack of insight often leads to issues with medication compliance, social withdrawal, and falls. Microscopically, microtubule associated protein *tau* accumulates, forming neurofibrillary tangles, so that pathogically PSP may be more closely related to Alzheimer's disease rather than PD.[10]

Dementia with Lewy bodies (DLB) is a relatively new diagnostic entity that is the second most common cause of dementia after Alzheimer's disease. [11] DLB presents with prominent mental symptoms that often overshadow the movement disorder. Visual hallucinations (VH) develop insidiously and are very similar to the well-formed, complex medication-induced VH in PD. In contrast to PD, VH in DLB develop in the absence of dopaminergic medication exposure or with relatively low doses. Delusions revolving around spousal infidelity as well as neighbors, friends, or relatives stealing from them are also common. Striking cognitive fluctuations differentiate DLB from other causes of dementia. Patients may be relatively intact at one moment and minutes later become confused, disoriented, psychotic, or obtunded.

When present, several secondary features help to confirm the diagnosis. Repeated falls occur due to postural instability. Syncope and transient loss of consciousness may mimic seizures, stroke, transient ischemic attack, or a cardiac event and often prompt repeated evaluations or hospitalizations. DLB patients may be very sensitive to dopamine receptor blockers and can develop delirium or akinetic-rigid crises with neuroleptic treatment. For this reason, only antipsychotics such as quetiapine or clozapine should be considered when treating psychosis in DLB.

Both PD and DLB have in common the characteristic pathological inclusion called the Lewy body (LB), cytoplasmic inclusions containing the synaptic protein α-synuclein. In DLB, LB are present throughout the brainstem, limbic regions, and cortex, leading to the pathological term "diffuse Lewy body disease."

Multiple system atrophy (MSA) is a clinical term used to refer to three formerly distinct parkinsonian conditions, Shy-Drager syndrome (SDS), olivopontocerebellar atrophy (OPCA), and striatonigral denegeration (SND). The currently accepted designations are MSA-A (autonomic form) for SDS, MSA-C (cerebellar form) for OPCA, and MSA-P (parkinsonian form) for SND. Autonomic features include orthostatic hypotension, bowel or bladder incontinence, and sexual dysfunction. Cerebellar features include dysarthria, gait ataxia, and limb incoordination. In practice, there is often overlap between the syndromes.[12]

Although the response to levodopa in MSA is generally limited, some patients with MSA may experience partial benefit and should be tried on levodopa at least once. At the same time, even if there is a response, side effects such as facial dystonia, orthostasis or nausea may limit treatment. Secondary features suggestive of the diagnosis include early sexual dysfunction which may precede the diagnosis of MSA by many years, stridor, REM behavior disorder and obstructive sleep apnea due to brainstem respiratory and sleep center dysfunction.

Pathologically, all three syndromes share a common pathological finding of cytoplasmic inclusions containing α-synuclein in glial cells. The clinical phenotype is largely determined by the location of pathology, autonomic centers in the brainstem, cervical and sacral spinal cords are affected primarily in MSA-A. In MSA-C, the medulla, pons, and cerebellum are primarily affected and in MSA-P, the substantia nigra and the striatum.

Corticobasal ganglionic degeneration (CBD) is a condition that may present with either parkinsonism or dementia. Pathologically, it resembles Alzheimer's disease and frontotemporal dementia rather than Parkinson's disease. The classic corticobasal syndrome consists of asymmetric parkinsonism with prominent limb rigidity, dystonic posturing, and a gait disorder. There may be myoclonic jerks, cognitive impairment involving frontal lobe function, memory systems, or visuospatial systems. One of the most distinctive features of the syndrome is limb apraxia, or inability to perform a voluntary movement that is not due to muscle weakness, sensory loss, or ataxia. With time, the so-called alien limb phenomenon may develop in which the limb may assume unusual postures, wander in space, or seem out of the control of the person. Over time, rigidity and dementia predominate.[13]

In clinical practice, the most common secondary forms of parkinsonism that one needs to consider are vascular parkinsonism, drug-induced parkinsonism, and normal pressure hydrocephalus (NPH).

Cerebrovascular disease is a relatively common cause of parkinsonism, occurring as a result of both strategically placed lacunar infarctions in the basal ganglia or diffuse white matter disease. Patients may present with abrupt onset of a gait disorder or "lower body" parkinsonism. A stepwise pattern of progression is often a clue to recurrent small vessel ischemic events. Levodopa is not typically effective, but should be attempted for both diagnostic and therapeutic purposes. Cerebrovascular risk factors, a history of stroke or transient neurological events, cognitive disturbance, or gait apraxia are often present.[14]

Parkinsonism due to chronic antipsychotic treatment is a potentially reversible syndrome that may be identical to idiopathic PD. The risk of parkinsonism due to antipsychotic medications is dose dependent and increases in the elderly. With the exception of clozapine, no antipsychotic is free of this risk. Other medications that potentially may induce parkinsonism include antiemetics such as metoclopramide or prochlorperazine due to their dopamine blocking capabilities, dopamine depleting agents such as reserpine or tetrabenazine, and lithium. MPTP (1-methyl-4-phenyl-1, 2,3,6-tetrahydropyridine), a compound that causes selective nigrostriatal degeneration, was discovered after it led to acute parkinsonism in a group of college students experimenting with heroin.[15] In addition to MPTP, other toxins associated with parkinsonism include manganese[16] and carbon monoxide.[17]

Treatment of PD

Treatment overview

Symptomatic treatment is typically initiated when patients begin to experience social or functional disability. Factors to consider when deciding to initiate treatment include primary symptom complex, age, functional status, comorbid medical conditions, and cognitive status. A wide range of medications with proven symptomatic effects exist for PD, including monoamine oxidase inhibitors (MAOI), anticholinergic agents, amantadine, catechol-O-methyltransferase (COMT) inhibitors, dopamine agonists, and levodopa (see Table 17.6).

Both selegiline and rasagiline irreversibly inhibit MAO type B resulting in modest enhancement of striatal dopamine levels. Side effects may include insomnia and orthostatic hypotension. One of the first agents studied for its potential neuroprotective effects was Selegiline, an irreversible MAO-B inhibitor with antioxidant properties. In the landmark DATATOP (deprenyl and tocopherol antioxidative therapy of parkinsonism) study, selegiline treatment

Table 17.6 Medications for the symptomatic treatment of PD

Medication	Mechanism of action	Typical therapeutic dosage
Selegiline	MAO-B inhibitor	5 mg–10 mg a day
Rasagiline	MAO-B inhibitor	1 mg once daily
Trihexyphenidyl	Anticholinergic	.5 mg to 2 mg three times daily
Amantadine	NMDA antagonist	200 mg two to three times a day
Pramipexole	Dopamine agonist	0.5 to 1.5 mg three times daily
Ropinirole	Dopamine agonist	1 mg to 8 mg three times daily
Rotigotine	Dopamine agonist (transdermal patch)	1 mg to 8 mg once daily
Apomorphine	Dopamine agonist (subcutaneous injection)	0.2–0.6 mL injections as needed for OFF periods
Levodopa	Repletes endogenous dopamine deficiency	150 mg–1500 mg daily (divided doses)
Entacapone	COMT inhibitor	200 mg three to five times daily with levodopa

was found to delay disability and the need for levodopa therapy.[18] However, the effect was deemed to be at least partly symptomatic, and a clear neuroprotective benefit was never demonstrated.

Anticholinergic agents such as benztropine and trihexyphenidyl were among the first treatments for PD. They have moderate effects on tremor, rigidity, and dystonia; however, side effects such as urinary retention, cognitive impairment, delirium, dry mouth, and blurred vision limit their use in the elderly.[19]

Amantadine, originally developed for use against influenza, is a tricyclic amine with multiple putative mechanisms including enhancing dopamine release, inhibition of dopamine reuptake, antimuscarinic effects, and N-methyl D-aspartate (NMDA) receptor antagonism. In addition to its use in early PD, antidyskinetic properties make it useful for advanced patients with motor fluctuations. Amantadine is generally well tolerated, but lower extremity edema and hallucinations may complicate treatment. In patients with renal insufficiency, dose adjustments need to be made based on creatinine clearance since amantadine is renally excreted.

Dopamine agonists directly stimulate striatal dopamine receptors and are used both in early PD and as an adjunct in advanced patients with motor fluctuations. Ropinirole, pramipexole, rotigotine, and subcutaneous apomorphine are available in the United States. Subcutaneous apomorphine injections has been available in the United States for the treatment of refractory *off* periods. The various non-ergot agonists have similar efficacy and side effects common to the class include nausea, lightheadedness, pedal edema, hallucinations, and sedation. Most adverse effects are dose-related and can be avoided by slow titration of the drug. The ergot agonists (e.g., bromocriptine and pergolide) carry the additional risk of retroperitoneal fibrosis and Raynaud's phenomenon. Furthermore, cardiac valvular abnormalities attributed to pergolide led to its withdrawal from the US market.[20] Long-term experience with the agonists, particularly pramipexole and ropinirole, has revealed that dopamine agonist use may be linked to compulsive behaviors such as gambling, binge eating, spending, and hypersexuality.[21]

The initial studies of ropinirole and pramipexole monotherapy compared to levodopa have both demonstrated reduced motor fluctuations and dyskinesias compared to levodopa therapy.[22, 23] However, a recent longitudinal study suggested that the development of motor fluctuations and dyskinesias are not associated with the duration of exposure to levodopa, but are associated with duration of disease and dose of levodopa. [24] Longitudinal experience with use of dopamine agonists either as monotherapy or adjunctive therapy has revealed that symptom control tends to be poorer with dopamine agonists and side effects are often more common on dopamine agonists.[25, 26]

251

Despite the recent advances in pharmacotherapy, levodopa remains the most time-honored and effective treatment for symptoms of PD. The majority of PD patients will attain significant, long-lasting benefit from levodopa superior to any of the previously mentioned agents. It is well tolerated and effective at a large dose range as long as it is administered with a peripheral decarboxylase inhibitor (e.g., carbidopa). Without such an inhibitor, large doses of levodopa would be required to provide a benefit that in turn would lead to intolerable peripheral side effects of dopamine such as orthostatic hypotension, nausea, and emesis. In the United States, carbidopa is combined with levodopa in various formulations (10/100, 25/100, 25/250) and marketed as Sinemet* allowing for flexible dosing. The half-life of Sinemet is approximately 90 minutes, so that multiple daily doses are necessary. We typically start with 1/2 of a 25/100 tablet three times daily, increasing over a few weeks to 1–2 tablets three times daily. Central nervous system side effects such as sedation, insomnia, visual hallucinations, confusion, or psychosis are more likely to occur in the elderly (>80 years of age) or in later stages of PD (see Table 17.7).

For convenience, medication dosing may be scheduled around meal times. However, because levodopa absorption occurs in the duodenum through a saturable amino acid transporter, bioavailability may be limited by meals containing large protein content. To maximize bioavailability, fluctuating patients should be instructed to take levodopa on an empty stomach (i.e., at least 45 minutes before a meal or one to two hours after a meal).

Controlled or extended release Sinemet (CR/ER)* has a half-life of approximately three hours, but with a slower onset of action, and decreased bioavailability. Sinemet CR* comes in 25/100 and 50/200 formulations. In early disease, CR can be dosed twice a day and is often used at bedtime to prevent wearing off upon awakening. Clinicians should be aware that Sinemet CR translates to less regular Sinemet during conversion from one to the other (100 mg regular Sinemet is equivalent to 133 mg of CR Sinemet). Two treatments aimed at improving the efficacy of levodopa have just recently been introduced in the United States. Rytary©, a carbidopa/levodopa extended release capsule, contains immediate acting and long acting beads of levodopa that provide a longer duration of effect. Clinical trials to date have shown a favorable pharmacologic profile which tends to reduce *off* time, increase *on* time without troublesome dyskinesia due to its improved half life.[27]

Levodopa intestinal gel has been available in the European Union for nearly a decade and was just introduced in the United States as Duopa©. The intestinal gel can be infused continuously up to 16 hours a day through a gastrostomy with a jejunal extension. Studies have shown less intrasubject variability in plasma concentration of levodopa and improved ON time with similar amounts of dyskinesia. The major adverse events surround the placement of the PEG-J tube and PEG site irritation. In addition, there are reports of emerging neuropathy that has been hypothesized to be related to the intestinal infusion and nutrient malabsorption.[28–30]

Medical treatment of advanced disease

Initially, the dose range and therapeutic window of levodopa is wide and low doses of levodopa have sustained benefits for several years. However, the dosage often needs to be increased (as high as 1,000 mg–1,500 mg) to maintain a stable level of function.

With chronic treatment, at least half of patients on dopaminergic therapy develop motor complications or response fluctuations.[31] As the disease progresses, levodopa's therapeutic window becomes narrowed, leading to clinically apparent fluctuations from *on* (levodopa is working) to *off* (levodopa is not working). In other words, the dose-response curve in advanced disease mirrors the short half-life of levodopa.

Table 17.7 Management of psychosis and hallucinations

- Exclude infection or other intercurrent illness that may cause a delirium

- Obtain detailed medication history with emphasis on recent additions (dosage changes, withdrawals, or possible ingestions)

- Withdraw medications in this order:

  Anticholinergics
  Amantadine
  Selegiline/rasagiline
  Dopamine agonists
  COMT inhibitors
  If troubling hallucinations persist, then consider decreasing levodopa dosage

- Trial of quetiapine

- Clozapine for refractory psychosis

Several types of response fluctuations exist. The duration of the response may progressively shorten (*wearing-off*), responses may become unpredictable (*on-off* phenomenon), painful limb dystonia may occur when wearing off and dyskinesias, an overexpression of movement, may develop. In addition, visceral (abdominal, chest pains, shortness of breath), autonomic, and neuropsychiatric symptoms (euphoria, dysphoria, panic/anxiety) may occur with response fluctuations. Dosing intervals may need to be shortened to one to two hours to maintain symptom control.

Strategies at this point focus on maximizing *on* time and minimizing *off* time, dyskinesias, and side effects. The development of fluctuations may be related to a combination of progressive loss of striatal dopamine storage capacity, pulsatile stimulation of striatal receptors, and receptor hypersensitivity.[32] Therefore, it follows that strategies that minimize pulsatile stimulation may prevent the development of motor complications.

Increased dosing frequency is the most basic therapeutic maneuver, but it is limited by the patient's ability to handle frequent round-the-clock dosing and levodopa failures. Use of Sinemet CR may prolong *on* time, but in our experience, unpredictable responses can occur in advanced patients. Furthermore, direct comparison of Sinemet CR to regular Sinemet has shown no major difference in the incidence of dyskinesia and motor complications.[33]

Dopamine agonists are effective in reducing *off* time, improving *on* function, and reducing levodopa dosages. However, adverse effects such as dyskinesias and hallucinations are more common. Amantadine has been shown to have anti-dyskinetic properties.

Catechol-o-methyltransferase (COMT) inhibitors – tolcapone and entacapone – inhibit the breakdown of levodopa in the periphery and central nervous systems and enhance central nervous system availability of levodopa. Since the action of COMT inhibitors is dependent on the presence of levodopa, COMT inhibitors have no effect on parkinsonian symptoms if levodopa is not administered. Entacapone significantly increases the area under the curve and the half-life of levodopa without increasing maximal plasma concentrations. Specific side effects of entacapone include severe diarrhea and an orange discoloration of urine. Both entacapone and tolcapone have been shown to improve motor fluctuations by reducing *wearing-off* and *off* time and increasing *on* time.[34, 35] Tolcapone is not commonly used due to rare cases of fulminant hepatitis associated with its use.[36]

A clinical algorithm

In summary, the medical treatment of PD has advanced dramatically in the last decade, but it is limited by the progression of the disease. To date, no definite disease modifying therapies exist, and the current state of treatment rests primarily on a symptom-based approach.

For patients with mild early symptoms below the age of 65, we typically use a "bottom-up" approach. We begin treatment of mild PD with a dopamine agonist or MAO-inhibitor either alone or in combination. Mild symptoms are often adequately controlled for several months to years on these agents and delaying levodopa treatment may delay the onset of response fluctuations and dyskinesias.

For patients over the age of 65, the incidence of motor complications is low and side effects of agonists are more common and may outweigh the benefits. In this population, we advocate a "top-down approach" starting with carbidopa/levodopa (25/100 mg), using the lowest effective dose possible. The dose may be increased by half- to whole-tablet increments as needed. There is no fixed dosage ceiling, although 1,000 mg of levodopa is generally considered adequate to control symptoms in the majority of mild to moderate patients.

Mild predictable *wearing-off* is easily addressed by increasing the frequency of dosing. However, compliance becomes an issue when levodopa is dosed every two to three hours. Entacapone (200 mg) can be added to each dose of levodopa to increase the duration of the response, thus increasing daily *on* time. A concomitant reduction in levodopa dosage by 15%–30% is recommended if the patient is at the high end of the therapeutic window.

The response to levodopa may become more unpredictable with advancing disease. Response failures may occur with absent or delayed onset of action, sudden or unpredictable *off*. The addition of a low-dose dopamine agonist is often useful in patients with complex or unpredictable motor complications as long as dyskinesias, visual hallucinations, and other levodopa-related side effects are manageable.

In a subset of patients, the secondary nonmotor symptoms of PD can become quite disabling. Often increasing dopaminergic therapy is not effective. Table 17.8 outlines some of the most common

Table 17.8 Nonmotor symptoms of PD and therapeutic strategies [52]

Symptom	Nonpharmacologic	Pharmacologic
Constipation	Increasing dietary fiber and fluid intake Regular exercise Discontinue anticholinergics	Osmotic macrogel (polyethylene glycol) Stool softeners (docusate) Stimulant laxative (bisacodyl), enemas
Drooling	Speech evaluation and therapy	Botulinum toxin injections Peripheral anticholinergic agent (e.g., glycopyrrolate)
Dysarthria/hypophonia	Speech therapy (Lee Silverman technique)	If *off* symptom, increase dopaminergic therapy
Dysphagia	Dysphagia evaluation Soft-mechanical diet Schedule meals with *on* time Gastrostomy	If *off* symptom, increase dopaminergic therapy
Freezing	Physical/occupational therapy for gait training Visual cues	If *off* symptom, increase dopaminergic therapy Droxidopa
Postural instability/falls	Physical/occupational therapy for gait training or home safety evaluation Cane, walker, wheelchair, or other form of assistance Evaluation for orthostasis	If *off* symptom, increase dopaminergic therapy
Male impotence	Review medications Evaluate for diabetes or underlying endocrine disorder Urological evaluation	Sildefanil (Level C) Alprostadil (intracavernous injections or intraurethral suppository)
Orthostasis	Elevate head of bed 10–30 degrees Encourage dietary salt intake Compression stockings	Discontinue potential hypotensive drugs Salt-retaining mineralocorticoid (e.g., fludrocortisone) Pressors (e.g., midodrine, ephedrine)
Overactive bladder	Avoid bedtime fluid intake Exclude infection, prostatitis, or other urological problems	Antimuscarinic agents (oxybutynin, tolteridine, imipramine)
Seborrheic dermatitis	Regular scalp or face washing with light moisturizer, humidifier, sunlight	Coal tar or selenium-based shampoos Topical steroids
Excessive daytime sleepiness and fatigue	Review medications (limit anticholinergics and dopamine agonists) Recommend good sleep hygiene	Modafinil Methylphenidate
Insomnia	Review medications	Increase evening levodopa/carbidopa Melatonin
Periodic limb movements of sleep		Increase evening levodopa/carbidopa Trial non-ergot dopamine agonists
REM sleep behavioral disorder		Melatonin Clonazepam

Table 17.8 (cont.)

Symptom	Nonpharmacologic	Pharmacologic
Depression	Review medications	SSRI, SNRI, tricyclic antidepressants ECT
Anxiety	Review medications	Modify anti-parkinsonian drug therapy to limit *off* time Antidepressant or benzodiazepine
Dementia	Rule out reversible causes of dementia Rule out pseudodementia Eliminate anticholinergics, dopamine agonists, amantadine, and selegiline Encourage exercise and social interactions	Donepezil Rivastigmine Memantine

nonmotor symptoms of PD and the accepted therapeutic strategies.

Surgical therapy

Deep brain stimulation (DBS) therapy has been the standard surgical therapy for medically advanced Parkinson's disease since it was FDA approved in 2003. The procedure was a natural extension of the previous lesioning techniques performed from the 1960s through the 1980s. Electrodes are stereotactically implanted into one of two locations in the basal ganglia, the globus pallidus interna (GPi) or the subthalamic nucleus (STN). The electrodes are then connected to a pulse generator implanted into the chest wall. The current devices manufactured by Medtronic, Inc., allow for a wide variety of physician and patient controls to allow for personalized symptom control.

More than a decade's worth of experience has defined specific selection criteria and outcomes/expectations of the surgery. DBS is highly effective for patients with advanced PD who continue to respond to levodopa or other dopaminergic agents, but who do not have adequate hours of good function (*on* time), suffer from prolonged periods of immobility or tremor (*off* time), medication induced dyskinesia, and other medication side effects. The appropriate candidate should have idiopathic PD with disabling symptoms that are responsive to levodopa, be free of cognitive or neuropsychological illness, have the emotional capabilities and social support to cope with a potentially life-altering surgery, and the often frequent and lengthy visits required after surgery. Although no firm age cut-off has been determined, most DBS specialists feel that patients older than 75 years of age tend to respond less well to the rigors of surgery and incur greater risk due to medical comorbidities and cognitive status.[37]

Randomized controlled trials reveal that DBS reduces *off* time, increases *on* time, reduces dyskinesia and medication requirements, and improves not only PD motor scores, but also quality of life scores. Complications unique to DBS include electrical malfunction, lead fracture, battery replacement (every one to five years), lengthy programming sessions, hardware infection, skin erosion, intracerebral hemorrhage or infarct.

Although the exact mechanism of DBS is not known, it is believed that high frequency electrical stimulation blocks or inhibits the stimulation target, which rebalances the basal ganglia circuitry. Ongoing studies continue to investigate the appropriate timing of surgery, the preferred location (STN versus GPi), optimal stimulation paradigms, device, and surgical techniques.[38]

Natural history

Since the advent of levodopa, mortality in early PD has been dramatically reduced. The mean duration of disease prior to levodopa discovery was 9.4 years and the mean age at death was 67 years. Hoehn and Yahr reported a mortality rate of 2.9 times that expected for an age-matched population. Since the introduction of levodopa, Hoehn reported a mortality ratio of 1.5 and other studies have found similar rates.[39] It is possible that surgical treatments may further improve mortality; however, there is limited data on how DBS affects the natural history of PD.[40] The mean

255

duration of symptoms is reported to be approximately 13 years, and the mean age of death is approximately 73 years. The DATATOP study found that increased symmetry of parkinsonism at presentation, early gait impairment, and rapid clinical decline portended a worse prognosis.[41] The most common cause of death in PD patients is cardiovascular disease, and the second most common cause of death is pneumonia.[42]

Although PD is associated with a shortened life-span, the diagnosis is not typically considered "terminal." Uncertainty about when to discuss end of life planning exists in part due to the lack of guidelines. Typically, the discussion of advanced directives, alternate means of nutrition (i.e., PEG), alternate living situations, and caregiver options are highly individual and based on the person's support systems in place, and family/patient's level of comfort.

A recent survey study showed that 94% of PD patients wanted to discuss prognosis and treatment options early. Most wanted their family members to be present during these discussions. Approximately half wanted to discuss advanced care documents early in the disease, while the others rather defer these discussions until their condition progresses.[43] Therefore, health-care providers should ask patients about their preferences and offer discussion periodically, preferably before an acute crisis such as a hospitalization occurs.

Gait disorders

General concepts

Gait impairment is a significant cause of morbidity and mortality in the elderly. As many as 15%–20% of patients over the age of 65 will suffer from gait impairment, often requiring an assistive device. This number increases with age, with an estimated 40%–50% of those over 85 years, and up to 70% in those over 90 years.[44] Falls from gait impairment represent the most common cause of injury in the elderly;[45] 30% of all elderly will have at least one fall annually, with the risk as high as 50% for those over 80 years. Institutionalization or hospitalization 50% of long-term care residents will have at least one fall annually.[46]

Normal locomotion depends on intact motor and sensory systems to maintain equilibrium and balance. The sensory inputs from vestibular, peripheral nervous, and visual systems are integrated by the cortex, cerebellum, and basal ganglia. The body also uses anticipatory and reactive postural reflexes to maintain equilibrium in response to environmental changes. Disruptions or lesions in any of these structures may result in gait impairment.

Historically, slowed gait has been considered a natural part of the aging process; however, this is no longer thought to be true. Some of the common changes seen with advancing age include bent posture, slower pace, shortened stride, increased time in double support phase, truncal and limb rigidity, widened base, and en bloc turning.[47] For the majority of elderly patients, gait speed declines by 12%–16% each decade, stride length shortens, and step frequency increases. The time in double support phase (when both feet are on the ground) increases from 18% in younger patients to 26% by age 70.[48] What distinguishes the so-called senile gait of the elderly and a true pathological gait is often controversial. In general, a disabling gait (one that causes functional impairment), no matter what the age, should be investigated thoroughly for a potentially reversible cause.

Differential diagnosis

Most gait disorders develop insidiously and may go unnoticed by the patient. Caregiver reports are often necessary for an accurate history. Patients may describe gait impairment in general terms such as "I'm off balance" or "I feel weak." Caregivers may narrow the differential by reporting that the patient appears "drunk" (suggesting cerebellar ataxia) or that the feet appear "frozen to the ground" (suggesting an extrapyramidal gait disorder).

Obtaining associated symptoms and signs are key to localizing the lesion and narrowing the differential (see Table 17.9). Patients with sensory neuropathy causing ataxia often complain of distal paresthesias and sensory loss. Sensory ataxia is classically associated with more difficulty at night or in the dark, when visual input is limited. Lumbar nerve root compromise generally causes radicular, radiating back or leg pain and would generally not cause gait impairment unless multiple lumbar root levels are affected. Myelopathy or spinal cord compression is often associated with muscle weakness and spasticity unless the pathology affects the dorsal columns in which sensory symptoms predominate. Concomitant memory and cognitive issues suggest a cerebral cause such as normal pressure hydrocephalus, while dysarthria depending on its quality suggests cerebellar, basal

Table 17.9 Localization by associated signs and symptoms

Sign	Diagnoses to consider
Dementia, cognitive impairment, urinary incontinence	Normal pressure hydrocephalus
Nystagmus	Vestibular, cerebellar, or brain stem dysfunction
Dysarthria	Cerebellar, basal ganglia, or corticobulbar dysfunction
Rigidity, tremor, bradykinesia	Parkinsonism
Hyperreflexia, spasticity with Babinski signs	Corticospinal tract disease
Sensory loss, paresthesias, hyporeflexia	Peripheral neuropathy
Dizziness, vertigo	Vestibular disease

ganglia, or hemispheric disease. Vestibular disorders such as labyrinthitis or Meniere's disease are often recognized more by the disequilibrium or vertigo that they cause rather than the gait impairment. Extrapyramidal disorders may initially lead to a primary gait disorder, but inevitably associated features such as tremor, rigidity, and bradykinesia emerge. Sudden gait failure generally implies a catastrophic medical illness, such as stroke, medication toxicity, infection, meningitis, or myocardial infarction.

Examination

A general gait screen should be incorporated into every encounter and begins by simply watching a patient enter or exit the examination room. Features of gait that should be observed include stance, base, initiation, velocity, stride length, cadence, fluidity of movements, and deviation. Patients should be observed walking normally, in tandem, and briefly on heels and toes to assess for distal muscle strength. Romberg testing and pull testing should also be performed to assess for postural stability.

A person with a normal gait pattern will hold their body erect, head straight, feet slightly apart, and both arms hanging loosely at the sides and moving forward easily with the opposite leg. Hips and legs flex with each step, while the ankle dorsiflexes. The heel strikes the ground first, moving smoothly along the sole and

pushing off with the toes. Stride length should be equal with each step. Some abnormalities may only be elicited through gait testing with obstacles or distractions: such as walking through a doorway, or over objects on the floor. Examination of footwear for pattern of wear may also be useful.

The get-up-and-go test is a timed test in which the patient is observed rising from a chair, walking three meters, turning around, and returning to the chair. A score of less than 10 seconds is considered normal, greater than 14 seconds is abnormal, while a time greater than 20 seconds indicates severe gait impairment. Although useful as a screen of functional capabilities, this test cannot distinguish between different causes of a gait disorder (described in Table 17.10).

Evaluation

In most cases, careful history and simple observation of the patient in motion using the above techniques can help to narrow the differential.

The laboratory evaluation will depend on the initial presentation, findings on physical exam, and may include: complete blood count, metabolic panel, fasting blood glucose, glycosylated hemoglobin, erythrocyte sedimentation rate (ESR), rapid plasma reagin (RPR), thyroid stimulating hormone (TSH), vitamin B12, folic acid levels, and brain imaging with computed tomography (CT). Additional testing if indicated may consist of magnetic resonance imaging (MRI) to evaluate structural degeneration or lesions, electromyography (EMG) and nerve conduction study (NCS) to evaluate the peripheral nervous system. Specialized gait labs staffed by neurologists, physical medicine specialists, or physical and occupational therapists may help to define a gait disorder and to clarify its etiology (see Table 17.11).

Gait patterns and select etiologies

Parkinson's disease and parkinsonism lead to a slow gait with shortened stride length and low step height that is often described as shuffling. When trying to walk faster, patients with parkinsonism tend to increase step speed out of proportion to stride length or step height. In the earliest stages of PD, gait impairment is very subtle with patients noting dragging of one leg, difficulty getting in and out of a car or low seat. The typical posture of a patient with PD consists

Table 17.10 Gait patterns and classification

Type of gait	Description	Associated signs	Causes
Parkinsonian	Short-stepped, shuffling, with hips, knees, and spine flexed, festination, en bloc turns	Bradykinesia, rigidity, postural instability, rest tremor, reduced arm swing	Parkinson's disease, and atypical or secondary forms of parkinsonism
Frontal gait disorder (gait apraxia)	Magnetic, start and turn hesitation, freezing, *marche petit pas*	Frontal lobe signs, dementia, incontinence	Normal pressure hydrocephalus, multi-infarct state, frontal lobe degeneration
Sensory ataxia	Unsteady, worse without visual input and at night.	Romberg sign present, impaired position and vibratory sensation, distal sensory loss	Sensory neuropathy, neuronopathy, dorsal column dysfunction
Cerebellar ataxia	Wide based, staggering, impaired tandem gait	Dysmetria, dysarthria, dysdiadochokinesia, postural instability, Romberg sign present, nystagmus, titubation, impaired check, rebound, intention tremor	Cerebellar degeneration, stroke, drug or alcohol intoxication, thiamine and B12 deficiency, multiple sclerosis
Vestibular ataxia	Unsteady but with narrow base and relatively normal stride, falling to one side, postural instability	Vertigo, nausea, unidirectional nystagmus, normal sensation, reflexes, strength	Acute labrynthitis, Meniere's disease
Steppage gait	Resulting from foot drop, excessive flexion of hips and knees when walking, foot slapping, tripping	Atrophy of distal leg muscles, loss of ankle jerks, distal sensory loss, weakness, and foot drop	Motor neuropathy
Waddling gait	Wide based, bilateral circumduction of leg, excessive lumbar lordosis, symmetric	Weakness of proximal muscles and hip girdle use arms to get up from chair	Myopathy, muscular dystrophy
Antalgic gait	Limping, unable to bear full weight, hesitant	Pain worsening with movement and weight-bearing	Degenerative joint disease, trauma
Hemiparetic	Extension and circumduction of weak and spastic leg, flexed arm	Face, arm, and leg weakness, hyperreflexia, extensor plantar response	Hemispheric or brainstem lesion
Paraparetic	Stiff appearing, extension of knees and ankles, adduction, scissoring both legs	Bilateral leg weakness, hyperreflexia, spasticity, extensor plantar responses	Spinal cord lesion or bilateral cerebral lesions
Dystonic	Extension of great toe (striatal toe), excessive inversion and plantar flexion of foot, excessive flexion of hip, spine deformity, hunched back ("dromedary gait") abducted shoulders, extension of arms, pronation at elbow	Worse with the action of walking, may improve when walking backwards	Inherited, acquired (i.e., post-stroke), or idiopathic

Table 17.10 (cont.)

Type of gait	Description	Associated signs	Causes
Choreic	Irregular, dancelike, widened base, exaggerated movements, lurching quality	Choreoathetic movements of upper extremities	Huntington's disease, levodopa induced dyskinesia
Cautious gait	Wide-based, careful, slow, "walking on ice," arms and legs abducted, en bloc turns	Associated with anxiety, fear of falling or open spaces	Post-fall syndrome, visual impairment, deconditioning
Psychogenic	Bizarre and nonphysiologic gait, rare fall or injury, wide sways with spontaneous ability to recover, "astasia abasia"	Give-way weakness, absence of objective neurological signs	Factitious, somatoform disorders, or malingering

Table 17.11 Gait disorders

Maneuver/condition	Finding	Implication
Sitting	Unable to sit upright	Profound imbalance and /or weakness
	Titubation (truncal or head tremor)	Cerebellar disease
	Leaning to one side	Hemiparesis or basal ganglia disorder
Rising from chair	Unable to rise without using arms to push off	Proximal muscle weakness (myopathy), arthritis, or basal ganglia disorder
Standing	Wide based stance	Cerebellar disease, dorsal column dysfunction
	Stiff neck and head, avoiding motion	Vestibular disease, shoulder or neck pain,
	Unstable with sternal nudge	Back problems or neurologic problems
Gait	Freezing or start hesitation	Parkinsonism
	Reduced arm swing	Parkinsonism
	Involuntary movements	Huntington's disease, basal ganglia disease
Turning	Widened base, multiple short steps without pivoting	Cerebellar disease, hemiparesis, reduced proprioception
	En bloc turns	Parkinsonism, cautious gait, frontal lobe gait
Romberg sign	Sway/instability with eyes closed	Impaired proprioception

of flexion of the neck, elbows, waist, and knees. Hesitation and freezing may occur upon initiating gait, turning, and maneuvering through a doorway. Festination refers to the short accelerating steps that occur when the center of gravity is ahead of the patients, leading to forward propulsion, and the need for legs to race to catch-up with the upper body. When making a turn, the upper and lower body move as a unit, with decreased arm swing and hip rotation, so-called en-bloc turning. Loss of postural stability is generally a late manifestation of idiopathic PD (>10 years symptom duration), but an early sign in atypical and secondary forms of parkinsonism (<5–10 years symptom duration).

Frontal lesions lead to a gait pattern similar to a parkinsonian gait. However in contrast to a parkinsonian gait, the gait often appears clumsy, ataxic, and unsteady with difficulty initiating gait. Patients with frontal lesions tend to hold their trunk upright, appear stiff, have a wide-based gait, and show prolonged time in double support phase.[49] Patients are prone to falling backward. A frontal gait may also appear "magnetic," referring to the appearance that the feet are stuck to the ground. The lower body is predominantly involved, so that arm swing is preserved and may even be exaggerated when a patient attempts to "release" the legs from the ground. Gait initiation fails, but patients show improvement with continued walking. The term "gait apraxia" is used to describe the fact that gait is impaired despite preserved sensation, muscle strength, and leg movements not related to walking. Associated frontal lobe signs, such as primitive reflexes (e.g., snout, grasp, or suck), cognitive impairment, or disinhibited behaviors may be present.

Frontal gait impairment is thought to arise due to a disconnection between frontal, basal ganglia, brainstem, and spinal cord gait centers. A wide variety of pathological conditions lead to frontal lobe dysfunction including normal pressure hydrocephalus (NPH), diffuse cerebrovascular disease, and frontal lobe degenerative conditions such as frontotemporal dementia (FTD), or progressive supranuclear palsy (PSP).

Communicating, or NPH, is an often misunderstood and potentially underdiagnosed entity. Early recognition of the condition is imperative since it may be reversible in the proper clinical setting. Classically, NPH is associated with the triad of gait impairment, urinary incontinence, and dementia. However, the full triad is not always present. Furthermore, the course may be relatively chronic and progressive mimicking a neurodegenerative disorder, acute or subacute mimicking a vascular insult, or static. Gait impairment is usually the first symptom that develops, with memory and urinary symptoms following later. The gait is often wide-based, unsteady, with small short steps and feet barely lifting off of the floor.

The diagnosis of NPH relies on high clinical suspicion, and the finding of enlarged ventricles on brain imaging (CT or MRI). It is important to differentiate between ventricular enlargement due to hydrocephalus and so-called hydrocephalus *ex vacuo* resulting from cerebral atrophy. This latter entity is characterized by both ventricular enlargement and increased sulcal size, and occurs as a result of neurodegenerative diseases and aging. In addition, communicating hydrocephalus needs to be differentiated from obstructive hydrocephalus, which is caused by an obstruction along the ventricular system.

Confirmatory testing includes a large volume lumbar puncture (the so-called tap test), which involves removal of 30 mL–40 mL of spinal fluid with careful examination of gait and cognitive function before and after the procedure. A patient with NPH will have a dramatic response to the procedure. Although a positive response to the tap test confirms the diagnosis, in practice, issues that may confound the test include: inability to remove a sufficient volume of spinal fluid, a clinical exam that is not sensitive to detect subtle improvements, delayed improvement, and placebo response.[50]

Patients with an indeterminate response may benefit from observation with a three-day lumbar drain placed by a neurosurgeon. The procedure increases the ability to detect responders and often helps to confirm the potential benefit of controlled drainage of fluid, before resorting to a permanent shunt. A ventriculoperitoneal shunt is the definitive treatment of choice, although other procedures such as third ventriculostomy may be considered by the surgeon.

Cerebellar lesions cause gait ataxia in combination with a wide variety of signs and symptoms. The gait is jerky, clumsy, and unsteady. The stance and base are broad-based. There is often truncal sway when sitting or standing. Patients are aware of the imbalance and take great effort to ambulate. Lurching of the body may occur as the patient overcompensates to maintain balance. Stepping, direction, distance, and timing are irregular. Step height and stride length are reduced. Tandem gait is impaired due to improper response to postural sway.

Patients with cerebellar dysfunction demonstrate dysmetria with past-pointing on finger-to-nose testing. Speech becomes ataxic or scanning with variations in rhythm, volume, and pitch. Rapid alternating movements display impaired rhythm, or dysdiadochokinesia, which is demonstrated by rapid tapping of the hand or foot. In the geriatric population, acute cerebellar ataxia is generally due to a vascular insult while chronic progressive ataxia is likely due to a neurodegenerative process. Subacute ataxia may be related to infection, nutritional deficiency, or autoimmune disorder. In the geriatric population, acute or subacute ataxia without a structural cause on MRI is suggestive of paraneoplastic cerebellar degeneration (PCD). Hereditary spinocerebellar ataxias (SCA) are marked by an autosomal dominant pattern of inheritance, onset in the third to fifth decades, and progressive loss of function.

Proper examination for a Romberg sign (RS) consists of having the patient stand with feet together and eyes open. Therefore, testing for RS would be impractical, if the patient is unsteady with eyes open.

Corticospinal tract lesions anywhere along its course from the cerebrum to spinal cord will cause weakness and spasticity. Spasticity is defined as increased tone to passive range of motion. Bilateral corticospinal tract lesions caused by spinal cord injury or cerebral palsy will lead to a spastic gait or "scissoring" gait. Both legs are spastic, extended, and internally rotated. The hips adduct excessively.

Hemiparetic gait is caused by a unilateral lesion of the corticospinal tract, most commonly occurring after a stroke. The weak leg is spastic, stiff, and extended and circumducts or makes an arc so that the foot can clear the ground. The weak arm is usually flexed at the elbow, and pulled towards the chest.

Waddling gait is associated with weakness of hip girdle muscles leading to the dropping of the pelvis toward the swinging leg, and compensatory lean towards the standing leg.

Sensory ataxia occurs when dorsal column or large fiber sensory loss occurs. A Romberg sign is often present. Steppage gait occurs as a result of foot drop as the knee and hip flex excessively to compensate for foot drop. Slapping of the feet to the ground may occur as well.

Cautious gait is commonly observed in the elderly who have suffered a fall, usually a severe accidental fall resulting in injury. Acute anxiety develops surrounding the risk of falling again. Physical activity is often decreased, and agoraphobia may develop. The appearance of the gait mimics the gait of a normal person walking on ice. The arms are tense, stance is wide-based, the body turns en bloc. Once a patient has found physical support, the gait is improved.

Treatment

Treatment of gait disorders involves addressing reversible causes and treating chronic medical conditions that exacerbate the gait problems. Physical and occupational therapy can improve strength, balance, and confidence. Medications should always be evaluated with special attention to psychotropic medications, and anticholinergic or antihistaminergic agents. Other treatment modalities include assistive devices, adaptive equipment training, drivers training, and nutritional counseling. Although not rigorously studied, exercise programs such as pilates, yoga, and tai chi would intuitively improve balance and gait.

Besides dopaminergic agents for Parkinson's disease and ventriculoperitoneal shunting for NPH, there are very few specific pharmacological agents for gait disorders. Amantadine, buspirone, and acetazolamide have shown mixed results in patients with cerebellar ataxia.[51]

References

1. Schneider SA, Deuschl G. The treatment of tremor. *Neurotherapeutics* 2014; **11**: 128–38.

2. Zesiewicz TA, Elble R, Louis ED, et al. Practice parameter: therapies for essential tremor: report of the Quality Standards Subcommittee of the American Academy of Neurology. *Neurology* 2005; **64**:2008–20.

3. Koller W, Pahwa R, Busenbark K, et al. High-frequency unilateral thalamic stimulation in the treatment of essential and parkinsonian tremor. *Ann Neurol* 1997; **42**:292–9.

4. Schuurman PR, Bosch DA, Bossuyt PM, et al. A comparison of continuous thalamic stimulation and thalamotomy for suppression of severe tremor. *N Engl J Med* 2000; **342**:461–8.

5. Deuschl G, Bain P, Brin M. Consensus statement of the Movement Disorder Society on Tremor: ad hoc scientific committee. *Mov Disord* 1998; **13**(Suppl 3):2–23.

6. Tyrer P, Alexander MS, Regan A, Lee I. An extrapyramidal syndrome after lithium therapy. *Br J Psychiatry* 1980; **136**:191–4.

7. Niethammer M, Ford B, Permanent lithium-induced cerebellar toxicity: three cases and review of literature. *Mov Disord* 2007; **22**:570–3.

8. Baumann C. Epidemiology, diagnosis and differential diagnosis in Parkinson's disease tremor. *Parkinsonism and Related Disorders* 2012; **18**(Suppl 1):S90–92.

9. Hughes AJ, Daniel SE, Blankson S, Lees AJ. A clinicopathologic study of 100 cases of Parkinson's disease. *Arch Neurol* 1993; **50**:140–8.

10. Respondek G, Stamelou M, Kurz C, et al. The phenotypic spectrum of progressive supranuclear palsy: a retrospective multicenter study of 100 definite cases. *Mov Disord*. 2014 Dec;**29**(14):1758–66.

11. Cummings JL. Reconsidering diagnostic criteria for dementia with lewy bodies. Highlights from the Third International Workshop on Dementia with Lewy Bodies and Parkinson's Disease Dementia, September 17–20, 2003, Newcastle Upon Tyne, United Kingdom. *Rev Neurol Dis* 2004 Winter;**1**(1):31–4.

12. Wenning GK, Geser F, Krismer F, et al. The natural history of multiple system atrophy: a prospective European cohort study. *Lancet Neurol* 2013 Mar;**12**(3):264–74.

13. Armstrong MJ, Litvan I, Lang AE, et al. Criteria for the diagnosis of corticobasal degeneration. *Neurology* 2013 Jan 29;**80**(5):496–503.

14. Winikates J, Jankovic J. Clinical correlates of vascular parkinsonism. *Arch Neurol* 1999; **56**:98–102.

15. Langston JW, Ballard P. Parkinsonism induced by 1-methyl-4-phenyl-1,2,3,6-tetrahydropyridine (MPTP): implications for treatment and the pathogenesis of Parkinson's disease. *Can J Neurol Sci* 1984; **11**:160–5.

16. Olanow CW. Manganese-induced parkinsonism and Parkinson's disease. *Ann N Y Acad Sci* 2004; **1012**:209–23.

17. Klawans HL, Stein RW, Tanner CM, Goetz CG. A pure parkinsonian syndrome following acute carbon monoxide intoxication. *Arch Neurol* 1982; **39**:302–4.

18. Parkinson Study Group. Effects of tocopherol and deprenyl on the progression of disability in early Parkinson's disease. *N Engl J Med* 1993; **328**:176–83.

19. Shults CW, Oakes D, Kieburtz K, et al. Effects of coenzyme Q10 in early Parkinson disease: evidence of slowing of the functional decline. *Arch Neurol* 2002; **59**:1541–50.

20. Whone AL, Watts RL, Stoessl AJ, et al. Slower progression of Parkinson's disease with ropinirole versus levodopa: the REAL-PET study. *Ann Neurol* 2003; **54**:93–101.

21. Parkinson Study Group. Dopamine transporter brain imaging to assess the effects of pramipexole vs. levodopa on Parkinson disease progression. *JAMA* 2002; **287**:1653–61.

22. Parkinson Study Group. A controlled trial of rasagiline in early Parkinson disease: the TEMPO Study. *Arch Neurol* 2002; **59**:1937–43.

23. Calne DB. The role of various forms of treatment in the management of Parkinson's disease. *Clin Neuropharmacol* 1982; **5**(Suppl 1):S38–43.

24. Pritchett AM, Morrison JF, Edwards WD, et al. Valvular heart disease in patients taking pergolide. *Mayo Clin Proc* 2002; **77**:1280–6.

25. Voon V, Sohr M, Lang AE, et al. Impulse control disorders in Parkinson disease: a multicenter case–control study. *Ann Neurol.* 2011 Jun;**69**(6):986–96.

26. Rascol O, Brooks DJ, Korczyn AD, et al. A five-year study of the incidence of dyskinesia in patients with early Parkinson's disease who were treated with ropinirole or levodopa: 056 study group. *N Engl J Med* 2000; **342**: 1484–91.

27. Parkinson Study Group. Pramipexole vs levodopa as initial treatment for Parkinson disease: a randomized controlled trial. Parkinson Study Group. *JAMA* 2000; **284**:1931–8.

28. Cilia R, Akpalu A, Sarfo FS, et al. "The modern pre-levodopa era of Parkinson's disease: insights into motor complications from sub-Saharan Africa." *Brain 137* 2014;**10**:2731–42.

29. Stowe RL, Ives NJ, Clarke C, et al. Dopamine agonist therapy in early Parkinson's disease. *Cochrane Database Syst Rev* 2008;2:CD006564.

30. PD MED Collaborative Group. Long-term effectiveness of dopamine agonists and monoamine oxidase B inhibitors compared with levodopa as initial treatment for Parkinson's disease (PD MED): a large, open-label, pragmatic randomised trial.*The Lancet* 2014;**384**(9949):1196–205.

31. Hauser RA, Hsu A, Kell S, et al. Extended-release carbidopa-levodopa (IPX066) compared with immediate-release carbidopa-levodopa in patients with Parkinson's disease and motor fluctuations: a phase 3 randomised, double-blind trial. *Lancet Neurol* 2013;**12**(4):346–56.

32. Fernandez HH, Standaert DG, Hauser RA, et al. Levodopa-carbidopa intestinal gel in advanced Parkinson's disease: final 12-month, open-label results. *Mov Disord* 2015 Apr;**30**(4):500–9.

33. Zibetti M, Merola A, Artusi CA, et al. Levodopa/carbidopa intestinal gel infusion in advanced Parkinson's disease: a 7-year experience. *Eur J Neurol* 2014 Feb;**21**(2):312–18.

34. Uncini A, Eleopra R, Onofrj M. Polyneuropathy associated with duodenal infusion of levodopa in Parkinson's disease: features, pathogenesis and management. *J Neurol Neurosurg Psychiatry* 2015 May;**86**(5):490–5.

35. Rinne UK, Rinne JO, Rinne JK, et al. Brain receptor changes in Parkinson's disease in relation to the disease process and treatment. *J Neural Transm Suppl* 1983; **18**:279–86.

36. Lew MF, Kricorian G. Results from a 2-year centralized tolcapone liver enzyme monitoring program. *Clin Neuropharmacol* 2007 Sep–Oct;**30**(5):281–6.

37. Martinez-Ramirez D, Okun MS. Rationale and clinical pearls for primary care doctors referring patients for deep brain stimulation. *Gerontology* 2014;**60**(1):38–48.

38. Perestelo-Pérez L, Rivero-Santana A, Pérez-Ramos J, et al. Deep brain stimulation in Parkinson's disease: meta-analysis of randomized controlled trials. *J Neurol* 2014 Nov;**261**(11):2051–60.

39. Mouradian MM, Heuser IJ, Baronti F, Chase TN. Modification of central dopaminergic mechanisms by continuous levodopa therapy for advanced Parkinson's disease. *Ann Neurol* 1990; **27**:18–23.

40. Block G, Liss C, Reines S, et al. Comparison of immediate-release and controlled release carbidopa/levodopa in Parkinson's disease: a multicenter 5-year study. The CR First Study Group. *Eur Neurol* 1997;**37**:23–7.

41. Nutt JG, Woodward WR, Beckner RM, et al. Effect of peripheral catechol-O-methyltransferase inhibition on the pharmacokinetics and pharmacodynamics of levodopa in parkinsonian patients. *Neurology* 1994;**44**:913–9.

42. Parkinson Study Group. Entacapone improves motor fluctuations in levodopa-treated Parkinson's disease patients. *Ann Neurol* 1997;**42**:747–55.

43. Rajput AH, Martin W, Saint-Hilaire MH, Dorflinger E, Pedder S. Tolcapone improves motor function in parkinsonian patients with the "wearing-off" phenomenon: a double-blind, placebo-controlled, multicenter trial. *Neurology* 1997;**49**:1066–71.

44. Pourfar M, Feigin A, Eidelberg D. Natural history. In: Factor SA, Weiner WJ, editors, *Parkinson's Disease: Diagnosis and Clinical Management*. 2nd ed. New York: Demos; 2008: 127–33.

45. Ostergaard K, Aa Sunde N. Evolution of Parkinson's disease during 4 years of bilateral deep brain stimulation of the subthalamic nucleus. *Mov Disord* 2006;**21**:624–631.

46. Marras C, McDermott MP, Rochon PA, et al. Survival in Parkinson disease: thirteen-year follow-up of the DATATOP cohort. *Neurology* 2005;**64**(1):87–93.

47. Tuck K, Brod L, Nutt J, Fromme EK. Preferences of patients with Parkinson. *American Journal of Hospice & Palliative Medicine* 2015;**32**(1):68–77.

48. Verghese J, Le Valley A, Hall CB, et al. Epidemiology of gait disorders in community-residing older adults. *Journal of American Geriatric Society* 2006;**54**:255–61.

49. Sudarsky LR. Gait impairment and falls. In: Samuels S and Feske S, eds. *Office Practice of Neurology*. Philadelphia: Churchill Livingstone; 2003: 25.

50. Marmarou A, Black P, Bergsneider M, et al. Guidelines for management of idiopathic normal pressure hydrocephalus: progress to date. *Acta Neurochir Suppl* 2005;**95**:237–40.

51. Perlman SL. Ataxias. *Clin Geriatr Med* 2006; **22**:859–77.

52. Zesiewicz TA, Sullivan KL, Arnulf I, et al. Practice parameter: treatment of nonmotor symptoms of Parkinson disease: report of the Quality Standards Subcommittee of the American Academy of Neurology. *Neurology* 2010;**74**(11):924–31.

57. Ruzicka E, Jankovic JJ. Disorders of gait. In: Jankovic J and Tolosa E, eds. *Parkinsons Disease and Movement Disorders*. Philadelphia: Lippincott Williams & Wilkins; 2007: 409.

58. Mouton CP, Espino DV. Health screening in older women. *Am Fam Physician* 1999;**59**(7):1835–42.

59. Barak Y, Wagenaar RC, Holt KG. Gait characteristic of elderly people with a history of falls: a dynamic approach. *Phys Ther* 2006 **86**:1501–10.

60. Gilman S. *Merritt's Neurology*. 10th ed. Philadelphia: Lippincott Williams & Wilkins, 2000.

61. Ondo W. Gait and balance disorders. *Med Clin N Am* 2003;**87**(4): 793–801.

62. Hyndman D, Ashburn A, Yardley L, Stack E. Interference between balance, gait, and cognitive task performance among people with stroke living in the community. *Disability and Rehabilitation*. 2006;**28**(13–14):849–56.

63. Nutt JG. Abnormalities of posture and movement. In: Cassel CK, Cohen HJ, Larson EB, et al. (eds). *Geriatric Medicine*. 3rd ed. New York: Spring-Verlag; 1997: 939–48.

64. Factora R, Luciano M. Normal pressure hydrocephalus: diagnosis and new approaches to treatment. *Clin Geriatr Med* 2006;**22**:645–57.

65. Kanade RV, van Deursen RWM, Harding K, Price P. Walking performance in people with diabetic neuropathy: benefits and threats. *Diabetologia* 2006;**49**:1747–54.

Chapter 18

Sleep disorders in the elderly*

Joseph M. Dzierzewski, PhD, Juan C. Rodriguez, MD, and
Cathy Alessi, MD

Introduction

Sleep disorders in late life are often unrecognized, underdiagnosed, and poorly treated. Epidemiological evidence suggests that over 50% of older people suffer from one of several different sleep disorders, many of which carry serious negative physical, mental, and social consequences.[1, 2] This chapter will focus on the two most common sleep disorders in older patients – insomnia and sleep apnea. Both disorders will be described in terms of epidemiology, diagnosis, and treatment management. Contextual factors that complicate the diagnosis and management of sleep disorders in late life will be reviewed with the aim of providing practical information for the medical professional working with older patients.

Healthy sleep

Although disturbed sleep is a common complaint, sleep disorders are not an inevitable event in late life, and many older adults maintain good sleep into the last decades of life. There are, however, noticeable and normal changes in sleep timing, sleep architecture, and sleep quantity that occur throughout the lifespan.[3, 4] Older adults often display an advanced circadian tendency, exhibiting an earlier sleep initiation and an earlier wake-up time. Sleep architecture changes with advanced age and includes spending an increased proportion of time, compared to younger adults, in stages N1 and N2 sleep (i.e., the lighter

stages of sleep) and a decreased proportion of time in stage N3 sleep (i.e., a deeper stage of sleep) and rapid eye movement (REM) sleep. These architecture changes reflect a relative decrease in deep, restorative sleep and an increase in light, transitory sleep. Lastly, older adults tend to spend slightly less time asleep than their younger counterparts. These changes are considered normal in late life and do not indicate a sleep disorder.

Insomnia

Insomnia is the subjective complaint of difficulty initiating sleep, maintaining sleep, or early morning awakenings that must occur at a minimum of three nights per week for three months and be related to significant daytime impairments such as difficulty concentrating, mood disturbances, or fatigue.[5] Key concepts in the definition are the subjective nature of both the sleep complaint and the subsequent daytime consequences. The insomnia complaint need not occur in isolation from other clinical disorders. Insomnia is commonly comorbid with other health conditions and/or other sleep disorders, and this co-occurrence does not preclude an insomnia diagnosis or treatment.

Current estimates suggest the prevalence of insomnia is as high as 60% in older adult community-based samples, and higher still in institutional settings. Prevalence rates tend to be higher in older individuals with multiple physical and psychiatric conditions, and higher among older women than men.[3, 6] There is evidence to suggest that the higher prevalence rates of insomnia among older adults are a direct consequence of the physical and mental health comorbidities of aging, rather than a consequence of aging itself.[7] Whether or not insomnia develops as a result of common disorders of aging or the aging process, it still necessitates an independent diagnosis and focused treatment plan.

---

* This work was supported by UCLA Claude D. Pepper Older Americans Independence Center (NIA 5P30 AG028748), NIH/NCATS UCLA CTSI (UL1TR000124), and VA Advanced Geriatrics Fellowship Program, and the Geriatric Research, Education, and Clinical Center (GRECC), VA Greater Los Angeles Healthcare System.

Reichel's Care of the Elderly, *7th Edition*, ed. Jan Busby-Whitehead *et al.* Published by Cambridge University Press.
© Cambridge University Press 2016.

In older adults, insomnia is most often experienced as a chronic condition (i.e., three months or longer), with the average length of insomnia complaints in older adults lasting several years.[11] Negative consequences of insomnia in late life include: decreased quality of life, risk for falls, psychological and physical difficulties, vast economic and social costs, risk for nursing home placement, and mortality.[8–10]

Diagnosis

Given the high prevalence rates of insomnia in older adults and the serious negative consequences of poor sleep, the routine examination of older patients by their primary care physician or geriatrician should include questions aimed at determining satisfaction with sleep. Asking about sleep satisfaction and sleep-related daytime impairment could highlight the need for additional inquiry. Formal insomnia diagnosis requires a structured clinical interview.

The clinical interview should focus on probable predisposing factors, precipitating factors, and perpetuating factors.[12] Predisposing factors include those that may increase an older adult's likelihood of experiencing poor sleep, such as poor physical and mental health, family history of insomnia, or low socioeconomic status. Precipitating factors include recent life events (e.g., depressive episode, hospitalization, loss of a loved one, moving residences) that may initially hasten an insomnia disorder. Perpetuating factors include all contextual, emotional, and behavioral influences that may sustain an insomnia disorder.

Did you know ...?

The 3P Model of insomnia is very useful for the conceptualization, diagnosis, and treatment of late life insomnia.[9]
- Predisposing factors are all things that increase an older adult's likelihood of experiencing insomnia.
- Precipitating factors are all things that may initially cause an insomnia disorder to occur.
- Perpetuating factors are all things that sustain an insomnia disorder.

Perpetuating factors are the focus of psychological treatment approaches, whereas pharmacotherapy tends to target symptoms alone.

Further tools to aid in insomnia diagnosis include validated self-report questionnaires. Examples include the Insomnia Severity Index and the Pittsburgh Sleep Quality Index.[13, 14] Both questionnaires should take less than five minutes to complete, and could be implemented within routine medical visits. Although both instruments have the potential to aid in insomnia diagnosis, some older patients may find the retrospective recall of sleep to be onerous. A prospective self-report measure of sleep (i.e., a daily sleep diary) can capture very useful information regarding sleep timing, quantity, and quality across consecutive days. However, the use of a sleep diary requires daily monitoring by the patient and a return visit to their provider in one to two weeks. As such, the use of a daily sleep diary may not be practical for the clinical diagnosis of late life insomnia by a primary care physician or geriatrician. More expensive, objective measures of sleep, including wrist actigraphy and polysomnography, are not indicated for routine use in the diagnosis of insomnia in older adults.

Treatment

Treatment of late life insomnia can involve either pharmacological agents, psychological strategies, or both. Given that psychological treatment is safe and has outperformed both pharmacotherapy and combined psychological/pharmacotherapy in head-to-head trials, psychological techniques should be considered as initial treatment.[15, 16]

Psychological interventions

Psychological interventions for insomnia encompass a variety of different techniques, including: sleep education, cognitive therapy, sleep hygiene, relaxation strategies, stimulus control, sleep restriction, and multicomponent treatment packages (often termed cognitive-behavioral treatment for insomnia, or CBTI). Sleep is largely behaviorally regulated, with a strong homeostatic biological drive and circadian component. Interventions with a foundation in behavioral theory and practice have been proven quite effective in the management of insomnia.

Did you know ...?
- Sleep hygiene recommendations are the most commonly used nonpharmacological treatment approach to the management of insomnia.
- There is no evidence to support use of sleep hygiene alone for insomnia management.
- In fact, sleep researchers often use sleep hygiene recommendations as the control or placebo condition in psychological intervention research.

Stimulus control is a behavioral strategy based on classical conditioning principles that aim to increase the response of sleep associated with the stimulus of the bed and bedroom. There is strong evidence in support of stimulus control for insomnia in late life.[17,18] Sleep restriction is a behavioral strategy aimed at increasing the homeostatic sleep drive and strengthening the circadian signal strength through more closely aligning time spent in bed to actual time spent asleep. There is strong evidence in support of sleep restriction for insomnia in late life.[17, 18] Sleep education (e.g., providing older patients with information regarding normal age-related changes in sleep), cognitive therapy (e.g., examining the evidence for commonly held dysfunctional beliefs and attitudes about sleep), and sleep hygiene (e.g., avoiding and/or limiting caffeine, nicotine, and alcohol consumption) have little empirical evidence to support their use as stand-alone treatment options for insomnia in older adults. These three techniques are better suited for use in combination with other psychological treatment strategies. Relaxation strategies may prove beneficial in isolation in improving the sleep of older adults. However, like the preceding strategies, relaxation techniques may be better suited for use in combination with other psychological treatments.

CBTI has the strongest empirical grounding of all available behavioral treatment options for insomnia in older adults.[17, 18] CBTI is a combination treatment for insomnia typically consisting of stimulus control, sleep restriction, and sleep education. CBTI has been demonstrated to result in large improvements in perceived sleep in older adults with insomnia, and older adults prefer CBTI to sedative hypnotics. The typical delivery of CBTI involves one-on-one, face-to-face delivery in four to six weekly (or biweekly) sessions, each lasting between 30 minutes and 60 minutes. CBTI has been successfully delivered in as little as one to two 30-minute sessions, in group formats, and over virtual communication lines. Although commonly delivered by specially trained clinical psychologists, CBTI has been successfully administered by supervised nurse practitioners, mental health nurses, and over web-based platforms.[19] The overwhelming confluence of the evidence leads to CBTI as the recommended frontline treatment for insomnia in older adults. See Table 18.1 for a comprehensive listing of psychological treatment options for insomnia in late life.

Pharmacotherapy

Although sedative hypnotic medications are the most commonly prescribed treatment approach for insomnia in older patients, medication treatment for late life insomnia should be used in the minority of patients. The fact that older adults are more than twice as likely to be prescribed medication treatment for insomnia as younger adults is particularly concerning, given the increased risk for drug side effects, drug interactions, tolerance and dependence, and lack of empirical evidence supporting long-term use in older patients.[20] Short-term pharmacotherapy may be indicated in situations of acute insomnia, but in older adults with chronic insomnia, sedative hypnotics should be used with great caution. When the decision is made to prescribe a sedative hypnotic to an older patient, the smallest effective dose with the lowest risk of adverse effects should be prescribed for the shortest duration of time

The commonly used sedative hypnotic medications can be broadly grouped into three categories: (1) short-, intermediate-, and long-acting benzodiazepines, (2) nonbenzodiazepines or "z-drugs," and (3) sedating antidepressants. See Table 18.2 for a detailed listing of specific drugs. In general, long-acting benzodiazepines should not be used with older adults due to increased risks of daytime sedation, falls, and confusion.[21] Short- or intermediate-acting benzodiazepines are preferable for patients with a primary complaint of sleep maintenance difficulties. The nonbenzodiazepines are a relatively newer group of sedating hypnotic medications. The nonbenzodiazepines have a shorter duration of action than the benzodiazepines, are believed to carry a lower side-effect profile, and appear to be well tolerated in late life; however, there is limited evidence pertaining directly to use of most nonbenzodiazepines specifically in older patients. Sedating antidepressants are often used off-label for their sedative hypnotic effects, though very little empirical evidence supports the use of sedating antidepressants as hypnotic agents in older adults. Additionally, agents with anticholinergic side effects should be avoided.

Sleep apnea

Sleep apnea is a breathing disorder characterized by a reduction (hypopnea) or absence (apnea) of airflow during sleep. When this phenomenon is secondary to a reduced respiratory effort, it is termed "central sleep

Table 18.1 Psychological treatment approaches for insomnia in older adults

Technique	Level of support
Sleep education	
Information regarding normal sleep changes with age. Aimed at normalizing current sleep, improving expectations, and reducing anxiety.	Low*; not an evidence-based practice**; not a recommendation.[†]
Cognitive therapy	
Maladaptive thoughts, beliefs, and attitudes can negatively impact sleep. Challenging these thoughts can help promote sleep through a reduction in sleep disruptive thoughts and emotions.	Low*; not an evidence-based practice**; not a recommendation.[†]
Sleep hygiene	
Instruction to avoid or limit sleep disruptive substances and behaviors, including caffeine, alcohol, nicotine, exercising, and heavy meals at night.	Low*; not an evidence-based practice**; not a recommendation.[†]
Relaxation strategies	
Active or passive relaxation techniques all aimed at reducing physiological or mental arousal that may be interfering with sleep.	Moderate*; not an evidence-based practice**; standard recommendation.[†]
Stimulus control	
Behavioral technique based on classical conditioning principles. Instructs an individual to limit use of the bed to sleep and sex, and to limit the amount of time spent awake in bed.	Strong*; not an evidence-based practice**; standard recommendation.[†]
Sleep restriction	
Behavioral strategy aimed at matching the amount of time one spends in bed with the actual amount of time asleep. A consistent sleep schedule and time in bed is collaboratively prescribed and adjusted as needed.	Strong*; evidence-based practice**; guideline recommendation.[†]
Multicomponent treatment packages	
Combine several individual components into a treatment package. Usually consist of stimulus control, sleep restriction, and sleep education. Sometimes include cognitive therapy, relaxation techniques, or sleep hygiene recommendations.	Strong*; evidence-based practice**; standard recommendation.[†]

* Based on authors' critical review of empirical evidence and clinical practice with older adults.

** Criteria for an intervention to be considered evidence-based include 50% of the outcome measures must demonstrate significant treatment effects with between-group effect sizes of at least 0.20.[14]

† American Academy of Sleep Medicine (AASM) practice parameters.[15]

apnea" (CSA). More frequent is obstructive sleep apnea (OSA), in which the respiratory effort persists during the episodes of hypoventilation.

The prevalence of sleep apnea increases with age, with rates up to 40% being reported in people older than 65 years old.[22] Sleep apnea is more common in men and in patients with multiple comorbidities,

especially dementia and obesity. In CSA the absence of respiratory effort is secondary to neurological conditions (e.g., stroke), heart failure, or drugs and substances that depress the central nervous system (e.g., opioids). In OSA, the repetitive obstructions of the upper airway are secondary to anatomical factors such as obesity and/or reduced activation of the dilatory

Table 18.2 Medications commonly used for insomnia in older adults

Generic name	Drug class	Initial dosage (mg)	Usual dosage	Half-life (in hours)	Comments
Eszopiclone	Short-acting nonbenzodiazepine	1	1–2	6	Approved for long-term use (not specific to older patients); may cause unpleasant taste and headache
Zolpidem	Short-acting nonbenzodiazepine	5	6.25	3	Little daytime carryover or rebound insomnia; risk of nocturnal behaviors
Zaleplon	Short-acting nonbenzodiazepine	5	5–10	1	Little daytime carryover or rebound insomnia
Temazepam	Intermediate-acting benzodiazepine	7.5	7.5–15	8.8	Psychomotor impairment; risk of falls
Ramelteon	Melatonin receptor agonist	8	8	2.6	Little rebound insomnia or withdrawal; dizziness, myalgia, and headaches
Doxepin	Sedating antidepressant	3	3–6	15.3	Should not be taken within 3 hours of eating; anticholinergic effects
Trazodone	Sedating antidepressant	25	25–150	2–4	Off-label use; insomnia + depression; low anticholinergic effects; orthostatic hypotension
Mirtazapine	Sedating antidepressant	7.5	7.5–45	31–39	Off-label use; insomnia + depression; increased appetite, weight gain, headache; akathisia

muscles of the airway (e.g., under the effect of alcohol or sedative drugs). Patients incur frequent episodes of hypoxia and hypercapnia during sleep resulting from these breathing pauses.

Associations between sleep apnea and medical and neuropsychiatric conditions are abundant, and include hypertension, coronary artery disease, depression, car accidents, cognitive impairment, stroke, and mortality.[23, 24] A healthy older adult with sleep apnea usually complains of headache (typically in the morning), daytime sleepiness, irritability, fatigue, and impotence in men. Medically compromised patients who perform few daytime activities or those with cognitive impairment may present with subtle manifestations or may even be asymptomatic. Bed partners should be interviewed, as they can describe snoring, gasping, choking, apnea episodes, or irritability. Although common findings at the physical exam include hypertension and obesity, the latter is less frequent in older patients.[25] A crowded oral pharynx may also be seen.

Diagnosis

Clinical findings are neither specific nor sensitive enough to diagnose sleep apnea. Some clinical prediction rules are useful for screening purposes (e.g., STOP-BANG).[26] The gold standard for the diagnosis of sleep apnea is in-laboratory polysomnography. The American Academy of Sleep Medicine recommends the measurement of the sleep stages (electroencephalogram), muscular activity, nasal airflow, oxygen saturation, electrocardiogram, snoring, body position, and limb movements.[27] A more convenient and feasible diagnostic alternative is the use of portable monitors at home, most of which record nasal airflow, respiratory movements, and arterial oxygenation. These tests have shown a high correlation with polysomnography, especially for moderate and severe cases, but are not recommended in patients with multiple comorbidities or when CSA or other sleep disorders are suspected. The diagnosis is based upon the average number of hypopneas and apneas per hour (apnea hypopnea index, or AHI). Sleep apnea is classified as mild (AHI 5–15), moderate (AHI 16–30), or severe (AHI >30). Coexisting sleep apnea and insomnia may be common in older adults. (See Figure 18.1.)

Did you know…?

Sleep apnea can be easily screened for during routine clinical care using the STOP-BANG questionnaire:[18]

1. Do you SNORE loudly (louder than talking or loud enough to be heard through closed doors)?
2. Do you often feel TIRED, fatigued, or sleepy during daytime?
3. Has anyone OBSERVED you stop breathing during your sleep?
4. Do you have or are you being treated for high blood PRESSURE?
5. Body mass index (BMI) more than 35?
6. AGE over 50 years old?
7. NECK circumference >15.75 inches?
8. Male GENDER?

≥ 3 yes answers: high-risk for obstructive sleep apnea

Treatment

General treatment recommendations for older patients diagnosed with OSA include avoidance of sedative drugs and alcohol, exercise, and the consumption of a hypocaloric diet to reduce weight and control blood pressure. In some cases, a short nap before long driving periods may be recommended if excessive daytime sleepiness is present.[28, 29] Positive airway pressure (PAP) used to keep the airway open during sleep episodes is the first-line therapy for patients with moderate or severe OSA. This therapy has been demonstrated to improve sleep quality, daytime symptoms, blood pressure, ventricular ejection fraction, and cognitive function. [28] Observational studies have reported that PAP reduces the risk of stroke, cardiovascular disease, and mortality in older patients.[30, 31] Good adherence to PAP therapy (defined as >4 hours of use per night on 70% of nights) may be a challenge to older patients.

Continuous PAP (CPAP) is the most commonly used type of PAP device. CPAP provides a fixed pressure of air during the breathing cycle. There are more advanced devices (e.g., BiPAP or APAP) that can provide different levels of pressure and may be better tolerated by some patients. Other measures that can improve patient compliance to PAP therapy are the use of humidifiers, proper fitting of a correct interface (e.g., nasal or facial mask), and concomitant

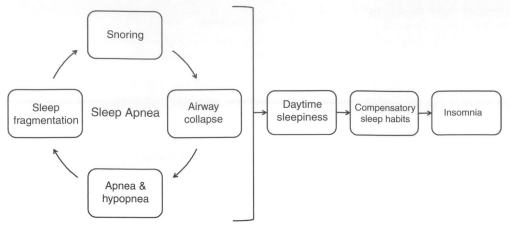

Figure 18.1 Hypothesized relationship between sleep apnea and the development of insomnia. The model illustrates that sleep apnea can cause daytime sleepiness, which in turn may relate to an individual engaging in compensatory sleep habits, which can lead to insomnia symptoms.

psychological cognitive behavioral therapy. A multidisciplinary approach is vital, especially at the beginning of the treatment. Long-term adherence is best predicted by use during the first week of therapy.[32]

There are several alternatives for patients who reject or do not adhere to PAP therapy. Oral appliances (i.e., mandibular advancement devices) move the jaw forward with the goal of reducing obstruction of the airway. Nose valves attempt to increase airway pressure through closing during expiration. Surgical procedures (e.g., uvulopalatopharyngoplasty) remove excess tissue in the upper airway. The effectiveness evidence and availability of these options is scarce, and most empirical studies have excluded older adults.[28]

Contextual factors

Hospitalization, institutionalization, and dementia are common in late life and are associated with increased rates of sleep disorders when compared to that seen in community-dwelling older adults. Sleep disorders in these contexts are reviewed in the following paragraphs.

Sleep disorders in the hospital

Sleep disorders are frequent and generally underrecognized in the hospital. Research has shown that patients tend to underestimate their total sleep time in hospitals, while nurses overestimate how long patients sleep.[33] Abnormalities in electroencephalogram patterns and plasma levels of melatonin have been observed among hospitalized patients. These

alterations may occur during sepsis or inadequate light exposure, but the underlying mechanisms behind these observations are not completely understood.[34]

There are many potential factors leading to the increased prevalence of insomnia in hospitalized older adults. Acute pulmonary and cardiac diseases may interfere with the normal breathing cycle, generate dyspnea and cough, and lead to subsequent problems during sleep. Other symptoms that are also common in the hospital setting and may disrupt sleep are pain, delirium, and anxiety. Hospital-related environmental factors that interrupt sleep are noise, light, an unfamiliar bed, administration of medications, and the measurement of vital signs during the night. These disruptors are much more frequent in intensive care units.

The overall prevalence of sleep apnea in the hospital setting is unknown; however, in specific populations such as stroke patients it is as high as 60%.[35] Adverse outcomes are more frequent in patients with sleep apnea and include intra- and postoperative complications, prolonged length of stay, and possibly increased mortality.[36, 37] Screening questionnaires can be used to assess the risk of undiagnosed sleep apnea in hospitalized patients. Some recommendations for patients at risk are to reduce the doses of neuromuscular blockers, avoid opioids, assume a semi-upright sleeping position in bed, peripheral oxygen monitoring, oxygen supplementation, and the use of PAP therapy. Empirical evidence to support these strategies is limited. Those patients who have been previously prescribed PAP therapy should use it during the hospital stay.

Sleep disorders in the nursing home

Sleep disorders are more frequent in nursing home residents than in community-dwelling older people. Sleep/wake patterns are altered in most residents. A typical sleep presentation includes several episodes of napping during the day, coupled with fragmented sleep at night. Factors associated with these findings are older age and presence of medical and psychiatric diseases. Institutionalized older people present with a high prevalence of comorbidities and geriatric syndromes, such as frailty, depression, heart failure, urinary incontinence, and dementia. As in the hospital, environmental factors (e.g., lack of exposure to sunlight and physical activity, increased amount of time spent in bed during the day, and the use of medications with effects on the central nervous system) also contribute to the occurrence of sleep disorders. Some of the negative consequences ascribed to sleep disorders in this population are poorer self-rated quality of life, reduced involvement in social activities, and increased mortality.[38, 39]

A multidimensional intervention should be considered to treat sleep disorders in nursing homes. Nonpharmacological measures such as increased light exposure (e.g., bright light boxes) and physical activity participation may have modest benefit. Nighttime reductions in noise and light should be attempted. Adherence of nursing home staff to these recommendations can prove difficult. Cognitive behavioral strategies have been demonstrated to improve the subjective sleep quality of older adults in nursing homes.[40] Sedative hypnotic medications may have a small benefit in improving sleep of residents, but considering the side effects, risks, and complex metabolism of these drugs in frail older adults, they should be avoided if possible.[41]

Sleep disorders and dementia

Sleep disorders are frequent and have a great impact on patients with dementia. Sleep disorders are associated with loss of function, cognitive impairment, and an increased burden in caregivers.[42] Disturbed sleep is a frequently cited reason for institutionalization.

> **Did you know …?**
>
> In addition to insomnia and sleep apnea, older adults may present with the following sleep disorders:
> 1. Advanced phase disorder: a systematic shift in sleep timing to an earlier sleep initiation and rise time.
> 2. REM behavior disorder: movement or acting out of dreams during sleep; much more common in people with Parkinson's disease.
> 3. Restless legs syndrome: uncomfortable sensations in the legs that occur with rest/inactivity.

Sundowning is a particularly salient sleep-related disturbance in older adults with dementia. Sundowning is an altered behavioral state (e.g., delirium, anxiety, agitation, wandering) of a patient with dementia, in which the symptoms are characteristically more intense during the evening and at night. Biological and environmental factors have been suggested to explain this phenomenon. Conversely, some authors have proposed that sundowning is the result of more exhausted caregivers' perceptions at the end of the day.[42]

In a patient with dementia, a comprehensive evaluation of not only the patient but also the environment should be performed to identify the potential causes of the sleep disorder. Special attention is necessary regarding the use of caffeine, alcohol, or any medication that may interfere with sleep. Common clinical findings in healthy older adults could be subtle or absent in patients with dementia. For example, delirium could be the only clinical manifestation of sleep apnea in dementia patients and should trigger further evaluation in patients with risk factors mentioned above. Pain and mood disorders could also be precipitating factors of the sleep disorder and may be more difficult to evaluate in patients with cognitive impairment.

Identifying and treating the underlying causal factors of the sleep disorder in conjunction with sleep-focused interventions could be effective in improving sleep patterns in older adults with dementia. Light exposure, physical exercise, stimulus control, sleep restriction, and behavioral activation/social activities should always be considered as first-line therapy. A recent meta-analysis of sleep medications for patients with Alzheimer's disease reported that trazodone in low doses (50 mg) improves total nocturnal sleep time and sleep efficiency, whereas there was no benefit for melatonin or ramelteon. There is a lack of evidence for use of most sedative hypnotic drugs in patients with Alzheimer's disease (e.g., benzodiazepines, nonbenzodiazepines hypnotics, other antidepressants, and antipsychotics agents). [43] Given the increased risk of falls and cognitive decline with benzodiazepines and increased mortality with antipsychotics agents in patients with dementia, a thoughtful risk/benefit evaluation should be performed and discussed with the patient and caregivers before considering these drugs.

Conclusions

Sleep disorders are a very common occurrence in late life. These sleep disorders are associated with serious negative physical, mental, and social consequences. Insomnia and sleep apnea are particularly important conditions in older adults, and may coexist. Although good sleep is often taken for granted, poor sleep can be very deleterious to the general health and quality of life of older patients. Recognition and appropriate management of sleep problems in older adults is essential.

References

1. Foley DJ, Monjan AA, Brown SL, et al. Sleep complaints among elderly persons: an epidemiological study of 3 communities. *Sleep*. 1995;**18**:425–432.

2. Mellinger GD, Balter MB, Uhlenhuth EH. Insomnia and its treatment: prevalence and correlates. *Arch Gen Psychiatry*. 1985;**42**:225–232.

3. Morgan K. Sleep and aging. In: Lichstein K, Morin C, eds. *Treatment of Late Life Insomnia*. Thousand Oaks, CA: Sage Publications, 2000.

4. Floyd JA, Medler SM, Ager JW, et al. Age-related changes in initiation and maintenance of sleep: a meta-analysis. *Res Nurs Health*. 2000;**23**:106–117.

5. Diagnostic Classification Steering Committee TMJC. *International Classification of Sleep Disorders*, 3rd edition. Rochester, NY: American Academy of Sleep Medicine, 2014.

6. Ford DE, Kamerow DB. Epidemiological study of the sleep disturbances and psychiatric disorders. *JAMA*. 1989;**262**:1479–1484.

7. Vitiello MV, Moe KE, Prinz PN. Sleep complaints cosegregate with illness in older adults: clinical research informed by and informing epidemiological studies of sleep. *J Psychosom Res*. 2002;**53**:555–559.

8. Bloom HG, Ahmed I, Alessi CA, et al. Evidence-based recommendations for the assessment and management of sleep disorders in older persons. *J Am Geriatr Soc*. 2009;**57**:761–789.

9. Rodriguez JC, Dzierzewski, JM, Alessi, CA. Sleep problems in the elderly. *Med Clin North Am*. 2015;**99**:431–439.

10. Roth T. Insomnia: Definition, prevalence, etiology, and consequences. *J Clin Sleep Med*. 2007;**3**:S7–S10.

11. Dzierzewski JM, O'Brien E, Kay DB, et al. Tackling sleeplessness: psychological treatment options for insomnia in older adults. *Nat Sci Sleep*. 2010;**2**:47–61.

12. Spielman AJ, Caruso LS, Glovinsky PB. A behavioral perspective on insomnia treatment. *Psychiat Clinics of N Amer*. 1987;**10**:541–553.

13. Bastien CH, Vallieres A, Morin CM. Validation of the Insomnia Severity Index as an outcome measure for insomnia research. *Sleep Med*. 2001;**2**:297–307.

14. Buysse DJ, Reynolds CFI, Monk TH, et al. The Pittsburgh Sleep Quality Index: a new instrument for psychiatric practice and research. *Psychiatry Res*. 1989;**28**(2):193–213.

15. Morin CM, Colecchi C, Stone J, et al. Behavioral and pharmacological therapies for late life insomnia: a randomized controlled trial. *JAMA*. 1999;**281**:991–999.

16. Sivertsen B, Omvik S, Pallesen S, et al. Cognitive behavioral therapy vs zopiclone for treatment of chronic primary insomnia in older adults. *JAMA*. 2006;**295**:2851–2858.

17. McCurry SM, Logsdon RG, Teri L, et al. Evidence-based psychological treatments for insomnia in older adults. *Psychol Aging*. 2007;**22**:18–27.

18. Morgenthaler T, Kramer M, Alessi CA, et al. Practice parameters for the psychological and behavioral treatment of insomnia: an update. An American Academy of Sleep Medicine report. *Sleep*. 2006;**29**:1415–1419.

19. Siebern AT, Manber R. New developments in cognitive behavioral therapy as the first-line treatment of insomnia. *Psychol Res Behav Manag*. 2011;**4**:21–28.

20. Stewart R, Besset A, Bebbington P, et al. Insomnia comorbidity and impact and hypnotic use by age group in a national survey population aged 16 to 74 years. *Sleep*. 2006;**29**:1391–1397.

21. Alessi CA. Sleep problems. In: Durso SC, Sullivan GM, eds. *Geriatrics Review Syllabus: A Core Curriculum in Geriatric Medicine*, 8th edition. New York: American Geriatrics Society, 2013: 316–339.

22. Young T, Peppard PE, Gottlieb DJ. Epidemiology of obstructive sleep apnea: a population health perspective. *Am J Respir Crit Care Med*. 2002;**165**:1217–1239.

23. George CFP. Sleep apnea, alertness, and motor vehicle crashes. *American Journal of Respiratory and Critical Care Medicine*. 2007;**176**(10):954–956.

24. Punjabi NM, Caffo BS, Goodwin JL, et al. Sleep-disordered breathing and mortality: a prospective cohort study. *PLoS Medicine*. 2009;**6**(8):e1000132.

25. Kales A, Cadieux RJ, Bixler EO, et al. Severe obstructive sleep apnea – I: onset, clinical course, and characteristics. *Journal of Chronic Diseases*. 1985;**38**(5):419–425.

26. Cowan DC, Allardice G, MacFarlane D, et al. Predicting sleep disordered breathing in outpatients with suspected OSA. *BMJ Open*. 2014;**4**:e004519.

27. Epstein LJ, Kristo D, Strollo PJ Jr, et al. Clinical guidelines for the evaluation, management and long-term care of obstructive sleep apnea in adults. *J Clin Sleep Med*. 2009;**15**:263–276.

28. Qaseem A, Holty JE, Owens DK, et al. Management of obstructive sleep apnea in adults: a clinical practice guideline from the American College of Physicians. *Annals of Internal Medicine*. 2013;**159**(7):471–483.

29. Strohl KP, Brown DB, Collop N, et al. An official American Thoracic Society Clinical Practice Guideline: sleep apnea, sleepiness, and driving risk in noncommercial drivers. An update of a 1994 Statement. *American Journal of Respiratory and Critical Care Medicine*. 2013;**187**(11):1259–1266.

30. Campos-Rodriguez F, Pena-Grinan N, Reyes-Nuñez N, et al. Mortality in obstructive sleep apnea-hypopnea patients treated with positive airway pressure. *Chest*. 2005;**128**:624–633.

31. Giles TL, Lasserson TJ, Smith BJ, et al. Continuous positive airway pressure for obstructive sleep apnoea in adults. *Cochrane Database Syst Rev*. 2006;**25**:CD001106.

32. Rosenthal L, Gerhardstein R, Lumley A, et al. CPAP therapy in patients with mild OSA: implementation and treatment outcome. *Sleep Medicine*. 2000;**1**(3);215–220.

33. Krahn LE, Lin SC, Wisbey J, et al. Assessing sleep in psychiatric inpatients: nurse and patient reports versus wrist actigraphy. *Ann Clin Psychiatry*. 1997;**9**:203–210.

34. Venkateshiah SB, Collop NA. Sleep and sleep disorders in the hospital. *Chest*. 2012;**141**:1337–1345.

35. Iranzo A, Santamaria J, Bereguer J, et al. Prevalence and clinical importance of sleep apnea in the first night after cerebral infarction. *Neurology*. 2002;**58**:911–916.

36. Kaw R, Chung F, Pasupuleti V, et al. Meta-analysis of the association between obstructive sleep apnoea and postoperative outcome. *British Journal of Anaesthesia*. 2012;**109**;897–906.

37. D'Apuzzo MR, Browne JA. Obstructive sleep apnea as a risk factor for postoperative complications after revision joint arthroplasty. *The Journal of Arthroplasty*. 2012;**27**(8):95–98.

38. Koch S, Haesler E, Tiziani A, Wilson J. Effectiveness of sleep management strategies for residents of aged care facilities: findings of a systematic review. *Journal of Clinical Nursing*. 2006;**15**(10):1267–1275.

39. Ancoli-Israel S, Klauber MR, Kripke DF, et al. Sleep apnea in female patients in a nursing home. Increased risk of mortality. *CHEST*. 1989;**96**(5):1054–1058.

40. Alessi CA, Martin JL, Webber AP, et al. Randomized, controlled trial of a nonpharmacological intervention to improve abnormal sleep/wake patterns in nursing home residents. *J Am Geriatr Soc*. 2005;**53**:803–810.

41. Koch S, Haesler E, Tiziani A, et al. Effectiveness of sleep management strategies for residents of aged care facilities: findings of a systematic review. *J Clin Nurs*. 2006;**15**:1267–1275.

42. Roth HL. Dementia and sleep. *Neurol Clin*. 2012;**30**:1213–1248.

43. McCleery J, Cohen DA, Sharpley AL. Pharmacotherapies for sleep disturbances in Alzheimer's disease. *Cochrane Database Syst Rev*. 2014;**3**:CD009178.

Chapter 19

Clinical geropsychiatry

Susan W. Lehmann, MD, and Peter V. Rabins, MD, MPH

Although most older people are mentally healthy, persons over the age of 65 are vulnerable to the same spectrum of psychiatric disorders as are younger people.[1] Community epidemiologic studies indicate that prevalence rates for major depressive disorders, panic disorders, and substance use disorders are lower in the elderly. However, the prevalence of phobic disorders does not change with age, and the prevalence of cognitive disorders and their associated psychiatric morbidity sharply increases with age.[2]

Psychiatric problems in the elderly are more common in certain settings. For instance, anxiety and depressive disorders are common among patients in medical clinics, and confusional states (delirium) are seen in approximately 25% of hospitalized patients on medical and surgical services.[3] In nursing homes and long-term care facilities, more than 50% of residents have been found to suffer from some sort of psychiatric problem, most commonly dementia, and behavioral problems and depression are common.[4] In all, there is a need for careful attention to psychiatric symptoms in the elderly, since compassionate and appropriate treatment improves both overall functioning and quality of life.

Evaluation

History

The evaluation of the older adult with a possible mental disorder begins, as does any medical evaluation, with a careful history. If the patient is accompanied by family members, it is helpful to meet with them also to facilitate obtaining a complete history and database. The history should focus on a thorough assessment of the reason for the appointment, including a careful determination of when symptoms first

appeared, how they have progressed over time, and accompanying features. In addition, the complete history should include the following:

1. *Family psychiatric history.* The clinician should inquire whether any blood relatives, especially first-degree relatives, have ever suffered from a mental disorder, suicide, or alcoholism or have been hospitalized in a psychiatric facility.

2. *Psychiatric history of the patient.* This should include any prior contact with psychiatrists or therapists, prior psychiatric hospitalizations, or previous treatment by any medical professional for mood problems or bad nerves.

3. *Medical history.* It is important to detail all prior hospitalizations and surgeries and any current medical conditions that continue to be a focus of treatment.

4. *Medications.* This should be a complete list of all medications, both prescription drugs and over-the-counter medications being taken by the patient, including dosages. Because many medications prescribed for a variety of medical conditions have psychiatric side effects, it is helpful to inquire about the length of time the patient has taken the medication and to pay particular attention to changes in medications prescribed shortly before the onset of the presenting psychiatric symptoms.

5. *Personal history.* This includes information about the patient's family of origin, siblings, childhood history, schooling (especially level of education), work history, adjustment to retirement, sexual history, marital history, and children. It is also important to inquire about the patient's living situation, including with whom he or she lives and the type of home (i.e., house or apartment, rented

Reichel's Care of the Elderly, *7th Edition*, ed. Jan Busby-Whitehead *et al.* Published by Cambridge University Press.
© Cambridge University Press 2016.

or owned). This is also a good time to ask about any structural aspects of the home that may pose problems for the patient, such as stairs, second floor bathrooms, tub, and showers.

6. *Patterns of alcohol use.* Problems of alcohol use occur in the elderly, as in younger persons, and may underlie symptoms of anxiety, depression, irritability, memory loss, sleep disturbance, sexual dysfunction, and paranoia. It is necessary to obtain information on the type of alcohol consumed, how frequently, and how much and to inquire about early-morning shakes, blackouts, alcohol-induced seizures, and prior episodes of detoxification and treatment.

Mental status examination

The heart of the psychiatric evaluation is the mental status examination, the here-and-now data gathering equivalent of the physical examination. It allows a systematic examination of the major aspects of the patient's mental state. Depending on the nature of the presenting complaint and the cooperativeness of the patient, certain areas of the mental status examination may be emphasized, whereas others may be only touched on briefly. The complete mental status examination, however, always includes attention to the following areas:

1. *General appearance.* This includes observation of neatness and personal hygiene, eye contact during the interview, and any abnormal movements, tremors, tics, or unusual behaviors.

2. *Speech.* This refers to the motor and linguistic forms of the patient's verbal language. It includes attention to the rate, rhythm, and loudness of the patient's speech and whether the patient's use of language is coherent, goal-oriented, logical, and easy to follow. Does the patient seem to jump from one idea to another with little connection between ideas? This is described as loose association and in an extreme form may be called flight of ideas. Some patients may have trouble sticking to the topic at hand and exhibit a tendency to wander off track (tangentially) but can be redirected to the issue being discussed. Obsessional patients may be inclined to be over-inclusive in detail (circumstantiality), sometimes losing sight of the forest for the trees. Aphasic patients have word-finding difficulty, paraphasias (made-up words), and nonfluent or fluent but content-free speech.

3. *Mood.* The assessment of mood involves both ascertainment of the patient's subjective description of his or her mood state and the clinician's objective observations of the patient's mood. Some depressed elderly patients report that they don't feel depressed yet use words such as "sad," "bewildered," or "drained" and appear tense, anxious, or withdrawn.

4. *Suicidal ideation.* It is important to ask any patient with a sad mood about suicidal thoughts. Contrary to popular myth, asking about suicidal thoughts does not increase the likelihood that a patient will follow through on such ideas. We distinguish between passive suicidal thoughts (i.e., wishing one were dead or would die) and active suicidal ideation (i.e., planning self-harm). Many depressed patients express passive wishes for death but are adamant that they would never attempt suicide for personal, religious, or family reasons.

5. *Abnormal thought content.*

   a. Hallucinations are sensory experiences that are perceived in the absence of a sensory stimulus. Auditory and visual hallucinations are most common, but tactile and olfactory hallucinations also occur in some disorders.

   b. Delusions are idiosyncratic, fixed, false beliefs that are not culturally determined or shared. Paranoid delusions and delusions of persecution are most common. Manic patients may have grandiose delusions about themselves and their abilities. Other types of delusions that may develop in older patients are delusional jealousy (falsely believing one's spouse has been unfaithful) and delusions of parasitosis (believing one's skin to be infested with worms or insects). Often the delusion seems plausible until further medical or social investigation reveals it to be unfounded. A distinguishing feature of delusions is that the patient cannot be persuaded that the belief is false despite evidence to the contrary.

   c. Obsessive thoughts are intrusive, repetitive, unwanted ideas that a person cannot stop from coming to mind.

   d. Compulsions are intrusive, repetitive, unwanted behaviors that a person cannot stop, although the person recognizes them as unnecessary, excessive, or foolish. Some examples are compulsive hand washing and checking behaviors.

e. Phobias are excessive specific fears that cause a person to avoid the dreaded situation.

6. *Cognitive assessment.* Every psychiatric evaluation of the older patient should include an assessment of cognitive functioning. Depending on the nature of the initial presenting complaint and the cooperativeness of the patient, this assessment may be fairly brief or detailed and focused. A basic cognitive screening should include level of alertness, attentiveness, orientation, short- and long-term memory, attention and concentration, naming ability and language comprehension, and abstract reasoning. If significant cognitive impairment is detected in one or more of these areas, further neuropsychological testing and/or laboratory testing may be warranted.

Specific conditions

Anxiety disorders

Anxiety is feelings of tension and distress that are distinct from sadness and that usually lack a stressful stimulus of such severity as to explain the feeling. It often has both somatic (physical) and psychological components. *Generalized anxiety disorder* is a condition marked by excessive worry and anxiety persisting for six months or more. It is accompanied by signs and symptoms of motor tension, including muscle aches or soreness, a feeling of restlessness, a feeling of shakiness, and reports of easy fatigability. In addition, there are feelings of being on edge, having difficulty concentrating and falling asleep, and being unusually irritable. At least three of these additional symptoms of motor tension must be present along with the subjective distress of constant worry to make the diagnosis of generalized anxiety disorder. Generalized anxiety disorder should be distinguished from a patient's report of feeling "anxious." The new development of a complaint of "anxiety" in an older person is most commonly caused by major depression. Generalized anxiety disorder, on the other hand, is usually lifelong, not episodic, and associated with the somatic and psychological accompanying symptoms previously described. *Panic disorder* is diagnosed when the patient reports discrete episodes (attacks) of intense fear and somatic anxiety symptoms that are both unprovoked and unexpected. The associated somatic symptoms include palpitations, sweating, trembling, shortness of breath, chest discomfort, lightheadedness, and abdominal distress. It is common for panic attacks to occur repeatedly in certain circumstances (e.g., in a grocery store). Specific phobias are clearly delineated fears of objects or situations that a person realizes are unrealistic but can nevertheless not resist. They sometimes occur in concert with panic attacks.

The anxiety disorders are among the most common psychologic problems identified in mental health surveys. Nonpharmacologic and pharmacologic therapies are usually used. Desensitization (gradually exposing the patient to the source of distress) coupled with relaxation in often effective. The most effective pharmacologic therapy is the use of antidepressants. There is no evidence that one antidepressant is better than another. Selective serotonin reuptake inhibitors (SSRIs), such as citalopram, sertraline, and fluoxetine, and selective noradrenergic/serotoninergic uptake inhibitors (SNRIs) such as venlafaxine and duloxetine, are effective for treating anxiety disorders. SSRIs are better tolerated with fewer side effects than tricyclic antidepressants.

Benzodiazepine compounds are also effective for anxiety disorders but, because of their addictive potential and side effects, are generally not prescribed as a first-line therapy. Short-acting benzodiazepines (e.g., alprazolam) have more abuse and addiction liability than longer-acting compounds (e.g., clonazepam), but the longer-acting compounds are more likely to accumulate and lead to sedation, functional impairment, and drowsiness. Buspirone is nonaddicting but appears to be less effective in the treatment of anxiety than benzodiazepine or antidepressants. If symptoms are severe and immediate results are desirable, the clinician may choose to initiate treatment with both an antidepressant and benzodiazepine and taper the benzodiazepine several weeks after the antidepressant begins to work.

Mixed anxiety and depression

Symptoms of anxiety and depression frequently co-occur. The clinician should make an effort to determine which is primary and to focus treatment on that set of symptoms. In our experience, depression is more frequently the primary disorder, but this is controversial. Features in the history suggesting that depression is primary include a history of episodic (prior) depressive episodes, a family history of depressive episodes, diurnal mood variation (i.e., a tendency for symptoms to be worse in the morning), self-blame, guilt, difficulty staying asleep in contrast to falling asleep, hopelessness, and mental somatization. Although anxiety disorders can begin de novo in late life, it is much more common for a depressive episode to appear for the first time in an older person. Because antidepressants are effective in both anxiety disorders and major depression, they should be the first-line treatment when the clinician is unsure which is primary.

Mood disorders

Mood disorders are the most frequently clinically diagnosed and the most treatable psychiatric disorders in older people.[5, 6] They encompass a spectrum of disorders ranging from adjustment disorder (in which an identified psychosocial stressor provokes a mild depressive reaction that impairs functioning) to psychotic major depression with hallucinations and/ or delusions to mania.

Major depression is characterized by a persistent diminution in three spheres of functioning: (a) mood, (b) vital sense (a sense of one's well-being and energy), and (c) attitude toward oneself (self-confidence). Depressed patients tend to have a more negative self-assessment than is usual for them, may be self-blaming, or can have excessive feelings of guilt, regret, or worthlessness. Patients with major depression experience loss of energy, disturbed sleep (usually insomnia and early morning awakening), diminished appetite and weight loss, difficulty thinking and concentrating, and a loss of interest and pleasure in activities that were once enjoyed. Ruminant thoughts of death and suicidal thoughts may occur during the course of a major depression. Elderly patients who are depressed often complain of physical rather than psychologic distress. Up to a third of older people who suffer from major depression do not describe their mood as depressed. Rather, they focus on feelings of weakness, lack of energy, and lack of motivation. Somatic complaints, including headaches, gastrointestinal disturbances, and body aches, are common. Occasionally, hallucinations and delusions occur. Such hallucinations and delusions tend to have a depressive theme and are consistent with low mood (e.g., the persecutory delusion that one deserves punishment; the delusion that one has no money, clothes, or insurance; and the delusion that one has a terrible illness that doctors cannot find).

Major depression can first occur at any point in the life span. It may occur as a single episode, but recurrence is common. The causation of major depression is complex, involving genetic, neurochemical, and psychologic factors. Although genetic transmission is poorly understood, it is clear that affective (mood) disorders tend to run in families and that there is a higher prevalence of affective disorders among the first-degree relatives of depressed individuals. The neurochemistry of depression is an active area of research focusing on abnormalities in adrenergic and serotonergic neurotransmitters in the brain. Many commonly prescribed medications, including steroids, reserpine, methyldopa, antiparkinsonian drugs, and β-adrenergic blockers, can cause depression. Depression is especially common in diseases of the brain. For example, 30%–60% of poststroke patients have a clinically significant episode of depression within six months to two years of the stroke. The incidence of poststroke depression has been found to be greatest among patients with strokes affecting the left anterior cerebral hemisphere.[7] Although major depression can occur in the absence of any precipitating event, psychologic issues such as recent loss (i.e., job, independence, social supports) and chronic medical illness play a contributing role in many cases.[8] Regardless of whether psychological factors provoke a depressive episode, they clearly can affect its course and outcomes. Supportive psychotherapy is an important part of the treatment of depression in conjunction with appropriate pharmacotherapy.

The psychopharmacologic treatment of major depression has advanced considerably in recent years, and many effective antidepressant medications are available. Tricyclic antidepressants are older drugs with well-established efficacy. Older persons do best when given antidepressant drugs with the least anticholinergic activity. Therefore, nortriptyline and desipramine are favored for older people. SSRIs, including fluoxetine, sertraline, and citalopram, are well tolerated by older patients. They have minimal anticholinergic effects and are not associated with blood pressure and heart rate changes. However, SSRIs can impair sleep even when taken in the morning. If this occurs, adding trazodone at bedtime can improve sleep. Nausea, another common side effect, may be dose related. Monoamine oxidase inhibitors can be given to older patients if prescribed cautiously. They may be indicated for difficult cases when other medications have failed.

Other antidepressants include buproprion, which has mild central nervous system-activating effects, minimal anticholinergic effects, and few cardiovascular side effects, but a higher risk of inducing seizures at higher doses; venlafaxine and duloxetine, which inhibit both norepinephrine and serotonin reuptake and have a side effect profile similar to those of the SSRI agents except that they can increase blood pressure; and mirtazapine, which has norandrogenic and serotonergic pharmacologic properties, is sedating, and stimulates appetite.

All antidepressants must be taken for a minimum of six to eight weeks at appropriate dosages before efficacy can be determined. To prevent relapse, they should be prescribed for a minimum of 6–12 months once the right dose and therapeutic response have been achieved.

Another effective treatment for serious depression is electroconvulsive therapy (ECT).[9, 10] ECT may be the first-line treatment of choice if the patient cannot eat or is refusing to eat and is at risk for dehydration. It may be used as a second-line treatment after one or two antidepressant trials have failed to improve symptoms adequately. There is no age limit to ECT, although several medical conditions are relative contraindications that must be evaluated case by case. Those include brain tumor, recent myocardial infarction, coronary artery disease, hypertensive cardiovascular disease, bronchopulmonary disease, and venous thrombosis. The only absolute contraindication for ECT is increased intracranial pressure, since ECT causes a rise in cerebrospinal fluid pressure that may lead to herniation. Relapse of major depression after ECT is high, and therefore it must be followed by maintenance antidepressant treatment.

Bipolar disorder is a lifelong recurrent disorder characterized by one of more manic episodes. There is often at least one prior episode of major depression. Recurrence can take the form of either mania or depression. Whereas most patients with bipolar disorder have their first episode of illness before age 50, late-onset mood disorder does occur.[11] Most patients with late-onset mania have had at least one episode of major depression, often 10–15 years earlier. There is a tendency for patients with late-onset bipolar disorder to have a lower incidence of positive family history of mood disorders. In addition, a number of studies of late-onset mania reveal a high rate of secondary mania, in which there is an association between onset of mania and known brain injury, especially affecting the right side of the brain, or another medical problem such as thyrotoxicosis or hypercortisolemia.

Patients having a manic episode usually have little need for sleep, are talkative, and may have loose associations in their speech. Hyperactivity, hypersexuality, overspending, and involvement in foolish or unwise endeavors are frequently seen. Patients usually have an inflated self-esteem and increased sense of well-being but may also be irritable and demanding to those around them. Frank grandiose delusions may develop, such as believing oneself to be chosen by God for a special mission.

The mainstay of treatment for mania is lithium pharmacotherapy, sometimes in combination with lose-dose antipsychotic medication. For patients who cannot tolerate lithium because of sensitivity to side effects or impaired renal function, divalproex sodium and carbamazepine are alternative mood-stabilizing agents. Although many patients enjoy long periods of remission, it is typical for episodes of illness to become more frequent with age. In addition, complicated clinical conditions such as mixed episodes, in which symptoms of mania and depression coexist, and rapid cycling, in which four or more mood episodes occur within 12 months, may develop. Because of the high recurrence rate, patients with bipolar disorder often require lifelong pharmacologic treatment and regular psychiatric monitoring.

Chronic depression is a persistent depressive condition lasting two years or longer and marked by a persistently low mood more days than not and at least two of the following: appetite change, insomnia, low energy, low self-esteem, poor concentration or difficulty making decisions, and hopelessness. It may be a milder depressive disorder than major depression in severity of individual symptoms, but the chronicity of the depressive symptoms can be disabling and demoralizing to the patient and may contribute to lowering functional capacities.[12] In addition, some patients with dysthymic disorder go on to develop a major depressive episode. In older people, dysthymic disorder often develops in the setting of physical disability, multiple medical problems, isolation, and loneliness. Many patients with a dysthymic disorder respond to treatment with an antidepressant. Supportive psychotherapy is a vital component of treatment, the goals being to increase social contacts and activity level and to improve self-esteem and outlook through an empathic therapeutic relationship.

Grief is not a mental disorder, and depressive symptoms are considered to be part of the normal bereavement process. Although persons vary in their response to losing a loved one, there are common predictable phases to grieving.[13] The initial response, which lasts several days, is characterized by shock, disbelief, and emotional numbing. This is often followed by prominent emotions, including anger and frustration, that evolve into periods of fluctuating despair, mourning, and wishing to be with the deceased. During the first three to six months following the death of a loved one, insomnia is common, as are frequent episodes of tearfulness, anxiety, and a loss of interest or pleasure in activities once enjoyed. Usually the intensity of symptoms begins to remit after the first 6–12 months; strong feelings of loss and mourning continue for one to two years, longer for some people. In addition, intense emotional feelings tend to return on the anniversary of the loved one's death and birthday and at holiday times. Transient hallucinations or a sense of presence of the deceased are common early in grief and normal.

It is unclear at what point a bereaved person should be referred for professional help or counseling. The support of family, friends, and clergy is sufficient to help most bereaved persons through the grieving process. Widow and widower support groups can also be helpful in readjusting to life without a spouse and increasing social contacts. When the bereaved person is overwhelmed by grief and unable to begin to return to usual activities or if grief is complicated by panic attacks, delusions, or suicidal thoughts, referral for psychiatric evaluation is indicated. Grief may trigger a full major depressive episode. Although sadness, disruption of sleep, and loss of motivation and interest may be part of an uncomplicated grief syndrome, feelings of guilt, worthlessness, and hopelessness are not part of grief and should signal concern that a major depression has developed and should be treated as outlined earlier.

Suicide

Suicide is the third leading cause of death due to injury among persons over age 65, after unintentional falls and motor vehicle accidents. Age-specific rates for suicide have consistently been higher among the elderly than for any other age group. Of particular concern are recent data from the National Center for Health Statistics (NCHS) of the Centers for Disease Control and Prevention which indicate that after decades of declining rates, the period from 1980 to 1992 saw a marked increase in the rate of suicide among persons aged 65 and older.[14] Of persons 65 and older, men accounted for 81% of the suicides. Rates were higher for divorced or widowed men. Other risk factors include depression, alcoholism, chemical dependency, physical illness, and social isolation. Older persons make fewer attempts per completed suicide than other age groups and tend to use violent means of suicide. Indeed, firearms were the most common method of suicide by both men and women over age 65.

Suicide cannot be predicted with complete accuracy, but the potential for suicide must be considered seriously by all health providers who care for the elderly. Particular attention must be paid to patients who are despondent, overwhelmed by the burdens of physical illness or disability, lack social support, drink alcohol excessively, or have made previous suicide attempts. Clinicians must become comfortable about asking their older patients about suicidal ideation and should not hesitate to seek psychiatric consultation for any patient who seems at high risk.

Personality disorder

Personality is the set of enduring traits that make each person unique. Traits are universally shared characteristics on which persons differ. They include patterns of perceiving and relating to one's self and one's social environment. For example, all people can be rated on their tendency for tidiness. People vary widely in this tendency, but for each person a certain degree of tidiness or lack thereof is characteristic. Personality disorders are diagnosed when a person falls at the extreme end of a normal distribution on a set of traits that commonly occur together. Personality disorders reflect enduring, inflexible, and maladaptive patterns of experience and behavior. For example, *dependent personality behavior* is characterized by an excessive need to be taken care of by others, which leads to difficulty in making independent everyday decisions. These persons lack confidence in their own judgment or abilities to do things on their own, and they often go to excessive lengths to obtain reassurance or support. *Antisocial personality disorder* is associated with repeated illegal actions, impulsivity, frequent lies, consistent irresponsibility, lack of remorse, and lack of concern toward others.

Obsessive-compulsive personality disorder is characterized by extreme perfectionism, rigidity, emotional inexpressiveness, excessive preoccupation with rules and details, and inflexibility. To satisfy a diagnosis of personality disorder, problems in these realms must be lifelong. Thus in the elderly a diagnosis of a personality disorder must reflect a pattern of behavior that has been present throughout adulthood and has caused problems for the person throughout his or her life.

Personality disorders complicate the care of the medically ill. Persons with *narcissistic personality disorder*, for example, are more likely to clash with health professionals, sometimes to the detriment of their well-being. Conversely, patients with obsessive-compulsive personality disorder may underreport symptoms, have very high expectations of their physicians, be inflexible, be unable to make decisions, and have difficulty accepting the lack of clear guidelines that sometimes occurs in medical conditions.

The physician who is aware that a personality disorder is underlying a problematic patient's behavior can avoid or alleviate problems by considering the patient's predispositions. Patients with prominent obsessional traits often need detailed discussions of proposed procedures and an extensive and specific discussion regarding the steps that are to be taken, the order in which they are to be taken, and the implications of the most likely outcomes. Whereas all patients need options and clear descriptions, patients with narcicisstic features often do best when information is presented in a reassuring, calm tone, a concise description of alternatives, a direct acknowledgment of emotional distress ("I know this is upsetting, but let me present the alternatives before we discuss them"), and frequent short visits. Patients with dependent personality disorder have difficulty following through with recommendations on their own and do better if important persons in their social support network are part of the treatment process.

Psychotic symptoms

Hallucinations (perceptions without a stimulus occurring in any of the five senses) and delusions (false ideas that are unshakable and persistent) occur in many medical and psychiatric disorders. The first step in their assessment is to determine whether a cognitive impairment (delirium or dementia) is present. The importance of this step is twofold. First, cognitive disorder is a common cause of hallucinations and delusions, and second, this recognition leads to the appropriate medical evaluation.

Hallucinations and delusions can also be caused by depression, schizophrenia, and delusional disorder. After a primary cognitive disorder has been ruled out, the next step is to assess for mood disorder. Self-deprecation, self-blame, hopelessness, loss of interest in usually enjoyed activities, somatic preoccupations, and complaints of sad mood all suggest the possibility that major depression is the cause of the psychotic symptoms.

Schizophrenia and *delusional disorder* are uncommon conditions, occurring in fewer than 1% of the population. They can present to medical practitioners with isolated somatic delusions (e.g., belief that someone is sending an electrical shock into the body or belief in a physical illness for which there is no evidence). By definition a *delusional disorder* is characterized by a single delusion occurring in the absence of cognitive impairment, mood impairment, and other psychiatric symptoms. *Schizophrenia* is an illness in which symptoms are present for at least six months, hallucinations and social dilapidation are predominant, and mood disorder criteria are not met. Although schizophrenia most commonly begins in early adulthood, it can begin in late life. Patients with late-onset schizophrenia frequently have paranoid delusions, social isolation, and hearing impairment.[15]

Lifelong schizophrenia has an associated cognitive decline (the original name was dementia praecox) characterized by progressive loss of social, occupational, and interpersonal skills. The cognitive impairment of schizophrenia typically impairs frontal-executive abilities, that is, reasoning, abstraction, planning, and adaptation to changing circumstances. The decline is usually slow. Prominent decline in cognition or function over a 6–12 month period, new onset language impairment such as paraphasic errors, new onset apraxias (inability to do motor tasks with intact strength) or agnosias (not recognizing familiar people or places), or a noticeable decline in memory over 6–12 months should trigger an evaluation for a cause of cognitive decline other than schizophrenia. A dramatic decline in alertness or cognition should always trigger an evaluation for delirium.

Psychiatric symptoms may arise from toxic effects of prescribed medication, such as carbidopa with levodopa (Sinemet) or steroids. In addition, isolated visual hallucinations (i.e., not accompanied by delusions, cognitive impairment, or mood disorder) sometimes occur in patients with a wide variety of visual disorders, such as glaucoma, cataracts, and retinal degeneration.[16] Finally, hallucinations and delusions may develop in the course of several neurologic diseases such as dementia, Huntington's disease, and Parkinson's disease.

The treatment of psychotic symptoms depends, in part, on the diagnosis of the underlying disorder. If the patient is delirious, all attempts should be made to correct the underlying abnormality and to avoid pharmacotherapy unless there are clear indications. So-called neuroleptic, psychotropic, or antipsychotic drugs are the treatment of choice when protection from harm makes pharmacotherapy necessary. Benzodiazepines should be avoided if possible. In dementia, reorientation and activity therapy should be tried first. Pharmacotherapy is appropriate when these symptoms increase the likelihood of harm to the patient or others or cause emotional distress to the patient. For mood disorder, several studies demonstrate that delusional major depression responds better to the combination of an antidepressant and neuroleptic than to an antidepressant alone.

Psychiatric treatment of irreversible cognitive disorders

Dementia and delirium are discussed in detail in Chapters 10 and 11. About 60% of patients with dementia have psychotic symptoms sometime in the course of a dementing illness. These noncognitive symptoms, which can interfere with the quality of life of the patient and caregiver, are often amenable to treatment. Nonpharmacologic, environmental therapy is most desirable because of the side effects of drugs, including a 60%–100% increase in mortality. Nondrug treatments include providing a structured environment, stimulating the patient at an appropriate level, redirection, and providing the level of care that the person needs. When hallucinations and delusions interfere with function, become distressing to the patient, or are dangerous to others, cautious low-dosage neuroleptic therapy is appropriate.

Some 15%–30% of patients with dementia also suffer from depression that interferes with function. Antidepressant drugs with low anticholinergic properties (e.g., nortriptyline, desipramine, SSRIs) are recommended although clinical trials have shown mixed results. Emotional support for both patient and caregiver is indicated in all cases. The physician should play an important role in educating the family, in managing specific behavioral and noncognitive symptoms, and in helping the families address their social, legal, and financial concerns.

Overview of treatment issues

Pharmacotherapy

Although older patients can benefit from the same psychopharmacologic agents as younger ones, the clinician must be aware both of changes in physiology and pharmacokinetics with age and of potential interactions with other medications. Prescribing psychotropic medication for older patients requires special considerations discussed in detail in other sources.[3] However, some important principles are outlined here.

Perhaps the most familiar axiom in prescribing for older adults is "start low and go slow." This means that for just about every medication, be it an anxiolytic, antipsychotic, or antidepressant, one should start at a low dose and titrate the dose up to a therapeutic dose slowly and gradually. A good rule of thumb is to allow at least five days between each dosage increase. This allows the patient to adjust to a new medication and to report any troublesome side effects before they become problematic.

Older patients are more sensitive to the anticholinergic effects of medication and therefore more likely than younger patients to develop delirium, constipation, urinary retention, dry mouth, and orthostatic hypotension. For these reasons, medications with the least anticholinergic effects are preferred when a choice of several agents is available.

Another important principle is to choose medications with shorter half-lives. Because of the changes in hepatic metabolism that occur with aging, the half-lives of most pharmacologic agents are prolonged in older people. This increases the likelihood that psychologically active metabolites will accumulate over time and cause toxicity. Obviously the problem is worsened if the original drug and/or its active metabolite or metabolites have long half-lives to begin with. Among benzodiazepines, for instance, lorazepam (half-life 16 hours) and oxazepam (half-life 8 hours) are better tolerated in older people than is diazepam (half-life 3 to 4 days). If a longer-acting benzodiazepine is required to manage severe anxiety or withdrawal from benzodiazepines, clonazepam (half-life 1 to 2 days) is useful.

Lithium carbonate deserves special mention, since it is nearly totally excreted in the kidneys. Because glomerular filtration rate and creatinine clearance decrease steadily with age, older patients are likely to develop lithium-induced tremor and delirium at low doses. Furthermore, recent studies seem to indicate that the therapeutic effects of lithium occur at lower blood levels in older patients than in younger ones. For all of these reasons, older patients require lower doses of lithium than younger patients, usually 150 mg daily to 300 mg twice a day.[1]

In general, the lowest dose of antipsychotic medication needed to control symptoms should be prescribed. In addition to their extrapyramidal and anticholinergic side effects, neuroleptics are likely to cause tardive dyskinesia in the elderly.

For most antidepressants, on the other hand, patients do best if the medication is within the therapeutic range regardless of age. Low-dose antidepressant treatment is likely to be inadequate to treat a major depressive episode. Because of wide variations in older persons' hepatic metabolism, it is impossible to predict the dose of antidepressant needed to achieve a therapeutic level, but often it is the same as for much younger persons. It is important to give an antidepressant an adequate trial length (four to six weeks minimum) at a therapeutic dose before deciding that the medication trial was a failure and changing to another antidepressant. Indeed, there is evidence for some antidepressants, such as fluoxetine, a longer trial period (six to eight weeks) may be necessary to establish maximum therapeutic benefits. Furthermore, to prevent relapse it is important that full-strength antidepressant therapy continue for 6–12 months once a therapeutic response has begun. Long-term antidepressant therapy is indicated for patients with recurrent depression.

Finally, as with all medications, it is important to consider drug interactions. Fluoxetine, for example, increases serum levels of digoxin, warfarin, and other protein-bound drugs. Tricyclic antidepressants and neuroleptics have hypotensive effects that can compound the effects of antihypertensive medications. Nonsteroidal anti-inflammatory drugs increase the plasma level of lithium and put an older person at risk for lithium toxicity. Thus, the older patients must

be carefully monitored while being treated with psychotropic medications to avoid both undertreatment and toxicity. Monoamine oxidase inhibitors should not be prescribed concomitantly with SSRIs or venlafaxine, and to avoid serotonin syndrome there should be a minimum two- to five-week washout period after one agent has been discontinued and the other type of antidepressant started. Serotonin syndrome is a serious, sometimes fatal, condition that is characterized by hyperthermia, rigidity, myoclonus, autonomic instability, and mental status changes.

Psychotherapy

Individual psychotherapy

Contrary to many prevailing myths, older patients do benefit from psychotherapy in the treatment of a variety of disorders.[17] For patients with depression, anxiety, and bereavement, psychotherapy is an important part of treatment even when pharmacotherapy is indicated. Through psychotherapy, older people can improve significantly in self-esteem, self-awareness, adaptation, and personal satisfaction. No one psychotherapeutic method works best with older people. We recommend a pluralistic approach that emphasizes life review and focuses on specific issues of concern. Many persons benefit from a focus on the development of problem-solving skills. Some patients benefit from a return to an active, creative life. Also, patients with anxiety disorders and phobias may benefit from a more cognitive-behavioral approach that stresses the importance of positive problem solving and teaches relaxation techniques.

Marital therapy

Marital or couples therapy is helpful for older people in several circumstances. Retirement and late-life illnesses can dramatically alter the dynamics of a marriage. Spouses who were used to busy but relatively independent work lives may find it an adjustment to be home together most of the time. Roles may change as one spouse does more or less of the cooking, shopping, and housekeeping. If one spouse is unable to drive because of health problems, this can put limitations on the lifestyles of both partners. Retirement also means living on a fixed income for most people, and these new financial constraints may pose an additional burden. In short, the reality of living "the golden years" often does not meet the expectations for this time of life. This may result in disappointment or resentment, especially if one spouse blames the other for preventing the fulfillment of the retirement dream. In addition, problems can develop between widowed or divorced elders involved in new relationships. Issues such as whether to live together or marry, how to combine finances, and how to deal with each other's adult children can put a strain on the relationship. While couples issues may be the presenting focus for treatment, usually they are not. Rather, these issues may emerge as the patient is beginning treatment for depression or anxiety. Short-term marital therapy can be very useful in defusing stressful situations, improving communications between partners, and fostering a more healthful adaptation to the couples' changing way of life.

Family assessment

Often other family issues come to light during the course of assessment and treatment of the older patient. For some, decreased functional abilities or illness raises dependence on adult children. This may necessitate moving in with adult children or moving closer geographically. When an elderly person develops dementia and/or other disabling medical illness, the spouse or adult child may become a primary caregiver and have to assume responsibilities for the impaired person's personal and financial care. Older patients may find that their grown children need them in new or different ways (e.g., because of illness or divorce on the part of the adult children).

These and other situations can produce family conflict and stress. It is very helpful to meet with all involved family members at least once to assess how various family members relate to one another, solve problems, deal with their changing family dynamics, and address the needs of the impaired elder person. These meetings can also be useful for teaching the family about the impaired older person's medications and illness, for mobilizing family and community resources, and for identifying others in the family who need support or counseling.

Barriers to treatment

There are many reasons older people often do not get the psychological treatment they need.[17] One common reason is that older people themselves are reluctant to see a psychiatrist because of embarrassment and negative attitudes. Although education is slowly changing society's outlook on mental illness and

mental health care, older people who grew up in the Depression or earlier may still believe one should solve one's own problems and "pick oneself up by the boot straps." To such persons, seeking help for psychologic problems is viewed as a sign of personal weakness. Other contributors to elders not receiving care for emotional problems include the negative attitude of their physician; the focus by patient, family, or physician on medical issues; and lack of transportation. These issues are best overcome by discussing them openly and reviewing the reasons a person is reluctant to seek help.

References

1. Stahl S. 2013. *Stahl's Essential Psychopharmacology*. 4th ed. Cambridge: Cambridge University Press.

2. Institute of Medicine. 2012. *The Mental Health Workforce for Geriatric Population*. Washington, DC: IOM Press.

3. Inouye SK, Bogardus ST, Charpentier PA, et al. 1999. A multicomponent intervention to prevent delirium in hospitalized patients. *NEJM*. **340**:669–74.

4. Rovner BW, Kalonek S, Filipp L, et al. 1986. Prevalence of mental illness in a community nursing home. *Am J Psychiatry*. **143**:1446–1449.

5. Blazer DG. 2001. *Depression in Late Life*. 3rd ed. St. Louis: Mosby-Year Book.

6. Blazer DG. 1994. Is depression more frequent in late life? *J Geriatr Psychiatry*. **2**:193–199.

7. Lipsey JR, Robinson RG, Pearlson GD, et al. 1985. The dexamethasone suppression test and mood following stroke. *Am J Psychiatry*. **142**:318–323.

8. Jorm A. 2000. Does old age reduce the risk of anxiety and depression? *Psychol Med*. **30**:11–22.

9. Philibert RA, Richards L, Lynch CF, et al. 1995. Effect of ECT on mortality and clinical outcome in geriatric unipolar depression. *J Clin Psychiatry*. **56**:390–394.

10. Stoppe A, Louza M, Moacyr, R, et al. 2006. Fixed high-dose ECT in the elderly with depression. *J ECT*. **22**:92–99.

11. Lehmann SW, Rabins PV. 2006. Factors related to hospitalization in elderly manic patients with early and late onset bipolar disorder. *Int J Geri Psych*. **21**: 1060–1064.

12. Blazer D, Hughes DC, George LK. 1987. The epidemiology of depression in an elderly community population. *Gerontologist*. **27**:281–287.

13. Bruce ML, Kim K, Leaf PJ. 1990. Depressive episodes and dysphoria resulting from conjugal bereavement in a prospective community sample. *Am J Psychiatry*. **147**:608–611.

14. Meehan PJ, Saltzman LE, Sattin RW. 1991. Suicides among older United States residents: epidemiologic characteristics and trends. *Am J Public Health*. **81**:1198–1200.

15. Howard R, Rabins PV, Seeman MV, et al. 2000. Late-onset schizophrenia and very-late-onset schizophrenia-like psychosis: an international consensus. *Am J Psychiatry*. **157**:172–178.

16. Holroyd S, Rabins PV, Finkelstein D, et al. 1994. Visual hallucinations in patients from an ophthalmology clinic and medical clinic population. *J Nerv Ment Dis*. **182**:272–276.

17. Myers WA. 1991. *New Techniques in the Psychotherapy of Older Patients*. Washington, DC: American Psychiatry Press.

Chapter 20

Unhealthy substance use in older adults

Alison A. Moore, MD, MPH, Lucia Loredana Dattoma, MD, Aaron Kaufman, MD, and Alexis N. Kuerbis, LCSW, PhD

Introduction

The population of older adults is rapidly growing, in large part due to the aging of the baby boomer generation who comprise 30% of the US population and the first of whom turned 65 years old in 2011.[1] This cohort engages in higher rates of alcohol and drug use compared to older cohorts,[2] and it also has a higher prevalence of substance use disorders and treatment admissions for substance use disorders.[3, 4] Although older adults use alcohol and illicit drugs at lower rates than younger adults, the sheer numbers of the older adult population and the aging of the baby boomer generation are expected to drive up the prevalence rates of substance use disorders among older adults.[3, 5] Because of these facts, it is increasingly understood that health-care professionals need to know how to identify, assess, and intervene in regard to substance use disorders among aging adults.

Prevalence of alcohol, tobacco, illicit and nonmedical prescription drug use, unhealthy use, and use disorders

Definitions

One of the challenges in the literature on substances is the multitude of terminology used to refer to various types of substance use. Here we will define "current use" as the use of substance within the past 12 months. "Unhealthy use" has been defined for alcohol as the use of alcohol that exceeds recommended drinking limits and includes a spectrum of risk.[6] At-risk or heavy use includes use that carries risk but has not resulted in harm. Problem drinking is the use of alcohol that has resulted in harm but does not meet *Diagnostic and Statistical Manual of Mental Disorders,*

Fifth Edition (DSM-5) criteria for an alcohol use disorder (AUD). All substance use disorders (SUD) now have the same diagnostic criteria using DSM-5 criteria (e.g., must meet 2 or more of 11 criteria).[7] For tobacco and illicit drugs, there is no recognized safe limit for use so any use of these substances would be considered unhealthy use. Finally, "nonmedical use of prescription-type drugs" is defined by the National Survey of Drug Use and Health as the use of these drugs without a prescription or use that occurs simply for the experience or feeling the drug causes.[3] Another definition that may be more relevant for older adults is use without a prescription, in greater amounts, more often or longer than prescribed, or for a reason other than a doctor said you should use them.[8]

Alcohol

Alcohol is the most commonly used substance among older adults.[8, 9] Although the amount of alcohol consumed declines with age,[10–13] and the prevalence of abstention increases with age, about 50% of adults aged 65 and older consume alcohol.[13, 14] Recommended guidelines for low-risk drinking from the National Institute on Alcohol Abuse and Alcoholism are that adults aged 65 and older drink no more than seven standard drinks (i.e., 12-oz beer, 4-to 5-oz glass of wine, 1.5-oz of 80-proof liquor) per week and no more than three drinks on any day.[15] Even these drinking thresholds many not be safe for older adults who have comorbid conditions that could be worsened or caused by any amount of alcohol use. Using these definitions, prevalence rates for those who exceed recommended drinking limits and are therefore considered unhealthy drinkers are estimated to be 10% for women and 12% for men aged

---

Reichel's Care of the Elderly, 7th Edition, ed. Jan Busby-Whitehead *et al.* Published by Cambridge University Press.
© Cambridge University Press 2016.

65 and older.[8, 14] Older adults have low rates of alcohol use disorders; approximately 1%–2% of persons aged 65 and older have a current diagnosis of alcohol abuse or dependence.[16] These rates are lower than younger persons due to the older adult maturing out of alcohol use disorders, increased mortality among those with longstanding AUDs, difficulty with accurate diagnosis, and diagnostic criteria being less well suited for older adults.

Tobacco

Approximately 12%–14% of adults aged 65 and older use tobacco.[17, 18] Data from the 2001–2002 National Epidemiologic Survey on Alcohol and Related Conditions (NESARC) indicate that 4% of this age group have a tobacco use disorder.[19] Tobacco and alcohol are frequently used together in both younger and older adult populations; 6% of older adults both drink alcohol and use tobacco. Those older adults who use tobacco are twice as likely to be binge drinkers.[18]

Illicit drugs

It is expected that the use of illicit drugs will rise among persons aged 65 and older in the United States. Data from the 2012 National Survey on Drug Use and Health (NSDUH) show that rates of past month use of illicit drugs doubled from 1.9%–3.4% to 3.6%–7.2% among those aged 50–65 in the 10-year period between 2002 and 2012.[3] Also, 19% of adults aged 65 and older in 2012 reported ever having using illicit drugs, whereas 48% of adults aged 60–64 reported this behavior. Among older adults who do use illicit substances, 12% meet the criteria for past year substance use disorder.[18] Cannabis is the most commonly used illicit drug (0.7% of those aged 65 and older compared to 3.9% of those 50–64) followed by cocaine (0.04% of those aged 65 and older compared to 0.7% of those 50–64).[18, 20]

Prescription drugs

In 2012, 2.9 million adults aged 50 and older reported nonmedical use of psychotherapeutic medication in the past year.[4] Using NSDUH, 1.4% of adults aged 50 and older used prescription opioids nonmedically in the past year, which was higher than sedatives, tranquilizers, and Stimulants (all <1%). [21] Benzodiazepines are the most commonly prescribed sedative medication for older adults, and

rates of their use among older adults range from 15% to 32%.[22] It is likely that nonmedical use of prescription drugs is underreported, as many older adults may not view use of medications for longer durations or at higher amounts than prescribed as a problem.

Older adult vulnerabilities

Although rates of substance use disorders and use of substances is lower among older adults compared to younger adults, aging is associated with specific risks for harm with substance use. Some risks are related to changes that occur with aging (e.g., changes in substance metabolism and distribution); however, the nature of some risks may vary considerably depending on the type and amount of the substance used (e.g., one drink a day for seven days vs. seven drinks on one day), the context in which it is used (e.g., a sedating substance such as alcohol used with other sedating substances like benzodiazepines), and the characteristics of the older person (e.g., cognitive impairment, gait disorder).

Alcohol

With increasing age, the percentage of lean body mass and total body water decrease; blood-brain barrier permeability and neuronal receptor sensitivity to alcohol in the brain increase.[23] Because of these changes, older adults have higher blood alcohol concentrations and increased brain sensitivity compared to younger adults given the same dose of alcohol.[24–30] Increases in morbidity and medication use also increase risks associated with alcohol.[31]

Tobacco

Older adults who use tobacco have higher risks for death, cardiac events, lung disease, cancer, and poorer physical function compared to younger adults.[32, 33] They are also less likely to think that smoking harms their health.[34]

Medications and illicit drugs

The same physiological changes that affect alcohol's effects among older adults pertain to other substances and increase their vulnerability to adverse effects from substances. In addition, older adults have an increased percentage of total body fat compared to younger adults, so fat soluble substances such as

Table 20.1 Risk factors related to unhealthy substance use in late life [37]

Physical risk factors	Psychiatric risk factors	Social risk factors
Male gender (for alcohol); female gender (for prescription drug)	Avoidance coping style	Caucasian race (for alcohol and prescription drugs)
Chronic pain	History of alcohol problems (for all substances)	Affluence
Physical disabilities or reduced mobility	Previous and/or concurrent substance use disorder (for all substances)	Bereavement
Transitions in care/living situations	Previous and/or concurrent psychiatric illness (for all substances)	Unexpected or forced retirement
Poor health status		Social isolation (living alone or with nonspousal others)
Chronic illness/multimorbidity		
Significant drug burden/ polypharmacy		

benzodiazepines have a longer duration of action in older adults compared to younger adults and have been associated with increased sedation and an increased risk for falls.[35] Other risks pertain to older adults with multimorbidity and multiple medication use. There is the potential for drug–drug interactions (e.g., benzodiazepine and opioid increase risk for confusion), and condition–drug interactions (e.g., gait impairment and sedative increase risk for falls). The increasing acceptance of marijuana use will pose unique risks in older adults. Marijuana may cause impairment of short-term memory; increased heart rate, respiratory rate, elevated blood pressure; and increased risk for heart attack.[36] These risks are likely to be heightened in older adults.

Risk factors for unhealthy substance use

Most research on correlates and predictors of unhealthy substance use among older adults has been conducted on alcohol and, to a lesser extent, on prescription drugs, but such factors may also apply to other substances. Table 20.1 lists some of the known and potential risk factors for older adults associated with the unhealthy use of alcohol and other substances.

Being male,[38] more affluent,[14, 39, 40] Caucasian,[38, 41] and young-old are consistently associated with exceeding recommended drinking limits among older adults. Female gender is associated with prescription drug abuse.[35]

Alcohol use has been associated with being in better overall health and abstention with poorer health.[38, 39] It has been suggested this is so because many abstainers stop drinking when they become sick. Older heavy drinkers have poorer physical and mental health compared to those older adults whose drinking does not exceed recommended limits.[24, 38, 42, 43] Some older adults drink alcohol to manage pain.[40]

Older adults who rely on avoidance to cope with stress have a greater likelihood of having a late-life alcohol use disorder compared to those who coped in other ways.[39] Similar to younger adults, older adults with past histories of an alcohol use disorder are at higher risk of a recurrence and/or heavy drinking.[39, 40]

Being other than married is associated with increased or unhealthy drinking in later life,[8, 38] while being socially engaged is also associated with drinking.[44] Particular life events or social transitions common in later life may heighten the risk of unhealthy substance use including bereavement, ill health, loneliness, retirement, and caregiving.[45–49]

Diagnosis of substance use disorders

The formal diagnosis of a substance use disorder generally relies on the criteria outlined by the DSM.[7, 50] Table 20.2 outlines several of the criteria used to diagnose SUD. Because of the biologic and social factors unique to older adults, these criteria may

Table 20.2 Substance use disorders (formerly substance abuse or dependence) criteria, from the *Diagnostic and Statistical Manual, Fifth Edition*, p. 49 [17, 37]

DSM-5 criterion for SUD	Consideration for older adults
A substance is often taken in larger amounts or over a longer period than was intended.	Cognitive impairment can prevent adequate self-monitoring. Substances may more greatly impair cognition among older adults than younger adults.
There is a persistent desire or unsuccessful efforts to cut down or control substance use.	Same as a general adult population
A great deal of time is spent in activities necessary to obtain the substance, use the substance, or recover from its effects.	Recovery from effects of a substance may be longer in older adults.
Craving or a strong desire to use the substance.	Older adults with entrenched habits may not recognize cravings in the same way as the general adult population.
Recurrent substance use resulting in a failure to fulfill major role obligations at work, school, or at home.	Role obligations may not exist for older adults in the same way as for younger adults, due to life stage transitions such as retirement. Role obligations more common in late life are caregiving for an ill spouse or family member, such as a grandchild.
Continued substance use despite having persistent or recurrent social or interpersonal problems caused or exacerbated by the effects of the substance.	Older adults may not realize the problems they experience are from substance use.
Important social, occupational, or recreational activities are given up or reduced because of substance use.	Older adults may engage in fewer activities regardless of substance use, making it difficult to detect.
Recurrent substance use in situations in which it is physically hazardous.	Older adults may not identify or understand that their use is hazardous, especially when using substances in smaller amounts.
Substance use is continued despite knowledge of having a persistent or recurrent physical or psychological problem that is likely to have been caused or exacerbated by the substance.	Older adults may not realize the problems they experience are from substance use.
Tolerance, as defined by either of the following: 1. A need for markedly increased amounts of the substance to achieve intoxication or the desired effect. 2. A markedly diminished effect with continued use of the same amount of the substance.	Due to increased sensitivity to substances as they age, older adults will appear to have a decrease rather than an increase in tolerance.
Withdrawal, as manifested by either of the following: 1. The characteristic withdrawal syndrome for the substance. 2. The substance or a close relative is taken to relieve or avoid withdrawal symptoms.	Withdrawal symptoms can manifest in ways that are more "subtle and protracted"[61]. Late onset substance users may not develop physiological dependence *or* non-problematic users of medications, such as benzodiazepines, may develop physiological dependence.

Note: A substance use disorder is defined as a medical disorder in which two or more of the above listed symptoms are occurring in the last 12 months.[7]
Source: Adapted from Barry, Blow and Oslin, 2002, p. 109.[61]

be less relevant to them and so present challenges for an accurate diagnosis.[12] For example, because of age-associated physiologic changes that increase the effects of alcohol and other substances, older adults generally experience a reduction in tolerance to substances. Also, interruption in social and occupational roles or other consequences of substance use may be less likely to occur or less noticeable in older adults. [51, 52] The criterion related to continued use despite persistent or recurrent problems may not apply to many older adults. Additionally, older adults and their health-care providers may not recognize that problems such as depression or falls are related to substance use.[12]

Screening and assessment

The US Preventive Services Task Force in 2013 reviewed the evidence and recommended that clinicians screen adults aged 18 or older for alcohol misuse and provide persons engaged in risky or hazardous drinking with brief behavioral counseling intervention to reduce alcohol misuse.[54] Despite this recommendation, older adults are less likely to be screened for substance use and less likely to have substance use and abuse identified compared to younger adults.[55, 56] Reasons for this include limited time to see older adults who have multimorbidity, stigma related to and discomfort assessing for addiction or unhealthy use, the similarity of the symptoms of alcohol and other substance use with illnesses common in older age,[57, 58] and the perception among older adults that symptoms experienced by the use of substances are part of normal aging rather than resulting from the substance itself.[59] Further, many older adults and their families view use of alcohol and other substances as being their one last pleasure, and a sense of time running out may reduce motivation to make changes in substance use.[60]

Potential indicators of unhealthy substance use

Several physical, cognitive, psychiatric, and social indicators for unhealthy substance use have been defined (see Table 20.3).[61, 57, 51]

When assessing older adults about substance use it is important to use a supportive, nonconfrontational approach rather than a more assertive style.[62–64] Further discussion of alcohol and other substance use should occur in the context of an overall assessment

and in reference to the presenting problem with the goal of health promotion and a complete understanding of their health behaviors.

Assessment should start with questions about substances. One approach to assessment is recommended by the US Department of Health and Human Services, and the National Institute on Alcohol Abuse and Alcoholism. In 2005, these organizations published an updated version *Helping Patients Who Drink Too Much: A Clinician's Guide*.[65] This approach has four steps: (1) ask about alcohol use; (2) assess for alcohol use disorders; (3) advise and assist; and (4) at followup, continue support. These steps may also be used for other substances.

Step 1: ask about substance use

The recommended question for alcohol use is the following: Do you sometimes drink beer, wine, or other alcoholic beverages? If no, stop; if yes, ask: "How many times in the past year have you had four or more drinks in a day?" (for those aged 65 and older). If no, it is recommended to give advice to stay within recommended drinking limits and/or to recommend lower limits if the person takes medications that may interact with alcohol and/or have a health conditions that alcohol may worsen. If yes, the person is an at-risk drinker and the person's weekly average of drinking should be assessed by asking: "On average, how many days a week do you have an alcoholic drink" and "On a typical day, how many drinks do you have?" Then multiply these two numbers to calculate the weekly average.

For other substances, the provider may ask about the quantity and frequencies of substances used and ask a specific question about nonmedical use of prescription drugs.

Step 2: assess for substance use disorders

Questions about symptoms of an SUD should be asked, and for older adults, additional questions should be asked to obtain information on risk factors for problematic use as well as reasons for use of the substance. An evaluation of safety of substance use in the context of the person's functional status, comorbid conditions, medication used, and symptoms should be performed.

Screening instruments

Brief screening tools can assess the level of risk caused by substances. Screening tools such as the Alcohol Use

Table 20.3 Potential indicators of unhealthy substance use [37]

Physical indicators	Cognitive indicators	Psychiatric indicators	Social indicators
Falls, bruises, and burns	Disorientation	Sleep disturbances, problems, or insomnia	Family problems
Poor hygiene or impaired self-care	Memory loss	Anxiety	Financial problems
Headaches	Recent difficulties in decision making	Depression	Legal problems
Incontinence	Overall cognitive impairment	Excessive mood swings	Social isolation
Increased tolerance to alcohol or medications or unusual response to medications			Running out of medication early
Poor nutrition			Borrowing medication from others
Idiopathic seizures			
Dizziness			
Sensory deficits			
Blackouts			
Chronic pain			

Disorders Identification Test (AUDIT);[66, 67] the Alcohol, Smoking, and Substance Involvement Screening Test (ASSIST);[68] and the Comorbidity-Alcohol Risk Evaluation Tool (CARET) [69–71] may also be used to assess quantity and frequency of use as well as level of risk. The AUDIT and the CARET have been validated in older adults. The CAGE [72, 73] and the Michigan Alcohol Screening Test-Geriatric Version (MAST-G) [74] have also been validated in older adults, but they do not include questions on quantity and frequency of substance use.

The CAGE and CAGE-AID

The CAGE questionnaire is the most common screening tool for alcohol misuse, and a version has been developed to assess for alcohol and other drugs called the CAGE-AID.[75, 76] Both of these tools have four questions. The CAGE-AID questions include (1) Have you ever felt that you could Cut down on your drinking or drug use? (2) Have people Annoyed you by criticizing your drinking or drug use? (3) Have you ever felt bad or Guilty about your drinking or drug use? (4) Have you ever had a drink or used drugs first

thing in the morning to steady your nerves or get rid of a hangover (Eye opener). Although the CAGE-AID has not been validated in older adults, the CAGE has with a sensitivity of 86% and specificity of 78% at a cut point of one positive question.[72, 73] One major limitation is the inability of the instrument to distinguish between current and lifetime problems.

The MAST-G and SMAST-G

The MAST-G[77] is designed to identify drinking problems for the older adult by modifying it from the Michigan Alcohol Screening Test. It contains 24 questions with yes/no responses; five or more positive responses indicate problematic use. It has good test characteristics, and it also has a short form – the SMAST-G – that has 10 questions with two positive responses indicating a problem with alcohol.[77]

The AUDIT

Developed by the World Health Organization (WHO), the AUDIT assesses for current alcohol problems.[66] It contains 10 questions about quantity and frequency of use, alcohol dependency, and consequences of alcohol abuse. Each of the questions is scored on a four-point continuum, with total scores ranging from 0 to 40. The cutoff threshold of five is used to indicate an alcohol problem in older adults.[67, 78]

The ASSIST

The ASSIST was also developed by WHO to screen for substances that may be abused including tobacco, alcohol, cannabis, cocaine, amphetamine type stimulants, inhalants, sedatives, hallucinogens, opioids, as well as another category.[68] It includes eight questions that identify the level of risk to guide decisions for intervention. For each substance, a score is calculated to indicate low (0–3), moderate (4–26), and high (27 or higher) risk use of the substance. It is not been validated in older adults.

The CARET

The CARET is a screening instrument that identifies older adults whose use of alcohol places them at risk for harm.[69–71] It is derived from another measure, the Short Alcohol Related Problems Survey.[79] It includes algorithms to identify at-risk drinkers within seven domains of risk: (1) amount of drinking, (2) episodic heavy drinking, (3) driving after drinking, (4) others being concerned about the respondent's drinking, (5) medical and psychiatric conditions, (6) symptoms that could be caused or worsened by alcohol, and (7) medications that could interact negatively with or whose efficacy could be diminished by alcohol. Respondents who have one positive response in any of the seven risk categories are considered at-risk drinkers. Because it includes items on medications and comorbid conditions common in older adults, it identifies older adults who would not be identified as at risk on other screening measures such as the AUDIT and MAST-G.

Interventions

A variety of treatment options exist for older adults. [51] Although there are a limited number of studies, older adults have demonstrated treatment outcomes as good as or better than those seen in younger age groups.[80–81] There are a spectrum of treatment interventions including brief interventions developed to address less severe substance use disorders and addiction specialty programs for those who are dependent on substances. However, there are few programs tailored specifically for older adults with substance use disorders,[82, 83] in part because their

utilization of such programs is lower than other age groups.[22]

Brief interventions

Brief interventions have been well studied in younger and older age groups, usually in primary care settings.[71, 84, 85] They have been tested primarily for alcohol and are proven to reduce drinking amount. They vary in frequency and length from a single five-minute session to multiple longer sessions. Their purpose is to provide education about the substance and how it might be harmful, enhance motivation to change, and connect severe users with more intensive treatments when needed. Most brief interventions use aspects of motivational interviewing (MI) or motivational enhancement therapy (MET),[86, 87] which encourage a patient-centered, nonjudgmental approach to discussing substance use and encouraging ambivalence by assisting the patient to identify the perceived pros and cons to making a change versus maintaining the status quo.[51] For older adults, the reasons for change may include maintaining independence, optimal health, and mental capacity.[58]

Step 3: advise and assist

Following the steps in the *NIAAA Guide*, when the screening (step 1) and assessment (step 2) of older individuals indicate they are either unhealthy drinkers or may have a substance use disorder, it is recommended that clinicians state their findings and make clear recommendations. For example, a clinician might say, "You are drinking more than is medically safe." Relate the advice to the patient's concerns and medical findings. You can then make a statement such as: "I strongly suggest you cut down (or quit) and I am willing to help. Are you ready to consider making a change to your substance use?" If yes, then help the patient set a goal and agree on a plan and provide educational material. If no, then encourage reflection about the substance use, what the patient likes and doesn't like about substance use, and reaffirm your willingness to help when the person is ready. For those who have a substance use disorder, it is advised that you recommend abstention and consider a referral to an addiction specialist. For both groups, arrange follow-up appointments.

Step 4: at follow-up, continue support

It is important to document substance use and review goals at each visit and determine if the patient was

291

able to meet and sustain the substance use goal. If yes, then reinforce and support continued adherence to recommendations. For those who are not dependent, renegotiate substance use goals if needed, encourage the patient to return, and rescreen regularly. For those who are dependent, ideally coordinate care with an addiction specialist, maintain medications for alcohol dependence for at least three months, and address coexisting disorders as needed.

If the patient has not been able to meet and sustain the substance use goal, then acknowledge that change is difficult, support any positive change, relate substance use to problems, and consider engaging significant others. For those without dependence, renegotiate goal and plan, and reassess diagnosis if the patient is unable to make change. For those with dependence, consider if not done already, referring to an addiction specialist or consulting with one, recommend a mutual help group, and prescribe a medication.

Interventions for substance use disorders

Psychosocial and behavioral treatments

More intensive behavioral interventions for SUDs include cognitive-behavioral therapy (CBT), abstinence-based treatments including individual and group counseling, peer support groups such as Alcoholics and Narcotics Anonymous, and residential treatment.

Two psychosocial and behavioral approaches have been studied with older adults: supportive therapeutic models (STM) [88] and cognitive-behavioral therapy (CBT).[62–64, 89, 90] STM models focus on developing support and coping for older adult substance abusers. CBT focuses on identifying and changing ways of thinking, feeling, and behaving that lead to problematic substance use.[91] The Substance Abuse and Mental Health Services Association published a treatment manual using CBT for older substance abusers.[12]

Medication interventions

A growing number of medications can be used for substance abuse disorders, but only a few have been tested in older adults.

Alcohol dependence

Naltrexone blocks opioid receptors and is the most well studied drug for SUDS in older adults.[81, 92, 93]

It can be given as a daily pill (50 mg) or as a monthly injection (380 mg). It has modest effects on risk for heavy drinking and relapse.[94] Because it blocks the effects of opiate-based pain medications, it cannot be given to those who require opioids. The most common adverse effect is nausea.

Acamprosate is an NMDA and GABA receptor modulator used to reduce craving and the pleasant effect of alcohol.[95, 96] The usual dose is 666 mg three times daily. It can reduce the rate of patients returning to drinking. It has not been tested in older adults. However, because of few reports of adverse effects across populations, it is considered relatively safe among older adults.[97] It is contraindicated in patients with renal failure.

Disulfiram is an aversive agent that causes flushing, headache, nausea, and palpitations when alcohol is consumed by increasing acetaldehyde levels.[95] It is generally not recommended in older adults, as it can cause low blood pressure, chest pain, shortness of breath, and even death.

Tobacco dependence

The most effective medications for smoking cessation include nicotine replacement therapy (NRT) (e.g., transdermal patch, gum, lozenge, inhaler, nasal spray), bupropion, and varenicline. The goal for NRT is to provide nicotine to a smoker without using tobacco, thereby relieving nicotine withdrawal symptoms as the smoker breaks the behavior of cigarette smoking. It is safe to use in patients with known cardiovascular disease.[98] Combining a short- and long-acting NRT has better efficacy than the use of a single product.[99]

Bupropion is believed to act by enhancing CNS noradrenergic and dopaminergic release. It is available as a sustained release form with the usual dose being 150 mg /day for three days, then 150 mg twice a day thereafter. It is recommended that treatment start one week before a smoker's quit date, and last 7–12 weeks. Most common side effects are insomnia, agitation, dry mouth, and headache. It is contraindicated in patients with seizure disorders and eating disorders such as anorexia nervosa and bulimia nervosa.

Varenicline is a partial nicotinic agonist that reduces the symptoms of nicotine withdrawal and reduces the rewarding aspects of cigarette smoking. [100, 101] It is given using the following schedule: days one to three, 0.5 mg daily; days four to seven, 0.5 mg twice daily; day eight and onward, 1 mg twice daily for 11 weeks. It is recommended that treatment start one week before target quit date. Common side effects are headache, insomnia, and nausea. It has not been tested in older adults.

Opioid dependence

Maintenance medications for opioid dependence include opioid agonist treatments including methadone and buprenorphine and opioid antagonist treatment, naltrexone. Agonists suppress craving and withdrawal symptoms. Antagonist treatments prevent the user from experiencing positive effects of opioids.

Methadone is usually provided daily in a controlled setting with direct observation of methadone ingestion by clinic personnel. Common side effects are constipation and sweating. Confusion and respiratory depression may be more common in older adults. QTc prolongation may also occur.

Buprenorphine, a partial opioid agonist, reduces illicit opioid use.[102] It may only be used by certified and specially trained clinicians. Patients must be abstinent from other opioids for at least 24 hours to prevent withdrawal. Constipation and sedation are common side effects.

Naltrexone dosing for opioid dependence is the same as for alcohol dependence, at 50 mg daily. Naltrexone maintenance is most effective in highly motivated patients.

Summary

Older adults are a fast growing population, and the emerging cohort of older adults are from the baby boomer generation who engage in unhealthy use of substances at higher rates than earlier cohorts. Although alcohol is likely to continue to be the most commonly used substance, use of illicit substances is growing. Because of age-related physiologic changes and an increase in comorbidity and medication use, older adults are more vulnerable to adverse effects of multiple substances, even at low doses. It can be more challenging to identify unhealthy substance use in older adults for a variety of reasons. One particular challenge is the difficulty discerning a consequence due to the substance from those of comorbid conditions and medications. There is some evidence that screening and interventions used widely in younger populations, primarily addressing unhealthy alcohol use, also work in older populations. Asking about use of substances is an important first step in identifying potential unhealthy substance use. However, the

health-care system is ill prepared for the coming population of aging substance users. We need to both develop a better understanding of and new approaches to manage unhealthy substance use in older adults.

References

1. US Census Bureau. Population profile of the United States. 2012.

2. Kerr WC, Greenfield TK, Bond J, et al. Age-period-cohort modelling of alcohol volume and heavy drinking days in the US National Alcohol Surveys: divergence in younger and older adult trends. *Addiction.* 2009 Jan;**104**(1):27–37. doi: 10.1111/j.1360-0443.2008.02391.x.

3. Substance Abuse and Mental Health Services Administration. Results from the 2012 National Survey on Drug Use and Health: Summary of national findings. NSDUH Series H-46, HHS Publication No. (SMA) 13–4795. Rockville, MD: Substance Abuse and Mental Health Services Administration; 2013.

4. Duncan DF, Nicholson T, White JB, et al. The baby boomer effect: changing patterns of substance abuse among adults ages 55 and older. *J Aging Soc Policy.* 2010 Jul;**22**(3):237–248. doi: 10.1080/08959420.2010.485511.

5. Cummings SM, Bride B, Rawlins-Shaw AM. Alcohol abuse treatment for older adults: a review of recent empirical research. *Journal of Evidence-Based Social Work.* 2006;**3**(1):79–99.

6. Saitz R. Unhealthy alcohol use. *New Eng J Med.* 2005;**352**(6):596–607.

7. American Psychiatric Association. *Diagnostic and Statistical Manual of Mental Disorders.* 5th ed. Arlington, VA: American Psychiatric Publishing; 2013.

8. Moore AA, Karno MP, Grella CE, et al. Alcohol, tobacco, and nonmedical drug use in older US adults: Data from the 2001/02 National Epidemiologic Survey of Alcohol and Related Conditions. *Journal of the American Geriatrics Society.* 2009;**57**(12):2275–2281.

9. Arndt S, Clayton R, Schultz S. Trends in substance abuse treatment 1998–2008: Increasing older adult first time admissions for illicit drugs. *American Journal of Geriatric Psychiatry.* 2011;**19**:704–711.

10. Moos RH, Schutte KK, Brennan PL, Moos BS. Older adults' alcohol consumption and late-life drinking problems: a 20-year perspective. *Addiction.* 2009;**104**:1293–1302.

11. Kirchner J, Zubritsky C, Cody M, et al. Alcohol consumption among older adults in primary care. *Journal of General Internal Medicine.* 2007;**22**:92–97.

12. Center for Substance Abuse Treatment. *Substance Abuse among Older Adults: Treatment Improvement Protocol*

(TIP) Series 26. Rockville, MD: Substance Abuse and Mental Health Services Administration; 1998.

13. Moore AA, Gould R, Reuben DB, et al. Longitudinal patterns and predictors of alcohol consumption in the United States. *American Journal of Public Health*. 2005;**95**(3):458–465.

14. Blazer DG, Wu L. The epidemiology of at risk and binge drinking among middle-aged and elderly community adults: National Survey on Drug Use and Health. *Am J Psychiat*. 2009;**166**:1162–1169.

15. National Institute on Alcohol Abuse and Alcoholism. *Rethinking Drinking*. NIH Publication No. 13–3770. Bethesda, MD: NIH; 2010.

16. Grant BF, Dawson DA, Stinson FS, et al. The 12-month prevalence and trends in DSM-IV alcohol abuse and dependence: United States, 1991–1992 and 2001–2002. *Drug Alcohol Depen*. 2004;**74**:223–234.

17. King BA, Dube SR, Tynan MA. Current tobacco use among adults in the United States: findings from the National Adult Tobacco Survey. *Am J Public Health*. 2012 Nov;**102**(11):e93–e100. doi: 10.2105/ AJPH.2012.301002. Epub 2012 Sep 20.

18. Wu LT, Blazer DG. Illicit and nonmedical drug use among older adults: a review. *J Aging Health*. 2011;**23**:481–504.

19. Lin JC, Karno MP, Grella CE, et al. Alcohol, tobacco, and nonmedical drug use disorders in US adults aged 65 years and older: data from the 2001–2002 National Epidemiologic Survey of Alcohol and Related Conditions. *Am J Geriatr Psychiatry*. 2011 Mar;**19** (3):292–9. doi: 10.1097/JGP.0b013e3181e898b4.

20. Blazer DG, Wu L. The epidemiology of substance use and disorders among middle aged and elderly community adults: national survey on drug use and health. *Am J Geriatr Psychiatry*. 2009;**17**:237–245.

21. Blazer DG, Wu L. Nonprescription use of pain relievers by middle-aged and elderly community-living adults: national survey on drug use and health. *J Am Geriatr Soc*. 2009;**57**:1252–1257.

22. Bartels SJ, Coakley EH, Zubritsky C, et al. Improving access to geriatric mental health services: a randomized trial comparing treatment engagement with integrated versus enhanced referral care for depression, anxiety, and at-risk alcohol use. *American Journal of Psychiatry*. 2004;**161**:1455–1462.

23. Kennedy GJ, Efremova I, Frazier A, Saba A. The emerging problems of alcohol and substance abuse in late life. *J Soc Distress Homel*. 1999;**8**(4):227–239.

24. Oslin DW. Alcohol use in late life: disability and comorbidity. *J Geriatr Psychiat Neur*. 2000;**13**:134–140.

25. Gilbertson R, Ceballos NA, Prather R, Nixon SJ. Effects of acute alcohol consumption in older and younger adults: perceived impairment versus psychomotor performance. *J Stud Alcohol Drugs*. 2009;**70**(2):242–252.

26. Blow FC, Barry KL. Older patients with at-risk and problem drinking patterns: new developments in brief interventions. *J Geriatr Psychiat Neur*. 2000;**13**:115–123.

27. Sklar AR, Gilbertson R, Boissoneault J, et al. Differential effects of moderate alcohol consumption on performance among older and younger adults. *Alcoholism: Clinical & Experimental Research*. 2012;**36** (12):2150–2156.

28. Linnoila M, Erwin CW, Cleveland WP, et al. Effects of alcohol on psychomotor performance of men and women. *J Stud Alcohol*. 1978;**39**:745–758.

29. Vestal RE, McGuire EA, Tobin JD, et al. Aging and ethanol metabolism. *Clin Pharmacol Ther*. 1977;**21**:343–354.

30. Moore AA, Whiteman EJ, Ward KT. Risks of combined alcohol/medication use in older adults. *Am J Geriatr Pharmacother*. 2007;**5**:64–74.

31. Moore AA, Morton SC, Beck JC, et al. A new paradigm for alcohol use in older persons. *Med Care*. 1999;**37**:165–179.

32. LaCroix AZ, Guralnik JM, Berkman LF, et al. Maintaining mobility in late life. II. Smoking, alcohol consumption, physical activity and body mass index. *American Journal of Epidemiology*. 1993;**137**(8):858–869.

33. LaCroix AZ, Omenn GS. Older adults and smoking. *Clinics in Geriatric Medicine*. 1992;**8**(1):69–87.

34. Rimer BK, Orleans CT, Keintz MK, et al. The older smoker: status, challenges and opportunities for intervention. *Chest*. 1990;**97**:547–53

35. Simoni-Wastila L, Yang HK. Psychoactive drug abuse in older adults. *American Journal of Geriatric Pharmacotherapy*. 2006;**4**(4):380–394.

36. National Institute on Drug Abuse. *Marijuana Abuse*. Bethesda, MD: National Institute on Drug Abuse; 2012.

37. Kuerbis A, Sacco P, Blazer DG, Moore AA. Substance abuse among older adults. *Clin Geriatr Med*. 2014 Aug;**30**(3):629–654. doi: 10.1016/j.cger.2014.04.008. Epub 2014 Jun 12.

38. Merrick EL, Horgan CM, Hodgkin D, et al. Unhealthy drinking patterns in older adults: prevalence and associated characteristics. *J AmGeriatr Soc*. 2008;**56**:214–223.

39. Platt A, Sloan FA, Costanzo P. Alcohol-consumption trajectories and associated characteristics among adults older than age 50. *J Stud Alcohol Drugs*. 2010;**71**:169–179.

40. Moos RH, Brennan PL, Schutte KK, Moos BS. Older adults' health and late-life drinking patterns: a 20-year perspective. *Aging Ment Health*. 2010;**14**(1):33–43.

41. Collins PM, Kayser K, Platt S. Conjoint marital therapy: a practitioner's approach to single-system evaluation. *Families in Society*. 1994;75:131–141.

42. Sacco P, Bucholz KK, Spitznagel EL. Alcohol use among older adults in the National Epidemiologic Survey on Alcohol and Related Conditions. *J Stud Alcohol Drugs*. 2009;70(6):829–838.

43. Balsa AI, Homer JF, Fleming MF, French MT. Alcohol consumption and health among elders. *Gerontologist*. 2008;48(5):622–636.

44. Adams WL. Alcohol use in the retirement communities. *J Am Geriatr Soc*. 1996;44:1082–1085.

45. Brennan PL, Schutte KK, Moos RH. Reciprocal relations between stressors and drinking behavior: a three-wave panel study of late middle-aged and older women and men. *Addiction*. 1999;94(5):737–749.

46. Center for Substance Abuse Treatment. *Substance Abuse Relapse Prevention for Older Adults: A Group Treatment Approach*. Rockville, MD: Substance Abuse and Mental Health Services Administration; 2005.

47. Myers JE, Harper MC. Evidence-based effective practices with older adults. *Journal of Counseling & Development*. 2004;82:207–218.

48. Laidlaw K, Pachana NA. Aging, mental health, and demographic change: challenges for psychotherapists. *Professional Psychology: Research and Practice*. 2009;40(6):601–608.

49. Kuerbis A, Sacco P. The impact of retirement on the drinking patterns of older adults: a review. *Addict Behav*. 2012;37:587–595.

50. American Psychiatric Association. *Diagnostic and Statistical Manual of Mental Disorders*. 4th ed., text revision ed. Washington, DC: Author; 2000.

51. Sacco P, Kuerbis A. Older adults. In: Vaughn MG, Perron BE, eds. *Social Work Practice in the Addictions*. New York: Springer; 2013:213–229.

52. Kuerbis A, Hagman BT, Sacco P. Functioning of alcohol use disorders criteria among middle-aged and older adults: Implications for DSM-5. *Substance Use & Misuse*. 2013;48(4):309–322.

53. Barry KL, Blow FC, Oslin DW. Substance abuse in older adults: review and recommendations for education and practice in medical settings. *Substance Abuse*. 2002;23(3 Suppl):109.

54. Moyer VA, US Preventive Services Task Force. Screening and behavioral counseling interventions in primary care to reduce alcohol misuse: US Preventive Services Task Force recommendation statement. *Ann Intern Med*. 2013 Aug 6;159(3):210–8. doi: 10.7326/0003-4819-159-3-201308060-00652.

55. Duru OK, Xu H, Tseng C-H, et al. Correlates of alcohol-related discussions between older adults and their physicians. *J AmGeriatr Soc*. 2010;58(12):2369–2374.

56. D'Amico EJ, Paddock SM, Burnam A, Kung FY. Identification of and guidance for problem drinking by general medical providers: results from a national survey. *Medical Care*. 2005;43(3):229–236.

57. Dar K. Alcohol use disorders in elderly people: fact or fiction? *Advances in Psychiatric Treatment*. 2006;12:173–181.

58. Barry KL, Oslin DW, Blow FC. *Alcohol Problems in Older Adults*. New York: Springer Publishing Company; 2001.

59. Rodin J. Aging and health: effects of the sense of control. *Science*. 1986;233:1271–1276.

60. Klein WC, Jess C. One last pleasure? Alcohol use among elderly people in nursing homes. *Health & Social Work*. 2002;27(3):193–203.

61. Barry KL, Blow FC, Oslin DW. Substance abuse in older adults: review and recommendations for education and practice in medical settings. *Substance Abuse*. 2002;23(3 Suppl):105–131.

62. Dupree LW, Broskowski H, Schonfeld L. The Gerontology Alcohol Project: a behavioral treatment program for elderly alcohol abusers. *Gerontologist*. 1984;24:510–516.

63. Schonfeld L, Dupree LW. Treatment approaches for older problem drinkers. *International Journal of the Addictions*. 1995;30(13–14):1819–1842.

64. Schonfeld L, Dupree LW, Dickson-Fuhrman E, et al. Cognitive-behavioral treatment of older veterans with substance abuse problems. *J Geriatr Psychol Neur*. 2000;13:124–128.

65. National Institute on Alcohol Abuse and Alcoholism. *Helping Patients Who Drink Too Much: A Clinician's Guide*. 2005 Edition. Bethesda, MD: Author; 2007.

66. Babor TF, Higgins-Biddle JC, Saunders JB, Monteiro MG. *The Alcohol Use Disorders Identification Test (AUDIT): Guidelines for Use in Primary Care*. 2nd ed. Geneva: Department of Mental Health and Substance Dependence, World Health Organization; 2001.

67. Piccinelli M, Tessari E, Bortolomasi M, et al. Efficacy of the alcohol use disorders identification test as a screening tool for hazardous alcohol intake and related disorders in primary care: a validity study. *British Medical Journal*. 1997;314(8):420–424.

68. Humeniuk R, Henry-Edwards S, Ali R, et al. *The Alcohol, Smoking, and Substance Involvement Screening Test (ASSIST)*. Geneva: World Health Organization; 2010.

69. Moore AA, Beck JC, Babor TF, et al. Beyond alcoholism: identifying older, at-risk drinkers in primary care. *J Stud Alcohol*. 2002;63(3):316–324.

70. Barnes AJ, Moore AA, Xu H, et al. Prevalence and correlates of at-risk drinking among older adults: the Project SHARE study. *JGIM*. 2010;**25**(8):840–846.

71. Moore AA, Blow FC, Hoffing M, et al. Primary care-based intervention to reduce at-risk drinking in older adults: a randomized controlled trial. *Addiction*. 2011;**106**(1):111–120.

72. Stewart D, Oslin DW. Recognition and treatment of late-life addictions in medical settings. *Journal of Clinical Geropsychology*. 2001;**7**(2):145–158.

73. Buchsbaum DG, Buchanan R, Welsh J, et al. Screening for drinking disorders in the elderly using the CAGE questionnaire. *J Am Geriatr Soc*. 1992;**40**:662–665.

74. Brennan PL, Nichol AC, Moos RH. Older and younger patients with substance use disorders: Outpatient mental health service use and functioning over a 12-month interval. *Psychol Addict Behav*. 2003;**17**(1):42–48.

75. Ewing JA. Detecting alcoholism: the CAGE questionnaire. *JAMA*. 1984 Oct 12;**252**(14):1905–7.

76. Brown RL, Rounds LA. Conjoint screening questionnaires for alcohol and other drug abuse. *Wisconsin Medical Journal*. 1995;**94**(3):135–140.

77. Barry KL, Blow FC. Screening, assessing and intervening for alcohol and medication misuse in older adults. In: Lichtenberg PA, ed. *Handbook of Assessment in Clinical Gerontology*. Burlington, MA: Elsevier; 2010:307–330.

78. O'Connell H, Chin A-V, Hamilton F, et al. A systematic review of the utility of self-report alcohol screening instruments in the elderly. *International Journal of Geriatric Psychiatry*. 2004;**19**:1074–1086.

79. Fink A, Morton SC, Beck JC, et al. The Alcohol-Related Problems Survey: identifying hazardous and harmful drinking in older primary care patients. *J Am Geriatr Soc*. 2002;**50**:1717–1722.

80. Brennan PL, Nichol AC, Moos RH. Older and younger patients with substance use disorders: outpatient mental health service use and functioning over a 12-month interval. *Psychol Addict Behav*. 2003;**17**(1):42–48.

81. Kuerbis AN, Sacco P. A review of existing treatments for substance abuse among the elderly and recommendations for future directions. *Substance Abuse: Research and Treatment*. 2013;**7**:13–37.

82. Han B, Gfroerer JC, Colliver JD, Penne MA. Substance use disorder among older adults in the United States in 2020. *Addiction*. 2009;**104**:88–96.

83. Schultz SK, Arndt S, Liesveld J. Locations of facilities with special programs for older substance abuse clients in the US. *International Journal of Geriatric Psychiatry*. 2003;**18**(9):839–843.

84. Fleming MF, Manwell LB, Barry KL, et al. Brief physician advice for alcohol problems in older adults: a randomized community-based trial. *Journal of Family Practice*. 1999;**48**(5):378–384.

85. Fink A, Elliot MN, Tsai M, Beck JC. An evaluation of an intervention to assist primary care physicians in screening and educating older patients who use alcohol. *J Am Geriatr Soc*. 2005;**53**:1937–1943.

86. Miller WR, Rollnick S. *Motivational Interviewing: Preparing People for Change*. 2nd ed. New York: The Guilford Press; 2002.

87. Miller WR, Zweben A, DiClemente CC, Rychtarik RG. *Motivational Enhancement Therapy Manual: A Clinical Research Guide for Therapists Treating Individuals with Alcohol Abuse and Dependence*. Rockville, MD: National Institute on Alcohol Abuse and Alcoholism; 1992.

88. Kofoed LL, Tolson RL, Atkinson RM, et al. Treatment compliance of older alcoholics: an elder-specific approach is superior to "mainstreaming." *J Stud Alcohol*. 1987;**48**:47–51.

89. Rice C, Longabaugh R, Beattie M, Noel N. Age group differences in response to treatment for problematic alcohol use. *Addiction*. 1993;**88**:1369–1375.

90. Schonfeld L, Dupree LW. Age-specific cognitive behavioral and self management treatment approaches. In: Gurnack AM, Atkinson RM, Osgood NJ, eds. *Treating Alcohol and Drug Abuse in the Elderly*. New York: Springer Publishing Company; 2002:109–130.

91. Rotgers F. Cognitive-behavioral theories of substance abuse. In: Rotgers F, Morgenstern J, Walters ST, eds. *Treating Substance Abuse: Theory and Technique*. 2nd ed. New York: The Guilford Press; 2003:166–189.

92. Oslin DW, Liberto JG, O'Brien J, et al. Naltrexone as an adjunctive treatment for older patients with alcohol dependence. *American Journal of Geriatric Psychiatry*. 1997;**5**(4):324–332.

93. Oslin DW, Pettinati H, Volpicelli JR. Alcoholism treatment adherence: older age predicts better adherence and drinking outcomes. *American Journal of Geriatric Psychiatry*. 2002;**10**(6):740–747.

94. Rösner S, Hackl-Herrwerth A, Leucht S, et al. Opioid antagonists for alcohol dependence. *Cochrane Database Syst Rev*. 2010;**12**:CD001867.

95. Barrick C, Connors GD. Relapse prevention and maintaining abstinence in older adults with alcohol-use disorders. *Drugs & Aging*. 2002;**19**(8):583–594.

96. Tempesta E, Janiri L, Bignamini A, et al. Acamprosate and relapse prevention in the treatment of alcohol dependence: a placebo controlled trial. *Pharmacopsychiatry*. 2000;**29**:27–29.

97. US National Library of Congress. *DailyMed*. 2013; http://dailymed.nlm.nih.gov/dailymed/about.cfm.

98. Hays JT, Ebbert JO. Adverse effects and tolerability of medications for the treatment of tobacco use and dependence. *Drugs.* 2010;**70**(18):2357–2372.

99. Smith SS, McCarthy DE, Japuntich SJ, et al. Comparative effectiveness of five smoking cessation pharmacotherapies in primary care clinics. *Arch Intern Med.* 2009;**169**(22):2148.

100. Keating GM, Lyseng-Williamson KA. Varenicline: a pharmacoeconomic review of its use as an aid to smoking cessation. *Pharmacoeconomics.* 2010;**28**(3):231–254.

101. Garrison GD, Dugan SE. Varenicline: a first-line treatment option for smoking cessation. *Clinical Therapeutics.* 2009;**31**(3):463–491.

102. Fudala PJ, Bridge TP, Herbert S, et al. Office-based treatment of opiate addiction with a sublingual-tablet formulation of buprenorphine and naloxone. *N Engl J Med.* 2003;**349**(10):949–958.

Chapter 21

Pulmonary issues in the elderly

Charles A. Austin, MD, and Shannon S. Carson, MD

Introduction

The majority of pulmonary disease processes observed in young patients are also observed in elderly populations. However, older people have numerous physiologic changes associated with aging that alter their response to these disease processes when compared to younger patients. Furthermore, they frequently have associated comorbidities that can complicate the management of respiratory conditions. This chapter will review aging physiology and the most commonly encountered pulmonary conditions.

Physiologic changes with aging

Numerous changes to the respiratory system occur naturally with aging. First, the chest wall stiffens. This is likely due to degenerative joint disease of the spine, kyphoscoliosis, and calcifications of the costal cartilages and chondrosternal junctions.[1] These changes lead to almost a one-third decrease in chest wall compliance.[2] With age, airway size decreases as elastic tissue is replaced by collagen.[3] Small airways collapse as end inspiration increases, leading to a greater amount of air trapping. The diaphragm becomes less efficient as well, resulting in increased work of breathing.[4]

The alveolar-arterial oxygen difference increases in older persons due to a variety of factors, including loss of alveolar surface area and an increase in ventilation-perfusion mismatch.[5] Despite these changes, elderly patients should not be hypoxic at sea level in the absence of disease.[6] They also should not have a significant increase in alveolar hypoventilation resulting in elevations of arterial pCO_2.[7] Either of these findings should prompt investigation into an underlying disease process.

Finally, geriatric patients can undergo a number of physiologic changes that decrease their natural mechanical defenses. The cough reflex is decreased as well as mucociliary clearance.[8] Elderly patients can also be susceptible to dysfunction of the swallowing mechanism from central nervous system disorders, primary swallowing dysfunction, or sedating medications, thus increasing the frequency of aspiration events.

Obstructive lung diseases

Obstructive lung diseases, including chronic obstructive pulmonary disease (COPD) and asthma, are diseases frequently encountered in the geriatric population. Approximately 11.6% of the US population 65 or older suffers from COPD.[9] Although fully reversible asthma may be seen in elderly patients,[10] it is less likely to be reversible in this population due to a diminished response to β-agonists with aging.[11] Therefore, this discussion will focus on COPD, as this is the more common geriatric entity.

Chronic obstructive pulmonary disease

The Global Initiative for Chronic Obstructive Lung Disease (GOLD) defines COPD as "a common preventable and treatable disease (that) is characterized by airflow limitation that is usually progressive and associated with an enhanced chronic inflammatory response in the airways and the lung to noxious particles or gases."[12] COPD is currently the third leading cause of death in the United States and an important source of morbidity. It is a significant contributor to health-care costs and utilization as well. Approximately 43% of patients with COPD visit a physician at least once yearly for COPD-related symptoms, and almost 18% either present to an

Reichel's Care of the Elderly, 7th Edition, ed. Jan Busby-Whitehead *et al*. Published by Cambridge University Press.
© Cambridge University Press 2016.

emergency department or are admitted to a hospital yearly for COPD-related complaints.[13]

COPD is primarily divided into two classifications: chronic bronchitis and emphysema. Chronic bronchitis is clinically defined as a chronic productive cough for at least three months in each of two successive years in a patient in which other causes of chronic cough have been excluded.[14] Emphysema is defined anatomically as the destruction of alveolar walls distal to the terminal bronchioles with permanent enlargement of the air spaces.[15] In clinical practice, however, the majority of patients have components of both disorders.

The diagnosis of COPD is made based on clinical suspicion with a history of chronic cough, dyspnea, or sputum production. Suspicion should be heightened if the patient is a smoker, as this is the primary risk factor for COPD. Approximately 80% of patients diagnosed with COPD have a history of smoking. The diagnosis is confirmed by spirometry with a ratio of forced expiratory volume in one second (FEV1) to forced vital capacity (FVC) of <70%. However, there is some controversy associated with this cut-off value in older persons, as the physiologic changes of aging can lead to measurable reductions in FEV1/FVC ratio.[16] The GOLD criteria further classify COPD severity according to FEV1 as follows: stage 1 is an FEV1 ≥80% of predicted; stage 2 is an FEV1 50%–<80% predicted; stage 3 is an FEV1 30%–<50% predicted; and stage 4 is an FEV1 <30% predicted.

Management of stable COPD

Treatment of COPD focuses both on chronic symptom control and on the management of acute exacerbations of COPD. Both of these treatment strategies have special considerations in the geriatric population. Management of stable disease is largely based on three factors: severity of obstruction, impact of symptoms, and frequency of exacerbations.[12] (See Table 21.1.) Treatments are managed in a stepwise manner with addition of medications as the disease severity increases.

The mildest form of COPD is GOLD category A disease, which is characterized by mild symptoms, FEV1 ≥50% predicted, and 0–1 exacerbations in the past year. Category A disease can usually be managed with a short-acting bronchodilator such as ipratropium or albuterol used as needed. (It is important to note that short-acting bronchodilators are

Table 21.1 Classes of COPD, diagnosis, and treatment

Disease class	Diagnosis requirements	Suggested treatment
A	Mild symptoms FEV ≥50% predicted 0–1 exacerbations in past year	Short-acting, prn, bronchodilator such as ipratropium or albuterol
B	Moderate or severe symptoms FEV1 ≥ 50% predicted 0–1 exacerbations in the past year	Daily treatment with LABA or LAMA Prn short-acting bronchodilator
C	Mild symptoms **AND** FEV1 <50% predicted **OR** ≥2 exacerbations per year	Daily treatment with LABA plus ICS **OR** LAMA Prn short-acting bronchodilator
D	Moderate to severe symptoms **AND** FEV1 <50% predicted **OR** ≥2 exacerbations per year	Consider daily treatment with LABA plus ICS plus LAMA Prn short-acting bronchodilator

recommended for use as needed in all categories of COPD severity.) Category B disease is characterized as having either moderate or severe symptoms, FEV1 ≥50% predicted, and 0–1 exacerbations in the past year. Category B patients benefit from a long-acting bronchodilator, including a long-acting beta agonist (LABA) such as salmeterol or a long-acting anti-muscarinic (LAMA) such as tiotropium.[17]

Patients with category C disease have mild symptoms but FEV1 <50% predicted or ≥2 exacerbations per year. They should also use a LABA in addition to an inhaled glucocorticoid (ICS) such as fluticasone or a LAMA.[18] Category D disease is the most severe and is characterized by moderate to severe symptoms and FEV1 <50% predicted or ≥2 exacerbations per year. These patients benefit from the same treatment regimens as patients with category C disease, but a combination of a LABA, ICS, and LAMA should be considered, as triple therapy may improve outcomes.[19]

In addition to medications, multiple nonpharmacologic interventions are helpful for these patients.

For seniors who continue to smoke, smoking cessation is paramount, since smoking leads to a more rapid decline in FEV1.[20] Cessation can be achieved with nicotine replacement therapy, buproprion, verenicline, or counseling. The highest success is seen with a combination of counseling and medications.[21] It is important to note that both buproprion and verenicline have significant potential side effects. Buproprion can lower the seizure threshold in patients. Verenicline can lead to neuropsychiatric changes in some patients and may increase the risk of adverse cardiovascular events in patients with known cardiovascular disease.[22] Unfortunately, to date, these agents have not been studied in the geriatric population.

Pulmonary rehabilitation should be prescribed for all patients with category B disease or greater, as it has been shown to improve symptoms, decrease mortality, and decrease health care utilization.[23] Patients with more severe disease who are hypoxemic at rest should be prescribed long-term supplemental oxygen therapy, which improves survival rates in these patients. Severe hypoxemia is defined as a PaO_2 ≤ 55 mmHg or a SaO_2 $\leq 88\%$.[24] Patients should also be assessed for severe oxygen desaturation during walking or during sleep.

Annual influenza vaccinations should be given to all patients with COPD; it has been shown to greatly reduce the incidence of flu in this population.[25] The pneumococcal polysaccharide vaccine should also be offered to all patients with COPD.

Acute exacerbations of COPD

An acute exacerbation of COPD is defined as an acute increase in baseline symptoms and can include increases in cough, sputum production, or dyspnea.[12] Exacerbations frequently require emergency department utilization and hospitalization, and if severe, can lead to respiratory failure and death. Approximately 75% of exacerbations are attributable to viral or bacterial infection.[26] Treatment goals include resolving the underlying cause and optimizing lung function, which can become greatly compromised during exacerbations.

Oxygen therapy should be utilized to target an arterial oxygen saturation of approximately 92%.[12] Noninvasive positive pressure ventilation (NPPV) should be utilized if necessary, particularly if the patient is suffering from hypercapneic respiratory failure, as this has been shown to decrease mortality.[27] If the patient fails NPPV or has a contraindication, invasive ventilation is indicated if in congruence with the patient's advance directives.

Pharmacologic interventions center on improving lung function. Inhaled short-acting bronchodilators are the primary intervention and should be used liberally. Glucocorticoids at doses equivalent to 40 mg–60 mg of prednisone improve symptoms and decrease hospital length of stay.[28] Oral medications can be used if the patient can take them. If the exacerbation is so severe that the patient cannot tolerate oral medications, IV medications should be used. There is debate about the optimal duration of glucocorticoid treatment, but recent literature supports a course of 5–14 days.[29] Finally, antibiotics with good respiratory coverage – such as a respiratory fluoroquinolone – should be used if the exacerbation is severe.[30] Both oral and IV routes are acceptable.

Special considerations for the geriatric population

The medications just discussed have a few adverse effects that should be considered in the geriatric patient. For inhaled medications, some systemic absorption does occur. For example, tiotropium may have as much as 25% systemic bioavailability.[31] Absorption of inhaled medications can lead to the same adverse reactions as would be observed from oral or intravenous drugs in the same classes. This can be amplified further by common comorbidities in the geriatric population, such as benign prostatic hypertrophy, which may precipitate urinary retention with the use of LAMAs.

Use of short-acting bronchodilators have not been demonstrated to increase the risk of acute MI.[32] However, tachycardia is a known side effect of these medications, so caution should be exercised when used in patients with known arrhythmias. Initiation of long-acting muscarinic antagonists should be monitored, as they can lead to urinary retention due to their anticholinergic effect.[33] Further, inhaled corticosteroids may increase the risk of pneumonia.[34] In the treatment of acute exacerbations, hyperglycemia severe enough to require intervention can be observed with the usage of systemic glucocorticoids.[28] Glucocorticoids and fluoroquinolones can also be deliriogenic, although this is much less common with fluoroquinolones.

Advance directives should be discussed with all patients with severe COPD, particularly if the patient has had acute exacerbations requiring hospitalization, as this is associated with a marked increase in mortality.[35] Patients on oxygen therapy are at an inherently increased risk of respiratory failure, so mechanical ventilation preferences should be clarified in these patients.

Pneumonia

Pneumonia is undoubtedly an important clinical entity, and geriatric practitioners should be comfortable with its diagnosis and management. It is the eighth leading cause of death in the United States,[36] and the 30-day mortality rate for community-acquired pneumonia (CAP) approaches 10%.[37] Further, elderly patients with pneumonia can frequently require hospital and even ICU admission.[38]

Diagnosis

The diagnosis of pneumonia can be difficult in the elderly patient, but it begins with clinical suspicion based on history and exam. Common signs and symptoms include cough, pleuritic chest pain, and dyspnea. On exam, fevers are frequently encountered, although this response may be blunted in the elderly. Altered mental status may occur in the elderly patient and may be the initial presentation of pneumonia. Tachypnea, tachycardia, hypoxia, crackles, or evidence of consolidation by egophony and percussion are also common.[39] It is important to note that geriatric patients are often taking beta blockers, thus tachycardia may be blunted as well. Plain film chest x-ray is recommended to confirm diagnosis if clinical suspicion is high. However, geriatric patients may lack characteristic x-ray findings.[40]

Pneumonia can be divided into four different classifications based on risks for infection with resistant organisms, and treatment largely depends on this classification. Hospital-acquired pneumonia (HAP) is not present on hospital admission but occurs ≥48 hours after admission. Ventilator-associated pneumonia (VAP) is a subclass of HAP that occurs ≥48 hours after intubation and mechanical ventilation. Health-care-associated pneumonia (HCAP) occurs in nonhospitalized patients who have had extensive contact with health care – defined as IV therapy, wound care, or IV chemotherapy – within the past 30 days; residence in a nursing home or other long-term care facility; hospitalization in the past 90 days for two or more days, or attendance at a hemodialysis clinic in the past 30 days.[41] Finally, community-acquired pneumonia (CAP) is a pneumonia that lacks any of these predisposing exposures. (See Table 21.2.)

Treatment

Antibiotic treatment for CAP consists of one of three regimens. (See Table 21.2.) Healthy patients with no comorbidities may be treated with a macrolide or doxycycline. Patients with comorbidities (chronic lung, heart disease, etc.) should be treated with either a respiratory fluoroquinolone or a beta-lactam plus a macrolide.[40] Elderly patients usually require one of the two latter treatments, since they frequently possess comorbid health conditions.

Treatment of HAP and VAP requires IV antibiotics initially and includes coverage for resistant Staphylococcus (MRSA) and pseudomonas organisms based on clinical suspicion. Vancomycin is frequently used first line for MRSA coverage, and multiple antibiotics including fourth generation cephalosporins, carbapenems, and piperacillin-tazobactam are used for pseudomonas coverage. For the patients at highest risk for resistant organisms, dual coverage with two different anti-pseudomonas agents is recommended.[41] Empiric antibiotic choices should be narrowed based upon culture and sensitivity of respiratory tract specimens.

Geriatricians should be familiar with the management of HCAP, as elderly patients with pneumonia commonly fall into this category. Antibiotic selection should be tailored based on severity of illness. Oral antibiotics have similar efficacy to IV antibiotics in nursing home patients who are not severely ill from HCAP.[42] For patients who are more severely ill, IV antibiotics should be used in a similar approach to the treatment of HAP and VAP. The decision to admit patients to the hospital for treatment of pneumonia is also based upon severity of illness. There are validated clinical scoring rules to offer guidance on hospital admission based upon risk of death from pneumonia. In the simplest terms, any patient age 65 or over presenting with community acquired pneumonia should be admitted to the hospital if they present with confusion or have a respiratory rate ≥30 or are hypotensive. Other risk factors that increase the

Table 21.2 Classifications and suggested treatments of pneumonia

Classification	Predisposing exposures	Antibiotic treatment
Hospital-acquired pneumonia (HAP)	Occurs ≥48 hours after admission	Vancomycin **plus** broad anti-pseudomonal agent (4th-generation cephalosporin, carbapenem or piperacillin-tazobactam) Consider dual coverage for Pseudomonas if resistance expected
Ventilator-associated pneumonia (VAP)	Occurs >48 hours post intubation	Vancomycin **plus** broad anti-pseudomonal agent (4th-generation cephalosporin, carbapenem or piperacillin-tazobactam) Consider dual coverage for pseudomonas if resistance expected
Health-care-associated pneumonia (HCAP)	IV therapy, wound care or chemotherapy in past 30 days Residence in long-term care or nursing facility Hospitalization in past 90 days for ≥2 days Hemodialysis in past 30 days	If severely ill: vancomycin **plus** broad anti-pseudomonal agent (4th-generation cephalosporin, carbapenem or piperacillin-tazobactam) Nursing home patients: Oral respiratory fluoroquinolone **OR** beta-lactam **plus** macrolide
Community-acquired pneumonia (CAP)	PNA contracted in absence of predisposing exposures	Patients with minimal comorbidities: macrolide **OR** doxycycline Patients with comorbidities: Oral respiratory fluoroquinolone **OR** beta-lactam **plus** macrolide

consideration for hospital admission in elderly patients include associated hypoxemia or acidosis, hyperglycemia, hypernatremia, anemia, pleural effusion, and severe underlying comorbidities.[43, 44] Finally, for nursing home patients with pneumonia and advanced dementia, goals of care should be clarified, as antimicrobial treatment has been shown to modestly prolong survival but not increase comfort.[45, 46]

Pulmonary embolism

Acute pulmonary embolism (PE) is a common malady among older persons, with an approximate prevalence of 400 per 100,000 patients who are ≥ 80 years old.[47] It carries a mortality rate of 30% if untreated.[48] Risk factors for PE include immobilization, stroke, paresis, malignancy, chronic heart disease, recent central venous catheter or pacemaker placement, autoimmune disease, and a history of prior venous thromboembolism (VTE).[49, 50] Additionally, obesity and hypertension have been identified as risk factors in women.[51] Geriatric

patients frequently suffer from one or many of these conditions, increasing their inherent PE risk.

Diagnosis

Due to its associated mortality, accurate and early diagnosis of PE is important. However, this is not always easily achieved, since the signs and symptoms are nonspecific and our current diagnostic tests are imperfect. Symptoms most commonly include the acute onset of dyspnea, pleuritic chest pain, and cough; and less commonly, hemoptysis. Signs include tachypnea, inspiratory crackles, and tachycardia.[52]

Multiple studies of laboratory and imaging modalities have been performed in an attempt to improve accuracy of PE diagnosis. The D-dimer is one laboratory test utilized in the diagnosis of PE. Its results can be available in minutes, which makes it appealing.[53] Further, if D-dimer is measured by ELISA testing, its sensitivity approaches 95%. However, its specificity is only 40%–68%.[53] Due to these characteristics, it has an excellent negative predictive value for patients whose pretest probability is low.

Pulmonary angiography is the gold standard for diagnosis of PE. However, there is an approximately 5% morbidity associated with this procedure.[54] For this reason, two other imaging modalities – spiral (helical) CT with IV contrast and the ventilation-perfusion (V/Q) scan – are routinely used in the diagnosis of PE. The V/Q scan has a high sensitivity for detecting PE in patients with a high pretest probability and a high-probability scan. It also has a high specificity to exclude PE in patients with a low pre-test probability and low-probability scan.[55] Spiral CT has similar performance characteristics in that it has good sensitivity in those with high pretest probability and a positive CT, and good specificity for those with low pretest probability and a negative CT.[56] Both scans are much less accurate in intermediate probability patients.

Overall, the current data support utilizing a combination of clinical probability, laboratory tests, and radiographic imaging. One widely used algorithm utilizes the modified Wells criteria to stratify patients into high- or low-risk for PE (Table 21.3).[57] For those deemed low risk for PE, with a Wells score <4, a D-dimer should be checked. A negative D-Dimer (<500 ng/mL) virtually excludes PE. A positive D-dimer should prompt further imaging with either CT or V/Q scans. A Wells score ≥4 suggesting high pretest probability should proceed to imaging without checking a D-dimer.[57] For those patients with inconclusive results based on this method, pulmonary angiogram should be considered (see Figure 21.1).

Table 21.3 Well's criteria for assessment of PE

Clinical cymptoms of DVT (leg swelling, palpable cord)	3.0
Other diagnoses less likely than PE	3.0
Heart rate >100	1.5
Immobilization (≥3 days) or surgery in prior four weeks	1.5
Previous DVT/ PE	1.5
Hemoptysis	1.0
Malignancy	1.0

Treatment

Anticoagulation is the mainstay of treatment and results in a decrease in mortality.[58] Parenteral anticoagulation should be initiated after diagnosis is

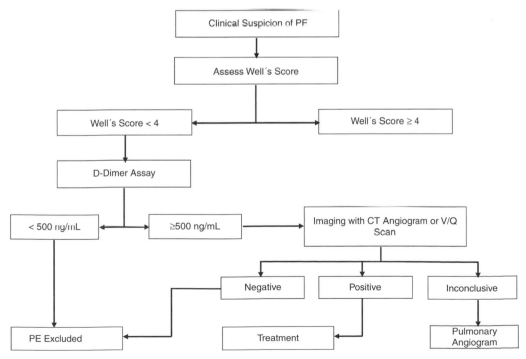

Figure 21.1 PE diagnosis algorithm.

made. At one time, options were limited to IV unfractionated heparin. Recently, however, low molecular weight heparin and subcutaneous fondaparinux have become the preferred initial treatmentsdue to comparable mortality rates with superior morbidity.[59, 60] After the initial treatment, patients are usually transitioned to oral agents. The 2012 American College of Chest Physicians recommendations suggest the usage of warfarin as the agent of choice.[61] However, newer oral agents such as dabigatran or rivaroxaban may be considered in the appropriate clinical scenarios. These agents have the advantage of not requiring routine blood testing. However, they do not have an effective reversal agent so should be used with caution if the patient has an increased risk for falls or propensity for bleeding. Duration of therapyis dependent on risk factors for a recurrent embolic event and whether or not these risk factors are modifiable.

Special considerations in the elderly

Diagnosis of PE can be complicated in elderly patients, as D-dimer is a nonspecific marker for inflammation and is frequently elevated in the elderly due to comorbidities. This can decrease specificity of the D-dimer test.[62] Renal function naturally decreases with age, so caution must be exercised when using IV contrast for CT scans in older patients. Low molecular weight heparin must also be used with caution in this group for the same reason since it is renally metabolized. Finally, patients >65 years old and those at risk for falls are at an increased risk of bleeding while on anticoagulation, so great caution should be exercised with usage of these drugs.[59]

Interstial lung diseases

Interstitial lung diseases (ILD) are a heterogenous group of diseases that ultimately result in chronic lung damage and scarring. The diseases affect people of various ages; some causes are identifiable while others are idiopathic. Most forms of ILD are uncommon in older persons with the exception of idiopathic pulmonary fibrosis (IPF). The prevalence of IPF in patients aged 75 or older has been estimated at 227 per 100,000 compared to 4 per 100,000 in the 18- to 34-year-old demographic.[63]

Diagnosis

Patients with IPF typically have dyspnea on exertion that has progressed over several years with an associated nonproductive cough. Fine crackles are frequently heard on lung exam,[64] and clubbing may been seen in later stages of disease.[65] In IPF, pulmonary function tests reveal a restrictive pattern, and severity of restriction correlates with worse disease.[66] Radiographic studies are vital for diagnosis. Plain film chest x-rays typically demonstrate reticular opacities with a basilar predominance.[67] High-resolution chest CT can demonstrate subpleural and bibasilar reticular opacities with honeycombing or bronchiectasis, which is often diagnostic of the disease.[68]

Treatment

IPF is a serious illness with a mean survival after diagnosis of 5.6 years.[69] Unfortunately, to date, no pharmacological intervention has been proven to be efficacious.[70] Therefore, treatment recommendations are based on consensus guidelines and largely consist of supportive care with oxygen therapy and pulmonary rehabilitation. Corticosteroids have been frequently utilized, but current data do not support their efficacy,[71] and current American Thoracic Society recommendations do not support corticosteroid monotherapy.[70] Other regimens such as a combination of prednisone, azathioprine, and N-acetylcysteine have been studied, but the most recent trial on this combination was stopped due to increased mortality with this regimen.[72] Pirfenidone, an anti-inflammatory agent, is approved for use in Europe, and the FDA is reviewing promising data from recent clinical trials in the United States.[73] A recent phase III trial of the tyrosine kinase inhibitor nintedanib showed marked improvement in decreasing progression of loss of FVC in idiopathic pulmonary fibrosis, although further research on the mortality benefit of this medication is needed.[74]

Given the current lack of effective treatment options, advance care planning discussions are paramount, especially in the elderly patient presenting with advanced disease. Guidelines recommend against mechanical ventilation in this progressive and irreversible disease process.[70] Patients and their families should be made aware of this after diagnosis and counseled accordingly.

Nontuberculous mycobacterium

In the past few years, more attention has been focused on the diagnosis and treatment of nontuberculous mycobacterium (NTM). This group includes mycobacterium avium complex (MAC) and can result in progressive pulmonary illness. Two-year prevalence has been estimated at 20 per 100,000 people in those over age 55. Median age of incidence is 66 years old with an increased prevalence in females.[75]

Presentation and diagnosis

Two different clinical presentations of pulmonary infection are observed. One is seen primarily in older white men with pre-existing lung disease such as COPD. The disease resembles *M. tuberculosis* (TB) infection in these patients, with cough and weight loss, but the symptoms are not usually as severe as in TB. It can also have similar radiographic findings as TB, with cavitary lung lesions.[76]

NTM infection is also seen in people without underlying lung disease. These patients are usually elderly, nonsmoking women.[77] They present with a persistent cough of unclear etiology, and nodules and bronchiectasis are typically seen on chest imaging.[78] Signs and symptoms are vague and nonspecific and include cough, fatigue, malaise, dyspnea, weakness, and, less commonly, hemoptysis. Diagnosis requires a combination of pulmonary symptoms, radiographic changes, and a positive culture from at least two separate sputum samples or from one bronchial lavage sample.[79]

Treatment

Therapy for slowly progressive NTM infection is not always indicated and should be based on disease severity, symptom burden, and the patients' wishes according to risks and benefits of therapy.[79] Treatment consists of multiple antibiotics and is usually recommended for at least one year. Patients with mild symptoms or significant other comorbidities, such as malignancy, may choose to forgo treatment. For those patients who do decide to undergo treatment, antibiotic susceptibility testing should be performed on the MAC isolates. The current recommended regimen consists of a daily combination of a macrolide, such as clarithromycin, plus rifampin plus ethambutol.[79] Treatment should continue until sputum cultures are consecutively negative for one year, if possible. It is important to note that an elderly patient undergoing treatment must be monitored closely, as these medications can have significant side effects to which the geriatric patient may be more prone due to the decline in metabolic clearance with aging. Gastrointestinal side effects and intolerance may be more pronounced in the older patients, necessitating dose reductions.

Sleep-related breathing disorders

Sleep-related breathing disorders refer to a variety of syndromes that result in either abnormal respiratory pattern such as apnea, or reduction in gas exchange during sleep. Between 12 and 18 million adults in the United States are affected with these disorders.[80] The most common two syndromes are obstructive sleep apnea (OSA) and central sleep apnea.

OSA is the most common of these disorders, with an estimated prevalence of 17% in men and 9% in women aged 50–70.[81] In addition to age and male gender, obesity is a significant risk factor, with obese individuals suffering up to a sixfold increased risk for OSA when compared to non-obese patients.[82] Smoking also increases risk significantly.[83] Presenting symptoms of OSA include daytime sleepiness, snoring, and witnessed apneas by a bed partner. Excessive sleepiness from OSA may result in daytime errors, and a threefold increase in motor vehicle crashes has been observed in patients with OSA.[84] OSA is a risk factor for systemic hypertension and multiple adverse cardiac effects, including coronary artery disease and arrhythmias.[85–87]

Diagnosis

Diagnosis is made via overnight polysomnography. Diagnosis is made when there are 15 or more apneas, hypopneas, or respiratory-effort-related awakenings per hour of sleep in asymptomatic patients or five or more events per hour in a patient with symptoms of disturbed sleep.[88] Diagnostic evaluation should be encouraged; the test is relatively safe, and treatment has large potential benefits on quality of life. Home sleep apnea testing is becoming increasingly available. Although it may be less informative than conventional polysomnography, it is less expensive and more convenient for patients.

Treatment

Treatment of choice of OSA is positive airway pressure therapy delivered via either continuous positive airway pressure (CPAP) or bilevel positive airway pressure (BIPAP) devices. Although improved morbidity and symptoms have been demonstrated with these therapies, no randomized controlled trial to date has demonstrated an improvement in mortality.[89] The pressure is titrated to the required setting during polysomnography either in a split-night fashion or with a second visit to the sleep laboratory. As with home diagnostic testing, out-of-center treatment with autotitrating positive pressure therapy is becoming available for patients with high pretest probability of uncomplicated, moderate OSA.

Critical care in the elderly

Elderly patients account for over 40% of patients in intensive care units (ICUs).[90] Despite the higher utilization of ICU resources by the elderly, age is frequently a factor in decisions to withhold aggressive therapies.[91] Many providers assume that geriatric patients have worse outcomes in the ICU when compared to younger patients. However, age itself is not nearly as important in predicting mortality risk as is severity of the acute illness and degree of underlying comorbidities.[92] Further, although many elderly survivors of critical illness are left with significant functional impairments, an overwhelming majority would choose to undergo ICU care again if necessary.[93] Therefore, the most important factor in whether an elderly person should be treated in an ICU setting is whether ICU treatment would be in congruence with the patient's wishes. This can be difficult to ascertain if the patient does not have advance care planning (ACP) documentation or if that documentation is ambiguous. These situations are best averted by being proactive with ACP in the outpatient setting.[94]

There are many important issues that should be considered when caring for elderly patients in the ICU. Delirium is common, with approximately 70% of elderly patients suffering from delirium during a hospitalization requiring ICU care.[95] It is defined as an acute change in mentation that results in inattention and either disorganized thinking or an altered level of consciousness. Delirium is an independent predictor of both increased inhospital mortality and prolonged hospitalization.[96] Diagnosis in the ICU is frequently made using convenient bedside tools such as the Confusion Assessment Method-ICU (CAM-ICU) assessment tool. Given the association of delirium with worse outcomes, prevention may be important. Potential strategies include orientation protocols, environmental modifications such as dimming the lights at night in order to preserve the sleep-wake cycle, and early mobilization. Minimization of long-acting sedatives such as lorazepam has also been proven to be an effective prevention strategy.[97] These interventions may not always be possible in the critically ill patient but should be implemented when possible. (See Chapter 11, "Recognition, Management, and Prevention of Delirium.")

Severe sepsis is one of the most common diagnoses leading to admission to critical care units, and elderly patients are at higher risk for hospitalization with severe sepsis than the general population. The yearly incidence of severe sepsis for patients over 80 years old is 26.2 per 1,000 compared to 3 per 1,000 overall. The incidence of severe sepsis in the elderly is expected to increase in the coming years as patients live longer with multiple comorbid conditions that increase the likelihood of sepsis, such as end-stage renal disease, COPD, cirrhosis, and malignancies.[98] Considering the high incidence of cardiac and renal dysfunction in the elderly, they benefit from early and aggressive resuscitation upon presentation with severe sepsis. Early appropriate antibiotics are also essential to good outcomes.

Geriatric patients are at higher risk for prolonged mechanical ventilation after acute illness.[99] Although recent strategies to improve mechanical ventilation liberation have improved the rates of prolonged ventilation, the most effective approach is still to avoid intubation when possible. Judicious use of noninvasive positive pressure ventilation in patients presenting with respiratory failure due to COPD or congestive heart failure reduces the incidence of mechanical ventilation and the risk of mortality.[27, 100]

Conclusion

Elderly patients suffer from the majority of pulmonary disease processes that are observed in young patients. However, due to their differing physiology and increased likelihood of comorbidities, older persons have numerous special diagnosis and treatment considerations. Practitioners should focus on utilizing the most effective therapies while minimizing potential harm to the patient. Further, one should make every effort to ensure that diagnosis and treatment strategies are in congruence with the patients' wishes.

References

1. Edge JR, Millard FJ, Reid L, Simon G. The radiographic appearances of the chest in persons of advanced age. *British Journal of Radiology.* 1964;**37**:769–74.

2. Estenne M, Yernault JC, De Troyer A. Rib cage and diaphragm-abdomen compliance in humans: effects of age and posture. *J Appl Physiol.* 1985;**59**:1842–8.

3. Bode FR, Dosman J, Martin RR, et al. Age and sex differences in lung elasticity, and in closing capacity in nonsmokers. *J Appl Physiol.* 1976;**41**:129–35.

4. Polkey MI, Harris ML, Hughes PD, et al. The contractile properties of the elderly human diaphragm. *American Journal of Respiratory and Critical Care Medicine.* 1997;**155**:1560–4.

5. Janssens JP. Aging of the respiratory system: impact on pulmonary function tests and adaptation to exertion. *Clinics in Chest Medicine.* 2005;**26**:469–84, vi–vii.

6. Crapo RO, Jensen RL, Hegewald M, Tashkin DP. Arterial blood gas reference values for sea level and an altitude of 1,400 meters. *American Journal of Respiratory and Critical Care Medicine.* 1999;**160**:1525–31.

7. Hardie JA, Vollmer WM, Buist AS, et al. Reference values for arterial blood gases in the elderly. *Chest.* 2004;**125**:2053–60.

8. Svartengren M, Falk R, Philipson K. Long-term clearance from small airways decreases with age. *European Respiratory Journal.* 2005;**26**:609–15.

9. Centers for Disease Control and Prevention. Chronic obstructive pulmonary disease among adults – United States, 2011. *MMWR.* 2012;**61**: 938–43.

10. Yunginger JW, Reed CE, O'Connell EJ, et al. A community-based study of the epidemiology of asthma: incidence rates, 1964–1983. *American Review of Respiratory Disease.* 1992;**146**:888–94.

11. Pfeifer MA, Weinberg CR, Cook D, et al. Differential changes of autonomic nervous system function with age in man. *American Journal of Medicine.* 1983;**75**:249–58.

12. Global strategy for the diagnosis, management, and prevention of chronic obstructive pulmonary disease. Revised 2014. Available at: www.goldcopd.org (accessed Apr 10, 2014).

13. Minino AM, Murphy SL, Xu J, Kochanek KD. Deaths: final data for 2008. *National vital Statistics Reports: from the Centers for Disease Control and Prevention, National Center for Health Statistics, National Vital Statistics System.* 2011;**59**: 1–126.

14. Celli BR, MacNee W, Force AET. Standards for the diagnosis and treatment of patients with COPD: a summary of the ATS/ERS position paper. *European Respiratory Journal.* 2004;**23**:932–46.

15. Rennard SI. COPD: overview of definitions, epidemiology, and factors influencing its development. *Chest.* 1998;**113**:235S–41S.

16. Mohamed Hoesein FA, Zanen P, Lammers JW. Lower limit of normal or FEV1/FVC <0.70 in diagnosing COPD: an evidence-based review. *Respiratory Medicine.* 2011;**105**:907–15.

17. Chong J, Karner C, Poole P. Tiotropium versus long-acting beta-agonists for stable chronic obstructive pulmonary disease. *Cochrane Database Syst Rev.* 2012;**9**:CD009157.

18. Calverley PM, Anderson JA, Celli B, et al. Salmeterol and fluticasone propionate and survival in chronic obstructive pulmonary disease. *N Engl J Med.* 2007;**356**:775–89.

19. Tashkin DP, Celli B, Senn S, et al. A 4-year trial of tiotropium in chronic obstructive pulmonary disease. *N Engl J Med.* 2008;**359**:1543–54.

20. Anthonisen NR, Connett JE, Murray RP. Smoking and lung function of Lung Health Study participants after 11 years. *American Journal of Respiratory and Critical Care Medicine.* 2002;**166**:675–9.

21. Warnier MJ, van Riet EE, Rutten FH, et al. Smoking cessation strategies in patients with COPD. *European Respiratory Journal.* 2013;**41**:727–34.

22. Rigotti NA, Pipe AL, Benowitz NL, et al. Efficacy and safety of varenicline for smoking cessation in patients with cardiovascular disease: a randomized trial. *Circulation.* 2010;**121**:221–9.

23. Puhan MA, Scharplatz M, Troosters T, Steurer J. Respiratory rehabilitation after acute exacerbation of COPD may reduce risk for readmission and mortality – a systematic review. *Respiratory Research.* 2005;**6**:54.

24. Qaseem A, Wilt TJ, Weinberger SE, et al. Diagnosis and management of stable chronic obstructive pulmonary disease: a clinical practice guideline update from the American College of Physicians, American College of Chest Physicians, American Thoracic Society, and European Respiratory Society. *Annals of Internal Medicine.* 2011;**155**:179–91.

25. Wongsurakiat P, Maranetra KN, Wasi C, Acute respiratory illness in patients with COPD and the effectiveness of influenza vaccination: a randomized controlled study. *Chest.* 2004;**125**:2011–20.

26. Sethi S, Murphy TF. Infection in the pathogenesis and course of chronic obstructive pulmonary disease. *N Engl J Med.* 2008;**359**:2355–65.

27. Ram FS, Picot J, Lightowler J, Wedzicha JA. Non-invasive positive pressure ventilation for treatment of respiratory failure due to exacerbations of chronic obstructive pulmonary disease. *Cochrane Database Syst Rev.* 2004;**3**:CD004104.

28. Niewoehner DE, Erbland ML, Deupree RH, et al. Effect of systemic glucocorticoids on exacerbations of chronic obstructive pulmonary disease: Department of Veterans Affairs Cooperative Study Group. *N Engl J Med.* 1999;**340**:1941–7.

29. Leuppi JD, Schuetz P, Bingisser R, et al. Short-term vs conventional glucocorticoid therapy in acute exacerbations of chronic obstructive pulmonary disease: the REDUCE randomized clinical trial. *JAMA.* 2013;**309**:2223–31.

30. Vollenweider DJ, Jarrett H, Steurer-Stey CA, Antibiotics for exacerbations of chronic obstructive pulmonary disease. *Cochrane Database Syst Rev.* 2012;**12**:CD010257.

31. Keam SJ, Keating GM. Tiotropium bromide: a review of its use as maintenance therapy in patients with COPD. *Treatments in Respiratory Medicine.* 2004;**3**:247–68.

32. Suissa S, Assimes T, Ernst P. Inhaled short acting beta agonist use in COPD and the risk of acute myocardial infarction. *Thorax.* 2003;**58**:43–6.

33. Kesten S, Jara M, Wentworth C, Lanes S. Pooled clinical trial analysis of tiotropium safety. *Chest.* 2006;**130**:1695–703.

34. Calverley PM, Stockley RA, Seemungal TA, et al. Reported pneumonia in patients with COPD: findings from the INSPIRE study. *Chest.* 2011;**139**:505–12.

35. Connors AF Jr, Dawson NV, Thomas C, et al. Outcomes following acute exacerbation of severe chronic obstructive lung disease. The SUPPORT investigators (Study to Understand Prognoses and Preferences for Outcomes and Risks of Treatments). *American Journal of Respiratory and Critical Care Medicine.* 1996;**154**:959–67.

36. File TM Jr, Marrie TJ. Burden of community-acquired pneumonia in North American adults. *Postgraduate Medicine* 2010;**122**:130–41.

37. Ruhnke GW, Coca-Perraillon M, Kitch BT, Cutler DM. Marked reduction in 30-day mortality among elderly patients with community-acquired pneumonia. *American Journal of Medicine.* 2011;**124**:171–8 e1.

38. Marrie TJ, Huang JQ. Epidemiology of community-acquired pneumonia in Edmonton, Alberta: an emergency department-based study. *Canadian Respiratory Journal.* 2005;**12**:139–42.

39. Metlay JP, Kapoor WN, Fine MJ. Does this patient have community-acquired pneumonia? Diagnosing pneumonia by history and physical examination. *JAMA.* 1997;**278**:1440–5.

40. Mandell LA, Wunderink RG, Anzueto A, et al. Infectious Diseases Society of America/American Thoracic Society consensus guidelines on the management of community-acquired pneumonia in adults. *Clinical Infectious Diseases.* 2007;**44** Suppl 2: S27–72.

41. American Thoracic Society and Infectious Diseases Society of America. Guidelines for the management of adults with hospital-acquired, ventilator-associated, and healthcare-associated pneumonia. *American Journal of Respiratory and Critical Care Medicine.* 2005;**171**:388–416.

42. Loeb M, Carusone SC, Goeree R, et al. Effect of a clinical pathway to reduce hospitalizations in nursing home residents with pneumonia: a randomized controlled trial. *JAMA.* 2006;**295**:2503–10.

43. Fine MJ, Auble TE, Yealy DM, et al. A prediction rule to identify low-risk patients with community-acquired pneumonia. *N Engl J Med.* 1997;**336**:243–50.

44. Lim WS, van der Eerden MM, Laing R, et al. Defining community acquired pneumonia severity on presentation to hospital: an international derivation and validation study. *Thorax.* 2003;**58**:377–82.

45. Givens JL, Jones RN, Shaffer ML, et al. Survival and comfort after treatment of pneumonia in advanced dementia. *Archives of Internal Medicine.* 2010;**170**:1102–7.

46. van der Steen JT, Lane P, Kowall NW, et al. Antibiotics and mortality in patients with lower respiratory infection and advanced dementia. *Journal of the American Medical Directors Association.* 2012;**13**:156–61.

47. Kroger K, Kupper-Nybelen J, Moerchel C, et al. Prevalence and economic burden of pulmonary embolism in Germany. *Vascular Medicine.* 2012;**17**:303–9.

48. Horlander KT, Mannino DM, Leeper KV. Pulmonary embolism mortality in the United States, 1979–1998: an analysis using multiple-cause mortality data. *Archives of Internal Medicine.* 2003;**163**:1711–7.

49. Heit JA, O'Fallon WM, Petterson TM, et al. Relative impact of risk factors for deep vein thrombosis and pulmonary embolism: a population-based study. *Archives of Internal Medicine.* 2002;**162**:1245–8.

50. Zoller B, Li X, Sundquist J, Sundquist K. Risk of pulmonary embolism in patients with autoimmune disorders: a nationwide follow-up study from Sweden. *Lancet.* 2012;**379**:244–9.

51. Goldhaber SZ, Grodstein F, Stampfer MJ, et al. A prospective study of risk factors for pulmonary embolism in women. *JAMA.* 1997;**277**:642–5.

52. Stein PD, Beemath A, Matta F, et al. Clinical characteristics of patients with acute pulmonary embolism: data from PIOPED II. *American Journal of Medicine.* 2007;**120**:871–9.

53. Stein PD, Hull RD, Patel KC, et al. D-dimer for the exclusion of acute venous thrombosis and pulmonary embolism: a systematic review. *Annals of Internal Medicine.* 2004;**140**:589–602.

54. Stein PD, Athanasoulis C, Alavi A, et al. Complications and validity of pulmonary angiography in acute pulmonary embolism. *Circulation.* 1992;**85**:462–8.

55. Investigators P. Value of the ventilation/perfusion scan in acute pulmonary embolism. Results of the

prospective investigation of pulmonary embolism diagnosis (PIOPED). *JAMA.* 1990;**263**:2753–9.

56. Stein PD, Fowler SE, Goodman LR, et al. Multidetector computed tomography for acute pulmonary embolism. *N Engl J Med.* 2006;**354**:2317–27.

57. van Belle A, Buller HR, Huisman MV, et al. Effectiveness of managing suspected pulmonary embolism using an algorithm combining clinical probability, D-dimer testing, and computed tomography. *JAMA.* 2006;**295**:172–9.

58. Kernohan RJ, Todd C. Heparin therapy in thromboembolic disease. *Lancet.* 1966;**1**:621–3.

59. Kearon C, Akl EA, Comerota AJ, et al. *Antithrombotic therapy for VTE disease: Antithrombotic Therapy and Prevention of Thrombosis,* 9th ed: American College of Chest Physicians Evidence-Based Clinical Practice Guidelines. *Chest* 2012;**141**:e419S–94S.

60. Van Dongen CJ, van den Belt AG, Prins MH, Lensing AW. Fixed dose subcutaneous low molecular weight heparins versus adjusted dose unfractionated heparin for venous thromboembolism. *Cochrane Database Syst Rev.* 2004;**4**:CD001100.

61. Van den Berghe G, de Zegher F, Bouillon R. Clinical review 95: acute and prolonged critical illness as different neuroendocrine paradigms. *J Clin Endocrinol Metab.* 1998;**83**:1827–34.

62. Righini M, Goehring C, Bounameaux H, Perrier A. Effects of age on the performance of common diagnostic tests for pulmonary embolism. *American Journal of Medicine.* 2000;**109**:357–61.

63. Raghu G, Weycker D, Edelsberg J, et al. Incidence and prevalence of idiopathic pulmonary fibrosis. *American Journal of Respiratory and Critical Care Medicine.* 2006;**174**:810–6.

64. Bohadana A, Izbicki G, Kraman SS. Fundamentals of lung auscultation. *New Eng J Med.* 2014;**370**:744–51.

65. Spicknall KE, Zirwas MJ, English JC 3rd. Clubbing: an update on diagnosis, differential diagnosis, pathophysiology, and clinical relevance. *Journal of the American Academy of Dermatology.* 2005;**52**:1020–8.

66. Chetta A, Marangio E, Olivieri D. Pulmonary function testing in interstitial lung diseases. *Respiration.* 2004;**71**:209–13.

67. Pipavath S, Godwin JD. Imaging of interstitial lung disease. *Clinics in Chest Medicine.* 2004;**25**:455–65, v–vi.

68. Wittram C, Mark EJ, McLoud TC. CT-histologic correlation of the ATS/ERS 2002 classification of idiopathic interstitial pneumonias. *Radiographics.* 2003;**23**:1057–71.

69. Carrington CB, Gaensler EA, Coutu RE, et al. Natural history and treated course of usual and desquamative interstitial pneumonia. *N Engl J Med.* 1978;**298**:801–9.

70. Raghu G, Collard HR, Egan JJ, et al. An official ATS/ERS/JRS/ALAT statement: idiopathic pulmonary fibrosis: evidence-based guidelines for diagnosis and management. *American Journal of Respiratory and Critical Care Medicine.* 2011;**183**:788–824.

71. Douglas WW, Ryu JH, Schroeder DR. Idiopathic pulmonary fibrosis: impact of oxygen and colchicine, prednisone, or no therapy on survival. *American Journal of Respiratory and Critical Care Medicine.* 2000;**161**:1172–8.

72. Idiopathic Pulmonary Fibrosis Clinical Research Network, Raghu G, Anstrom KJ, et al. Prednisone, azathioprine, and N-acetylcysteine for pulmonary fibrosis. *N Engl J Med.* 2012;**366**:1968–77.

73. King TE Jr, Bradford WZ, Castro-Bernardini S, et al. A phase 3 trial of pirfenidone in patients with idiopathic pulmonary fibrosis. *N Engl J Med.* 2014;**370**:2083–92.

74. Richeldi L, du Bois RM, Raghu G, et al. Efficacy and safety of Nintedanib in idiopathic pulmonary fibrosis. *N Engl J Med.* 2014;**370**:2071–82.

75. Winthrop KL, McNelley E, Kendall B, et al. Pulmonary nontuberculous mycobacterial disease prevalence and clinical features: an emerging public health disease. *American Journal of Respiratory and Critical Care Medicine.* 2010;**182**:977–82.

76. Teirstein AS, Damsker B, Kirschner PA, et al. Pulmonary infection with Mycobacterium avium-intracellulare: diagnosis, clinical patterns, treatment. *Mount Sinai Journal of Medicine.* 1990;**57**:209–15.

77. Reich JM, Johnson RE. Mycobacterium avium complex pulmonary disease presenting as an isolated lingular or middle lobe pattern: the Lady Windermere syndrome. *Chest.* 1992;**101**:1605–9.

78. Prince DS, Peterson DD, Steiner RM, et al. Infection with Mycobacterium avium complex in patients without predisposing conditions. *N Engl J Med.* 1989;**321**:863–8.

79. Griffith DE, Aksamit T, Brown-Elliott BA, et al. An official ATS/IDSA statement: diagnosis, treatment, and prevention of nontuberculous mycobacterial diseases. *American Journal of Respiratory and Critical Care Medicine.* 2007;**175**:367–416.

80. Young T, Palta M, Dempsey J, et al. Burden of sleep apnea: rationale, design, and major findings of the Wisconsin Sleep Cohort study. *WMJ: Official Publication of the State Medical Society of Wisconsin.* 2009;**108**:246–9.

81. Peppard PE, Young T, Barnet JH, et al. Increased prevalence of sleep-disordered breathing in adults. *American Journal of Epidemiology.* 2013;**177**:1006–14.

82. Peppard PE, Young T, Palta M, et al. Longitudinal study of moderate weight change and sleep-disordered breathing. *JAMA.* 2000;**284**:3015–21.

83. Wetter DW, Young TB, Bidwell TR, et al. Smoking as a risk factor for sleep-disordered breathing. *Archives of Internal Medicine.*1994;**154**:2219–24.

84. George CF. Sleep apnea, alertness, and motor vehicle crashes. *American Journal of Respiratory and Critical Care Medicine.* 2007;**176**:954–6.

85. Marin JM, Agusti A, Villar I, et al. Association between treated and untreated obstructive sleep apnea and risk of hypertension. *JAMA.* 2012;**307**:2169–76.

86. Marin JM, Carrizo SJ, Vicente E, Agusti AG. Long-term cardiovascular outcomes in men with obstructive sleep apnoea-hypopnoea with or without treatment with continuous positive airway pressure: an observational study. *Lancet.* 2005;**365**:1046–53.

87. Monahan K, Storfer-Isser A, Mehra R, et al. Triggering of nocturnal arrhythmias by sleep-disordered breathing events. *Journal of the American College of Cardiology.* 2009;**54**:1797–804.

88. Duchna HW. [Sleep-related breathing disorders–a second edition of the International Classification of Sleep Disorders (ICSD-2) of the American Academy of Sleep Medicine (AASM)]. *Pneumologie.* 2006;**60**:568–75.

89. Giles TL, Lasserson TJ, Smith BJ, et al. Continuous positive airways pressure for obstructive sleep apnoea in adults. *Cochrane Database Syst Rev.* 2006;**3**: CD001106.

90. Chelluri L, Grenvik A, Silverman M. Intensive care for critically ill elderly: mortality, costs, and quality of life. Review of the literature. *Archives of Internal Medicine.* 1995;**155**:1013–22.

91. Hamel MB, Teno JM, Goldman L, et al. Patient age and decisions to withhold life-sustaining treatments from seriously ill, hospitalized adults. SUPPORT Investigators. Study to Understand Prognoses and Preferences for Outcomes and Risks of Treatment. *Annals of Internal Medicine.* 1999;**130**:116–25.

92. Knaus WA, Wagner DP, Draper EA, et al. The APACHE III prognostic system: risk prediction of hospital mortality for critically ill hospitalized adults. *Chest.* 1991;**100**:1619–36.

93. Danis M, Patrick DL, Southerland LI, Green ML. Patients' and families' preferences for medical intensive care. *JAMA.* 1988;**260**:797–802.

94. Lynn J, Goldstein NE. Advance care planning for fatal chronic illness: avoiding commonplace errors and unwarranted suffering. *Annals of Internal Medicine.* 2003;**138**:812–8.

95. McNicoll L, Pisani MA, Zhang Y, et al. Delirium in the intensive care unit: occurrence and clinical course in older patients. *J Am Ger Soc.* 2003;**51**:591–8.

96. Thomason JW, Shintani A, Peterson JF, et al. Intensive care unit delirium is an independent predictor of longer hospital stay: a prospective analysis of 261 non-ventilated patients. *Critical Care.* 2005;**9**:R375–81.

97. Carson SS, Kress JP, Rodgers JE, et al. A randomized trial of intermittent lorazepam versus propofol with daily interruption in mechanically ventilated patients. *Critical Care Medicine.* 2006;**34**:1326–32.

98. Angus DC, Linde-Zwirble WT, Lidicker J, et al. Epidemiology of severe sepsis in the United States: analysis of incidence, outcome, and associated costs of care. *Critical Care Medicine.* 2001;**29**:1303–10.

99. Carson SS. Outcomes of prolonged mechanical ventilation. *Curr Opin Crit Care.* 2006;**12**:405–11.

100. Weng CL, Zhao YT, Liu QH, et al. Meta-analysis: noninvasive ventilation in acute cardiogenic pulmonary edema. *Annals of Internal Medicine.* 2010;**152**:590–600.

Chapter 22

Gastrointestinal disease in the elderly

Karen E. Hall, MD, PhD

The "scope" of the problem

Gastrointestinal symptoms are common in patients aged 65 and older and can range from mild self-limited episodes of constipation or acid reflux to life-threatening episodes of infectious colitis or bowel ischemia. According to data from the US Census Bureau in 2005, 45–50 million people over age 65 had at least one gastrointestinal (GI) complaint that impacted their daily life and that might result in a medical visit. Geriatric-aged patients may present with unusual or subtle symptoms of serious GI disease due to alterations in physiology with aging. This chapter highlights common GI problems in older patients, with an emphasis on practical management and goals of care in this population.

Disorders of the esophagus

Gastroesophageal reflux disease

Gastroesophageal reflux disease (GERD) is one of the more common GI disorders affecting the elderly.[1] Population studies have indicated that more than 20% of adults over age 65 have heartburn at least weekly. This may actually underestimate the true prevalence of GERD due to the finding that, while symptoms appear to decrease in intensity with age, the severity of reflux and the risk of complications increase. The ubiquitous use of proton pump inhibitors (PPIs) in clinical practice has probably resulted in treatment of unsuspected GERD, but chronic PPI use comes with its own set of problems, including accelerated osteoporosis, decreased efficacy of Plavix, and potential increase in risk of developing serious respiratory infections. Hence, there has been a recent focus on decreasing chronic use of PPIs in patients who do not appear to have an indication for their use.

Presentation

GERD is straightforward to diagnose if it presents with the classic symptoms of pyrosis (substernal burning with radiation to the mouth and throat) and sour regurgitation. Geriatric patients may present with more subtle symptoms, such as a chronic cough, difficult-to-control asthma, laryngitis, or recurrent chest pain. They may also be completely asymptomatic and present with a complication such as anemia or dysphagia due to dysmotility or stricture. Patients taking multiple medications – particularly nonsteroidal anti-inflammatory drugs (NSAIDs) or bisphosphonates – are at increased risk for pill-induced esophagitis or erosions, which can present with symptoms similar to GERD and should be investigated in a similar way.

Diagnosis

If GERD is suspected from the history, patients should be tested for anemia and low iron levels, which may be due to esophagitis. Upper endoscopy (EGD) should be performed in all patients with new-onset GERD over age 50, persistent symptoms of reflux despite medical therapy, patients with a history of acid reflux longer than five years, and those with possible complications from acid reflux. These groups have an increased risk of malignancy. EGD is safe to perform even in the very elderly frail patient – the main contraindication is end-stage chronic obstructive pulmonary disease (COPD) or other situation where sedation is contraindicated. Other testing is typically reserved for patients who do not respond to therapy or who have atypical symptoms. Patients presenting with hoarseness or cough that is suspected to be related to GERD can undergo ambulatory evaluation with a 24-hour pH monitoring after a negative workup (including EGD and other tests for

Reichel's Care of the Elderly, 7th Edition, ed. Jan Busby-Whitehead *et al.* Published by Cambridge University Press.
© Cambridge University Press 2016.

malignancy) and failure of empiric treatment with PPIs and lifestyle changes. Esophageal manometry is typically reserved for the elderly patient with a suspected motility disturbance or to rule out a motility disturbance prior to the consideration of reflux surgery.

Differential diagnosis

In older patients presenting with heartburn and dysphagia, malignancy in the esophagus and/or stomach should be considered and excluded. Patients with hoarseness and cough may require evaluation by imaging or referral to specialists to exclude oropharyngeal causes of vocal cord dysfunction such as stroke or malignancy.

Complications

Complications that have been associated with GERD include esophagitis, esophageal ulceration, bleeding, strictures, Barrett's esophagus, and esophageal adenocarcinoma, all of which are increased in patients over 65 years of age.[2]

Treatment and prevention

Treatment of GERD in the elderly is essentially the same as that in younger patients. Although the "step-up" approach of lifestyle changes followed by acid-reducing drugs may work, immediate initiation of a PPI with lifestyle modifications usually results in fewer office visits, a reduction in procedures, improved patient satisfaction, and reduced overall costs. Histamine$_2$ receptor antagonists (H$_2$RAs) are also effective for mild symptoms, and avoid the side effects of PPIs such as accelerated osteoporosis and drug interactions. (See Table 22.1.) Cimetidine is generally not recommended in older patients because of potential drug interactions and a higher incidence of adverse side effects compared with other H$_2$RAs. Although effective, chronic PPI use has been associated with an increased relative risk of osteoporosis of 1.97 with long-term use of PPIs (>7 years).[3] There have been reports of other concerns, such as decreased efficacy of clopidogrel anticoagulation for prophylaxis against coronary stent occlusion when clopidogrel is used in conjunction with PPIs. (See Table 22.2.)

For this reason, it is recommended to reevaluate the need for PPIs in patients who have been taking them for longer than six months or who had PPIs started for ulcer prophylaxis during hospitalization.

Table 22.1 Treatment of gastroesophageal reflux disease: a step-up approach

1. Lifestyle modifications

Eat smaller, more frequent meals.
Avoid chocolate, peppermint, and acidic foods (tomato juice, citrus juice) or foods that stimulate acid production (caffeine-containing foods).

Do not eat 3–4 hours before going to bed.

Minimize fats, alcohol, caffeine, and nicotine, especially at night.

Sleep with head of bed elevated 6 inches.

2. Antacid liquids or tablets

Mylanta, Maalox, Gaviscon, Tums, Rolaids

3. H$_2$RAs

Cimetidine (Tagamet; not routinely recommended in older patients because of increased incidence of drug interactions and delirium)

Famotidine (Pepcid; 20 mg qd or bid)

Nizatidine (Axid; 150 mg qd or bid)

Ranitidine (Zantac; 150 mg qd or bid)

4. Proton pump inhibitors

Esomeprazole (Nexium; 20 mg–40 mg qd)

Lansoprazole (Prevacid; 15 mg–30 mg qd)

Omeprazole (Prilosec; 20 mg–40 mg qd) – available OTC as Prilosec 20 mg

Pantoprazole (Protonix; 40 mg qd)

Rabeprazole (Aciphex; 20 mg qd)

5. Surgery

Laparoscopic fundoplication

Nissen fundoplication

H$_2$RAs – histamine$_2$ receptor antagonists

Antireflux surgery should be reserved for patients with severe refractory GERD with complications. Results from high-volume centers indicate that mortality and morbidity are not increased in patients over 70 who are deemed low surgical risk for complications. However, as in younger patients undergoing reflux surgery, there is an immediate decrease in patients with symptoms post-surgery to 10%–15%, yet some 60% of patients are taking acid suppressive medications 5–15 years later.

Dysphagia

Dysphagia, or difficulty swallowing, is a common complaint in older individuals.[4] (See Box 22.1.) Dysphagia is classified as oropharyngeal (transfer) or esophageal (transit).

Oropharyngeal dysphagia refers to impaired movement of liquids or solids from the oral cavity to the upper esophagus. Changes with aging affecting the ability to chew and swallow food include painful or diseased teeth, xerostomia (dry mouth), poorly fitting

Table 22.2 Reported complications of PPIs.

Osteoporosis
Small intestinal bacterial overgrowth
Increased susceptibility to infection with enteric pathogens

Traveler's diarrhea

C. difficile

Drug–drug interactions
Cytochrome P450 interaction with clopidogrel
Reduced absorption of Atazanavir
Increased susceptibility to aspiration pneumonia
Vitamin B12 and iron malabsorbtion
Increased risk of *Helicobacter pylori* gastritis
Acute interstitial nephritis

dentures, and loss of mandibular bone density. Muscle function slows with aging, resulting in slower transfer of food into the pharynx, and delayed relaxation of the upper esophageal sphincter (UES). The resultant inability to move food into the esophagus can cause penetration of food into the area above the vocal cords, and possibly aspiration into the trachea. Studies of normal healthy adults over age 85 demonstrate that approximately 10% have silent aspiration documented on barium cinefluoroscopy. Neuromuscular disorders affecting the tongue, soft palate, oropharynx, and upper esophageal sphincter such as cerebrovascular disease, Parkinson's disease, multiple sclerosis, Alzheimer's disease, and upper motor neuron diseases exacerbate the problem, as do muscular disorders such as myasthenia gravis, polymyositis, and amyloidosis. Finally, patients with a history of surgery or radiation to the oral cavity or neck are at risk for transfer dysphagia. This can occur many years later due to structuring or fibrosis in the irradiated muscles. In this group, recurrence of cancer should be part of the differential diagnosis.

Dysphagia occurring in the esophagus distal to the UES is transit dysphagia, and is even more common than transfer dysphagia. In a review of patients presenting with dysphagia in a primary care setting, the most common diagnoses were esophageal reflux (44%), benign strictures (36%), esophageal motility disorder (11%), neoplasm (6%), infectious esophagitis (2%), and achalasia (1%).

BOX 22.1 Dysphagia in the elderly patient

- Dysphagia in the elderly is common and should always be investigated
- Check history of smoking, alcohol use, review medications, do neurologic exam
- Dysphagia may be oropharyngeal (mostly caused by neurological disorders) or esophageal; the causes of esophageal dysphagia can generally be determined by history
- Common causes of dysphagia
  - Neuromuscular: strokes, Parkinson's disease, dementia
  - Mechanical: strictures, Zenker's diverticulum, Shatski's ring, tumors of the head, neck, esophagus
  - Motility: achalasia, paraneoplastic, diffuse esophageal spasm, hypertonic LES, diffuse motility disorder with ineffectual peristalsis
  - Inflammatory esophagitis: pill esophagitis, acid reflux, radiation, caustic ingestion
- Dysphagia is associated with aspiration, weight loss, and poor quality of life
- Patients considered for a feeding tube should be able to participate in the decision
- Esophageal cancer usually presents in an advanced stage in the elderly, with symptoms of progressive dysphagia and weight loss.
- Surveillance of Barrett's esophagus should be performed at one-to-three-year intervals to detect early adenocarcinoma

Presentation

Patients with oropharyngeal dysphagia typically cough, gag, choke, or aspirate their food during the initiation of a swallow. Patients may also complain of odynophagia, or painful swallowing. (See Table 22.3.) Those with transit dysphagia often complain of solid foods or liquids "sticking," "catching," or "hanging up" in their esophagus, and may point to their substernal area as the problem location. This does not always indicate the true location of the problem, as patients with distal esophageal obstruction may have sensations referred higher up in the chest. Using a series of questions, the cause of esophageal (transit) dysphagia can be identified in nearly 90% of cases. Dysphagia to solids usually reflects an underlying mechanical obstruction, whereas dysphagia to both liquids and solids starting simultaneously usually reflects an underlying neuromuscular disorder (motility disorder). It is helpful in this age group to ask about risk factors that predispose patients to infection, inflammation, or malignancy and whether the patient is experiencing odynophagia.

Table 22.3 Causes of odynophagia.

1. Medications

Tetracycline
Quinidine
Doxycycline
Alendronate
Iron
NSAIDs
ASA
Vitamin C
Potassium chloride

2. Infections

Viral (HSV, CMV, HIV, VZV)
Bacterial (Mycobacteria)
Fungal (*Candida, Asperigillus*)

3. Acid reflux disease

4. Miscellaneous

Ischemia
Chemotherapy
Radiation
Crohn's disease
Sarcoid

NSAIDs – nonsteroidal anti-inflammatory drugs; ASA – acetylsalicylic acid; HSV – herpes simplex virus; CMV – cytomegalovirus; VZV – varicella zoster virus.

Patients with odynophagia may have underlying infection (such as esophageal candidiasis) or obstruction. Use of steroid inhalers for COPD can result in yeast colonization of the mouth and throat. History of smoking or heavy alcohol use is associated with increased risk of squamous cell esophageal cancer. The physician should look for evidence of anemia and unintentional weight loss due to inability to eat, either of which could indicate a serious disorder such as malignancy. Finally, associated symptoms of chest pain or acid reflux should be elicited, as GERD is a risk for peptic strictures and development of Barrett's esophagus and subsequent adenocarcinoma.[2]

Diagnosis

In the elderly a barium esophagogram is often ordered as the initial test to evaluate dysphagia, but an EGD should also be performed to check for malignancy and take biopsies.[5] Patients with oropharyngeal symptoms of transit dysphagia should be evaluated by a speech-language pathologist who can coordinate a swallowing study (modified barium swallow or videofluoroscopy) using thin, thick, and solid food materials. If upper endoscopy is normal and complaints of dysphagia persist, then esophageal manometry should be performed. This is a safe and readily performed procedure that can accurately identify neuromuscular disorders that cause dysphagia.

Treatment

Treatment is directed toward the underlying disorder in addition to ensuring adequate nutrition and preventing aspiration. Patients with transfer dysphagia are taught which foods can be safely swallowed, proper swallowing techniques, and how to modify their posture to improve their swallowing. Patients with transit dysphagia due to decreased esophageal contractility and increased lower esophageal sphincter (LES) pressure (achalasia) may benefit from lower esophageal sphincter (LES) dilation or botulinum toxin injection. Drugs that decrease smooth muscle contractions (anticholinergics, calcium antagonists, nitrates) may decrease diffuse esophageal spasm. Laparoscopic Heller myotomy to open the LES has been performed in elderly patients with achalasia with reasonable safety and efficacy. If aspiration occurs or the nutritional status of the patient suffers, a feeding jejunostomy or gastrostomy should be considered. The patient should participate in the decision to proceed with a feeding tube as part of long-term

BOX 22.2 Peptic ulcer disease in the elderly

- Peptic ulcer disease is usually caused by NSAIDs or *H. pylori*.
- Complications of peptic ulcer disease are more common in the elderly and morbidity and mortality are higher in this age group.
  - PUD in the elderly may present without pain, particularly with NSAID use, and hemorrhage or perforation may be the first sign of an ulcer.
- Dyspepsia is a common complaint in the elderly and requires endoscopy to rule out ulcer or cancer.
- Consider depression as a cause of dyspepsia in an older patient with a negative workup and other symptoms of depression
  - A CT scan of the abdomen may be helpful to diagnose abdominal pain, as elderly patients often present with atypical symptoms of diseases such as cholecystitis, appendicitis, and renal stones
  - Mesenteric ischemia is a diagnosis often missed in older adults

management. Current recommendations are to avoid placing G tubes in demented patients, as those have not been shown to improve quality of life.

Disorders of the stomach

Peptic ulcer disease

Peptic ulcer disease (PUD) refers to both gastric ulcers (GUs) and duodenal ulcers (DUs). Approximately five million cases of PUD will occur this year in the United States, and the demographics are shifting towards an older age of presentation. This may be due to increased use of NSAIDs, *H. pylori* infection, and longer lifespan. The elderly are more likely to suffer complications of PUD, including hospitalization, need for blood transfusions, emergency surgery, and death. The two most common causes of PUD are NSAIDs and *H. pylori*.[6] (See Box 22.2.)

Presentation

Patients may have bleeding with hematemesis or coffee-ground emesis, or present with anemia. Elderly patients are less likely to have epigastric pain with PUD than younger patients, with as many as 50% of patients without significant pain from either a GU or a DU. Because elderly patients may have little or no symptoms of significant ulceration, complications such as perforation are also more common in this age group.[7]

Diagnosis

Patients should be asked about a history of PUD; their use of aspirin, NSAIDs, and warfarin; and previous diagnostic studies (upper GI series, testing for *H. pylori*). Upper endoscopy should be performed in older patients suspected of having PUD to identify the lesion, perform a biopsy in the stomach for *H. pylori*, rule out a malignancy, and initiate endoscopic therapy for a bleeding ulcer, if necessary.[8] Morbidity and mortality of GI bleeding is higher in patients over 70; this has been correlated with delayed endoscopy and continued hemorrhage causing hypotension and cardiac ischemia. Current recommendations in this population are to perform endoscopy within 12 hours of presentation if possible and transfuse if the hemoglobin falls below 7.

Treatment

If the patient is found to be *H. pylori* positive, double or triple antibiotic therapy should be started. In the case of a GU, healing should be documented eight to twelve weeks later, with follow-up EGD to make sure that the ulcer is not malignant. The most common issue is what to do about using ASA or NSAIDs in patients with prior ulceration or bleeding. Patients with a prior history of PUD who did not have a significant bleed, and who require chronic NSAID or aspirin use should be treated concurrently with a PPI or misoprostol. Both agents are effective in reducing the risk of PUD in chronic NSAID users, although, as a group, the PPIs are generally better tolerated than misoprostol. Older patients with serious complications such as hemorrhage or perforation should avoid NSAIDs and ASA, as risk of recurrent bleeding is so high, even with prophylaxis with PPIs or misoprostol, that it outweighs any potential benefit.

Dyspepsia

Dyspepsia is defined as chronic or recurrent pain or discomfort in the upper abdomen that is thought to

315

arise in the upper GI tract. It is exceedingly common in clinical practice, affecting an estimated 20%–30% of older adults. It can sometimes be difficult to distinguish abdominal pain due to gastric or esophageal irritation from colonic spasm, but the latter is usually "spasmodic" in that it waxes and wanes within minutes, whereas dyspepsia lasts for a longer time (hours). There is overlap with the symptoms of cholecystitis, and patients often end up being evaluated for gallbladder disease.

Presentation

Patients may complain of upper abdominal pain, nausea, bloating, early satiety, or reflux symptoms. It is important to distinguish patients with structural damage due to problems such as an ulcer from those with "functional" or non-ulcer dyspepsia, because treatment approaches are different.

Patients should be asked about unintentional weight loss, odynophagia, dysphagia, prior PUD, pancreatitis, biliary tract disease, bleeding, prior trauma, a family history of GI tract cancer, and evidence of blood loss or jaundice. *H. pylori* infection is a risk factor for PUD and accounts for a significant number of cases of dyspepsia in younger patients (aged <60). Older patients may be more likely to be infected but most are asymptomatic. Noninvasive tests for active *H. pylori* infection include urease breath testing and stool antigen. Patients undergoing endoscopy for dyspepsia should be tested for *H. pylori* and treated if positive.

Laboratory tests – including a CBC, erythrocyte sedimentation rate (ESR), liver function tests (LFTs), electrolytes, amylase, and lipase – should be performed. Older patients should be evaluated by upper endoscopy to rule out an ulcer or cancer rather than simply initiating treatment with triple therapy. If endoscopy is normal and symptoms persist, then it is reasonable to get a right upper quadrant (RUQ) ultrasonogram to check for evidence of cholecystitis (gallbladder wall thickening and fluid around the gallbladder). If this is normal and complaints persist, a solid-phase gastric emptying scan can be performed to check for gastroparesis. In an older patient with persistent symptoms, concerns about occult malignancy should prompt a CT scan of the abdomen with both oral and intravenous contrast if the patient's renal function will allow this.

Treatment

Patients with persistent dyspeptic symptoms and a normal evaluation are categorized as having non-ulcer dyspepsia. Although this is more often seen in patients younger than 65, there are geriatric patients who fall into this group. There is not much data to support the routine use of antacids, antimuscarinic agents, or sucralfate. Routine treatment with H_2RAs has shown a slight benefit, but better results have been obtained with the use of once-or twice-daily PPIs in patients with burning pain or pain relieved by food. This suggests that these patients likely have GERD or some effect of acid on gastroesophageal motility.

It is important to consider depression with somatization as a potential underlying cause of dyspepsia, as recent studies have shown a correlation between chronic abdominal pain and depression. The Rome III classification of gastrointestinal motility disorders is based on evidence that patients with chronic abdominal pain without irritable-bowel-type relief with defecation actually respond better to antidepressants than GI-directed medications such as PPIs. This is particularly worth remembering in older patients, as they may have somatic manifestations of depression, such as chest pain, abdominal pain, nausea, and early satiety. There are no controlled, published studies to date on the use of selective serotonin reuptake inhibitors in the treatment of dyspepsia in older patients; however, if the patient has other symptoms and signs of depression, use of SSRIs should be considered. Antidepressants that have been used to treat chronic pain include tricyclic antidepressants, fluoxetine, paroxetine, venlafaxine, and duloxetine.

Gastric cancer

In 2002, the number of new cases of gastric cancer diagnosed reached 900,000, with the highest incidence in China, Japan, Korea, and Eastern Europe; most were diagnosed in patients older than 60.[9] The incidence of gastric cancer is increasing in the elderly worldwide, while it is decreasing in younger cohorts. The overall five-year survival rate is estimated at 16%. Nearly 95% of gastric cancers are adenocarcinomas, followed by lymphoma at 4%. Gastrointestinal stromal tumors (GISTs), carcinoids, and sarcomas make up the remaining 1%. Risk factors for gastric cancer include chronic atrophic gastritis, *H. pylori*, pernicious anemia, family history of gastric cancer, partial

BOX 22.3 Gastric cancer

- Symptoms of gastric cancer are nonspecific, and diagnosis is often delayed.
- Gastric cancer is most common in China, Japan, Korean, and Eastern Europe, therefore consider this diagnosis in patients from those areas.
- MALT lymphoma, although uncommon, has a relatively good prognosis and appears to be sequelae of chronic *H. pylori* infection.
- Patients need continued endoscopic and EUS surveillance for at least five years after surgical resection of gastric cancer.

gastrectomy, tobacco use, alcohol use, and consumption of large quantities of salted or smoked foods containing nitrites and nitrates. (See Box 22.3.)

Diagnosis

Presenting symptoms of gastric cancer are often vague. Patients may complain of nausea, early satiety, epigastric fullness, intermittent vomiting, weight loss, and abdominal pain. Physical examination may reveal a mass, a succussion splash from gastric outlet obstruction, or evidence of peripheral lymphadenopathy. Unfortunately, by the time symptoms are severe or physical examination findings are apparent, patients usually have widespread disease.

Gastric cancer is best detected by upper endoscopy. CT scanning is useful to assess the depth of tumor invasion and the presence of lymphadenopathy. Both endoscopic ultrasonography and positron emission tomography scans are used to improve tumor staging. Mucosal-associated lymphoid tissue (MALT lymphoma), which is confined to the gastric mucosa, has the best prognosis of all gastric cancers. There appears to be an association between development of this tumor and infection with *H. pylori*, and treatment of *H.pylori* (if present) is the first-line treatment-grade MALT lymphoma. There are no specific lab tests for gastric cancer, although levels of CEA are often elevated, which can be useful to monitor efficacy of treatment.

Treatment

Surgical therapy offers the only cure for gastric cancer; however, the overall five-year survival is poor (20%–40%), and operative mortality high (15%–25%). Endoscopic resection of large masses, laser therapy, and stent placement may provide palliation for some patients with obstructive symptoms. Neo-adjuvant chemotherapy has been shown to improve survival. Palliative chemotherapy should be considered, as this has been shown to prolong survival and preserve quality of life. Both chemotherapy and radiation are used for treatment of high-grade MALT lymphoma. Patients undergoing surgery should have EGD and EUS surveillance at frequent intervals (at least yearly) until at least five years after surgery.

Disorders of the colon

Diarrhea

Patients with diarrhea most often complain of frequent stools (>3/day) or loose stools. However, other patients use the term "diarrhea" to describe fecal incontinence or fecal urgency. The etiology of acute diarrhea (lasting <2 weeks) in the elderly is similar to that of younger adults. Most cases of acute diarrhea are related to viral or bacterial infections, but it can also be caused by medications, medication interactions, or dietary supplements. *Clostridium difficile* colitis is more prevalent in the elderly because of more frequent hospitalizations, increased antibiotic use, and increased numbers of patients in institutional settings. *C. difficile* colonization in long-term care facilities has been estimated to be at least 50% in the United States. Chronic diarrhea, lasting more than two weeks, may result from fecal impaction, medications, irritable bowel syndrome, microscopic or lymphocytic colitis, inflammatory bowel disease, obstruction from colon cancer, malabsorption, small bowel bacterial overgrowth, thyrotoxicosis, or lymphoma. Patients with underlying neuromuscular disease such as Parkinson's disease who use anticholinergic medications that slow GI transit may be at much higher risk of small bowel bacterial overgrowth. (See Box 22.4.)

Lactase deficiency should be considered in elderly patients with diarrhea. Symptoms of bloating, abdominal distention, and loose stools usually begin in early adulthood, often worsening with age. Patients are usually aware that they are lactose intolerant; however, lactose intolerance can develop acutely after an episode of diarrhea due to other causes such as viral gastroenteritis. This usually resolves, but may take several weeks or months in some patients. Celiac disease is an increasingly recognized cause of diarrhea and bloating in older adults. Whether this is occurring

BOX 22.4 Diarrhea

Acute diarrhea is usually self-limited and caused by infections. Chronic diarrhea has many causes, and an extensive workup may be needed.
- Consider early hospitalization or admission to an observation unit for older patients with diarrhea due to increased risk of dehydration, falls, and inability to perform activities of daily living.
- Diverticulosis increases with age. Complications include bleeding, diverticulitis, and perforation.
- Most patients with diverticulitis respond to outpatient treatment. Elderly patients may develop abscess or perforation without significant peritonitis – consider early admission if decreased bowel sounds or WBC >12,000.
- Inflammatory bowel disease (IBD) may present for the first time in older people and is often more limited in distribution compared to younger patients.
- Treatment of IBD in older patients may be limited by side effects of immunosuppressive drugs and have higher risk of infection.
- Surgical treatment of IBD in the elderly has higher risk of morbidity.

de novo in later life or reflects chronic gluten intolerance is not clear. Uncommon causes of diarrhea include Whipple's disease, jejunal diverticulosis, bowel ischemia, amyloidosis, lymphoma, and scleroderma with bacterial overgrowth.

Diagnosis

A complete history and physical examination, including a rectal examination, may provide information on cause and direct further evaluation. Medication history may reveal a causative agent, and recent antibiotic use or hospitalization should trigger a workup for *C. difficile*. A history of weight loss raises the concern for malignancy, IBD, microcytic colitis, malabsorption, or thyrotoxicosis. Fluid status with orthostatic blood pressure measurement should be assessed in all elderly patients with diarrhea, because they are particularly susceptible to dehydration. Bloating and gas may indicate small bowel overgrowth, or even underlying celiac disease. Stool cultures should be obtained to exclude infection in patients with acute diarrhea, although routine stool cultures usually give a specific diagnosis in only 20%–30% of cases. This is likely due to the fact that most infectious diarrheas are due to viruses such as rotavirus and Norwalk agent.

For chronic diarrhea, qualitative or quantitative stool fat should be checked to detect steatorrhea, and a TSH should be performed. *C. difficile* toxin assay (toxin A and possibly B) should be obtained if there is a history of recent antibiotic use. Colonoscopy should be performed in patients with a history of weight loss, bloody diarrhea, and diarrhea lasting more than four weeks if deemed safe to do. Even if the colonoscopy appears grossly normal, an elderly patient with chronic diarrhea should be biopsied to rule out microscopic colitis, which has a much higher prevalence in older adults. X-rays and a CT scan of the abdomen may demonstrate bowel wall thickening with severe enteritis or colitis; they are also useful if complications such as perforation or abscess formation are suspected. In patients who are suspected to have small bowel bacterial overgrowth causing bloating and diarrhea, a positive breath hydrogen/methane test will confirm early fermentation of ingested sugars in the small bowel. Serum antibodies to tissue transglutamidase (tTG) are often positive in patients with celiac disease, with IgA tTG being the most sensitive and specific. Definitive diagnosis is made on demonstration of villous damage and atrophy in small bowel biopsies performed during upper endoscopy.

Treatment

Treatment of diarrhea is based on the underlying cause. In those with no evidence of sepsis and no blood in the stool, loperamide ($\leq$ 8/day) can be used and is effective in treating symptoms. Lomotil, which contains atropine, may cause confusion and toxicity in the elderly and should be avoided, as should antispasmodics such as dicylcomine. Bismuth subsalicylate, which has bactericidal action on common bacterial pathogens, can also be used. *C. difficile* should be treated with oral metronidazole for mild infections, and oral vancomycin for moderate to severe colitis or very ill patients. Elderly patients have a decreased response to metronidazole compared to younger patients (85% vs. 95%), and relapse of *C. difficile* diarrhea is more common in the older patient. Antidiarrhea agents should be avoided in *C.*

BOX 22.5 Gastrointestinal bleeding

- Gastrointestinal bleeding is more common in the elderly and is associated with a worse outcome.
- Increased risk for gastrointestinal bleeding with use of nonsteroidal anti-inflammatory drugs, warfarin, and the presence of *H. pylori*.
- Acute upper gastrointestinal bleeding usually presents with hematemesis, melena, or increased blood urea nitrogen–creatinine ratio.
- Chronic or slow upper gastrointestinal bleeding may present with anemia, melena, or a positive fecal occult blood test.
- Upper gastrointestinal endoscopy is usually performed first because two-thirds of acute GI bleeding originates in the upper GI tract.
- Lower gastrointestinal bleeding usually presents with hematochezia or a positive fecal occult blood test. Colonoscopy may be deferred to outpatient if patient is stable.
  - Use PPI prophylaxis in patients with a history of GI bleeding who must take aspirin for cardiac prophylaxis or NSAIDs.

difficile colitis due to the risk of precipitating ileus and toxic megacolon. In microscopic colitis, initial treatment with nonspecific antidiarrheal agents such as loperamide and bismuth subsalicylate should be tried. If this fails and symptoms are severe then the patient should be referred to a specialist. Budesonide has been shown to be effective.[10]

If small bowel overgrowth is present, then treatment with bismuth-containing medications may be helpful in mild cases. For severe small bowel overgrowth, treatment with 14–21 days of antibiotics to eradicate the bacteria is needed. If the underlying cause of slow intestinal transit is not addressed or is not treatable, then overgrowth is likely to recur. Elimination of gluten is the treatment for celiac disease, and has become easier with the increase in gluten-free foods. Medication review is often helpful in patients with refractory celiac disease, as medications have been shown to be an unsuspected source of gluten.

Diverticular disease

Diverticular disease has a high incidence in industrialized nations and increases with age, such that >60% of those older than 70 and nearly 80% of those older than 80 have diverticular out-pouchings of the colonic mucosa and submucosa. They are thought to develop because of increased colonic luminal pressures, particularly with constipation and straining. Diverticula are most commonly found on the left side of the colon. The majority of patients who have diverticula are asymptomatic. Approximately 15%–20% of older adults who have diverticulosis will have a

complication, among them diverticular bleeding or inflammation of a diverticulum (diverticulitis). (See Box 22.5.)

Diverticular bleeding

Diverticular bleeding is characterized by the sudden onset of painless hematochezia, which may be large in volume. Although most diverticula are present on the left side of the colon, 70% of diverticular bleeding comes from right-sided diverticulae.[8] Eighty percent of diverticular bleeding episodes stop spontaneously without requiring treatment. Patients should be hospitalized if bleeding persists, if they are hemodynamically unstable, or if blood loss compromises other organ systems. Older patients are at higher risk for poor outcomes with bleeding, and the threshold for hospitalization should be lower than in younger patients.

Diagnosis

Evaluation of lower GI bleeding usually involves colonoscopy to exclude sources of bleeding such as arteriovenous malformations (AVMs), ischemia, IBD, and cancer. Diverticular bleeding is often a diagnosis of exclusion in a patient with diverticuli, significant bleeding, and no other source found. (See Table 22.4.) If bleeding persists, a tagged RBC scan should be performed or, if necessary, angiography, for intervention to control bleeding. In refractory cases, surgical resection of the bleeding area may be required.

In uncomplicated diverticulitis, patients have lower abdominal pain, fever, and an elevated white blood cell count.[11] They may have diarrhea or may have decreased bowel movements due to spasm in the

Table 22.4 Causes of GI bleeding in the elderly

UGI bleeding	LGI bleeding
Gastric, duodenal or esophageal ulcer	Colonic diverticuli
Gastritis, duodenitis or esophagitis	Ischemic bowel disease
Esophageal varices	Inflammatory bowel disease
Mallory-Weiss tear	Angiodysplasia
Neoplasm	Infectious diarrhea
Telangiectasias	Radiation proctitis
Angiodysplasia	Postpolypectomy
	Hemorrhoids
	Stercoral ulcers

GI – gastrointestinal; UGI – upper GI; LGI – lower GI

> **BOX 22.6** Inflammatory bowel disease in the elderly
>
> - Inflammatory bowel disease (IBD) may present for the first time in older people and is often more limited in distribution compared to younger patients.
> - Treatment of IBD in older patients may be limited by side effects of immunosuppressive drugs and have higher risk of infection
> - Surgical treatment of IBD in the elderly has higher risk of morbidity.

inflamed colon. On physical examination there are no palpable abdominal masses or peritoneal signs. An abdominal radiograph should be performed to look for pneumoperitoneum. If there is no evidence of perforation or sepsis, treatment can be initiated in the outpatient setting with clear liquids for two to three days and oral antibiotics that should cover both anaerobes and gram-negative organisms. The patient should call the office in 24 hours and be seen 48–72 hours after the initial evaluation. If no improvement occurs, the patient should be hospitalized and have a CT scan of the abdomen performed.

Diverticulitis becomes complicated if an abscess, stricture, large volume bleeding, or fistula develops. In addition to presenting with tachycardia or hypotension, elderly patients may present with lethargy or confusion. Abdominal examination may reveal a mass in the left lower quadrant, with or without peritonitis; significant blood in the stool; or evidence of a draining fistula to the bladder, uterus, or skin. Patients with complicated diverticulitis require hospitalization.

Older patients with an episode of diverticulitis have approximately a 35% chance of a second episode occurring within the next five years. Patients with more than two episodes of diverticulitis in the same segment of colon should be referred to a surgeon for consideration of segmental resection, particularly if

they had a complicated hospitalization. Older patients tolerate elective resection with primary anastomosis well. Emergency colon resection has a higher morbidity and mortality in patients over 70 compared to younger patients, and diverting colostomy may be a better alternative in that situation.

Inflammatory bowel disease

Whereas the majority of patients with IBD are under age 65, approximately 10%–15% of all newly diagnosed cases of Crohn's disease and ulcerative colitis occur in patients over age 65.[12] Symptoms of Crohn's disease are similar to those in a younger population, although older patients with Crohn's disease may have fewer complaints of abdominal pain or cramps. This may be due to reduced visceral sensation or the concurrent use of multiple medications that may suppress pain or decrease intestinal motility. (See Box 22.6.)

Crohn's disease

Patients typically have a history of nonbloody diarrhea, unintentional weight loss, and fatigue. They may have symptoms and signs of anemia (pallor, shortness of breath, reduced exercise tolerance). Extra-intestinal manifestations of Crohn's disease commonly occur. These include joint effusions, oral ulcers, painful nodular lesions on the extremities (erythema nodosum), uveitis, and back pain secondary to sacroileitis. Although Crohn's disease may develop anywhere from the mouth to the anus, in elderly patients it is less likely than in younger patients to involve large portions of the GI tract. The correct diagnosis is often delayed in older patients because the GI symptoms of Crohn's disease may mimic other diseases, including infectious diarrhea, ischemic colitis, lactose intolerance, medication-induced diarrhea, diverticulitis, celiac disease, microscopic colitis, or bacterial overgrowth. Use of serologic antibody panels that detect autoantibodies in IBD can sometimes be helpful for diagnosis but are fairly expensive, and their use should probably be deferred to specialists in IBD treatment.

Ulcerative colitis

Ulcerative colitis (UC) usually presents with tenesmus and frequent bloody bowel movements. Extraintestinal manifestations of UC include dermatological manifestations such as pyoderma gangrenosum (round or oval lesions on the shins and forearms). Elderly patients with UC are more likely to have limited left-sided disease or proctitis compared with younger patients. The first attack of UC in an older patient is generally more severe and more likely to require steroids than in a younger patient. Of elderly patients with UC, approximately 15% will eventually require surgery. The diagnosis of either Crohn's or UC is made based on a thoughtful physical examination and history supplemented by appropriate laboratory studies and colonoscopy. Patients will require endoscopy for definitive diagnosis; however, this should be undertaken with caution in patients with severe colitis because of the risk of perforation. For Crohn's disease, CT enterography or small bowel radiography is used to look for small bowel involvement.

Patients should be followed by a gastroenterologist with expertise in treating IBD. There is limited data on the safety and efficacy of IBD treatment in patients over age 70, as few patients of that age have been included in trials of medications.

Colon cancer

The topic of colon cancer screening in older patients is a large one and is beyond the scope of this chapter to fully review. However there are some important take home points for medical providers who treat older patients that are worth reviewing. The incidence and prevalence of colon cancer increases with age, and the bulk of the diagnosed disease occurs in patients over age 65.

Colon cancer is one of the best understood malignancies in terms of the mechanism of transition from normal tissue to cancer, and there is strong evidence that screening and removal of precancerous growths decreases the risk of subsequent development of colon

Table 22.5 Indications for colonoscopy in older patients

Screening at age 50 and every 10 years afterward (if no lesions identified)

Shorter frequency of surveillance if risk factors:
First-degree family member with colon cancer
Personal history of colon cancer, colonic polyps, inflammatory bowel disease
History of breast cancer

Diagnostic colonoscopy if alarm symptoms present:
Hemeoccult positive stool on routine screening
New change in bowel habits
Anemia secondary to blood loss from the gastrointestinal tract
Hematochezia
Unintentional weight loss
New unexplained abdominal pain

cancer in older patients. The controversy in applying screening is primarily based on what techniques to use and how long to continue. Several recent consensus statements indicate that some type of screening should be done starting at age 50, and continuing as long as patients have an expectation of life expectancy of greater than five years. Life tables incorporating morbidity and functional status indicate that the utility of colon cancer screening diminishes to unacceptable levels between age 80 and 85 years of age. (See Table 22.5.)

Anorectal disorders

Constipation and fecal incontinence

Constipation is very common in older patients due to changes in the colonic motility with age, and superimposed risks such as immobility and medication use. (See Table 22.6.) Constipation is a risk for fecal impaction and resultant fecal incontinence. (See Box 22.7.)

Acute and chronic fecal incontinence occur commonly in elderly patients with comorbid conditions and are often socially embarrassing and incapacitating.[13, 14] Despite its adverse effect on patients' life and well-being, fecal incontinence is under-reported by older patients to physicians. The prevalence of fecal incontinence increases with age. Among community-residing people, the prevalence of fecal incontinence in older women is as high as 15% and in older men 10%. The prevalence is nearly 50% in patients in long-term care. Fecal incontinence is now the second

Table 22.6 Common causes of constipation

Constipation-predominant irritable bowel syndrome (abdominal pain relieved by defecation)
Slow colonic transit
Pelvic floor dysfunction (anismus, persistent puborectalis contraction)

Medication-induced:

Opiates	Anticholinergics
Calcium channel blockers	Antidepressants
Antipsychotics	Ganglion-blocking agents

Mechanical obstruction:

Cancer	Large rectocele
Volvulus	Intussusception
Stricture	Anal fissure
Extrinsic compression	
Descending perineum syndrome	

Neurological disorders:

Parkinson's disease	Spinal cord or sacral root tumors
Multiple sclerosis	Spinal cord injury
	Prior colon surgery with neurologic damage

Systemic disorders:

Hypothyroidism	Amyloid
Diabetes mellitus	Connective tissue disorders
Congestive heart failure	

Metabolic disorders:

Hypokalemia	Uremia
Hypophosphatemia	Hypercalcemia
Hypomagnesemia	

Miscellaneous:

Poor fluid intake
Immobility
Cognitive impairment
Autonomic neuropathy
Diminished rectal sensation

BOX 22.7 Constipation in the elderly

- Constipation is common in the elderly and requires careful assessment to rule out mechanical causes.
- New onset constipation that cannot be explained by acute illness or use of a culprit medication should be investigated with colonoscopy.
- Patients with multiple risk factors should start stimulant or osmotic laxatives prior to becoming obstipated (less than three stools per week). This requires a proactive approach if prescribing narcotics or other constipating medications.

leading cause of precipitating nursing home placement in the United States. Up to 7% of the elderly population has incontinence of solid or liquid stool at least once each week. Fecal incontinence is closely associated with urinary incontinence and constipation (i.e., the passage of infrequent, hard, or difficult-to-pass stools). Because overflow fecal incontinence with liquid stool is a common manifestation of constipation, the latter should always be considered in the workup of fecal incontinence. Usually the most difficult aspect of treating overflow fecal incontinence is convincing the patient and/or family that constipation is actually the problem, not diarrhea.

Diagnosis

Aging is associated with neuronal loss and changes in neuromuscular function that may predispose patients to constipation and difficulty with anorectal control.[15]

Medications, especially opioids and anticholinergic agents, are common causes of constipation.

The evaluation of constipation and fecal incontinence should include a review of the patient's cognitive status, a history of the circumstances of the incontinence episodes, abdominal and neurologic examination, and a rectal examination. Abdominal tenderness, bloating, or distention may indicate a fecal impaction. The presence of hard stool in the rectal vault may suggest a fecal impaction; however, a negative rectal examination does not rule out a proximal fecal impaction. With high impactions, an x-ray or CT scan of the abdomen may confirm fecal masses or stool backup. Mental status examination identifies the patient with dementia or delirium who may have lost self-toileting capacity. The absence of anal sphincter tone or anal wink may suggest denervation of the pudendal nerve (S2–4), resulting from a local or spinal cord lesion.

An abdominal plain film to assess fecal loading is helpful when fecal impaction is suspected and this can be done in the outpatient setting. Acute onset of incontinence should prompt examination to check for fecal impaction and spinal imaging to rule out cord compression. Anorectal manometry can objectively measure the resting pressure of the anal canal (predominantly from the IAS), tone and contractile pressures of the EAS, and sensation within the anorectal area. Pudendal nerve testing may be required in some patients. These studies are not usually feasible in bed-bound or very debilitated patients, and often the main focus in the latter is detecting fecal impaction and reviewing medications to check for those that may cause diarrhea or constipation.[16]

Treatment

The treatment of constipation and fecal impaction include disimpaction, bowel cleansing, modification of risk factors, and an effective maintenance regimen. (See Table 22.7.) Disimpaction should start with manual removal of stool and/or enemas, before administering an oral polyethylene glycol solution. Tap water enemas of 1 L–2 L may be needed. Milk and molasses (1 cup each) enemas that are both osmotic and mildly stimulating are often effective when tap water is not. Avoid magnesium citrate solutions and Fleet Phospho-soda enemas with inpatients with underlying cardiac or renal disease. Phosphate-containing oral solutions have been linked to development of phosphate nephropathy and are not recommended. Soapsuds enemas have a high risk of precipitating ischemic colitis and should not be used in elderly patients. Prevention of constipation and recurrent impaction involves risk factor modification including mobilization, good hydration and nutrition, and minimizing use of constipating medications. Scheduled toileting after breakfast may be helpful for patients with cognitive impairment. Add fiber supplements when bowel function has been regularized. Regular use of a stimulant laxative such as senna or Dulcolax, or use of hyperosmolar solutions such as polyethylene glycol (PEG) or lactulose may prevent severe constipation or impaction in high-risk patients. Intermittent use of glycerin or bisacodyl suppositories is warranted if patients have infrequent episodes of constipation, but if these have to be used more than once a week, the entire bowel regimen should be

Table 22.7 Treatment of constipation

Initial management

Increase fluid intake (most likely to be effective if dehydrated)

Exercise

Bowel training regimen (try to toilet when gastro-colic reflex active after meals)

Second-line therapy

Bulking agents (avoid as initial therapy in Parkinson's disease and severe constipation)

Stool softeners

Glycerin suppositories

Third-line therapy

Osmotic agents (milk of magnesia, lactulose, sorbitol)

PEG solutions (Miralax)

Stimulating agents (Senna, bisacodyl)

Fourth-line therapy

Tap water enema or milk and molasses enema (1/2 cup molasses; 1 liter milk)

Misoprostol, colchicine

Agents to avoid

Prokinetics (erythromycin, metoclopramide, cisapride)

Lubricating agents (oral mineral oil because of aspiration)

Routine use of enemas (increased risk of rectal perforation in the elderly)

PEG – polyethylene glycol

reviewed and adjusted. The role of other agents such as lubiprostone or probiotics is not clear; however, these could be used as an alternative for patients unable to take other laxatives. Lubiprostone has been studied in patients aged 70–75 and is effective at increasing stool frequency, but elderly patients also respond to much cheaper alternatives such as senna and PEG solution.

Colonic ischemia

The colon is more commonly affected by ischemia than the small bowel, due to the high prevalence of

BOX 22.8 Mesenteric ischemia

- Mesenteric ischemia is primarily a disease of the elderly, particularly those with underlying cardiovascular disorders.
- Acute mesenteric ischemia presents with pain out of proportion to physical findings and may be caused by an embolus, thrombus, or low-output state.
- Selective superior mesenteric artery angiography is required for diagnosis and, often, for treatment.
- Chronic mesenteric ischemia presents with postprandial pain (intestinal angina) and weight loss. It is seen in elderly patients with arteriosclerotic changes in the mesenteric circulation.
- Colonic ischemia presents with left lower quadrant pain and loose bloody stools. It is diagnosed by colonoscopy, but the findings may mimic infectious or inflammatory colitis.
  - Most patients with colonic ischemia recover with bowel rest, fluids, and IV antibiotics and do not require surgery.

silent occlusion of the inferior mesenteric artery (IMA) in older patients (shown in up to 10% of autopsies over age 80).[17, 18] The causes of colonic ischemia (CI) include acute and chronic mesenteric ischemia due to IMA thrombus or embolus, CHF, cardiac arrhythmias, shock, vasculitis, hematological disorders, infections, medications (NSAIDs, digitalis, vasopressin, pseudoephedrine, sumatriptan, cocaine, amphetamines, gold), constipation, surgery, and trauma. The usual site of ischemic damage is the splenic flexure in the so-called watershed area of the colon primarily supplied by the IMA. Most colonic ischemia is precipitated by low blood flow states caused by hypotension. The extent of injury can range from mild, reversible colopathy to gangrene or fulminant colitis. Abdominal aortic aneurysm repair is a well-known risk for acute CI, with up to 3% of elective repairs and 14% of emergent repair developing CI, usually due to SMA occlusion. This can result in small bowel ischemia as well, which has a very high mortality in older patients (>90%). Rapid recognition and reversal of the ischemia is essential in treating severe ischemic colitis or small bowel infarction. (See Box 22.8.)

Diagnosis

Patients with acute CI usually present with cramping lower left quadrant pain and loose, bloody stools. Blood loss significant enough to lead to hemodynamic instability is actually atypical of CI and suggests other diagnoses. Physical examination often reveals abdominal tenderness of variable severity over the location of the affected portion of bowel. Peritoneal signs may be transiently present in reversible CI; the persistence of these signs for several hours suggests transmural

infarction, thus surgical exploration should happen quickly.

Strictures, chronic colitis, gangrene resulting in perforation, and intra-abdominal sepsis are complications of CI. Chronic CI, which is probably a lot more common than previously thought, may present with diarrhea, left-sided abdominal cramps, and gas or bloating due to dysmotility caused by the mismatch of blood supply to demand. The symptoms can be slowly progressive and insidious, and patients have often been investigated for other causes of abdominal pain, bloating, and diarrhea. Endoscopy may show mild inflammation in the left colon near the splenic flexure, but the mucosa can appear relatively normal if the ischemia is slowly developing. Many patients are asymptomatic and found to have IMA occlusion with extensive collateral blood supply to the affected colon.

Stool cultures should be obtained to exclude infectious colitis. The patient with suspected CI who does not have peritoneal signs should have CT angiography and possibly careful sigmoidoscopy within 48 hours of symptom onset. Patients with peritoneal signs should undergo urgent/emergent surgical exploration. CT scans are normal in up to 66% of patients with chronic or slowly progressive CI but may show colonic thickening, mucosal edema, or pericolonic fluid and/or stranding suggestive of inflammation. Evaluation of the intestinal blood flow using doppler ultrasound may indicate an SMA occlusion; however, more invasive procedures such as MR angiogram or interventional angiography are often required. The latter allows treatment with thrombolytics or angioplasty if necessary. The greatest difficulty occurs in the initial recognition that ischemia is present rather than in establishing a definitive diagnosis of acute ischemia once it is in the differential. CI should be considered if the patient has had a "low flow state" with hypotension as this is the most common cause of CI in elderly patients.

Treatment

The patient with CI who does not have peritoneal signs should be treated with fluids, bowel rest, and broad-spectrum antibiotics. Hypotension should be aggressively reversed, underlying CHF or cardiac arrhythmias should be treated, and vasoconstricting medications should be stopped. The persistence of peritoneal signs should prompt surgical exploration. Recurrence of CI occurs in only 3%–10% of patients. Congenital or acquired thrombophilic states account for a significant percentage of ambulatory younger patients presenting with colonic ischemia, and should be tested in the elderly.[19] However, it is much less likely that these are the cause of intestinal ischemia.

Liver disease

Viral hepatitis

Hepatitis A occurs less frequently in the elderly than in the younger population, but the elderly may have a more severe course, with a higher risk of fulminant liver failure and death. (See Box 22.9.) International travel is the main risk factor, as more geriatric patients are traveling to endemic areas. Comorbidities and a decreased likelihood of liver transplantation contribute to the lower survival of older patients with fulminant disease. Older patients planning travel should

be tested for HAV antibody, and vaccinated if negative. This should be done two to three months prior to travel, as immunity may take four to six weeks to develop, and there is an increased likelihood that a second vaccination may be required in older patients due to decreased immune responsiveness.

Acute hepatitis B virus (HBV) infection is uncommon in the older population and often runs a mild and subclinical course. Symptoms, when present, include fever, malaise, arthralgias, myalgias, nausea, vomiting, abdominal pain, and jaundice.[20] Chronic hepatitis B is endemic in sub-Saharan Africa and the Far East, and should be screened in patients from high-risk areas, or in patients with known risk factors for acquisition (IV drug use, sexual exposure, and transfusions or blood products prior to 1980). PEG interferon-α, used to treat chronic HBV in patients with decompensated liver disease, may cause increased side effects in the elderly. Other viral suppressive agents such as entecavir and tenofovir are well tolerated in older patients. Patients diagnosed with chronic viral hepatitis should be referred to a hepatologist, and undergo a liver ultrasound to determine whether they have cirrhosis or masses that could be hepatocellular carcinoma. A noninvasive fibroscan may demonstrate fibrosis. The role of liver biopsy is controversial; however, biopsy is recommended for patients with significant elevation in liver enzymes or evidence of active viral replication.

Hepatitis C (HCV) is becoming more common in patients over age 65, as cohorts infected by exposure to IV drugs or blood products before 1990 are aging. Most patients with chronic hepatitis C are

---

BOX 22.9 Liver disease in older patients

- Elderly patients should be vaccinated against hepatitis A prior to international travel.
- Screen patients who have immigrated from endemic areas for chronic hepatitis B.
- Screen all patients born between 1945 and 1965 for hepatitis C.
- Nonalcoholic fatty liver disease (NAFLD) is the most common cause of elevated liver enzymes, and can progress to fibrosis and cirrhosis in 20% of patients.
- Alcohol is an underdiagnosed cause of liver disease in the elderly.

  - Both prescription and OTC/herbal drugs can cause elevated liver enzymes and liver damage: withdraw any culprit drug and monitor until enzymes normal.
  - Best candidates for treatment of hepatocellular carcinoma by surgical resection or liver transplantation have small tumors without vascular invasion, no portal hypertension, and normal liver function
  - Consider gallstones in patients with acute RUQ pain and fever. Laparoscopic cholecystectomy is well tolerated by stable elderly patients. Unstable patients should have cholecystotomy drainage followed by delayed cholecystectomy.

asymptomatic and are diagnosed after routine laboratory studies reveal elevated aminotransferase levels. Acute hepatitis C symptoms are similar to those seen in acute HBV. Older age at HCV infection is associated with increased rates of cirrho [21] Daily alcohol use worsens the prognosis. Because of the increasing prevalence of chronic hepatitis C in the geriatric population, recent guidelines indicate that all patients born between 1945 and 1965 should have a one-time screen for hepatitis C antibody. PEG interferon-α with ribavirin has been the standard treatment for chronic HCV infection. Heart disease, a common affliction in the elderly, is a relative contraindication to ribavirin therapy. Several new treatments have demonstrated a significant improvement in viral clearance compared to ribavirin alone. Decisions concerning treatment of chronic viral hepatitis in the elderly should take into account the expected lifespan of the patient, the likelihood of progression to cirrhosis, and the increased risk of side effects of treatment.

Drug-induced liver disease

Polypharmacy coupled with altered pharmacodynamics accounts for the increased incidence of drug-related hepatotoxicity in the elderly. NSAIDs, amiodarone, hepatic hydroxymethylglutaryl coenzyme A reductase inhibitors, and antituberculosis medications have been associated with hepatotoxicity in the elderly.[22] LFTs should be monitored in patients receiving these medications. Several herbal medications have been shown to cause liver injury, including kava, chaparral, black cohosh, herbalife, and germander. A complete list of herbal medications should be elicited from all older patients. Statin drugs often are associated with a modest elevation in transaminases, and if these remain <2× normal, studies have indicated a low risk of progression to liver damage. Usually the benefit of the statin in patients with hyperlipidemia, cardiac disease, diabetes, or metabolic syndrome far outweighs the risk, and patients should continue them unless enzymes continue to rise above 2× normal.

Hepatic ischemia

Steep elevations in aminotransferase levels after a hemodynamic insult are typical of hepatic ischemia. Risk factors include acute myocardial infarction, CHF, valvular heart disease, cardiac arrhythmias, cardiomyopathy, sepsis, trauma, and burns. The magnitude of the aminotransferase elevation does not correlate with the extent of liver injury and does not predict outcome. Most patients recover with observation and correction of hemodynamic instability and abnormal coagulation, with normalization of aminotransferase levels within 10 days.

Primary biliary cirrhosis

Up to 40% of patients with primary biliary cirrhosis are elderly. Women outnumber men by six to one. Patients present with fatigue, pruritus, and elevated alkaline phosphatase levels. Diagnosis is suggested by the presence of antimitochondrial antibody (AMA) in the appropriate clinical setting and is confirmed by liver biopsy. Treatment with ursodeoxycholic acid improves survival and delays the need for liver transplantation. As with all patients with fibrosis and cirrhosis, patients with PBC should avoid NSAIDs and alcohol. Doses of hepatically excreted drugs should be adjusted in patients with significant cholestatsis to avoid toxicity.

Hepatocellular carcinoma

More than 50% of patients with hepatocellular carcinoma (HCC) in the United States are elderly. Survival rates are significantly lower in patients diagnosed with HCC after the age of 65. Cirrhosis secondary to chronic HCV or HBV infection and alcoholic liver disease is the most frequent cause of HCC. HCC can present with acute onset of right upper quadrant pain, elevated alpha-fetoprotein (AFP) levels, or mass on imaging studies. Patients with hepatic cirrhosis should be screened with liver ultrasonography every six months for early detection of HCC. A CT scan of the abdomen is recommended every one to two years. Surgical resection in selected patients is the treatment of choice, if the tumor is small and there is no vascular invasion. Liver transplantation is indicated for patients with one tumor <5 cm, or up to three tumors <3 cm without vascular invasion. Unfortunately the mortality of liver transplantation increases over age 70, and five-year survival is lower. Patients who are poor surgical candidates may be treated with transarterial chemoembolization, one of the many mechanical ablation techniques, or systemic chemotherapy.

Biliary disease

Cholelithiasis

Age-related increases in cholesterol secretion in bile, combined with decreased bile acid secretion, lead to increased cholesterol saturation and, therefore, increased bile lithogenicity. Cholelithiasis is twice as common in women as in men, and is often asymptomatic and discovered during radiological studies of the abdomen performed for unrelated reasons. Each decade, 10%–25% of patients with asymptomatic gallstones will become symptomatic.[23] Symptomatic gallstone disease typically presents with RUQ pain, nausea, and vomiting. Diagnosis is suggested in the appropriate clinical setting by elevated alkaline phosphatase and bilirubin levels and is confirmed by ultrasonography. Diagnosis of gallstones in the biliary ducts is usually made using ultrasound, or magnetic resonance cholangiopancreaticogram (MRCP). The sensitivity of MRCP is lower in patients with biliary obstruction and cholestasis, therefore a negative test in a patient strongly suspected to have biliary stones should precipitate consideration of ERCP for definitive diagnosis and treatment.

Laparoscopic cholecystectomy is the treatment of choice for symptomatic cholelithiasis in the elderly; postoperative mortality and morbidity in selected elderly patients are comparable to that for younger patients if the procedure is performed when the patient is hemodynamically stable. Poor surgical candidates may be treated with endoscopic retrograde cholangiopancreatography (ERCP) with sphincterotomy, or ursodeoxycholic acid. Patients with Charcot's Triad (RUQ pain, fever, jaundice) likely have cholangitis and should undergo emergency ERCP as soon as possible to decompress the biliary system. Asymptomatic cholelithiasis should not be treated.

Cholecystitis

Common symptoms of gallbladder inflammation (cholecystitis) are often blunted in older patients or are mistaken for other disease processes. Symptoms consist of epigastric or RUQ pain, nausea, and vomiting. Fever and RUQ tenderness are present on physical examination. Elevations in serum bilirubin, alkaline phosphatase, aminotransferases, and white blood cell counts are characteristic. The diagnosis is made clinically and confirmed ultrasonographically.

Gangrene and necrosis of the gallbladder are more common in the elderly population and are associated with increased morbidity and mortality. Cholangitis or chronic cholecystitis are other frequent complications. Treatment of cholecystitis consists of stabilization with intravenous fluids, bowel rest, pain control, and broad-spectrum antibiotics followed by cholecystectomy. Older patients with acute cholecystitis frequently have significant comorbidities and hemodynamic or respiratory instability, and emergent cholecystectomy often carries a high risk of complications and death. Studies have shown that immediate percutaneous cholecystostomy, followed several weeks later by definitive surgery or ERCP, has less morbidity and mortality compared to urgent surgery.[24]

Gallbladder carcinoma is rare in the United States. Gallstone disease, female gender, and smoking are significant risk factors. The diagnosis is often made incidentally at surgery. The prognosis is poor.

Pancreatic disease

Acute pancreatitis

Gallstones, medications, and cancer account for a higher proportion of acute pancreatitis in the elderly compared with younger patients. Alcohol is a common precipitating factor in both age groups.[25, 26] Typical presenting symptoms include epigastric pain radiating to the back along with nausea and vomiting. The diagnosis is made by elevations in amylase and lipase levels. Elevated alkaline phosphatase and bilirubin levels suggest gallstone pancreatitis, which can be confirmed by abdominal ultrasonography or CT. Patients with altered mental status; hemodynamic instability; blood, urea, nitrogen (BUN) over 25; as well as those meeting three or more of Ranson's criteria should undergo a dynamic CT scan to rule out pancreatic necrosis. (See Table 22.8.) Patients with elevated BUN should be considered for ICU admission, as this has been shown to predict severe disease. Bowel rest, intravenous hydration, and pain control are the cornerstones of therapy for mild acute pancreatitis. Patients with pancreatic necrosis should be placed on broad-spectrum antibiotics, and CT-guided aspiration of necrotic areas to check for infection should be considered if symptoms do not improve after five to seven days. Surgical debridement or endoscopic debridement should be considered if infection is documented in the necrotic tissue. Morbidity and

Table 22.8 Ranson's criteria

On admission

1. Age >55 years

2. WBC count >16,000/μL

3. Serum glucose >200 mg/dL

4. Serum LDH >350 units/L

5. Serum AST >250 units/L

Over the first 48 hours

1. Increase in BUN exceeding 5 mg/dL

2. Arterial PO_2 <60 mm Hg

3. Hematocrit drop >10 percentage points

4. Serum calcium <8 mg/dL

5. Base deficit >4 mEq/L

6. Fluid sequestration exceeding 6L

Presence of three or more on admission predicts severe course with a sensitivity of 60%–80%.
WBC – white blood cell, LDH – lactate dehydrogenase, AST – aspartate aminotransferase, BUN – blood urea nitrogen, PO_2 – partial pressure of oxygen

mortality of laparoscopic cholecystectomy with pre-operative ERCP or intraoperative cholangiography are comparable to that for younger individuals. In patients who are poor surgical candidates, ERCP with sphincterotomy decreases the risk for recurrent gallstone pancreatitis.

Drug-induced pancreatitis can be caused by azathioprine, 6-mercaptopurine, estrogen, mesala-mine, furosemide, and angiotensin-converting enzyme inhibitors. Suspected medications should be stopped when pancreatitis is diagnosed. Other causes of pancreatitis, such as hyperlipidemia or hypercalce-mia, should be sought and treated.

Chronic pancreatitis

The diagnosis of chronic pancreatitis in elderly patients poses several difficulties. The structural changes commonly associated with chronic pancrea-titis (ductal irregularity or dilation, calcification, abnormal echogenicity) are also observed in aging patients without pancreatitis. Because pancreatic function is maintained in the elderly, functional test-ing may help in establishing the diagnosis. Treatment

consists of hydration, pain management, pancreatic enzyme replacement, and avoidance of alcohol.

Pancreatic cancer

Pancreatic cancer accounts for 5% of all cancer deaths in the United States. Painless jaundice, pruritus, and weight loss are common presenting symptoms. Elevated CA19–9 levels suggest the diagnosis. Abdominal imaging or demonstration of extrinsic compression of the bile duct during ERCP and/or a mass on endoscopic ultrasound (EUS) are usually confirmatory. Pancreaticoduodenectomy is the only treatment with any demonstrated benefit and should be offered to selected elderly patients with high overall fitness and low comorbidity. The prognosis of pan-creatic cancer remains grim.

Management of malnutrition and weight loss in older patients

Weight loss of 5% or more of usual body weight in the past month or 10% in the past six months is associated with increased morbidity and mortality in older patients.[27] The usual pattern of weight change during an individual's lifetime is character-ized by a gradual increase in weight that peaks in the fourth to fifth decade of life, followed by a period of stable weight and a gradual decline in weight thereafter from the sixth to seventh decades. (See Box 22.10.)

Diagnosis

Major indicators of poor nutritional status include weight loss over time, low weight for height (body mass index of 18.5 kg/m^2 or less), a loss of indepen-dence in two activities of daily living (e.g., bathing and dressing), reduction in midarm circumference to less than the 10th percentile of ideal, decreased triceps skinfold thickness to less than the 10th per-centile of ideal, and the presence of nutrition-related disorders (e.g., osteoporosis, vitamin B12 deficiency, or folate deficiency). A serum albumin level below 3.5 g/dL is generally the most reliable, although nonspecific, indicator of chronic malnutrition. Unexplained normocytic anemia, low serum trans-ferrin, low pre-albumin, and a very low serum cho-lesterol level (<160 mg/dL) are also seen in malnutrition.

BOX 22.10 Malnutrition and weight loss in older patients

- Malnutrition is a common problem in older patients and is often multifactorial.
- A detailed diet history is very helpful to determine whether the patient is unable to eat, or is unwilling or disinterested in eating.
- Depression is a common cause of involuntary weight loss in the elderly, as is cognitive impairment.
- Low albumin/pre-albumin and vitamin deficiencies are indicators of malnutrition.
- In addition to treating diseases associated with weight loss, interventions may need to address social isolation, ability to obtain and prepare meals, and cognitive impairment.
  - The decision to place a percutaneous gastrostomy tube should take into account the cognitive status and quality of life of the patient. Patients with advanced dementia, while at risk for weight loss, do not benefit from feeding tubes.

Treatment

If the gastrointestinal tract is functional, enteral nutrition is preferred over parenteral nutrition as it is safer, and enteric food provides trophic stimulus to the gastrointestinal tract.[28, 29] Patients who are unable to swallow or who cannot eat sufficiently to maintain adequate nutrition may be candidates for tube feeding. Nasogastric tubes are a short-term alternative; however, percutaneous gastrostomy tube placement is indicated when long-term tube feeding is anticipated for weeks to months or for patient comfort. Aspiration precautions (elevating the head of the bed, checking residuals) should be carefully observed because gastrostomy tube feeding does not prevent aspiration. Gastrostomy tube feedings are not recommended for patients with severe dementia, given the absence of data to show that tube feedings improve quality of life and overall clinical outcomes in such patients.

Total parenteral nutrition (TPN) is appropriate only in carefully selected older patients whose GI tract cannot be used. This includes patients with a nonfunctioning or obstructed GI tract, prolonged ileus, massive GI bleeding, severe malabsorbtion, persistent vomiting, high-output fistulas, severe pancreatitis or enterocolitis, peritonitis, and mesenteric ischemia. Complications of parenteral feeding include catheter-related thrombosis and sepsis, and elderly patients have a higher mortality on TPN than younger patients.

References

1. Becher A., Dent J. Systematic review: aging and gastro-oesophageal reflux disease symptoms, oesophageal function and reflux oesophagitis. *Aliment Pharmacol Ther.* 2011: **33**:442–54.

2. Morganstern B, Anandasabapathy S. GERD and Barrett's esophagus: diagnostic and management strategies in the geriatric population. *Geriatrics.* 2009. **64**:9–12.

3. Desilets AR, Asal NJ, Dunican KC. Considerations for the use of proton pump inhibitors in older adults. *Consult Pharm.* 2012; **27**:114–20.

4. Lee J, Anggiansah A, Anggiansah R. et al. Effects of age on the gastroesophageal junction, esophageal motility, and reflux disease. *Clin Gastroenterol Hepatol.* 2007; **5**:1392–8.

5. Esfandyari T, Potter JW, Vaczi MF. Dysphagia: a cost analysis of the diagnostic approach. *Am J Gastroenterol.* 2002: 97–2733–7.

6. Griffin MR: Epidemiology of nonsteroidal anti-inflammatory drug-associated gastrointestinal injury. *Am J Med* 1998;**104**: 23S.

7. Rosen AM: Gastrointestinal bleeding in the elderly. *Clin Geriatr Med* 1999;**15**: 511.

8. Farrell JJ, Friedman LS: gastrointestinal bleeding in the elderly. *Gastroenterol Clin North Am* 2001;**30**:377.

9. Saif MW, Makrilia N, Zalonis A, et al. Gastric cancer in the elderly: an overview. *Eur J Surg Oncol.* 2010; **36**:709–17.

10. Williams JJ, Beck PL, Andrews CN, et al. Microscopic colitis – a common cause of diarrhoea in older adults. *Age and Aging* 2010;**39**:162–8.

11. Stollman NH, et al. Diagnosis and management of diverticular disease of the colon in adults. *Am J Gastroenterology* 1999;**94**:3110–21.

12. Murad Y, Radi ZA, Murad M, Hall K. Inflammatory bowel disease in the geriatric population. *Front Biosci.* 2011 Jun;**1**(3):945–54.

13. Soffer EE, Hull T. Fecal incontinence: a practical approach to evaluation and treatment. *Am J Gastroenterology* 2000;**95**:1873–80.

14. Tariq SH. Fecal incontinence in older adults. *Clin Geriatr Med* 2007;**23**:857–69.

15. Mertz H, Naliboff B, Mayer EA. Symptoms and physiology in severe chronic constipation. *Am J Gastroenterology* 1999;**94**:131–8.

16. Stevens TK, Palmer RM. Fecal incontinence in long-term care patients. *Long-Term Care Interface* 2007;**8**:35–9.

17. Brandt LJ, Boley SJ AGA technical review on intestinal ischemia. *Gastroenterology* 2000;**118**:954.

18. Greenwald DA, Brandt LJ, Reinus JF. Ischemic bowel disease in the elderly. *Gastroenterol Clin North Am* 2001;**30**:445.

19. Koutroubakis IE, Sfiridaki A, Theodoropoulou A, et al. Role of acquired and hereditary thrombotic risk factors in colon ischemia of ambulatory patients. *Gastroenterology* 2001;**121**:561–5.

20. Befeler AS, Di Bisceglie AM. Infections of the liver: hepatitis B. *Infect Dis Clin North Am* 2000;**14**:617–32.

21. Lauer GM, Walker BD. Hepatitis C virus infection. *N Engl J Med* 2001;**345**:41–52.

22. Regev A, Schiff ER. Liver disease in the elderly. *Gastroenterol Clin North Am* 2001;**30**:547–63.

23. Affronti J. Biliary disease in the elderly patient. *Clin Geriatr Med* 1999;**15**: 571–8.

24. Spira RM, Nissan A, Zamir O, et al. Percutaneous transhepatic cholecystostomy and delayed laparoscopic cholecystectomy in critically ill patients with acute cholecystitis. *Am. J. Surg.* 2002; **183**:62–6.

25. Martin SP, Ulrich CD. Pancreatic disease in the elderly. *Clin Geriatr Med* 1999;**15**:579–605.

26. Ross SO, Forsmark CE. Pancreatic and biliary disorders in the elderly. *Gastroenterol Clin North Am* 2001;**30**:531–45.

27. Chapman IM. Weight loss in older persons. *Med Clin North Amer* 2011;**95**:579–93.

28. Jensen GL, McGee M, Binkley B. Nutrition in the elderly. *Gastroenterol Clin North Am* 2001;**30**: 313–34.

29. Meyyazhagan S, Palmer RM. Nutritional requirements with aging: prevention of disease. *Clin Geriatr Med* 2002;**18**:557–76.

Chapter 23

Serious infections in the elderly

David Alain Wohl, MD, and David van Duin, MD

Introduction

Although modern medicine has significantly reduced early death due to infection, diseases caused by infectious pathogens remain a major cause of illness and death among elderly persons.[1] Many of the most serious infectious diseases have a predilection for those at the extremes of age – individuals with relatively deficient immune function. In addition, infections common to persons of all ages can be devastating when they occur in those of more advanced age. Elderly individuals also are now commonly found in environments, such as hospitals and nursing facilities, where antibiotic-resistant organisms are prevalent and catheters and wounds breech the protection offered by an intact integument. On the other end of the functionality spectrum, many older individuals are active and may spend their postretirement years traveling to locales where they are exposed to exotic organisms. Many elders are also sexually active and may be at risk for sexually transmitted infections when establishing new intimate partnerships.[2]

Compounding their increase in risk of infection, older individuals may suffer from delays in diagnosis, as their infections often present atypically. Infectious diseases in older persons frequently occur without fever or leukocytosis and can be challenging to detect and localize – especially in those who suffer from cognitive impairments. Therefore, the diagnostic approach must be modified when the patient is elderly, and the clinician must appreciate the unique characteristics of this ever-increasing segment of our population in the United States.[3]

The elder host

Age-related changes have been described in various components of the immune system. Part of the increased burden of infections in elders may be due to changes in the adaptive and innate components of immunity: a negative correlation between age and immunity is observed in most studies.[4–6] Changes in innate immunity include decreases in T-cell activation by dendritic cells, cytotoxicity by natural killer cells, CD80 up-regulation, and TLR1/2 function.[7–10] The most generally accepted changes in the adaptive immune system are thymic involution and a resultant decrease in the output of naïve T-cells, and the accumulation of memory and CD28-null T-cells in the peripheral blood of elderly individuals.[4–6, 11–13] Vaccine responses become muted along with diminished delayed hypersensitivity in older persons. [14, 15] The important barriers to infection, such as skin and mucosal surfaces, also weaken. Skin becomes thinner and glandular secretions decrease and, along with age-related immune deficits, raise the risk for soft tissue infection and/or systemic spread.

A number of conditions associated with aging also enhance the risk of infectious diseases. These include diabetes mellitus, malignancies, chronic obstructive pulmonary disease, and bladder emptying disorders. As we age, the need for prosthetic joints and organ/tissue transplantation increases. Therefore, immunosuppressive drugs used to protect against transplant rejection or in the treatment of connective tissue diseases and other conditions are not uncommon in persons 50 years of age and older. Also, any malnutrition secondary to comorbid disease, poverty, poor dentition, or other causes of inadequate caloric intake further reduces host defenses against infection.

The environment

Approximately 5% of persons older than 65 reside in a nursing facility, but the rate increases to almost 20% by age 85 years.[16] In addition, many elderly individuals regularly attend clinics or require

Reichel's Care of the Elderly, 7th Edition, ed. Jan Busby-Whitehead *et al.* Published by Cambridge University Press.
© Cambridge University Press 2016.

Table 23.1 Factors increasing vulnerability to infectious diseases during aging

Host	Environment
Immunological	Nursing home residence
↓ Naïve T cells	Hospitalization
↓ CD8 + cells	Instrumentation
↓ IgM memory B cells	Exposure to drug-resistant organisms
↓ Toll-like receptor function	Exposure to endemic infectious diseases during travel
↓ NK cell cytotoxicity ↓ dendritic cell function	
Mechanical Skin thinning and breakdown	
↓ Glandular secretions	
↓ Cough reflex Poor dentition	
Systemic Cognitive impairment	
Malnutrition	
Tobacco use	
Poverty	

hospitalization at some point.[17] These encounters increase the risk of contact with infectious pathogens – including those resistant to antimicrobials (such as methicillin-resistant staphylococci) – exposure to outbreaks of endemic infections such as tuberculosis (TB), and nosocomial infectious diseases such as *Clostridium difficile*. The illnesses that attend advancing age often lead to instrumentation, catheterization, and surgery – each of which carries a risk of infection. Few hospital admissions of elderly patients do not include a urinary catheter or intravenous line, and many also entail even more invasive diagnostic and therapeutic procedures. Table 23.1 summarizes factors related to increased vulnerability to infection during aging.

Among more functional older patients, it is mandatory to take a complete travel and sexual risk behavior history. Older Americans comprise a significant proportion of those traveling domestically and internationally.[18] As highlighted in

Chapter 45, sexual activity may diminish as we age, but substantial numbers of persons in their later decades of life have sex, especially if their health is relatively good. New partnerships, such as after the death of a spouse, can risk sexually transmitted infections, and the clinician should never discount the possibility of such an infection based solely on the age of the patient. The Centers for Disease Control and Prevention and the US Preventive Services Task Force recommend that human immunodeficiency virus (HIV) testing should be ordered at least once for all persons seeking health care who are aged 13–65 years.[19] Many experts believe that testing should continue to be offered to those older than 65 years of age if they remain sexually active and at risk of acquiring HIV infection. Repeated testing is always warranted in persons with continued higher-risk behaviors.

Approach to the elderly patient with suspected infectious disease

The diagnosis of infectious diseases in elderly patients can be challenging. Classic features of some infections such as fever and leukocytosis may be absent in older individuals even during fulminant infection, dangerously delaying diagnosis.[20] Approximately 40% of older adults may not mount a febrile response to serious infection. [21] Therefore, small elevations in temperature above individual baseline should be concerning, and fevers of 38.3°C should be considered alarming.[22] Localizing symptoms of infection may be subtle, and impaired cognition because of dementia or as a manifestation of the infection may render the patient unable to describe symptoms accurately. Delirium, in particular, is common during infection in the elderly.[23] In addition, infections among older patients can present atypically with vague aches, anorexia, or confusion as the only indication that an acute illness is present. A high degree of suspicion for underlying infectious processes is necessary when older individuals present with such subtle changes. Failure to consider adequately the possibility of infection in the elderly patient and overreliance on indicators of infection that are more common among younger patients can lead to tragic misdiagnosis of potentially treatable conditions.

Major infectious diseases

Urinary tract infections

Infection of the urinary tract is the most common bacterial infection in older adults and is the major source of bacteremia in this population.[24] Urinary catheters – both urethral and condom types – greatly increase urinary tract infection (UTI) risk.[20] Furthermore, host factors – including neurogenic bladder, prostate enlargement in men, and vaginal atrophy and increased vaginal pH in women – can foster bacterial colonization that predisposes to UTI. [20] Frequent bladder emptying is protective against urinary infection but is often impaired in older patients. There are multiple factors that lead to poor bladder emptying in the elderly, including an increased volume of urine required to sense a need to void, as well as reduced urinary flow because of poor fluid intake, obstruction, and/or decreased bladder contractility.[25]

Clinical manifestations/diagnosis

Classic symptoms of UTI such as dysuria, urinary frequency and urgency, suprapubic tenderness, and fever are telltale when present. As mentioned previously, however, some or all of these symptoms may be absent despite serious UTI. Atypical presentation of UTI with nausea, vomiting, dehydration, and confusion is common.[26, 27] Urinalysis of a clean catch urine specimen demonstrating pyuria, increased leukocyte esterase, and nitrite is highly suggestive in the setting of the aforementioned clinical presentations. Confirmation of infection with urine culture also permits guidance of antibiotic therapy. Blood culture should be obtained in patients who have more concerning acute illness in order to assess for sepsis.

Quantitative clean catch urine culture revealing 100,000 CFU/mL or greater (for women, confirmed on repeated testing) in persons without symptoms of UTI is considered evidence of asymptomatic bacteriuria. Asymptomatic bacteriuria is common in elderly patients, especially women, and has been linked to institutionalization, bladder-emptying disorders, diabetes, and prior UTI.[28]

Management

Gram-negative organisms are the most commonly cultured UTI pathogens, and empiric therapy should be broadly directed toward these organisms until culture results return.[26, 29] Patients with indwelling urinary catheters are also at increased risk for *Enterococcus*, and in such patients, coverage of this Gram-positive organism, such as with ampicillin given resistance to cephalosporins, may be prudent. Detection of *Staphylococcus aureus* in the urine raises concern for endovascular infection, such as endocarditis, because this organism is often spread to the urine hematogenously. Echocardiography and blood cultures are indicated when *S. aureus* is retrieved from clean catch urine specimen.

Treatment of asymptomatic bacteriuria has not been demonstrated to have an impact on morbidity or mortality and is not recommended.[24] Removal of urinary catheters should be considered and the need for such catheters regularly assessed. Following antibacterial treatment, typically for 7–14 days, repeated urine analysis and culture can be obtained to demonstrate clearing of the organism and resolution of pyuria.

Candida is not infrequently encountered in the urine of elderly hospitalized patients, especially those treated with broad-spectrum antibacterials. In most cases, treatment is unnecessary; however, in patients who are immunocompromised, exhibit symptoms of UTI, or are in need of urological instrumentation, treatment of candiduria should be strongly considered.

Bacterial pneumonia

Respiratory infections are a leading cause of infectious-disease-associated deaths among older individuals and can be acquired in the community or at nursing/medical facilities.[1] A number of factors conspire to raise the risk of pneumonia in the elderly, including a decline in pulmonary function, diminished cough reflex, reduced mucociliary transport, and decreased lung elasticity.[16, 30, 31] These mechanical factors lead to trapping of air, diminished ability to clear oral secretions, and colonization of the pharynx with pathogenic bacteria.[31] Aspiration of such secretions is a major cause of pneumonia among elderly patients with impaired swallowing and/or cognition and is exacerbated by poor dentition. Prior or current smoking and its sequelae, including chronic obstructive pulmonary disease, further enhance the risk of respiratory infections among older patients.

Clinical manifestations/diagnosis

As with other infections in the elderly, pneumonia may not be heralded by the usual signs and symptoms.

333

Cough may not be prominent, fever can be absent or mild, and shortness of breath subtle. Nonspecific symptoms of confusion or other mental status change, lethargy, and falling may be the only indications that something is amiss.[32, 33] A high index of suspicion is required, and a chest radiograph should be obtained when the physician is confronted with such changes. X-rays often reveal an infiltrative process, but the absence of an infiltrate on the film does not preclude pneumonia, as dehydration may minimize radiographic evidence of infection.[34] The presence of a cavity suggests anaerobic abscess, TB, or mycotic infection. Sputum analysis, although potentially valuable in the identification of causative organisms, is rarely obtainable, as older individuals may be unable to cooperate with specimen collection or expectorate. When respiratory secretions can be obtained, Gram stain and routine bacterial culture should be performed. Blood cultures may also yield an organism associated with pneumonia. Other non-invasive or minimally invasive studies to be considered include multiplex polymerase chain reaction (PCR) for respiratory viruses on nasopharyngeal cells, obtained by either swabbing the nasopharynx or performing lavage. In addition, urinary antigen testing for *Streptococcus pneumoniae* is now available. In select cases, testing for *Legionella pneumophila* and/or *Histoplasma capsulatum* should be considered by urinary antigen testing. Pulse oximetry and, in some cases, arterial blood gas level should be measured to assess oxygenation status. Viral and other atypical pneumonias, malignancy, and pulmonary embolus should also be considered in the differential diagnosis of the older patient in whom pneumonia is suspected.

Management

Treatment of bacterial pneumonia should be guided by sputum Gram stain and culture. Given the difficulty of establishing a specific bacterial cause of pneumonia via sputum analysis and the seriousness of such infections in elderly patients, empiric therapy directed at the likely culprits is prudent and recommended. [35] Delay in the initiation of therapy risks progression of disease; therefore, treatment should begin within hours of presentation.[36] In community-acquired pneumonia, *Streptococcus pneumoniae*, *Hemophilus influenza*, enteric Gram-negative bacilli, influenza, and other respiratory viruses are most common; however, *S. aureus* and atypical organisms such as *Mycoplasma, Legionella*, and *Chlamydia* also occur. [37] Patients residing in nursing homes more commonly experience pneumonia caused by the enteric Gram-negative organisms, oral aerobes and anaerobes, and *S. aureus*.[16] These organisms (see Table 23.2) are responsible for the lion's share of pneumonia in the hospitalized patient, but more unusual organisms (including *Acinetobacter* and *Pseudomonas*) may also cause disease. Obviously, those patients who are more ill and those unable to

Table 23.2 Causes of pneumonia in the elderly [2]

Community acquired	Nursing facility associated	Hospital associated
S. pneumonia	Enteric Gram-negative bacilli	Enteric Gram-negative bacilli
H. influenzae	Oral aerobes and anaerobes	Oral aerobes and anaerobes
Enteric Gram-negative bacilli	*S. aureus*	*S. aureus*
S. aureus	*S. pneumonia*	*S. pneumonia*
Legionella pneumophila	*H. influenzae*	*Legionella pneumophila*
Mycoplasma pneumoniae	*Moraxella catarrhalis*	*Moraxella catarrhalis*
Chlamydia pneumoniae	Influenza	*Pseudomonas* spp.
Influenza	Other respiratory viruses	*Acinetobacter* spp.
Respiratory syncytial virus		*Stenotrophomonas* spp.
Other respiratory viruses		Influenza
Pneumocystis jiroveci		Other respiratory viruses

tolerate oral intake require inpatient care and intravenous administration of antibiotics. Treatment of most bacterial pneumonia lasts for 7–14 days.

Antibiotic choice must be guided by host and environmental factors such as concomitant illnesses, risk of aspiration, and the setting in which the patient resides.[35] Broader coverage – taking into account drug-resistant organisms and anaerobes – is typically indicated in institutionalized patients compared with those who live at home who may be able to be treated initially with an antipneumococcal fluoroquinolone, third-generation cephalosporin, or macrolide, depending on local drug susceptibility patterns. There is likely a spectrum of risk for drug-resistant bacterial infection spanning from living at home to assisted-living facilities to nursing homes and skilled nursing facilities, and the attendant risk with each setting may influence selection of treatment. In general, the level of independence for activities of daily living as well as the exposures to the healthcare system and specifically antibiotic exposure will determine the risk for multidrug resistance.

Detection of a specific organism can lead to the narrowing of antibiotic therapy. Failure to detect improvement during therapy may indicate that the selected therapy is suboptimal and that a change in antibiotics is required. In such cases, the presence of underlying immunodeficiency, such as that from HIV infection, and atypical infections caused by fungi or *P. jiroveci* (formerly *carinii*), should be considered.

Patients with pneumonia who are moderately to severely ill should be hospitalized. Findings associated with poor prognosis in elderly patients with community-acquired pneumonia include PaO_2 <60 mm Hg, O_2 saturation <90%, altered mental status, heart rate higher than 125 beats/minute, respiratory rate higher than 30/min, hypo- or hyperthermia, leukocytosis or leukopenia, anemia, hyponatremia, hyperglycemia, multilobar infiltrates, and pleural effusion.[20] In addition, older patients with pneumonia and significant comorbid diseases such as malignancy, immunodeficiency, renal or hepatic insufficiency, or cardiovascular disease may also require inpatient monitoring.

The risk of pneumococcal pneumonia can be reduced by vaccination. Patients who are naïve to the pneumococcal conjugate 13-valent (PCV13) should receive a single dose of PCV13. For those who received pneumococcal polysaccharide vaccine-23 (PPSV23), PCV13 should be administered at least one year after the last PPSV23 dose.[38]

Influenza

Influenza is a cause of viral pneumonia, occurring generally in the winter months in the United States. Recent data suggest that the virus thrives in cool temperatures with limited humidity, accounting for its seasonality.[39] Community and institutional acquisition occur under these conditions because this is a highly infectious virus with an incubation period of only two to three days. The infection and its complications can be lethal in elderly individuals.

Clinical manifestations/diagnosis

As in bacterial pneumonia, elderly patients with influenza may present atypically, with the triad of cough, fever, and acute onset less evident than mental status alteration, generalized malaise, and other nonspecific complaints.[40] Among patients living in confined settings, the report of a similar illness or actual influenza among other residents or staff is an important epidemiological clue. Secondary bacterial infection with streptococci or staphylococci occurs and typically manifests as a period of worsening of disease after an initial improvement. The chest radiograph may demonstrate bilateral infiltrates – suggestive of a viral pneumonia. Definitive diagnosis is made on nasopharyngeal samples through rapid antigen testing or through PCR testing. The benefit of point-of-care rapid antigen testing must be seriously weighed against a decreased sensitivity.[41]

In travelers returning from Asia or the Middle East, it is important to assess for infection with more virulent strains of influenza or with coronaviruses such as severe acute respiratory syndrome (SARS) or Middle East respiratory syndrome (MERS).

Management

Antiviral drugs active against influenza include the adamantine derivatives, amantadine and rimantadine, and neuraminidase inhibitors such as oseltamivir and zanamivir.[42, 43] The adamantine derivatives are only active against influenza A and do not cover influenza B strains. Currently, adamantine derivatives are of very limited use, given the widespread resistance found in circulating strains of the most recent influenza seasons. Also, they are associated with

335

reversible adverse effects involving the central nervous system, such as anxiety, concentration issues, nervousness, and insomnia.

Neuraminidase inhibitors are the drug of choice to treat influenza. Starting treatment early after the onset of symptoms is key to maximum efficacy. However, in elderly patients who are ill or need to be hospitalized, treatment should not be withheld even if several days have passed since symptom onset.

Both oseltamivir and zanamivir can be used as prophylaxis in institutionalized elderly patients in outbreak situations. Per guidelines from the Infectious Disease Society of America, when more than two institutional residents manifest signs and symptoms of influenza-like illness within 72 hours of each other, testing for influenza should occur. When influenza viruses are circulating in the community, even one positive laboratory result in conjunction with other compatible illnesses on the unit indicates that an outbreak of influenza is occurring. In these outbreaks, all residents – not just those on the floor or ward where the first cases have occurred – should receive chemoprophylaxis, regardless of vaccination status. Quarantining of cases does not appear to be a useful strategy.

The most effective method of preventing influenza and reducing its impact on morbidity and mortality of older adults is vaccination. The multi-valent inactivated influenza vaccine is recommended annually for those 65 years and older and younger individuals with chronic medical conditions or who reside in confined settings.[44, 45] The vaccine contains killed virus and cannot cause influenza. Unfortunately, the influence of aging on the immune system is associated with a decreased vaccine response to influenza.[8, 46, 47] Therefore, individuals such as health-care workers who have frequent contact with high-risk older adults should also be vaccinated annually.

Pulmonary tuberculosis

More than half the cases of tuberculosis (TB) in the United States are diagnosed in individuals 65 years of age or older.[48] Age-related waning of cellular immunity, comorbid conditions, immunosuppressant medications, and malnutrition increase the risk of reactivation of latent TB in the elderly. In addition, failure to administer isoniazid to older individuals with a positive tuberculin skin test because of fears of hepatotoxicity may also increase the risk of future reactivation of TB. Primary acquisition of TB also

occurs among the elderly, and transmission of TB within nursing facilities is well documented.[49]

Clinical manifestations/diagnosis

Pulmonary TB presents generally as a nonacute illness characterized by weight loss, fever, night sweats, and cough. Some patients may have hemoptysis. Nonspecific constitutional complaints may mask the more classic symptoms, and the diagnosis of TB should be considered in elderly persons with "failure to thrive." Chest radiographs, tuberculin skin testing and sputum stain, and culture are the foundations of the diagnostic workup for pulmonary TB. Chest films may reveal an area of infiltration – often in the upper lobes – or a cavitary lesion, but patterns similar to bacterial pneumonia can also be seen.[50] The diagnosis is made microbiologically with the culture of sputum for *Mycobacterium tuberculosis*. The specimen should undergo an acid-fast stain and be plated on specialized media. Unfortunately, sputum may be difficult to collect, and it may take six weeks for the culture to grow sufficiently. In some cases, bronchoscopy may be required to obtain specimens for stain and culture. Given the difficulty of establishing a quick diagnosis, empiric therapy is a consideration when suspicion of TB is high, such as in a patient with a classic chest film and a positive tuberculin skin test. Rapid tests for TB are now available; these molecular assays may be of use in some patients.[51] They are generally used to confirm the presence of TB in respiratory specimens that reveal acid-fast bacilli (AFB). The use of these assays in AFB-negative smears, although not approved for such use by the US Food and Drug Administration (FDA), is tempting in cases in which TB is suspected despite the smear result, and a positive result would be considered strong evidence of the infection.

Tuberculin skin testing is useful for determining prior exposure to TB. As the test relies on cellular immune responses, the false-negative rate of the test increases during advanced age. In some individuals, skin testing itself can boost immune responses to tuberculin such that repeated testing will become positive, giving the appearance of a conversion in the test from initially negative to positive.[52] In settings where skin testing for TB is performed on a regular basis, a two-step procedure at initial intake is advisable. If the initial reaction is negative, a repeated skin test is done two to three weeks later, and the second result is considered final. Bacillus-Calmette-Guérin vaccination may produce skin reactions to tuberculin. For those who received the vaccine as a child, the cross-reactivity to the skin testing should wane by adulthood and not be a significant factor in elderly individuals. Those who receive Bacillus-Calmette-Guérin vaccination as adults should have skin testing done several months after vaccination to establish a baseline test reaction size. Subsequent skin testing can be compared with this baseline result, and increases of more than 15 mm should be considered positive in persons older than 35 years of age.

Gamma-interferon assays of blood are also used to detect latent TB and are now available through commercial laboratories.[53, 54] There are limited data on the accuracy of this assay in the elderly, but a positive result indicates prior exposure. The Centers for Disease Control and Prevention have published recommendations regarding the use of the interferon-γ assay QuantiFeron-TB Gold. They state that the test can be used in all circumstances in which tuberculin skin testing is performed.[55]

All patients with either latent or active TB, regardless of age, should be tested for HIV infection.

Management

The therapeutic management of pulmonary TB in the elderly patient is not different from that in younger patients.[56] As discussed previously, empiric therapy for TB may be considered in patients with an illness consistent with pulmonary TB, especially when the sputum reveals acid-fast bacilli. Drug therapy typically consists of four drugs (isoniazid, rifampin, pyrazinamide, and ethambutol) administered for two months. Provided drug susceptibility testing indicates sensitivity to isoniazid and rifampin, treatment can be whittled down to these two agents for the remainder of the course. As polypharmacy is common in many elderly patients, care must be taken to avoid drug–drug interactions between anti-TB and other medications. Monitoring for drug toxicity, especially changes in hepatic transaminases (alanine aminotransferase and aspartate aminotransferase), is prudent. In general, aspartate aminotransferase or alanine aminotransferase elevations up to five times normal can be tolerated if the patient is free of hepatitis symptoms and up to three times normal if there are signs or symptoms of liver toxicity.[57] When treatment-limiting hepatic toxicity occurs, expert consultation should be sought so that reintroduction

of therapy can be considered. Because of the risk of optic neuritis, patients receiving ethambutol should have a baseline ophthalmology evaluation and be questioned monthly regarding visual disturbances. Monthly ocular evaluations are recommended for patients taking doses greater than 15 mg/kg–25 mg/kg, patients receiving the drug for longer than two months, and any patient with renal insufficiency.

Latent TB should be treated in elderly individuals.[57, 58] In one study, the risk of isoniazid-associated hepatotoxicity increased with age and was 2.3% among those aged 50 years or older.[59] More recent data indicate the risk of isoniazid-related hepatitis was generally rare, with only one case per 1,000 persons; however, the incidence was not analyzed according to age.[60] Current guidelines recommend that age not be considered when deciding to treat latent TB.[58] Importantly, alcohol raises the risk of the isoniazid-related hepatitis, and all patients on this drug need to be warned to abstain. Peripheral neuropathy, which occurs in up to 2% of patients taking isoniazid, can be prevented by pyridoxine supplementation.[61, 62]

Herpes zoster

Herpes zoster, or shingles, is a common condition associated with advancing age. It is also a commonly misunderstood disease by both patients and clinicians. The causative organism is the varicella zoster virus (VZV). This virus is the same one that causes chickenpox in younger persons and, like all herpes viruses, remains latent within the body following initial infection. In the case of VZV, the virus resides in the dorsal root ganglion, where it can remain without causing illness. With diminished immune function subsequent to aging, drugs, or illness, the virus can be activated and lead to the clinical syndrome known as shingles.[63]

Clinical manifestations/diagnosis

As opposed to the indistinct, if not misleading, presentation of other infectious diseases in the elderly, herpes zoster almost always announces itself with a constellation of classic symptoms. The illness starts with a two- to seven-day prodrome of tingling and pain at the site where soon thereafter an erythematous rash emerges in an area restricted to one or two adjacent dermatomal regions and does not usually cross the midline.[63] The rash matures quickly, first becoming papular and then vesicular coincident with an increased intensity of pain and burning. Within two weeks, the lesions crust and begin to fade; however, they may leave permanent scars. Serious systemic illness is rare, although fever, weakness, and anorexia can occur. Involvement of multiple dermatomes, crossing of the midline by lesions, and continued emergence of new lesions suggest more profound immunodeficiency.[63–65]

Although the clinical presentation is usually sufficient to establish the diagnosis of herpes zoster, laboratory confirmation can be achieved by testing of the vesicle fluid for the presence of VZV, either via viral culture, polymerase chain reaction, or Tzanck smear.

Unusually, herpes zoster can involve the eye, either externally or at the retina. Zoster lesions at the tip of the nose are an indication of involvement of cranial nerve V. Myelitis and encephalitis are rare, but serious, complications. The most common complication of shingles is postherpetic neuralgia (PHN). Continued pain and hypersensitivity at the area of the rash continues during PHN and can last up to a year.[66]

Management

A number of oral antivirals – including acyclovir, valacyclovir, and famciclovir – are active against VZV and can be used to reduce the duration of illness.[63] These are most effective in reducing the time to lesion crusting and acute pain resolution when initiated within 72 hours of the onset of the rash. Prompt valacyclovir and famciclovir treatment may also shorten the duration of PHN. Treatment with antivirals should continue until crusting of all the lesions occurs – generally 7–10 days. The addition of corticosteroids has not been shown to prevent PHN, and should not be administered.

Persons with active lesions are infectious and can transmit VZV to those who have not previously been exposed to or vaccinated against the virus. Persons with a clear history of chickenpox are at no risk of infection (even if pregnant) and need not take any special precautions regarding VZV. Crusting of the lesions is associated with a marked reduction in infectiousness.

The management of PHN is often difficult. Topical therapies (including anesthetics) and capsaicin can be used; however, systemic therapy with narcotics, anticonvulsant drugs (e.g., gabapentin), or antidepressants (e.g., nortriptyline, amitriptyline, desipramine, and

sertraline) may be required.[67] Intransigent cases of PHN should be referred to a pain management specialist.

As described in Chapter 35, prevention of herpes zoster is possible with a newly FDA-approved zoster vaccine. This vaccine contains a much higher concentration of the attenuated virus as compared to the vaccine used for immunizing previously uninfected individuals. It is approved for use in immunocompetent persons without a history of shingles who are older than 50 years of age.[67–69] The Advisory Committee on Immunization Practices recommends its use in immunocompetent adults older than 60.[38] A mild varicella rash can occur as an adverse effect of the vaccine. The efficacy of the vaccine to prevent shingles ranges from 70% in the 50–59 year age group to 38% in persons aged 70 years or older. In addition, the vaccine is efficacious at preventing the dreaded complication of post-herpetic neuralgia, with an efficacy of around 67% in all age groups.[70]

Methicillin-resistant *Staphylococcus aureus*

Methicillin-resistant *S. aureus* (MRSA) is a major cause of nosocomial infections, including skin and soft tissue infections, septicemia, endovascular infections, and infections of indwelling catheters or implanted prosthetic devices.[71] The spread of MRSA in health-care settings has had a significant impact on both clinical outcomes and health costs. [72] Hospital stays are prolonged, and mortality is higher among those with this infection. Risk factors associated with hospital-acquired MRSA include prolonged hospitalization (often more than 14 days), preceding antimicrobial therapy (especially with cephalosporins or fluoroquinolones), presence in an intensive care unit or burn unit, hemodialysis, surgical site infection, and proximity to a patient colonized or infected with MRSA.[72] As many, if not most, hospital inpatients are elderly, MRSA can be considered a major infection in this population. Furthermore, there is a great potential for the spread of MRSA within nursing facilities, given the high rates of colonization with the organism among residents of such facilities.

Recently, community-acquired (CA) MRSA infections are becoming more common. Studies performed between 1997 and 2001 demonstrated that 12%–22% of all staphylococcal isolates in patients presenting from community settings were methicillin resistant.

[73] In a study performed in 2004, 59% of staphylococcal isolates obtained strictly from skin and soft tissue infections were characterized as CA-MRSA. [74] Risk factors that have been associated with CA-MRSA infection include African-American race, HIV infection, antibiotic therapy within the past six months, and skin trauma.[75]

Clinical presentation/diagnosis

MRSA colonizes the nasal mucosa and oropharynx but may also be found on the skin. Colonization itself does not cause illness, but it does increase the risk of subsequent disease from the organism. The clinical manifestations of MRSA infection are protean and include skin and soft tissue infections, pneumonia, endovascular infections, and joint infections.[71, 72] CA-MRSA frequently presents as a boil or skin abscess that is painful and erythematous. Clinically, it is impossible to distinguish between MRSA and other bacterial causes of these infections. Culture of the organism from infected tissue or blood is the basis of diagnosis. Given the aggressive nature of many staphylococcal infections, however, a high level of suspicion should be maintained in the presence of predisposing conditions such as defects in phagocytic function and diabetes mellitus.

As mentioned previously, a common error in the management of endovascular infections caused by *S. aureus* is the assumption that detection of this organism in the urine indicates only a UTI. Isolation of this organism in the urine should prompt evaluation for the presence of endocarditis or other endovascular infection, as this organism commonly enters the genitourinary system hematogenously.

Management

Antibiotics and drainage of infected material are the mainstays of therapy. Skin and soft tissue abscesses require surgical drainage and adjunctive antibiotic therapy. Nonsurgically managed MRSA infections require appropriate antibiotic therapy. There are different drug susceptibility profiles for MRSA seen in hospital compared with community-acquired isolates. [76] There is also a difference in patterns of drug resistance depending on geography. It is, therefore, important to tailor treatment according to regional antibiotic susceptibility patterns (see Table 23.3). In some cases, drugs such as trimethoprim-sulfamethoxazole and doxycycline can be used to treat a drained abscess. Other infections resulting from MRSA may require more active agents against the organism.

In general, vancomycin is active against MRSA. There are reports of some strains of *S. aureus* with reduced susceptibility to vancomycin, but these are rare, show only intermediate resistance to the drug, and retain susceptibility to the newer classes of antistaphylococcal antibiotics: the oxazolidinones, quinupristin/dalfopristin, the cyclic lipopeptide daptomycin, and the glycylcycline tigecycline.[77] These alternatives are typically used when vancomycin is not tolerated.

Newer approaches to therapy involve decolonization to prevent person-to-person transmission and to break the cycle of recurrent outbreaks of MRSA skin and soft tissue infections in a single individual. Currently no clear consensus guidelines exist, and evidence from controlled trials is limited; however, general measures include intranasal mupirocin, topical antiseptic washes (i.e., chlorhexidine gluconate) during daily showers, and weekly Clorox baths (approximately 0.25 cups per bath with a 10-minute soak). One recent encouraging study utilized a triple approach with an oral regimen of rifampin and doxycycline, intranasal 2% mupirocin ointment, and 2% chlorhexidine gluconate for washing.[78] In that study, 112 hospitalized patients who were colonized with MRSA were randomized to receive either this decolonization therapy for seven days or no treatment. Of those treated, 74% had negative MRSA cultures at three months, whereas only 32% of those who were not treated were culture negative at follow-up. Eight months later, 54% of those who were treated remained culture negative. This same study found that in patients who were colonized with mupirocin-resistant *S. aureus* at baseline, treatment was nine times more likely to fail.

Personal hygiene measures include keeping nails trimmed short and scrubbed daily with soap, single use only of bath towels and garments, and washing clothes in hot water. If a single patient has recurrent MRSA outbreaks, then often oral antibiotics are used in conjunction. Also, all members of the household should be treated with the general decolonization measures. Hand washing and other infection control measures are essential to prevent the spread of MRSA, especially in institutionalized settings.

Summary

The diagnosis and management of infectious diseases in older persons can be challenging. Clinicians must be familiar with the differences in clinical presentation among older and younger patients. In addition, it

Table 23.3 Antibiotic options for MRSA

Antibiotic	Route	Indications	Routine dose	Major side effects
Trimethoprim-sulfamethoxazole (septra, bactrim)	PO, IV	Skin and soft tissue infections. Not specifically FDA approved for infections resulting from MRSA.	2 double-strength tablets (160 mg TMP/ 800 mg SMX) po bid	Anemia, neutropenia, rash, pruritus, Stevens-Johnson syndrome. Not recommended during the third trimester of pregnancy.
Minocycline (minocin) and doxycycline (doryx)	PO	Skin and soft tissue infections. Not specifically FDA approved for infections resulting from MRSA.	100 mg po bid	Photosensitivity, rash. Not recommended for use during pregnancy.
Clindamycin (cleocin)	PO, IV	Skin and soft tissue infections, bone infections. Not specifically FDA approved for infections resulting from MRSA.	300–600 mg po tid-qid	Rash, *Clostridium difficile* colitis
Rifampin (rifampicin)	PO	Should not be used as a single agent. May be used in combination for treatment and eradication of MRSA.	600 mg po qd	Rash, liver inflammation. High frequency of drug–drug interactions.
Vancomycin (vancocin)	IV	Endocarditis, bacteremia, bone/joint infections.	1000 mg q12h	Hypersensitivity reactions, red man syndrome.
Quinupristin – dalfopristin (synercid)	IV	Skin and soft tissue infections.	7.5 mg/kg q8–12h	Arthralgias, myalgias.
Linezolid (zyvox)	IV, PO	Skin and soft tissue infections, pneumonia.	600 mg q12h	Bone marrow suppression. *Note:* Not recommended for routine oral use because of potential for inducing resistance and/or toxicity, and high cost.
Daptomycin (cubicin)	IV	Skin and soft tissue infections. Right-sided endocarditis, bacteremia.	4–6 mg/kg qday	Myopathy. *Note:* Not active in pneumonia.
Ceftaroline (teflaro)	IV	Skin and soft tissue infections, pneumonia.	600 mg q12h	Rash, diarrhea, nausea.
Tigecycline (tygacil)	IV	Skin and soft tissue infections. Intra-abdominal infections, pneumonia.	100 mg loading dose followed by 50 mg q12h	**Black box warning for increased mortality.** Nausea, vomiting, headache, liver inflammation.

is important that subtle indicators of serious infection and impending clinical decompensation such as hypothermia or leukopenia not be missed. Timely therapeutic intervention when infection is suspected is essential, as a delay in appropriate treatment – even for a few hours – can have devastating consequences.

As the population in the United States continues to age, familiarity with the clinical presentation, diagnosis, and management of the major serious infections of elderly individuals becomes an increasingly critical component of general medicine and primary care.

References

1. Heron MP, Smith BL. Deaths: leading causes for 2003. *National Vital Statistics Reports* 2007 March 15;**55**:1–92

2. Hyde Z, Flicker L, Hankey GJ, et al. Prevalence of sexual activity and associated factors in men aged 75 to 95 years: a cohort study. *Annals of Internal Medicine* 2010;**153**(11):693–702.

3. Van Duin D. Diagnostic challenges and opportunities in older adults with infectious diseases. *Clinical Infectious Diseases: an official publication of the Infectious Diseases Society of America* 2012;**54**(7):973–8.

4. Grubeck-Loebenstein B, Wick G. The aging of the immune system. *Adv Immunol* 2002;**80**:243–84.

5. Linton PJ, Dorshkind K. Age-related changes in lymphocyte development and function. *Nat Immunol* 2004;**5**:133–9.

6. Aspinall R. Age-related changes in the function of T cells. *Microsc Res Tech* 2003;**62**:508–13.

7. Plackett TP, Boehmer ED, Faunce DE, Kovacs EJ. Aging and innate immune cells. *J Leukoc Biol* 2004;**76**:291–9.

8. Van Duin D, Allore HG, Mohanty S, et al. Prevaccine determination of the expression of costimulatory B7 molecules in activated monocytes predicts influenza vaccine responses in young and older adults. *J Infect Dis* 2007;**195**(11):1590–7.

9. Van Duin D, Mohanty S, Thomas V, et al. Age-associated defect in human TLR-1/2 function. *J Immunol* 2007;**178**(2):970–5.

10. Van Duin D, Shaw AC. Toll-like receptors in older adults. *J Am Geriatr Soc* 2007;**55**(9):1438–44.

11. Davenport RJ. Immunity challenge. *Sci Aging Knowledge Environ* 2003;**23**:1–6.

12. Vallejo AN. CD28 extinction in human T cells: altered functions and the program of T-cell senescence. *Immunological Reviews* 2005;**205**(1):158–69.

13. Posnett DN, Sinha R, Kabak S, Russo C. Clonal populations of T cells in normal elderly humans: the T cell equivalent to "benign monoclonal gammapathy." *J Expl Med* 1994;**179**:609–18.

14. Howells CHL, Vesselinova Jenkins CK, Evans AD, et al. Influenza vaccination and mortality from bronchopneumonia in the elderly. *Lancet* 1975;**1**:381–3.

15. Ammann AJ, Schiffman G, Austrian R. The antibody responses to pneumococcal capsular polysaccharides in the aged. *Proc Soc Exp Biol Med* 1980;**164**:312–6.

16. Htwe TH, Mushtaq A, Robinson SB, et al. Infections in the elderly. *Infect Clin N Am* 2007;**21**(3):711–43.

17. Greenberg S. Administration on Aging: Profile of older Americans: 2005;30. Available at: www.aoa.acl.gov/Aging_Statistics/Profile/2005/2005profile.pdf (accessed February 4, 2016).

18. www.aarp.org/research/ppi/liv-com2/resources/nhts-AARP-ppi-liv-com (accessed September 23, 2014).

19. Branson BM, Handsfield HH, Lampe MA, et al. Revised recommendations for HIV testing of adults, adolescents, and pregnant women in health-care settings. *MMWR* 2006;**55**(RR-14):1–17.

20. Mouton CP, Bazaldua OV. Common infections in older adults. *Am Fam Physician* 2001;**63**:257–68.

21. Yoshikawa TT, Norman DC. Fever in the elderly. *Infect Med* 1998;**15**:704–6.

22. Norman DC. Special infectious disease problems in geriatrics. *Clin Geriatr* 1999;(Suppl 1):3–5.

23. Fraser D. Assessing the elderly for infections. *J Gerontol Nurs* 1997;**23**:5–10.

24. Yoshikawa TT. Ambulatory management of common infections in elderly patients. *Infect Med* 1991;**20**:37–43.

25. Pfisterer MH, Griffiths DJ, Schaefer W, et al. The effect of age on lower urinary tract function: a study in women. *J Am Geriatr Soc* 2006;**54**:405–12.

26. McCue JD. Treatment of urinary tract infections in long-term care facilities: advice, guidelines and algorithms. *Clin Geriatr* 1999;(Suppl):11–7.

27. Nicolle LE. Urinary tract infection in long-term-care facility residents. *Clin Infect Dis* 2000;**31**:757–61.

28. Zhanel GG, Harding G. K., Guay D. R. Asymptomatic bacteriuria. Which patients should be treated? *Arch Intern Med* 1990;**150**:1389–96.

29. Lienderrozos HJ. Urinary tract infections: management rationale for uncomplicated cystitis. *Clin Fam Pract* 2004;**6**:157–73.

30. Meyer KC. Lung infections and aging. *Ageing Res Rev* 2004;**3**:55–67.

31. Meyer KC. Aging. *Proc Am Thorac Soc* 2005;**2**:433–9.

32. Venkatesan P, Gladman J., MacFarlane J., et al. A hospital study of community acquired pneumonia in the elderly. *Thorax* 1990;**17**:254–8.

33. Riquelme R, Torres AWI, Ebiary M., et al. Community-acquired pneumonia in the elderly. *Am J Respir Crit Care Med* 1997;**156**:1908–14.

34. Hash R, Stephens J., Laurens M., et al. The relationship between volume status, hydration, and radiographic findings in the diagnosis of community-acquired pneumonia. *J Fam Pract* 2000;**49**:833–7.

35. Loeb M. Pneumonia in older persons. *Clin Infect Dis* 2003;**37**:1335–9.

36. Meehan T, Fine M, Krumholz H, et al. Quality of care, process, and outcomes in elderly patients with pneumonia. *JAMA* 1997;**278**:2080–4.

37. Ruiz M, Ewing S, Marcos M, et al. Etiology of community-acquired pneumonia: impact of age, comorbidity, and severity. *Am J Respir Crit Care Med* 1999;**160**:397–405.

38. General recommendations on immunization: recommendations of the Advisory Committee on Immunization Practices (ACIP). *MMWR Recommendations and Reports* 2011;**60**: 1–64.

39. Lowen AC, Mubareka S, Steel J, Palese P. Influenza virus transmission is dependent on relative humidity and temperature. *PLoS Pathogens* 2007 Oct 19;**3** (10):1470–6.

40. Govaert TME, Dinant GJ, Aretz K, et al. The predictive value of influenza symptomatology in elderly people. *Fam Pract* 1998;**15**:16–22.

41. Talbot HK, Falsey AR. The diagnosis of viral respiratory disease in older adults. *Clin Infect Dis* 2010;**50**(5):747–51.

42. Winquist AG, Fukada K, Bridges CB, Cox NJ. Neuraminidase inhibitors for treatment of influenza A and B infections. *MMWR* 1999;**48**(RR-14):1–9.

43. Kuhle C, Evans JM. Prevention and treatment of influenza infections in the elderly. *Clin Geriatr* 1999;**7**(2):27–35.

44. Centers for Disease Control and Prevention. Recommendations of the Advisory Committee on Immunization Practices (ACIP), 2007–2008. Available at: www.cdc.gov/flu/professionals/acip (accessed June 1, 2008).

45. Gross PA, Hermogenes AW, Sacks HS, et al. The efficacy of influenza vaccine in elderly persons: a meta-analysis and review of the literature. *Ann Intern Med* 1995;**123**:518–27.

46. Panda A, Qian F, Mohanty S, et al. Age-associated decrease in TLR function in primary human dendritic cells predicts influenza vaccine response. *J Immunol* 2010;**184**(5):2518–27.

47. Goronzy JJ, Fulbright JW, Crowson CS, et al. Value of immunological markers in predicting responsiveness to influenza vaccination in elderly individuals. *J Virol* 2001;**75**(24):12182–7.

48. Dutt AK, Stead WW. Tuberculosis in the elderly. *Med Clin North Am* 1993;**77**:1353–68.

49. Zevallos M, Justman JE. Tuberculosis in the elderly. *Clin Geriatr Med* 2003;**19**:121–38.

50. Imperato J, Sanchez LD. Pulmonary emergencies in the elderly. *Emerg Med Clin N Am* 2006;**24**:317–38.

51. American Thoracic Society Workshop. Rapid diagnostic tests for tuberculosis: what is the appropriate use? *Am J Respir Crit Care Med* 1997 May;**155**(5):1804–14.

52. Menzies D. Interpretation of repeated tuberculin tests. *Boosting, Conversion, and Reversion* 1999;**159**:15–21.

53. Pai M, Riley LW, Colford JM Jr. Interferon-gamma assays in the immunodiagnosis of tuberculosis: a systematic review. *Lancet Infect Dis* 2004;**4**:761–76.

54. Menzies D, Pai M, Comstock G. Meta-analysis: new tests for the diagnosis of latent tuberculosis infection: areas of uncertainty and recommendations for research. *Ann Intern Med* 2007;**146**:340–54.

55. Mazurek GH, Jereb J, Lobue P, et al. Guidelines for using the QuantiFERON-TB Gold test for detecting Mycobacterium tuberculosis infection, United States. *MMWR* 2005;**54**:49–55.

56. Bass J, Farer L, Hopewell P, et al. Treatment of tuberculosis and tuberculosis infection in adults and children. American Thoracic Society and the Centers for Disease Control and Prevention. *Am J Respir Crit Care Med* 1994;**149**:1359–74.

57. Blumberg HM, Burman WJ, Chaisson RE, et al. American Thoracic Society/Centers for Disease Control and Prevention/Infectious Diseases Society of America. Treatment of tuberculosis. *Am J Respir Crit Care Med* 2003;**167**:603–62.

58. Jasmer RM, Nahid P, Hopewell PC. Clinical practice: latent tuberculosis infection. *N Engl J Med* 2002;**347**:1860–6.

59. Kopanoff DE, Snider DE Jr, Caras GJ. Isoniazid-related hepatitis: a US Public Health Service Cooperative Surveillance Study. *Am Rev Respir Dis* 1978;**117**:991–1001.

60. Nolan CM, Goldberg SV, Buskin SE. Hepatotoxicity associated with isoniazid preventive therapy: a 7-year survey from a public health tuberculosis clinic. *JAMA* 1999;**281**:1014–18.

61. Oestreicher R, Dressler SH, Middlebrook G. Peripheral neuritis in tuberculous patients treated with isoniazid. *Am Rev Tuberc* 1954;**70**:504–8.

62. Snider DE Jr. Pyridoxine supplementation during isoniazid therapy. *Tubercle* 1980;**61**:191–6.

63. Dworkin RH, Johnson RW, Breuer J, et al. Recommendations for the management of herpes zoster. *Clin Infect Dis* 2007;**44**:S1–44.

64. Weinberg JM, Vafaie J, Scheinfeld NS. Skin infections in the elderly. *Dermatol Clin* 2004;**22**:51–61.

65. Heininger U, Seward J. Varicella. *Lancet* 2006;**368**:1365–76.

66. Schmader KE, Studenski S. Are current therapies useful for the prevention of postherpetic neuralgia? A critical analysis of the literature. *J Gen Intern Med* 1989;**4**(2):83–9.

67. Kost RG, Straus SE. Postherpetic neuralgia – pathogenesis, treatment and prevention. *N Engl J Med* 1996;**335**:32–42.

68. Kimberlin D, Whitley RJ. Varicella-zoster vaccine for the prevention of herpes zoster. *N Engl J Med* 2007;**356**:1338–43.

69. Oxman MN, Levin MJ, Johnson GR, et al. A vaccine to prevent herpes zoster and post-herpetic neuralgia in older adults. *N Engl J Med* 2005;**352**(22):2271–84.

70. Cohen JI. Clinical practice: Herpes zoster. *N Engl J Med* 2013;**369**(3):255–63.

71. Crossley KB, Archer GL. *The* Staphylococci *in Human Disease*. New York: Churchill Livingstone, 1997.

72. Kaplan AH. *Staphylococci* infections. *Netter's Internal Medicine*. Teterboro, NJ: Icon Learning Systems, 2003.

73. Chambers HF. The changing epidemiology of *Staphylococcus aureus*? *Emerg Infect Dis* 2001;7:178–82.

74. Moran GJ, Krishnadasan A, Gorwitz RJ, et al. Methicillin-resistant *S. aureus* infections among patients in the emergency department. *N Engl J Med* 2006;**355**: 666–74.

75. Centers for Disease Control and Prevention. Outbreaks of community-associated methicillin-resistant *Staphylococcus aureus* skin infections – Los Angeles County, California, 2002–2003. *MMWR* 2003;**52**:88.

76. Foster TJ. The *Staphylococcus aureus* "superbug." *J Clin Invest* 2004;**114**:1693–6.

77. Liu C, Chambers HF. *Staphylococcus aureus* with heterogeneous resistance to vancomycin: epidemiology, clinical significance, and critical assessment of diagnostic methods. *Antimicrob Agents Chemother* 2003;**47**:3040–5.

78. Simor A, Phillips E, McGeer A, et al. Randomized controlled trial of chlorhexidine gluconate for washing, intranasal mupirocin, and rifampin and doxycycline versus no treatment for the eradication of methicillin-resistant *Staphylococcus aureus* colonization. *Clin Infect Dis* 2007;**44**:178–85.

Chapter 24

Human immunodeficiency virus in the elderly

Christina Prather, MD, and David Alain Wohl, MD

Introduction

The human immunodeficiency virus (HIV) epidemic began as a fatal illness among young gay men but has now matured into a chronic disease that increasingly affects older men and women. One in five persons living with HIV is aged 55 or older, according to the Centers for Disease Control and Prevention (CDC), and it is expected that in the coming years over half of those infected with HIV in the United States will be older than 50.[1, 2] The graying of the HIV epidemic reflects two major phenomena: the dramatic increase in the life expectancy of HIV-positive individuals following advances in HIV therapeutics, and newly acquired infections among older men and women.[3]

The challenges associated with normal aging are often compounded for elder HIV-infected individuals given their increased risks for HIV-related illnesses, comorbid conditions, polypharmacy, poverty, and stigmatization. Clinicians must therefore be attuned to the evolving and special needs of HIV-infected patients as they age.

Epidemiology of HIV in older adults

Even as new infections among young men are on the rise, a significant proportion of people living with HIV infection in the United States are 50 years old or older (Figure 24.1) [1, 2] – a demographic group that is the fastest growing subset of patients with HIV in the nation.[3] Advances in HIV treatment, particularly the advent of potent combination antiretroviral therapy (ART), have led to dramatically increased survival and quality of life for HIV-infected individuals. The life expectancy for those infected with the virus is now close to that of the general population.[4] As described in this chapter, older persons may also acquire HIV, typically via unprotected sex, further increasing the pool of HIV-positive persons in this age category.

Screening and diagnosis

Missed opportunities for screening: is it HIV or is it aging?

Detection of HIV infection is the obvious starting point for prevention and treatment. However, older individuals are less likely to be screened for HIV infection compared to younger people, and as a consequence they present later and with more advanced disease.[5, 6] The diagnosis is also obscured when symptoms and signs of immunodeficiency in older adults mimic normal aging or other medical problems that are common in the elderly.[7] Awareness of symptoms and signs associated with HIV infection, both acute and chronic, increases the likelihood of proper testing being performed, and the identification of patients who will benefit from early treatment, counseling, and other interventions to avert further transmission.

Routine HIV testing

The CDC and the US Preventive Services Task Force recommend routine, voluntary opt-out HIV screening for all adults ages 13–64 regardless of risk factors. [8, 9] Although there remains an important role for a detailed sexual and substance use history, screening independently of risks improves identification of HIV-infected individuals. It is notable that these recommendations do not include routine testing in persons 65 years of age or older despite the hesitation

---

Reichel's Care of the Elderly, *7th Edition*, ed. Jan Busby-Whitehead *et al.* Published by Cambridge University Press.
© Cambridge University Press 2016.

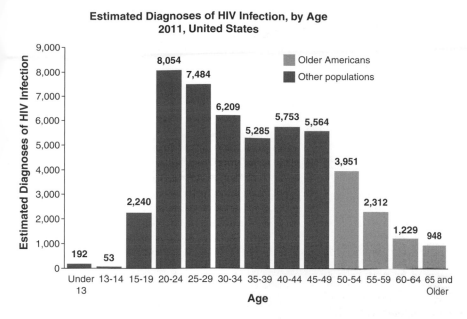

Figure 24.1 Estimated diagnoses of HIV infection by age, 2011, United States. (A black-and-white version of this figure will appear in some formats. For the color version, please refer to the plate section.)

of adults and their providers to correctly appreciate risk factors for infection.[5, 6] Many experts (these authors included) recommend extending routine HIV screening beyond the age of 65 years. Clinicians must appreciate that older persons can be sexually active, and should be comfortable and adept at taking a sexual and substance use history from older patients [10]

HIV testing relies on detection of antibodies to HIV, the virus itself, or both.[11] The fourth-generation assay that is now recommended by the CDC for universal use is a combination HIV antibody and antigen (p24 antigen) assay that detects antibodies to both HIV-1 and HIV-2. It is commercially available and in wide use. This test reduces the window period from acquisition of HIV to laboratory detection of infection to 4–12 days (Figure 24.2). Negative results can be considered conclusive unless a potential exposure to HIV occurred within the two weeks prior to the test. If the antibody/antigen screen is positive, follow-up testing including a nucleic acid test for HIV RNA is performed.

Acute HIV infection is symptomatic in most cases and may present as fever, generalized lymphadenopathy, viral exantham, and severe fatigue. As these are nonspecific symptoms especially during flu season, a careful history should be taken to assess for possible HIV exposure. Although the fourth-generation HIV Ag/Ab test reduces the window period between infection and test positivity, when acute HIV is suspected, an HIV RNA test is most appropriate.

Clinical characteristics

At diagnosis, older adults present with characteristics of more advanced or severe HIV disease compared with younger adults.[12] They consistently have a lower median CD4+ cell count at the time of diagnosis, and a greater proportion have an acquired immune deficiency syndrome (AIDS) defining diagnosis at or within three months prior to presenting for HIV care.[13] Delayed testing due to a low clinical suspicion for HIV infection contributes to advanced presentation at time of diagnosis. While HIV disease can present in myriad ways, certain clinical situations should prompt HIV testing (Table 24.1).

Infections

A number of opportunistic infections are associated with the immune deficiency that characterizes progressive HIV disease. Development of any of these is a clarion call for HIV screening. Among these are oral or esophageal candidiasis (thrush), varicella zoster infections, bacterial pneumonia, and pyomyositis. More pathognomonic for AIDS are rarer conditions such as pneumocystis pneumonia, cryptococcal meningitis, toxoplasmosis encephalitis, cytomegalovirus (CMV) retinitis or enteritis, and disseminated mycobacterium avium complex. Pneumocystis pneumonia is associated with late diagnosis of HIV/AIDS and may be unrecognized, with catastrophic consequences. It classically presents with progressive

345

Table 24.1 Major indications for HIV testing

Risk factors	Infections	Noninfectious conditions	Laboratory/clinical abnormalities
Sex with a partner who is known to be HIV-infected	Hepatitis B or C infection	Diffuse lymphadenopathy	Albumin/globulin ratio of <1.0
Men who have sex with men	Opportunistic infections such as pneumocystis, toxoplasmosis, cryptococcal disease, cytomegalovirus disease	Hairy leukoplakia of the tongue	Anemia
Multiple sex partners	Active or latent tuberculosis	Non-Hodgkin's lymphoma and CNS lymphoma	Lymphopenia
Commercial sex or trading sex for goods or services	Other sexually transmitted infections including herpes simplex, syphilis, gonorrhea, and chlamydia	Kaposi's sarcoma	Thrombocytopenia
History of injection drug use	Recurrent pneumonia	High-grade cervical dysplasia	Renal insufficiency
Transfusion of blood or blood products prior to	Thrush or candidiasis	Severe psoriasis	Unexplained weight loss
	Varicella zoster	Seborrheic dermatitis	Night sweats
	Pyomyositis,	Extensive molluscum	
	Recurrent bacterial infections	Ano-genital condylmoata	

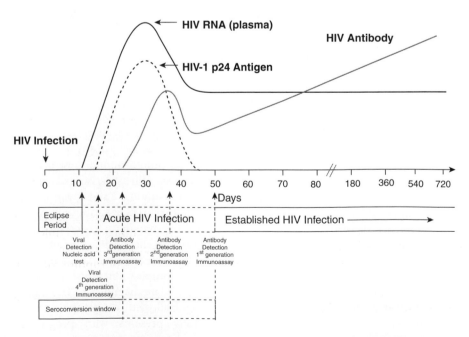

Figure 24.2 Sequence of appearance of laboratory markers of HIV-1 infection.

symptoms of cough (productive of scant, white/gray sputum), dyspnea, hypoxia, and diffuse pulmonary infiltrates, although radiographic findings can be minimal even in the face of severe respiratory compromise.

Recurrent bacterial pneumonia, skin and soft tissue infections with MRSA or other bacteria, and perirectal abscess or fistula may also be the presenting manifestations of HIV infection.

In most of the world, tuberculosis is the most common and lethal opportunistic condition complicating AIDS. All patients with either active tuberculosis or latent infection, as determined by a positive purified protein derivative (PPD) test or blood interferon gamma release assay, should be tested for HIV infection. Those diagnosed with other sexually transmitted infections such as gonorrhea, chlamydia, syphilis, hepatitis C virus (HCV), and hepatitis B virus (HBV) are almost by definition at risk for HIV infection.

Neurologic conditions

Neuropathy and dementia, although common in elderly patients, are also prevalent in those with HIV infection.[14–16] HIV-associated dementia classically presents with early behavioral changes and occasionally includes focal neurologic findings such as isolated weakness or aphasia. Peripheral neuropathy in the setting of HIV can present as a painful distal sensory process, or may appear almost indistinguishable from diabetic neuropathy. Early antiretroviral medications have left a legacy of peripheral neuropathy that produces burning, persistent pain and loss of sensation, posing risks for foot sores and infection; newer medications are less likely to cause nerve disease.

HIV-related toxoplasmosis, progressive multifocal leukoencephalopathy, bacterial and viral meningitis, and acute HIV headache continue to pose diagnostic and management challenges.

Malignancies

The immune system provides surveillance not only for infectious pathogens but also malignant cells. As such, deficiencies in immune function are associated with increased risk of neoplasm, particularly those that have a viral etiology.[17] In the setting of HIV, a number of cancers are more common, including non-Hodgkin's lymphomas, lung cancer, central nervous system lymphomas, testicular cancer, and

Kaposi's sarcoma. Cancers due to human papilloma virus (HPV) – including those involving the anus, vulva, or mouth – are also seen more commonly in men and women with HIV infection. Detection of any of these malignancies should prompt HIV testing.

Other conditions

Symptoms of acute HIV: fatigue, headache, weight loss, diffuse lymphadenopathy . . .

A number of dermatologic conditions are associated with HIV infection, including severe psoriasis, seborrheic dermatitis, common warts, condylomata acuminata, molluscum contagiosum, and purigo nodularis. Oral hairy leukoplakia is a viral mediated nonmalignant condition affecting the lateral aspects of the tongue and presents as a shiny white tiger-striping that is not easily removed. Leukoplakia and erythroplakia are oral premalignant conditions that should prompt monitoring and referral.

Laboratory abnormalities

Common but nonspecific laboratory findings in persons with advanced HIV infection include anemia, thrombocytopenia, and leucopenia, specifically lymphopenia. An increase in globulin is often seen in HIV-positive patients.[18] Isolated thrombocytopenia can be seen in persons with HIV infection and/or advanced viral hepatitis.

Aging process and HIV infection

There is growing concern that HIV-infected persons experience aging differently than those without the virus.[19] A number of studies document comorbidities and frailty rates that are higher among HIV-infected men and women compared to uninfected controls.[19–22] In a comparison of a large cohort of HIV-infected and uninfected patients receiving care at two Boston hospitals, those infected with HIV had an almost twofold greater risk of acute myocardial infarction than uninfected patients, with the difference between the groups increasing at older ages.[23] Other studies have demonstrated an increase in carotid artery intima-media thickness, coronary artery calcium deposition, and non-calcified coronary plaque (increased risk of rupture compared to noncalcified plaque) in HIV-infected persons.[24, 25] HIV-infected men and women have also relatively high rates of diminished bone density and nontraumatic fractures, as well as neurocognitive impairment.[26, 27] An analysis of data collected during the Men's AIDS Cohort Study (MACS), a large multi-center longitudinal observational study of HIV-infected and uninfected men who have sex with men (MSM) in the United States, found significantly higher rates of frailty (defined as having ≥3 of the following: low grip strength; slow four-meter walking speed; low physical activity; exhaustion; and unintentional weight loss of >10 pounds) among the HIV-positive men at each decade of life past 50 years of age.[28]

That HIV-infected individuals experience conditions associated with aging at rates that exceed those uninfected should not be a surprise, given the higher rates of smoking, substance abuse, poverty, and similar factors among those living with the virus. Studies that adjust for such confounders typically find that the associations between HIV and comorbidity are attenuated.[25] However, several lines of data strongly suggest that HIV infection and its treatment do have a direct role in age-related disease. In general, markers of immune activation are elevated in HIV-infected patients, as are those that assess inflammation.[29, 30] Such markers of inflammation, including C-reactive protein (CRP), interleukin 6 (IL-6), and D-dimer have been associated with mortality and non-AIDS morbidity in HIV-positive cohorts.[31] Similarly, altered gut integrity has been demonstrated in HIV-infected persons, leading to microbial translocation – an additional contributor to the inflammatory state. [32] Common coinfections in HIV-infected patients, such as hepatitis C virus (HCV) and CMV, may also play a role by triggering additional immune activation and inflammation.[33] Further, there is evidence that traditional risk factors for disease, such as smoking, may have a greater impact on cardiovascular and pulmonary health among HIV-infected patients than those uninfected.[34]

HIV therapies have led to profound improvements in survival and quality of life but may have long-term consequences. LDL cholesterol and triglyceride levels are increased by many commonly used antiretrovirals; abacavir and protease inhibitors have been associated with an increased risk of CVD in some but not all large cohort studies.[35, 36] Renal complications develop in a small but significant minority of patients treated with tenofovir; it can also reduce bone density. Tenofovir can rarely cause

Fanconi syndrome, but it can also exacerbate preexisting renal disease. All patients who take this very effective antiretroviral should be monitored with serum creatinine and urine protein/creatinine ratio every three to six months. The renal effects of tenofovir are magnified because it is excreted by renal tubules and can accumulate and cause additional toxicity if renal function is impaired. Despite these concerns, accumulated data, including examination of treatment interruptions, make clear that uncontrolled HIV itself presents a greater risk for CVD, renal, hepatic, and other end-organ diseases, trumping any contributions by ART.[37, 38]

Management considerations

With HIV-infection now a long-term chronic condition for most patients, the management of this disease has started to shift toward primary care providers. Although many patients rely on their HIV specialist to attend to their general health needs, or see both a specialist and a primary care clinician, others have their HIV care provided by their primary care clinic. The clinician responsible for managing HIV, whether specialist or generalist, must be well versed in HIV care including relevant guidelines regarding HIV treatment and opportunistic infection prophylaxis.[47] Clinics providing HIV care must also be prepared to handle psychosocial aspects of HIV management.

Regardless of specialty of the clinician, the provision of HIV care must address HIV and related diseases as a syndrome, in the method familiar to geriatrics. Implementing geriatric principles in HIV care has a particular role in managing treatment regimens and polypharmacy. Older patients require close surveillance for liver, renal, metabolic, endocrine, and hematologic abnormalities while on ART, with special attention paid to drug interactions between ART and medications for other conditions (Table 24.2).

Select conditions of particular importance in the management of the aging HIV-infected patient are discussed later in the following paragraphs. In addition, more general health maintenance of older patients, such as cancer screening and immunizations, must also be attended to.

Cardiovascular disease

As described earlier, HIV-infected adults are at increased risk for CVD, including heart disease and stroke, and have increased subclinical CVD related to

Table 24.2 Characteristics of older (≥50 years) adults relative to younger adults with HIV

- More severe disease course
- Less desirable health indices at diagnosis, including lower CD4+ counts and higher HIV RNA levels
- Shorter AIDS-free intervals and greater risk of opportunistic infections
- Earlier development of certain malignancies
- Higher daily medication and pill burden
- Higher rates of HIV treatment response
- Greater rates of HIV therapy adherence and persistence

age-matched controls. The etiology for this is unclear, but traditional and HIV-related risk factors are likely at play. Given that advanced age is a well-recognized risk factor for CVD, additional subclinical disease suggests the need for awareness of CVD risk in HIV-infected persons.

The management of risk factors for CVD can reduce clinical disease incidence for HIV-infected patients. A recent study from investigators at Kaiser Permanente in California found that over the past several years, the rates for stroke and myocardial infarction for HIV-positive patients has approached that of uninfected members – a reduction attributed to more aggressive risk factor management and earlier initiation of ART to control viremia.[39] Overall, these are reassuring outcomes for HIV-infected patients and punctuate the need to address well-recognized risk factors associated with cardiovascular disease such as obesity, hypertension, tobacco and substance use, and dyslipidemia.

Some underappreciated risks include renal disease, depression, and toxic levels of stress and trauma. In a Veterans Aging Cohort Study (VACS) reviewing 81,000 patients with HIV, renal disease (GFR <30) was associated with a hazard ratio of 5 for development of heart failure.[40] This group has also highlighted the importance of anemia as a harbinger of very poor outcomes among HIV-infected patients. [41] In another study from the VA, depression, which has increased prevalence in HIV-infected patients,[42, 43] was independently associated with heart failure and myocardial infarction, with a 31% increased risk above other known risk factors.[44] In addition to depression, stress and psychological

trauma, both common in the HIV population, have been linked to adverse health outcomes and may influence CVD risk.[45, 46]

At present, the recommended management of CVD risk follows that for those without HIV infection, although some HIV clinicians favor a more aggressive approach. Drug–drug interactions, especially between statins and ART (e.g., lovastatin and simvastatin are contraindicated with protease inhibitors), must be recognized and drug selection and dosing adjusted accordingly.[47]

Renal disease

The 2009 Medical Monitoring Project evaluated the prevalence of chronic kidney disease (CKD) in the HIV-infected population and emphasized the importance of recognizing impaired renal function. These data estimated that age older than 60 years was associated with a hazard ratio (HR) of 7.8 for development of CKD, defined in this study as glomerular filtration rate (GFR) <60 mL/min/1.73 m^2 using the MDRD. [48] Other risk factors for CKD were female gender (HR: 1.4), longer duration of HIV infection (HR: 1.4), CD4 <350 cells/mm^3 (HR: 1.6), and AIDS (HR: 2.1). Causes of renal impairment in the setting of HIV infection include the virus itself. HIV replicates in the kidney, and moderate HIV-associated nephropathy improves with the start of HIV medications. Tenofovir can cause a Fanconi's syndrome characterized by proteinuria, glycosuria, and phosphate wasting. This adverse effect accounts for less than 5% of cases of acute kidney injury in HIV-positive patients and is usually reversible.[49] The protease inhibitor atazanavir can crystalize in the urine and form kidney stones.[50] Non-HIV-related etiologies of renal problems include hypertension, diabetes, and nonsteroidal anti-inflammatory use.

Recognition of CKD in the HIV-infected population is important, given the major role of renal function in medication clearance and the resultant risk of drug toxicity from pharmacologic treatment for HIV and other comorbidities.

Liver disease

Hepatitis is an important predictor of mortality in the HIV-infected population; liver disease in HIV-infected patients is associated with increased hospitalization, morbidity, and mortality.[51] Risk for liver disease in HIV-infected patients is multifactorial.

Infection with hepatitis B and C, alcohol use, diabetes, and rapid weight gain all contribute. Fatty liver disease is not uncommon. Additionally, older patients are more likely to have end-stage liver disease compared with younger patients due to longer or more rapid courses of hepatitis infection. Hepatotoxicity due to multidrug ART is rare but can occur. Awareness of the presence of liver disease is important for providers when managing complicated medication regimens with hepatic clearance as well as for anticipating prognosis. Referral for treatment of hepatitis C with direct acting agents is essential in HIV patients; staging of disease and vaccination against hepatitis A and B are responsibilities of the primary care physician. Screening for hepatitis B should be initiated as soon as HIV is diagnosed, and management or referral should be initiated as soon as possible, because hepatitis B–related cirrhosis and hepatocellular carcinoma in HIV-infected patients are significantly more common in the older patient. Treatment of hepatitis B in HIV-infected patients requires two nucleoside agents, as compared to only one in most non-HIV-infected patients. Screening for hepatocellular carcinoma (HCC) in the older patient involves liver ultrasound every six months.

Bone health and fractures

Low bone mineral density (BMD) is prevalent in HIV-infected persons. Bone loss may be due to ART, as well as traditional osteoporosis risk factors such as low levels of vitamin D, low body mass, alcohol use, corticosteroids, and proton pump inhibitors. Fracture rates in the HIV-infected population are estimated to be 30%–70% higher than in age-matched controls.[52] In older patients, this can greatly impact function and independence.

ART initiation is associated with a sharp decline in BMD.[53] Patients may experience a decrease in BMD from 2% to 6% over the first two years after initiation of ART, a decline that is similar to that experienced as a result of menopause and is independent of the ART regimen selected. Recent research suggests that supplementation with vitamin D and calcium may attenuate bone loss.[54] In a clinical trial of 165 patients started on efavirenz/emtricitabine/tenofovir, bone loss at the hip was 50% lower in the group receiving 4,000 IU of vitamin D and 1,000 mg of calcium daily. Supplementation with daily calcium

(1,000 mg–1,500 mg) and vitamin D (800 IU–1,000 IU) for all HIV-infected patients has been suggested, although this has not been incorporated into treatment guidelines.[52]

Screening for bone disease with dual-energy x-ray absorptiometry (DXA) is currently recommended for women ≥ 65 years old, men ≥ 70 years old, and any person with a fragility fracture regardless of age.[55] If additional risk factors are present, DXA scanning should be considered at earlier ages. Currently, HIV infection is not considered a risk factor for bone loss; however, some experts recommend DXA for all HIV-infected postmenopausal women, as well as men ≥ 50 years old, due to the high incidence of BMD in this population.[52]

Treatment recommendations for bone loss are consistent with those published by the National Osteoporosis Foundation.[55] Briefly, patients who have a T-score at the hip, femoral neck, or lumbar spine less than or equal to –2.5 or have a history of fragility fracture, should be considered for pharmacologic treatment. Patients should be reevaluated every two to five years based on the proximity of their results to treatment thresholds. Fracture risk should be calculated for all patients with osteopenia, using the World Health Organization (WHO) Fracture Risk Assessment Tool (FRAX) to further determine potential candidates for pharmacologic treatment.[56] As with all patients with severe bone disease, rheumatologists and endocrinologists play a significant role in comanaging these patients, in part because HIV is associated with hypogonadism at a higher rate than in non-HIV-infected persons

Psychiatric illness

HIV-positive older adults have higher rates of depression and poorer cognitive function compared to HIV-negative age-matched adults.[57] Untreated depression is a predictor of nonadherence to treatment and portends adverse effects on overall morbidity and mortality.[58] As older patients with HIV infection have inherently more severe disease and complications from comorbidities, identifying barriers to ART adherence is essential. When evaluating patients for depression, providers must consider concomitant HIV-associated dementia (HAD), which can often present with apathy, lethargy, and social withdrawal.[59] Although depressive symptoms should be appropriately treated, patients with symptoms concerning for neurocognitive impairment require further evaluation.

In addition to depressive disorders, anxiety, panic, and substance abuse disorders are prominent in HIV-positive patients regardless of age. Estimates predict that 18% of older HIV-infected adults experience anxiety disorders and 30% of older HIV-infected adults continue to use illicit substances.[60] Medications utilized to treat any psychiatric illness should be closely evaluated with regard to their metabolism by the cytochrome P450 3A4 isoenzyme system, which is strongly inhibited by protease inhibitors, a backbone in HIV treatment regimens.[61] Benzodiazepines, already recognized in the geriatric patient population as potentially harmful, in particular are potentially dangerous, especially when utilized in the long-acting form.

Cognitive impairment, HAND, and peripheral neuropathy

Nearly 50% of HIV-infected adults demonstrate impaired performance on neuropsychological testing consistent with cognitive impairment.[14, 15] Only a quarter of these patients endorse symptoms, and only half of symptomatic patients will meet diagnostic criteria for HIV-associated dementia (HAD).[14] Although few patients meet criteria for HAD, many demonstrate functional impairment due to cognitive dysfunction and meet criteria for HIV-associated neurocognitive disorder (HAND). HAND and HAD predominantly affect subcortical processes, which manifest through impaired executive and frontal lobe functions. Patients typically endorse difficulty completing tasks, maintaining attention, and learning new material, as well as difficulty with balance and motor coordination.[15] On cognitive testing, HAND manifests as impaired attention and concentration, psychomotor slowing, executive dysfunction, and impaired recall and learning. Visuospatial and semantic abilities are spared.[50] Patients may have depression, impaired manual dexterity, gait disturbance, and impaired information retrieval.[16] Patients with HAND demonstrate difficulty with ART adherence, making screening and identification of cognitive impairment imperative for successful treatment. HIV patients with advanced disease may develop progressive multifocal leukoencephalopathy, which requires management modalities familiar in geriatric medicine, including physical and occupational therapy, incontinence supplies, safety evaluations, and advance directives.

Currently, there are no established consensus recommendations for particular screening tools to utilize in this population. The Montreal Cognitive Assessment fares well given its evaluation of executive and other higher cognitive abilities; however, validation studies are lacking. The Mini-Mental State Exam fails to address domains primarily impaired in HAND and should not be used for screening. Both the HIV Dementia Scale and International HIV Dementia Scale are well validated to detect HAND; however, they are limited by their inability to detect clinically significant impairment that is not severe.[61, 62] A review by Valcour et al. extensively reviewed screening instruments specific for use in the HIV population and may serve as a useful reference.[63] Regardless of the screening method utilized, providers should recognize that cognitive impairment in HIV is prevalent and presents with changes in behavior, motor, and cognitive domains.

Both HIV and some of the older antiretroviral medications rarely in use today can cause peripheral neuropathy. This may manifest as numbness of the distal extremities, similar to diabetic sensory neuropathy or be painful with burning and tingling. Treatment of peripheral neuropathy in the setting of HIV is similar to that of diabetic neuropathy and range from topical treatment such as capsaicin or lidocaine to antiepileptic medications such as gabapentin. In some cases, careful administration of narcotics is required.

Functional decline

HIV-infected adults experience functional limitations earlier than HIV-negative adults.[64] In addition to high rates of multimorbidity, HIV-infected older adults often lack social and familial support at the time of functional decline. Fragile social networks are a limitation for many older adults who need assistance in order to maintain independence.[65] Nearly 70% of HIV-infected older adults live alone and are estranged from family and friends due to their HIV/AIDS diagnosis.[66] As the population of HIV-infected adults ages and experiences complications of multimorbidity, adverse effects of treatment, and premature aging, consideration of the role of available caregivers, or lack thereof, is important for helping patients manage functional decline.

ART-associated adverse events and the importance of polypharmacy

Although ART is overall beneficial in the older HIV-infected patient, reducing progression of AIDS and reducing mortality, it can be associated with toxicity in this population. Reductions in drug clearance due to renal and hepatic impairment can lead to drug accumulation and heighten risk of adverse effects.

In addition, polypharmacy can result in significant drug–drug interactions between ART and other indicated medications. Awareness of the potential for such interactions is essential. An online database of potential drug interactions with ART can be found at www.HIV-druginteractions.org, at Micromedex, and at hivinsite.ucsf.edu.

ART adherence

Older adults demonstrate greater adherence to ART compared with the younger HIV-infected population. [67] However, risk of cognitive impairment increases with age and is a legitimate concern when managing HIV-positive adults due to its potential impact on treatment adherence. Older patients with detectable viral loads are twice as likely to have cognitive impairment as similarly aged patients with undetectable viral loads; this may serve as an indicator to clinicians that patients need to be evaluated for treatment adherence.[68] Providers should also be aware that patients with depression and other psychiatric disorders are at increased risk for nonadherence and should be evaluated to assess compliance with treatment.

Prevention

Minimizing disease transmission remains a core tenet of HIV education and patient care; however, elderly patients remain at risk for new infections, in part due to lack of patient and provider education. There were only 49,274 new HIV infections reported in 2011, and 9% (4,489) occurred in patients 55 and older; this is increased from 5% of new infections reported in 2010 (2,500).[69] Although older adults engage in risky behaviors, lack of perceived risk leads to failure to adopt safer practices.[70] Sexual activity among older adults is consistently underestimated. Sexual activity does decrease with age and is less commonly reported by women, but a study of 3,005 adults in the United States aged 57 to 85 emphasizes the importance of recognizing ongoing sexual activity.

Overall, 73% of respondents aged 57–64, 53% of respondents aged 65–74, and 26% of respondents aged 75–85 reported sexual activity in the preceding 12 months.[10] Sexual activity in this sample correlated with overall health and self-reported well-being.

Male-with-male unprotected sex is the chief risk factor in older men and accounted for 60% of new infections in 2010. Due to social stigmatization, many older men have decreased self-identification with their sexuality and are in denial about their increased risk of HIV. Heterosexual contact and intravenous drug use are the second and third risk factors, accounting for 23% and 14% of infections, respectively. During this same time period, 82% of older women were infected through heterosexual contact, and intravenous drug use accounted for 18%.[1]

In addition to risk factors related to sexual activity, older adults are at increased risk for infection due to a variety of physical and psychosocial factors including:

- less knowledge about HIV
- less education about HIV prevention
- denial regarding their own risk factors for HIV infection
- a sense of false security about risk because they are in monogamous or "nearly monogamous" relationships
- decreased screening due to lack of patient and provider awareness of HIV risk factors and prevalence
- decreased screening due to provider discomfort asking about sexual activity and habits
- increased risk of stigmatization and lack of social support in the community once diagnosed with HIV
- increased susceptibility to new infection due to age-related immune compromise
- increased transmission risk in postmenopausal women due to age-related vaginal wall dryness and thinning from estrogen loss
- decreased condom use due to lack of concern for pregnancy
- decreased condom use due to erectile dysfunction [71, 72]

HIV prevention and health education materials targeted to older persons are lacking and must counter the challenge of stigmatization and lack of social support that elders may encounter.[73] Older adults self-identify stigmatization due to HIV status more often than younger adults and are less likely to disclose their HIV status to relatives, partners, church members, or neighbors.[74] Further barriers to educating older adults about HIV may exist at the level of the medical provider. Literature suggests that even when older adults had questions and were willing to discuss these issues with their health-care providers, they were uncomfortable broaching the subject without the conversation being initiated by their provider.[71] Only 38% of men and 22% of women reported discussing sex with a physician after the age of 50.[10] Physician recognition of HIV risk factors and the existence of social supports are essential not only for individualized HIV care and acceptance of HIV-infected patients in the community, they play an important role in minimizing exposures to new infection.

Summary

1. The population of older adults with HIV in the United States and worldwide is increasing, due to aging of the HIV-infected population as well as new infections in adults 50 years of age and older.

2. Older adults have more advanced HIV at the time of presentation compared to younger patients. A low suspicion for HIV infection contributes to delayed diagnosis.

3. Older adults are less knowledgeable about HIV compared with younger adults and are less likely to ask providers about sexual health or HIV. Older adults also tend to lack community support and may be stigmatized due to HIV diagnosis.

4. HIV infection should be considered when patients present with new dementia or neurologic findings and if laboratory studies are significant for unexplained elevated protein, lymphopenia, or anemia.

5. Older HIV-infected adults have a high level of comorbidity and are at risk for functional decline.

6. ART should be prescribed to older adults. Awareness of drug metabolism should guide drug selection, monitoring for adverse effects, and consideration of avoidable drug interactions.

7. Older adults have robust virologic responses to treatment and delayed but similar immunologic responses compared to younger patients. Despite this, they have increased progression to AIDS within the first year of presentation.

Recommended additional resources

Patient and provider education on HIV

University of North Carolina Center for Aging and Health. HIV/AIDS in Older Adults. Available at: www.med.unc.edu/aging/elderhiv/act.htm.

Provider education on HIV

"HIV Infection in the Elderly" by Kelly Gebo and Amy Justice. In: *Current Infectious Disease Reports*. 2009;11(3):246–254.

Primary care guidelines for managing HIV

"Primary Care Guidelines for the Management of Persons Infected with HIV: 2013 Update" by the HIV Medicine Association of the Infectious Diseases Society of America. Available at: www.idsociety.org. *Clinical Infectious Disease*. 2014;58(1):1–10.

Monitoring antiretroviral medications

"HIV Infection in the Elderly" by Nancy Nguyen and Mark Holodniy. Available at: *Clinical Interventions in Aging*. 2008;3(3):453–472.

World Health Organization Consolidated Guidelines on the Use of Antiretroviral Drugs for Treating and Preventing HIV Infection. Available at: www.who.int/hiv/en.

References

1. Centers for Disease Control. HIV among older Americans, 2013. Available at: www.cdc.gov/hiv/risk/age/olderamericans/index.html (accessed December 4, 2014).

2. O'Keefe KJ, Scheer S, Chen MJ, et al. People fifty years or older now account for the majority of AIDS cases in San Francisco, California, 2010. *AIDS Care*. 2013;25(9):1145–8.

3. CDC. HIV Surveillance Report, 2011. Available at: www.cdc.gov/hiv/library/reports/surveillance/2011/surveillance_Report_vol_23.html (accessed December 4, 2014).

4. Samji H, Cescon A, Hogg RS, et al. Closing the gap: increases in life expectancy among treated HIV-positive individuals in the United States and Canada. *PLoS One*. 2013 Dec 18;8(12):e81355.

5. Luther VP, Wilkin AM. HIV infection in older adults. *Clin Geriatr Med*. 2007 Aug;23(3):567–83, vii.

6. Illa L, Brickman A, Saint-Jean G, et al. Sexual risk behaviors in late middle age and older HIV seropositive adults. *AIDS Behav*. 2008 Nov;12(6):935–42.

7. Lekas HM, Schrimshaw EW, Siegel K. Pathways to HIV testing among adults aged fifty and older with HIV/AIDS. *AIDS Care*. 2005 Aug;**17**(6):674–87.

8. Branson BM, Handsfield HH, Lampe MA, et al. Revised recommendations for HIV testing of adults, adolescents, and pregnant women in health-care settings. *MMWR Recomm Rep*. 2006 Sep 22;**55**(RR-14):1–17.

9. US Preventive Services Task Force. AHRQ publication number 12–05173-EF-3. April 2013. Available at: www.cdc.gov/nchhstp/preventionthroughhealthcare/preventiveservices/hivaids.htm (accessed February 4, 2016).

10. Lindau ST, Schumm LP, Laumann EO, et al. A study of sexuality and health among older adults in the United States. *N Engl J Med*. 2007 Aug 23;**357**(8):762–74.

11. CDC and APHL. Laboratory testing for the diagnosis of HIV infection: updated recommendations. Version June 27, 2014. Available at: http://stacks.cdc.gov/view/cdc/23447 (accessed February 4, 2016).

12. Stoff DM, Khalsa JH, Monjan A, Portegies P. Introduction: HIV/AIDS and Aging. *AIDS*. 2004 Jan 1;**18**(Suppl 1):S1–2.

13. Observational HIV Epidemiological Research Europe (COHERE) Study Group, Sabin CA, Smith CJ, et al. Response to combination antiretroviral therapy: variation by age. *AIDS*. 2008 Jul 31;**22**(12):1463–73.

14. Heaton RK, Franklin DR, Ellis RJ, et al. HIV-associated neurocognitive disorders before and during the era of combination antiretroviral therapy: differences in rates, nature, and predictors. *J Neurovirol*. 2011 Feb;**17**(1):3–16.

15. Ances BM, Ellis RJ. Dementia and neurocognitive disorders due to HIV-1 infection. *Semin Neurol*. 2007 Feb;**27**(1):86–92.

16. McArthur JC, Haughey N, Gartner S, et al. Human immunodeficiency virus-associated dementia: an evolving disease. *J Neurovirol*. 2003 Apr;**9**(2):205–21.

17. Engels EA, Biggar RJ, Hall HI, et al. Cancer risk in people infected with human immunodeficiency virus in the United States. *Int J Cancer*. 2008;**123**:187–94.

18. Szerlip MA, DeSalvo KB, Szerlip HM. Predictors of HIV-infection in older adults. *J Aging Health*. 2005 Jun;**17**(3):293–304.

19. Guaraldi G, Orlando G, Zona S, et al. Premature age-related comorbidities among HIV-infected persons compared with the general population. *Clin Infect Dis*. 2011 Dec;**53**(11):1120–6.

20. Goulet JL, Fultz SL, Rimland D, et al. Aging and infectious diseases: do patterns of comorbidity vary by HIV status, age, and HIV severity? *Clin Infect Dis*. 2007;**45**:1593–1601.

21. Losina E, Linas B, Hyle E, et al. Projecting 10-year, 20-year, and lifetime risks of cardiovascular disease in HIV+ individuals in the US: competing risks and premature aging. *Program and abstracts of the 20th Conference on Retroviruses and Opportunistic Infections*; March 3–6, 2013; Atlanta, GA. Abstract 747.

22. Bhavan KP, Kampalath VN, Overton ET. The aging of the HIV epidemic. *Curr HIV/AIDS Rep*. 2008;**5**:150–8.

23. Triant VA, Lee H, Hadigan C, Grinspoon SK. Increased acute myocardial infarction rates and cardiovascular risk factors among patients with human immunodeficiency virus disease. *J Clin Endocrinol Metab*. 2007 Jul;**92**(7):2506–12.

24. Johnsen S, Dolan SE, Fitch KV, et al. Carotid intimal medial thickness in human immunodeficiency virus-infected women: effects of protease inhibitor use, cardiac risk factors, and the metabolic syndrome. *J Clin Endocrinol Metab*. 2006 Dec;**91**(12):4916–24.

25. Post WS, Budoff M, Kingsley L, et al. Associations between HIV infection and subclinical coronary atherosclerosis. *Ann Intern Med* 2014 Apr 1;**160**(7):458–67.

26. Bedimo R, Zhang S, Drechsler H, et al. Osteoporotic fracture risk associated with cumulative exposure to tenofovir and other antiretroviral agents. Program and abstracts of the 6th International AIDS Society Conference on HIV Pathogenesis, Treatment, and Prevention; July 17–20, 2011; Rome, Italy. Abstract MoAB0101.

27. Gebo KA, Justice A. HIV infection in the elderly. *Curr Infect Dis Rep*. 2009 May;**11**(3):246–54.

28. Margolick J, Detels R, Phair J, et al. Earlier occurrence of the frailty phenotype in HIV+ men than HIV- men: the MACS. *Program and abstracts of the 18th Conference on Retroviruses and Opportunistic Infections*; February 27–March 2, 2011; Boston, MA. Abstract 794.

29. Deeks SG, Lewin SR, Havlir DV. The end of AIDS: HIV infection as a chronic disease. *Lancet*. 2013 Nov 2;**382**(9903):1525–33.

30. Hunt PW, Martin JN, Sinclair E, et al. T cell activation is associated with lower CD4+ T cell gains in human immunodeficiency virus-infected patients with sustained viral suppression during antiretroviral therapy. *J Infect Dis*. 2003 May 15;**187**(10):1534–43.

31. Sandler NG, Wand H, Roque A, et al. Plasma levels of soluble CD14 independently predict mortality in HIV infection. *J Infect Dis*. 2011 Mar 15;**203**(6):780–90.

32. Brenchley JM, Prince DA, Schacker TW, et al. Microbial translocation is a cause of systemic immune activation in chronic HIV infection. *Nat Med*. 2006 Dec;**12**(12):1365–71.

33. Hunt PW, Martin JN, Sinclair E, et al. Valganciclovir reduces T cell activation in HIV-infected individuals

with incomplete CD4+ T cell recovery on antiretroviral therapy. *J Infect Dis.* 2011 May 15;**203**(10):1474–83.

34. Fitch KV, Looby SE, Rope A, et al. Effects of aging and smoking on carotid intima-media thickness in HIV-infection. *AIDS.* 2013 Jan 2;**27**(1):49–57.

35. Sabin C, Reiss P, Ryom L, et al. Is there continued evidence for an association between abacavir and myocardial infarction risk? *Program and abstracts of the 21st Conference on Retroviruses and Opportunistic Infections*; March 3–6, 2013; Boston, MA. Abstract 747LB.

36. Lichtenstein KA, Armon C, Buchacz K, et al; HIV Outpatient Study (HOPS) Investigators. Low CD4+ T cell count is a risk factor for cardiovascular disease events in the HIV outpatient study. *Clin Infect Dis.* 2010;**51**:435–47.

37. Lichtenstein KA, Armon C, Buchacz K, et al. Initiation of antiretroviral therapy at CD4 cell counts ≥350 cells/mm3 does not increase incidence or risk of peripheral neuropathy, anemia, or renal insufficiency. *J Acquir Immune DeficSyndr.* 2008;**47**(1):27–35.

38. Strategies for Management of Antiretroviral Therapy (SMART) Study Group. CD4+ count-guided interruption of antiretroviral treatment. *N Engl J Med.* 2006 Nov 30;**355**(22):2283–96.

39. Klein DB, Leyden WA, Chao CR, et al. No difference in incidence of myocardial infarction for HIV+ and HIV-individuals in recent years. Program and abstracts of the 21st Conference on Retroviruses and Opportunistic Infections; March 3–6, 2013; Boston, MA. Abstract 737.

40. Llibre JM, Falco V, Tural C, et al. The changing face of HIV/AIDS in treated patients. *Curr HIV Res.* 2009 Jul;**7**(4):365–77.

41. Justice AC, McGinnis KA, Skanderson M, et al.; VACS Project Team. Towards a combined prognostic index for survival in HIV infection: the role of "non-HIV" biomarkers. *HIV Med.* 2010 Feb;**11**(2):143–51.

42. White JR, Chang CH, Butt AA, et al. Depression and HIV are risk factors for incident heart failure among veterans [CROI abstract 726]. In Special Issue: Abstracts from the 2014 Conference on Retroviruses and Opportunistic Infections. *Top Antivir Med.* 2014;**22**(e-1):369–70.

43. Atkinson JH, Heaton RK, Patterson TL, et al. Two-year prospective study of major depressive disorder in HIV-infected men. *J Affect Disord.* 2008 Jun;**108**(3):225–34.

44. Khambaty T, Stewart JC, Gupta SK, et al. Depression predicts incident myocardial infarction in HIV+ veterans: Veterans Aging Cohort Study [CROI abstract 735]. In Special Issue: Abstracts from the 2014 Conference on Retroviruses and Opportunistic Infections. *Top Antivir Med.* 2014;**22**(3-1):375.

45. Batten SV, Aslan M, Maciejewski PK, Mazure CM. Childhood maltreatment as a risk factor for adult cardiovascular disease and depression. *J Clin Psychiatry.* 2004 Feb;**65**(2):249–54.

46. Dale S, Franklin G, Kelso R, et al. Childhood sexual abuse, traditional gender roles, and coronary heart disease risk among women with HIV. Second International Workshop on HIV & Women; 2012. Abstract P_14.

47. Panel on Antiretroviral Guidelines for Adults and Adolescents. Guidelines for the use of antiretroviral agents in HIV-1-infected adults and adolescents. Department of Health and Human Services. Available at: http://aidsinfo.nih.gov/ContentFiles/Adultand AdolescentGL.pdf (accessed December 4, 2014).

48. Garg S, Furlow-Parmley C, Frazier E, et al. Prevalence of chronic kidney disease among HIV+ adults in care in the US: medical monitoring Project 2009. [CROI abstract 809]. *Program and abstracts of the 20th Conference on Retroviruses and Opportunistic Infections.* March 3–6, 2013; Atlanta, GA.

49. Wyatt CM. Antiretroviral therapy and the kidney. *Top Antivir Med.* 2014 Jun–Jul;**22**(3):655–8.

50. Rockwood N, Mandalia S, Bower M, et al. Ritonavir-boosted atazanavir exposure is associated with an increased rate of renal stones compared with efavirenz, ritonavir-boosted lopinavir and ritonavir-boosted darunavir. *AIDS.* 2011 Aug 24;**25**(13):1671–3.

51. Gebo KA, Diener-West M, Moore RD. Hospitalization rates differ by hepatitis C satus in an urban HIV cohort. *J Acquir Immune Defic Syndr.* 2003 Oct 1;**34**(2):165–73.

52. McCommey GA, Tebas P, Shane E, et al. Bone disease in HIV infection: a practical review and recommendations for HIV care providers. *Clin Infect Dis.* 2010 Oct 15;**51**(8):937–46.

53. Tebas P, Powderly WG, Claxton S, et al. Accelerated bone mineral loss in HIV-infected patients receiving potent antiretroviral therapy. *AIDS.* 2000 Mar 10;**14**(4):F63–7.

54. Overton ET, Chan ES, Brown TT, et al. High-dose vitamin D and calcium attenuates bone loss with ART initiation: results from ACTG A5280 [CROI abstract 133]. In Special Issue: Abstracts from the 2014 Conference on Retroviruses and Opportunistic Infections. *Top Antivir Med.* 2014;**22**(e-1):66–7.

55. National Osteoporosis Foundation. *Clinician's Guide to Prevention and Treatment of Osteoporosis.* Washington, DC: National Osteoporosis Foundation; 2010.

56. University of Sheffield U. FRAX WHO Fracture Risk Assessment Tool. Available at: www.shef.ac.uk/FRAX/tool.aspx (accessed December 4, 2014).

57. Skapik JL, Treisman GJ. HIV, psychiatric comorbidity, and aging. *Clinical Geriatrics.* 2007(15):26–36.

58. Gonzalez JS, Batchelder AW, Psaros C, Safren SA. Depression and HIV/AIDS treatment nonadherence: a review and meta-analysis. *J Acquir Immune Defic Syndr*. 2011 Oct 1;**58**(2):181–7.

59. Goodkin K. Psychiatric aspects of HIV spectrum disease. *Focus Psychiatry Review*. 2007;**7**(3):303–10.

60. Zanjani F, Saboe K, Oslin D. Age difference in rates of mental health/substance abuse and behavioral care in HIV-positive adults. *AIDS Patient Care Stds*. 2007 May;**21**(5):347–55.

61. Work Group for HIV and Aging Consensus Project. Summary report from the Human Immunodeficiency Virus and Aging Consensus Project: treatment strategies for clinicians managing older individuals with the human immunodeficiency virus. *J Am Geriatr Soc*. 2012 May;**60**(5):974–9.

62. Power C, Selnes OA, Grim JA, McArthur JC. HIV Dementia Scale: a rapid screening test. *J Acquir Immune Defic Syndr Hum Retrovirol*. 1995 Mar 1;**8**(3):273–8.

63. Valcour V, Paul R, Chiao S, et al. Screening for cognitive impairment in human immunodeficiency virus. *Clin Infect Dis*. 2011 Oct;**53**(8):836–42.

64. Oursler KK, Sorkin JD, Smith BA, Katzel LI. Reduced aerobic capacity and physical functioning in older HIV-infected men. *AIDS Res Hum Retroviruses*. 2006 Nov;**22**(11):1113–21.

65. Shippy RA, Karpiak SE. The aging HIV/AIDS population: fragile social networks. *Aging Ment Health*. 2005 May;**9**(3):246–54.

66. Brennan DJ, Emlet CA, Eady A. HIV, sexual health, and psychosocial issues among older adults living with HIV in North America. *Ageing International*. 2011;**36**(3):313–33.

67. Silverberg MJ, Leyden W, Horberg MA, et al. Older age and the response to and tolerability of antiretroviral therapy. *Arch Intern Med*. 2007 Apr 9;**167**(7):684–91.

68. Vance DE, Burrage JW. Promoting successful cognitive aging in adults with HIV: strategies for intervention. *J Gerontol Nurs*. 2006 Nov;**32**(11):34–41

69. Centers for Disease Control. HIV surveillance report: diagnoses of HIV infection and AIDS in the United States and dependent areas, 2011. Available at: www.cdc.gov/hiv/statistics/basics (accessed December 4, 2014).

70. Goodroad BK. HIV and AIDS in people older than 50: a continuing concern. *J Gerontol Nurs*. 2003 Apr;**29**(4):18–24.

71. Linsk NL. HIV among older adults: age-specific issues in prevention and treatment. *AIDS Read*. 2000 Jul;**10**(7):430–40.

72. Skiest DJ, Keiser P. Human immunodeficiency virus infection in patients older than 50 years: a survey of primary care physicians' beliefs, practices, and knowledge. *Arch Fam Med*. 1997 May–Jun;**6**(3):289–94.

73. Orel NA, Wright JM, Wagner J. Scarcity of HIV/AIDS risk-reduction materials targeting the needs of older adults among state departments of public health. *Gerontologist*. 2004 Oct;**44**(5):693–6.

74. Centers for Disease Control and Prevention. HIV-related knowledge and stigma: United States, 2000. *MMWR*. 2000;**49**(RR47):1062–4.

Chapter 25

Renal disorders in the elderly

William D. Sirover, MD, Brooke Salzman, MD, and
Christopher B. McFadden, MD

Introduction

Kidney anatomy and function change with increasing age. A large cohort trial noted the decline in creatinine clearance of 1 mL/min/year beginning in the fifth decade of life.[1] These changes may begin to occur at the age of 40, if not before.[2] Pathologically, glomerulosclerosis of cortical glomeruli is a common finding in elderly subjects.[3] Clinically, elderly subjects develop a number of alterations in renal function related to change in renal blood flow, loss of glomeruli and changes in tubular function. Such changes in renal function include a reduced ability to raise glomerular filtration rate (GFR) during times of stress and a reduction in renal dilution and concentration abilities.[4–7] These changes have the potential to increase the risk of acute kidney injury and electrolyte imbalances as well as lead to long-term abnormalities in kidney function. To what extent long-term abnormalities in kidney function represent normal aging or a disease state is an area of debate.

Chronic kidney disease

Chronic kidney disease (CKD) is a five-tier disease state based on abnormalities in kidney function and/or other urinary abnormalities such as microscopic hematuria or proteinuria for three or more months. An equation designed from the Modification of Diet in Renal Disease Study (MDRD) uses age, sex, gender, race, and serum creatinine to estimate GFR.[8] CKD affects 10%–13% of the adult US population.[9] A large number of elderly subjects fall into stage 3 CKD because of the impact of their age, and this may label them with an inappropriate disease state. [10, 11] The level of proteinuria becomes very important in determining prognosis. Finally, muscle mass declines in older age and creatinine would be expected to decrease. Practically speaking then, healthcare providers need to recognize how different levels of kidney function can be associated with a creatinine of 1.2 mg/dL. Table 25.1 illustrates this point.

Most CKD patients do not progress to end-stage renal disease (ESRD) because of intrinsic CKD stability as well as the high rate of cardiovascular and noncardiovascular mortality in this population.[12–15] Proposals exist to more clearly distinguish elderly subjects with stage 3 CKD who are more likely to have progressive disease from those whose renal dysfunction appears less progressive and more age related.[11] Consequently, a growing body of literature supports the use of stage 3A and stage 3B to define those patients who have an eGFR of 45–60 and 30–44 mL/min, respectively. In the absence of proteinuria or other signs of inflammatory kidney disease, it is not expected that patients with stage 3A disease will progress.[16] The CKD EPI (Chronic Kidney Disease Epidemiology Collaboration) formula and the MDRD equation both estimate GFR, but the CKD-EPI formula classifies fewer individuals as having kidney disease.[17] This formula may be more specific for identifying renal dysfunction in the geriatric population, although studies are ongoing.

Table 25.1 Estimated GFR with a serum creatinine of 1.2 mg/dL among different individuals

Based on 4 variable eGFR formula (Levey, AS, Annals, 1999); (results per 1.73 m^2 BSA)	
80-year-old African-American male	71 mL/min
80-year-old Caucasion female	43 mL/min
40-year-old Caucasian male	67 mL/min
40-year-old African-American female	60 mL/min

Reichel's Care of the Elderly, 7th Edition, ed. Jan Busby-Whitehead *et al.* Published by Cambridge University Press.
© Cambridge University Press 2016.

Table 25.2 Common chronic kidney disease etiologies in elderly patients

Disease	UA findings
Atherosclerotic renal vascular disease protein	Negative blood, negative to trace
Glomerular	Variable blood, moderate to large protein
Membranous	Variable blood, moderate to large protein
Diabetic nephrosclerosis	
Focal segmental glomerlosclerosis	Variable blood, moderate to large protein
Light chain depostion disease (myeloma)	Variable blood, small to moderate protein
Myeloma cast nephropathy	Variable blood, small to moderate protein
Obstructive uropathy	Variable blood, negative to small protein

Dipstick result may be falsely low due to nonalbumin proteins.

A broad variety of disease states can lead to chronic kidney disease. As much as possible, delineating the cause of disease is important in order to predict which patients are at higher risk of progression. Table 25.2 lists causes of abnormal kidney function commonly seen in elderly patients and the associated urinary findings seen for each. Other diseases that patients have experienced in the past may result in abnormal kidney function. One classic example is reflux nephropathy as a child manifesting as subtle renal dysfunction in an adult. The pathologic finding that differentiates advancing kidney disease from previous renal injury is glomerulosclerosis. In examples such as this, particularly with limited proteinuria, a biopsy is usually not pursued if it is not felt to alter therapy. As a general rule, kidney disease progression is less likely to occur in diseases without inflammation (hematuria) or significant glomerular disease (proteinuria).

Determining the cause of CKD in elderly subjects is no different than nonelderly subjects and involves a thorough medical history, physical examination, and evaluation of the urine. Important considerations include a history of frequent urinary infections (particularly as a child) suggestive of reflux nephropathy, symptoms and signs of a connective tissue disease or vasculitis, use of NSAIDs (which may lead to temporary renal dysfunction due to reduced blood flow or chronic interstitial nephritis), or suggestions of significant peripheral vascular disease. The latter may be suggestive of atherosclerotic renal vascular disease. As noted in Table 25.2, a UA without blood or protein rules out most glomerular disease except those related to myeloma. For this reason, all elderly subjects with unexplained kidney disease should have at least one spot urine protein (not albumin) to urine creatinine ratio in order to exclude proteinuria. Spot urine protein/creatinine ratios provide enough information to assess proteinuria levels and, as a result, a 24-hour urine collection is no longer required. However, the urine protein to creatinine ratio *cannot* be assessed with a traditional office dipstick for protein, as the office dipstick only reacts to urinary albumin.

Despite the high prevalence of kidney disease in the United States, only a small number of patients progress to ESRD. This relates to the stability of most cases of CKD as well as the large burden of cardiovascular disease in this population.[18] Additional complications related to kidney disease include anemia, metabolic acidosis, hypertension, and CKD mineral-bone disorder (MBD) manifested as hyperparathyroidism and hyperphosphatemia. Prospective well-designed studies support the treatment of metabolic acidosis and hypertension, although the traditional goal blood pressure of 130/80 mm Hg has been replaced with 140/90 mm Hg.[19, 20] The treatment of anemia and CKD mineral bone disorder is based on guidelines with less prospective based evidence.[21, 22] A workshop recently reviewed the challenges to treating elderly subjects with CKD and areas in which focus should occur.[23] Major challenges identified by this group included best methods to differentiate age-related declines in kidney function from more aggressive disease states, the lack of prospective studies in the large population of elderly patients with CKD, and unique situation of elderly patients with CKD. For example, elderly CKD patients with less aggressive kidney disease, as shown by a lack of proteinuria, may not benefit from earlier referral to a nephrologist as would a younger patient.[24]

Acute kidney injury

Acute kidney injury (AKI) commonly occurs in elderly patients. Although the same differential diagnosis applies to patients of all ages, elderly patients are more prone to AKI due to several characteristics of the aging kidney. As mentioned earlier, anatomic and physiologic changes in the kidneys of elderly patients can have important consequences. Anatomically, kidney size diminishes with age.[25] This change is associated with microscopic findings that show decreased glomeruli number, glomerulosclerosis, tubulointerstitial fibrosis, and intimal thickening of arteries and arterioles.[26–28] With aging, muscle mass decreases. A creatinine in the normal reference range may be inappropriately high and could be indicative of AKI. Age-associated renal atrophy results in diminished capability to withstand pathologic insults and increased likelihood of developing AKI.

In addition, renal blood flow can decrease by 50% by the age of 80.[29] This decrease may be due, in part, to a reduction in prostaglandin and dopamine levels. [30] Nitric oxide (NO), a vasodilator that balances decreases of renal perfusion may be reduced in older adults.[31] In animal models of AKI, aged rats appear to be more sensitive to lowering of NO levels.[32] Overall, mechanisms needed to maintain renal blood flow to prevent renal injury may be significantly reduced with aging.[33] Additionally, NSAIDs, which are commonly administered to elderly patients, may further counteract these vasodilatory intrinsic compensatory processes.[34]

The algorithm for diagnosis of AKI begins by differentiating between prerenal, renal, and postrenal causes. Renal, or intrinsic renal causes, are divided in to acute tubular necrosis (ATN), AIN, glomerulopathies, vasculitis, and intratubular obstruction that can be seen, for instance, in uric acid nephropathy. In the inpatient setting, prerenal reasons can cause up to 30% of cases of AKI.[35, 36] Factors complicating AKI in the elderly patient include decrease in thirst sensation, impairment of urinary concentrating ability and concomitant diuretic usage.[37–39] Physiologic changes associated with the aging kidney may contribute to the development of AKI. For instance, (1) sodium reabsorption in the loop of Henle decreases with aging and (2) plasma renin and aldosterone levels also decrease.[33] This latter change causes less collecting tubule sodium reabsorption. With sodium loss from the body, hypovolemia may develop and could lead to AKI. Consistent with this pathophysiologic development, Macias et al. showed that when placed on low-sodium diets, elderly patients have higher urinary sodium levels compared to younger patients.[40]

A more common cause of AKI in the hospitalized setting is acute tubular necrosis (ATN), which occurs in up to 48% of cases in patients 65 years old and greater.[36] Sepsis is the most frequent cause of ATN. [41] ATN can also be caused by contrast dye and medications. In particular, NSAIDs are frequently recognized as the source of ATN.[34] Of note, contrast nephropathy can occur in 17% of elderly patients administered contrast dye during cardiac catheterization as compared to in 9.1% of the general population receiving contrast dye during cardiac catheterization. [42, 43] ATN due to contrast nephropathy is more common in the setting of CKD, diabetic nephropathy, hypovolemia, and use of ace inhibitors or angiotensin receptor blockers.[44, 45] In general, a less common cause of AKI is rapidly progressive glomerulonephritis. However, it occurs most in those 65 and older. The incidence is 60 cases per million in patients 65–74 years old.[46] Advancing age is not a contraindication for immunosuppression therapy.[47–50] Other less common causes of intrinsic renal disease to be considered as causes of AKI are interstitial nephritis and other glomerulopathies.

Lastly, from an intrinsic renal disease perspective, atherosclerotic vascular renal disease occurs in 42% of elderly patients.[51] Atheroembolic disease as a cause of AKI should be thought of in cases of aortic procedures, angiography, thrombolysis, and anticoagulation.[52–55] The remainder of AKI cases is due to post-renal causes. Post-renal causes include intrinsic ureteral obstruction (i.e., calculi, blood clots), extrinsic ureteral obstruction (i.e., malignancy), bladder outlet obstruction (i.e., prostatic hypertrophy), and urethral obstruction (i.e., stricture).[33]

As part of the AKI evaluation, urine indices including a random urine sodium are often obtained. Owing to increases in urinary sodium, in early stages of prerenal azotemia due to hypovolemia, urine sodium may be higher than the classical threshold of 20 meq/L.[33] Renal biopsy can be beneficial when intrinsic renal disease is suspected and the specific cause remains uncertain. Findings may alter management as histologic findings may indicate a disease different from the one suspected based on clinical grounds;[56] renal biopsy may directly influence treatment.[57]

Consistent with the anatomic and physiologic issues mentioned earlier, age has been independently associated with AKI.[58] After developing AKI, renal recovery has been reported in 43%–67% of patients. [41] The need for chronic dialysis has ranged from 2.7%–6% [59]. In another study, dialysis dependence was studied in 425 patients who needed hemodialysis after developing AKI due to ATN. Fifty-three percent of patients survived, of which 57% had complete recovery of renal function, 33% had creatinine levels >1.3 and <3 mg/dL, and 10% continued to have creatinine levels >3 mg/dL.[60] Although degree of illness, history of chronic kidney disease, and cause of CKD can affect the occurrence of renal recovery in the setting of AKI, the study of age as a prognostic factor has produced contradictory results.[41, 61–63] In terms of mortality, age has not been shown to be an associated factor in elderly patients.[62]

The preceding studies detail AKI in elderly inpatients. Feest et al. reported AKI risk in the outpatient setting.[64] In a large, community-based study, the incidence of AKI rose substantially with age. The annual incidence of AKI was 17 per million in adults <50 years old and increased with age to a yearly incidence of 949 per million in adults 80–89 years old. Medical causes included hypovolemia (34% of cases), and second most common was prostatic obstruction (25% of cases).

Hypertension in elderly subjects

A number of mechanisms lead to increased blood pressure in elderly subjects. First, systolic blood pressure increases with age, independent of CKD status, due to stiffening of vessels over time. A consequence of this is the frequent finding of isolated systolic hypertension and a large pulse pressure. In addition, CKD leads to elevations in sympathetic tone and hormones of the renin-angiotensin activating system. The major clinical consequence is increased vasoconstriction and increased sodium absorption in the kidney. Key medication classes directed at these dysfunctional physiologic systems include diuretics, ace-inhibitors, aldosterone antagonists, and beta blockers. Although beta blockers reduce renin levels, they are also associated with significant fatigue and, in the absence of clear cardiac indications, should not be first-line agents for blood pressure control.[20]

Recent blood pressure guidelines suggest that in the absence of chronic disease, blood pressure treatment targets in subjects over the age of 60 should be <150/90 mm Hg. This is largely based on the HYVET trial; importantly, nearly 30% of subjects in a subset of this trial had white coat HTN.[65] Consequently, a low threshold should be used to investigate for white coat hypertension by home BP monitoring or ambulatory blood pressure monitoring. Additional factors to consider in the elderly population include the potential need to reduce BP medications over time due to changes in diet and weight loss with advancing age, the need to monitor for orthostatic hypotension regularly, and the challenge of treating patients with isolated high systolic blood pressures.[66] Although patients with isolated high systolic blood pressures are at high risk for vascular events, lowering DBP to less than 55 mg Hg may lead to symptoms of cerebral, renal, or peripheral underperfusion.[67]

Fluid and electrolyte disorders associated with the aging kidney

Hyponatremia has been reported to occur in 20% of elderly patients, compared to 5% in all patients.[68] Hyponatremia risk increases with age.[69, 70] The syndrome of inappropriate antidiuretic hormone (SIADH) was found to be the etiology in 73.6% of normovolemic elderly patients.[71] Elderly patients treated with thiazide diuretics, bupropion, and SSRIs are more prone to become hyponatremic.[72–74] Consequences of hyponatremia may lead to gait disturbance, secondary falls and fracture risk.[75, 76] Intracellular sodium in bone can serve as a sodium reservoir and can be released in hyponatremia; resultant osteoporosis may further increase risk for fractures.[77] Also, regression analysis revealed that anemia is independently associated with hyponatremia and consideration should be given to monitoring hemoglobin levels in patients with this electrolyte abnormality.[78]

On the other side of the spectrum, hypernatremia also increases with age, with the most common cause due to bacterial infections.[79, 80] Decreased thirst response in elderly patients is a contributing factor. Azotemia may further exacerbate hypernatremia, as blood urea nitrogen (BUN) may act as an osmotic agent to increase free water urinary losses. Assuring a patient's access to water and/or administering free water may be necessary to avoid hypernatremia in clinical situations when dehydration can occur.

Hyperkalemia in the elderly is exacerbated by medication use. Risk of hyperkalemia increases in patients treated with ace inhibitors. Furthermore, aldosterone antagonist use is another cause. This risk was studied in patients already on an ace inhibitor for treatment of congestive heart failure. In patients greater than 75 years of age, with a mean creatinine clearance of 39 mL/min, the addition of this medication class was associated with a 36% incidence of a potassium level greater than 5.5 meq/L and 11% incidence of a potassium level greater than 6 meq/L.[81] Furthermore, hypokalemia can also frequently occur with diuretic use.[82] In elderly patients with a mean age of 68 years, the hazard ratio for all-cause mortality in patients with hypokalemia, compared to normokalemia, was 1.56 (CI 1.25–1.95, p <0.001).[83]

End-stage renal disease

Most patients with ESRD in the United States receive dialysis in the form of in-center hemodialysis, while peritoneal dialysis is used far less frequently. Nonetheless, if patients can follow and comply with necessary instructions, home renal replacement is the preferred modality either in the form of peritoneal dialysis or home-hemodialysis. This view is driven by improved health outcomes in patients on home modalities and potential cost savings. However, such outcomes have not been demonstrated in older populations.

Older adults comprise a significant percentage of those on dialysis, as the mean age for all patients initiating dialysis in 2011 was 62.7 years.[84] The ideal time to initiate dialysis is not clear. One randomized trial, involving over 800 patients with a mean age of 60, compared initiation of dialysis at a creatinine clearance of 5–7 mL/min to a creatinine clearance of 10–14 mL/min, as determined by the Cockcroft Gault equation. This trial found that late initiation of dialysis did not lead to worse outcomes.[85] However, most patients in the late-initiation group actually started dialysis earlier than planned due to the development of ESRD-related symptoms. Ultimately, this study suggests that dialysis initiation should be based on an assessment of the patients' symptoms, not only their creatinine or eGFR.

In frail elderly patients, dialysis initiation may lead to a downward spiral in health quality and unnecessary pain and suffering.[86] Defining expectations and goals of dialysis before initiation is critical in the frail elderly patient with advanced CKD. A model predicting mortality in the six-month period following dialysis initiation, based on a large group of elderly French patients, has been prospectively validated in a similar population and may be useful in discussion of imminent mortality.[87] Interestingly, increasing age was not associated with a worse outcome in this model though other known CV risk factors were. Guidelines from the nephrology community

exist in regards to the importance of shared decision making about dialysis initiation and, at times, withdrawal.[88] Generally, this cites substantial neurologic injury without hopeful recovery as an example of when dialysis would be inappropriate or when withdrawal from dialysis should be considered.

Access for dialysis is essential in any patient with ESRD; all subjects with advanced, progressive CKD who may be candidates for dialysis should discuss preferred dialysis modalities with their nephrology care providers. Nonetheless, the elderly represent a population where the commonly prescribed "fistula first" philosophy of obtaining dialysis access prior to dialysis initiation may not be ideal for all patients, especially those with high surgical risk.[89, 90] In this setting, tunneled dialysis catheters may have a role despite their known increased risk of infection. It is now recognized that brachial and subclavian accesses should be avoided in any patients who may subsequently need an arteriovenous fistula or graft (AVF or AVG). Venous stenosis has been reported to occur in upward of 30% of patients receiving a PICC line.[91]

Age over 65 years is not a contraindication to transplantation, and experience is growing with transplantation in the elderly population. Between 2002 and 2012, the percentage of patients on the kidney transplant wait list between the age of 65 and 74 increased from 11.1% to 18.1%.[92] From a practical perspective, elderly dialysis patients who have a potential living related donor are much more likely to complete the transplant process before associated comorbid conditions disqualify them from transplantation.

Polypharmacy

Older adults are the largest consumers of prescription medications.[91] Polypharmacy is highly prevalent in older populations due to the increased number of chronic conditions associated with aging that require multiple medications for adequate treatment, such as hypertension, arthritis, heart disease, cancer, and diabetes.[92] A survey study of 2,976 community-residing adults aged 57–85 reported that at least 29% used at least five prescription medications concurrently. [93] Polypharmacy can be defined by the absolute number of medications, such as five or more medications, but there is no consensus regarding what this number should be.[92] Therefore, polypharmacy may be more simply defined by the utilization of more medications than are clinically indicated.[94, 95] Polypharmacy raises the risk for drug-related problems including adverse drug events (ADEs), drug–drug interactions, drug–disease interactions, medication cascade effects, and nonadherence with medications. Other significant adverse outcomes associated with polypharmacy involve increased hospital admissions and emergency room visits, nursing home placement, hypoglycemia, falls and fractures, pneumonia, malnutrition, mobility impairments, and death.[94–96] Medications commonly implicated for causing adverse drug events associated with visits to the emergency room in older adults include warfarin, insulin, and digoxin.[97]

Decreases in renal function associated with aging are due to both physiologic changes in the kidney (as discussed previously) as well as the presence of multiple chronic conditions and numerous medications. These alterations in kidney function can greatly impact the pharmacokinetics and pharmcodynamics of medications, such as reducing the excretion of drugs and their metabolites. The common coexistence of reduced renal function and polypharmacy renders older patients particularly vulnerable to medication-related problems, alterations in drug metabolism, and susceptibility to adverse drug events. The prevalence of potentially inappropriate medication prescribing in elderly patients with CKD is high.[98] Various tools, such as the Beers Criteria, have been developed to help identify and avoid such medications.[99] Studies have also observed significant correlations between polypharmacy and the occurrence of acute renal failure in hospitalized patients.[100] Inadequate dosing adjustment in renally excreted drugs is one of the main causes of drug-related problems.[101]

A careful review of medications and minimization of drug–drug interactions and potentially inappropriate medications is critically important in the older population, especially those with reduced renal function. Whenever possible, dosing should be based either on drug levels or titration to clinical effect, with consideration to the aging kidney.[102] Because lean body mass decreases with aging, the serum creatinine level is a poor indicator of, and tends to overestimate, the creatinine clearance in older adults. Therefore, rather than relying on the serum creatinine, the Cockroft-Gault formula should be used to estimate creatinine clearance in older adults.[103]

References

1. Lindeman RD, Tobin JD, Shock NW. Association between blood pressure and the rate of decline in renal function with age. *Kidney Int* 1984;**26**:861–8.

2. Coresh J, Astor BC, Greene T, et al. Prevalence of chronic kidney disease and decreased kidney function in the adult US population: Third National Health and Nutrition Examination Survey. *Am J Kidney Dis* 2003;**41**:1–12.

3. Kaplan C, Pasternack B, Shah H, Gallo G. Age-related incidence of sclerotic glomeruli in human kidneys. *Am J Pathol* 1975;**80**:227–34.

4. Weidmann P, De Myttenaere-Bursztein S, Maxwell MH, de Lima J. Effect on aging on plasma renin and aldosterone in normal man. *Kidney Int* 1975;**8**:325–33.

5. Preisser L, Teillet L, Aliotti S, et al. Downregulation of aquaporin-2 and -3 in aging kidney is independent of V(2) vasopressin receptor. *Am J Physiol Renal Physiol* 2000;**279**:F144–52.

6. Fliser D, Zeier M, Nowack R, Ritz E. Renal functional reserve in healthy elderly subjects. *J Am Soc Nephrol* 1993;**3**:1371–7.

7. Corman B, Barrault MB, Klingler C, et al. Renin gene expression in the aging kidney: effect of sodium restriction. *Mech Ageing Dev* 1995;**84**:1–13.

8. Levey AS, Bosch JP, Lewis JB, et al. A more accurate method to estimate glomerular filtration rate from serum creatinine: a new prediction equation. Modification of diet in renal disease study group. *Ann Intern Med.* 1999;**130**:461–70.

9. Coresh J, Selvin E, Stevens LA, et al. Prevalence of chronic kidney disease in the United States. *JAMA* 2007;**298**:2038–47.

10. Glassock RJ, Winearls C. Screening for CKD with eGFR: doubts and dangers. *Clin J Am Soc Nephrol* 2008;**3**:1563–8.

11. Winearls CG, Glassock RJ. Classification of chronic kidney disease in the elderly: pitfalls and errors. *Nephron Clin Pract* 2011;**119**(Suppl 1):c2–4.

12. Go AS, Chertow GM, Fan D, et al. Chronic kidney disease and the risks of death, cardiovascular events, and hospitalization. *N Engl J Med* 2004;**351**:1296–305.

13. Henry RM, Kostense PJ, Bos G, et al. Mild renal insufficiency is associated with increased cardiovascular mortality: the Hoorn Study. *Kidney Int* 2002;**62**:1402–7.

14. Deo R, Fyr CL, Fried LF, et al. Kidney dysfunction and fatal cardiovascular disease–an association independent of atherosclerotic events: results from the Health, Aging, and Body Composition (Health ABC) study. *Am Heart J* 2008;**155**:62–8.

15. Fried LF, Katz R, Sarnak MJ, et al. Kidney function as a predictor of noncardiovascular mortality. *J Am Soc Nephrol* 2005;**16**:3728–35.

16. Minutolo R, Lapi F, Chiodini P, et al. Risk of ESRD and death in patients with CKD not referred to a nephrologist: a 7-year prospective study. *Clin J Am Soc Nephrol* 2014;**9**(9):1586–93.

17. White SL, Polkinghorne KR, Atkins RC, Chadban SJ. Comparison of the prevalence and mortality risk of CKD in Australia using the CKD Epidemiology Collaboration (CKD-EPI) and Modification of Diet in Renal Disease (MDRD) Study GFR estimating equations: the AusDiab (Australian Diabetes, Obesity and Lifestyle) Study. *Am J Kidney Dis* 2010;**55**(4):660–70.

18. Briasoulis A, Bakris GL. Chronic kidney disease as a coronary artery disease risk equivalent. *Current Cardiology Reports* 2013;**15**:340.

19. de Brito-Ashurst I, Varagunam M, Raftery MJ, Yaqoob MM. Bicarbonate supplementation slows progression of CKD and improves nutritional status. *J Am Soc Nephrol* 2009;**20**:2075–84.

20. James PA, Oparil S, Carter BL, et al. 2014 evidence-based guideline for the management of high blood pressure in adults: report from the panel members appointed to the Eighth Joint National Committee (JNC 8). *JAMA* 2014;**311**(5):507–20.

21. Locatelli F, Del Vecchio L. Optimizing the management of renal anemia: challenges and new opportunities. *Kidney Int Suppl* 2008;**74**:S33–7.

22. KDIGO clinical practice guideline for the diagnosis, evaluation, prevention, and treatment of Chronic Kidney Disease-Mineral and Bone Disorder (CKD-MBD). *Kidney Int Suppl* 2009:S1–130.

23. Anderson S, Halter JB, Hazzard WR, et al. Prediction, progression, and outcomes of chronic kidney disease in older adults. *J Am Soc Nephrol* 2009;**20**:1199–209.

24. Martinez-Ramirez HR, Jalomo-Martinez B, Cortes-Sanabria L, et al. Renal function preservation in type 2 diabetes mellitus patients with early nephropathy: a comparative prospective cohort study between primary health care doctors and a nephrologist. *Am J Kidney Dis* 2006;**47**:78–87.

25. Emamian SA, Nielsen MB, Pedersen JF, Ytte L. Sonographic evaluation of renal appearance in 665 adult volunteers. Correlation with age and obesity. *Acta Radiologica* 1993;**34**:482–5.

26. Thomas SE, Anderson S, Gordon KL, et al. Tubulointerstitial disease in aging: evidence for underlying peritubular capillary damage, a potential role for renal ischemia. *J Am Soc Nephrol* 1998;**9**:231–42.

27. Abrass CK, Adcox MJ, Raugi GJ. Aging-associated changes in renal extracellular matrix. *Am J Pathol* 1995;**146**:742–52.

28. Hoy WE, Douglas-Denton RN, Hughson MD, et al. A stereological study of glomerular number and volume: preliminary findings in a multiracial study of kidneys at autopsy. *Kidney Int Suppl* 2003:S31–7.

29. Hollenberg NK, Adams DF, Solomon HS, et al. Senescence and the renal vasculature in normal man. *Circ Res* 1974;**34**:309–16.

30. Kuhlik F, Epstein F, Elahi D, et al. Urinary prostaglandin E2 and dopamine response to water loading in young and elderly humans. *Gertatr Nephrol Urol* 1995;**5**:79–83.

31. Rivas-Cabanero L, Rodriguez-Barbero A, Arevalo M, Lopez-Novoa JM. Effect of NG-nitro-L-arginine methyl ester on nephrotoxicity induced by gentamicin in rats. *Nephron* 1995;**71**:203–7.

32. Reckelhoff JF, Manning RD Jr. Role of endothelium-derived nitric oxide in control of renal microvasculature in aging male rats. *American Journal of Physiology* 1993;**265**:R1126–31.

33. Macias-Nunez JF, Lopez-Novoa JM, Martinez-Maldonado M. Acute renal failure in the aged. *Semin Nephrol* 1996;**16**:330–8.

34. Kleinknecht D, Landais P, Goldfarb B. Pathophysiology and clinical aspects of drug-induced tubular necrosis in man. *Contrib Nephrol* 1987;**55**:145–58.

35. Liano F, Pascual J. Epidemiology of acute renal failure: a prospective, multicenter, community-based study. Madrid Acute Renal Failure Study Group. *Kidney Int* 1996;**50**:811–8.

36. Pascual J, Liano F. Causes and prognosis of acute renal failure in the very old. Madrid Acute Renal Failure Study Group. *J Am Geriatr Soc* 1998;**46**:721–5.

37. Sands JM. Urine-concentrating ability in the aging kidney. *Sci Aging Knowledge Environ* 2003;**24**:PE15.

38. Kenney WL, Chiu P. Influence of age on thirst and fluid intake. *Med Sci Sports Exerc* 2001;**33**:1524–32.

39. van Kraaij DJ, Jansen RW, Gribnau FW, Hoefnagels WH. Diuretic therapy in elderly heart failure patients with and without left ventricular systolic dysfunction. *Drugs Aging* 2000;**16**:289–300.

40. Macias Nunez JF, Garcia Iglesias C, Bondia Roman A, et al. Renal handling of sodium in old people: a functional study. *Age Ageing* 1978;**7**:178–81.

41. Cheung CM, Ponnusamy A, Anderton JG. Management of acute renal failure in the elderly patient: a clinician's guide. *Drugs Aging* 2008;**25**:455–76.

42. Rich MW, Crecelius CA. Incidence, risk factors, and clinical course of acute renal insufficiency after cardiac catheterization in patients 70 years of age or older: a prospective study. *Archives of Internal Medicine* 1990;**150**:1237–42.

43. Ivanes F, Isorni MA, Halimi JM, et al. Predictive factors of contrast-induced nephropathy in patients undergoing primary coronary angioplasty. *Arch Cardiovasc Dis* 2014;**107**:424–32.

44. Davidson CJ, Hlatky M, Morris KG, et al. Cardiovascular and renal toxicity of a nonionic radiographic contrast agent after cardiac catheterization: a prospective trial. *Ann Intern Med* 1989;**110**:119–24.

45. Lautin EM, Freeman NJ, Schoenfeld AH, et al. Radiocontrast-associated renal dysfunction: incidence and risk factors. *AJR Am J Roentgenol* 1991;**157**:49–58.

46. Watts RA, Lane SE, Bentham G, Scott DG. Epidemiology of systemic vasculitis: a ten-year study in the United Kingdom. *Arthritis Rheum* 2000;**43**:414–9.

47. Nachman PH, Hogan SL, Jennette JC, Falk RJ. Treatment response and relapse in antineutrophil cytoplasmic autoantibody-associated microscopic polyangiitis and glomerulonephritis. *J Am Soc Nephrol* 1996;**7**:33–9.

48. Cole E, Cattran D, Magil A, et al. A prospective randomized trial of plasma exchange as additive therapy in idiopathic crescentic glomerulonephritis. The Canadian Apheresis Study Group. *Am J Kidney Dis* 1992;**20**:261–9.

49. Mekhail TM, Hoffman GS. Longterm outcome of Wegener's granulomatosis in patients with renal disease requiring dialysis. *J Rheumatol* 2000;**27**:1237–40.

50. Jayne D, Rasmussen N, Andrassy K, et al. A randomized trial of maintenance therapy for vasculitis associated with antineutrophil cytoplasmic autoantibodies. *N Engl J Med* 2003;**349**:36–44.

51. Schwartz CJ, White TA. Stenosis of renal artery: an unselected necropsy study. *BMJ* 1964;**2**:1415–21.

52. Thadhani RI, Camargo CA Jr, Xavier RJ, et al. Atheroembolic renal failure after invasive procedures. Natural history based on 52 histologically proven cases. *Medicine (Baltimore)* 1995;**74**:350–8.

53. Gupta BK, Spinowitz BS, Charytan C, Wahl SJ. Cholesterol crystal embolization-associated renal failure after therapy with recombinant tissue-type plasminogen activator. *Am J Kidney Dis* 1993;**21**:659–62.

54. Hyman BT, Landas SK, Ashman RF, et al. Warfarin-related purple toes syndrome and cholesterol microembolization. *Am J Med* 1987;**82**:1233–7.

55. Fukumoto Y, Tsutsui H, Tsuchihashi M, et al. Cholesterol Embolism Study I: the incidence and risk factors of cholesterol embolization syndrome, a complication of cardiac catheterization: a prospective study. *J Am Coll Cardiol* 2003;**42**:211–6.

56. Haas M, Spargo BH, Wit EJ, Meehan SM. Etiologies and outcome of acute renal insufficiency in older adults: a renal biopsy study of 259 cases. *Am J Kidney Dis* 2000;**35**:433–47.

57. Moutzouris DA, Herlitz L, Appel GB, et al. Renal biopsy in the very elderly. *Clin J Am Soc Nephrol* 2009;**4**:1073–82.

58. Groeneveld AB, Tran DD, van der Meulen J, et al. Acute renal failure in the medical intensive care unit: predisposing, complicating factors and outcome. *Nephron* 1991;**59**:602–10.

59. Gentric A, Cledes J. Immediate and long-term prognosis in acute renal failure in the elderly. *Nephrol Dial Transplant* 1991;**6**:86–90.

60. Schiffl H. Renal recovery from acute tubular necrosis requiring renal replacement therapy: a prospective study in critically ill patients. *Nephrol Dial Transplant* 2006;**21**:1248–52.

61. Bhandari S, Turney JH. Survivors of acute renal failure who do not recover renal function. *QJM* 1996;**89**:415–21.

62. Liano F, Felipe C, Tenorio MT, et al. Long-term outcome of acute tubular necrosis: a contribution to its natural history. *Kidney Int* 2007;**71**:679–86.

63. Chertow GM, Soroko SH, Paganini EP, et al. Mortality after acute renal failure: models for prognostic stratification and risk adjustment. *Kidney Int* 2006;**70**:1120–6.

64. Feest TG, Round A, Hamad S. Incidence of severe acute renal failure in adults: results of a community based study. *BMJ* 1993;**306**:481–3.

65. Bulpitt CJ, Beckett N, Peters R, et al. Does white coat hypertension require treatment over age 80? Results of the hypertension in the very elderly trial ambulatory blood pressure side project. *Hypertension* 2013;**61**:89–94.

66. Pickering TG, Hall JE, Appel LJ, et al. Recommendations for blood pressure measurement in humans and experimental animals: part 1: blood pressure measurement in humans: a statement for professionals from the Subcommittee of Professional and Public Education of the American Heart Association Council on High Blood Pressure Research. *Circulation* 2005;**111**:697–716.

67. Cruickshank JM. Coronary flow reserve and the J curve relation between diastolic blood pressure and myocardial infarction. *BMJ* 1988;**297**:1227–30.

68. Kumar S, Berl T. Sodium. *Lancet* 1998;**352**:220–8.

69. Kleinfeld M, Casimir M, Borra S. Hyponatremia as observed in a chronic disease facility. *J Am Geriatr Soc* 1979;**27**:156–61.

70. Liamis G, Rodenburg EM, Hofman A, et al. Electrolyte disorders in community subjects: prevalence and risk factors. *Am J Med* 2013;**126**:256–63.

71. Shapiro DS, Sonnenblick M, Galperin I, et al. Severe hyponatraemia in elderly hospitalized patients:

prevalence, aetiology and outcome. *Internal Medicine Journal* 2010;**40**:574–80.

72. Bigaillon C, El Jahiri Y, Garcia C, et al. [Inappropriate ADH secretion-induced hyponatremia and associated with paroxetine use]. *Rev Med Interne* 2007;**28**:642–4.

73. Kim CS, Choi JS, Bae EH, Kim SW. Hyponatremia associated with bupropion. *Electrolyte Blood Press* 2011;**9**:23–6.

74. Rodenburg EM, Hoorn EJ, Ruiter R, et al. Thiazide-associated hyponatremia: a population-based study. *Am J Kidney Dis* 2013;**62**:67–72.

75. Renneboog B, Musch W, Vandemergel X, et al. Mild chronic hyponatremia is associated with falls, unsteadiness, and attention deficits. *Am J Med* 2006;**119**:71 e1–8.

76. Gankam Kengne F, Andres C, Sattar L, et al. Mild hyponatremia and risk of fracture in the ambulatory elderly. *QJM* 2008;**101**:583–8.

77. Barsony J, Sugimura Y, Verbalis JG. Osteoclast response to low extracellular sodium and the mechanism of hyponatremia-induced bone loss. *J Biol Chem* 2011;**286**:10864–75.

78. Tseng CK, Lin CH, Hsu HS, et al. In addition to malnutrition and renal function impairment, anemia is associated with hyponatremia in the elderly. *Arch Gerontol Geriatr* 2012;**55**:77 81.

79. Hawkins RC. Age and gender as risk factors for hyponatremia and hypernatremia. *Clin Chim Acta* 2003;**337**:169–72.

80. Borra SI, Beredo R, Kleinfeld M. Hypernatremia in the aging: causes, manifestations, and outcome. *J Natl Med Assoc* 1995;**87**:220–4.

81. Dinsdale C, Wani M, Steward J, O'Mahony MS. Tolerability of spironolactone as adjunctive treatment for heart failure in patients over 75 years of age. *Age Ageing* 2005;**34**:395–8.

82. Passarelli MC, Jacob-Filho W, Figueras A. Adverse drug reactions in an elderly hospitalised population: inappropriate prescription is a leading cause. *Drugs Aging* 2005;**22**:767–77.

83. Bowling CB, Pitt B, Ahmed MI, et al. Hypokalemia and outcomes in patients with chronic heart failure and chronic kidney disease: findings from propensity-matched studies. *Circ Heart Fail* 2010;**3**:253–60.

84. USRD. *USRDS 2013 Annual Data Report: Atlas of Chronic Kidney Disease and End-Stage Renal Disease in the United States*. Bethesda, MD: National Institutes of Health, National Institute of Diabetes and Digestive and Kidney Diseases, 2013. Available at: www.usrds.org/2013/pdf/v1_00_intro_13.pdf (accessed 14 November 2015).

85. Cooper BA, Branley P, Bulfone L, et al. A randomized, controlled trial of early versus late initiation of dialysis. *N Engl J Med* 2010;**363**:609–19.

86. Steinman TI. The older patient with end-stage renal disease: is chronic dialysis the best option? *Semin Dial* 2012;**25**:602–5.

87. Couchoud C, Labeeuw M, Moranne O, et al. A clinical score to predict 6-month prognosis in elderly patients starting dialysis for end-stage renal disease. *Nephrol Dial Transplant* 2009;**24**:1553–61.

88. Moss AH. Revised dialysis clinical practice guideline promotes more informed decision-making. *Clin J Am Soc Nephrol* 2010;**5**:2380–3.

89. O'Hare AM. Vascular access for hemodialysis in older adults: a "patient first" approach. *J Am Soc Nephrol* 2013;**24**:1187–90.

90. DeSilva RN, Patibandla BK, Vin Y, et al. Fistula first is not always the best strategy for the elderly. *J Am Soc Nephrol* 2013;**24**:1297–304.

91. Abdullah BJ, Mohammad N, Sangkar JV, et al. Incidence of upper limb venous thrombosis associated with peripherally inserted central catheters (PICC). *British Journal of Radiology* 2005;**78**:596–600.

92. *OPTN/SRTR 2012 Annual Data Report*. Rockville, MD: Department of Health and Human Services, Health Resources and Services Administration 2014. Available at: http://onlinelibrary.wiley.com/doi/10.11 11/ajt.v14.s1/issuetoc (accessed 14 November 2015).

Chapter 26

Urological issues in older adults

Tomas L. Griebling, MD, MPH, FACS, FGSA, AGSF

Introduction

Urological problems are extremely common in older adults. The prevalence of many urological disorders increases with advancing age in both men and women. Estimates indicate that approximately 20% of all primary care visits include some type of urological complaint. In fact, the specialty of urology ranks third, behind only ophthalmology and cardiology, in the total annual number of outpatient clinical visits by older Medicare recipients in the United States. These trends hold steady even when stratifying for ages older than either 75 or 85. There is a critical need for more clinicians across all specialties focused on care of older adults.[1] This chapter addresses the evaluation and management of many of the common urological conditions seen in older adults. Several topics relevant to urology are also covered in more detail in other chapters including urinary incontinence (Chapter 27), sexuality and sexual health (Chapter 45), and prostate cancer (Chapter 38).

Hematuria

Hematuria is a common urological condition seen in people of all ages. The condition may be gross or microscopic, and it may be episodic or persistent. Any episode of gross hematuria should be considered abnormal. On microscopic urinalysis, the generally accepted upper limit of normal is zero to three red blood cells per high-powered field.[2] Because it is a common presenting sign for many types of genitourinary pathology, elderly patients with gross or persistent microhematuria should undergo a thorough evaluation including upper urinary tract imaging and cystourethroscopy. The common sources of hematuria in older adults are summarized in Table 26.1. Computed tomography

Table 26.1 Causes of hematuria in older adults

Benign conditions
Stones
Urinary tract infections (UTI)
Pyelonephritis
Glomerular diseases of the kidney

Inflammatory conditions
Prostatitis
Cystitis
Urethritis

Malignant conditions
Bladder cancer
    Transitional cell carcinoma
    Squamous cell carcinoma
    Carcinoma in situ
Ureteral cancer
Renal cancer
    Renal cell carcinoma
    Transitional cell carcinoma
    Prostate cancer
    Urethral cancer

(CT) has become the preferred imaging modality for detection of urological abnormalities in patients with hematuria.[3] If possible, the study should be done both without and with intravenous contrast provided the patient's baseline renal function is adequate. The non-contrast images are particularly useful to evaluate for stones. After contrast administration, immediate and delayed images are obtained. These help to delineate renal function and anatomy, the course and caliber of

Reichel's Care of the Elderly, 7th Edition, ed. Jan Busby-Whitehead *et al.* Published by Cambridge University Press.
© Cambridge University Press 2016.

the ureters, and the general anatomy of the bladder. Delayed images are useful to identify hydronephrosis and potential ureteral obstruction.

Although larger lesions in the bladder may be identifiable on CT imaging or ultrasound, smaller mucosal lesions may not be evident on these studies. Therefore, cystourethroscopy must be considered an essential part of the complete urological evaluation for hematuria. Bladder cancers, particularly transitional cell carcinomas, usually start in the urothelium and are often visible as papillary lesions on cystoscopy. Carcinoma in situ is a particularly aggressive form of bladder cancer that may initially present with either microscopic or gross hematuria. On cystoscopy, this usually appears as a red, velvety patch in the urothelium. Histological examination of bladder biopsies and cytological examination of either voided urine or bladder washing specimens may be useful to help diagnose bladder malignancies. In the United States, transitional cell carcinoma is the most common form of bladder cancer in older adults, and cigarette smoking is one of the most common risk factors.

Although an episode of gross hematuria can be quite distressing for the patient, emergency evaluation is not usually necessary. The exceptions are patients experiencing clot retention with difficulty passing urine or patients requiring blood transfusions for anemia secondary to the hematuria. Cystourethroscopy with clot evacuation may be required in these cases. If a specific bleeding site is identified, electrocoagulation may be useful. In many cases, a specific source cannot be identified. In cases of persistent gross hematuria, chemical coagulation with bladder infusions of dilute alum or formalin may be required.

In older patients with renal insufficiency, a plain x-ray of the kidneys, ureters, and bladder and renal ultrasound can be performed as the initial imaging evaluation. This should be supplemented with cystourethroscopy and retrograde ureteropyelography to look for abnormalities in the ureters or renal collecting systems. Filling defects may indicate some type of space-occupying lesion such as a stone, tumor, polyp, fungus ball, blood clot, or stricture.

Acute conditions such as urinary tract infection (UTI), prostatitis, or stone passage may be associated with hematuria. Urinalysis should be repeated after these conditions have been treated, and, if hematuria persists, then urological consultation for further evaluation should be obtained. Hematuria is also frequently seen in elderly patients receiving chronic

anticoagulation therapy; however, these individuals still require a complete urological evaluation because 15%–20% will be found to have significant underlying genitourinary pathology.

If an older adult patient has persistent microhematuria despite a negative urological evaluation with upper tract imaging, cystourethroscopy, and cytology, then referral to a nephrologist to evaluate for possible glomerular bleeding would be warranted. This is particularly true in patients with a history of either proteinuria or hypertension.[2]

Hematospermia

Hematospermia, blood in the ejaculate, is occasionally seen in older men. Although it is most commonly idiopathic and benign, it may be an indication of other underlying genitourinary pathological conditions such as prostatitis or prostate cancer.[4] Bleeding from dilated capillary vessels in the prostate may also cause hematospermia. In some cases, this may be triggered by excessive physical exertion or vigorous sexual activity. Evaluation, including a thorough history taking and physical examination, may help to identify the cause of the condition. Additional tests that may be useful include cystourethroscopy, transrectal ultrasound, prostate biopsy, and determination of prostate-specific antigen (PSA) levels. Oral administration of 5-α-reductase inhibitors may be useful in treatment of hematospermia or hematuria caused by dilation of prostatic capillaries. These medications cause shrinkage of the prostate and can reduce bleeding from these small blood vessels.

Urinary tract infections

Bacteriuria and UTI are among the most common urological diagnoses in older adults. The estimated lifetime risk for development of a UTI in women is greater than 50%, and the associated costs are staggering. In the year 2000, the estimated overall annual expenditures for UTI care in the United States were $2.47 billion for women, and $1.03 billion for men.[5, 6] Epidemiological studies indicate that the incidence and prevalence of UTIs increases with advancing age.[7] Although seen in both sexes, a higher proportion of women are affected, with a ratio of 3:1. Various age-related physiological changes may predispose older adults to UTIs. These include hormonal and vaginal changes associated with menopause, alterations in cognitive function, prostate disease, and changes in bladder physiology.

Asymptomatic bacteriuria should be differentiated from symptomatic UTI. Symptomatic UTIs should be treated in patients of any age. Diagnosis should be confirmed with urinalysis and urine cultures. Determination of drug sensitivity on urine culture is important to ensure that appropriate antibiotic therapy has been administered. This is particularly important given the increased rates of drug resistance seen with many common bacteria. Typical symptoms of acute UTI include fever, dysuria, urinary urgency and frequency, burning with urination, and suprapubic discomfort. Elderly patients may not develop these symptoms because of normal alterations in overall immune status associated with aging. Older adults may exhibit other symptoms resulting from UTI including lethargy, anorexia, or confusion. In elderly patients with new onset of delirium, a urinalysis and urine culture should be checked to determine if a UTI is present.

Antibiotic therapy for acute UTI is usually administered as an oral preparation. Uncomplicated UTI may be treated with simple, low-cost antibiotics such as amoxicillin or ampicillin, nitrofurantoin, or trimethoprim-sulfamethoxazole. In patients who are allergic to these compounds, cephalosporins or doxycycline may be used as second-line therapy. Fluoroquinolones are usually reserved for complicated UTIs including those associated with concomitant stone disease, pyelonephritis, or sepsis. The choice of appropriate antibiotic therapy should of course be guided by the patient's overall medical condition, renal function status, and the results of the antibiotic sensitivity profile for the specific organism. The duration of therapy generally ranges from three to seven days, and is dependent on a variety of factors including overall complexity of the infection and response to therapy. Intravenous antibiotic therapy may be required in cases of severe infection, pyelonephritis, or urosepsis.

The most common organisms seen in elderly patients with UTI include Gram-negative bacteria such as *Escherichia coli, Pseudomonas, Klebsiella*, and *Proteus*. The most common Gram-positive organisms seen in older adults with UTI include *Staphylococcus aureus*, and *Enterococcus*.[8] In patients with recurrent, culture-documented UTI, a clinical investigation to search for a nidus of infection is warranted. Common causes of recurrent infection include

urolithiasis or other foreign body, chronic urinary retention, and vesicoureteral reflux. Treatment of the underlying condition may lead to resolution or a decrease in the frequency of UTIs.

Asymptomatic bacteriuria is quite common, particularly in elderly women. This is seen both in community-dwelling and institutionalized elders. In a community-based, cross-sectional analysis of 432 people aged 80 or older, 19.0% of the women and 5.8% of the men were found to have asymptomatic bacteriuria.[9] In this study, urinary incontinence, reduced mobility, and systemic estrogen replacement therapy were identified as independent risk factors for asymptomatic bacteriuria in women. There is general consensus that asymptomatic bacteriuria need not be treated with antibiotic therapy.

UTIs associated with systemic bacteremia in elderly patients carry a high risk of morbidity and mortality. In a retrospective study of 191 patients aged 75–105 years with concomitant positive urine and blood cultures, the in-hospital mortality rate was 33%.[8] A variety of factors associated with impaired physical and cognitive function were associated with increased mortality; however, advanced age itself was not identified as a significant risk factor in this particular study. Other studies have confirmed that mental status changes and a history of frequent UTIs may be associated with increased mortality in elderly patients with UTI.[10]

The role of impaired bladder emptying in development of UTI in older adults has been somewhat controversial. Intuitively, it makes sense that increased postvoid residual urine volume may be associated with UTI. The data, however, have been somewhat conflicting on this topic. A recent retrospective analysis of 101 stroke patients admitted for inpatient rehabilitation demonstrated that a finding of two or more postvoid residual urine volumes of 150 mL or more was independently associated with an increased risk of UTI.[11]

Impaired nutritional status may also be associated with an increased propensity for elderly patients to develop UTIs. In a study of 185 hospitalized older adults (mean age 81.6 ± 0.6 years), malnutrition was associated with an increased rate of nosocomial infections, including UTIs.[12]

Indwelling catheterization is clearly associated with an increased risk of UTI in older adults. Intermittent catheterization is preferred, if possible, in patients who have problems with urinary retention.

Indwelling catheters should be used only if absolutely necessary. A recently published study examined the rates of UTI observed in a group of 277 elderly patients who had an indwelling urinary catheter placed in the emergency room at the time of hospital admission.[13] Overall, 28% of these patients were diagnosed with a UTI during their hospitalization; however, 69% of these individuals either had a UTI diagnosed in the emergency room or had clinically significant bacteriuria ($\geq 10^5$ organisms/mL) prior to the catheter placement. Therefore, 9% of the patients who had an indwelling catheter placed developed a new UTI during hospitalization.

Several treatments may be helpful to prevent development of UTIs in susceptible older adults. Increased hydration may be helpful to decrease bacterial adherence to the urothelium of the bladder and urethra. Vaginal estrogen replacement may help to prevent development of UTI in postmenopausal women with atrophic vaginitis. Estrogen helps to acidify the vaginal fluid that facilitates growth of *Lactobacillus* sp., the natural vaginal flora. *Lactobacillus* is an important component of the natural host–defense mechanism, which helps prevent overgrowth of pathogenic bacteria associated with UTI. The estrogen is administered vaginally to enhance absorption in the vaginal and periurethral tissues. Even in patients already on systemic estrogen therapy, additional vaginal administration may be required to reach appropriate local tissue levels. Administration approximately three times weekly is usually sufficient. Exogenous estrogen administration is typically contraindicated in women with a history of uterine or breast cancer. However, oncologists may permit vaginal estrogen use in select women with a history of breast cancer, particularly if the tumor was estrogen receptor negative.

Cranberries (*Vaccinium macrocarpon*) have long been considered a preventive agent for UTIs, and consumption of cranberry juice has been associated with decreased rates of UTI in elderly patients.[14] This is most likely because of acidification of the urine and the azo ring chemistry found in the cranberries that prevents bacterial adherence to the urothelium. If patients are going to use cranberry to help prevent UTI, they should be counseled to look for products containing a high percentage of real juice rather than water. Cranberry tablets may be substituted for juice in diabetic patients or those on a reduced calorie diet. However, newer data suggests that cranberry supplementation may not be particularly effective in all older adults patients to prevent UTI, and differences in outcomes may be due to underlying risk of infection.[15]

Urinary catheters

In general, the use of indwelling urinary catheters should be avoided if at all possible.[16] Indwelling catheters can be associated with significant potential complications including UTIs, urosepsis, and stone formation. Care should be taken to remove the catheter as soon as feasible, and to monitor the patient for signs and symptoms of UTI. With extended time, chronic catheter irritation may lead to squamous metaplasia of the bladder epithelium and squamous cell carcinoma of the bladder.

If chronic indwelling catheter use is required, suprapubic catheter drainage is usually preferred over urethral catheterization. The suprapubic catheter may be easier for caregivers to change and is often more comfortable for patients. In patients who are sexually active, a suprapubic catheter is helpful because it moves the catheter away from the genitals. Chronic urethral catheterization may also lead to urethral or bladder neck erosion and subsequent urinary incontinence. Urinary leakage around an indwelling catheter is usually caused by either catheter blockage or bladder spasms. Gentle irrigation of the catheter with sterile saline can be used to relieve obstruction from urinary sediment. Placement of larger catheters should be avoided because this will only serve to dilate the urethra or suprapubic tract and will not correct the underlying problem. With time, the use of larger catheters may lead to urethral or bladder neck erosion and worsening urinary incontinence. Treatment of urinary incontinence in patients with this type of urethral erosion may be quite difficult and often involves major surgery such as a cystectomy with urinary diversion or augmentation enterocystoplasty with closure of the bladder neck.

Antimuscarinics or other medications for treatment of detrusor overactivity may be useful to diminish bladder spasms. The most common medications used in the treatment of overactive bladder including dosages and potential side effects are listed in Table 26.2. Care should be taken when prescribing these agents in older adults, and the patient and family or caregivers should be instructed to watch closely for any signs of side effects.

Table 26.2 Medications for overactive bladder

Medications	Typical dosages
Antimuscarinics	
Oxybutynin	5 mg twice daily to four times daily (maximum dose 30 mg total per day)
Oxybutynin (time released)	5, 10, or 15 mg once daily
Oxybutynin (transdermal patch)	3.9 mg/day, patch changed twice weekly
Oxybutynin (transdermal gel)	1 packet topically daily
Tolterodine	1 or 2 mg twice daily
Tolterodine (time released)	4 mg once daily
Darifenacin	7.5 or 15 mg once daily
Solifenacin	5 or 10 mg once daily
Fesoterodine	4 or 8 mg once daily
β-3 agonists	25 or 50 mg once daily
Mirabegron	
Potential side effects of anticholinergic medications	
Dry mouth	
Constipation	
Confusion	
Blurry vision	
Headache	
Tachycardia	
Prolongation of QT interval on electrocardiogram	
Potential side effects of β-3 agonists	
Hypertension	

Stone disease

Approximately 20% of all adults will develop urinary stone disease at some point in their lives. In general, rates of stone formation and passage do not differ in elderly patients compared with the general population.[17] Patients with a history of stone disease are at significantly increased risk for development of recurrent stone episodes. One of the primary risk factors for stone disease is inadequate hydration, which is often seen in older adults. Epidemiological and health care utilization analysis revealed that Medicare beneficiaries with a diagnosis of stone disease had a 2.5- to 3-fold higher rate of inpatient hospitalization for the condition compared with younger patients.[17] This study also demonstrated that rates of outpatient hospital and office visits for evaluation and treatment of stone disease increased by 29% and 41%, respectively, among Medicare beneficiaries between 1992 and 1998.

Small stones (<5 mm) can often be treated effectively with increased hydration and oral analgesics. In many cases, the stones will pass spontaneously. Administration of oral alpha-blocker medications such as tamsulosin may lead to relaxation of ureteral smooth muscle, which can aid in spontaneous stone passage with peristalsis. Patients are encouraged to collect and strain their urine to capture the stones for chemical analysis. Larger stones often require surgical intervention for treatment. Cystoscopy and ureteral stent placement may be required to bypass an obstructing stone and help relieve renal colic. Indications for stent insertion include upper tract obstruction, particularly with significant urinary infection or bacteriuria, a solitary functioning kidney, underlying renal insufficiency, or intractable nausea, vomiting, or pain. Subsequent surgical treatment may include ureteroscopy with stone fragmentation and removal or extracorporeal shock wave lithotripsy. Percutaneous nephrostolithotomy may be required for large stones in the renal pelvis or calyces. Outcomes for surgical intervention with percutaneous nephrostolithotomy or shock wave lithotripsy are quite favorable for older adults, and overall results are comparable with data from younger patients.

Stone composition may also change with advancing age. Alterations in stone chemistry in older adults may be related to associated changes in vitamin D and calcium metabolism, which can be affected by age-related physiological changes. The overall proportion of uric acid stones also appears to increase with advancing age.[18] This may be related to a progressive defect in urine ammoniagenesis, which is observed with aging, and which leads to a low urinary pH observed in patients who form uric acid stones. In addition, there is evidence that diabetic patients tend to have a higher incidence of uric acid stone production compared with nondiabetics.[19]

This may help explain the higher rates of uric acid stone production observed in older adults, who also have a greater tendency to have diabetes mellitus or a history of gout.

Rates of stone recurrence appear to be similar in older adults compared with younger individuals.[20] In a review of 209 stone patients older than 65, calcium oxalate and calcium phosphate were the most common types of stones observed. Elderly patients accounted for 9.6% of the total population in this study; however, the older patients demonstrated a significantly higher rate of uric acid stone formation compared with the younger patients. Hyperuricosuria and hypercalcuria appear to be common in older patients with recurrent stone disease.

Urological malignancies

The incidence and prevalence of most of the urological malignancies increase with advancing age. In some cases, there may be differences in the type or progression of cancer compared with younger patients. For a more detailed discussion regarding evaluation and management of cancers in older adults, refer to Chapter 38.

Prostate cancer

Prostate cancer is the most common nonskin cancer diagnosed in men, and the second leading cause of cancer deaths behind lung cancer. It is estimated that approximately 220,800 new cases of prostate cancer will be diagnosed in the United States in 2015, and approximately 27,540 men will die of the disease.[21] The incidence and prevalence of prostate cancer both increase with age. In general, prostate cancer is a slow-growing disease, and many men will die of other comorbid conditions rather than of prostate cancer itself. In patients with clinically organ-confined disease, treatment with curative intent by using either radical prostatectomy or radiation therapy may be utilized. Although there is no specific age limitation, curative treatment is most often considered for those men with a predicted life expectancy of at least 10 additional years. In men with metastatic disease or in those who are not deemed to be surgical candidates, hormonal therapy with androgen deprivation may be used to slow the progression of the disease. For additional information on the evaluation and treatment of prostate cancer in elderly men, refer to Chapter 38.

Routine screening for prostate cancer in elderly men is controversial. In younger men, the American Urological Association recommends screening with an annual serum PSA level and a digital rectal examination.[22] Guidelines suggest starting screening at the age of 50 years, and at 40 years for men considered to be at high risk for prostate cancer. These would include African-American men and those with a family history of prostate cancer. However other groups including the US Preventive Services Task Force do not recommend routine prostate cancer screening.[23] Specific age cut-offs at which to discontinue screening have not been definitively established. In general, routine prostate cancer screening in elderly men with a predicted life expectancy of less than 10 years is not indicated.[24] Decisions to screen for prostate cancer in elderly men should be tailored to each patient's specific clinical situation with consideration of overall health and other comorbid disease. Targeted diagnostic evaluation, which is conceptually different from screening, may be indicated in select elderly men based on other symptoms and health conditions.

Bladder cancer

Bladder cancer often presents initially with either gross painless hematuria or persistent microhematuria. In the United States, the most common type of bladder cancer is transitional cell carcinoma. On cystoscopic examination, this usually appears as either a papillary or sessile tumor of the bladder mucosa. Carcinoma in situ is a particularly aggressive form of bladder cancer. Cystoscopically, this typically appears as a velvety red patch in the bladder mucosa. Bladder wash cytology and biopsies are needed to help establish the diagnosis.

Treatment of bladder cancer is dependent on the grade and stage of the tumor. Low-grade tumors that do not invade into the muscular layer of the bladder are usually treated with endoscopic resection. Tumor recurrence occurs in up to 70% of patients, and careful postoperative follow-up is essential for proper treatment. Follow-up consists of repeated cystoscopy and cytology every three months for two years, every four months for two years, every six months for two years, and then annually. Adjuvant therapy with intravesical administration of Bacillus-Calmette-Guérin (BCG) or mitomycin-C may be used to help decrease tumor recurrence. High-grade noninvasive tumors may also be treated with a combination of surgical resection and intravesical chemotherapy.

Invasion of tumor into the muscularis propria is an ominous finding and is associated with a high risk of disease progression. The mainstay of therapy is radical cystectomy in women or cystoprostatectomy in men. This is a major surgical procedure that is associated with significant risk of morbidity and mortality. Recent studies indicate that elderly patients can safely undergo this type of surgery, although the risks and potential benefits need to be carefully considered for each individual patient.[25] Options for urinary diversion include both continent and noncontinent reconstruction procedures.[26] The traditional diversion is an ileal conduit, which is brought to the skin as a urinary stoma. The urine drains continuously into an ostomy bag that is secured directly to the skin. Methods for continent urinary diversion include either a catheterizable internal pouch made of detubularized bowel, which the patient drains several times daily using intermittent catheterization through a stoma in the abdominal wall, or an orthotopic neobladder. The neobladder is also a pouch made of detubularized bowel but it is anastomosed directly to the urethra. The patient voids per urethra to empty the neobladder, although some patients do need to do periodic intermittent catheterization to completely drain the reservoir. Because the orthotopic diversion relies on the external urinary sphincter for continence, many patients experience some urinary leakage particularly during their sleep.

Urethral cancer

Primary malignant tumors of the urethra are rare and occur more commonly in women than men. Patients usually present with hematuria or difficulty with urination. The tumor is often palpable on bimanual pelvic examination. Cystoscopy and biopsy are used to help confirm the diagnosis. Treatment consists of excision, and possible adjuvant chemotherapy or radiation.

Kidney cancer

Cancers of the kidney account for approximately 3%–5% of all diagnosed malignancies in both men and women.[21] The most common types of kidney cancer include renal cell carcinomas, which originate in the renal parenchyma, and transitional cell carcinomas, which originate in the transitional epithelium of the renal collecting system. Early treatment is essential to prevent development of metastatic disease beyond the kidney. For renal cell carcinomas, partial

nephrectomy using either open or laparoscopic and robotic surgery may be considered if the tumor is amenable to resection to spare as many functional nephrons as possible to preserve renal function. Recent advances in therapeutic methodology have made techniques such as cryotherapy and radio-frequency ablation of renal tumors minimally invasive options for some patients. These types of therapies may be particularly useful in elderly patients who may not be candidates for more invasive surgery, even with laparoscopic or robotic methods. Radical nephrectomy may be required if the tumor is large, if there is involvement of tumor in the renal vein or vena cava, or the tumor is anatomically not amenable to a nephron-sparing approach. The overall health and potential longevity of the patient must be carefully considered in each case.

Nephroureterectomy has been the traditional treatment for transitional cell carcinomas of the renal collecting system. The ureter is removed because the tumor usually involves a field change within the tissue, and subsequent recurrences in the ureter are extremely common (>70%). Nephron-sparing options including endoscopic tumor resection with administration of chemotherapeutic or immunotherapeutic agents into the renal collecting system. These may be viable options in patients who are not candidates to undergo more involved surgery.

Testis cancer

Testis cancer is a relatively uncommon malignancy, accounting for approximately 1% of all cancers diagnosed in males.[21, 27] Testis cancers can present at any point in a man's life, although the types of cancer differ significantly by patient age. In infants and children, yolk sac tumors and embryonal cell carcinomas are the most common. In young men between the ages of 15 and 35 years, testis cancer is actually the most common solid malignancy, and ranks behind only the leukemias and lymphomas in overall incidence. The most common forms of testis cancer in young men include seminomas and nonseminomatous germ cell tumors. In contrast, the most common testicular tumors in elderly men are lymphomas. These tend to be aggressive tumors and are generally managed with systemic chemotherapy or a combination of chemotherapy and radiation. Recurrence is common, occurring in up to 80% of patients.[28] Extranodal recurrence is not uncommon and may involve the central nervous system. Chemotherapy can be useful in some cases of testicular lymphoma.

Benign disorders of the prostate

Prostate diseases are among the most common urological conditions that affect older men. The primary nonmalignant conditions affecting the prostate gland in older men include benign prostatic hyperplasia (BPH) and prostatitis.

Benign prostatic hyperplasia

The prostate gland secretes fluid that helps form the ejaculate and provides nutrient factors required for the function and survival of sperm. Benign enlargement of the prostate gland typically begins at approximately 40–50 years of age.[29] This enlargement is driven by the presence of serum testosterone. Proliferation of both the stromal and the epithelial components of the prostate gland can occur in cases of BPH. The effect of prostatic enlargement is variable. Some men experience few symptoms; however, many men develop obstructive voiding symptoms including urinary frequency, hesitancy, nocturia, and a slow urinary stream. Nocturia can be particularly bothersome for some men.[30] Data have shown that experiencing two or more episodes of nocturia each night leads to substantial impairment in overall and health-related quality of life.[30] Other men experience chronic difficulty emptying the bladder or acute urinary retention. In some cases, men may also experience irritative voiding symptoms with urinary urgency or urge incontinence. Pain is uncommon unless men have acute urinary retention or need to strain to urinate. Prostate size does not always correlate with symptoms. In fact, some men with relatively small prostate glands have severe symptoms, particularly if the median lobe of the prostate gland is involved. Voiding symptoms associated with BPH can have a significantly negative impact on both overall and health-related quality of life.[31, 32] Fortunately, there are a wide variety of both surgical and nonsurgical therapies for BPH that can be quite effective in relieving these bothersome symptoms. These are outlined in Table 26.3. In addition, quality indicators for evaluation and management of BPH in vulnerable elderly men have recently been established.[33]

Medical therapies

Currently, there are three main categories of drugs used for the pharmacological treatment of BPH. These include the α-adrenergic antagonists, the 5-α-reductase inhibitors, and nutritional supplements and

Table 26.3 Treatment options for BPH

Medical therapies	
α-adrenergic antagonists	
Nonselective	
Terazosin (Hytrin)	1–10 mg PO at bedtime (must titrate dose)
Doxazosin (Cardura)	1–8 mg PO at bedtime (must titrate dose)
Selective	
Tamsulosin (Flomax)	0.4–0.8 mg PO at bedtime
Alfuzosin (Uroxatral)	10 mg PO once daily
5-α-reductase inhibitors	
Finasteride (Proscar)	5 mg PO once daily
Dutasteride (Avodart)	0.5 mg PO once daily
Surgical therapies	
Transurethral resection of the prostate (TURP)	
Transurethral incision of the prostate (TUIP)	
Open suprapubic prostatectomy	
Open retropubic (nonradical) prostatectomy	
Minimally invasive therapies	
Transurethral photovaporization (PVP)	
Transurethral needle ablation (TUNA)	
High-intensity focused ultrasound (HIFU)	
Transurethral microwave thermotherapy (TMT)	
Lasers (various)	
Prostatic stents	

phytotherapies. The α-adrenergic antagonists include terazosin (Hytrin), doxazosin (Cardura), tamsulosin (Flomax), and alfuzosin (Uroxatral). These drugs act by blocking α-adrenergic receptors in the tissue of the prostatic urethra and bladder neck. This leads to a relaxation of smooth muscle in these tissues, which causes a decrease in outlet resistance. These drugs have been shown to work well, particularly in men with smaller prostate glands.[34] The medications are usually prescribed once daily at bedtime. This helps to reduce some of the potential side effects of the medication including orthostatic hypotension. The more selective medications tamsulosin and alfuzosin appear to have less overall side effects compared to the older, less selective medications in this class.[34] Men should be warned to rise slowly and make sure they have their balance before getting up from bed. This is particularly true for men who have nocturia and get up to go to the toilet in the night. There have been associations reported between α-blocker therapy and erectile dysfunction in older men.[35, 36] Another potential side effect of this class of drugs is the floppy-iris syndrome.[37] The medications may cause relaxation of the smooth muscle in the iris of the eyes. This can become a problem if the medication is not discontinued prior to cataract surgery. The condition causes intraoperative billowing of the iris musculature with risk of prolapse and progressive miosis. Men taking these medications must advise their ophthalmologist prior to any surgical interventions.

The 5-α-reductase inhibitors act by blocking the enzyme that helps catalyze the conversion of testosterone into dihydrotestosterone. Limiting the amount of circulating dihydrotestosterone leads to a shrinking of the prostate gland, although the full effect may not be seen for several months after starting the medication.[38] The two main drugs in this category include finasteride (Proscar) and dutasteride (Avodart). These medications generally work better in men with larger prostate glands. The potential side effects include decrease in libido and development of gynecomastia or breast discomfort. The drugs will also cause an approximate 50% reduction in circulating serum PSA. It is recommended that a PSA level be checked prior to initiating these medications. After starting a 5-α-reductase inhibitor, observed PSA levels should be doubled to determine the actual PSA for a given patient.

Several recent studies have suggested that using a combination of an α-adrenergic antagonist and a 5-α-reductase inhibitor may have better overall efficacy compared with monotherapy, particularly for men with larger prostates or more severe voiding symptoms.[39, 40] Whereas this dual therapy may be beneficial for some patients, the potential side effects and additive costs of these medications must also be considered.

A number of natural remedies and plant extracts have gained popularity for the treatment of the symptoms of BPH. The most widely used preparation is saw palmetto (*Serenoa repens*). The exact mechanism of action is unknown, but theories suggest it may be similar to either 5-α-reductase inhibitors or other hormonally active agents. To date, there have been relatively few studies examining the efficacy of these types of preparations, particularly in elderly men. These agents are available in health food stores without a prescription. It is difficult to counsel patients about the safety and efficacy of these types of treatments because of the overall paucity of data. These phytotherapeutic agents are also not subject to regulation by the US Food and Drug Administration (FDA), and there may be significant variations between products and even between batches of the same product.

The roles of micronutrients and other nutritional components have recently attracted attention as a potential option for treatment and perhaps prevention of BPH.[41, 42] Research data are limited, particularly for elderly men; however, this is a rapidly growing area of both basic science and clinical research. Zinc has long been advocated as a mineral important for prostate health. Other agents being examined for their potential influence on prostate physiology include lycopenes, bioflavonoids including soy, and selenium. If these types of nutritional agents show a clinically significant effect in either treating BPH or preventing clinically significant symptoms, it may alter the ways in which this disorder is managed.

Surgery

Surgical treatment may be required in some patients, particularly if medical therapy has not been clinically successful. The traditional options for surgery include open surgical removal of the prostate through either a suprapubic or retropubic approach or transurethral resection. Open surgery is still used in men with very large prostate glands (>100 g). For most men, transurethral surgery has replaced open surgery as the technique of choice, because of lower overall morbidity and mortality and improved recovery. Transurethral resection of the prostate (TURP) remains the gold standard to which all other forms of therapy are compared. The main risks of TURP include bleeding and infection and development of hyponatremia from absorption of hypotonic irrigation solution during surgery. Recent technical advances have led to development of surgical systems that can utilize isotonic saline for intraoperative irrigation. This has reduced the incidence of the post-TURP hyponatremia syndrome and the associated morbidity of the procedure. Another potential side effect is the development of retrograde ejaculation after TURP. In men with a smaller prostate or with an elevated bladder neck, a transurethral incision of the prostate may help to avoid this potential complication.

Minimally invasive therapies

A number of minimally invasive surgical therapies have been developed to treat symptomatic BPH.[43, 44] Examples include transurethral photovaporization of the prostate (PVP), transurethral needle ablation of the prostate (TUNA), which utilizes radio-frequency energy, high-intensity focused ultrasound (HIFU), or transurethral microwave thermotherapy (TMT), which heats the prostate leading to subsequent sloughing of the treated tissue. Several different techniques using various laser energy methods have also been developed. Intraurethral prostatic stents have been developed for treatment of mild-to-moderate BPH.[45] These devices are placed across the prostatic urethra and function to push open the urethral lumen with a radial springlike configuration. The overall popularity of urethral stents for routine management of BPH has declined because of associated complications including erosion, migration, or stricture. Removal can be difficult as the components of the stent become incorporated in the epithelium of the urethra. Nonetheless, these devices could be useful in highly select patients, such as frail elderly men with diminished life expectancy who may be too ill to undergo a more involved procedure.[46]

Many of these current minimally invasive options do offer potential advantages in elderly patients. Some can be performed with the patient receiving a local anesthetic in the outpatient office setting. This obviates the need for general or regional anesthesia, which may be advantageous for older adults with multiple comorbidities. Some offer a significant reduction in the potential for perioperative bleeding, which is associated with the traditional TURP. This can be beneficial for elderly patients who may have undergone anticoagulation therapy for treatment of cardiovascular disease. Although each of the minimally invasive treatments show promise in clinical trials and with short-term follow-up, the long-term efficacy of each has yet to be fully determined.

Prostatitis

Several different forms of infection and inflammation can affect the prostate. These include acute prostatitis, chronic prostatitis, and prostatodynia. Although the precise prevalence of prostatitis is unclear and varies among studies, recent epidemiological data suggest an overall prevalence of 2%–10% in adult men.[47, 48] These studies suggested there are preliminary data that may indicate causal associations between a history of prostatitis and subsequent development of either BPH or prostate cancer. The clinical impact of prostatitis in elderly men is significant, and inpatient hospitalization rates to treat prostatitis in Medicare beneficiaries range from 2 to 2.5 times higher compared with younger men.[6, 49]

Acute bacterial prostatitis is most often associated with a rapid onset of symptoms including fever, chills, irritative voiding symptoms with frequency and urgency, dysuria, and pelvic or perineal pain. Because of a generalized decrease in immune function, elderly men may not mount a full symptomatic response and the clinical findings may be more subtle. The cause is usually from an ascending infection with bacteria from the distal urethra. This may be exacerbated by sexual activity or urethral instrumentation such as cystoscopy or catheter insertion. Rectal examination will usually reveal a swollen and tender prostate. Prostate massage should *not* be performed if acute bacterial prostatitis is suspected, because this can lead to systemic dissemination of bacteria and subsequent urosepsis. Urine cultures should be obtained to identify the organism involved in the infection and to help guide antibiotic therapy. If the patient is acutely ill, hospitalization with intravenous antibiotic administration may be necessary. Acute urinary retention may need to be treated with suprapubic tube insertion. Urethral catheterization should be avoided to prevent development of urosepsis. Oral antibiotic therapy is usually continued for four weeks. The most common antibiotics used for this are doxycycline or the fluoroquinolones because they can achieve adequate tissue concentrations in the prostate. CT examination may be useful to identify prostatic abscesses that would require surgical drainage.

Chronic prostatitis occurs more commonly than acute prostatitis in elderly men.[50] Typical symptoms include urinary urgency and frequency, dysuria, nocturia, low back pain, scrotal or perineal discomfort, or suprapubic pain. Findings on rectal examination can be variable. Some men will have significant tenderness or swelling of the prostate gland but others will not. Secretions obtained from prostatic massage may be helpful to establish the diagnosis. Microscopic examination may reveal bacteria or white blood cells. A urine culture should be obtained to help guide antibiotic selection. Initial therapy with approximately two weeks of antibiotic agents is indicated, although longer courses of antibiotics may be necessary. Avoiding dietary irritants such as caffeine, alcohol, or carbonated beverages may also be helpful.

Prostatodynia refers to a syndrome in which patients have symptoms suggestive of acute or chronic prostatitis without objective clinical findings. Pain is one of the hallmarks of this condition. Antibiotics often do not help to alleviate symptoms in these patients. Other causes of chronic pelvic pain should be considered such as interstitial cystitis, a chronic inflammatory condition of the urinary bladder that can cause similar symptoms. Treatment may be difficult and needs to be individualized for each patient. Anti-inflammatory agents, antihistamines, α-adrenergic antagonists, and pain medications may be useful. Conservative therapies with pelvic floor relaxation techniques or biofeedback therapy may also be of some benefit.

Penile disorders

In addition to penile cancers, a wide variety of benign conditions may affect the male genitalia. Many of these are inflammatory conditions, and these may be influenced by both anatomical factors and other comorbid conditions such as diabetes mellitus.

Phimosis

Phimosis is a condition characterized by narrowing of the foreskin, which makes retraction of the foreskin difficult or impossible. This may lead to pain and inflammation and may be associated with difficult voiding for some patients. Some dermatological conditions such as lichen sclerosis and balanitis xerotica obliterans (BXO) may increase the incidence of development of phimosis and potentially penile cancer.[51, 52] Surgical treatment with either a dorsal slit or circumcision may be needed to treat the condition.

Paraphimosis

In paraphimosis, the foreskin is retracted and becomes trapped behind the coronal sulcus. Tissue edema and swelling occurs that prevents the foreskin from reducing back over the glans penis. This can be quite painful, and, if left untreated, may lead to tissue necrosis or significant infection.[53] One of the most common causes of paraphimosis is retraction of the foreskin for placement of a urinary catheter or other manipulation of the penis, with failure to properly reduce the foreskin back to anatomical position after the procedure. It may also occur following sexual intercourse if the foreskin is not returned to anatomical position covering the glans penis. Manual reduction of a paraphimosis should be attempted and may require the use of a penile block with injectable local anesthetic. Once an adequate anesthetic level is obtained, gentle pressure can be applied circumferentially to the penis to help reduce tissue edema. The thumbs are then placed on the sides of the glans penis, and the first two forefingers of each hand are used to pull the foreskin back down past the coronal sulcus and over the glans. If this is unsuccessful, surgical reduction with a dorsal slit or circumcision may be required. Treatment should be considered a urological emergency.

Balanoposthitis

Balanoposthitis or balanitis is an inflammatory condition of the glans penis that may also involve the adjacent foreskin. The condition is frequently associated with diabetes mellitus and may be more common in men whose blood glucose levels are poorly controlled. An evaluation for diabetes should be performed in previously undiagnosed men with an episode of balanitis. Treatment of the condition includes cleansing of the glans penis with mild soap and water, and subsequent application of topical antifungal ointment. Limited administration of topical steroids may also be helpful to reduce inflammation. Oral antifungal agents may be necessary to help completely resolve any infection. If the condition does not improve with topical treatments or oral medication, then surgical intervention with circumcision may be required.

BXO is a specific type of balanitis that may be chronic and difficult to eradicate. In this condition, the tissue becomes firm and sclerotic in response to inflammation. Some studies have identified an association between BXO and an increased risk of developing penile cancers such as squamous cell carcinoma.[52]

Peyronie's disease

One of the more common benign conditions of the penis is Peyronie's disease.[54] This condition is characterized by development of a painful lump within the tissue of the penis associated with curvature of the penile shaft toward the lesion with erection. The condition is caused by a fibrous plaque in the tunica albuginea, the dense connective tissue that forms the outer layers of the corpus cavernosum of the penis. The fibrous plaque prevents stretching of this tissue with erection, which causes the penile curvature toward the side of the lesion. The condition may cause painful erections and may lead to significant erectile dysfunction.[55] Originally described more than a century ago, the exact etiology of the condition is still unknown, although research suggests that prior tissue trauma from vigorous sexual activity and systemic vascular disease may be risk factors.[56]

Treatment of Peyronie's disease can be difficult, and a variety of different therapies have been tried with variable success.[54, 55] Oral anti-inflammatory agents, including vitamin E, colchicine, and p-aminobenzoate (Potaba), have been useful in some men and may reduce the pain associated with both erection and the plaques themselves. Plaque injection with verapamil, interferon, and steroids has been used with variable success. In 2013, the FDA approved the use of injectable collagenase clostridium histolyticum (Xiaflex) for treatment of Peyronie's disease.[57] This acts to break down the collagen plaque through an enzymatic reaction. Several treatments may be necessary to yield clinical improvement. Surgical excision of the plaques can also be performed, although this may require tissue grafting to replace the tunica albuginea, which is removed. Depending on the technique used, this may also result in foreshortening of the penile shaft length. Placement of a penile prosthesis at the time of plaque excision may be necessary to help treat the associated erectile dysfunction.

Scrotal disorders

In addition to testis cancer, several benign conditions of the scrotum can occur in elderly men. These can be quite bothersome for patients and often require additional evaluation and treatment.

Epididymitis

Acute epididymitis is one of the most common scrotal problems seen in older men.[48] This is usually caused by a bacterial infection and may be associated with recent urinary tract instrumentation or chronic urethral catheter use. The condition often occurs in conjunction with other genitourinary infections including acute cystitis or prostatitis. Symptoms include swelling of the affected hemiscrotum with pain and swelling of the involved epididymis. Patients may also experience systemic symptoms of fever, chills, and malaise. If the cause of the patient's symptoms is unclear, a scrotal ultrasound can be helpful to establish the diagnosis. Epididymitis is typically associated with increased arterial blood flow to the epididymis in response to the acute inflammation. A urine culture should be obtained to help guide choice of antibiotic therapy, although empiric treatment should be administered prior to obtaining the final culture results. Scrotal support, bed rest, and topical application of ice packs can provide symptomatic relief.

Hydrocele

A hydrocele is caused by collection of fluid surrounding the testicle. It is usually associated with an anatomical defect of the layers of the tunica vaginalis. Diffuse scrotal enlargement is the most common presenting symptom, and this usually occurs gradually. Hydroceles are typically not painful unless there is an associated infection. In many cases, symptoms have been present for months or years before the patient seeks medical attention. Rapid development of hydrocele may be an indication of an underlying scrotal malignancy and appropriate clinical evaluation should be performed. With larger hydroceles, the volume of fluid surrounding the testicle may prevent palpation of the gonad. Positive transillumination of the scrotum is a clinical hallmark of the condition. Scrotal ultrasound may also be useful to establish the diagnosis.

Treatment is usually based on symptoms. Smaller asymptomatic hydroceles may be watched conservatively and often do not need additional therapy. Larger hydroceles can be bothersome for the patient and frequently interfere with walking or dressing. Although aspiration of the hydrocele fluid has been described, this is usually temporary and is associated with an increased risk of scrotal infection. Excision of the hydrocele is often effective and can be done with the patient receiving local or regional anesthetic on an outpatient basis.[58, 59] Hydroceles are sometimes associated with an inguinal hernia, which may also require surgical repair.

Spermatocele

Another common cystic enlargement in the scrotum is a spermatocele. These can vary in size and are located adjacent to the testicle, which is usually palpably normal. Spermatoceles typically transilluminate, but differ from hydroceles by the lack of excess fluid surrounding the testis. Spermatoceles are more common in men who have undergone prior vasectomy for control of fertility. In most cases, spermatoceles are asymptomatic and require no additional therapy beyond education and reassurance. Excision is often performed for enlarging or painful spermatoceles.[58]

Varicocele

A varicocele is caused by dilation of the veins of the pampiniform plexus. Patients experience a swelling of the veins in the spermatic cord and may feel a sense of heaviness or fullness in the hemiscrotum. Varicoceles are often unilateral and are most common on the left because the left gonadal vein drains into the left renal vein. In contrast, the right gonadal vein drains directly into the inferior vena cava, which is larger and thus less prone to causing venous obstruction and varicocele. Approximately 15% of all adult males have some degree of varicocele. In younger men, varicoceles may be associated with infertility and impaired sperm quality. Many varicoceles are asymptomatic and they often develop over months or years. Rapid development of a varicocele or presence of an isolated right-sided varicocele should prompt clinical and radiographic evaluation for a possible retroperitoneal mass or renal tumor. Tumor thrombus into the vena cava from a renal cell carcinoma or venous obstruction from extrinsic compression by a pelvic mass may cause rapid development of a varicocele. Asymptomatic varicoceles in older adults do not require treatment. If the varicocele is large or painful, excision or radiographic embolization may be performed; however, the patient must be counseled that treatment might not improve symptoms of scrotal pain.

Testicular torsion

Testicular torsion occurs when the testis rotates on its vascular axis, leading to arterial compromise. The onset of symptoms is usually sudden and includes pain and swelling of the associated hemiscrotum. Scrotal ultrasound with vascular Doppler imaging is useful to help establish the correct diagnosis. This condition is considered a urological emergency, and surgical intervention is indicated if the torsion cannot be manually reduced. Detorsion and fixation of the testis in the scrotum should be performed within four hours of the onset of symptoms to help improve clinical outcomes. If treatment is significantly delayed, the decreased arterial flow may result in tissue necrosis and loss of the testicle. Torsion of the testicle is rare in elderly men, and more often occurs in infants, children, and adolescents.

Scrotal edema

Benign scrotal edema is a very common condition seen in older men, particularly in the acute hospital setting. Patients with vascular disease, hypertension, ascites, congestive heart failure, and pulmonary edema are at increased risk for developing scrotal edema. Excess fluid accumulates in the most dependent areas including the legs and feet, the presacral tissues, and the scrotum. The condition is usually painless. In some cases of severe scrotal swelling, urination may be difficult because of compression of the urethra and penis. This may require placement of a urinary catheter. Treatment typically involves conservative therapy with scrotal elevation and support, and ice packs if the patient has pain. Diuretics may be indicated to treat underlying conditions such as congestive heart failure or pulmonary edema. The scrotal swelling will typically resolve with time once the underlying cause has been adequately treated.

Urethral strictures

Urethral strictures are scars that develop in the urethra that may lead to narrowing or even obliteration of the urethral lumen. Historically, sexually transmitted diseases (STDs) such as gonorrhea were a major cause of urethral stricture disease. They are now most often associated with a history of urethral or pelvic trauma. Traumatic urethral instrumentation increases the risk for development of a urethral stricture. In men who have undergone radical prostatectomy for prostate cancer or transurethral resection of the prostate (TURP) for BPH, scarring may develop at the junction between the urethra and bladder, leading to a bladder neck contracture. Urethral strictures are most often treated surgically; however, in some cases of mild strictures, urethral dilation may be adequate.[60] Urethral strictures are uncommon in women, and urethral dilation is not typically indicated unless an instrument cannot be passed easily during surgery. There are no data to support the routine use of urethral dilation in women for the treatment of voiding dysfunction.

Benign disorders of the lower female urinary tract

Urethral caruncle

Urethral caruncles typically present as benign, polypoid lesions of the distal urethra and are most often seen in postmenopausal women. These are usually small lesions, although in some cases they can reach up to 1 cm–2 cm in diameter. The etiology is unknown but may be related to urethral prolapse and chronic irritation associated with estrogen deficiency. In some patients the lesion may be painful or may bleed to the touch. Care must be taken to differentiate urethral caruncles, which are typically soft and mobile, from urethral carcinomas, which are typically firm or hard and more fixed in position. Excisional biopsy may be performed if there is a question about the histological composition. In most cases, urethral caruncles can be treated nonsurgically with warm Sitz baths and antiinflammatory medications. Topical estrogen can be quite useful and helps to shrink the lesions. Complete resolution may be observed with continued estrogen application. Excision is indicated only if more conservative therapy is ineffective or if the patient experiences clinically significant voiding dysfunction from obstruction.[61]

Urethral diverticulum

A urethral diverticulum is an outpouching of the anterior urethra in women that may be associated with significant lower urinary tract symptoms. The classic clinical triad includes dysuria, dyspareunia, and postvoid dribbling. Although the exact etiology is unknown, theories include obstruction of paraurethral ducts with development of an inclusion cyst in the wall of the urethra. Subsequent spontaneous drainage of the cyst cavity into the urethral lumen leads to development of an epithelialized tract between the diverticulum and the urethra. Congenital abnormalities can also lead to a thinning of the anterior urethral wall, which in turn could cause development of an opening between the diverticular space and the urethra. Physical examination usually reveals a soft tissue bulge in the suburethral area in the vagina. These are often tender to palpation because of the trapping of infected urine or sediment in the diverticular sac. Radiographic examination with voiding cystourethrography or pelvic magnetic resonance imaging may be helpful to establish the correct diagnosis. Excision including removal of the entire diverticular sac is indicated for symptomatic diverticula.[62] In some cases, the diverticular sac may be quite close to the external urethral sphincter, and care must be taken not to injure this structure during surgery because this could lead to urinary incontinence. If the opening to the diverticulum is small, the urethra may be repaired primarily; however, a vascularized pedicle flap may be necessary to repair larger defects in the anterior urethra.

Genitourinary fistulae

A fistula is defined as a connection between two hollow organs or between a hollow organ and the skin. Fistulae can occur in the genitourinary tract in older adults, often resulting from other underlying conditions or after treatment for these conditions. The most common types of fistulae involving the urinary system in older women include vesicovaginal fistulae between the bladder and vagina and vesicoenteric fistulae between the bladder and bowel. In developed countries, most vesicovaginal fistulae are iatrogenic and related to prior pelvic surgery such as hysterectomy. Colonic diverticular disease leads to an increased risk of vesicocolonic fistulae. Inflammatory bowel disorders such as Crohn's disease increase the risk of fistulae between the bladder and small intestine. Other risk factors for development of fistula include prior pelvic surgery or radiation or a history of pelvic malignancy. With a vesicovaginal fistula, women typically experience continuous urinary leakage from the vaginal vault. Chronic UTI with enteric bacteria is the most common problem associated with vesicoenteric or vesicocolonic fistulae. These associated symptoms may have a strong negative influence on quality of life. Evaluation includes identification of the type and location of the fistula tract by using physical examination, endoscopy, and imaging. Biopsy should be performed if there is a history of malignancy to check for possible recurrent disease. Treatment is most often surgical with excision of the fistula tract and repair of the effected organs.[63]

Atrophic vaginitis

In postmenopausal women, the decrease in vaginal estrogen levels may be associated with tissue changes in the vaginal mucosa. The most common condition is atrophic vaginitis, which may involve variable degrees of tissue inflammation. On clinical examination, the tissue appears pale and thin with loss of natural rugations. Patients may experience pelvic pain or dryness. Women who are sexually active may complain of dyspareunia. Unless contraindicated by a history of breast or uterine cancer, topical estrogen replacement is indicated to help reduce symptoms.

Pelvic organ prolapse

Various forms of pelvic organ prolapse are common in elderly women. Loss of anterior pelvic floor support results in a protrusion of the bladder into the vaginal vault, which is referred to as a cystocele. A rectocele occurs if the posterior aspect of the vaginal wall is involved. In an enterocele, the apex of the vaginal vault is prolapsed. These entities may occur alone or in combination. Pessaries can be used to reduce the prolapse and provide a nonsurgical form of therapy for some patients. In some cases, surgical repair may be indicated. Additional information on pelvic organ prolapse is provided in Chapter 28 on gynecological disorders in elderly women.

Sexual health

Assessment and treatment of sexual disorders is an important part of health care for many older adults. Several comorbid conditions that are common in older adults can have significant negative influence on sexual health including diabetes, hypertension, heart disease, and vascular insufficiency. Urinary incontinence can negatively influence sexual activity in both men and women.[64, 65]

Sexually transmitted diseases (STDs) can occur in older adults, and patients with clinical symptoms or those who are at risk should be screened for STDs as indicated.[66] Older adults have generally not been targeted in public health campaigns for prevention of STDs including human immunodeficiency virus

(HIV). This is changing, however, and there is an increased awareness that older adults may need education for prevention and treatment of STDs. Some clinical trials are also now focusing on therapy for STDs and HIV in older adults.[67] Issues related to sexual health are discussed in more detail in Chapter 45.

Conclusion

A wide variety of urological conditions occur in older adults. Because of associated symptoms such as urinary incontinence, infection, or pain, these may have a significant negative influence on activities and health-related quality of life. Appropriate evaluation and treatment are important for effective management. Successful treatment may lead to reduction or elimination of symptoms and significant improvements in quality of life for elderly patients.[68]

References

1. Bragg E, Hansen JC. A revelation of numbers: will America's eldercare workforce be ready to care for an aging America? *Generations.* 2011;**34**(4):11–19.

2. Davis R, Jones JS, Barocas DA, et al. Diagnosis, evaluation and follow-up of asymptomatic microhematuria (AMH) in adults: AUA guideline. *J Urol.* 2012;**18**(6 Suppl):2473–2481.

3. Cowan NC. CT urography for hematuria. *Nat Rev Urol.* 2012;**9**(4):218–226.

4. Zargooshi J, Nourizad S, Vaziri S, et al. Hematospermia: long-term outcome in 165 patients. *Int J Impot Res.* 2014;**26**(3):83–86.

5. Griebling TL. Urologic Diseases in America Project: trends in resource use for urinary tract infections in women. *J Urol.* 2005;**173**:1281–1287.

6. Griebling TL. Urologic Diseases in America Project: trends in resource use for urinary tract infections in men. *J Urol.* 2005;**173**:1288–1294.

7. Eriksson I, Gustafson Y, Fagerström L, Olofsson B. Prevalence and factors associated with urinary tract infections (UTIs) in very old women. *Arch Gerontol Geriatr.* 2010;**50**(2):132–135.

8. Tal S, Guller V, Levi S, et al. Profile and prognosis of febrile elderly patients with bacteremic urinary tract infection. *J Infect.* 2005;**50**:296–305.

9. Rodhe N, Mölstad S, Englund L, et al. Asymptomatic bacteriuria in a population of elderly residents living in a community setting: prevalence, characteristics and associated factors. *Fam Pract.* 2006;**23**:303–307.

10. Ginde AA, Rhee SH, Katz ED. Predictors of outcome in geriatric patients with urinary tract infections. *J Emerg Med.* 2004;**27**:101–108.

11. Dromerick AW, Edwards DF. Relation of postvoid residual to urinary tract infection during stroke rehabilitation. *Arch Phys Med Rehabil.* 2003;**84**:1369–1372.

12. Paillaud E, Herbaud S, Caillet P, et al. Relations between under-nutrition and nosocomial infections in elderly patients. *Age Ageing.* 2005;**34**:619–625.

13. Hazelett SE, Tsai M, Gareri M, Allen K. The association between indwelling urinary catheter use in the elderly and urinary tract infection in acute care. *BMC Geriatr.* 2006;**6**:15.

14. Henig YS, Leahy MM. Cranberry juice and urinary-tract health: science supports folklore. *Nutrition.* 2000;**16**:684–687.

15. Caljouw MA, van den Hout WB, Putter H, et al. Effectiveness of cranberry capsules to prevent urinary tract infections in vulnerable older persons: a double-blind randomized placebo-controlled trial in long-term care facilities. *J Am Geriatr Soc.* 2014;**62**(1):103–110.

16. Parsons BA, Narshi A, Drake MJ. Success rates for learning intermittent self-catheterisation according to age and gender. *Int Urol Nephrol.* 2012;**44**(4):1127–1131.

17. Pearle MS, Calhoun EA, Curhan GC, et al. Urologic Diseases in America Project: urolithiasis. *J Urol.* 2005;**173**:848–857.

18. Daudon M, Doré JC, Jungers P, et al. Changes in stone composition according to age and gender of patients: a multivariate epidemiological approach. *Urol Res.* 2004;**32**:241–247.

19. Wong YV, Cook P, Somani BK. The association of metabolic syndrome and urolithiasis. *Int J Endocrinol.* 2015;**2015**:570674.

20. Usui Y, Matsuzaki S, Matsushita K, et al. Urolithiasis in geriatric patients. *Tokai J Exp Clin Med.* 2003;**28**:81–87.

21. Siegel RL, Miller KD, Jemal A. Cancer statistics, 2015. *CA Cancer J Clin.* 2015;**65**:5–29.

22. Gupta M, McCauley J, Farkas A, et al. Clinical practice guidelines on prostate cancer: a critical appraisal. *J Urol.* 2015;**193**(4):1153–1158.

23. US Preventive Services Task Force. Screening for prostate cancer: US Preventive Services Task Force recommendation statement. *Ann Intern Med.* 2008;**148**:185–191.

24. Walter LC, Bertenthal D, Lindquist K, Konety BR. PSA screening among elderly men with limited life expectancies. *JAMA.* 2006;**296**:2336–2342.

25. Fontana PP, Gregorio SA, Rivas JG, et al. Perioperative and survival outcomes of laparoscopic radical cystectomy for bladder cancer in patients over 70 years. *Cent European J Urol.* 2015;**68**(1):24–29.

26. Deliveliotis C, Papatsoris A, Chrisofos M, et al. Urinary diversion in high-risk elderly patients: modified cutaneous ureterostomy or ileal conduit? *Urology.* 2005;**66**:299–304.

27. Wheater MJ, Manners J, Nolan L, et al. The clinical features and management of testicular germ cell tumours in patients aged 60 years and older. *BJU Int.* 2011;**108**:1794–1799.

28. Fonseca R, Habermann TM, Colgan JP, et al. Testicular lymphoma is associated with a high incidence of extranodal recurrence. *Cancer.* 2000;**88**:154–161.

29. Fitzpatrick JM. The natural history of benign prostatic hyperplasia. *BJU Int.* 2006;**97**(Suppl 2):3–6.

30. Tikkinen KA, Auvinen A, Johnson TM 2nd, et al: A systematic evaluation of factors associated with nocturia: the population-based FINNO study. *Am J Epidemiol.* 2009;**170**:361–368.

31. Perchon LFG, Pintarelli VL, Bezerra E, et al.Quality of life in elderly men with aging symptoms and lower urinary tract symptoms (LUTS). *Neurourol Urodyn.* 2011;**30**:515–519.

32. DuBeau CE. The aging lower urinary tract. *J Urol.* 2006;**175**:S11–S15.

33. Saigal CS. Quality indicators for benign prostatic hyperplasia in vulnerable elders. *J Amer Geriatr Soc.* 2007;**55**:S253 S257.

34. Resnick MI, Roehrborn CG. Rapid onset of action with alfuzosin 10 mg once daily in men with benign prostatic hyperplasia: a randomized, placebo-controlled trial. *Prostate Cancer Prostatic Dis.* 2007;**10**:155–159.

35. Giuliano F. Impact of medical treatments for benign prostatic hyperplasia on sexual function. *BJU Int.* 2006;**97**(Suppl 2):34–38.

36. Van Dijk MM, de la Rosette JJ, Michel MC. Effects of alpha(1)-adrenoceptor antagonists on male sexual function. *Drugs.* 2006;**66**:287–301.

37. Friedman AH. Tamsulosin and the intraoperative floppy iris syndrome. *JAMA.* 2009;**301**:2044–2045.

38. Roehrborn CG, Bruskewitz R, Nickel JC, et al. Sustained decrease in incidence of acute urinary retention and surgery with finasteride for 6 years in men with benign prostatic hyperplasia. *J Urol.* 2004;**171**:1194–1198.

39. Roehrborn CG, Siami P, Barkin J, et al. The effects of dutasteride, tamsulosin and combination therapy in lower urinary tract symptoms in men with benign prostatic hyperplasia and prostatic enlargement: 2-year results from the CombAT Study. *J Urol.* 2008;**179**(2):616–621.

40. Wang X, Wang X, Li S, et al. Comparative effectiveness of oral drug therapies for lower urinary tract symptoms due to benign prostatic hyperplasia: a systematic

review and network meta-analysis. *PLoS One.* 2014;**9**(9):e107593.

41 Espinosa G. Nutrition and benign prostatic hyperplasia. *Curr Opin Urol.* 2013;**23**(1):38–41.

42. Poon KS, McVary KT. Dietary patterns, supplement use, and the risk of benign prostatic hyperplasia. *Curr Urol Rep.* 2009;**10**(4):279–286.

43. Hoffman RM, Monga M, Elliot SP, et al. Microwave thermotherapy for benign prostatic hyperplasia. *Cochrane Database Syst Rev.* 2007;**17**:CD004135.

44. Aagaard MF, Niebuhr MH, Jacobsen JD, Krøyer Nielsen K. Transurethral microwave thermotherapy treatment of chronic urinary retention in patients unsuitable for surgery. *Scand J Urol.* 2014;**48**(3):290–294.

45. Bozkurt IH, Yalcinkaya F, Sertcelik MN, et al. A good alternative to indwelling catheter owing to benign prostate hyperplasia in elderly: Memotherm prostatic stent. *Urology.* 2013;**82**:1004–1007.

46. Ogiste JS, Cooper K, Kaplan SA. Are stents still a useful therapy for benign prostatic hyperplasia? *Curr Opin Urol.* 2003;**13**:51–57.

47. Krieger JN, Riley DE, Cheah PY, et al. Epidemiology of prostatitis: new evidence for a world-wide problem. *World J Urol.* 2003;**21**:70–74.

48. Nickel JC, Teichman JMH, Gregore M, et al. Prevalence, diagnosis, characterization, and treatment of prostatitis, interstitial cystitis, and epididymitis in outpatient urologic practice: the Canadian PIE Study. *Urology.* 2005;**66**:935–940.

49. Suskind AM, Berry SH, Ewing BA, et al. The prevalence and overlap of interstitial cystitis / bladder pain syndrome and chronic prostatitis/chronic pelvic pain syndrome in men: results of the RAND Interstitial Cystitis Epidemiology Male Study. *J Urol.* 2013;**189**(1):141–145.

50. Wagenlehner FM, Weidner W, Pilatz A, Naber KG. Urinary tract infections and bacterial prostatitis in men. *Curr Opin Infect Dis.* 2014;**27**(1):97–101.

51. Fistarol SK, Itin PH. Diagnosis and treatment of lichen sclerosus: an update. *Am J Clin Dermatol.* 2013;**14**(1):27–47.

52. Philippou P, Shabbir M, Ralph DJ, et al. Genital lichen sclerosus/balanitis xerotica obliterans in men with penile carcinoma: a critical analysis. *BJU Int.* 2013;**111**(6):970–976.

53. Williams JC, Morrison PM, Richardson JR. Paraphimosis in elderly men. *Am J Emerg Med.* 1995;**13**:351–353.

54. Miner MM, Seftel AD. Peyronie's disease: epidemiology, diagnosis and management. *Curr Med Res Opin.* 2014;**30**(1):113–120.

55. Garaffa G, Trost LW, Serefoglu EC, et al. Understanding the course of Peyronie's disease. *Int J Clin Pract.* 2013;**67**(8):781–788.

56. Bjekic MD, Vlajinac HD, Sipetic SB, Marinkovic JM. Risk factors for Peyronie's disease: a case-control study. *BJU Int.* 2006;**97**:570–574.

57. Alwaal A, Hussein AA, Zaid UB, Lue TF. Management of Peyronie's disease after collagenase (Xiaflex*). *Curr Drug Targets.* 2015;**16**(5):484–494.

58. Kiddoo DA, Wollin TA, Mador DR. A population based assessment of complications following outpatient hydrocelectomy and spermatocelectomy. *J Urol.* 2004;**171**:746–748.

59. Menon VS, Sheridan WG. Benign scrotal pathology: should all patients undergo surgery? *BJU Int.* 2001;**88**:251–254.

60. Barbagli G, Palminteri E, Lazzeri M, et al. Long-term outcomes of urethroplasty after failed urethrotomy versus primary repair. *J Urol.* 2001;**165**:1918–1919.

61. Ozkurkcugil C, Ozkan L, Tarcan T. The effect of asymptomatic urethral caruncle on micturition in women with urinary incontinence. *Korean J Urol.* 2010;**51**:257–259.

62. Ljungqvist L, Peeker R, Fall M. Female urethral diverticulum: 26-year followup of a large series. *J Urol.* 2007;**177**:219–224.

63. Wong MJ, Wong K, Rezvan A, et al. Urogenital fistula. *Female Pelvic Med Reconstr Surg.* 2012;**18**(2):71–78.

64. Tannenbaum C, Corcos J, Assalian P. The relationship between sexual activity and urinary incontinence in older women. *J Am Geriatr Soc.* 2006;**54**:1220–1224.

65. Griebling TL. The impact of urinary incontinence on sexual health in older adults. *J Am Geriatr Soc.* 2006;**54**:1290–1292.

66. Wilson MM. Sexually transmitted diseases. *Clin Geriatr Med.* 2003;**19**:637–655.

67. Greene M, Justice AC, Lampiris HW, Valcour V. Management of human immunodeficiency virus infection in advanced age. *JAMA.* 2013;**309**(13):1397–1405.

68. Gerharz EW, Emberton M. Quality of life research in urology. *World J Urol.* 1999;**17**:191–192.

Chapter 27

Urinary incontinence and fecal incontinence

Alayne D. Markland, DO, MSc, Theodore M. Johnson II, MD, MPH, Mary H. Palmer, PhD, RN-C, and Jan Busby-Whitehead, MD, CMD

Urinary incontinence (UI), the involuntary loss of urine, has a prevalence of 40% in older women and about 22% in older men.[1] Fecal incontinence (FI), the involuntary loss of bowel or accidental bowel leakage, has a lower prevalence than UI, but is equally prevalent in older men and women, 8%–17%. Dual incontinence, both UI and FI, is present in 10% of the older male and female community-dwelling population, according to data in the United States (see Figure 27.1).[1]

Only approximately one-third of incontinent women have UI or FI to such a degree that they viewed it as a significant bother.[2] Twelve percent of older women report severe or very severe UI. Frequent or severe UI and FI can have a devastating impact on people's lives, leading to social withdrawal and depression and contributing to the decision to go into a nursing home.[3] Leaking small amounts of urine and/or bowel can often be managed by wearing pads and has only a modest impact on quality of life.

UI and FI prevalence increases with age in older men and women compared to younger age groups (<65 years). Older men may have increases in UI and FI prevalence with age similar to older women, as shown in Figure 27.2. The loss of continence will not always occur with aging. Many specific age-related changes, such as functional impairments in mobility, dexterity, cognition, and reduction in bladder and bowel capacity and sensation, contribute to UI and FI. Other established risk factors that are not age related include obesity and parity in women for UI and FI. The strongest single risk factor for UI in men other than age is prostatectomy or transurethral resection.[2] Stool consistency is a strong risk factor for FI in men and women.

An estimated 60% of people with UI and FI who are identified through surveys have not reported their incontinence to a health care provider,[4] perhaps because they are embarrassed or believe nothing can be done to help.[5] This is unfortunate because UI and FI are curable in many and can be managed in most cases.[6] Health-care providers, therefore, should specifically ask about incontinence.

Physiological mechanism for continence, micturition, and defecation

Innervation of the lower urinary tract system and the anorectal area is under cholinergic, adrenergic, and somatic control. The early phase of bladder accommodation is mediated by β-adrenergic receptors in the bladder dome. Bladder and lower rectal contraction is mediated by cholinergic (parasympathetic) activity, whereas relaxation of the urethral and anal internal and external sphincters is mediated by adrenergic (sympathetic) pathways in the pudendal nerve via a spinal reflex mediated by the S2–S4 sacral nerve roots. Normal bladder capacity is 300 mL–600 mL. Less is known about normal bowel capacity, given the wide variations in compliance of the recto-sigmoid region.

Central nervous system control of bladder and bowel sphincter function is mostly inhibitory; that is, reflex bladder and bowel contractions are actively inhibited until a socially appropriate time and place to urinate and/or defecate is found. This inhibition occurs through neural linkages from the sensorimotor cortex of the frontal lobes to the brainstem, cerebellum, thalamus, and spinal cord. Micturition and defecation normally involve a conscious disinhibition of bladder and/or bowel contractions. Thus, stroke and other neurological processes can result in UI and FI because of loss of central cortical inhibition. Excessive

Reichel's Care of the Elderly, 7th Edition, ed. Jan Busby-Whitehead *et al.* Published by Cambridge University Press.
© Cambridge University Press 2016.

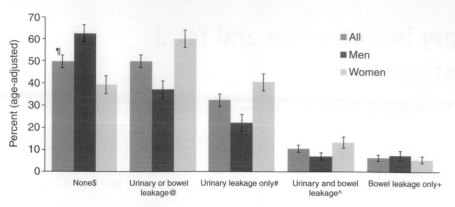

Figure 27.1 and 27.2 Prevalence of UI, FI, and DI among older community-dwelling adults in the United States. (A black-and-white version of these figures will appear in some formats. For the color version, please refer to the plate section.)

¶ - 95% confidence interval

$ - Persons who answered "Never" to each question about frequency of urinary leakage and accidental bowel leakage of mucus, liquid stool, or solid stool.

@ - Persons who reported urinary leakage or accidental bowel leakage of mucus, liquid stool, or solid stool.

- Persons who reported a urinary leakage and answered "Never" to each question about frequency of accidental bowel leakage or mucus, liquid stool, or solid stool.

^- Persons who reported a urinary leakage and accidental bowel leakage of mucus, liquid stool, or solid stool.

+ - Persons who answered "Never" to the question about frequency of urinary leakage, and reported accidental bowel leakage of mucus, liquid stool, or solid stool

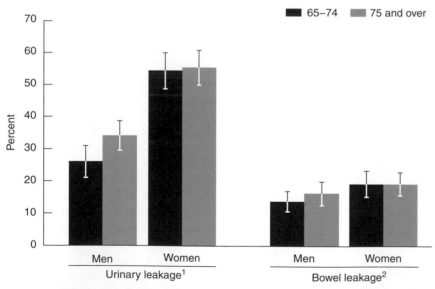

I 95% confidence interval.

[1]Persons who reported a urinary leakage.

[2]Persons who reported accidental bowel leakage of mucus, liquid stool, or solid stool.

bladder filling may overcome higher cortical inhibitory inputs, resulting in the involuntary contraction of the bladder via the reflex arc (referred to as uninhibited bladder contractions). Less is known about the central process of defecation in comparison to micturition.

The urethra and anus are composed of internal (smooth muscle) and external (striated muscle) sphincters. Somatic innervation through the pudendal nerve allows voluntary contraction of the external sphincter and pelvic floor musculature that protects against urine and bowel loss from sudden increases in abdominal pressure. Voluntary contraction of the external urethral muscle also reflexively inhibits bladder contraction and can interrupt voiding. Voluntary contraction of the external anal muscles can also inhibit bowel wall contraction and delay defecation.

Continence depends on voluntary inhibition of reflex bladder and bowel contraction and intermittent, as needed, voluntary contraction of the striated pelvic floor muscles to counter increases in intra-abdominal pressure. Micturition and defecation require voluntary disinhibition of bladder and bowel contractions, which reflexly leads to relaxation of both the internal and external urethral sphincters.

Classification for urinary and fecal incontinence

Transient incontinence is defined as new leaking of sudden onset that is generally associated with an acute medical or surgical illness or drug therapy, and it is usually reversible with resolution of the underlying problem. "Functional incontinence" is another term that has been used for this condition. Causes of transient urinary and fecal incontinence are diverse (Table 27.1). Drug side effects contribute greatly to this problem; therefore, a review of prescription and over-the-counter medications is extremely important.

Established urinary and fecal incontinence are usually chronic, require investigation, and are amenable to treatment in many cases. There are four types of established urinary incontinence: stress, urge, mixed incontinence, and overflow (also termed "chronic urinary retention" and "incontinence with a high postvoid residual") (see Table 27.2).

Urgency urinary incontinence

Urgency incontinence results from unsuppressed bladder contractions (detrusor instability). These uninhibited contractions are associated with an irresistible urge to void and usually result in loss of a large volume (>100 mL). Patients with urgency incontinence may also have symptoms of urgency, frequent urination, and nocturia, which is called overactive bladder (OAB). By definition, to have OAB, one must have urinary urgency

Table 27.1 Identification of reversible conditions that may cause or contribute to urinary incontinence and fecal incontinence

Conditions affecting the lower urinary tract and anorectal area

Urinary tract infection (symptomatic with frequency, urgency, dysuria)

Atrophic vaginitis or urethritis

Prostatectomy

Stool impaction

Radiation treatments for cancer – prostate, colon, cervical

Hemorrhoidectomy

Drug side effects that may contribute to UI and FI

Diuretics: polyuria, frequency, urgency

Caffeine: aggravation or precipitation of UI and FI (bowel stimulation)

Anticholinergic agents: urinary retention, overflow incontinence, constipation

Psychotropic medications

Antidepressants: anticholinergic actions, sedation, diarrhea

Antipsychotics: anticholinergic actions, sedation, immobility, rigidity, constipation

Sedatives, hypnotics, CNS depressants: sedation, delirium, immobility, muscle relaxation

Opioid analgesics: urinary retention, constipation, fecal impaction, sedation, delirium

α-adrenergic blockers: urethral relaxation

α-adrenergic agonists: urinary retention (found in many cold and diet over-the-counter preparations)

$\beta3$-adrenergic agonists: urinary retention

Calcium channel blockers: urinary retention, constipation

Alcohol: polyuria, frequency, urgency, diarrhea, sedation, delirium, immobility
Digoxin: diarrhea if serum levels elevated
Metformin: diarrhea
Colchine: diarrhea
Nonsteroidal anti-inflammatory medications: constipation

385

Table 27.1 (cont.)

Increased urine production

Metabolic disorders (hyperglycemia, hypercalcemia)

Excess fluid intake

Volume overload

Venous insufficiency with edema

Congestive heart failure

Increased stool production and loose stool

Malabsorption syndromes, including lactose intolerance

Irritable bowel syndrome

Inflammatory bowel diseases

Impaired ability or willingness to reach the toilet

Delirium

Chronic illness, injury; restraint that interferes with mobility

Psychological disorders

CNS – central nervous system
Source: Modified from Fantl et al.[6]

Table 27.2 Types of urinary incontinence and characteristics

UI type	Characteristics
Urgency UI	Often occurs with a strong urgency sensation and uninhibited detrusor (bladder) contraction Large volume leakage
Stress UI	Hypermobile urethra Internal sphincter insufficiency Reduced pelvic floor musculature
	May also be secondary to trauma (e.g., obstetrical) or surgery (e.g., prostatectomy)
	Small or large amounts of leakage may occur
Overflow UI	More common in older adults with impaired mobility and functional impairments (e.g., long-term care residents)
	Usually involves prostatic enlargement in men and prolapse in women
	Worsened with medications with anticholinergic side effects
	May need to treat constipation symptoms

without a urinary tract infection (UTI). "Detrusor hyperreflexia" is a term describing unsuppressed bladder contractions associated with a neurological disorder. Any damage to the structural integrity of the cholinergic inhibitory center of the central nervous system, or the afferent innervation from the lower spinal cord where the reflex arc is located, can cause detrusor hyperreflexia. Processes such as Alzheimer's disease, cerebrovascular atherosclerosis, multiple sclerosis, Parkinson's disease, spinal cord tumors or transection, and cervical spondylosis (among others) may result in UI by this mechanism.[6]

Stress urinary incontinence

Stress UI occurs in women more than men and results from a hypermobile urethra, internal sphincter insufficiency, or reduced support by the pelvic floor musculature in the bladder outlet. Multiple childbirths, gynecological surgery, and decreased effects of estrogen on pelvic tissues, vasculature, and urethral mucosa are possible causes. Sphincter weakness may also be the result of urethral inflammation, neurological disease, radiation therapy, or α-blocker drugs. In men, stress incontinence may occur following prostatectomy. Patients are likely to complain of losing small amounts of urine with coughing, straining, lifting, or changing posture. Some men following prostatectomy will have constant urinary dribbling.

Overflow urinary incontinence (bladder outlet obstruction and neurogenic bladder)

Bladder outlet obstruction is more common in men than women, and it occurs primarily because of benign prostatic hypertrophy (BPH) or prostatic enlargement, prostatic neoplasm, or urethral stricture. BPH may result in lower urinary tract symptoms (LUTS) such as frequency, urgency, nocturia, hesitancy, or weak urinary stream. In women, urethral stricture or severe bladder prolapse may also impede urine flow. In both men and women, partial obstruction may become complete obstruction with the use of anticholinergic or α-agonist pharmacological agents, or with severe constipation. "Atonic" and "neurogenic bladder" are terms describing impaired bladder contractions resulting from low spinal cord lesions, diabetic or alcoholic neuropathy, and/or intake of muscle relaxants, opioids, or antidepressants. The usual clinical presentation of bladder outlet obstruction or neurogenic bladder is constant dribbling or leaking associated with an enlarged, palpable bladder. The physical examination finding of a grossly enlarged bladder is very specific, but poorly sensitive for establishing the diagnosis of outlet obstruction. Patients generally strain to urinate, and voluntarily and involuntarily voided urine volumes are frequently small.

Urge, passive, and mixed fecal incontinence

Types of FI are similar to UI and include urge, passive, mixed (urge and passive), and overflow fecal incontinence. Seepage and staining can also be types of passive fecal incontinence. Seepage can also occur with fecal impaction and severe constipation. Accidental bowel leakage is the preferred terminology to use when discussing FI with patients.[7] (See Table 27.3.)

Fecal incontinence and fecal impaction

FI can result from constipation with stool impaction and may be more common in certain frail, older populations. In a recent study, 81% of residents in long-term care settings had symptoms of constipation and FI.[8] However, the true prevalence of impaction and FI in nursing home residents and home-care settings has not been clearly identified. Since constipation with FI is difficult to diagnose, treatments should target constipation.

Incontinence evaluation

History

Evaluation should begin with a detailed history of the nature, severity, and burden of incontinence and identifying the most easily remedied contributing causes. An incontinence diary for urination or defecation filled out before the patient's visit is helpful. A history of leakage occurring with specific activities or before/after toileting can also help determine the type of incontinence. Questionnaires may also be used to help determine the predominant symptoms associated with urinary leakage.[9]

Table 27.3 Types of fecal incontinence and characteristics

FI type	Characteristics
Urgency FI	Often occurs with a strong urgency sensation to have a bowel movement Liquid stool or diarrhea often associated with the inability to hold stool in the rectal vault
Passive FI	Accidental bowel leakage without the sensation of the need to defecate
	May not be able to differentiate passing gas from having a bowel movement
	May also involve seepage after a bowel movement Staining may also be a type of passive accidental bowel leakage
Overflow FI	More common in older adults with impaired mobility and functional impairments (e.g., long-term care residents)
	May also involve seepage or smaller amounts of stool loss around an impaction
	Associated with symptoms of constipation
	May need to treat constipation symptoms to improve FI

Important items of the medical history include data about childbirth, pelvic surgery, cancer, neurological disease, diabetes mellitus, congestive heart failure, pelvic floor radiation, prior hemorrhoid surgery, and previous treatment of UI or FI. Specific questions should be asked about prescription and over-the-counter medication use, alcohol use, and fluid intake, along with food sensitivities (e.g., lactose intolerance). Inquiries should be made about the physical layout of the patient's residence and whether impaired mobility limits access to toilet facilities. The patient should bring a bag containing all prescription and nonprescription drugs to the clinic so that medications that may contribute to incontinence can be identified.

Physical examination and diagnostic testing

The physical examination should focus on the abdomen and urogenital area and the central and

387

peripheral nervous systems. The abdominal examination is insensitive for a high postvoid residual (PVR) or in chronic urinary retention, but gross bladder distention (e.g., >500 mL) can usually be detected. In acute urinary retention, the distended bladder is a firm, midline mass that originates from the pelvis and is dull to percussion. The rectal examination may reveal fecal impaction, a pelvic mass, external hemorrhoids, or an enlarged prostate gland. It is very important to assess perianal sensation and the patient's ability to contract and relax the anal sphincter voluntarily. An abnormal clinical sign can suggest serious lumbosacral disease, possibly requiring emergency treatment. In women, a pelvic examination is indicated to assess urethral, uterine, or bladder prolapse and to evaluate the patient for any pelvic mass. A gray, dry vaginal mucosa is suggestive of atrophic vaginitis.

The most important diagnostic distinction is between overflow urinary and fecal incontinence and the other types of UI or FI. Most studies show a poor correlation between the underlying cause and the patient's symptoms. Urinary and fecal incontinence that results from several causes (mixed incontinence) in older people limits the usefulness of evaluation algorithms based on symptoms and signs alone.[10]

Diagnostic tests for incontinence

Selected tests are recommended for the evaluation of patients with urinary leakage. On initial evaluation, a urinalysis and/or a urine culture, if indicated, should be done. Properly collected clean catch urine is adequate for culture even for nursing home residents,[11] although some persons will require an in-and-out catheterization to obtain an appropriate specimen. Further evaluation may be indicated for older patients with even transient hematuria, as the risk of malignancy is appreciable.[12]

Tests for blood urea nitrogen (BUN), creatinine, glucose, and calcium are recommended if compromised renal function or polyuria is suspected in patients not taking diuretics.[6] The PVR urine volume should be measured in all patients with symptoms of incontinence. This can be done by inserting, in sterile fashion, a No.14 French straight catheter into the bladder. Caution is indicated for patients with outflow obstruction, as a single catheterization may cause infection. Alternatively, a bladder ultrasound scan may be obtained 5–10 minutes after the

patient has voided. The portable ultrasound scan has been shown to be highly reliable, especially at low and very high bladder volumes.[13, 14] Although the definition of a high PVR is controversial, a volume of 200 mL or more suggests either outlet obstruction or neurogenic bladder and is an indication for further urological evaluation.[15] Clinical tests for stress incontinence in women may be useful if urine leakage is present on pelvic examination. Such tests include a supine cough stress test and other types of pad testing for cough or strain induced urinary leakage.[16]

Laboratory tests for causes of loose stool may include evaluation for infectious causes of diarrhea and malabsorption syndromes (including *Clostridium difficile* evaluation, fat malabsorption, and the presence of leukocytes). Other testing could involve serum tests to evaluate for celiac disease.

Formal urodynamic testing

After the basic evaluation, treatment for the presumed type of incontinence should be initiated, unless there is need for further evaluation. Further evaluation may be indicated for the following: failure of initial treatment, a history of surgery or radiotherapy, marked prolapse on physical examination, PVR greater than 200 mL, inability to pass a catheter, or patients considering more invasive treatment options who desire further evaluation.[15] Common urodynamic tests that provide more detailed diagnostic information include urine flowmetry, voiding cystourethrography, multichannel cystometrogram, pressure-flow study, urethral pressure profile measurement, and sphincter electromyography.[6]

Specialized tests for fecal incontinence

Specialized testing for FI may be indicated if other warning signs are present, such as hematochezia, a family history of colon cancer/inflammatory bowel disease, anemia, positive fecal occult blood test, unexplained weight loss ≥10 pounds, constipation that is refractory to treatment, and new onset constipation/diarrhea without evidence of potential primary cause. If these symptoms are present, colonoscopy may be needed to evaluate for colonic lesions, mass or obstruction, volvulus, megacolon, strictures, or mucosal biopsy. Abdominal radiographs may indicate significant stool retention in the colon and suggest the diagnosis of megacolon, a volvulus, or a mass lesion.

Abdominal ultrasound could be ordered if acute or chronic cholecystitis symptoms are suspected as a potential cause for the change in bowel symptoms.

Evaluation may be needed to identify anatomic abnormalities or factors such as external or internal anal sphincter tears or scarring, rectal sphincter muscle weakness, or pelvic floor dyssynergia. Three types of specialized testing may help with the diagnosis and etiology of FI symptoms.[17] Although findings from these tests may identify specific treatments, few have been evaluated for cost-effectiveness.

1. Anorectal manometry measures internal and external anal sphincter pressure at rest and during contraction. High-resolution manometry may also be considered. Sensation and rectal capacity can also be evaluated with a rectal balloon. Balloon expulsion tests can be used with anorectal manometry to evaluate pelvic floor dyssynergia and other defecation disorders.

2. Two- or three-dimensional endoanal ultrasound evaluates structural defects in the external or internal anal sphincters. Often, scarring or thinning of the muscle layers can also be detected. Endoanal ultrasound is done to evaluate patients with FI.

3. Defecography evaluates the defecatory process after a barium paste is inserted rectally and the patient defecates under fluoroscopy. Defecography can assess rectal emptying or structural abnormalities in the pelvic floor, like obstruction or the presence of a rectocele.

Treatments for UI and FI

Accurate diagnosis of UI and FI is essential for appropriate treatment. Any cause of transient incontinence identified during evaluation should be addressed specifically. Behavioral, pharmacological, and surgical therapies are all effective in older people (see Table 27.4). It is generally advisable to begin a treatment regimen with the least risk and burden to the patient and caregiver. In all types of incontinence, except those characterized by an obstructive process or poor bladder contractility, behavioral techniques should be considered as first-line therapy unless the patient has a specific preference for another type of therapy.[6]

Management of UI and FI in long-term care settings differs from management in the ambulatory care setting for two principal reasons. First, comorbidities such as dementia and mobility impairment are more frequent and more severe in the long-term care

setting, and these complicate management. Second, in the outpatient setting, behavioral interventions can be implemented by the patients themselves or by highly motivated caregivers who are usually family members. In long-term care, these interventions are implemented by nursing assistants whose motivation may be compromised by high patient-to-staff ratios. For these reasons, treatment of UI in the long-term care setting is discussed separately.

Ambulatory care treatment of UI

Successful treatment of functional incontinence relies on the recognition that physical, pharmacological, psychological, and environmental problems coexist that can cause or worsen UI. Providing the patient with assistive devices such as a urinal or bedside commode; reassessing drug indications, doses, and schedules; treating depression; addressing hostility; eliminating barriers in the path to the toilet; and removing restraints may improve incontinence dramatically. A visit to the patient's home by a visiting nurse and discussion with family members can be very helpful in identifying barriers to continence and implementing simple changes that improve continence. Treatments that are specific to each type of UI are discussed in the following sections.

Urgency incontinence

The treatment of urge incontinence entails designing interventions to decrease or block uninhibited bladder contractions, improve bladder capacity, and prolong the time from symptoms of urgency to voiding. Effective strategies include (1) dietary and lifestyle changes, (2) behavioral training (timed voiding), and (3) drugs to reduce bladder contractions.

Dietary management

Self-monitoring techniques such as reducing caffeine and alcohol intake, management of constipation, and drinking an adequate intake of fluids throughout the day, but decreasing fluid intake close to bedtime, have been shown to be helpful in reducing UI in women.[18]

Behavioral treatment

The primary behavioral treatment for UI or OAB is timed voiding. The rationale for this treatment is that patients with urge incontinence may void too

389

Table 27.4 Therapeutic modalities in urinary incontinence

Type of incontinence	Recommended therapies
Urgency urinary incontinence	Diet and fluid management
	Behavioral therapy: Timed/scheduled voiding
	Pelvic muscle exercises with or without biofeedback
	Drug therapy:
	Anticholinergic agents:
	Oxybutynin (IR 2.5–5 mg qd to tid; ER 5–30 mg qd; 3.8-mg TD patch changed 2×/wk)
	Tolterodine (IR 1–2 mg bid; 2–4 mg qd ER)
	Fesoterodine (4–8 mg qd)
	Trospium (20 mg qd to bid)
	Solifenacin (5–10 mg qd)
	Darifenacin (7.5–15 mg qd)
	Beta-3-agonist agent:
	Mirabegron (25–50 mg qd)
Stress urinary incontinence	Pelvic muscle exercises with or without biofeedback
	Behavioral therapy: Timed voiding
	Surgery: Referral for consultation for minimally invasive surgeries
Neurogenic urinary incontinence	*Management:* Intermittent catheterization
Functional urinary incontinence	Correct underlying cause
Fecal incontinence	
Urgency and passive fecal incontinence	*Behavioral therapy:* Pelvic floor muscle therapy with or without biofeedback
	Timed or scheduled toileting to improve bowel habits
	Drug therapy (to manage stool consistency):
	Loperamide (2–4 mg daily), may use less if needed
	Psyllium fiber (1–3 teaspoons daily), may use more or less if needed
	Cholestyramine powder (1 packet or 3 gm daily) – use 10–20 minutes prior to meals
	Injectable therapy: Dextranomer and sodium hyaluronate
Overflow fecal incontinence	*Surgery:* Referral for consultation if indicated *Management:* Correct underlying causes for constipation

Treatments recommended for management of urinary incontinence are adapted from the Agency for Health Care Policy and Research (AHCPR) 1996 clinical practice guideline "Urinary Incontinence in Adults," with updated drug recommendations.
Source: Modified from Fantl et al.[6]

frequently and may gradually develop an intolerance for bladder filling. The treatment is to instruct the patient to void at fixed, short intervals such as every 30 minutes and to increase gradually the duration of the interval to two to three hours. Patients are encouraged to resist the urge to void between these intervals. Timed voiding may be combined with pelvic floor muscle exercises to strengthen the pelvic floor muscles, and patients may be taught to contract pelvic floor muscles when they experience an urge to void to reflexly inhibit bladder contractions.[19] A typical regimen for pelvic muscle exercises is described later under treatments for stress incontinence.

Pharmacological therapy

Anticholinergic agents have been the mainstay of pharmacologic therapy for patients with urgency and mixed incontinence, along with OAB. Newer drugs are also available. In general, systematic reviews have found that extended release formulations of the anticholinergic agents have fewer side effects than the immediate release formulations for the treatment of UI and OAB.[20]

Oxybutynin has both anticholinergic and smooth muscle relaxant properties. Studies with the immediate release (IR) formulation have shown a 15%–58% greater reduction in urge UI compared with placebo. The extended release (ER) and transdermal (TD) formulations have similar efficacy. The initial dosage for IR demonstrated to be effective in clinical trials is 2.5 mg–5 mg three times a day, although some elderly patients benefit from only 2.5 mg daily. The initial dosage for the ER formulation is 5 mg daily and can be titrated up to 30 mg daily. The 3.8-mg TD patch is applied twice weekly and is now available over the counter. Up to 50% of patients in clinical trials of the IR medication had side effects such as dry mouth and constipation that limited therapy. The ER and TD formulations are associated with a lower rate of dry mouth. Narrow-angle glaucoma and urinary retention are contraindications for treatment with oxybutynin.

Tolterodine, a muscarinic receptor antagonist, was found to be as effective as oxybutynin in double-blind studies, and it had a lower incidence and decreased severity of the side effect of dry mouth. As with oxybutynin, tolterodine should not be used in patients with narrow-angle glaucoma or urinary retention.

Trospium is a nonselective muscarinic receptor antagonist metabolized in the kidneys for treatment of the OAB symptom complex of urgency, frequency, and incontinence. The dose for older persons and those with renal impairment is 20 mg daily. Trospium must be taken on an empty stomach.

Solifenacin and darifenacin are more selective muscarinic receptor (M3) antagonists. These drugs were also approved for treatment of OAB symptoms. Initial dosage of solifenacin is 5 mg, which may be titrated to 10 mg, and the dose of darifenacin is 7.5 mg–15 mg daily. Studies have not shown these drugs to be associated with a clear increase in efficacy or decrease in side effects compared with other anticholinergic drugs such as tolterodine.

Fesoterodine, an isomer of tolterodine, is approved for the treatment of OAB and UI. Data suggests that even frail, older adults may have some benefit from this medication from a randomized, controlled trial done specifically in this population.[21]

As of July 2012, a nonselective beta-3 adrenoreceptor agonist (beta 3-AR), mirabegron, was approved by the FDA as the first agent in this newest category of pharmaceutical treatment for OAB and UI in men and women. Reductions in dose (from 50 mg to 25 mg daily) are recommended for patients with liver and renal impairment. Mirabegron is not indicated for patients with severe liver impairment or uncontrolled hypertension.

For all older patients taking anticholinergic drugs, the lowest dose possible that is efficacious should be prescribed. PVRs should be monitored on a regular schedule to identify urinary retention that causes worsening of incontinence. In these cases, the drug dose should be reduced, and in severe cases, discontinued.

Sacral nerve stimulation with percutaneous tibial nerve stimulation

Percutaneous tibial nerve stimulation (PTNS) has emerged as a viable, minimally invasive, low-risk, and relatively low-cost option for management of OAB and UI. PTNS has comparable efficacy to bladder drug treatments with fewer side effects. Percutaneous electrical stimulation of the tibial nerve (PTNS) appears to facilitate neuromodulation via the sacral S3 nerves. The posterior tibial nerve contains mixed sensory motor nerve fibers that originate from L4 through S3 nerve roots involving nerves that provide sensory and motor control of the pelvic floor and viscera. The site of stimulation in PTNS, posterior and superior to the medial malleolus (inner ankle), is an acupuncture point ("sanyinjiao" or "spleen-6") in traditional Chinese acupuncture. PTNS is an office-based procedure that is currently done weekly for 10 to 12 weeks.

Recently, new surgical approaches have been developed for urge incontinence that remains unresponsive to medical and behavioral treatment. Discussion of these treatments is beyond the scope of this chapter.

Stress incontinence (sphincter insufficiency/pelvic floor muscle weakness)

Behavioral treatment

The rationale behind behavioral treatments for stress incontinence is that this type of incontinence results from transient increases of bladder pressure above urethral pressure, which can be corrected by strengthening the external urethral sphincter muscle so that urethral sphincter pressure is higher or by elevating the bladder neck. The simplest and least costly behavioral technique is referred to as pelvic floor muscle training (PFMT), or Kegel exercises.[22] These are often taught verbally by instructing patients to squeeze the pelvic floor muscles as if they are holding back urine or holding back a bowel movement but to keep their abdominal wall muscles relaxed (i.e., to avoid inappropriate increases in intraabdominal pressure that may increase the likelihood of stress incontinence). These instructions may include the suggestion that patients place a hand on the abdomen to detect abdominal wall contraction or that they continue to breathe while squeezing pelvic floor muscles. Patients are instructed to squeeze pelvic floor muscles and hold a maximum squeeze for 3–10 seconds, with 10-second rest periods in between squeezes. They are told to perform 20–30 squeezes, three to five times a day for at least 8–12 weeks.

The literature on PFMT and exercise has demonstrated that it is effective for reducing stress, urge, and mixed urinary incontinence in most outpatients who cooperate with training. Cochrane Database systematic reviews concluded that there is grade A evidence for PFMT and that it should be offered as first-line treatment to women with stress, urge, or mixed

incontinence.[23] Less research has been conducted with men. However, a recent randomized trial of an exercise-based behavioral training program for men with persistent post-prostatectomy incontinence demonstrated a 51% reduction in incontinent episodes, significantly greater than the 24% reduction in the control group.[24]

The initial instruction in pelvic floor muscle exercises should be done during a digital rectal or pelvic examination: With the examining finger in the anal canal or vagina, the therapist instructs the patient to squeeze the pelvic floor muscles and provides verbal feedback on whether she is squeezing correctly. The examiner can also place a hand on the abdominus rectus muscles to detect inappropriate contractions. Biofeedback may also be used to teach pelvic floor muscle exercises in the treatment of stress UI. Although this may be helpful to many patients, studies have generally shown no significant difference in efficacy between Kegel exercise training alone and biofeedback.

An alternative treatment for stress UI in women is to wear pessaries in the vagina to elevate the bladder neck. In theory, this accomplishes the same thing as a bladder suspension continence surgery; elevating the bladder neck makes the angle between the bladder and the urethra more acute so that bladder filling mechanically pinches off the urethral opening. Pessaries come in various sizes and shapes and should be selected based on effectiveness and patient preference/comfort following a therapeutic trial. Referral to a nurse clinical specialist experienced in the use of pessaries should be considered.

Drug treatment

Estrogen has direct effects on urethral mucosa and periurethral tissues and increases the number and responsiveness of α-receptors in women. Vaginally applied estrogen cream, ring, or tablets may improve stress and mixed UI. The duration of topical estrogen application has not yet been established; however, several large studies have shown that oral estrogen or estrogen plus progesterone worsens stress, urge, or mixed UI.[25] Based on these data, oral estrogen is not recommended as treatment for UI.

Surgical management

When conservative therapy has failed, surgery may be appropriate. In women with urethral hypermobility of the bladder neck and stress UI, the use of minimally invasive surgeries with transvaginal tape (TVT) are outpatient surgical procedures with a low complication rate.[26]

Overflow incontinence (neurogenic bladder)

Neurogenic bladder is a potentially life-threatening condition because it increases the risk of reflux of bacteria to the kidneys. In patients with severe neurological deficits, intermittent clean catheterization every two to four hours by the patient or caregiver is often the best management. If this is not possible or practical, an indwelling catheter may be necessary. The use of chronic indwelling catheters is generally not encouraged because of the frequency of complications, including urolithiasis, symptomatic bacteriuria, periurethral abscess, and acute pyelonephritis. Appropriate management of an indwelling catheter depends on proper insertion using sterile technique and maintaining a closed sterile system. Urethral cleansing, routine bladder irrigation, and prophylactic antibiotic therapy should be avoided, as these procedures do not prevent bladder colonization and are likely to result in the selection of resistant organisms.[27]

For patients with mild overflow incontinence, a prompted voiding schedule (reminding the patient to void every two to three hours) may be beneficial. Overflow incontinence resulting from a hyporeflexic bladder is generally poorly responsive to behavioral or pharmacological therapy. Surgery is not indicated.

Outflow obstruction

Use of a questionnaire, such as the American Urological Association Symptom Inventory, is useful in deciding on initial treatment for men with BPH.[28] Men with milder symptoms can be managed by watchful waiting. For men with moderate-to-severe symptoms, medications are often the treatment of choice. Current medication approaches for BPH include α-antagonists (such as doxazosin, terazosin, and tamsulosin) that reduce the dynamic component of prostatic obstruction; 5-α reductase inhibitors (such as finasteride and dutasteride), which shrink the prostate gland; and more recent use of phosphodiesterase inhibitors (sildenafil, tadalafil, vardenafil, etc.), which may regulate smooth muscle tone in the prostate gland. These can be used in combination to treat moderate to severe symptoms. There is a growing use of minimally invasive surgical techniques that have proved efficacious for BPH other than transurethral resection of the prostate (TURP). Women may present with bladder outlet obstruction secondary to pelvic organ prolapse, specifically anterior compartment prolapse or cystocele. This may require surgical repair. In these patients, full evaluation, including urodynamic testing prior to surgery, may be indicated to rule out coexisting causes of incontinence.

Treatment of fecal incontinence

Initial treatments for FI includes conservative measures (dietary modifications, bowel habit training, and pelvic floor muscle training with or without biofeedback and electrical stimulation),[29] and pharmacologic treatments (constipating and/or stool bulking agents).[30, 31] Conservative therapies are often combined and improve mild FI by 50%–95%, depending on the modality used.[29] When FI is not responding to initial treatments, perianal injectable bulking agents and sacral neuromodulation (surgical and nonsurgical) may be considered.[31, 32]

Dietary and behavioral interventions for fecal incontinence

Dietary modifications should focus on avoiding triggers for loose stool such as lactose-containing products. Increasing dietary or supplementary fiber may improve loose stool and decrease diarrhea by bulking the stool. Solid stool may be easier to retain in the rectum. Recent data suggests that fiber treatment may be beneficial for FI.[33] Bowel habit training and scheduled toileting with or without laxatives to empty the rectum may help those with cognitive or mobility problems.

Biofeedback

Biofeedback involves a trained provider who utilizes an instrument with visual or auditory feedback on the proper control of voluntary muscle contraction and relaxation of the external anal sphincter and recognition of anal sphincter sensation.[29] Strength training, sensory training, and coordinated training (strength and sensory) occur in most biofeedback protocols for FI. The goal is improved external anal sphincter muscle contraction in response to rectal sensation or distention. For success, patients who undergo biofeedback treatment need to have awareness of their defecation symptoms and be able to actively participate during the office-based treatments and a home exercise program.

Pharmacologic treatment

The most commonly used pharmacologic treatments involve antidiarrheal drugs for diarrhea-associated FI, such as loperamide and diphenoxylate plus atropine. [30] No antidiarrheal drugs have specific approval for the treatment of FI in the United States. In clinical studies for these drugs for FI treatment, more people on an antidiarrheal drug as compared to placebo reported constipation, abdominal pain, diarrhea, headache, and nausea. Given the anticholinergic properties of diphenoxylate plus atropine, this treatment should be avoided in older adults. Treatment of constipation-associated FI with laxatives can be effective, especially in long-term care settings, when used with other behavioral interventions.

Occasionally, when antidiarrheal drugs are not effective for improving diarrhea-associated FI, a trial with cholestyramine is warranted. Cholestyramine is a bile salt binding medication used to lower cholesterol and can reduce diarrhea associated with the production of excess bile acid salts. Limited data exists on the use of this medication specifically for FI.

Injectable agents

When conservative measures for FI fail, a new minimally invasive injectable agent has been approved. An office-based procedure involves the perianal injection of dextranoner microspheres and hyaluronic acid. Initial data are promising for reduced FI episodes, but more long-term data is needed. Studies involving other injectable agents into the perianal area have not had significant improvements in FI episodes.[31]

Sacral neuromodulation

Percutaneous tibial nerve stimulation (PTNS) and a surgically implanted device, Interstim™, involve the treatment of FI by stimulating the sacral nerves that help control defecation. PTNS is an office-based procedure to indirectly stimulate the sacral nerves through the posterior tibial nerve and is the same treatment mentioned earlier for UI. A small, acupuncture-sized needle is inserted into the medial aspect of the lower extremity and attached to a stimulation device. Often, 12 weeks of treatment are needed to see improvement in symptoms. Data from adequately powered randomized controlled trials for PTNS treatment for FI are ongoing and will add significantly to the evidence.[34]

A surgically implanted neuromodulation device (Interstim™) has been approved in Europe since 1994 and is approved in the United States for refractory FI. This surgically implanted device stimulates the sacral nerves (at S3) and has shown improvement in symptoms compared to conservative measures.[31]

Other surgical approaches

Other surgical therapies include anal sphincter repairs, artificial bowel sphincter implant, and colostomy. Overlapping sphincteroplasty can be used to repair a torn anal sphincter, which most commonly results from an obstetrical injury and can be an occult finding in older women. Although short-term benefits may exist, longer-term data on outcomes is needed. Use of an artificial bowel sphincter has significant associated morbidity, and colostomy is essentially used as a salvage procedure.

Managing UI and FI with absorbent pads and continence products

Absorbent pads and other continence products are designed for management rather than treatment of UI and FI. Although evaluation and treatment are recommended, many patients will either depend on continence products exclusively or will use absorbent pads for security in circumstances where they are fearful of incontinence.

Disposable absorbent pads typically consist of a superabsorbent layer surrounded by an outer barrier and an inner membrane that conducts moisture away from the skin. They are supplied both as small pads to be worn in undergarments by patients who typically experience small-volume leakage or as briefs worn in place of undergarments by patients who at least occasionally have large-volume leakage of urine. For men with light incontinence, pads may be constructed as pouches or in the shape of a shield or leaf that surrounds the penis. Pads are also available specifically for accidental bowel leakage.

For men, sheaths made of latex or plastic, as a condom, that can be attached around the penis and that connect via tubing to a collection bag are more commonly used than absorbent pads. Sheaths are associated with a higher incidence of UTIs than pads, although this risk can be minimized by ensuring that the connection between the sheath and collection device does not kink or become obstructed. Other risks associated with sheaths are allergic reactions to latex, irritation, and compression from sheath binding straps.

Treatment in long-term care facilities

Prevalence estimates of UI from MDS data in both men and women aged 65 and older residing in long-term care facilities range from 30% to 77% with up to 60% also having FI.[1] The prevalence of UI reported in a recent population-based study involving 95,911 older nursing home residents from eight southeastern states was 65% on admission, suggesting that the majority of nursing home residents are incontinent. [35] It is possible to decrease the frequency and severity of UI in at least half of incontinent long-term care patients through prompted voiding, but this approach is rarely used in long-term care facilities, because the financial and staff resources needed to implement this program are seen as prohibitive. Prompted voiding may also have some benefit for adults with constipation and FI in long-term care settings.[7] For the most part, in nursing homes UI and FI are managed rather than treated or prevented, usually by placing absorbent pads on beds or chairs or by keeping residents in absorbent undergarments and changing these two to three times per day.

Behavioral treatment for UI and FI

Prompted voiding is the behavioral program that has been most thoroughly evaluated.[7, 36] A staff member approaches each incontinent resident every two hours (or at intervals individualized to each patient) and asks the resident if he or she would like assistance to get to the toilet. Assistance is provided if needed, and staff is instructed to encourage patients to void/defecate and to praise them for success at remaining continent between prompts. Increasing fluid intake and exercise may also be included. In a large number of studies, this approach reduced the severity of UI (the proportion of times checked that the patient was found to be wet) by approximately 50% overall, although relatively few patients become fully continent. When prompts were no longer provided, the rate of UI quickly returned to its former level. Moreover, approximately half of nursing home

residents do not benefit because of the severity of cognitive impairment or other functional limitations. A trial period may be indicated to focus prompted voiding techniques on those who respond.

Management studies have shown that the average time required to assist a patient to the toilet to urinate greatly exceeds the time required to change absorbent undergarments or bed pads and linens.[37]

Summary

Incontinence – both UI and FI – remains a common, underreported, and vexing problem in older patients that can lead to social isolation. New therapeutic options using behavioral, pharmacological, and surgical approaches can lead to symptomatic improvements or cure for this important clinical problem and increased quality of life for the older patient.

References

1. Gorina Y, Schappert S, Bercovitz A, et al. Prevalence of incontinence among older Americans. *National Center for Health Statistics. Vital Health Stat.* 2014;3(36):1–24.

2. Hannestad YS, Rortveit G, Sandvik H, Hunskaar S. A community-based epidemiological survey of female urinary incontinence: the Norwegian EPINCONT study. Epidemiology of Incontinence in the County of Nord-Trondelag. *J Clin Epidemiol.* 2000;53:1150–1157.

3. Thom DH, Haan MN, Van Den Eeden SK. Medically recognized urinary incontinence and risks of hospitalization, nursing home admission and mortality. *Age Ageing.* 1997;26:367–374.

4. Burgio KL, Ives DG, Locher JL, et al. Treatment seeking for urinary incontinence in older adults. *J Am Geriatr Soc.* 1994;42:208–212.

5. Umlauf MG, Goode S, Burgio KL. Psychosocial issues in geriatric urology: problems in treatment and treatment seeking. *Urol Clin N Am.* 1996;23:127–136.

6. Fantl JA, Newman DK, Colling J, et al. Urinary incontinence in adults: Acute and chronic management. *Clinical practice guideline 2 (1996 Update). AHCPR* 96–0682. 3–1–1996. Rockville, MD: US Department of Health and Human Services, Public Health Service, Agency for Health Care Policy and Research.

7. Schnelle JF, Leung FW, Rao SS, et al. A controlled trial of an intervention to improve urinary and FI and constipation. *J Am Geriatr Soc.* 2010;58(8):1504–1511.

8. Brown HW, Wexner SD, Segall MM, et al. Accidental bowel leakage in the mature women's health study: prevalence and predictors. *Int J Clin Pract.* 2012 Nov;66 (11):1101–1108.

9. Brown JS, Bradley CS, Subak LL, et al. Diagnostic Aspects of Incontinence Study (DAISy) Research

Group: the sensitivity and specificity of a simple test to distinguish between urge and stress urinary incontinence. *Ann Intern Med.* 2006 16;**144**(10):715–723.

10. DuBeau CE, Resnick NM. Evaluation of the causes and severity of geriatric incontinence. A critical appraisal. *Urol Clin N Am.* 1991;**18**:243–256.

11. Ouslander JG, Schapira M, Schnelle JF. Urine specimen collection from incontinent female nursing home residents. *J Am Geriatr Soc.* 1995;**43**:279–281.

12. www.auanet.org/education/guidelines/asymptomatic-microhematuria.cfm (accessed January 2016).

13. Ouslander JG, Simmons S, Tuico E, et al. Use of a portable ultrasound device to measure post-void residual volume among incontinent nursing home residents. *J Am Geriatr Soc.* 1994;**42**:1189–1192.

14. Goode PS, Locher JL, Bryant RL, et al. Measurement of postvoid residual urine with portable transabdominal bladder ultrasound scanner and urethral catheterization. *Int Urogynecol J Pelvic Floor Dysfunct.* 2000;**11**(5):296–300.

15. www.auanet.org/education/guidelines/adult-urody namics.cfm (accessed January 2016).

16. Holroyd-Leduc JM, Tannenbaum C, Thorpe KE, Straus SE. What type of urinary incontinence does this woman have? *JAMA.* 2008 Mar 26;**299**(12):1446–1456.

17. Rao SS. Advances in diagnostic assessment of fecal incontinence and dyssynergic defecation. *Clin Gastroenterol Hepatol.* 2010 Nov; 8 (11):910–918.

18. Kincade JE, Dougherty MC, Carlson JR, et al. Randomized clinical trial of efficacy of self-monitoring techniques to treat urinary incontinence in women. *Neurourol Urodyn.* 2007;**26**:507–511.

19. Nygaard IE, Kreder KJ, Lepic MM, et al. Efficacy of pelvic floor muscle exercises in women with stress, urge, and mixed urinary incontinence. *Am J Obstet Gynecol.* 1996;**174**:120–125.

20. Hartmann K, McPheeters M, Biller D, et al. Treatment of overactive bladder in women. Evidence Report/ Technology Assessment No.187 (Prepared by the Vanderbilt Evidence-based Practice Center under Contract No. 290–2007-10065-I) AHRQ Publication No. 09-E017. Rockville, MD: Agency for Healthcare Research and Quality. August 2009.

21. Dubeau CE, Kraus SR, Griebling TL, et al. Effect of fesoterodine in vulnerable elderly subjects with urgency incontinence: a double-blind, placebo controlled trial. *J Urol.* 2014 Feb;**191**(2):395–404.

22. Kegel AH. Progressive resistance exercise in the functional restoration of the perineal muscles. *Am J Obstet Gynecol.* 1948;**56**:238–248.

23. Hay-Smith EJC, Dumoulin C. Pelvic floor muscle training versus no treatment, or inactive control treatments, for urinary incontinence in women. *Cochrane Database Syst Rev.* 2006 Jan 25;**1**:CD005654.

24. Goode PS, Burgio KL, Johnson TM 2nd, et al. Behavioral therapy with or without biofeedback and pelvic floor electrical stimulation for persistent postprostatectomy incontinence: a randomized controlled trial. *JAMA.* 2011 Jan 12;**305**(2):151–159.

25. Hendrix SL, Cochrane BB, Nygaard IE, et al. Effects of estrogen with and without progestin on urinary incontinence. *JAMA.* 2005;**293**:935–948.

26. Ogah J, Cody DJ, Rogerson L. Minimally invasive synthetic suburethral sling operations for stress urinary incontinence in women: a short version Cochrane review. *Neurourol Urodyn.* 2011 Mar;**30**(3):284–291.

27. Gould CV, Umscheid CA, Agarwal RK, et al. *Guideline for prevention of catheter-associated urinary tract infections 2009.* Atlanta, GA: Centers for Disease Control and Prevention. 2009.

28. Svatek R, Roche V, Thornberg J, Zimmern P. Normative values for the American Urological Association Symptom Index (AUA-7) and short form Urogenital Distress Inventory (UDI-6) in patients 65 and older presenting for non-urological care. *Neurourol Urodyn.* 2005;**24**:606–610.

29. Norton C, Cody JD. Biofeedback and/or sphincter exercises for the treatment of faecal incontinence in adults. *Cochrane Database Syst Rev.* 2012 Jul 11;7: CD002111.

30. Omar MI, Alexander CE. Drug treatment for faecal incontinence in adults. *Cochrane Database Syst Rev.* 2013 Jun 11;**6**:CD002116.

31. Maeda Y, Laurberg S, Norton C. Perianal injectable bulking agents as treatment for faecal incontinence in adults. *Cochrane Database Syst Rev.* 2013 Feb 28;**2**: CD007959.

32. Brown SR, Wadhawan H, Nelson RL. Surgery for faecal incontinence in adults. *Cochrane Database Syst Rev.* 2013 Jul 2;7:CD001757.

33. Bliss DZ, Jung HJ, Savik K, et al. Supplementation with dietary fiber improves fecal incontinence. *Nurs Res.* Jul–Aug 2001;**50**(4):203–213.

34. Horrocks EJ, Thin N, Thaha MA, et al. Systematic review of tibial nerve stimulation to treat faecal incontinence. *Br J Surg.* 2014 Apr;**101**(5):457–468.

35. Boyington JE, Howard DL, Carter-Edwards L, et al. Differences in resident characteristics and prevalence of urinary incontinence in nursing homes

in the southeastern United States. *Nurs Res.* 2007;**56**:97–107.

36. Schnelle JF. Treatment of urinary incontinence in nursing home patients by prompted voiding. *J Am Geriatr Soc.* 1990;**38**:356–360.

37. Schnelle JF, Keeler E, Hays RD, et al. A cost and value analysis of two interventions with incontinent nursing home residents. *J Am Geriatr Soc.* 1995;**43**:1112–1117.

Gynecologic issues in the elderly

Michele Q. Zawora, MD, and Christine Hsieh, MD

Introduction

Gynecologic concerns remain common throughout the lifespan. This chapter focuses on the presentation, workup, and appropriate treatment of the most common concerns of elderly females: vulvovaginitis and other conditions, gynecologic-specific cancers, pelvic floor prolapse, postmenopausal symptoms, and sexual dysfunction. Urogynecologic conditions and osteoporosis are covered in other chapters.

The approach to the geriatric patient should be based individually on functional status and patient goals. Frail elders should be managed with quality of life and maintenance of function as the top priorities. When evaluating any elder patient, the clinician must recognize how capacity limitations including cognitive, physical, emotional, and social dysfunction may affect the assessment process. Patients with cognitive impairment may not be able to provide the clinician with pertinent details and history. Frail elders with mobility concerns and/or chronic pain and disability may have difficulty ambulating in the room, ascending exam tables, and lying on the table in the typical lithotomy position without pain or assistance. Vision and hearing impairments are common in older adults, and clinicians must adapt their interviewing and exam techniques to accommodate patient needs. The clinician should speak slowly and clearly; limit interruptions, distractions, and outside noise; and ensure that any hearing or visual aids are available and being used. Providing the patient with enough time to relate their history and concerns, repeating information throughout the visit, and providing written materials at the end of the visit promotes understanding and adherence to the treatment recommendations and follow-up plans.

Elderly patients are less likely to report symptoms than younger patients, particularly when pertaining to gynecologic concerns and sexual dysfunction. Careful attention to risk factors with sensitive history taking is an important part of health and wellness in the aging female.[1] A thorough sexual history includes lifetime and current partners, previous exposures to sexually transmitted infections (STIs), sexual practices, and any sexuality concerns of the patient.[2, 3]

Specific adjustments can be made during the physical exam: providing lower and/or adjustable tables for osteoarthritic stiffness, pain, and decreased range of motion in hips, knees, and spine; and providing extra pillows for those with cervical disc disease or kyphosis and congestive heart failure. Some may benefit from topical lidocaine creams to avoid tenderness and pain during more invasive vaginal exams.[4] A gentle internal exam, using a smaller width speculum in cases of severe atrophy, is recommended for patient comfort.

Vulvovaginitis and other conditions

Vulvovaginitis

Vulvovaginitis is a common complaint in the postmenopausal female. The lack of estrogen and the normal aging process leads to increased irritation of the vaginal tissue, along with increased susceptibility for trauma and infection. The three most common causes of vulvovaginitis complaints are atrophy, candidiasis, and lichen sclerosis.

Atrophic changes of the vulvovaginal area are very common following menopause, when the decreased presence of estrogen leads to thinning of the vaginal tissue. Physical findings include atrophic vaginal tissue that may be pale, smooth, and shiny; erythematous and friable with petechiae; loss of natural ruggae; and introital stenosis.[5] Intravaginal lubricants and long-term use of moisturizers can be helpful in

Reichel's Care of the Elderly, *7th Edition*, ed. Jan Busby-Whitehead *et al.* Published by Cambridge University Press.
© Cambridge University Press 2016.

treating mild to moderate symptoms.[6–8] Topical estrogen creams are the most effective at treating severe postmenopausal atrophic vaginitis.[6–9] It should be noted that unopposed systemic estrogen has been shown to increase risk of endometrial cancer; however, the risk is lower in topical formulation and does not require concurrent treatment with progesterone.[6, 7]

Vulvovagnitis caused by *Candida* infection, candidiasis, presents similarly in patients of all ages, with complaints of pruritus, irritation, and discharge. Physical findings include inflammation, erythema, along with a discharge demonstrating buds and hyphae on microscopy. Treatment is similar for all age groups, including several different antifungals in topical or suppository formulations, or with a single dose of fluconazole in oral form.[3]

Lichen sclerosis may present with thin, white "cigarette paper" patches and can be treated with topical steroids.[1] Patients with this diagnosis should be examined annually, as lichen sclerosis has been associated with certain cancers. Biopsy is indicated in any of the following findings: asymmetry, border irregularity, color variation, sudden change, bleeding, nonhealing ulceration, persistence, and lack of firm diagnosis.[4]

Pruritus

The differential for pruritus without discharge is large and includes primary dermatologic conditions, as well as manifestations of systemic illnesses. (See Table 28.1 for a full differential diagnosis.) A complete history should be obtained, including use of topical creams, lotions, detergents, and bath products. Any ulcerations or lesions may warrant biopsy to rule out vulvar intraepithelial neoplasia (VIN) or squamous cell carcinoma.

Vaginal discharge

Any vaginal discharge should be evaluated by pelvic exam, vaginal pH, and wet prep, with screening and culture for STIs when indicated. The three most common causes of vaginal discharge are caused by bacterial vaginosis, trichomoniasis, and candidiasis. Bacterial vaginosis occurs when various anaerobes replace normal vaginal flora. Treatment for bacterial vaginosis is the same in elderly as in younger patients, with either oral metronidazole or clindamycin, or topical metronidazole.[10] Trichomonas may cause

Table 28.1 Differential diagnosis of pruritis without discharge [1]

Dermatitis
Vulvar intraepithelial neoplasia (VIN)
Cancer
Lichen sclerosis
Squamous cell hyperplasia
Hypoestrogenic atrophic vaginitis
Mechanical irritation and wetness from urinary incontinence
Dermatoses (lichen sclerosis, lichen planus, psoriasis, contact and seborrheic dermatitis)
Sexually transmitted infections (STIs)
Systemic causes • Uremia • Hepatic disease • Diabetes • Thyroid disease • Lymphomas/leukemias • Graft versus host disease

foul-smelling discharge and may be treated with single 2-g dose of metronidazole. Candidiasis presents with irritation, pruritus, and/or discharge and may be treated as previously discussed.[10] The differential diagnosis for chronic vaginal discharge includes desquamative inflammatory vaginitis, chronic endometritis with malodorous purulent discharge, vesicovaginal fistula or enterovaginal fistula following bowel inflammation and injury as in cases of diverticulitis.[1, 4]

Vulvodynia

Vulvodynia is pain or discomfort of the vulva. Typically women describe a burning, stinging, irritation, or rawness. Vulvodynia without evidence of infection, dermatologic conditions, or vagina atrophy can be treated with topical lidocaine and low-dose antidepressants. There is weak evidence that a low oxalate diet may reduce symptoms.[1]

Bleeding

All postmenopausal bleeding requires a workup to rule out endometrial cancers. Benign causes of vaginal bleeding include atrophic endometrium, cervicitis, cervical or endometrial polyps, hormone therapy (HT), endometriosis, leiomyomas, vaginal atrophy and friability.[11] The workup should include a full history, medications including HTs (i.e., tamoxifen), a complete exam to evaluate for causes of bleeding other than vaginal (i.e., hematuria or rectal bleeding); an ultrasound to evaluate endometrial lining, and an in-office endometrial biopsy if the endometrial lining is abnormal. Hysteroscopy with D&C may be indicated in refractory or inconclusive cases and would warrant referral to a gynecology specialist.[1]

Sexually transmitted infections

The elderly are at increased risk of contracting STIs. The number of elderly patients with HIV has been slowly increasing.[10] There has been an overall increased incidence across all age groups of chlamydia, gonorrhea, and syphilis since 2011.[10] The Centers for Disease Control and Prevention (CDC) reports 3.4/100,000 new cases of chlamydia in men over age 65, and 2.2/100,000 new cases in women over age 65. Gonorrhea cases have shown a 4% increase since 2011, accounting for 537/100,000 men over 65 years and 105/100,000 women over 65 years. The incidence of syphilis has increased by 11% since 2011, with 138/100,000 new cases in patients over 65 years.[10]

Age-related vaginal atrophy creates micro-tears in the vaginal mucosa allowing bacteria more access, while a waning immune response makes those tears more susceptible to infection. Clinicians should encourage open communication between sexual partners and educate the patient about safer sex techniques, including use of latex condoms and limiting the number of partners, to reduce the risk of infection and illness. Any presence of rash, blisters, or discharge should be evaluated right away.[2]

Gynecological cancers

Advancing age, frailty, and cancer screening

Frailty should be considered in the risk and benefit profile when deciding whether to screen for cancer in the older adult. The utility of cancer screening may decrease with increasing age and frailty. Upper age limit for cancer screening varies from different organizations such as the American Cancer Society (ACS),

the US Preventive Services Task Force (USPSTF), and the American College of Obstetricians and Gynecologists (ACOG), due to limited research data in the older geriatric population. Cancer screening is generally not recommended for women with less than five years' life expectancy.[12]

Vulvar cancer

Cancers of the vulva usually present with persistent itching and a vulvar mass.[13] Vulvar cancer accounts for approximately 5% of gynecologic malignancies, and occurs most frequently in women 65–75 years old.[14] The most common cancer is vulvar squamous cell carcinoma. Melanoma accounts for 2%– 9% of vulvar cancers.[15] Warty appearing lesions such as verrucous carcinoma may also occur in postmenopausal women. Precancerous lesions include vulvar intraepithelial neoplasia, which is associated with human papillomavirus (HPV) infection. Suspicious lesions in the vulva should undergo biopsy to confirm diagnosis. Treatment for vulvar cancer is primarily surgical resection. Surgery also determines the extent of disease and the need for additional radiation or chemotherapy.[13]

Vaginal cancer

Vaginal cancers typically present with painless bleeding. Primary vaginal cancers account for only 3% of gynecologic malignancies.[14] Squamous cell carcinoma is the most common histologic type and occurs in older women. Melanoma may also rarely occur in older women. Vaginal cancers can be metastatic from other primary sources such as the cervix, rectum, and ovary.[16] Risk factors for primary vaginal cancers include persistent HPV infection, multiple sexual partners, early age at first intercourse, and prior anogenital malignancy.[17] Although a Papanicolaou (Pap) smear may occasionally detect abnormal cells from the vagina, the diagnosis of vaginal cancer usually occurs with direct visualization of the vagina and biopsy of the suspected lesion. Treatment for vaginal cancer is primarily surgical excision or radiation based on disease stage and patient factors.[18]

Cervical cancer

The presentation for cervical cancer is usually postcoital bleeding and vaginal discharge or spotting. Cervical cancer is the third most common gynecologic malignancy in the United States, although cervical cancer deaths in the United States have decreased overall due to increased cervical cancer screening. [14] HPV acquired mainly through sexual transmission has been found to be the oncogenic pathogen that causes cervical cancer. Risk factors that increase exposure to HPV include early sexual activity, multiple partners, and STIs. Immunosuppression and smoking are also associated with increased risk of cervical cancer. Twenty-five percent of new cases of cervical cancer are diagnosed in women over the age of 65.[19] Updated cervical cancer screening guidelines from ACOG and ACS recommend screening older women over the age of 30 every three years with cytology or, preferably, every five years with cytology and HPV DNA co-testing.[20, 21] Guidelines from ACOG, ACS, and the USPSTF recommend to stop screening for cervical cancer in women over the age of 65 who have had a history of adequate cervical cancer screening.[20–22] Adequate cervical cancer screening is defined by these current guidelines as having had three consecutive negative cytology results or two consecutive negative co-testing (cytology and HPV testing) results within the past 10 years, with the most recent test done within five years.[20–22] Women who have had a total hysterectomy with removal of the cervix for benign lesions such as uterine fibroids do not require further screening.[20–22] Most new cases of cervical cancer occur in women who have never had a Pap smear or have not had one for many years.[23] The ACS recommends screening for women who have not been previously screened or in whom screening information is not available. The ACS and ACOG also recommend continued screening for women with precancer lesions such as CIN2 or higher for at least 20 years after regression or treatment.[20, 21] The result of abnormal Pap screening or presence of high-risk HPV strains 16 and 18 as well as persistence of any high-risk HPV type for one year must be confirmed by colposcopy and biopsy of abnormal areas on the cervix. Treatment depends on the extent of the precancerous or cancerous lesion. Low-grade intraepithelial lesions may require only close monitoring or cryosurgery. Loop electrosurgical excision procedure (LEEP), laser, and cold knife conizations are used in women at high risk for cervical cancer with high-grade intraepithelial lesions. Radical hysterectomy and/or radiation therapy is the treatment for women with invasive cervical cancer.[24]

Endometrial cancer

Endometrial cancers commonly present with postmenopausal bleeding, and for this reason it is generally diagnosed in the early stages. Endometrial cancer is the most common gynecologic cancer in the United States. The lifetime incidence is 2.5% in the United States.[14] The majority of cases occur in postmenopausal women aged 50 and older. The most common type of uterine cancer is adenocarcinoma of the endometrium (lining of the uterus).[25] Endometrial cancer is estrogen responsive, so the greatest risk factor is exposure to excess estrogen therapy either exogenous or endogenous. The use of unopposed exogenous estrogen such as with hormone replacement therapy without progestin causes endometrial hyperplasia, which can lead to endometrial cancer. The use of tamoxifen, which is a selective estrogen receptor modulator, increases the risk of endometrial cancer in postmenopausal women.[26] Other risk factors associated with increased excessive endogenous estrogen include obesity, early menarche, late menopause, and nulliparity.[27] Women with hereditary nonpolyposis colorectal cancer (HNPCC) have a high risk – up to 40%–60% lifetime risk – of developing endometrial cancer.[28] These women develop endometrial cancer at an earlier age. Prolonged oral contraceptive use and cigarette smoking protect against endometrial cancer. [29, 30] Increased physical activity, coffee, and green tea consumption have also been associated with decreased risk of endometrial cancer.[31–33] Endometrial cancer, when diagnosed in the early stages, has an approximately 90% survival rate.[34] Endometrial biopsy, measurement of the endometrial stripe thickness on ultrasound, or hysteroscopy can be used to evaluate for endometrial cancer in women who present with postmenopausal bleeding.[35] Treatment of endometrial cancer usually includes surgery for total hysterectomy, bilateral salpingo-oopherectomy, and peritoneal washings. Then depending on the staging of endometrial cancer, radiation and chemotherapy is used in women with metastatic disease.[25]

Ovarian cancer

Ovarian cancer is often detected at advanced stages due to a lack of early symptoms. It is the second most common gynecologic cancer, but it has the highest death rate of all the gynecologic cancers with an overall five-year survival rate for white and black

American women of 46% and 37%, respectively.[14] Many women with ovarian cancer in the early stages may be asymptomatic or have vague complaints of abdominal fullness, early satiety, nausea, constipation, gas, pelvic pressure, and low back pain. Clinicians need to have a high index of suspicion in these women to evaluate for ovarian cancer. Women with advanced disease may present with weight loss, intra-abdominal mass, or intestinal obstruction. Currently available screening tests have not proven to be beneficial for screening low-risk, asymptomatic women. ACOG recommends annual pelvic examination to evaluate for ovarian mass.[36] The USPSTF recommends against screening for ovarian cancer in asymptomatic women. However, women with a family history for breast and ovarian cancer should be considered for genetic counseling to evaluate their potential risks. Women with BRCA1 and 2 genetic mutations and Lynch syndrome (hereditary nonpolyposis colon cancer) are at an increased risk of ovarian cancer.[37] Advancing age, race, nulliparity, infertility, and history of endometrial or breast cancer have been associated with an increased risk of ovarian cancer. Multiparity, breastfeeding, and previous use of oral contraceptives have been linked to reduced risk of ovarian cancer.[38] The cancer antigen-125 (CA-125) is a tumor marker for epithelial ovarian cancer, which is the most common type of tumor in women older than 50. The CA-125 level is used for monitoring women with known ovarian cancer, but it is not sensitive or specific for use in screening in asymptomatic women.[39] Although an adnexal mass discovered in a postmenopausal woman is suspicious for ovarian cancer, benign ovarian cysts are not uncommon.[40] Women who have an adnexal mass palpated on pelvic examination should have diagnostic imaging performed initially with transvaginal ultrasonography. Ultrasound characteristics such as complex masses with cystic and solid components, septated cysts, thick cyst walls, and free fluid in the pelvis are concerning for malignancy.[41] Simple cysts up to 10 cm have lower likelihood of malignancy. The majority will resolve spontaneously and can usually be followed by serial transvaginal ultrasonography.[42] Gadolinium-enhanced magnetic resonance imaging is more specific compared to ultrasonography and may be used for further evaluation of concerning ovarian masses.[43] In postmenopausal women with a pelvic mass, a CA-125 may be helpful in predicting a higher likelihood of a malignant versus benign tumor.

[36] Serum tumor markers should be used together with transvaginal ultrasonography to identify ovarian masses at high risk for malignancy.[44] Current treatment for ovarian cancer includes aggressive debulking surgery and chemotherapy.[45]

Pelvic organ prolapse

Pelvic organ prolapse is an underdiagnosed condition but a common problem for older women. Symptoms can affect women's quality of life by altering their function and activity. Women living with prolapse reported feeling self-conscious and isolated; they also reported a loss of interest in activities and avoidance of intimacy because of embarrassment or discomfort.[46] Pelvic organ prolapse is the descent of one or more of the pelvic organs such as the uterus, bladder, or rectum into or beyond the vagina. This can cause a sensation of pressure or bulge in the vagina and is associated with difficulty voiding (urinary incontinence or retention) or difficulty having bowel movements (fecal incontinence or constipation).[47] Some women may be asymptomatic, and the condition is visualized during pelvic examination. The causes for pelvic floor musculature weakening leading to pelvic organ prolapse are not well understood but may be multifactorial due to childbirth, aging and decreased estrogen levels, and increased intraabdominal pressure from straining with bowel movements and obesity.[47] Treatment for pelvic organ prolapse is based on the severity of symptoms. The Pelvic Organ Prolapse Quantitation (POPQ) system is commonly used to grade the degree of prolapse.[48] Asymptomatic women may require only observation. Conservative management begins with pelvic floor muscle strengthening via Kegel exercises.[49] Another nonsurgical option is the vaginal pessary, which supports the pelvic organs when fitted appropriately and can improve symptoms.[49] In general, the pessary can be left in place and removed every three months in the clinician's office for cleaning and inspection of the vagina. However, if symptoms are severe and conservative management is not effective, surgical repair may be warranted.[47]

Postmenopausal symptoms

Postmenopausal symptoms remain common late into the lifecycle. The most common symptoms reported are hot flashes (occurring in up to 75% of women), vaginal dryness, poor sleep, and dyspareunia.

Systemic HT is still considered the most effective treatment option for women experiencing postmenopausal symptoms [Grade I Recommendation (insufficient evidence to recommend for or against)].[8, 50] The Women's Health Initiative study data revealed significant adverse events and side effects for many women taking HT and prompted many women to cease treatment. Many clinicians have avoided its use due to these potential negative findings. Further analysis of the data has revealed more information regarding the use of HT. Understanding the potential risk factors for each type of hormone therapy allows the clinician and patient to individualize treatment of symptoms incorporating quality of life, individualized risk factors, and goals of therapy.[9, 51] See Table 28.2 for more information regarding the risks and benefits of HT.

General evidence has shown that the duration of therapy for combined estrogen progesterone therapy (EPT) should be limited to three to five years due to an increased risk of breast cancer with more prolonged use.[9, 51] Estrogen therapy (ET) remains the most effective treatment of symptoms of vulvar and vaginal atrophy; however, ET should be delivered in a low-dose, local vaginal preparation.[9, 51] Although systemic/oral ET carries risk for venous thromboembolism (VTE), the risk is very low with topical vaginal preparations (evidence grade III).[6] Low-dose and ultra-low-dose ET have better risk profiles; however, it may decrease effectiveness of treating symptoms (evidence grade I).[8]

If the clinician and patient decide to choose HT, the goal should be to individualize care with the lowest effective dose for the shortest duration needed to relieve vasomotor symptoms (evidence grade I).[8] Phytoestrogens and bioidenticals may carry the same cardiovascular disease (CVD) risk as hormonal therapy. They are not FDA regulated and are not recommended for menopausal symptoms.[11]

Specific recommendations:

1. Vasomotor symptoms

   a. Mild vasomotor symptoms may be managed with lifestyle modifications, including: reducing core body temperature, regular exercise, weight management, smoking cessation, and avoidance of certain triggers such as hot drinks and alcohol (evidence grade I).[8, 50]

   b. Systemic HT with either ET or EPT is the most effective therapy for vasomotor symptoms (evidence grade I).[8, 9]

   c. Alternative, nonhormonal therapies can be considered and include antidepressants (selective serotonin reuptake inhibitors, serotonin-norepinephrine reuptake inhibitors), gabapentin, and bellergal (evidence grade I).[8, 50] All medications come with side effects, and therapy should be individualized based on the patient's history and risk factors.

   d. There is no data to support the use of alternative medications: progestin-only, testosterone, or compounded bioidentical hormones, phytoestrogens, or herbal supplements (evidence grade I).[8, 50]

2. Vaginal and vulvar atrophy

   a. First-line treatment for symptomatic vulvovaginal atrophy (VVA) include nonhormonal lubricants with intercourse and regular use of long-acting vaginal moisturizers (evidence grade I).[6–8]

   b. Moderate to severe VVA and those cases that are not effectively managed with nonhormonal topical options should be treated with low-dose vaginal ET. For patients with VVA and other symptoms, low-dose oral therapy can be considered (evidence grade II).[6–9]

   c. Topical vaginal ET can be continued for as long as symptoms are bothersome (evidence grade III).[6]

   d. Progestin co-therapy is not required for vaginal ET (evidence grade III).[6, 7]

3. Dyspareunia

   a. Long-acting vaginal moisturizers are effective for treating dyspareunia (evidence grade I).[7]

   b. Vaginal ET is an effective treatment for those with atrophic changes (evidence grade I).[52]

Sexuality and sexual dysfunction

Sexuality and a healthy sex life are part of overall quality of life. Clinicians should become adept at asking about sexuality and any concerns that their patients have in a sensitive manner. Elderly patients are less likely to bring up their concerns, so integrating screening into regular interview questions and normalizing the conversation will help. The clinician should discuss normal age-related physiologic changes, address how medications and chronic medical conditions can affect sexual function, and teach about safer sex practices as well as protection from

Table 28.2 Risks and benefits of hormone therapy [51]

Benefits

1. Vasomotor symptoms

   - Estrogen therapy (ET) with or with progesterone remains the most effective treatment of vasomotor symptoms.
   - Most systemic HT are FDA approved, except for ultralow dose transdermal HT.

2. Vaginal symptoms

   - ET remains the most effective treatment of moderate to severe vulvovaginal atrophy.
   - Many systemic HT and local vaginal ET products are FDA approved; however, low-dose systemic preparations may be less effective.
   - Local ET is the treatment of choice for those women who only have vaginal symptoms. Concomitant use of progesterone is not indicated for vaginal local ET.

3. Sexual function

   - Use of ET to treat sexual dysfunction is not supported by the evidence.
   - However, treatment with local ET may help with sexual satisfaction due to improvements in lubrication and blood flow.
   - HT is not recommended for diminished libido or other forms of sexual dysfunction.

Risks

1. Cardiovascular effects

   - Coronary heart disease (CHD)

     - Findings inconsistent. ET may reduce CHD risk if initiated in younger women shortly after menopause, but may increase CHD risk if started more than 10 years after menopause.
     - Effect may be due to reduced accumulation of coronary artery calcium deposits.

   - Venous thromboembolism (VTE)

     - Oral HT increases the risk of VTE. This risk returns to baseline soon after discontinuation.

   - Stroke

     - Estrogen progesterone therapy (EPT) and ET may increase the risk of stroke. Findings are inconsistent; however, risk rapidly decreases after discontinuation of HT.

2. Endometrial cancer

   - Unopposed systemic ET in those with an intact uterus increases the risk of endometrial cancer. The risk is sustained after discontinuation.
   - Concomitant use of progesterone is recommended only in those with an intact uterus.

3. Breast cancer

   - EPT use longer than three to five years increases the risk of breast cancer.
   - May promote proliferation of preexisting cancers.
   - Risk may be higher when started early in menopause.

4. Ovarian cancer

   - Findings are inconsistent.
   - Observational data indicates an association between prolonged HT use and increased ovarian cancer risk.

STIs and abuse.[53] The most common medications that are linked to sexual dysfunction are selective serotonin reuptake inhibitors (SSRIs).[52]

Healthy adults remain sexually active throughout life. One national study revealed that older adults reported having sex an average of two to four times per month. Another study looking at men over the age of 80 years reported 29% of the study participants were having at least weekly sex, while 38% were not sexually active.[2] When asking patients about sexual activity, keep in mind that 2.5%–3% of older adults report having two or more sexual partners in the last year, so screening for STIs is still indicated.[2] In addition, screening for sexual abuse is indicated in older adults, both independent-living and those residing in long-term care facilities. Patients with cognitive impairment may not be able to consent to sexual activity and are at risk for abuse.[2, 53]

Most sexual dysfunction in the elderly female is caused by lack of natural lubrication. Dyspareunia is common and thought to be due to atrophic changes that happen in the absence of estrogen.[1] The *Diagnostic and Statistical Manual of Mental Disorders, Fourth Edition* (DSM-IV) classifies three different female categories of sexual dysfunction: hypoactive sexual desire disorder (HSDD), female sexual arousal disorder, and female orgasmic disorder.[1]

Most female concerns are related to normal, age-related atrophic changes, which can be treated with water-based lubricants or low-dose vaginal estrogen creams (evidence grade II).[53] A biopsychosocial assessment of both partners is recommended prior to treatment of woman's sexual dysfunction if not related to inadequate lubrication (evidence grade III).[7]

Benign breast disease

Mastalgia, or breast pain, is a common complaint of women of any age. A full evaluation of this complaint in a postmenopausal woman will include a clinical breast exam, along with selective imaging. The differential diagnosis for mastalgia must include angina, cholecystitis, hiatal hernia or reflux, zoster, radiculopathy, or costochondritis. If the breast exam reveals a mass, lymphadenopathy, skin changes, or discharge, further workup for malignancy is warranted.[4] (See Chapter 38 for more details regarding breast cancer.)

In the patient with a normal exam and pain as a complaint, mammogram is indicated in those that are due for screening. Ultrasound is indicated for those with a unilateral, persistent source of pain. In those patients with normal ultrasound and mammogram, reassurance that there is no evidence of breast cancer is often the best course of treatment. Assess the pain severity, frequency, and change over time, offering nonpharmacologic and/or pharmacologic options to help alleviate persistent, bothersome pain symptoms. Nonpharmacologic methods include proper-fitting support bras, massage, hot and cold packs, and certain lifestyle modifications, including smoking cessation,

stress reduction, and caffeine reduction. Evening primrose oil has shown some improvement in breast pain for both cyclic and noncyclic causes of mastalgia, and due to low incidence of side effects, may be an alternative option for the postmenopausal female. Pharmacologic options first include eliminating or reducing medications that may be leading to the mastalgia: HT/ET/EPT and spironolactone in heart failure patients. Although ibuprofen may be beneficial, cautious use of NSAIDs is recommended in the elderly population. Acetaminophen may be a safer alternative. Should the patient have refractory pain or present with additional symptoms and findings on exam, consultation with a gynecologist or breast specialist is indicated.[54]

References

1. Sultana C. Geriatric gynecology. In: Arenson C, Busby-Whitehead J, Brummel-Smith K, et al., editors. *Reichel's Care of the Elderly, Clinical Aspects of Aging.* 6th ed. Cambridge: Cambridge University Press; 2009.

2. Letvak S, Schoder D. Sexually transmitted diseases in the elderly: what you need to know: the young aren't the only ones at risk for STDs. *Geriatric Nursing.* 1996;**17** (4):156–160. doi:10.1016/S0197-4572(96)80063 2.

3. Centers for Disease Control and Prevention (CDC). Clinical prevention guidance. In: Sexually transmitted diseases treatment guidelines, 2010. *MMWR Recomm Rep.* 2010 Dec 17;**59**(RR-12):2–8. Available at: www.gu ideline.gov/content.aspx?id=25577&search=sexually+tr ansmitted+infections (accessed November 14, 2015).

4. Miller KL, Baraldi CA. Geriatric gynecology: promoting health and avoiding harm. *Am J Obstet Gynecol.* 2012 Nov;**207**(5):355–367. Available at: http://dx.doi.org/10.1016/j.ajog.2012.04.014 (accessed November 14, 2015).

5. Bachmann GA, Nevadunsky NS. Diagnosis and Treatment of Atrophic Vaginitis. *Am Fam Physician.* 2000 May 15;**61**(10):3090–3096.

6. Management of symptomatic vulvovaginal atrophy: 2013 position statement of the North American Menopause Society. *Menopause.* 2013 Sep;**20**(9):888–902.

7. Urogenital health. In: Menopause and osteoporosis update 2009. *J Obstet Gynaecol Can.* 2009 Jan;**31**(1 Suppl 1):S27–S30. Available at: http://sogc.org/wp-content/u ploads/2013/01/Menopause_JOGC-Jan_09.pdf (accessed November 14, 2015).

8. American College of Obstetricians and Gynecologists (ACOG). *Management of Menopausal Symptoms.* Washington, DC: American College of Obstetricians and Gynecologists (ACOG); 2014 Jan. 15 (ACOG Practice Bulletin No. 141). Available at: www.guideline

.gov/content.aspx?id=47751&search=postmenopausal +symptoms (accessed November 14, 2015).

9. North American Menopause Society. The 2012 hormone therapy position statement of the North American Menopause Society. *Menopause*. 2012 Mar;**19**(3):257–271.

10. Centers for Disease Control and Prevention. *Sexually Transmitted Disease Surveillance* 2012. Atlanta: CDC. Available at: www.cdc.gov/std/stats12 (accessed November 14, 2015).

11. Perkins KE, King MC. Geriatric gynecology. *Emerg Med Clin N Am*. 2012;**30**(4):1007–1019.

12. Walter LC, Covinsky KE. Cancer screening in elderly patients: a framework for individualized decision making. *JAMA* 2001;**285**(21):2750–2756.

13. Canavan TP, Cohen D. Vulvar cancer. *Am Fam Physician* 2002;**66**(7):1269–1274.

14. Jemal A, Siegel R, Xu J, Ward E. Cancer statistics, 2010. *CA Cancer J Clin* 2010;**60**(5):277–300.

15. Johnson TL, Kumar NB, White CD, Morley GW. Prognostic features of vulvar melanoma: a clinicopathologic analysis. *Int J Gynecol Pathol* 1986;**5**(2):110–118.

16. Creasman WT, Phillips JL, Menck HR. The National Cancer Data Base report on cancer of the vagina. *Cancer* 1998;**83**(5):1033–1040.

17. Daling JR, Madeleine MM, Schwartz SM, et al. A population-based study of squamous cell vaginal cancer: HPV and cofactors. *Gynecol Oncol* 2002;**84**(2):263–270.

18. Lee LJ, Jhingran A, Kidd E, et al. ACR appropriateness criteria management of vaginal cancer. *Oncology Journal, Gynecologic Cancers* 2013. Available at: www.cancernetwork.com/oncology-journal/acr-appropriateness-criteria-management-vaginal-cancer/page/0/1 (accessed September 16, 2014).

19. Cervical cancer. *NIH Consensus Statement*. 1996;**14**:1–38. Available at: consensus.nih.gov/1996/1996CervicalCanc er102PDF.pdf (accessed August 11, 2014).

20. American College of Obstetricians and Gynecologists. ACOG Practice Bulletin No. 131. Screening for cervical cancer. *Obstet Gynecol*. 2012;**120**(5):1222–1238.

21. Saslow D, Solomon D, Lawson HW, et al. American Cancer Society, American Society for Colposcopy and Cervical Pathology, and American Society for Clinical Pathology screening guidelines for the prevention and early detection of cervical cancer. *CA Cancer J Clin*. 2012;**62**(3):147–172.

22. US Preventive Services Task Force. Screening for Cervical Cancer: Recommendation Statement. *Am Fam Physician*. 2012;**86**(6):555–559.

23. Vesco KK, Whitlock EP, Eder M, et al. Risk factors and other epidemiologic considerations for cervical cancer screening: a narrative review for the US Preventive Services Task Force. *Ann Intern Med*. 2011;**155**(10):698–705.

24. American College of Obstetricians and Gynecologists. ACOG Practice Bulletin No. 35. Diagnosis and treatment of cervical carcinomas. *Obstet Gynecol*. 2002;**78**(1):79–91.

25. Sorosky JI. Endometrial cancer. *Obstet Gynecol* 2012;**120**(2 Pt 1):383–397.

26. Swerdlow AJ, Jones ME. British Tamoxifen Second Cancer Study Group. Tamoxifen treatment for breast cancer and risk of endometrial cancer: a case-control study. *J Natl Cancer Inst* 2005;**97**(5)375–384.

27. Brinton LA, Berman ML, Mortel R, et al. Reproductive, menstrual and medical risk factors for endometrial cancer: results from a case control study. *Am J Obstet Gynecol* 1992;**167**(5):1317–1325.

28. Lancaster JM, Powell CM, Kauff ND, et al. Society of Gynecologic Oncologists Education Committee statement on risk assessment for inherited gynecologic cancer predispositions. *Gynecol Oncol* 2007;**107**(2):159–162.

29. Mueck AO, Seeger H, Rabe T. Hormonal contraception and risk of endometrial cancer: a systematic review. *Endocr Relat Cancer* 2010;**17**(4):R263–R271.

30. Zhou B, Yang L, Sun Q, et al. Cigarette smoking and the risk of endometrial cancer: a meta-analysis. *Am J Med* 2008;**121**(6):501–508.

31. Moore SC, Gierach GL, Schatzkin A, Matthews CE. Physical activity, sedentary behaviours, and the prevention of endometrial cancer. *Br J Cancer* 2010; **103**(7):933–938.

32. Yu X, Bao Z, Zou J, Dong J. Coffee consumption and risk of cancers: a meta-analysis of cohort studies. *BMC Cancer* 2011;**11**:96.

33. Tang NP, Li H, Qiu YL, et al. Tea consumption and risk of endometrial cancer: a metaanalysis. *Am J Obstet Gynecol* 2009;**201**(6):605.

34. Von Greunigen VE, Karlen JR. Carcinoma of the endometrium. *Am Fam Phys* 1995;**51**(6):1531–1536.

35. Buchanan EM, Weinstein LC, Hillson C. Endometrial Cancer. *Am Fam Phys* 2009;**80**(10):1075–1080.

36. American College of Obstetricians and Gynecologists. ACOG Committee Opinion No. 280. The role of the generalist obstetrician-gynecologist in the early detection of ovarian cancer. *Obstet Gynecol*. 2002;**100**(6):1413–1416.

37. US Preventive Services Task Force. Screening for ovarian cancer: reaffirmation recommendation statement. *Ann Intern Med* 2012;**157**(12):900–904.

38. Tortolero-Luna G, Mitchell MF, Rhodes-Morris HE. Epidemiology and screening for ovarian cancer. *Obstet Gynecol Clin North Am* 1994;**21**(1):1–23.

39. Teneriello MG, Park RC. Early detection of ovarian cancer. *CA Cancer J Clin* 1995;**45**(2):71–87.

40. McDonald JM, Modesitt SC. The incidental postmenopausal adnexal mass. *Clin Obstet Gynecol* 2006;**49**(3):506–516.

41. Roett M, Evans P. Ovarian cancer: an overview. *Am Fam Physician* 2009;**361**:170–177.

42. Modesitt SC, Pavlik EJ, Ueland FR, et al. Risk of malignancy in unilocular ovarian cystic tumors less than 10 centimeters in diameter. *Obstet Gynecol* 2003;**102**(3):594–599.

43. Komatsu T, Konisha I, Mandai M, et al. Adnexal masses: transvaginal US and gadolinium-enhanced MR imaging assessment of intratumoral structure. *Radiology* 1996;**198**(1):109–115.

44. van Nagell JR Jr, Hoff JT. Transvaginal ultrasonagraphy in ovarian cancer screening: current perspectives. *Int J Womens Health* 2013;**6**: 25–33.

45. NIH consensus conference. Ovarian cancer: screening, treatment, and follow-up. Development Panel on Ovarian Cancer. *JAMA* 1995;**273**(6):491–497.

46. Lowder JL, Ghetti C, Nikolajski C, et al. Body image perceptions in women with pelvic organ prolapse: a qualitative study. *Am J Obstet Gynecol* 2011;**204**(5):411.e1–5.

47. Jelovsek JE, Maher C, Barber MD. Pelvic organ prolapse. *Lancet* 2007;**369**(9566):1027–1038.

48. Bump RC, Mattiasson A, Bo K, et al. The standardization of terminology of female pelvic organ prolapse and pelvic floor dysfunction. *Am J Obstet Gynecol*. 1996;**175**(1):10–17.

49. Culligan PJ. Nonsurgical management of pelvic organ prolapse. *Obstet Gynecol* 2012;**119**(4):852–860.

50. Vasomotor symptoms. In: Menopause and osteoporosis update 2009. *J Obstet Gynaecol Can.* 2009 Jan;**31**(1 Suppl 1):S9–S10.

51. North American Menopause Society. The 2012 hormone therapy position statement of the North American Menopause Society. *Menopause.* 2012 Mar;**19**(3):257–271. doi:10.1097/gme.0b013e31824b970a.

52. American College of Obstetricians and Gynecologists (ACOG). *Female Sexual Dysfunction.* Washington, DC: American College of Obstetricians and Gynecologists (ACOG); 2011 Apr: 12 p. (ACOG Practice Bulletin No. 119). Available at: www.guideline.gov/content.aspx?id=32672&search=postmenopausal+symptoms (accessed November 14, 2015).

53. Wallace Kazer M. Issues regarding sexuality. In: Boltz M, Capezuti E, Fulmer T, Zwicker D, editors. *Evidence-based Geriatric Nursing Protocols for Best Practice.* 4th ed. New York, NY: Springer Publishing Company; 2012: 500–515. Available at: www.guideline.gov/content.aspx?id=43928&search=sexual+dysfunction (accessed November 14, 2015).

54. *Health Care Guideline: Diagnosis of Breast Disease*, 14th ed. January 2012. Available at: www.icsi.org/_asset/v9l91q/DxBrDis.pdf (accessed November 14, 2015).

Chapter 29

Endocrine disorders in the elderly

Swaytha Yalamanchi, MD, Laila S. Tabatabai, MD, and
Kendall F. Moseley, MD

Introduction

Dysfunction of the endocrine glands can occur at any point in the life cycle. Although many endocrine diseases will present with classic signs and symptoms, atypical presentation of hormonal dysregulation can make diagnosis in the elderly particularly challenging. Normal physiologic changes associated with aging, as well as medical comorbidities and medications, may all cloud the identification of endocrine dysfunction in this complicated population. As such, the diagnosis of endocrinopathies in the elderly population requires a careful medical history, detailed physical exam, rational biochemical workup, and if necessary, directed imaging. Management of endocrine disorders can be equally complex. Many endocrine disorders are treated with medications that may complicate an already-lengthy list, causing unwanted side effects or even drug–drug interactions. If therapy includes possible surgical referral, careful assessment of the risk–benefit ratio and candidacy of the elderly patient is imperative. Endocrine guidelines have been designed to assist the clinician with accurate diagnosis and rational therapeutic decision making; however, guidelines cannot supplant the need for patient-centered care in this vulnerable population in whom disorders of the endocrine glands fail to adhere to "textbook" scenarios.

Parathyroid disease and other diseases of calcium metabolism

Primary hyperparathyroidism

Parathyroid hormone (PTH)-mediated hypercalcemia is often an incidental finding on routine laboratory assessment. Primary hyperparathyroidism (PHPT) is the most common cause of hypercalcemia and occurs in 1 in 1,000 persons in the United States. The incidence of PHPT peaks in the seventh decade of life. More than 80% of patients with PHPT are considered asymptomatic at the time of diagnosis. [1] Classic symptoms of the disease include nephrolithiasis and bone disease (osteoporosis, osteitis fibrosa cystica). Other symptoms of PHPT are often vague, nonspecific, and may overlap with common complaints among elderly patients. These include easy fatigability, myalgias, bone pain, depressed affect, abdominal cramping or constipation, weakness, headaches, irritability, forgetfulness, difficulty rising from a chair. Laboratory findings in PHPT universally include hypercalcemia as well as inappropriately normal or high serum PTH levels. Additional studies may show low serum phosphate, hypercalciuria, high levels of renal cyclic adenosine monophosphate (cAMP), and enhanced markers of bone resorption.

Patients with confirmed PHPT who are symptomatic should undergo parathyroidectomy. Unfortunately, the distinction between symptomatic and asymptomatic patients is rarely well defined. A careful history for onset of symptoms compared to trajectory of serum calcium may be helpful in challenging cases. If a patient is not clearly symptomatic, guidelines should be followed to determine management.[2] Specifically, parathyroidectomy is indicated in asymptomatic patients with PHPT who meet any one of the following conditions: (1) serum calcium concentration of 1.0 mg/dL or more above the upper limit of normal; (2) creatinine clearance that is reduced to <60 mL/min; (3) bone density at the hip, lumbar spine, or distal radius that is more than 2.5 standard deviations below peak bone mass (T score ≤−2.5) and/or previous fragility fracture; (4) age less than 50 years.

Reichel's Care of the Elderly, 7th Edition, ed. Jan Busby-Whitehead *et al.* Published by Cambridge University Press.
© Cambridge University Press 2016.

The type of surgical intervention is dictated by the number of parathyroid glands involved. PHPT is most often caused by a single adenoma (80%–85%) or four-gland hyperplasia (10%–15%).[1] It is rarely part of hereditary syndromes such as multiple endocrine neoplasia types 1 and 2A. Neck imaging is not necessary for diagnosis of PHPT, but it should be ordered if surgery is indicated. Localization of the overactive gland(s) can decrease the invasiveness and morbidity of surgery. Both sestamibi scan and neck ultrasound are useful for localization.[3] Parathyroidectomy should be performed by an experienced surgeon who uses intraoperative PTH monitoring. Surgery is associated with a cure rate of 95%–98%. There is a low rate (1%–3%) of complications, including laryngeal-nerve palsy and postoperative hypocalcemia, particularly when vitamin D is not replete prior to surgery. Successful parathyroidectomy is followed by a prompt normalization of the PTH level, serum and urinary calcium levels, and gradual increases in bone mineral density (up to 10% over the course of several years).

In elderly patients who are asymptomatic and have serum calcium concentrations <1.0 mg/dL above the upper limit of normal, parathyroidectomy can be deferred. Surveillance should include monitoring with yearly measurement of serum creatinine, calcium, and bone mineral density. Although counterintuitive, calcium intake through dietary sources or supplements should reach 1,000 mg daily for skeletal protection. Vitamin D deficiency often coexists with PHPT and should be actively managed to prevent additional bone loss and superimposed secondary hyperparathyroidism. Vitamin D should be repleted to levels ≥20 ng/mL both prior to surgery and with conservative management. In elderly patients who meet criteria for parathyroidectomy but are medically unfit for surgery or do not wish to have surgery, medical management with cinacalcet may be effective. Unfortunately, cinacalcet does not improve bone mineral density, and there is no data on its effects on nephrolithiasis. In patients with PHPT who are medically unfit for surgery and have low bone mineral density, bisphosphonates may have a dual benefit of improving bone density and lowering calcium levels.[5]

Vitamin D deficiency

Vitamin D is predictive of a wide variety of clinical outcomes related to mortality, cardiovascular health, cognitive function, muscle and bone health, and multiple sclerosis. The prevalence of vitamin D deficiency in persons over the age of 65 has been estimated at 50%, although this is highly variable and dependent on geographic location and socioeconomic, clinical, and other factors.[6] Further complicating this statistic is the lack of consensus regarding the definition of "deficiency." Although the Institute of Medicine defines sufficient as serum 25-hydroxy vitamin D above 20 ng/mL (50 nmol/L), many organizations – including the Endocrine Society, National Osteoporosis Foundation, and American Geriatric Society – recommend that the elderly maintain a minimum serum level of 30 ng/mL (75 nmol/L) to reduce the risk of falls and fracture.[7–9] Elderly and institutionalized patients are at risk for vitamin D deficiency due to age-related decline in renal function and skin structure modifications that affect vitamin D production. Low sunlight exposure, female sex, dark skin pigmentation, malnutrition, and obesity are also risk factors for vitamin D deficiency.[10]

A 2005 Cochrane review concluded that calcium and vitamin D treatment in frail elderly people who are confined to institutions reduces hip and vertebral fractures.[11] A meta-analysis of randomized controlled trials investigating oral vitamin D with or without calcium concluded that vitamin D 700 IU–800 IU per day reduces the risk of hip and nonvertebral fractures in ambulatory or institutionalized elderly individuals, whereas 400 IU per day was insufficient for fracture protection. For individuals with vitamin D deficiency on lab testing, high-dose repletion in the form of weekly ergocalciferol 50,000 IU may be necessary for several weeks. In some, ergocalciferol every other week standing has been shown to effectively maintain serum levels. Vitamin D deficiency has been implicated as a cause of bone pain, weakness, impaired cognition, low mood, and fatigue. Repletion may improve these symptoms, although data have not been definitive.

Secondary and tertiary hyperparathyroidism

Secondary hyperparathyroidism is diagnosed in the setting of elevated PTH with concurrent normo- or hypocalcemia. The most common causes of secondary hyperparathyroidism in the elderly are vitamin D deficiency and chronic kidney disease (CKD). PTH increases in CKD as an adaptive response to declining glomerular filtration rate (GFR). Produced in the kidney, circulating 1,25-dihydroxyvitamin D levels begin to decrease in stage 2 CKD and continue to fall with ongoing renal insufficiency. As GFR decreases below 60 mL/min/1.73m^2 , phosphate is retained in the kidney and stimulates synthesis and secretion of PTH. Hypocalcemia develops as the GFR decreases below 50 mL/min/1.73 m^2, further stimulating release of PTH.

Chronic secondary hyperparathyroidism of any cause can result in bone loss and fractures, cardiovascular disease, and increased mortality. Elderly patients with secondary hyperparathyroidism due to CKD should be followed by a nephrologist and/or endocrinologist for implementation of calcium, vitamin D, and cinacalcet and/or calcitriol therapy to lower PTH levels.[12] If left untreated, secondary hyperparathyroidism may evolve into tertiary disease in which parathyroid glands begin to function autonomously. This phenomenon is most commonly observed in those with longstanding renal disease or hemodialysis patients. Laboratory studies in tertiary hyperparathyroidism mimic those of primary disease with elevations in serum calcium and PTH levels. If pharmacotherapy is not effective in controlling serum calcium and PTH levels, subtotal parathyroidectomy may be necessary.

Hypercalcemia of malignancy

In the elderly population, hypercalcemia in the presence of a low or suppressed PTH level should always prompt screening for occult malignancy. Parathyroid hormone–related protein (PTHrP) has been identified as the most common cause of hypercalcemia in patients with nonmetastatic solid tumors. PTHrP elevations are seen most commonly in squamous cell carcinoma (lung, head, neck), breast, prostate, renal, and bladder cancers.[13] Patients with non-Hodgkin's lymphoma, chronic myeloid leukemia, and adult T-cell leukemia may also have elevated PTHrP levels. The two other major mechanisms of hypercalcemia of malignancy are (1) osteolytic metastases with local release of cytokines (including osteoclast-activating factors), and (2) tumor production of 1,25-dihydroxyvitamin D (calcitriol). Osteolytic metastases account for approximately one-fifth of cases of hypercalcemia of malignancy due to bone destruction by osteoclasts and occur in solid tumors with bone metastases and multiple myeloma. In lymphoma, hypercalcemia may be due to increased and

PTH-independent production of 1,25-dihydroxyvitamin D (calcitriol), increased intestinal calcium absorption, and bone resorption. In most cases, treatment of the underlying malignancy improves serum calcium levels; occasionally, antiresorptive medications or steroids are also needed.

Hypoparathyroidism

Congenital hypoparathyroidism is usually part of a genetic syndrome detected early in life. In elderly patients, new onset hypoparathyroidism is more likely to be iatrogenic. Acquired hypoparathyroidism is often due to inadvertent removal of the parathyroid glands or irreversible damage to their blood supply during thyroidectomy, parathyroidectomy, or neck dissection surgery. Patients may present with perioral numbness and tingling, tetany, hypotension, and arrhythmias, depending on the acuity of serum calcium declines. In the outpatient setting, these patients are treated with high-dose calcium and/or and calcitriol, with the goal albumin-corrected calcium level at the lower end of normal range (8.0 mg/dL–8.5 mg/dL) to prevent nephrolithiasis.

Disorders of the thyroid gland

Hypothyroidism

The most common form of hypothyroidism is due to autoimmune disease (Hashimoto's) in which circulating thyroid antibodies damage the thyroid gland over time, impairing its ability to make thyroid hormone. Hypothyroidism may also result from surgical removal of the thyroid or radiation therapy. The symptoms of hypothyroidism can be nebulous and similar to those occurring in natural aging. These include fatigue, cold intolerance, constipation, dry skin and hair, weight gain, and impaired concentration. It is important to consider depression and anemia in these patients as well, since all three conditions share the same symptoms and are commonly diagnosed in the elderly.[14] Measurement of serum thyrotropin (TSH) should be used to screen for an underactive thyroid gland. The anterior pituitary releases TSH in response to decreased circulating levels of free thyroxine (FT4) and free tri-iodothyronine (FT3) inadequately produced by the thyroid gland. Overt hypothyroidism is defined by elevated TSH with frankly low FT4 levels. There has been some debate as to whether the reference range for normal

TSH should be adjusted for age. It is well known that TSH increases with each decade of life despite maintenance of circulating thyroid hormone. Some studies have shown that elderly individuals with high TSH and lower FT4 have a prolonged survival, suggestive that changes in thyroid function are adaptive mechanisms to conserve energy expenditure with age.[15]

Overt hypothyroidism requires treatment with thyroid hormone to alleviate symptoms and prevent progression to myxedema, an endocrine emergency characterized by undetectable thyroid hormone levels, obtundation, hypothermia, and decreased cardiac output that can progress to heart failure.[16] Patients with established hypothyroidism should be treated with synthetic L-thyroxine (T4), which is peripherally converted in peripheral tissues to FT3, the active form of thyroid hormone. L-thyroxine is typically administered as a once-daily dose of 1.6 ug/kg. A recent clinical trial demonstrated that starting with full-dose L-thyroxine is safe and effective in asymptomatic patients with hypothyroidism, including the elderly.[17] TSH levels should be monitored six weeks after initiation of L-thyroxine and at six-week intervals after any dose adjustments. After dose stabilization, TSH levels can be monitored annually. The most common complications of L-thyroxine therapy in the elderly are myocardial ischemia, arrhythmias (usually atrial fibrillation), and bone loss. The risk of these complications can be minimized by avoiding TSH suppression below the normal range.

Subclinical hypothyroidism

Subclinical hypothyroidism is defined by elevated TSH with normal FT4 levels. This condition can occur with the progression of autoimmune disease or temporarily in the setting of thyroiditis. In contrast to overt hypothyroidism, there are no clearly established indications for treatment of subclinical hypothyroidism in the elderly. Possible, although contentious, reasons to treat subclinical hypothyroidism may include alleviating hypothyroid symptoms, preventing progression to overt hypothyroidism if antibodies are present, and possibly reducing the risk of cardiovascular and all-cause mortality.[18] The majority of trials of L-thyroxine in elderly patients with subclinical hypothyroidism showed no improvement in symptoms. In patients with subclinical hypothyroidism, the combination of TSH >10 uIU/mL and thyroid antibody positivity has been linked to increased risk of progression to overt hypothyroidism. There is insufficient evidence to suggest that treatment of subclinical hypothyroidism reduces cardiovascular complications in the elderly. [19, 20] A very small number of trials in patients with subclinical hypothyroidism have shown increased risk of congestive heart failure, cardiovascular mortality, and all-cause mortality.

Given limited data supporting the treatment of subclinical disease, current guidelines recommend L-thyroxine therapy (LT4) only when serum TSH concentrations are >10 uIU/mL in the setting of normal FT4.[21] Treatment should be considered in patients with serum TSH concentrations above a laboratory's normal reference range but below 10 uIU/mL on the basis of individual factors, including symptoms, thyroid antibody positivity, or evidence of atherosclerotic cardiovascular disease. Treatment of subclinical hypothyroidism usually requires only 50 ug–75 ug of L-thyroxine daily; TSH levels should be monitored six weeks after initiating therapy. Elderly patients with cardiovascular disease should start with even lower doses, LT4 12.5 ug–25 ug daily.

Hyperthyroidism

Hyperthyroidism is defined by low TSH levels and frankly elevated FT4 and/or T3 levels. Elderly patients with hyperthyroidism are more likely to present with cardiovascular symptoms (tachycardia, atrial fibrillation), dyspnea, edema, weakness, and weight loss and are less likely to present with tremor or nervousness. Hyperthyroidism in the elderly is often termed "apathetic," as the classic hyperactive symptoms are often absent. Overt hyperthyroidism is associated with increased cardiovascular risk, osteoporosis, and mortality in the elderly. Compared to younger patients, a higher proportion of elderly patients with hyperthyroidism have toxic multinodular goiter. Thyrotoxicosis can also be due to autoimmune stimulation of the thyroid gland (Graves' disease), thyroiditis, or iodine-containing medications (namely amiodarone).[22] Given the broad differential of hyperthyroidism, neck examination is a key component of the physical exam. Multiple thyroid nodules may suggest toxic multinodular goiter, whereas a single thyroid nodule could be an autonomous toxic nodule. Presence of a diffuse goiter may suggest Graves' disease, although many elderly patients with Graves' disease may have a nonpalpable thyroid gland. A tender thyroid gland suggests subacute (granulomatous) thyroiditis.

Neck ultrasound and radioactive iodine (RAI) uptake and scan should be performed in patients with suppressed TSH and nodule(s) on examination. Toxic nodules that appear "hot" on nuclear medicine testing can be definitively treated with radioactive iodine, though thionamide treatment can be temporizing. Nodules seen on neck ultrasound but "cold" on scan should be biopsied to rule out thyroid cancer. If RAI scanning shows diminished radiotracer uptake and poor gland visibility, subacute or subclinical thyroiditis should be suspected. Subacute thyroiditis can occur transiently following an upper respiratory illness and is associated with neck pain. The condition can be treated with NSAIDs and/or a short course of prednisone. Subclinical, painless thyroiditis is thought to be autoimmune mediated and does not typically require therapy. Both subacute and subclinical thyroiditis can be associated with a hypothyroid phase that follows hyperthyroidism. In some cases, the hypothyroidism does not resolve and requires lifelong LT4 therapy. As such, TSH and free T4 should be monitored closely every six weeks.

Graves' disease will show diffuse RAI uptake and increased vascularity on neck ultrasound. Graves' disease can be initially treated with thionamides (methimazole, PTU), as remission can occur within the first year in 20%–30% of patients. Unless contraindicated, methimazole is preferred over PTU, given its once daily dosing. Starting dose depends on the severity of thyrotoxicosis, but is usually 10 mg–15 mg daily for mild Graves' disease. Beta blockers are also recommended in Graves' disease, if appropriate. Thyroid function tests with TSH, free T4, and total T3 should be monitored every six weeks in Graves' patients, with adjustment of methimazole dose to achieve normal free T4 and total T3 levels and a TSH in the detectable range. If Graves' does not go into remission with methimazole treatment for a year or becomes difficult to control, RAI treatment should be pursued. In cases where RAI is required to manage hyperthyroidism, resultant hypothyroidism should be anticipated and managed accordingly.[16]

Amiodarone is an iodine-containing antiarrhythmic medication that can cause thyrotoxicosis in one of two ways: amiodarone-induced thyrotoxicosis (AIT) type 1 is iodine-induced and occurs in individuals with autoimmune thyroid disease or thyroid nodules; AIT type 2 is destructive thyroiditis caused by toxic effects of amiodarone on follicular thyroid cells. It is important to obtain a thyroid ultrasound in these patients to distinguish which type of AIT exists, as the treatment is different for the two conditions. AIT type 1 is treated with thionamides, radioactive iodine, or surgery, if necessary. AIT type 2 is treated with steroids. A baseline TSH should be checked in all patients prior to initiating amiodarone and monitored at least yearly.

Subclinical hyperthyroidism

Subclinical hyperthyroidism is defined by low TSH levels and normal FT4 and total T3 levels. It is important to distinguish this condition from nonthyroidal illness or "euthyroid sick syndrome," which can be due to chronic or critical illness. Euthyroid sick syndrome is characterized by low or normal TSH, low or normal FT4, and low total T3 and FT3. This condition is common in the elderly and affects up to one-third of critically ill hospitalized patients.[23, 24] The failure of TSH to rise in response to low thyroid hormone levels in critical illness is due in part to central hypothyroidism from alterations in the hypothalamic-pituitary-thyroid axis. Euthyroid sick syndrome is usually transient and does not require treatment, as the laboratory findings normalize when the underlying illness has resolved.

Many studies have shown that subclinical hyperthyroidism has adverse effects on cardiovascular health and bone mass in patients >65 years. It has been linked to a threefold increased risk of atrial fibrillation in the elderly. For treatment purposes, a clinical consensus group with representatives from the Endocrine Society, American Thyroid Association, and American Association of Clinical Endocrinologists has recommended that elderly patients with TSH <0.1 uIU/mL undergo diagnostic testing and begin treatment for the causative condition. Elderly men and women with TSH in the 0.1–0.5 uIU/mL range should also be treated, as they are at increased risk of cardiac arrhythmia and bone loss.[25]

Thyroid nodules

Almost 50% of patients >65 years of age have thyroid nodules on ultrasound examination, the prevalence confirmed by autopsy studies. Greater than 95% of thyroid nodules are benign. Elderly patients with palpable thyroid nodules should be evaluated with thyroid ultrasound, as the incidence of thyroid cancer increases with age. Those with thyroid nodule(s) and suppressed TSH should have 24-hour radioactive iodine uptake and scan (as detailed earlier), to identify hyperfunctioning, "hot" nodule(s). Hyperfunctioning nodules rarely harbor malignancy, and cytologic evaluation is rarely necessary.

Elderly patients with thyroid nodules should be evaluated by an endocrinologist to determine if biopsy with fine-needle aspiration (FNA) is indicated. In general, nodules measuring 1.0 cm or larger with suspicious features (hypoechoic, microcalcifications, increased vascularity, infiltrating margins, etc.) should undergo biopsy. All patients with abnormal cervical lymph nodes detected on exam or ultrasound and thyroid nodule(s) should also undergo FNA. Spongiform and mixed cystic-solid nodules do not require FNA biopsy unless they are 2.0 cm or larger in size. If biopsy reveals a benign nodule or nodules, patients can be followed every one to two years with thyroid ultrasound for changes in size or character, in which case repeat biopsy or surgical removal may be warranted.[26]

Thyroid cancer

Differentiated thyroid carcinoma has a good prognosis if detected early and treated with thyroidectomy (and radioactive iodine, if indicated). However, patients older than 65 often have more aggressive disease with multiple, larger tumors and more advanced-stage disease, nonpapillary histology, and extrathyroidal extension. Anaplastic thyroid carcinoma, which carries the worst prognosis among thyroid cancers, presents almost exclusively after the age of 60 years. If biopsy of a thyroid nodule reveals thyroid cancer cells or findings suspicious for thyroid cancer, thyroidectomy should be performed. Total thyroidectomy is generally recommended if the primary thyroid carcinoma is >1 cm; there are contralateral thyroid nodules present, or regional or distant metastases are present, the patient has a personal history of radiation therapy to the head and neck, or the patient has first-degree family history of differentiated thyroid cancer. Older patients (age >45 years) should also undergo total thyroidectomy even with tumors <1 cm–1.5 cm, because of higher recurrence rates in this age group.[26] Age by itself is not a contraindication to thyroidectomy. Studies have shown no difference in complication rates (permanent hypoparathyroidism, recurrent laryngeal nerve

palsy, etc.) between older and younger patients who undergo thyroidectomy for thyroid cancer.[27] Treatment decisions to include thyroidectomy, neck dissection, radioactive iodine remnant ablation, TSH suppression, and ongoing follow-up should be made by an experienced endocrinologist and thyroid surgeon.

Disorders of the pituitary gland

Hypopituitarism

The incidence of hypopituitarism in the adult general population (mean age of diagnosis 50 years; range 18–79 years) has been estimated at 4.2 cases per 100,000. [28] Pituitary adenomas, particularly nonfunctional pituitary adenomas, are the most common cause of hypopituitarism in the elderly, with an incidence of 7%–9.9% in this population.[29–31] The incidence of pituitary adenomas in the elderly is increasing, likely related to the increasing frequency of neuroimaging in this population. Pituitary adenomas are nonfunctional in 65%–84% of cases, with the most common functional pituitary adenomas secreting growth hormone (GH, 17%), prolactin (4.5%–10%), and adrenocorticotropic hormone (ACTH, 0%–6%). Gonadotrophic adenomas, which are usually included in the non-functional pituitary adenoma group, tend to increase with age, particularly over the age of 50.[32] Other causes of hypopituitarism include nonadenomatous tumors such as craniopharyngiomas, meningiomas, gliomas, and metastases, as well as infiltrative lesions such as hemochromatosis, granulomatous diseases, histiocytosis and autoimmune lymphocytic hypophysitis. Pituitary apoplexy, surgery and radiation can result in hypopituitarism up to 10 years following therapy.[33]

Clinical manifestations of either partial or complete hypopituitarism may be nonspecific and attributed to the natural aging process or related comorbidities. Pituitary tumors are incidentally discovered on imaging in approximately 5%–15% of elderly patients. Due to the predominance of nonfunctioning pituitary adenomas, clinical symptoms are often associated with local mass effect on the optic chiasm resulting in visual impairment. Due to age-related decline in visual acuity, cataracts, and macular degeneration, the link between visual symptoms and pituitary pathology may be misdiagnosed in up to 20% of cases. Other manifestations of mass effect – including headaches, cranial nerve palsy due to cavernous sinus invasion or pituitary apoplexy, and opthalmoplegia – are less common.[34]

Symptoms of hormonal deficits are less commonly recognized as a presenting feature of pituitary tumors, largely due to their nonspecific nature and overlap with those related to aging and medical comorbidities. However, with thorough preoperative evaluations, rates of symptoms at presentation can be identified in up to 50% of individuals.[35] Hyponatremia, whether due to age-related changes in vasopressin secretion or adrenal insufficiency, can be a presenting feature of hypopituitarism in up to 9.5% of cases in the elderly.[36] Conversely, diabetes insipidus is unlikely to be due to a pituitary adenoma and is more commonly seen in cases of craniopharyngioma, lymphocytic hypophysitis, infiltrative disease, or pituitary metastases.[35]

Biochemical hormonal assessment with cortisol, IGF-1, free T4, and prolactin levels, as well as neuroradiological imaging with a pituitary-protocol MRI with baseline visual field testing are important components of the diagnosis of hypopituitarism at any age. However, the diagnosis of pituitary dysfunction in the elderly individual poses specific challenges. There are morphologic changes in the hypothalamus and pituitary in addition to age-related declines in GH, androgens, and estrogen that must be considered. Additional illnesses and medications may further confound assessment. Classically, acquired hypopituitarism progresses such that GH deficiency appears first, followed by hypogonadotrophic hypogonadism and subsequently thyroid and/or adrenal insufficiency.[35]

Growth hormone deficiency is diagnosed on the basis of subnormal serum insulin-like growth factor 1 (IGF-1) levels measured against gender and age-specific norms. GH deficiency is then confirmed with a glucagon stimulation test. In the setting of acromegaly, documentation of elevated IGF-1 levels should be followed by confirmatory oral glucose tolerance testing with measurement of growth hormone levels. [35] Assessment of central hypogonadism in the elderly man is made on the basis of 8 AM testosterone levels in the setting of low LH and FSH levels. Prolactinomas typically present as macroadenomas (>2 cm) in the elderly. There may be associated hypogonadism in men as well as galactorrhea. Prolactin levels may be elevated as a side effect of several medications used commonly in the elderly, including antipsychotic agents. Nonfunctional pituitary adenomas

may also result in modest elevations in prolactin levels due to stalk compression. The diagnosis of central hypothyroidism can be made on the basis of low plasma free T4 levels in the setting of thyroid stimulating hormone (TSH) levels in the low or inappropriate-normal range. Adrenal insufficiency is diagnosed based on low morning serum cortisol levels with confirmatory subnormal response to the 250 mcg ACTH stimulation test (<18 mcg/dL).

When selecting the appropriate treatment for pituitary tumors, whether surgical or medical, it is important to consider the impact of mass effect, hormonal deficits, and hormonal excess. Transsphenoidal surgery is regarded as both safe and successful in the elderly in the hands of an experienced neurosurgical team. Studies show no increase in perioperative morality or severe anesthesiologic complications in individuals aged 65 and older. The most frequent postoperative complications include diabetes insipidus and cerebrospinal fluid leak.[31, 37] Transsphenoidal surgery is also the treatment of choice for elderly patients with visual disturbances due to nonfunctioning pituitary adenomas. More than 70% of individuals will demonstrate postoperative visual improvement, although a small percentage may develop visual deterioration due to hemorrhagic or ischemic damage.[31] The indication for surgical intervention in nonfunctional sellar masses without visual impairment is less clear. Conservative interval monitoring with laboratory studies and imaging may be a reasonable option and should be considered in those at high surgical risk.[35]

Hormonal replacement in elderly patients with hypopituitarism can be complicated and requires addressing each of the impaired axes. For ACTH deficiency, cortisol replacement regimens must be tailored to achieve hemodynamic stability while avoiding overtreatment that could adversely impact bone health and metabolism. It is of paramount importance to ensure that individuals with ACTH deficiency wear a medical alert tag and are aware of the need to contact their physician for dose adjustments in acute illness or prior to invasive procedures. Thyroid hormone should be started at low dose and uptitrated gradually to a goal of 1.3 +/–0.2 mcg/kg/day.[38] In hypopituitarism, dosing is titrated to free T4 levels and not to TSH levels. Further, prior to initiating thyroid hormone replacement, central adrenal insufficiency should be identified and treated to avoid precipitating an adrenal crisis.

Indications for replacement of testosterone and growth hormone in cases of hypopituitarism are less well established, particularly in the elderly population. Testosterone replacement therapy has important implications for maintaining lean body mass, bone mineralization, erythropoiesis, and sense of well-being. However, recent studies have revealed a possible link between testosterone replacement and increased cardiovascular risk in older men. Testosterone initiations should take place after carefully assessing the risk–benefit ratio for the individual in question. Deficiency in growth hormone is associated with visceral obesity, insulin resistance with impaired glucose tolerance, and dyslipidemia. In the absence of contraindications such as malignancy or proliferative diabetic retinopathy, growth hormone replacement may be beneficial in select cases. Lower-dose therapy is typically required in the elderly, and IGF-1 levels should be closely monitored.[34, 35]

Ectopic ACTH production

Clinical assessment, physical exam, and laboratory findings suggestive of Cushing's syndrome in the absence of a pituitary or adrenal adenoma are rare in the elderly. Similar to Cushing's syndrome of other etiologies, the most common clinical manifestations of ectopic ACTH production include muscle weakness, change in body weight, hypertension, hirsutism, low bone mineral density, and hypokalemia.[39] Distinction of ectopic ACTH secretion from Cushing's disease can be quite difficult. Typically, the high-dose dexamethasone suppression test is the first-line test, followed by intrapetrosal sphenoid sinus sampling. Identifying the source of ACTH secretion can be equally challenging. Bronchial carcinoid tumors, small cell lung carcinoma, and gastroenteric pancreatic tumors may all secrete ACTH. Because pulmonary tumors are often a source of ectopic ACTH production, computed tomography (CT) chest is the most useful form of imaging, with either CT or magnetic resonance imaging (MRI) of the abdomen/pelvis as the next step. Treatment includes surgical removal of the tumor and/or medical therapy.[40]

Disorders of the adrenal glands

Adrenal nodules

Among one of the more common "incidentalomas," adrenal nodules are often detected in imaging tests ordered for the workup of other conditions. The prevalence of adrenal nodules increases with age, ranging from 0.2% among individuals 20–39 years of age to 7% in individuals over the age of 70.[41] Although often benign, adrenal nodules may be functional and/or malignant. Thus, further evaluation of the incidentaloma is often warranted. In the general population, nonfunctional adenomas are the most common (80%), followed by cortisol-producing tumors (Cushing's syndrome), pheochromocytomas, aldosteronomas, adrenocortical carcinoma, and metastatic disease, respectively.[42–44]

Important diagnostic information may be gleaned from adrenal protocol CT. Features suggestive, but not diagnostic, of malignancy include size >6 cm, irregular borders, lack of homogeneity, calcifications, and washout of contrast after 15 minutes less than 40%. Unless CT findings are clearly characteristics of benign findings such as a myelolipoma or cyst, lesions ≥4 cm should be resected to rule out adrenal cortical carcinoma.[42, 45, 46] In general, FNA of adrenal nodules is recommended only if there is high suspicion for metastatic disease or infection and if biochemical assessment for functional adenomas (i.e. pheochromocytoma) is negative. For those lesions less than 4 cm, guidelines from the American Association of Clinical Endocrinologists and the American Association of Endocrine Surgeons recommend that patients with an adrenal incidentaloma undergo clinical and biochemical evaluation for hyperaldosteronism (if hypertensive), as well as for the presence of a pheochromocytoma and hypercortisolism.[42] The evaluation of each of these entities will be described in further detail.

Primary aldosteronism

All patients with hypertension and adrenal nodules should be screened for primary aldosteronism (PA). PA encompasses a group of disorders characterized by inappropriately high and relatively autonomous aldosterone production that is nonsuppressible by sodium loading. PA is most commonly caused by an adrenal adenoma, unilateral or bilateral adrenal hyperplasia, or less commonly, glucocorticoid-remediable aldosteronism.[47] Diagnosis of PA has important implications for patients, as evidence suggests that these individuals have higher cardiovascular morbidity and mortality than age- and sex-matched patients with essential hypertension and the same degree of blood pressure elevation.[47–49] Although a minority of patients present with hypokalemia, normokalemic hypertension is the most common presentation of hyperaldosteronism.[50] Screening for PA includes measurement of plasma renin activity (PRA) and aldosterone levels. An aldosterone level of 15 ng/dL or greater in conjunction with plasma aldosterone to PRA ratio of 20 or greater is suggestive of aldosterone excess. Unfortunately, there are many medications that can confound laboratory studies. Patients should be taken off of spironolactone, epleronone, amiloride, triamterene, potassium-wasting diuretics, and products derived from licorice root for at least four weeks prior to testing. If results are nondiagnostic and suspicion for PA remains high, it may be necessary to replace other antihypertensives – including alpha-adrenergic blockers, central alpha-2-agonists, nonsteroidal anti-inflammatory drugs, angiotensin-converting enzyme inhibitors, angiotensin receptor blockers, renin inhibitors, and dihydropyridine calcium channel antagonists.[47, 48] Confirmatory testing is recommended with aldosterone-suppression testing using oral sodium loading, saline infusion, fludrocortisone suppression, or captopril challenge.

Given the high incidence of adrenal nodules in the elderly, all individuals older than 40 years of age should undergo adrenal vein sampling if surgical intervention is considered to confirm laterality. In individuals with evidence of unilateral PA, whether it is due an aldosterone-producing adenoma or unilateral adrenal hyperplasia, laparoscopic adrenalectomy should be offered to all patients after a careful consideration of surgical risks. Nonsurgical candidates are best served with a mineralocorticoid receptor antagonist such as spironolactone or eplerenone. After surgery, approximately 50% of individuals maintain blood pressure <140/90 mm Hg without antihypertensive drugs. However, among the most common reasons for persistent hypertension after adrenalectomy are older age and longer duration of disease.[47]

Pheochromocytoma

In the general population, pheochromocytomas constitute approximately 4%–7% of adrenal incidentalomas.[45] Pheochromocytomas are diagnosed most frequently in the fourth and fifth decades with occurrences in approximately 9%–27% of patients aged 60 and older. Despite textbook symptomatology, only 10% of patients 12–85 years of age will present with the classic triad of headaches, sweating, and

palpitations; further, 12.5% patients are normotensive at the time of diagnosis.[51] Other less common signs and symptoms of pheochromocytomas include tremors, pallor, dyspnea, generalized weakness, anxiety attacks, orthostatic hypotension, visual blurring, papilledema, weight loss, polyuria, polydipsia, constipation, and psychiatric disorders. However, older patients with pheochromocytoma may be less likely to experience classic symptoms of sympathetic overactivity and catecholamine excess.[52] This may be attributed to decreased baroreceptor function and slowed responsiveness to catecholamines with aging, as well as concurrent comorbidities and medications. Catecholamine excess leading to myocardial injury and cardiomyopathy are of particular concern in this vulnerable age group.[52, 53]

Appropriate screening includes measurement of plasma free metanephrines as well as 24-hour urinary metanephrines and normetanephrines. Management is surgical, but should be postponed until liberalization of fluid and salt intake and initiation of alpha-adrenergic blockade for at least one to two weeks preoperatively to minimize risk of intraoperative hemodynamic instability. Either phenoxybenzamine or doxazosin is appropriate, with titration to the goal of normotensive blood pressure readings and mild orthostasis. Beta blockade may be initiated only after adequate alpha blockade if the patient demonstrates persistent tachycardia or arrhythmias. Patients require close hemodynamic monitoring intra- and postoperatively.[54]

Cushing's syndrome

Patients with cortisol-producing adrenal adenomas, Cushing's disease, or ectopic ACTH secretion may present with either subclinical or overt Cushing's syndrome. The scope of this section will be limited to cortisol-producing adrenal adenomas. Of the functional adrenal incidentalomas, cortisol production is the most common at approximately 5.3%.[43] Symptoms of Cushing's syndrome may overlap with those seen in normal aging to include truncal weight gain, sarcopenia, hypertension, glucose intolerance, fatigue, depression, sleep disturbances, easy bruisability, or osteoporosis. The Endocrine Society guidelines recommend that the diagnosis of Cushing's syndrome is likely if two out of the three following tests are positive: 24-hour urine free cortisol, late night salivary cortisol, and dexamethasone suppression

(1 mg overnight or 2 mg two-day test).[55] An important consideration in the elderly population when selecting appropriate testing is how concomitant medications will affect cortisol levels and rate of clearance of dexamethasone. For example, medications such as phenobarbital, phenytoin, carbamazepine, primidone, rifampin, and pioglitazone may accelerate the metabolism of dexamethasone. In contrast, aprepitant/fosaprepitant, fluoxetine, and dilitazem may decrease dexamethasone metabolism. Similarly, carbamazepine and fenofibrate are examples of medications that may affect 24-hour urinary cortisol results.[55]

In the appropriate candidate, surgical management of a cortisol-secreting adenoma involves laparoscopic adrenalectomy. Postoperatively, all patients require initiation of steroid replacement therapy until the hypothalamus-pituitary-adrenal (HPA) axis recovers. For those with multiple comorbidities, the benefit of surgery may not outweigh the associated risks. In these cases, medical therapy for Cushing's syndrome will require treating the end-organ damage associated with cortisol excess (i.e., increased bone resorption, hypertension, etc.). The degree of cortisol secretion from the adenoma may also be tempered with medications and should be instituted in conjunction with an experienced endocrinologist.

Adrenal insufficiency

Adrenal insufficiency (AI) may be broadly categorized as primary or secondary, depending on whether disease originates in the adrenal glands (primary) versus the hypothalamus or pituitary (secondary); the diagnosis of primary adrenal insufficiency peaks in the fourth decade of life, and secondary adrenal insufficiency in the sixth decade.[56] AI, irrespective of etiology, is up to six times higher in the elderly, possibly related to decreased responsiveness of the HPA axis.[57] The most common causes of secondary adrenal insufficiency are iatrogenic and include long-standing steroid use (systemic or topical), megestrol acetate, ketorolac, opiate drugs, antipsychotic drugs (chlorpromazine), and antidepressants (imipramine). Though less commonly observed in the elderly, primary disease may occur as a result of anticoagulants precipitating bilateral adrenal hemorrhage. Other broad, but important, etiologic categories of primary AI include infection (HIV-1, CMV, tuberculosis, candidiasis, and histoplasmosis), metastatic disease, infiltrative disorders (amyloidosis, hemochromatosis

and sarcoidosis), infarct due to coagulation disorders, and autoimmune disease.[58]

AI may be a difficult clinical diagnosis to make in the elderly given that symptoms of chronic adrenal insufficiency may be nonspecific, classically including weakness, fatigue, anorexia, abdominal pain, nausea, vomiting, constipation or diarrhea, postural dizziness, myalgias, and arthralgias. Altered sensorium, abdominal pain, and fever together with severe hypotension may be seen in the setting of adrenal crisis, a medical emergency.[56–59] In the absence of exogenous steroid administration, basal cortisol levels of ≥15 mcg/dL–19 mcg/dL rule out AI, whereas 8 AM cortisol levels ≤3 mcg/dL are virtually diagnostic and are made using ACTH testing. As noted briefly earlier, for this stimulation test, serum cortisol is measured prior to and 60 minutes following an intramuscular injection of cosyntropin 250 mcg. A serum cortisol peak greater than 18 mcg/dL indicates an appropriate response.[58] However, mild adrenal insufficiency may be missed by the 250-mcg test; if suspicion for AI is high, a 1-mcg cosyntropin test may be a more sensitive measure to establish the diagnosis of AI.[58–60]

Treatment for AI includes glucocorticoid replacement, generally in the form of hydrocortisone. To mimic physiologic secretion of cortisol, hydrocortisone is taken twice daily with half to two-thirds of the total dose (generally 15 mg–25 mg) given in the morning and the remaining dose in mid-afternoon. Mineralocorticoid replacement, necessary only in primary adrenal insufficiency, includes fludrocortisone 0.05 mg–0.2 mg in the morning with optional dehydroepiandrosterone replacement (25 mg–50 mg).[58, 59] In contrast, adrenal crisis should be managed with IV fluid resuscitation and immediate IV hydrocortisone at a dose of 100 mg followed by 100 mg–200 mg every 24 hours with close cardiac monitoring.[58] If there is concern for coexisting hypothyroidism, glucocorticoid replacement should precede levothyroxine therapy.

References

1. Pyram R, Mahajan G, Gliwa A. Primary hyperparathyroidism: Skeletal and non-skeletal effects, diagnosis and management. *Maturitas*. 2011;**70**(3):246–255.

2. Bilezikian JP, Khan AA, Potts JT Jr. Third International Workshop on the Management of Asymptomatic Primary Hyperthyroidism. Guidelines for the management of asymptomatic primary

hyperparathyroidism: Summary statement from the third international workshop. *J Clin Endocrinol Metab.* 2009;**94**(2):335–339.

3. Boonen S, Vanderschueren D, Pelemans W, Bouillon R. Primary hyperparathyroidism: Diagnosis and management in the older individual. *Eur J Endocrinol.* 2004;**151**(3):297–304.

4. Grant P, Velusamy A. What is the best way of assessing neurocognitive dysfunction in patients with primary hyperparathyroidism? *J Clin Endocrinol Metab.* 2014;**99**(1):49–55.

5. Marcocci C, Cetani F. Clinical practice: primary hyperparathyroidism. *N Engl J Med.* 2011;**365**(25):2389–2397.

6. Cesari M, Incalzi RA, Zamboni V, Pahor M. Vitamin D hormone: a multitude of actions potentially influencing the physical function decline in older persons. *Geriatr Gerontol Int.* 2011;**11**(2):133–142.

7. Holick MF, Binkley NC, Bischoff-Ferrari HA, et al. Evaluation, treatment, and prevention of vitamin D deficiency: an endocrine society clinical practice guideline. *J Clin Endocrinol Metab.* 2011;**96**(7):1911–1930.

8. Dawson-Hughes B, Mithal A, Bonjour JP, et al. IOF position statement: vitamin D recommendations for older adults. *Osteoporos Int.* 2010;**21**(7):1151–1154.

9. American Geriatrics Society Workgroup on Vitamin D Supplementation for Older Adults. Recommendations abstracted from the American geriatrics society consensus statement on vitamin D for prevention of falls and their consequences. *J Am Geriatr Soc.* 2013;**62**:147–152.

10. Malik R. Vitamin D and secondary hyperparathyroidism in the institutionalized elderly: a literature review. *J Nutr Elder.* 2007;**26**(3–4):119–138.

11. Avenell A, Gillespie WJ, Gillespie LD, O'Connell DL. Vitamin D and vitamin D analogues for preventing fractures associated with involutional and post-menopausal osteoporosis. *Cochrane Database Syst Rev.* 2005;3:CD000227.

12. Fraser WD. Hyperparathyroidism. *Lancet.* 2009;**374**(9684):145–158.

13. McCauley LK, Martin TJ. Twenty-five years of PTHrP progress: from cancer hormone to multifunctional cytokine. *J Bone Miner Res.* 2012;**27**(6):1231–1239.

14. Bensenor IM, Olmos RD, Lotufo PA. Hypothyroidism in the elderly: diagnosis and management. *Clin Interv Aging.* 2012;7:97–111.

15. Boelaert K. Thyroid dysfunction in the elderly. *Nat Rev Endocrinol.* 2013;**9**(4):194–204.

16. Papaleontiou M, Haymart MR. Approach to and treatment of thyroid disorders in the elderly. *Med Clin North Am.* 2012;**96**(2):297–310.

17. Roos A, Linn-Rasker SP, van Domburg RT, et al. The starting dose of levothyroxine in primary hypothyroidism treatment: a prospective, randomized, double-blind trial. *Arch Intern Med.* 2005;**165**(15):1714–1720.

18. Pasqualetti G, Tognini S, Polini A, et al. Is subclinical hypothyroidism a cardiovascular risk factor in the elderly? *J Clin Endocrinol Metab.* 2013;**98**(6):2256–2266.

19. Collet TH, Gussekloo J, Bauer DC, et al. Subclinical hyperthyroidism and the risk of coronary heart disease and mortality. *Arch Intern Med.* 2012;**172**(10):799–809.

20. Biondi B, Cooper DS. The clinical significance of subclinical thyroid dysfunction. *Endocr Rev.* 2008;**29**(1):76–131.

21. Garber JR, Cobin RH, Gharib H, et al. Clinical practice guidelines for hypothyroidism in adults: Cosponsored by the American Association of Clinical Endocrinologists and the American Thyroid Association. *Endocr Pract.* 2012;**18**(6):988–1028.

22. Visser WE, Visser TJ, Peeters RP. Thyroid disorders in older adults. *Endocrinol Metab Clin North Am.* 2013;**42**(2):287–303.

23. De Alfieri W, Nistico F, Borgogni T, et al. Thyroid hormones as predictors of short- and long-term mortality in very old hospitalized patients. *J Gerontol A Biol Sci Med Sci.* 2013;**68**(9):1122–1128.

24. Iglesias P, Ridruejo E, Munoz A, et al. Thyroid function tests and mortality in aged hospitalized patients: a 7-year prospective observational study. *J Clin Endocrinol Metab.* 2013;**98**(12):4683–4690.

25. Cooper DS. Approach to the patient with subclinical hyperthyroidism. *J Clin Endocrinol Metab.* 2007;**92**(1):3–9.

26. American Thyroid Association (ATA) Guidelines Taskforce on Thyroid Nodules and Differentiated Thyroid Cancer, Cooper DS, Doherty GM, et al. Revised American Thyroid Association management guidelines for patients with thyroid nodules and differentiated thyroid cancer. *Thyroid.* 2009;**19**(11):1167–1214.

27. Gervasi R, Orlando G, Lerose MA, et al. Thyroid surgery in geriatric patients: a literature review. *BMC Surg.* 2012;**12**(Suppl 1):S16.

28. Regal M, Paramo C, Sierra SM, Garcia-Mayor RV. Prevalence and incidence of hypopituitarism in an adult Caucasian population in northwestern Spain. *Clin Endocrinol (Oxf)* 2001 Dec;**55**(6):735–740.

29. Ferrante L, Trillo G, Ramundo E, et al. Surgical treatment of pituitary tumors in the elderly: clinical outcome and long-term follow-up. *J Neurooncol* 2002 Nov;**60**(2):185–191.

30. Barzaghi LR, Losa M, Giovanelli M, Mortini P. Complications of transsphenoidal surgery in patients with pituitary adenoma: experience at a single centre. *Acta Neurochir (Wien)* 2007;**149**(9):877–885; discussion 885–886.

31. Hong J, Ding X, Lu Y. Clinical analysis of 103 elderly patients with pituitary adenomas: transsphenoidal surgery and follow-up. *J Clin Neurosci* 2008 Oct;**15**(10):1091–1095.

32. Minniti G, Esposito V, Piccirilli M, et al. Diagnosis and management of pituitary tumours in the elderly: a review based on personal experience and evidence of literature. *Eur J Endocrinol* 2005 Dec;**153**(6):723–735.

33. Ascoli P, Cavagnini F. Hypopituitarism. *Pituitary* 2006;**9**(4):335–342.

34. Foppiani L, Ruelle A, Bandelloni R, et al. Hypopituitarism in the elderly: multifaceted clinical and biochemical presentation. *Curr Aging Sci* 2008 Mar;**1**(1):42–50.

35. Minniti G, Esposito V, Piccirilli M, et al. Diagnosis and management of pituitary tumours in the elderly: a review based on personal experience and evidence of literature. *Eur J Endocrinol* 2005 Dec;**153**(6):723–735.

36. Turner HE, Adams CB, Wass JA. Pituitary tumours in the elderly: a 20 year experience. *Eur J Endocrinol* 1999 May;**140**(5):383–389.

37. Locatelli M, Bertani G, Carrabba G, et al. The transsphenoidal resection of pituitary adenomas in elderly patients and surgical risk. *Pituitary* 2013 Jun;**16**(2):146–151.

38. Ferretti E, Persani L, Jaffrain-Rea ML, et al. Evaluation of the adequacy of levothyroxine replacement therapy in patients with central hypothyroidism. *J Clin Endocrinol Metab* 1999 Mar;**84**(3):924–929.

39. Ilias I, Torpy DJ, Pacak K, et al. Cushing's syndrome due to ectopic corticotropin secretion: twenty years' experience at the National Institutes of Health. *J Clin Endocrinol Metab* 2005 Aug;**90**(8):4955–4962.

40. Isidori AM, Kaltsas GA, Pozza C, et al. The ectopic adrenocorticotropin syndrome: clinical features, diagnosis, management, and long-term follow-up. *J Clin Endocrinol Metab* 2006 Feb;**91**(2):371–377.

41. Herrera MF, Grant CS, van Heerden JA, et al. Incidentally discovered adrenal tumors: an institutional perspective. *Surgery* 1991 Dec;**110**(6):1014–1021.

42. Zeiger MA, Thompson GB, Duh QY, et al. American Association of Clinical Endocrinologists and American Association of Endocrine Surgeons Medical Guidelines for the Management of Adrenal Incidentalomas: executive summary of recommendations. *Endocr Pract* 2009 Jul–Aug;**15**(5):450–453.

43. Young WF Jr. Management approaches to adrenal incidentalomas: a view from Rochester, Minnesota. *Endocrinol Metab Clin North Am* 2000 Mar;**29**(1):159–185, x.

44. Grumbach MM, Biller BM, Braunstein GD, et al. Management of the clinically inapparent adrenal mass ("incidentaloma"). *Ann Intern Med* 2003 Mar 4;**138**(5):424–429.

45. Nieman LK. Approach to the patient with an adrenal incidentaloma. *J Clin Endocrinol Metab* 2010 Sep;**95**(9):4106–4113.

46. Lo CY, van Heerden JA, Grant CS, et al. Adrenal surgery in the elderly: too risky? *World J Surg* 1996 Mar–Apr;**20**(3):368–373; discussion 374.

47. Funder JW, Carey RM, Fardella C, et al. Case detection, diagnosis, and treatment of patients with primary aldosteronism: an endocrine society clinical practice guideline. *J Clin Endocrinol Metab* 2008 Sep;**93**(9):3266–3281.

48. Stowasser M, Sharman J, Leano R, et al. Evidence for abnormal left ventricular structure and function in normotensive individuals with familial hyperaldosteronism type I. *J Clin Endocrinol Metab* 2005 Sep;**90**(9):5070–5076.

49. Milliez P, Girerd X, Plouin PF, et al. Evidence for an increased rate of cardiovascular events in patients with primary aldosteronism. *J Am Coll Cardiol* 2005 Apr 19;**45**(8):1243–1248.

50. Mulatero P, Stowasser M, Loh KC, et al. Increased diagnosis of primary aldosteronism, including surgically correctable forms, in centers from five continents. *J Clin Endocrinol Metab* 2004 Mar;**89**(3):1045–1050.

51. Kopetschke R, Slisko M, Kilisli A, et al. Frequent incidental discovery of phaeochromocytoma: data from a German cohort of 201 phaeochromocytoma. *Eur J Endocrinol* 2009 Aug;**161**(2):355–361.

52. Lenders JW, Eisenhofer G, Mannelli M, Pacak K. Phaeochromocytoma. *Lancet* 2005 Aug 20–26;**366**(9486):665–675.

53. Khoo JJ, Au VS, Chen RY. Recurrent urosepsis and cardiogenic shock in an elderly patient with pheochromocytoma. *Case Rep Endocrinol* 2011;**2011**:759523.

54. Pacak K. Preoperative management of the pheochromocytoma patient. *J Clin Endocrinol Metab* 2007 Nov;**92**(11):4069–4079.

55. Nieman LK, Biller BM, Findling JW, et al. The diagnosis of Cushing's syndrome: an Endocrine Society Clinical Practice Guideline. *J Clin Endocrinol Metab* 2008 May;**93**(5):1526–1540.

56. Arlt W, Allolio B. Adrenal insufficiency. *Lancet* 2003 May 31;**361**(9372):1881–1893.

57. Chen YC, Chen YC, Chou LF, et al. Adrenal insufficiency in the elderly: a nationwide study of hospitalizations in Taiwan. *Tohoku J Exp Med* 2010 Aug;**221**(4):281–285.

58. Bornstein SR. Predisposing factors for adrenal insufficiency. *N Engl J Med* 2009 May 28;**360**(22):2328–2339.

59. Oelkers W. Adrenal insufficiency. *N Engl J Med* 1996 Oct 17;**335**(16):1206–1212.

60. Magnotti M, Shimshi M. Diagnosing adrenal insufficiency: which test is best–the 1-microg or the 250-microg cosyntropin stimulation test? *Endocr Pract* 2008 Mar;**14**(2):233–238.

Chapter 30

Diabetes mellitus in the older adult

Lisa B. Caruso, MD, MPH

Introduction

Diabetes mellitus (DM) is a dominant chronic disease in the older adult population in the United States as well as in many other countries of the world. The prevalence of DM in the future is only expected to grow with the increase in the population of older adults, the prevalence of obesity, and physical inactivity. Clinicians are faced with many unique challenges when caring for this older diabetic population. The clinician's major challenges are (1) to avoid symptoms and complications of hyper- and hypoglycemia, (2) to minimize or delay micro- and macrovascular complications, if possible, and (3) to maximize daily functioning. Underlying these challenges is the realization that the geriatric population is a heterogeneous one. Goals of care and treatment decisions may vary, depending more on the patient's functional abilities and on other comorbidities or coexisting geriatric syndromes, and less on the chronological age of the patient. This chapter will focus on specific aspects of diabetes care in the older adult.

Epidemiology

An estimated 11.2 million people or 25.9% of those 65 years of age or older in the United States are afflicted with DM, the majority of whom have type 2 disease. [1] About 40% of adult Americans with diabetes are 65 or older with an approximately even split between men and women. DM is more prevalent in minority groups. After adjusting for population age differences, Native Americans are 2.1 times as likely, non-Hispanic blacks and Hispanics are 1.7 times as likely, and Asian Americans are 1.2 times as likely to have DM as non-Hispanic whites. The direct costs of medical care are great with almost $176 billion being spent in 2012, with about 59% on older adults with DM.[2]

The majority of this expense is for inpatient costs, with higher admission rates and longer lengths of stay. Most hospitalizations for chronic complications of DM are attributed to the care of cardiovascular conditions. As the US population ages, the absolute number of older persons with diabetes will continue to rise for at least three reasons: (1) older adults are more likely to develop diabetes, (2) there will be an increased percentage of the population of older adults in minority groups, and (3) older adults with DM are living longer.[3] If methods of detection improve, the numbers of clinically recognized diabetes in older adults may rise even further, since 27.8% of all ages were undiagnosed in 2012.[1]

Diagnosis

Although the "poly" symptoms (polydipsia, polyuria, and polyphagia) are considered by many to be pathognomonic of diabetes, this is often not true in older persons for several reasons. First, these symptoms are nonspecific and may be due to other conditions, such as urinary difficulties or diuretic use. Second, they may not be present due to age-related or disease-related changes in organ function. For example, thirst mechanisms often become impaired with age. Third, they may be masked by other conditions. Thus, relying on them will result in both false positives and false negatives. The challenge to the clinician is to maintain a high level of suspicion, yet be prudent with glucose testing.

To improve the predictive power of glucose testing, criteria for the diagnosis of diabetes were revised by the Expert Committee on the Diagnosis and Classification of Diabetes Mellitus in 1997.[4] Due to consistent correlation between A1c and complications related to diabetes and improved standardization of the A1c assay, the 2009 International Expert

Reichel's Care of the Elderly, *7th Edition*, ed. Jan Busby-Whitehead *et al.* Published by Cambridge University Press.
© Cambridge University Press 2016.

Committee recommended that the A1c assay supplant glucose testing as the first-line diagnostic test for diabetes. The current American Diabetes Association (ADA) criteria for the diagnosis of DM are (1) A1c $\geq 6.5\%$, or (2) a fasting plasma glucose level of 126 mg/dL or greater, or (3) an elevation in plasma glucose to ≥ 200 mg/dL two hours following a 75-gram oral glucose tolerance test, or (4) symptoms of diabetes and a random glucose level of ≥ 200 mg/dL.[5] The diagnosis should be confirmed by abnormal glucose levels on a different day unless the patient has obvious hyperglycemia.

The majority of elderly diabetics are classified as either type 1 or type 2. Type 1 diabetics require insulin and are ketosis prone. Type 2 diabetics are insulin resistant and ketosis resistant. Many elderly type 1 diabetics who started insulin in the 1930s are still alive; therefore, when caring for a diabetic patient, it is important to establish when and how the diagnosis of diabetes was made in order to institute proper therapy and to anticipate the types of complications that are likely to develop.

Screening

As with other conditions, screening for diabetes would be indicated if the treatment of asymptomatic patients resulted in better outcomes, if the burden of suffering associated with it were high, and if the screening test were sensitive and specific, simple and inexpensive, safe, and acceptable for both patients and practitioners.[6] Although no one would argue that the burdens associated with diabetes are great, the US Preventive Services Task Force recommends screening for type 2 diabetes in asymptomatic adults with sustained blood pressure over 135/80 mm Hg despite only moderate evidence (B level) that screening improves outcomes.[7] The ADA, in the Standards of Medical Care in Diabetes – 2014, recommends screening for diabetes in asymptomatic adults every three years who are overweight or obese with a body mass index (BMI) ≥ 25 kg/m^2 and who have one additional risk factor for diabetes, also B level evidence. [8] The ADA recommends screening using fasting plasma glucose (FPG), A1c, or the 2-hour 75-gram oral glucose tolerance test. Once diabetes has been detected clinically, screening for complications, specifically for retinopathy and foot lesions, can be effective in reducing morbidity, as will be discussed.

Management

To the elderly person, receiving the diagnosis of diabetes may evoke multiple emotions including dread, fear, and sadness. Not only are complications devastating, but following complex dietary, medication, and monitoring regimens can be overwhelming. Daily functional, nutritional, and medical assistance from professional and lay caregivers is often necessary when patients are physically and/or cognitively impaired. When developing a treatment plan with the older diabetic patient, it is important to customize the plan to the individual and involve the patient in his or her own self-care, to the extent that this is possible, and to be sensitive to the patient's perception of his or her quality of life, as it is affected by various therapeutic interventions.

The concept of *collaborative management* has received attention as a mechanism to better care for patients with chronic diseases such as diabetes. Collaborative management consists of (1) defining problems from the perspective of the patient and physician, (2) targeting key problems, goal setting, and planning methods to achieve goals, (3) creating patient education and support services, and (4) evaluating patient progress in a frequent and regular follow-up plan.[9] These elements can be implemented in a variety of practice models from the small group practice to the large health maintenance organization. It is important for all the members of the health-care team to provide as much education to the patient as possible in order to make the patient an active participant in his or her own diabetic management. Evidence suggests that interventions targeted at improving the diabetes care delivery system and promoting diabetes self-management lead to improved patient outcomes and metabolic control.[10, 11]

In 2003, the first guidelines for improving the care of the older adult with diabetes were created by the California Health Care Foundation (CHCF) and the American Geriatrics Society (AGS).[12] These published guidelines were the first to stress the importance of setting individualized goals of care using the best evidence available for the very heterogeneous group of older adults with diabetes. In 2012, the ADA convened a Consensus Development Conference on Diabetes and Older Adults to address questions about diabetes care in those adults ≥ 65 years old for which evidence from clinical trials is often lacking.[13] The guidelines also included recommendations for individualizing management

Table 30.1 Components of care of the older adult with diabetes: 2013 update

- Aspirin
- Smoking
- Hypertension
- Glycemic control
- Lipid management
- Eye care
- Foot care
- Nephropathy screening
- Diabetes mellitus self-management education and support (DSME)
- Depression
- Polypharmacy
- Cognitive impairment
- Urinary incontinence
- Injurious falls
- Pain

of diabetes in the older adult considering eight geriatric syndromes, or conditions, for which there is evidence or strong consensus opinion that persons with diabetes are at greater risk. The conditions include cognitive dysfunction, functional impairment, falls and fractures, polypharmacy, depression, vision and hearing impairment, pain, and urinary incontinence. Most recently in 2013, the American Geriatrics Society Expert Panel on the Care of Older Adults with Diabetes Mellitus updated the previous CHCF/AGS guidelines from 2003.[14] Table 30.1 summarizes the key components of diabetes management.

The remaining sections of this chapter will elaborate on diet and weight loss, exercise, smoking, glycemic control and therapy, monitoring, managing cardiovascular risk factors (specifically hypertension and hyperlipidemia), aspirin use, eye care, foot care, and nephropathy screening. More specific information on the screening for and management of the preceding geriatric syndromes can be found in other chapters of this book.

Diet and weight loss

In general, diabetes is closely related to being overweight or obese, although a subset of older patients is either of normal weight or underweight.[15] What constitutes an optimal diabetic diet for older persons has not yet been determined, but weight loss, even if modest, in obese older persons can improve metabolic control, thereby reducing symptoms of hyperglycemia.

Achieving weight loss and metabolic control is not easy. Lifelong dietary habits are difficult to change, as are notions of what constitutes a "healthy" diet. This may be compounded by the fact that older patients frequently must rely on someone else for food acquisition and preparation. They may live in households where food preferences are disparate. Limited financial resources may interfere with patients' procuring appropriate foods, such as fresh fruits and vegetables. Furthermore, weight loss can be considered a syndrome that correlates with increased mortality in a certain subset of older adults. It can signify progression of underlying comorbidities (i.e., dementia or malignancy) and is not always a desirable outcome.

Weight loss in obese diabetics should be attempted to improve insulin sensitivity. A registered dietitian or nutritionist should be an active member of the diabetes management team to assist the patient and/or caregiver in creating an individualized diet plan. Although a recent systematic review was unable to find strong evidence for an ideal percentage of carbohydrates, fats and proteins in an individual's diet with diabetes,[16] calorie consumption should be consistent with weight management goals. When weight loss is not possible, the best strategy for many patients should focus on achieving a balanced diet of all three macronutrients that includes high-fiber unprocessed carbohydrates, more unsaturated fats than saturated or trans fats, and leaner meats and meat alternatives for protein.[17] The amount of protein in the diet has not been shown to be associated with proteinuria or worsening glomerular filtration rate (GFR). Adequate fluid intake of non–sucrose containing beverages is also important. This alone may help to reduce glucose levels and will correct mild volume contraction related to osmotic diuresis.

Older diabetics living in long-term care facilities must have diets appropriate to prevent or correct malnutrition. The ADA recommends serving regular, unrestricted meals to institutionalized older adults with diabetes.[13] It is important for such patients to enjoy meal time to satisfy nutritional needs as well as to contribute to their quality of life.

Exercise

Weight maintenance and glycemic control may be added benefits of regular exercise, specifically with resistance training. Physical activity has been found to increase insulin sensitivity of muscle and other tissues that have insulin receptors. Other cardiovascular risk factors (e.g., hyperlipidemia and hypertension) may be reduced by regular exercise as well. Self-esteem, risk of falls, and quality of life may also improve. However, exercise in the older diabetic may not be without substantial risk. Exercise can exacerbate angina or ischemia in a patient with underlying cardiovascular disease. The presence of peripheral neuropathy may result in soft tissue or musculoskeletal injuries. Symptomatic hypoglycemia can also occur, especially in patients taking oral hypoglycemic drugs. The ADA recommends that type 2 diabetics who want to begin an exercise program "more vigorous than brisk walking" undergo an assessment for cardiovascular disease and for other conditions, such as uncontrolled hypertension, neuropathy, and retinopathy, which may increase the risks of harm from the exercise program.[18] Older adults with diabetes should also monitor their glucose levels following any workout.

Smoking

Although rates of cigarette smoking decline with age, an important subset of smokers survives to old age. Recent evidence suggests that the hazards of cigarette smoking for men and women, particularly with respect to cardiovascular mortality, extend into later life. Furthermore, the risk of death from cardiovascular disease for former smokers is similar to that of never smokers, independent of age at which people quit.[19] Taken together, these data should compel clinicians to work with their older diabetic smokers to help them to quit.

Glycemic control

Establishing individualized goals of therapy are of great importance when treating older adults with diabetes. In certain patients, such as the frail, demented nursing home resident with sporadic eating habits, controlling symptoms of hypoglycemia or hyperglycemia is more important than preventing macrovascular and microvascular complications of diabetes. Other older, more active patients with longer life expectancies may benefit from tighter glucose control. The benefits of improved glycemic control in reducing microvascular complications of diabetes, such as retinopathy and nephropathy, are seen at approximately eight years, according to the UK Prospective

Diabetes Study (UKPDS) which excluded participants ≥ 65 years.[20]

To date, there is limited evidence from clinical trials that establishes recommendations for glycemic targets in adults ≥ 75 years. However, three recent trials were specifically designed to examine the independent effects of intensive glycemic control on cardiovascular disease (CVD) and mortality in middle-aged and older adults with diabetes. The Action to Control Cardiovascular Risk in Diabetes (ACCORD) trial randomized adults with a mean age of 62.2 years to intensive glycemic control (A1c <6%) or standard therapy (A1c 7%–7.9%).[21] The study was stopped after 3.5 years of follow up due to excessive deaths from any cause in the intensive group and no reduction in outcomes related to CVD. Hypoglycemia requiring assistance, greater polypharmacy, and other adverse treatment events were more common in the intensive group.

The Action in Diabetes and Vascular Disease: Preterax and Diamicron MR Controlled Evaluation (ADVANCE) trial was also designed to test the effect of intensive glycemic control (A1c <6.5%) on major cardiovascular events in subjects with diabetes ≥ 55 years.[22] Contrary to the results of the ACCORD trial, during a median follow-up of five years, there was no statistically significant difference in mortality or in macrovascular events in the intensive group compared to standard therapy, but there was a significant relative risk reduction in new or worsened nephropathy in the intensive group (RRR 21; 95% CI 7–34.)

The Veterans Affairs Diabetes Trial (VADT) randomized a sample of older veterans with uncontrolled type 2 diabetes (A1c ≥ 7.5%) to intensive or standard therapy aiming to reduce A1c levels in the intensive group by 1.5%.[23] Followed for a median of 5.6 years, the results were similar to the ADVANCE trial; there was no statistically significant difference in major cardiovascular events or death but there was found to be a reduction in the progression of albuminuria in the intensive group.

Whereas no independent effect of intensive glycemic control on cardiovascular events has been shown in the preceding randomized controlled trials, several cohort studies have examined the association between A1c values and mortality and cardiac events in adults with type 2 diabetes ≥ 50 years.[24, 25] It appears that there is a ∪-shaped curve with lower mortality between 6.0% and 9.0% compared to ≤ 6.0% and

$\geq 11\%$. Given new evidence to support some loosening of glycemic targets, the 2013 update of the AGS Expert Panel on the Care of Older Adults with Diabetes Mellitus recommends A1c values between 7.5% and 8.0%. For older adults with "few comorbidities and good functional status," A1c values of 7.0%–7.5% may be appropriate, while for those with "multiple comorbidities, poor health, and limited life expectancy," A1c values of 8.0%–9.0% are acceptable.[17]

Dietary modifications, exercise, and weight loss, if appropriate, are recommended for elderly diabetics. As lifestyle modification is often difficult especially for the clinically complex older adult, engaging the help of a Certified Diabetes Educator, specialty physician care, or group adult education classes can improve the patient's chances for success. Individualized education may be especially helpful for non-English speaking and culturally diverse older adults.[26] Drug therapy is warranted if the combination of diet, exercise, and weight loss are not successful in reaching glycemic control and if benefits outweigh potential risks of treatment.

Therapy

Multiple oral hypoglycemic agents are currently available including (1) the biguanide, metformin; (2) the sulfonylureas, such as glipizide, glyburide, and glimepiride; (3) the meglitinides, nateglinide and repaglinide; (4) the thiazolidinediones, pioglitazone and rosiglitazone; 5) the dipeptidyl peptidase-4 (DPP-4) inhibitors, sitagliptin, saxagliptin, linagliptin, and alogliptin; (6) the sodium-glucose cotransporter-2 (SGLT2) inhibitors, canagliflozin and dapagliflozin; and (7) the alpha-glucosidase inhibitors, acarbose and miglitol. Oral agents are easy to use and are frequently preferred by patients but vary significantly in cost and side-effect profiles (Table 30.2).

For reasons of low tolerability and limited effects on A1c values, SGLT2 inhibitors and alpha-glucosidase inhibitors are not often used in older adults and will not be discussed in detail here. The SGLT2 inhibitors work in the kidney to block reabsorption of glucose increasing glucosuria, which can lead to urinary tract and yeast infections, although alpha-glucosidase inhibitors block the breakdown of starch in the intestine leading to the significant side effects of intestinal gas and bloating. Pramlintide, an amylin mimetic, and exenatide, a glucagon-like peptide 1 (GLP-1) agonist and incretin mimetic, both decrease

postprandial plasma glucose and suppress glucagon secretion and are administered subcutaneously before meals, but will also not be discussed here given their limited use. Multiple types of insulin are available, giving clinicians even more tools to individualize therapy for older adults.

Biguanides

The only biguanide currently available in the United States is metformin, which is considered initial therapy in type 2 diabetes. It is approved for oral treatment either alone or in combination with a sulfonylurea or insulin. Metformin is a unique treatment for diabetes in that it suppresses hepatic glucose production and improves insulin sensitivity to promote glucose uptake at the cellular level. Therefore, the drug alone does not cause hypoglycemia. It also has a positive effect on lipids by lowering triglycerides and LDL cholesterol, does not contribute to weight gain in the obese patient, and may even assist with weight loss. Data from the UKPDS showed a decrease in macrovascular complications of diabetes and in overall mortality in obese patients with newly diagnosed diabetes taking metformin independent of glucose control compared with patients on only dietary changes and with patients on a sulfonylurea after 10 years of follow-up.[27]

Given the cardiovascular benefits and side-effect profile that does not include hypoglycemia, metformin is an excellent first choice for the management of diabetes in the older adult. While age should not be a contraindication to the use of metformin, renal function should be monitored closely during treatment. It should be used with caution in patients with impaired glomerular filtration rates, probably less than 30 mL/min–60 ml/min, although there is no evidence to support a specific cut-off. It should probably be avoided in patients with conditions associated with renal insufficiency (e.g., hepatic or cardiac failure) and in patients with renal failure who are more susceptible to lactic acidosis. Drug clearance decreases with increase in age independent of renal function,[28] so low to moderate doses, 500 mg/day –2,000 mg/day, should be used in older adults. Side effects include nausea, vomiting, anorexia, diarrhea, most of which resolve within a few weeks and can be avoided with slowly titrating up the dose.

Contraindications to the use of metformin are drug hypersensitivity, administration of iodinated contrast dye in radiological studies, metabolic

Table 30.2 Selected oral hypoglycemic agents for use in older adults

Class	Medication	Dosage schedule	Mechanism of action	Side effects
Biguanide	Metformin (Glucophage®)	Two or three times daily	Decreases glucose release from the liver	Bloating, gas, dyspepsia, loss of appetite in first few weeks. Not for use if liver or kidney problems. Will not cause hypoglycemia. May help with weight loss.
Sulfonylurea	Glipizide (Glucotrol®), glyburide (Micronase®, Diabeta®), glimepiride (Amaryl®)	Once or twice daily	Stimulates pancreas to secrete more insulin	Hypoglycemia, sometimes rash or dyspepsia, weight gain
Meglitinide	Nateglinide (Starlix®), repaglinide (Prandin®)	Rapid onset of action and short acting, so must be taken with each meal two, three or four times daily	Stimulates pancreas to secrete insulin after a meal	Hypoglycemia, but less likely than sulfonylureas
Thiazolidinediones	Pioglitizone (Actos®), rosiglitazone (Avandia®)	Once or twice daily	Sensitizes tissues to insulin	Fluid retention, so increased risk of heart failure, macular edema, bone loss in women, weight gain. Not for use if severe heart failure or liver failure.
Dipeptidyl peptidase-4 (DPP-4) inhibitors	Sitagliptin (Januvia®), saxagliptin (Onglyza®), linagliptin (Tradjenta®), alogliptin	Once daily	Increases insulin secretion after a meal	Dyspepsia, diarrhea, pharyngitis, nasal congestion. Will not cause hypoglycemia.
Sodium-glucose cotransporter-2 (SGLT2) inhibitors	Canagliflozin (Invokana®), dapagliflozin (Farxiga®), empagliflozin (Jardinance®)	Once daily	Blocks re-uptake of glucose by the kidneys thereby increasing loss of glucose in the urine	Potential dehydration, vaginal and penile yeast infections, urinary tract infections
Alpha-glucosidase inhibitors	Acarbose (Precose®), miglitol (Glyset®)	Short acting, so must be taken with each meal	Slows absorption of carbohydrates	Bloating, gas, diarrhea, abdominal pain in first few weeks of use, may cause elevations of transaminases

acidosis, and renal impairment (in men, a serum creatinine concentration >1.5 mg/dL and in women, a serum creatinine concentration >1.4 mg/dL). The drug should be stopped two days prior to radiological procedures involving contrast dyes. The most serious potential side effect of metformin is lactic acidosis but this is a much less common problem than with the

biguanide phenformin, which is no longer available. Since the biguanides inhibit lactate metabolism, increased concentrations of the drug due to renal insufficiency can cause lactic acidosis. However, a Cochrane Collaboration meta-analysis of both prospective comparative and observational cohorts found that lactic acidosis occurs as often in patients with diabetes who are metformin-users as in non-metformin users.[29] The trials included 24% of patients over age 65 years, whereas 46% of the trials allowed inclusion of patients with renal insufficiency, defined as a creatinine >1.5 mg/dL. No trial listed any cases of lactic acidosis, but it was not clear how many patients with standard contraindications were included in the trials. A separate trial of 393 diabetic patients on metformin followed for four years with at least one contraindication to its use reported no cases of lactic acidosis either. All participants in this trial had creatinine levels of 1.5 mg/dL –2.5 mg/dL.[30]

Sulfonylureas

The sulfonylurea drugs are the most frequently prescribed and least expensive agents for treating hyperglycemia. They are generally efficacious especially in patients who are not obese and within the first two to five years after diagnosis. Given that their mechanism of action is to stimulate the beta cells to produce more insulin, their loss of efficacy with time is probably due to a progressive diminution in pancreatic beta cell function and increased insulin resistance. The sulfonylureas may contribute to modest weight gain probably due to the effect of increased circulating insulin.

All sulfonylureas are now available in generic form and are reasonably priced. The choice of sulfonylurea should take into account the following considerations. First, since all are metabolized at least in part by the liver, they should be used with care in patients with severe liver disease. Second, renal insufficiency and normal decline in kidney function will prolong the half-lives of the sulfonylureas. Third, because of its long half-life (36 hours), a risk factor for hypoglycemia, and its propensity to cause hyponatremia, chlorpropamide should be avoided in older persons. Fourth, longer acting sulfonylureas, such as glyburide, have the highest risk of hypoglycemia in older adults, and should be avoided.[31] Glipizide is preferable because it does not have any active metabolites and has a half-life of two to five hours. It must be taken 30 minutes before meals so as not to delay absorption.

Meglitinides

Nateglinide and repaglinide act similarly to the sulfonylureas in stimulating the pancreatic insulin release, but are very short acting, with half-lives of 1–1.5 hours. For this reason, they are less likely than sulfonylureas to cause hypoglycemia. These agents can be used when patients have erratic eating habits, such as those with dementia. The medication can be administered with a meal or held if the meal is not eaten. However, dosing schedules of two or three times daily add to the pill burden in older adults.

Thiazolidinediones

The agents rosiglitizone and pioglitizone are peroxisome proliferator-activated receptor-gamma (PPAR-γ) agonists. Activation of PPAR-γ receptors regulates gene transcription involved in lipid metabolism and in glucose production, transport, and utilization, thus decreasing peripheral insulin resistance.

The pharmacokinetics of these drugs do not appear to be altered by age. The thiazolidinediones (TZDs) have been used in trials alone as well as in combination with sulfonylureas or insulin. They have been shown to significantly improve glucose control in older patients with diabetes.[32] These drugs do increase the risk for fluid retention and should not be used in patients with New York Heart Association class III or IV heart failure.[33] Troglizazone, the first of these agents to be approved for use in the United States, was removed from the market due to its association with hepatic failure. Therefore serum transaminase levels should be checked at the start of therapy, and periodically thereafter. Therapy should be stopped if the patient exhibits signs or symptoms of liver disease or if the transaminases are elevated to three times normal.

There has been some controversy as to the safety of the TZDs. The TZDs have been associated with macular edema,[34] bone loss,[35] and increased fracture risk in women.[36] Rosiglitazone has been implicated in increasing the risk of myocardial infarction and death from cardiovascular causes in a meta-analysis of 42 randomized controlled trials. [37] Methodological limitations of the study somewhat weaken the conclusions, but this preliminary evidence should stimulate further review of original source data. Pioglitazone, on the other hand, may have a protective effect in reducing the risk of myocardial infarctions in patients with diabetes and existing macrovascular disease.[38] Although the use of the TZDs in combination with other oral agents may delay the transition to or addition of insulin therapy, individuals' risks for known side effects on this class of agents must be weighed against potential benefits.

Dipeptidyl peptidase-4 inhibitors

The dipeptidyl peptidase-4 (DPP-4) inhibitors approved in the United Stateds are sitagliptin, saxagliptin, linagliptin, and alogliptin. This class of oral hypoglycemic agents increases incretin levels, an intestinal hormone which inhibits glucagon release, thus lowering blood glucose levels. Although expensive, they have an intermediate effect on A1c levels but low risk of hypoglycemia and are well tolerated, giving them advantages for use in frail elderly. In 2013, there were reports of pancreatitis and pancreatic cancer in patients taking DPP-4 inhibitors and GLP-1 agonists, raising the question of a causal association. On review of human and animal data by the US Food and Drug Administration (FDA) and the European Medicines Agency (EMA), evidence of a causal association was "inconsistent with current data" but both agencies have implemented strategies for continued monitoring of the safety of the DPP-4 inhibitors and the GLP-1 agonists.[39]

Insulins

Insulin therapy may be needed to achieve metabolic control and may be preferable to oral agents in some patients. The decision to treat with insulin must include an assessment of patients' beliefs about insulin and the potential for its safe use. For example, since most older patients have type 2 disease, they are likely to have had experiences with other family members or friends with diabetes. Insulin therapy is frequently instituted after several years of diagnosed disease duration, at a time when disease complications may be manifest. Thus, the development of worsening complications may be falsely attributed to the insulin itself and fears should be explored with patients. In addition, visual and cognitive function and manual dexterity require careful evaluation if patients will be administering the insulin themselves. If not, the adequacy of informal or formal supports to consistently and safely manage insulin therapy must be reviewed.

Insulin therapy is frequently instituted in the hospital setting, when a diagnosis of diabetes is first made in conjunction with an admission for an acute infectious illness or for a complication, or when a patient is admitted for complicated hyperglycemia (e.g., for the diabetic hyperosmolar state or ketoacidosis). Even patients admitted to the hospital on oral agents may be transitioned to insulin to achieve better glycemic control. Randomized controlled trials have shown that intensive glucose control in critically ill adults requiring intensive care unit settings decreases mortality, sepsis, new dialysis, blood transfusions, and critical illness-related polyneuropathy.[40] Observational studies of noncritically ill general medical and surgical patients have found an association between hyperglycemia and poor clinical outcomes, making glycemic control with insulin the standard of care in many hospital settings.[41] Although there is limited evidence supporting exact targets, the ADA and the American Association of Clinical Endocrinologists have proposed pre-meal glucose ≤ 140 mg/dL and all glucose ≤ 180 mg/dL.[42, 43] These targets may be loosened in an older population to avoid hypoglycemia, being mindful that the sequelae of hyperglycemia includes dehydration, glycosuria, and higher risk of infection associated with glucose ≥ 180 mg/dL. Given the differences in diet, physical activity, and stress levels that exist in the hospital as compared to the home setting, particular attention should be paid to monitoring the transition from hospital to home. This is a time when serious hyperglycemia or hypoglycemia is likely to occur, either because of changes in these factors or because of misunderstandings about dosing and the technical aspects of insulin administration.

When exogenous insulin is used as sole therapy for older diabetics, its dosage and injection schedule should be individualized to each patient's needs. In addition, many insulin formulations are distributed in the form of pens where the patient dials in the desired dose that is then administered. Pens are quite useful for older adults with vision or manual dexterity problems. The ideal insulin regimen should have a low risk of hypoglycemia while still controlling symptoms of hyperglycemia. Newer basal insulins, such as glargine and detemir, have no peak and an action duration of 24 hours. When these are combined with rapid acting insulin, such as lispro or aspart, prior to meals, glycemic goals for fasting and postprandial states can be achieved. However, older adults with physical and cognitive impairments may not be able to monitor plasma glucose and/or self-administer different types and doses of insulin reliably. A starting dose of 10 units or 0.2 units/kg/day of a basal or intermediate-acting insulin (NPH) minimizes the risk of hypoglycemia. Adding a dose before dinner or at bedtime will help to lower fasting blood glucose values. Additional doses of short-acting insulin can be given with or between the NPH in order to control hyperglycemia.

Insulin regimens should be tailored according to the individual patient's response as well as to his or her acceptance of the regimen. The use of sliding scale insulin should be avoided. Standardized protocols contribute to the risk of hyperglycemia and hypoglycemia and, as per the 2012 Beers Criteria, sliding scale insulin is associated with hypoglycemia without managing hyperglycemia across all sites of care for older adults.[44]

Monitoring

Although self-monitoring of blood glucose is safe and relatively easy for most patients to manage, its use has not been studied systematically in older persons. The main reasons to consider glucose monitoring in older patients are (1) to prevent the development of hypoglycemia in patients treated with hypoglycemic medications, particularly during times of illness or when medication changes are planned; and (2) to guide adjustments of hypoglycemic therapy in conjunction with hemoglobin A1c levels. The hemoglobin A1c reflects glucose levels over the previous 8–12 weeks and is therefore useful in monitoring glycemic control over time.

Cardiovascular risk factors

While diabetes was ranked as the sixth leading cause of death in American adults 65 years and older in 2010,[45] about two-thirds of deaths in adults with diabetes are due to heart disease or stroke. Mutable risk factors for cardiovascular disease (CVD) include hypertension, hyperlipidemia, smoking, and obesity. Embedded in the known CVD risk factors is the insulin resistance syndrome, otherwise known as the *metabolic syndrome*, which is a group of conditions that collectively increases an individual's risk of developing coronary artery disease and diabetes. The syndrome includes the presence of three of the five following conditions: abdominal obesity, elevated triglycerides, low HDL, hypertension, and higher than normal fasting glucose.[46] The underlying defect in the metabolic syndrome is insulin resistance in adipose and muscle tissue resulting in high circulating insulin levels.

There is strong evidence to support the goal of achieving moderate blood pressure targets in order to lower the risk of heart disease and stroke in older adults with diabetes. Society recommendations from the ADA, the Eighth Joint National Committee

(JNC8), and the American College of Physicians (ACP) range from <130/80 mmHg to <140/90 mmHg.[47–49] Most trials, however, have enrolled study participants who are middle-aged to young-old aged (65–75 years old) such that benefits to the older age groups has been inferred. In the ACCORD-BP study, lowering systolic blood pressure below 120 mmHg was not associated with a lower risk of major adverse cardiovascular events but was associated with a decreased risk of stroke.[50] Older adults with diabetes as a group may be most likely to benefit in terms of decreased CVD morbidity and mortality given their decreased life expectancy compared with persons of the same age without diabetes. Reductions in macrovascular endpoints from treating hypertension in controlled studies are seen at approximately two to five years.[51, 52]

The choice of antihypertensive therapy should be guided by side-effect profile, ease of administration, and cost, as diuretics, angiotensin-converting enzyme inhibitors (ACEIs), angiotensin-receptor blockers (ARBs), beta blockers, and calcium channel blockers are comparable in their impact on reducing cardiovascular morbidity and mortality. The ARBs have the added benefit of slowing serum creatinine rise, decreasing proteinuria, and reducing the development of end-stage renal disease in patients with type 2 diabetes.[53] This is an important consideration since at least 20% of type 2 patients will develop nephropathy. Careful attention should be paid to electrolyte, renal function, and potassium levels when beginning therapy or changing doses with diuretics, ACEIs, and ARBs. An additional advantage of using ACEIs or ARBs is that they do not cause or exacerbate urinary incontinence, constipation, lipid abnormalities, or hyperglycemia.

Based on new guidelines from the American College of Cardiology and the American Heart Association, it is recommended that all adults (aged 40–75 years) with diabetes be considered for moderate intensity treatment with a statin for primary prevention of CVD.[54] Moderate intensity is defined as an LDL-C reduction of 30%–50%. The 3-hydroxy-3-methylglutaryl coenzyme A reductase inhibitors (statins) are the preferred pharmacological therapy. Statins have some gastrointestinal side effects, but minimal drug–drug interactions. Liver transaminases and creatinine kinase levels should be checked prior to starting therapy, but if normal, no further testing is required unless the patient experiences muscle symptoms. Given that there is limited evidence supporting the benefit of statin therapy in older diabetics >75 years for primary prevention of CVD, statins should be discontinued in this age group. For secondary prevention, there is evidence that moderate-intensity statin therapy can be beneficial in CVD risk reduction in adults >75 years. Decisions for treatment should be based on life expectancy, goals of care, and potential for harm over benefit. Niacin should be avoided since it can worsen glycemic control.

Aspirin therapy should be used in patients with diabetes and known CVD in doses of 81 mg–325 mg daily to decrease the risk of another cardiovascular event. The question still remains as to whether low- or high-dose aspirin is better for secondary prevention, and is a trial recently approved by Patient-Centered Outcomes Research Institute to be administered through the National Patient-Centered Clinical Research Network. However, the risk of gastrointestinal bleeding in older adults taking aspirin is 1–10 in 1,000 annually and probably increases with age and dose.[55] Therefore, given the risk for harm of bleeding from gastrointestinal or other sources (i.e., intracranial) and limited evidence for efficacy in primary prevention for reducing the risk for cardiovascular events, current recommendations are to not prescribe aspirin therapy for these individuals unless their 10-year risk of CVD is ≥10%.[14] Further studies are needed to better understand the role of aspirin for primary prevention of CVD in this group of patients.

Eye disease

Given the critical importance of visual function to overall functional independence, eye disease in older diabetics deserves critical attention by clinicians. Data from the 2011 National Health Interview Survey indicate that among diabetics aged 65 years and older, almost 20% have serious trouble seeing, even with glasses.[56] This is due, not only to the ravages of diabetic retinopathy, but also because older diabetics are likely to have comorbid eye conditions, namely cataracts, glaucoma, and macular degeneration. The risk of developing diabetic retinopathy increases with duration of disease and with poor glucose control. Nearly all of type 1 diabetics and more than 60% of type 2 diabetics have retinopathy after 20 years. Because patients with type 2 disease frequently have had their disease for some time prior to diagnosis, over one third may already have retinopathy at the time they are diagnosed.[57]

Retinopathy may be manifested by preproliferative background changes, nonproliferative retinopathy, or by more severe proliferative changes. Because of the high likelihood of finding preexisting retinopathy, all newly diagnosed diabetics should be referred for ophthalmologic evaluation, not only for the presence of retinopathy, but also for the presence of cataracts and glaucoma. This evaluation should include a comprehensive and dilated-eye examination by an ophthalmologist or an optometrist, since even in the best hands, dilated ophthalmoscopy only has a sensitivity of about 80% for detecting proliferative retinopathy.[58] In addition, there is strong evidence from two randomized controlled trials showing that diagnosis and treatment of diabetic retinopathy reduces its progression and visual loss.[59, 60] The AGS and the ADA have published guidelines stating that if the initial dilated-eye exam is normal, the frequency of eye exams should be every two years. Higher-risk individuals such as those with A1c values ≥8% or blood pressure ≥140/90 mmHg should be screened at least annually. This strategy, of course, demands that careful attention be given to ensuring that older patients are followed carefully (1) to avoid missing vision changes due to other eye diseases common in this group and (2) to monitor blood pressure and A1c.

Foot care

For diabetic patients advancing in age, the risk of amputation increases. In 2009, the lower extremity amputation rate per 1,000 persons with diabetes was 3.1 among persons aged less than 65 years, 3.5 among persons aged 65–74, and 3.7 among persons aged 75 years or older.[61] The rate of amputation for people with diabetes is 10 times higher than for people without diabetes. Of those with diabetes, blacks are almost twice as likely as whites to undergo a lower extremity amputation (4.5 versus 2.3 per 1,000 persons with diabetes). Amputation rates are also twice as high in men as in women with diabetes (4.1 versus 2.2 per 1,000 persons with diabetes).[62] In addition to the monetary costs of amputations, they obviously have a profound effect on patients' mobility and may precipitate institutionalization.

Older adults with diabetes are at increased risk of developing foot ulcers due to peripheral arterial disease, sensory neuropathy, and joint malformations. Resulting gait abnormalities from these problems can lead to falls and trauma. Prevention of diabetic foot ulcers would lead to reductions in amputation rates. One case-control study demonstrated that lack of patient education is an additional important risk factor for amputation.[63] It is well known that patients do not engage in preventive care of their feet and that physicians infrequently examine diabetics' feet. Improved self-care and physician attention to foot abnormalities, however, can be achieved relatively easily and inexpensively, resulting in reduction of foot lesions in one randomized controlled trial.[64] More recently, a Cochrane Collaboration review found mixed results on the effect of patient education for the prevention of diabetic foot ulceration.[65] Even without better evidence, patients should be instructed in self-examination methods, nail and callus care, washing techniques, and what constitutes appropriate footwear. Since many older persons have fungal infections of their nails and may not be able to safely cut them, referral to a podiatrist is a prudent strategy.

For their part, health-care providers should perform a comprehensive foot exam at least annually, although there is no evidence to support this interval of screening. The foot examination can be used to reinforce important patient foot care behaviors. The exam should include (1) an assessment of vascular perfusion by palpation of the lower extremity pulses, (2) a neurological exam to assess sensorimotor deficits using the Semmes-Weinstein 5.07 (10-g) monofilament, (3) an assessment of skin integrity, and (4) a musculoskeletal exam to evaluate range of motion of the foot and ankle as well as bony abnormalities.[16] Although there is still much to learn about the prevention and treatment of diabetic foot lesions, successful implementation of these strategies is a reasonable place to start.

Nephropathy screening

Diabetes is the leading cause of end-stage renal disease. Evidence from the UKPDS has shown that glycemic and blood pressure control provide protection from advancing renal disease. Albuminuria ($\geq$30 mg/24 hrs) is an early sign of diabetic nephropathy and is associated with an increase in cardiovascular mortality.[66, 67] The simplest test for albuminuria is a spot urine albumin-to-creatinine ratio where normal is accepted as <30 μgm albumin/mg creatinine. Since it may be helpful for risk assessment, testing for albuminuria should be performed at diagnosis of type 2 diabetes, then yearly in its absence. Once a patient has albuminuria, there is little evidence to support continued monitoring.

Both ACEIs and ARBs slow the progression of albuminuria. ACEIs have the added benefit of reducing cardiovascular events and should be used in diabetics with hypertension if there are no side effects such as hyperkalemia or acute kidney injury.

Cognitive function

Compared with age-matched controls, older adults with diabetes are more likely than their nondiabetic counterparts to perform more poorly on cognitive tests,[68, 69] and they are twice as likely to develop dementia.[70] One systematic review found consistent deficits in verbal memory in diabetics compared to nondiabetics despite significant heterogeneity among the methods of the studies reviewed.[71] These changes are similar to those associated with normal aging, but whether they are manifestations of an accelerated aging process or occur via other mechanisms is not clear. There may be adverse effects on cognition from hyper- and hypoglycemia and hyper-and hypo-osmolar states furthering the importance of maintaining metabolic stability. Older diabetics are also more likely to have strokes, which also predisposes these patients to cognitive deficits and further necessitates treatment of other modifiable risk factors such as hypertension. Because of diabetes-related changes in cognitive function and the increased likelihood of dementia with age, periodic assessment of cognitive function in older diabetics is essential. This can serve to reassure the "worried well" who may have concerns about memory problems, and to identify early those beginning to experience subtle difficulties. Careful attention to these issues may uncover adverse drug effects, other metabolic derangements (e.g., hypothyroidism), or depression and will identify those who may need additional help from clinicians and family or friends in adhering to complex treatment regimens.

Comorbidity

By virtue of their having diabetes and having manifestations of the complications previously described, as well as by virtue of being older, older type 2 diabetic patients are likely to have considerable coexisting disease. Due to the fact that these patients take several medications, the likelihood that they may have diminished organ function (especially renal function), and decreased physiologic reserve together mean that they are at an increased risk of adverse drug effects. Careful attention therefore needs to be paid to avoiding drug–drug interactions. In addition, since compliance with medications is known to diminish as the number of medications and the complexity of the regimen increases, thought needs to be given to ways of decreasing the total number of medications (e.g., using one medication for multiple indications).

Family considerations

There is growing evidence that families play significant roles in the management of older persons with chronic disease in addition to the well-known role that they play in the general daily care of frail older persons.[72] A study of 357 family members of diabetic patients 70 years of age or older demonstrated that over half (71% were spouses) participated in the patients' diabetes care.[73] If patients are having difficulty adhering to treatment regimens, if they rely on family members for certain activities (e.g., food preparation, management of medications), or if they have functional disabilities, their family members or other caregivers need to be educated about diabetes and receive instruction and support in methods of management.

Summary and conclusions

Diabetes is a common condition in older persons and is associated with considerable economic and personal costs. Attention to the prevention and management of cardiovascular, eye, and foot disease is therefore critical. The risks and benefits of tight glycemic control will vary for a given individual depending on cognitive status, functional status, and life expectancy. Although reducing blood glucose levels to values that eliminate hyperglycemic symptoms while minimizing the potential for hypoglycemic reactions should be attempted, and cardiovascular risk factors treated, equal attention should be given to preventing eye and foot complications, where screening and treatment interventions also have known efficacy.

References

1. Centers for Disease Control and Prevention. National Diabetes Statistics Report: Estimates of Diabetes and Its Burden in the United States, 2014. Atlanta, GA: US Department of Health and Human Services; 2014.

2. American Diabetes Association. Economic costs of diabetes in the US in 2012. *Diabetes Care* 2013;**36**:1033–46.

3. Boyle JP, Thompson TJ, Gregg EW, et al. Projection of the year 2050 burden of diabetes in the US adult population: dynamic modeling of incidence, mortality, and prediabetes prevalence. *Population Health Metrics* 2010:**8**:29.

4. The Expert Committee on the Diagnosis and Classification of Diabetes Mellitus: Report of the Expert Committee on the Diagnosis and Classification of Diabetes Mellitus. *Diabetes Care* 1997;20;1183–97.

5. American Diabetes Association. Standards of medical care in diabetes – 2014. *Diabetes Care* 2014;**37**:S14–S80.

6. Fletcher RH, Fletcher SW, Wagner EH. *Clinical Epidemiology – The Essentials*. Baltimore: Williams & Wilkins, 1982.

7. Screening for Type 2 Diabetes Mellitus in Adults, Topic Page. US Preventive Services Task Force. www.uspreventiveservicestaskforce.org/uspstf/uspsdiab.htm, accessed September 28, 2014.

8. American Diabetes Association. Standards of medical care in diabetes – 2014. *Diabetes Care* 2014;**37**:S14-S80.

9. Von Korff M, Gruman J, Schaefer J, et al. Collaborative management of chronic illness. *Ann Intern Med* 1997;**127**:136–45.

10. Renders, CM, Valk GD, Griffin SJ, et al. Interventions to improve the management of diabetes in primary care, outpatient, and community settings; a systematic review. *Diabetes Care* 2001;**24**:1821–33.

11. Caruso LC, Clough-Gorr KM, Silliman RA. Improving quality of care for urban elders with diabetes and cardiovascular disease. *J Am Geriatr Soc* 2007;**55**:1656–62.

12. California Healthcare Foundation/American Geriatrics Society Panel in Improving Care for Elders with Diabetes. Guidelines for improving the care of the older person with diabetes mellitus. *J Am Geriatr Soc* 2003;**51**: 265–80.

13. Kirkman MS, Briscoe VJ, Clark N, et al. Diabetes in older adults: a consensus report. *J Am Geriatr Soc* 2012;**60**;2343–56.

14. American Geriatrics Society Expert Panel on the Care of Older Adults with Diabetes Mellitus. Guidelines abstracted from the American Geriatrics Society guidelines for improving the care of older adults with diabetes mellitus: 2013 update. *J Am Geriatr Soc* 2013;**61**:2020–26.

15. National Heart, Lung, and Blood Institute. *Clinical Guidelines on the Identification, Evaluation and Treatment of Overweight and Obesity in Adult*. Bethesda, MD: National Institutes of Health, 1998.

16. Wheeler ML, Dunbar SA, Jaacks LM, et al. Macronutrients, food groups, and eating patterns in the management of diabetes: a systematic review of the literature, 2010. *Diabetes Care* 2012;**35**:434–45.

17. Evert AB, Boucher JL, Cypress M, et al. Nutrition therapy recommendations for the management of adults with diabetes. *Diabetes Care* 2013;**36**:3821–42.

18. American Diabetes Association. Position statement: standards of medical care in diabetes–2007. *Diabetes Care* 2007;**30**:S4–S41.

19. LaCroix AZ, Lang J, Scherr P, et al. Smoking and mortality among older men and women in three communities. *N Engl J Med* 1991;**324**:1619–25.

20. United Kingdom Prospective Diabetes Study (UKPDS) Group. Intensive blood-glucose control with sulphonylureas or insulin compared with conventional treatment and risk of complications in patients with type 2 diabetes (UKPDS 33). *Lancet* 1998;**352**:837–53.

21. Gerstein HC, Miller ME, Byington RP, et al. Action to control cardiovascular risk in diabetes study group: effects of intensive glucose lowering in type 2 diabetes. *N Engl J Med* 2008;**358**:2545–59.

22. Patel A, MacMahon S, Chalmers J, et al. ADVANCE Collaborative Group: intensive blood glucose control and vascular outcomes in patients with type 2 diabetes. *N Engl J Med* 2008;**358**:2560–72.

23. Duckworth W, Abraira C, Moritz T, et al. Investigators of the VADT: glucose control and vascular complications in veterans with type 2 diabetes. *N Engl J Med* 2009;**360**:129–39.

24. Currie CJ, Peters JR, Tynan A, et al. Survival as a function of HbA(1c) in people with type 2 diabetes: a retrospective cohort study. *Lancet* 2010;**375**:481–89.

25. Huang ES, Liu Jy, Moffet HH, et al. Glycemic control, complications, and death in older diabetic patients: the Diabetes and Aging Study. *Diabetes Care* 2011;**34**:1329–36.

26. California Healthcare Foundation/American Geriatrics Society Panel on Improving Care for Elders with Diabetes. Guidelines for improving the care of the older person with diabetes mellitus. *J Am Geriatr Soc* 2003;**51**:S265–S280.

27. United Kingdom Prospective Diabetes Study (UKPDS) Group. Effect of intensive blood-glucose control with metformin on complications in overweight patients with type 2 diabetes (UKPDS 34). *Lancet* 1998;**352**:854–65.

28. Sambol NC, Chiang J, Lin ET, et al. Kidney function and age are both predictors of pharmacokinetics of metformin. *J Clin Pharmacol* 1995;**35**:1094–1102.

29. Salpeter S, Greyber E, Pasternak G, et al. Risk of fatal and nonfatal lactic acidosis with metformin use in type 2 diabetes mellitus. *Cochrane Database Syst Rev* 2006;**1**: CD002967 [update of *Cochrane Database Syst Rev* 2003;2:CD002967; PMID: 12804446].

30. Rachmani R, Slavachevski I, Levi Z, et al. Metformin in patients with type 2 diabetes mellitus: reconsideration of traditional contraindications. *Eur J Int Med* 2002;**13**:428–33.

31. American Geriatrics Society. Beers Criteria Update Expert Panel. American Geriatrics Society updated Beers Criteria for potentially inappropriate medication use in older adults. *J Am Geriatr Soc* 2012;**60**:616–31.

32. Rajagopalan R, Perez A, Ye Z, et al. Pioglitazone is effective therapy for elderly patients with type 2 diabetes mellitus. *Drugs Aging* 2004;**21**:259–71.

33. Nesto RW, Bell D, Bonow RO, et al. Thiazolidinedione use, fluid retention and congestive heart failure; a consensus statement from the American Heart Association and American Diabetes Association. *Diabetes Care* 2004;**27**:256–63.

34. Kendall C, Wooltorton E. Rosiglitazone (Avandia) and macular edema. *CMAJ* 2006;**174**:623.

35. Schwartz AV, Sellmeyer DE, Vittinghoff E, et al. Thiazolidinedione use and bone loss in older diabetic adults. *J Clin Endocrinol Metab* 2006;**91**:3349–54.

36. Kahn SE, Haffner SM, Heise MA, et al. Glycemic durability of rosiglitazone, metformin, or glyburide monotherapy. *N Engl J Med* 2006;**355**:2427–43.

37. Nissen SE, Wolski K. Effect of rosiglitazone on the risk of myocardial infarction and death from cardiovascular causes. *N Engl J Med* 2007;**356**:2457–71.

38. Dormandy JA, Charbonnel B, Eckland J, et al. Secondary prevention of macrovascular events in patients with type 2 diabetes in the PROactive Study (Prospective pioglitazone clinical trial in macrovascular events): a randomized trial. *Lancet* 2005;**366**:1279–1289.

39. Egan AG, Blind E, Dunder K, et al. Pancreatic safety of incretin-based drugs – FDA and EMA assessment. *N Engl J Med* 2014;**370**:794–97.

40. Van den Berghe G, Wouters p, Weekers F, et al. Intensive insulin therapy in the critically ill patients. *N Engl J Med* 2001;**345**:1359–67.

41. ACE/ADA Task Force on Inpatient Diabetes. American College of Endocrinology and American Diabetes Association Consensus Statement on Inpatient Diabetes and Glycemic Control. *Diabetes Care* 2006;**29**:1955–62.

42. Moghissi ES, Korytkowski MT, DiNardo M, et al. American Association of Clinical Endocrinologists and American Diabetes Association consensus statement on inpatient glycemic control. *Diabetes Care* 2009;**32**:1119–31.

43. Umpierrez GE, Hellman R, Korytkowski MT, et al. Management of hyperglycemia in hospitalized patients in non-critical care setting: an endocrine society clinical practice guideline. *J Clin Endocrinol Metab* 2012;**97**:16–38.

44. The American Geriatrics Society 2012 Beers Criteria Update Expert Panel. American Geriatrics Society updated Beers Criteria for potentially inappropriate medication use in older adults. *J Am Geriatr Soc* 2012;**60**:616–31.

45. www.cdc.gov/nchs/data/nvsr/nvsr62/nvsr62_06.pdf (accessed September 28, 2014).

46. Expert Panel on Detection, Evaluatoin, and Treatment of High Blood Cholesterol in Adults. Executive summary of the third report of the National Cholesterol Education Program (NCEP) Expert Panel on Detection, Evaluation, and Treatment of High Blood Cholesterol in Adults (Adult Treatment Panel III). *JAMA* 2001; **285**: 2486–97.

47. American Diabetes Association. Standards of medical care in diabetes – 2014. *Diabetes Care* 2014;**37**:S14–S80.

48. James PA, Oparil S, Carter BL, et al. 2014 evidence-based guideline for the management of high blood pressure in adults: report from the panel members appointed to the Eighth Joint National Committee (JNC8). *JAMA* 2014;**311**:507–20.

49. Snow V, Weiss KB, Mottur-Pilson C, et al. The evidence base for tight blood pressure control in the management of type 2 diabetes mellitus. *Ann Intern Med* 2003;**138**:587–92.

50. Cushman WC, Evans GW, Byington RP, et al. ACCORD Study Group: effects of intensive blood-pressure control in type 2 diabetes mellitus. *N Engl J Med* 2010;**362**:1575–85.

51. Curb JD, Pressel SL, Cutler JA, et al. Effect of diuretic-based antihypertensive treatment on cardiovascular disease risk in older diabetic patients with isolated systolic hypertension: Systolic Hypertension in the Elderly Program Cooperative Research Group. *JAMA* 1996;**276**:1886–92.

52. United Kingdom Prospective Diabetes Study (UKPDS) Group. Tight blood pressure control and risk of macrovascular and microvascular complications in type 2 diabetes (UKPDS 38). *BMJ* 1998;**317**:703–713.

53. Brenner BM, Cooper ME, de Zeeuw D, et al. Effects of losartan on renal and cardiovascular outcomes in patients with type 2 diabetes and nephropathy. *N Engl J Med* 2001;**345**:861–69.

54. Stone NJ, Robinson JG, Lichtenstein AH, et al. ACC/AHA Prevention Guideline: 2013 ACC/AHA guideline on the treatment of blood cholesterol to reduce atherosclerotic cardiovascular risk in adults. *Circulation* 2014;**129**:S1–S45.

55. Hernandes-Diaz S, Garcia Rodriguez LA. Cardioprotective aspirin users and their excess risk of upper gastrointestinal complications. *BMC Med* 2006;**300**:2134–41.

56. www.cdc.gov/diabetes/statistics/visual/fig3.htm, accessed September 28, 2014.

57. Kohner EM, Aldington SJ, Stratton IM, et al. United Kingdom Prospective Diabetes Study, 30: diabetic retinopathy at diagnosis of non-insulin-dependent diabetes mellitus and associated risk factors. *Archives of Ophthalmology* 1998;**116**:297-303.

58. Singer DE, Nathan DM, Fogel HA, et al. Screening for diabetic retinopathy. *Ann Intern Med* 1992;**116**:660–71.

59. Early Treatment Diabetic Retinopathy Study Research Group. Photocoagulation treatment of proliferative diabetic retinopathy: the second report of diabetic retinopathy study findings. *Ophthalmology* 1978;**85**:82–106.

60. Early Treatment Diabetic Retinopathy Study Research Group. Photocoagulation for diabetic macular edema: Early Treatment Diabetic Retinopathy Study report number 1. *Arch Ophthalmol* 1985;**103**:1796–1806.

61. www.cdc.gov/diabetes/statistics/lea/fig4.htm (accessed September 28, 2014).

62. www.cdc.gov/diabetes/statistics/lea/index.htm (accessed September 28, 2014).

63. Reiber GE, Pecoraro RE, Koepsell TD. Risk factors for amputation in patients with diabetes mellitus: a case-control study. *Ann Inter Med* 1992;**117**:97–105.

64. Litzelman DK, Slemenda CW, Langefeld CD, et al. Reduction of lower extremity clinical abnormalities in patients with non-insulin-dependent diabetes mellitus: a randomized, controlled trial. *Ann Intern Med* 1993;**119**:36–41.

65. Dorresteijn JA, Kriegsman DM, Assendelft WJ, et al. Patient education for preventing diabetic foot ulceration. *Cochrane Database Syst Rev* 2012 Oct 17;**10**: CD001488.

66. Garg JP, Bakris GL. Microalbuminuria: marker of vascular dysfunction, risk factor for cardiovascular disease. *Vasc Med* 2002;**7**:35–43.

67. Klausen K, Borch-Johnsen K, Feldt-Rasmussen B, et al. Very low levels of microalbuminuria are associated with increased risk of coronary heart disease and death independently of renal function, hypertension, and diabetes. *Circulation* 2004;**110**:32–35.

68. Logroscino G, Kang, JH, Grodstein F. Prospective study of type 2 diabetes and cognitive decline in women aged 70–81 years. *BMJ* 2004;**328**:548.

69. Bent N, Rabbitt P, Metcalfe D. Diabetes mellitus and the rate of cognitive ageing. *Br J Clin Psychol* 2000;**39**:349–62.

70. Lu FP, Lin KP, Kuo HK. Diabetes and the risk of multi-system aging phenotypes: a systematic review and meta-analysis. *PLoS ONE* 2009;**4**:e4144.

71. Strachan MWJ, Deary IJ, Ewing FME, et al. Is type II diabetes associated with an increased risk of cognitive dysfunction? *Diabetes Care* 1997;**20**:438–45.

72. Wolff JL, Kasper JD. Caregivers of frail elders: updating a national profile. *Gerontologist* 2006;**46**:344–56.

73. Silliman RA, Bhatti S, Khan A, et al. The care of older persons with diabetes mellitus: families and primary care physicians. *J Am Geriatr Soc* 1996;**44**:1314–21.

Chapter 31

Lipid management in older patients

Phil Mendys, PharmD, FAHA, CPP, Ross J. Simpson, Jr., MD, PhD, and Murrium I Sadaf, MD

Overview

This chapter will review issues related to the management of lipid disorders for cardiovascular disease (CVD) risk reduction in older patients. Because lipid metabolism and regulation do not vary greatly between younger and older people, age-related influences on cardiovascular risk and lipoprotein-mediated disease processes will be our central focus. Risk assessment and patient selection, as outlined in the 2013 American College of Cardiology/American Heart Association (ACC/AHA) guidelines, will also be reviewed.[1]

Age and cardiovascular risk

Clinicians typically approach the task of assessing cardiovascular risk by focusing on patients' age as an obvious "nonmodifiable risk factor." The Framingham risk score estimates a 10-year absolute risk for CVD events; age contributes enormously to the end result and is the greatest contributor to absolute cardiovascular risk. Multiple observations have concluded that atherosclerosis is a process that begins in early life.[2, 3] Compelling work by Hobbs and others focused on identifying the variant of the PCSK-9 gene has supported the concept that even a moderate reduction of low-density lipoprotein cholesterol (LDL-C) over a lifetime can result in a lowering of coronary events.[4] Their hypothesis that LDL-C might be sufficient and necessary for the cause and progression of atherosclerosis points to a lower threshold of benefit, one that was presaged by Brown and Goldstein.[5] The concept of lifetime exposure was further supported by the analysis by Ferrence et al. in which they speculated that a delay of statin therapy until later in life results in a nearly threefold increase in cardiovascular events.[6]

Advanced age reflects an increased duration of exposure to various risk factors and an accumulation of coronary disease burden.[7] The Framingham Risk Score is less robust in elderly people (>70 years of age). A comparison of the risk factor counting method as outlined in the National Cholesterol Education Program Guidelines to a multivariate analysis demonstrated that these guidelines underestimated risk among at least 10% of persons with fewer than two risk factors. Those *misclassified* as low risk were older and more likely to be male.[8] This issue was addressed in 2013 ACA/AHA Task Force on Practice Guidelines, which derived risk equations from community-based cohorts focusing on first hard atherosclerotic cardiovascular disease (ASCVD) event to predict 10-year risk in non-Hispanic African American and non-Hispanic white men and women aged 40 to 70.[1]

Recognizing that age is such a powerful predictor for risk of heart disease, clinicians should address common modifiable risk factors in older patients such as LDL-C in order to slow the development of subclinical disease. Many elderly people are eligible for secondary prevention, and many others qualify as high-risk primary prevention. Treatment of older people has been summarized as follows:

- The purpose of treating risk factors is to prevent morbid and mortal cardiovascular events and to decrease the disease burden of atherosclerosis in individuals and in communities.
- Current guidelines on pharmacologic therapy of hypertension and hypercholesterolemia are based on algorithms estimating the five- or ten-year absolute risk of morbid and mortal events.
- Age is the strongest determinant of absolute risk. New algorithms have improved precision of risk calculation by including modifiable risk factors

Reichel's Care of the Elderly, 7th Edition, ed. Jan Busby-Whitehead *et al*. Published by Cambridge University Press. © Cambridge University Press 2016.

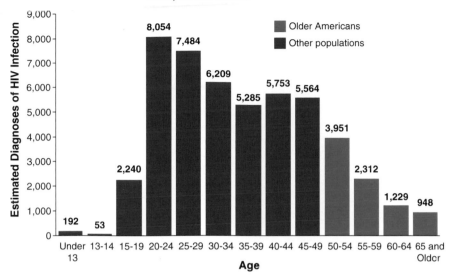

Estimated Diagnoses of HIV Infection, by Age
2011, United States

Figure 24.1 Estimated diagnoses of HIV infection by age, 2011, United States. (A black-and-white version of this figure will appear in some formats.)

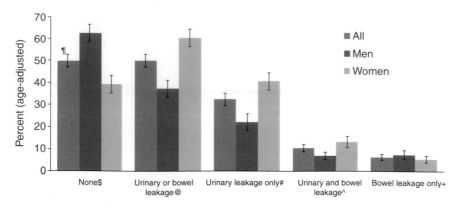

¶ - 95% confidence interval

$ - Persons who answered "Never" to each question about frequency of urinary leakage and accidental bowel leakage of mucus, liquid stool, or solid stool.

@ - Persons who reported urinary leakage or accidental bowel leakage of mucus, liquid stool, or solid stool.

- Persons who reported a urinary leakage and answered "Never" to each question about frequency of accidental bowel leakage or mucus, liquid stool, or solid stool.

^- Persons who reported a urinary leakage and accidental bowel leakage of mucus, liquid stool, or solid stool.

+ - Persons who answered "Never" to the question about frequency of urinary leakage, and reported accidental bowel leakage of mucus, liquid stool, or solid stool

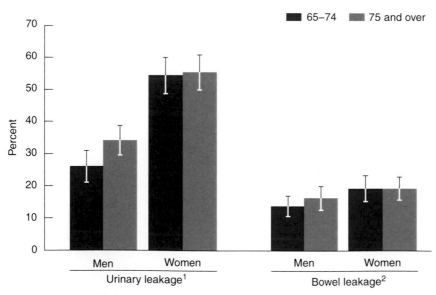

I 95% confidence interval.

[1]Persons who reported a urinary leakage.

[2]Persons who reported accidental bowel leakage of mucus, liquid stool, or solid stool.

Figure 27.1 and 27.2 Prevalence of UI, FI, and DI among older community-dwelling adults in the United States. (A black-and-white version of these figures will appear in some formats.)

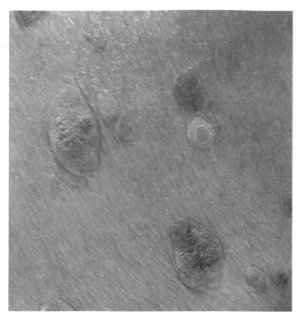

Figure 35.1 Seborrheic keratoses: stuck-on, waxy, crumbling, hyperpigmented papules and plaques. (A black-and-white version of this figure will appear in some formats.)

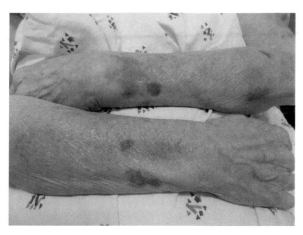

Figure 35.2 Actinic purpura: purpura classically located on the forearm with absence of yellow-green hues. (A black-and-white version of this figure will appear in some formats.)

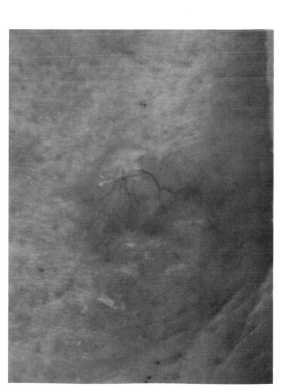

Figure 35.3 Basal cell carcinoma: pearly papule in the retro-auricular area with arborizing telangiectasias. (A black-and-white version of this figure will appear in some formats.)

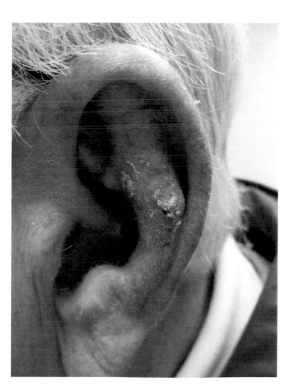

Figure 35.4 Squamous cell carcinoma: crusted nodule on the antihelix, a high-risk location. (A black-and-white version of this figure will appear in some formats.)

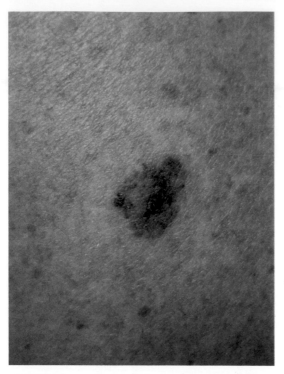

Figure 35.5 Superficial spreading melanoma: irregularly shaped, pigmented plaque with variegated pigment. (A black-and-white version of this figure will appear in some formats.)

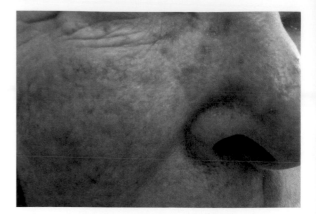

Figure 35.6 Rosacea: erythema, telangiectasias, and scattered papules and pustules. (A black-and-white version of this figure will appear in some formats.)

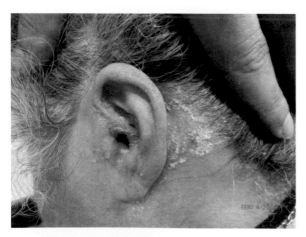

Figure 35.7 Seborrheic dermatitis: erythematous plaques that are flaky, adherent, and slightly greasy affecting the scalp, ear, and retroauricular sulcus. (A black-and-white version of this figure will appear in some formats.)

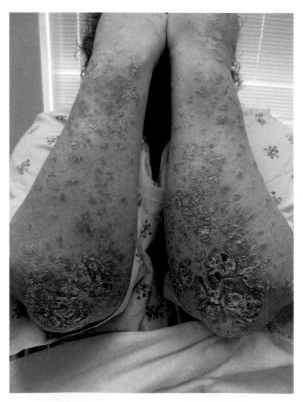

Figure 35.8 Psoriasis: scaly, erythematous plaques with a predilection for extensor surfaces. (A black-and-white version of this figure will appear in some formats.)

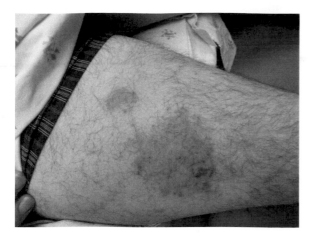

Figure 35.9 Nummular dermatitis: annular, slightly scaly, with pruritic plaques on the extremities. (A black-and-white version of this figure will appear in some formats.)

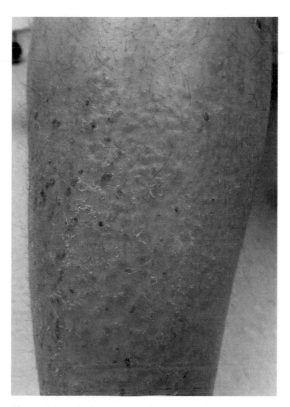

Figure 35.10 Lichen simplex chronicus: thick, excoriated, lichenified plaque on the lower leg at a site of frequent scratching due to contact dermatitis. (A black-and-white version of this figure will appear in some formats.)

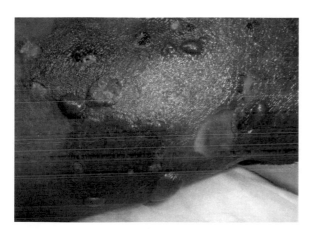

Figure 35.11 Bullous pemphigoid: widespread, tense bullae erupting diffusely on the trunk and extremities. Shallow ulcers are present where bullae have ruptured. (A black-and-white version of this figure will appear in some formats.)

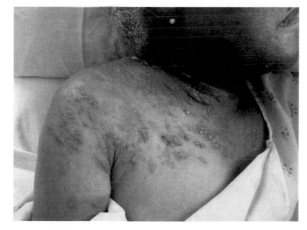

Figure 35.12 Herpes zoster: clustered vesicles on an erythematous base in a dermatomal distribution. Note the sharp demarcation at midline. (A black-and-white version of this figure will appear in some formats.)

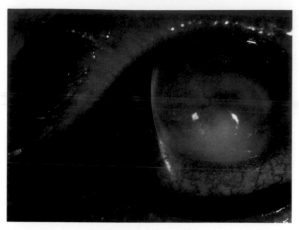

Figure 39.2 Infectious keratitis; noted features include mattering of the eyelashes, injected conjunctiva, corneal haze, and hypopyon (anterior chamber collection of white blood cells). (A black-and-white version of this figure will appear in some formats.)

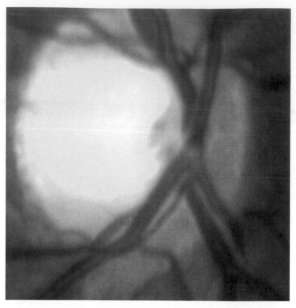

Figure 39.3 Glaucomatous cupping of the optic nerve; a loss of the nerve fiber layer is noted temporally. (A black-and-white version of this figure will appear in some formats.)

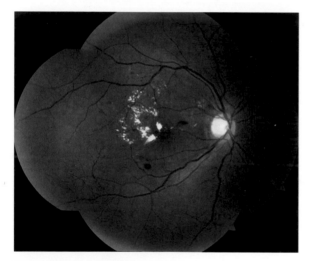

Figure 39.4 Nonproliferative diabetic retinopathy; noted features include dot and flame hemorrhages, microaneurysms, and hard exudates throughout the fundus. (A black-and-white version of this figure will appear in some formats.)

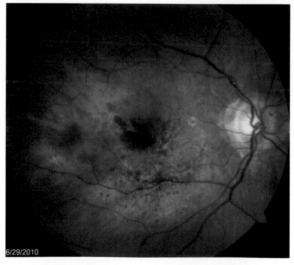

Figure 39.5 Wet age-related macular degeneration; subretinal hemorrhage denotes the choroidal neovascularization. (A black-and -white version of this figure will appear in some formats.)

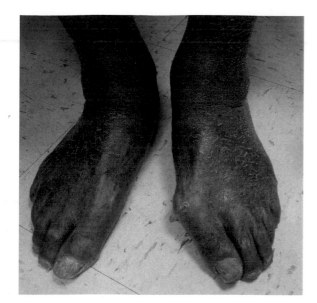

Figure 42.1 Feet of an older adult showing many of the conditions that can happen with aging. Xerosis is present on both legs and feet. Onychomycosis is present bilaterally. Hallux valgus (bunion) is noted on the left foot. Digiti flexus (hammertoe) is present in the right second toe. (A black-and-white version of this figure will appear in some formats.)

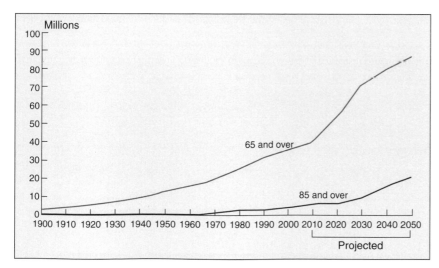

Figure 53.1 Number of people aged 65 and over, by age group in selected years 1900–2010. *Note:* Data for 2020–2050 are projections of the population. *Reference population:* These data refer to the resident population. *Source:* US Census Bureau, Decennial Census and Projections. (A black-and-white version of this figure will appear in some formats.)

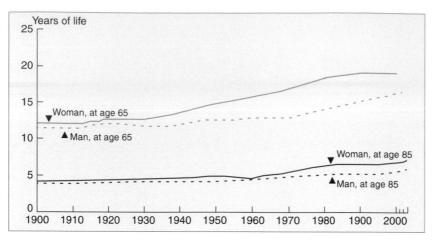

Figure 53.2 Life expectancy at ages 65 and 85 years, by gender, in selected years 1900–2009. *Reference population:* These data refer to the resident population. *Source:* Centers for Disease Control and Prevention, National Center for Health Statistics, National Vital Statistics System. (A black-and-white version of this figure will appear in some formats.)

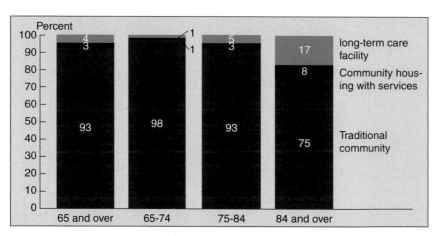

Figure 53.3 Percentage of Medicare enrollees aged 65 and over residing in selected residential settings, by age group, 2010. *Note:* Community housing with services applies to respondents who reported they lived in retirement communities or apartments, senior citizen housing, continuing care retirement facilities, assisted-living facilities, staged living communities, board-and-care facilities/homes, and other similar situations, *and* who reported they had access to one or more of the following services through their place of residence: meal preparation, cleaning or housekeeping services, laundry services, help with medications. Respondents were asked about access to these services but not whether they actually used the services. A residence is considered a long-term care facility if it is certified by Medicare or Medicaid; or it has three or more beds and is licensed as a nursing home or other long-term care facility and provides at least one personal care service, or provides 24-hour, 7-days-a-week supervision by a caregiver. *Reference population:* These data refer to Medicare enrollees. *Source:* Centers for Medicare and Medicaid Services. Medicare Current Beneficiary Survey. (A black-and-white version of this figure will appear in some formats.)

(such as total and high density lipoprotein cholesterol, systolic blood pressure, diabetes, and current smoking status) in addition to age.

- Functional and structural cardiovascular abnormalities are caused by risk factors and precede the occurrence of morbid and mortal events.
- Prevention of these asymptomatic functional and structural abnormalities by controlling all risk factors will result in the prevention of cardiovascular events.
- Age should be removed from the algorithms used to decide whether to treat risk factors.[9]

It is clear from clinical trials that both younger and older patients who are at risk for atherosclerotic events benefit from intensive lipid-lowering therapy for both primary and secondary prevention. Ultimately, treatments should be based on a comprehensive assessment of overall cardiovascular risk, life expectancy, and patient preference, not just chronologic age.

Lessons from observational data

The incidence of coronary disease in individuals over 65 years of age is high. The middle of the 1990s saw the publication of numerous analyses questioning the predictive value of cholesterol in determining cardiovascular risk in older patients. However, in a study including patients from 52 countries (INTERHEART), the two most important predictors of coronary disease mortality were total cholesterol and smoking. In fact, abnormal lipid profiles, as determined by an Apolipoprotein A/Apolioprotein B ratio, were the most important population attributable risk in both younger and older individuals.[10] The 2013 ACC/AHA Cardiovascular Risk Guidelines supported assessment of coronary artery calcium scoring, high sensitivity C-reactive protein, ApoB, creatinine, and micro-albuminuria as the most useful marker in improving risk assessment in the intermediate risk group.[1] The purpose of the Cardiovascular Health Study (CHS) was to address the uncertainty of the risks of smoking and cholesterol in predicting overall cardiovascular risk in older patients. The ankle brachial blood pressure, carotid artery stenosis and wall thickness, electrocardiographic and echocardiographic abnormalities, and positive responses to the Rose angina and claudication questionnaire were found to be significant predictors of CVD in both

men and women. At present, these measures are readily accessible to clinicians and can add greatly to the assessment of patients at risk for cardiovascular events.[11] The combination of these assessments with the demonstrated benefit of current preventive therapies is an effective strategy to reduce the incidence of and mortality associated with CVD in older patients. The importance of the CHS was to build a better understanding of the specific risk issues in managing older people and overcome some of the historical bias in the medical community to manage cardiovascular risk, particularly high cholesterol. Current standards have changed to keep up with the generation of additional evidence and risk assessment strategies.

2013 ACC/AHA guideline on the treatment of blood cholesterol to reduce atherosclerotic cardiovascular risk in adults

Recent ACC/AHA guidelines, based upon evidence from 27 randomized clinical trials, outline optimal goals for LDL-C and HDL C levels in both primary and secondary prevention and evaluate the efficacy of statins (or HMG-CoA reductase inhibitors) as the drug of choice to achieve LDL C reductions in individuals with clinical ASCVD, LDL-C $\geq$190 mg/dL, comorbid diabetes or with estimated risk of ASCVD of $\geq$7.5%.[1] Rather than titrating medications toward a target LDL-C and HDL-C, the guidelines recommend the use of the 10-year risk of ASCVD and LDL-C 70 mg/dL–189 mg/dL levels to determine initiation of low-, moderate-, or high-dose statins. Guidelines support the continuation of moderate dose statins in people over the age of 75 years for secondary prevention, but caution is warranted due to comorbidities and the risk for polypharmacy in older adults. Although the 2013 guideline for cholesterol management has been the subject of debate, it is critically important for clinicians to appreciate the context for which they were written:

Guidelines attempt to define practices that meet the needs of patients in most circumstances and are not a replacement for clinical judgment. *The ultimate decision about care of a particular patient must be made by the healthcare provider and patient in light of the circumstances presented by that patient.* As a result, situations might arise in which deviations from these

437

guidelines may be appropriate. These considerations notwithstanding, in caring for most patients, clinicians can employ the recommendations confidently to reduce the risks of atherosclerotic cardiovascular disease events. [1, our emphasis]

Given the potential for a significant absolute risk reduction, statins can also be used for primary prevention in persons aged 70 years with an increased 10-year risk of ASCVD. These new guidelines would increase new statin prescriptions by 12.8 million as compared to Adult Treatment Panel (ATP) III guidelines, and most of this increase in prescriptions would be for primary prevention in adults aged 60–75 years.[12]

Clinical trials and duration of therapy

Numerous clinical trials demonstrate benefits of lowering LDL-C in older persons with established CHD. Increased levels of LDL-C carry predictive power for the development of CHD in older persons as well as younger individuals. Implications from several recent clinical studies with an even broader range of baseline risk of cardiovascular disease influenced the NCEP ATP III panel to revise thinking on the intensity of treatment.[13] As reported in the Cardiovascular Health Study in 2002, the use of statin therapy in study participants at baseline who were 65 years or older and free of cardiovascular disease resulted in a 56% lower risk of CV events and 44% lower all-cause mortality.[14] Although the value of lipid lowering in older patients with known coronary disease is evident, the decision to manage risk has been modified in the current guidelines. Since relatively few individuals older than 75 were included in randomized clinical trials of high- versus moderate-intensity statin therapy, there was not clear evidence of an additional reduction in ASCVD events from utilizing higher doses of statins. Most of the benefit in older patients was seen in moderate-intensity statin trials; thus, moderate-intensity statin therapy should be considered for individuals older than 75 with *clinical* ASCVD. This should be considered in the context of potential for adverse effects and drug-drug interactions as well as patient choice and access to medicines.[1]

We are often asked, "How long will I be on this medication?" In more medical terms, do the benefits we see with the clinical trials last a lifetime? The answer, of course, is not known, but it would seem to lie in what we know and believe about the role of LDL-C in causing cardiovascular disease and the probability that lowering LDL-C with statins stabilizes or prevents atherosclerosis progression and limits atherosclerosis. We have strong indications that the benefit of long-term statin therapy occurs and persists in older as well as in younger and middle-aged individuals. In the 10-year follow-up of the Simvastatin Survival Study, a reduction in mortality from coronary disease, with no increase in death from cancer or other causes, in the simvastatin-treated group was noted.[15] Follow-up from the Heart Protection Study further supported this observation that ongoing lipid lowering treatment with a statin confers benefits over time without an increased risk of non-cardiovascular mortality.[16]

The Cholesterol Treatment Trialist Collaboration meta-analysis of 27 statin therapy trials demonstrated even a substantial risk reduction among low-risk patients with a five-year risk of a coronary event of less than 10% – a reduction comparable to the event reductions seen in higher-risk groups. Again, there was no compromise in safety related to cancer or other non-cardiovascular mortality over the long term. Although the most common concern for patients is muscle-related side effects, as referenced in this meta-analysis, statin therapy is associated with a small increased risk of myopathy (excess incidence of about 0.05% over 5 years) and, more rarely, of rhabdomyolysis (excess incidence of about 0.01% over 5 years).[38] The risks of myopathy are typically dose-related but, with the exception of simvastatin 80 mg daily (or lower doses in Asian populations), intensive statin regimens have not been shown to result in substantial myopathy risks.[17]

A recent report from Thompson et al. concluded that the long-term adverse events related to statin therapy – including myopathy, central nervous system effects, and the occurrence of diabetes – appear to be low but that the cumulative risk needs further study.[18]

Primary prevention in older patients

Two out of three first major coronary events occur in persons over the age of 65. Many older persons with advanced coronary atherosclerosis are asymptomatic and require further assessment – as well as clinical judgment – to determine a proper risk/benefit estimate. Given that CHD deaths account for one-half of all CHD events in older patients and the assumption that statin therapy reduces risk for all CHD categories by approximately one-third, there is likely mortality benefits of lipid lowering of 50% in older patients.[11] Recent guidelines also strongly support the use of low, moderate, or high dose statins for risk reduction based on their LDL-C levels at initiation of therapy and ten-year ASCVD risk.[1] Based on this construct, the prospects for reducing clinical CHD in the older patients by LDL-C lowering are good.

The first specific prevention trial to evaluate the role of lipid lowering with statins in older patients (aged 70–82) was the Prospective Study of Pravastatin in the Elderly (PROSPER). Older men ($n = 2,804$) and women ($n = 3,000$) at high risk of developing cardiovascular disease and stroke were randomized to placebo or 40 mg pravastatin. Patients were evaluated over an average of 3.2 years and assessed based on a composite endpoint of major coronary events, including nonfatal MI and CHD death. Each endpoint was reduced with treatment by 19% and 24%, respectively. Although no reduction in stroke occurred in the treatment group, there was a 25% reduction in transient ischemic events. These results support the notion that the benefits of statin therapy could be safely extended to older persons.[13]

A more contemporary trial in evaluating the possible role of lipid lowering in at-risk patients was completed in a large hypertensive population. The Anglo Scandinavian Cardiac Outcomes Trial – Lipid-Lowering Arm (ASCOT-LLA) program evaluated more than 10,000 patients aged 40–79 (average 63 years of age) with at least three risk factors in addition to high blood pressure. Patients were randomly assigned to either atorvastatin 10 mg or placebo. The original study design was to provide follow-up for an average of five years, but the trial was stopped at a median follow-up of 3.3 years due to a marked reduction of events in the treatment group. Treatment with atorvastatin resulted in a reduction in the incidence of fatal and nonfatal stroke by 27% ($p = 0.024$), total cardiovascular events by 21% ($p = 0.0005$), and total coronary events by 29% ($p = 0.0005$).[13]

Another recent randomized trial evaluated the role of rosuvastatin as a lipid lowering agent in primary prevention in elderly persons with high C-reactive protein and low LDL-C levels. This double-blinded trial, based on a secondary analysis of the Justification for the Use of statin in Prevention:

an Intervention Trial Evaluating Rosuvastatin (JUPITER) trial, randomized patients to rousuvastatin 20 mg or placebo. Participant profiles differed from the original JUPITER trial participants in that among more than 17,000 patients, 32% were aged 70 years or older. These patients were predominantly female and more likely to be hypertensive as compared to younger participants enrolled in the JUPITER trial.[19]

The primary endpoint of this study was occurrence of first major cardiovascular event or death from components of primary endpoints. Inclusion criteria included LDL-C level at screening of 130 mg/dL and C-reactive protein level of 2.0 mg/L at the beginning of the study. LDL-C was reduced to half (54 mg/dL) and C-reactive protein was reduced by 36%–37% in the treatment group as compared to placebo at twelve months. An absolute reduction of 48% or more was seen in the primary endpoint in the participant group treated with 20 mg rousuvastatin. Although the trial was stopped early, assessment of cumulative risks in the treatment group continued for up to four years. Statistically, the number needed to treat (NNT) to prevent one cardiovascular event or death in adults over 70 years was 24 (95% CI: 15 to 57) as compared to 36 (95% CI: 23 to 77) in younger individuals, thus indicating the relative benefit in treating older patients based on age.[19]

The results of both PROSPER and ASCOT support the efficacy of statin therapy in older, high-risk persons without established CVD. In addition, there is evidence that the absolute benefit and risk reduction seen in older patients treated with statin therapy for primary prevention of cardiovascular events is greater than that in younger patients.

Secondary prevention in older persons with established CVD

Early landmark trials using both simvastatin (Scandinavian Simvastatin Survival Study [4S]) and pravastatin (Cholesterol and Recurrent Events [CARE] trial) helped to establish the benefit of cholesterol lowering in a wide range of patients with established coronary disease.[20, 21] Both of these studies also demonstrated a treatment benefit in patients greater than 60 years of age. In the LIPID (Long-term Intervention with Pravastatin in Ischemic Disease) Study, an analysis of the comparative effects of pravastatin on CVD outcomes in patients with

CHD who are 65 years of age or older compared with those in patients 31–64 years of age was performed. Whereas older patients were at greater risk for death, MI, unstable angina, and stroke than younger patients, pravastatin reduced the risk for all CV events to the same degree. Given that older patients are at greater risk than younger patients for these events, the absolute benefit of treatment is significantly greater in older patients. For every 1,000 people treated over six years, pravastatin prevented 45 deaths and 133 major cardiovascular events in older patients compared with the prevention of 22 deaths and 107 major cardiovascular events in younger patients.[22]

A Bayesian meta-analysis of statin use in elderly patients aged 62–82 was undertaken using data for secondary prevention in elders from nine clinical trials, including the 4S, CARE, and Heart Protection Study. It was shown that statins reduced all-cause mortality by 22% over five years (RR 0.78; 95% CI 0.65 to 0.89), mortality due to CHD by 30% (RR 0.70; 95% CI 0.53 to 0.83), nonfatal MI by 26% (RR 0.75; 95% CI 0.56 to 0.94), and revascularization as consequence of disease progression by 30% (RR 0.70; 95% CI 0.53 to 0.83). To save one life, the NNT with statins was 28 (95% CI 15 to 56).[23]

Atherosclerotic cardiovascular disease

The definition of heart disease in the 2013 guidelines was expanded as the expert panel was charged with updating the clinical practice recommendations. For this guideline, ASCVD includes CHD, stroke, and peripheral arterial disease (PAD), all of which have been considered "CAD equivalents" and linked to atherosclerosis.[1] PAD has become an established CHD equivalent as outlined in various epidemiological studies and as represented in the current ACC/AHA treatment guidelines. Given the increased risk for all-cause and cardiovascular mortality, individuals with PAD – regardless of age – should be aggressively managed with respect to coexisting risk factors.[24]

Although the benefits of cholesterol lowering on coronary disease events have been established, cholesterol was traditionally considered a poor predictor of stroke. Moreover, the results of treatment studies in the pre-statin era were inconclusive. Recently, high serum cholesterol was identified as a predictor of risk in patients with ischemic stroke.[25] Given that almost 30% of the 700,000 strokes that occur each year are recurrent events, it is critical that we identify the risk and determinants of recurrent stroke and review the evidence base to support improved outcomes in this patient population. Recent studies, such as the Heart Protection Study, have shown encouraging results in reducing the risk of coronary events in this patient group; however, among those patients with preexisting cerebrovascular disease, the incidence of stroke was not significantly reduced. The first trial to demonstrate a reduction in stroke risk in non-coronary disease patients with a history of cerebrovascular events (stroke, TIA) associated with statin therapy has been published. The Stroke Prevention by Aggressive Reduction in Cholesterol Levels (SPARCL) included more than 4,700 patients with a prior history of stroke or TIA within six months before study entry. These individuals had no known history of CHD and baseline LDL between 100 mg/dL and 190 mg/dL. After treatment assignment of either placebo or atorvastatin 80 mg, patients were followed for a median period of 4.9 years. In patients with a recent stroke or TIA, treatment with 80 mg of atorvastatin per day decreased the risk of stroke, major coronary events, and revascularization procedures. These results support the initiation of atorvastatin treatment soon after a stroke or TIA.[26]

Therapeutic lifestyle changes in the elderly

As in prior clinical recommendations, the recent AHA/ACC guidelines continue to emphasize the importance of lifestyle modification (i.e., adhering to a heart healthy diet, regular exercise habits, avoidance of tobacco products, and maintenance of a healthy weight) as a critical component of health promotion and ASCVD risk reduction prior to and in concert with the use of cholesterol-lowering drug therapies. Healthy diet or lifestyle modifications were recommended as background therapy for the RCTs of cholesterol-lowering drug therapy.[1] The 2013 Lifestyle Management Work Group Guideline for lifestyle recommendations for healthy adults identifies patterns of nutrition rather than specific diets such as the DASH (Dietary Approach to Stop Hypertension) or Mediterranean diets. These "patterns" include an emphasis on intake of fruits, vegetables and whole grains. Sources of proteins should include low-fat dairy products, poultry, fish, and legumes. Individuals should also limit intake of sweets, sugar-sweetened beverages, red meats, and overall calorie intake from saturated fat.[27] Plant stanols/sterols (2 gm/day) and up to 25 mg of soluble fiber can aid in lowering LDL-C, which could be used alone or in conjunction with appropriate pharmacotherapy.[7]

In terms of physical activity, older patients are quite a heterogeneous group; many have one or more chronic illnesses to manage. The 2008 Physical Activity Guidelines for Americans endorses regular physical activity as a key to healthy aging. Although the 2013 AHA/ACC Lifestyle Management Guideline suggests two and a half hours per week of moderate-intensity exercise, an individual approach should be outlined to support as much physical activity as patients' abilities and conditions allow.[28]

Pharmacological therapy for lipid management in older patients

We have established that the decision to treat a patient should be predicated on the assessment of baseline risk. LDL cholesterol has been established as the primary target of treatment in reducing cardiovascular risk. Although the use of therapeutic lifestyle change, including LDL-lowering dietary options (plant stanols/sterols and increased viscous fiber), will achieve the therapeutic goal in many at-risk persons, drug treatment options add greatly to our ability to achieve treatment objectives: to reduce ASCVD risk and improve patient outcomes.

Statins

As emphasized in the 2013 AHA/ACC guidelines, the statin class has evidence derived from multiple randomized clinical trials as well as meta-analyses to inform clinical decision making. The statins, which have been used clinically for more than 25 years, provide critical support in reducing ASCVD risk, as well as improving the outcomes in those patients with known coronary disease. Currently statins are considered as first-line treatment because of their ability to safely and effectively lower LDL cholesterol up to 60%. [1] Onset of effect is generally within four to six weeks, which allows a reasonable time for patient follow-up. The extensive clinical experience with statins has helped to identify patient characteristics and monitoring strategies that enhance the safe use of high- and

moderate-intensity statin therapy. There are multiple patient characteristics that may influence but not serve as absolute contraindications regarding statin safety, including multiple or serious comorbidities, impaired renal or hepatic function, history of previous statin intolerance or muscle disorders, concomitant use of drugs affecting statin metabolism, a history of hemorrhagic stroke, and age over 75. It should be emphasized that age and history of hemorrhagic stroke are not absolute contraindications to therapy. There is also data suggesting that Asian ancestry may also influence the initial choice of statin intensity due to differences in pharmacokinetics.[1] As referenced, among the several factors that may predispose patients to increased risk of myopathy is age. This may be due to a number of features such as co-morbidities, polypharmacy, or an age-related decline in renal function.

Despite the fact that statins may differ in their ability to lower LDL cholesterol levels and inhibit HMG-CoA reductase, the risk of severe myotoxic events does not appear to be associated with LDL-C lowering potency.[29] Routine measurement of creatine kinase in individuals receiving statin therapy is not recommended; however, it may be considered for those with "increased risk for adverse muscle events. Such individuals include those with a personal or family history of statin intolerance or muscle disease, clinical presentation, or concomitant drug therapy that might increase the likelihood of myopathy."[1] It may be useful in clinical practice to make a baseline estimate of muscle symptoms prior to initiating treatment and then compare the assessment upon follow-up with the patient at subsequent encounters.

The most comprehensive age-based analysis of safety for a statin was a pooled analysis of more than 50 clinical trials for atorvastatin that compared four different dosages of active drug to placebo in 5,437 patients older than 65 years (range of mean age 71–74), of which almost half of those studied were female (42%). This included a large number of individuals on either the 10 mg ($n = 2,042$) or the 80 mg dose ($n = 1,698$), along with a comparison group of almost 1,000 placebo-treated individuals. Serious adverse events (AEs) were rare ($\leq 1\%$), and rates of discontinuation due to treatment AEs were low between treatment doses and placebo (2.1% vs. 1.7%). At the maximum dose, elevations of liver enzymes (AST/ALT) were higher than placebo

441

(3.2% vs. ≤0.9%). Treatment-associated myalgia was low and no patient experienced persistent elevated creatine kinase of greater than 10 times upper limits of normal.[30]

The European Society of Cardiology conducted a large-scale systematic review of 14 primary prevention trials ($n = 46,262$) to assess the proportion of side effects directly attributable to statin therapy in an attempt to aid clinicians and patients in making decisions on a future course of therapy. Analysis showed an increase in type II diabetes by absolute risk of 0.5% ($p = 0.012$) while decreasing mortality by the same extent: 0.5% ($p = 0.003$). The study also looked at 15 RCTs (37,618 participants) for secondary prevention, and statins decreased mortality by 1.4% ($p < 0.001$). Asymptomatic increase in liver transaminase was seen 0.4% times more frequently in both primary and secondary prevention groups than the placebo group. Current guidelines highlight the very small increase in cases of new onset diabetes (0.1 excess cases per 100 on moderate-dose statin treatment and 0.3 excess cases per 100 on high-dose statin treatment), myopathy, and hemorrhagic stroke (~0.01 excess cases per 100), making statins a relatively safe choice for the management of ASCVD risk.[31]

Non-statins

A number of agents/classes have an impact on the lipid profile, but beyond the statins, there is limited data on their impact on cardiovascular events. Even in trials in which statins were combined with non-statins, there was little to no added benefit. Given the interpretation of the 2013 ACC/AHA guidelines, clinicians treating high-risk patients who have a less-than-anticipated response to statins, who are unable to tolerate a less-than-recommended intensity of a statin, or who are completely statin-intolerant may consider the addition of a non-statin cholesterol-lowering therapy. High-risk individuals include those individuals with known vascular disease including stroke or TIA, those with LDL–C ≥190 mg/dL, and those with diabetes.[1]

Limitations of treatment in the older patient

Older patients generally do not receive evidence-based therapies for atherosclerosis-related disease on par with their younger counterparts. That being said, there are certainly real limitations of treatment in this age group. Statins, for example, are contraindicated in patients with active liver disease or unexplained persistent elevations of serum transaminases. Although cases of rhabdomyolysis are rare with statin treatment, patients should promptly report muscle pain, tenderness, or weakness. The clinician should review these patients carefully for possible concomitant physiological compromise, including renal status, and the potential for drug–drug interactions as a contributor to risk for rhabdomyolysis. Other pharmacological approaches also have specific limitations in this age group. Bile acid resins often interfere with absorption of other drugs and are difficult to dose. Fibrates carry warnings on their use in patients with compromised renal function, as well as distinct risk benefit considerations when used in combinations with statins. Sound judgment and a review of specific agents should be made in all patients, particularly older patients who are likely to be on multiple medications and may have age-related physiological compromise.

Beyond risk assessment, there may be other factors that come into play in older persons that affect the decision to employ LDL-lowering drugs. Ultimately, as with patients of any age, individualized therapy should match the needs of each specific patient.

Adherence: making medicines work

Official guidelines offer a framework to address many specific patient care challenges, yet there are often issues up to and beyond the patient–physician encounter that impact the optimization of outcomes and quality of care. Adherence to treatment is one such issue. Poor adherence to all therapies across all age groups represents a significant challenge to the health-care system, leading to suboptimal outcomes and increased costs from additional emergency room visits and hospitalizations. Nonadherence to pharmacological therapies for chronic conditions such as hypertension, diabetes, and cardiovascular disease in the elderly (which is frequently complex and includes on average five to eight different medications daily) is estimated at between 14% and 77%.[32]

Older patients may require additional support for medication management and monitoring. Based on a study of elders enrolled in two separate managed care plans, the primary challenges were related to the failure to prescribe appropriate medications, monitoring treatment, providing adequate education, and supporting continuity of treatment among providers. Quality improvement in this regard should focus on errors of omission in which the underuse of potentially beneficial medications manifests potential harm. These omissions may arise from the provider belief that there is insufficient evidence of clinical benefit associated with underrepresentation of older patients in clinical trials, concerns regarding polypharmacy, and substantial financial barriers with insufficient insurance coverage of outpatient prescription drugs.[33]

Underutilization and nonadherence with lipid-lowering therapies

The beneficial role of statins in secondary prevention is well documented for patients of all age groups. However, in a recently published retrospective cohort study of more than 75,000 patients older than 65, the use of statin therapy declined with increasing age. This treatment paradox suggested that despite an annual 1% increase in mortality risk, there was a greater than 6% decline in the use of preventive therapy. Other reviews as well have commented on the relative "clinical inertia" with respect to using statins in older patients.[34, 35, 36]

Additional studies have assessed the specific challenges in using statins in older patients. In a retrospective cohort analysis of more than 34,000 New Jersey Medicaid patients, Brenner and colleagues described a rapid decline in statin persistence in use in older patients. Unlike data reported in clinical trials, this analysis found that after five years, only 26% of patients were still taking their prescribed regimens. Several predictors of poor persistence were identified as age (>75 years), socioeconomic factors, issues of ethnicity, and depression. These findings supported the concept that strategies for improved adherence require early intervention and specific targeting of high-risk groups.[37]

A meta-analysis conducted by Mann and colleagues reviewed 22 cohort studies to find predictors of statin nonadherence. They found age >70 (odds of nonadherence 0.46; 95% CI 0.38 to 0.57), female gender (odds of nonadherence 1.07; 95% CI 1.04 to 1.11), and lower income (odds of nonadherence 1.18 95% CI 1.10 to 1.28) to be associated with decreased adherence. Cardiovascular disease (odds of nonadherence 0.68; 95% CI 0.66 to 0.78) and other comorbidities, including hypertension and diabetes, led to increased

adherence to therapy[38]. Frequent lipid testing and lower out of pocket costs appeared to increase adherence, but the number of studies was too small for a firm finding. Thus, this review clearly outlines the complex nature of nonadherence – especially in the elderly population – as there is no sole contributor. Rather, many socioeconomic factors, health-care utilization resources, and co-morbid medical conditions play a role.[39]

The challenge of improving adherence in elderly patients as well as in all patient groups is clear. A recent series of articles support the Institute of Medicine report indicating that much of the care gap between recommended care and actual levels of chronic disease is attributable to medication non-adherence. Although a systems approach must be recognized and acted upon by providers, payers, insurers, and policy makers, there are steps individual clinicians and teams can take to improve adherence.[40]

For example, providers should acknowledge self-efficacy, or the awareness that an individual patient has the confidence and belief in his or her ability to take medicine properly. This is related to the issue of patients' knowledge of their disease and, in the case of cardiovascular disease, an awareness of risk factors. Patients who understand the benefits/necessity of their treatment and have fewer concerns about the risk of prescribed drugs, have better self-reported adherence rates. Lastly, there is a clear benefit of a trusting patient-provider relationship, in which the patient has trust in the care decisions being provided by the clinician. At the time of the patient visit, providers should learn to identify specific patient characteristics, including age, number and complexities of regimen, motivation, and knowledge. If clinical judgment suggests a risk for nonadherence, caregivers should attempt to intervene early and establish continuity within the practice as well as among providers.[32, 40]

Conclusion

Appropriate lipid management in older patients provides an important opportunity to address cardiovascular risk. Statins have proven to be the drug of choice in recent years because of their lipid-lowering effects and relatively safe drug profile. Whereas the most recently published guidelines may have modified the clinical approach to risk assessment and management, the critical issue of a patient-centered focus remains entirely relevant as we consider cardiovascular risk in older patients. As health-care providers acknowledge the higher absolute risk of cardiovascular disease in older patients, they should also acknowledge the benefits of currently appropriate diagnostic and treatment modalities. Although guidelines and randomized clinical trials help inform our approach to patient care, the clinician's clinical judgment, experience, and patient centeredness will help truly improve outcomes.

References

1. Stone N, Robinson J, Lichtenstein AH, et al. 2013 ACC/ AHA guideline on the treatment of blood cholesterol to reduce atherosclerotic cardiovascular risk in adults: a report of the American College of Cardiology/American Heart Association Task Force on Practice Guidelines. *Circulation* 2014;**129**:51–545.

2. Enos WF, Holmes RH, Beyer J. Coronary disease among United States soldiers killed in action in Korea. *JAMA* 1953;**152**:1090–3.

3. Berenson GS, Wattigney WA, Tracy RE, et al. Atherosclerosis of the aorta and coronary arteries and cardiovascular risk factors in persons ages 6 to 30 years and studied at necropsy (the Bogalusa Heart Study). *American Journal of Cardiology* 1992;**70**:851–8.

4. Cohen JC, Boerwinkle E, Mosley TH Jr, Hobbs HH. Sequence variations in PCSK9, low LDL, and protection against coronary heart disease. *N Eng J Med.* 2006;**354** (12):1264–72.

5. Brown M, Goldstein J. Lowering LDL – not only how low, but how long? *Science* 2006;**311**(5768):1721–3.

6. Ference BA, Yoo W, Alesh I, et al. Effect of long-term exposure to lower low-density lipoprotein cholesterol beginning early in life on the risk of coronary heart disease: a Mendelian randomization analysis. *J Am Coll Cardiol.* 2012;**60**(25):2631–9.

7. National Cholesterol Education Program; National Heart, Lung, and Blood Institute; National Institutes of Health. *Detection, Evaluation, and Treatment of High Blood Cholesterol in Adults (Adult Treatment Panel III) Final Report.* NIH Publication No. 02–5215. Bethesda, MD: National Cholesterol Education Program, National Heart, Lung, and Blood Institute, National Institutes of Health, 2002.

8. Persell SD, Lloyd-Jones DM, Baker DW. National Cholesterol Education Program risk assessment and potential for risk misclassification. *Prev Med.* 2006;**43**(5):368–71.

9. Kostis JB. Disputation on the use of age in determining the need for treatment of hypercholesterolemia and hypertension. *J Clin Hypertension* 2006;**8**(7):519–20.

10. Yusuf S, Hawken S, Ounpuu S, et al. Effect of potentially modifiable risk factors associated with myocardial infarction in 52 countries (the INTERHEARTstudy): case-control study. *Lancet* 2004;**364**:937–52.

11. Kuller LH, Arnold AM. 10-year follow-up of subclinical cardiovascular disease and risk of coronary heart disease in the Cardiovascular Health Study. *Arch Intern Med.* 2006;**166**:71–8.

12. Pencina MJ, Navar-Boggan AM, D'Agostino RB Sr, et al. Application of new cholesterol guidelines to a population-based sample. *N Engl J Med.* 2014;**370**:1422–31.

13. Grundy SM, Cleeman JI. Implications of recent clinical trials for the National Cholesterol Education Program Adult Treatment Panel III Guidelines. *J Am Coll Cardiol.* 2004;**44**:720–32.

14. LeMaitre R, Psaty BM, Heckbert SR, et al. Therapy with hydroxylmethylglutaryl coenzyme A reductase inhibitors (statins) and associated risk of incident cardiovascular events in older adults: evidence from the Cardiovascular Health Study. *Arch Int Med.* 2002;**162**:1395–1400.

15. Strandberg TE, Pyörälä K, Cook TJ, et al. Mortality and incidence of cancer during 10-year follow-up of the Scandinavian Simvastatin Survival Study (4S). *Lancet* 2004;**364**(9436):771–7.

16. Bulbulia R, Armitage J. Does the benefit from statin therapy extend beyond 5 years? *Curr Atheroscler Rep.* 2013;**15**(2):297.

17. Cholesterol Treatment Trialists' (CTT) Collaborators, Mihaylova B, Emberson J, et al. The effects of lowering LDL cholesterol with statin therapy in people at low risk of vascular disease: meta-analysis of individual data from 27 randomised trials. *Lancet* 2012;**380**(9841):581–90.

18. Huddy K, Dhesi P, Thompson PD. Do the frequencies of adverse events increase, decrease, or stay the same with long-term use of statins? *Curr Atheroscler Rep.* 2013;**15**(2):301.

19. Glynn RJ, Koenig W, Nordestgaard B. Rosuvastatin for primary prevention in older individuals with high C-reactive protein and low LDL levels: exploratory analysis of a randomized trial. *Ann Intern Med.* 2010;**152**(8):488–96, W174.

20. Pederson T, for the Scandinavian Simvastatin Survival Study Group.Randomised trial of cholesterol lowering in 4444 patients with coronary heart disease: the Scandinavian Simvastatin Survival Study (4S). *Lancet* 1994; **344**(8934);1383–9.

21. Sacks FM, Pfeffer MA, Moye LA, et al., for the Cholesterol and Recurrent Events Trial Investigators. The effect of pravastatin on coronary events after myocardial infarction in patients with average cholesterol levels. *N Engl J Med.* 1996;**335**:1001–9.

22. Hunt D, Young P, Simes J, et al. Benefits of pravastatin on cardiovascular events and mortality in older patients with coronary heart disease are equal to or exceed those seen in younger patients: results from the LIPID trial. *Ann Intern Med.* 2001;**134**:931–40.

23. Afilalo J, Duque G, Steele R, et al. Statins for secondary prevention in elderly patients: a hierarchical bayesian meta-analysis. *J Am Coll Cardiol.* 2008;**51**(1):37–45.

24. Aronow WS. Drug treatment of peripheral arterial disease in the elderly. *Drugs Aging* 2006;**23**(1):1–12.

25. Sacco R, Adams R, Albers G, et al. Guidelines for prevention of stroke in patients with ischemic stroke or transient ischemic attack: a statement for healthcare professionals from the American Heart Association/ American Stroke Association Council on Stroke. *Stroke.* 2006;**37**:577–617.

26. The Stroke Prevention by Aggressive Reduction in Cholesterol Levels (SPARCL) Investigators. High-dose atorvastatin after stroke or transient ischemic attack. *N Engl J Med.* 2006;**355**:549–59.

27. Eckel R, Jakicic J, Ard J, et al. 2013 AHA/ACC guideline on lifestyle management to reduce cardiovascular risk. *Circulation.* 2014;**129**(25 Suppl 2):S76–S99.

28. US Department of Health and Human Services. *2008 Physical Activity Guidelines for Americans.* Washington, DC: US Department of Health and Human Services; 2008:1–61. Available at: www.health.gov/PAGuidelines.

29. Rosenson RS. Current overview of statin-induced myopathy. *Am J Med.* 2004;**116**:408–16.

30. Hey-Hadavi JH, Kuntze D, Luo D. Tolerability of atorvastatin in a population aged > or = 65 years: a retrospective pooled analysis of results from fifty randomized clinical trials. *Am J Geriatr Pharmacother.* 2006;**4**:112–22.

31. Finegold J, Manisty C, Goldacre B, et al. What proportion of symptomatic side effects in patients taking statins are genuinely caused by the drug? Systematic review of randomized placebo-controlled trials to aid individual patient choice. *Eur J Prevent Cardiol.* 2014;**21**(4):464–74.

32. Chia L, Schlenk EA. Effect of personal and cultural beliefs on medication adherence in the elderly. *Drugs Aging* 2006;**23**(3):191–202.

33. Higashi T, Shekelle PG, Solomon DH, et al. The quality of pharmacologic care for vulnerable older patients. *Ann Intern Med.* 2004;**140**:714–20.

34. Ayanian JZ, Landrum MB, McNeil BJ. Use of cholesterol-lowering therapy by elderly adults after myocardial infarction. *Arch Intern Med.* 2002;**162**:1013–19.

35. Ko DT, Mamdani M, Alter D. Lipid-lowering therapy with statins in high-risk elderly patients: the treatment-risk paradox. *JAMA* 2004;**291**:1864–70.

36. Dewilde S, Carey IM, Bremner SA, et al. Evolution of statin prescribing 1994–2001: a case of agism but not of sexism? *Heart* 2003;**89**:417–21.

37. Brenner JS, Glynn RJ, Mogun H, et al. Long-term persistence in use of statin therapy in elderly patients. *JAMA* 2002;**288**:445–56.

38 O'Connor P. Improving medication adherence: challenges for physicians, payers, and policy makers. *Arch Intern Med.* 2006;**166**:1802–4.

39. Munn M, Woodard M, Munter P. Predictors of non-adherence to statins: a systematic review and meta-analysis. *Ann Pharmacother.* 2010;**44**(9):1410–21.

40. Osterberg L, Blaschke T. Adherence to medication. *N Engl J Med.* 2005;**353**:487–97.

445

Osteoporosis and other metabolic bone disorders

Michele F. Bellantoni, MD, CMD

Aging and bone health

Peak bone mass achieved at about age 25 years is largely determined by genetic factors, although extreme malnutrition, impaired reproductive status, paralysis, and severe chronic illness may cause a significantly lower peak bone mass. Bone is an active organ with a normal physiology of removing older bone and replacing with new matrix to achieve tensile strength through a three-dimensional architecture of cross-linked and calcified proteins.

Aging is associated with reductions in the synthesis of new bone matrix proteins, while menopausal reductions in sex and adrenal hormones for women result in accelerated resorption of existing bone. Age-related male endocrine changes have less clinical impact as men have greater peak bone mass than woman and sex steroid decreases occur more gradually than menopausal endocrine changes. Reductions in sun exposure and inadequate vitamin D intake place some older adults at risk for impaired bone mineralization.

Osteoporosis is the common disorder of compromised bone architecture and reduced tensile strength that contributes greatly to fractures with aging, estimated to occur in half of Caucasian women and one in five men.[1] Although osteoporosis is less common in African Americans, those with osteoporosis have the same fracture risks as Caucasians. Fractures result when weakened bone is overloaded, often by falls or lifting heavy objects.

Hip fractures are a significant consequence of osteoporosis and are associated with excess mortality, ranging from 8% to 36% at one year, with higher mortality in men than in women. Vertebral and pelvic fractures contribute to gait disorders and can cause disabling back or pelvic pain. Severe kyphosis resulting from vertebral fractures in addition to age-related degenerative changes of the spine may contribute to restrictive lung disease, impaired bowel function, and limited mobility.

Osteoporosis screening

The US Preventive Services Task Force (USPSTF) recommends bone mineral density testing for women >65 years of age, and for younger adult women who have fracture risks comparable to those of an otherwise healthy 65-year-old woman,[2] estimated by the World Health Organization (WHO) Fracture Assessment Tool as a 10-year risk of about 9.3% (forearm, shoulder, clinical spine, and hip fracture). However, the Women's Health Initiative Study reported in 2014 that a Simple Calculated Osteoporosis Risk Estimate (SCORE) >7 or an Osteoporosis Self-Assessment Tool calculated as $0.2 \times$ (weight in kg − age in years) < 2 were more predictive of low bone density for postmenopausal women aged 50–64 than the Fracture Risk Assessment >9.3%.[3]

The National Osteoporosis Foundation recommends bone mineral density testing in men >70 years of age,[4] although the USPSTF cites insufficient data to recommend screening bone density in men.[2] All agree that postmenopausal women and men over age 50 who experience a low-impact adult fracture of the hip, spine, pelvis, humerus, or forearm should undergo bone mineral density testing and consideration for osteoporosis drug therapies.

Medical conditions and certain drug therapies are associated with bone loss (Table 32.1). Fall risk is a consideration when determining need for bone mineral density testing. Fall risks are associated with neurologic conditions that impair gait and balance, cardiac conditions that predispose to orthostasis, and

---

Reichel's Care of the Elderly, *7th Edition*, ed. Jan Busby-Whitehead *et al.* Published by Cambridge University Press.
© Cambridge University Press 2016.

Table 32.1 Medical conditions and therapies associated with bone loss

Endocrine	Gastrointestinal	Hematologic	Neurologic	Other
Diabetes mellitus	Celiac disease	Monoclonal gammopathy	Stroke	Familial hypercalciuria
Central obesity	Inflammatory bowel diseases	Systemic mastocytosis	Parkinson's disease	Chronic kidney disease
Hyperparathyroidism	Short gut syndrome	Chemotherapy	Antiseizure medications	Rheumatoid arthritis
Thyrotoxicosis	Bariatric surgery	Radiation therapy		Systemic steroid therapy
Cushing syndrome	Chronic anti-acid therapy			

musculoskeletal conditions that impair gait such as degenerative and inflammatory arthritis and degenerative spine.

Dual energy x-ray absorptiometry is considered the most cost-effective bone mineral density technique,[5] although for older adults, degenerative changes of the spine may give falsely elevated results. The proximal radius and hip are two additional sites for clinical measurement. The WHO defines osteoporosis using only the mean lumbar spine (at least two vertebral bodies), total hip, proximal femur, and proximal radius bone sites. Osteoporosis is defined by bone density criteria as bone mineral density of at least one of these bone sites more than 2.5 standard deviations below normal gender peak specific bone mass (T score ≤ -2.5). Normal bone density is defined by the WHO as a bone density greater than one standard deviation below normal peak bone mass, (T score ≥ -1.0), with osteopenia T score between -1 and -2.5.

Although other technologies exist to measure bone density, dual energy x-ray absorptiometry is preferred based on access, radiation exposure, and cost. Quantitative CT scanning has greater radiation exposure and cost; ultrasound techniques, while portable and low cost, limit the bone sites for measurement and cannot be used for serial monitoring of osteoporosis treatments.

The clinical history and physical exam determine the need for additional diagnostic studies beyond bone densitometry. For example, a bone density that is significantly below that expected for age and gender in the setting of comorbid conditions of migraine syndrome and GI symptoms of bloating may prompt

studies for celiac disease. Evaluation of hypercalcemia or renal calculi associated with osteoporosis includes serum intact parathyroid hormone and 24-hour urine collection to assess for hypercalciuria.

Without additional clinical findings of comorbid medical conditions, further diagnostic studies before offering drug therapies for postmenopausal or age-related osteoporosis include assessment of renal function, serum calcium, and serum 25-hydroxyvitamin D3.

Osteoporosis treatments

Bone health nutrition

A heart healthy diet may not meet the nutritional needs for bone health because fresh fruits, vegetables, and lean meats contain small amounts of calcium and vitamin D. The addition of low- and no-fat dairy products, plant milk (such as soy and almond milk), calcium-fortified beverages (such as calcium-fortified fruit juices), and foods such as breakfast cereals can achieve a bone healthy diet without compromising cardiovascular health. Optimal calcium intake is 1,000 mg elemental calcium daily through dietary sources, although older adults taking loop diuretics may require 1,200 mg to account for calcium loss resulting from diuresis. In contrast, thiazide diuretics conserve calcium from renal loss.

For those who cannot obtain adequate calcium intake through diet alone, calcium supplements are available in various formulations – tablets, soft chews, gummies, and dissolvable powders – but may cause gas, bloating, and constipation to a greater extent than dietary sources. Anti-acid drugs, such as H2 blockers and proton pump inhibitors, impair digestion of calcium, although calcium citrate supplements do not require gastric acid for digestion. Clinical trials have demonstrated an association among calcium supplementation and increased risk of cardiovascular disease;[6] however, a systematic review considering benefits/risks of adequate calcium and vitamin D intake in treating osteoporosis concluded that adequate, but not excessive, supplementation of bone nutrients is appropriate osteoporosis management for those with comorbid cardiovascular conditions.[7]

Vitamin D deficiency in the elderly can result in deep bone and muscle pain, muscle weakness, hyperesthesia, as well as fractures from brittle bone that lacks calcium deposition, called osteomalacia. Vitamin D is the hormone that facilitates calcium absorption from the gut. Changes in skin metabolism and decreased sun exposure are thought to contribute to vitamin D deficiency in older adults. Daily intake of 800 units of vitamin D is adequate to prevent vitamin D deficiency for most older adults, with higher dose supplements needed for those with GI malabsorption, including those with acquired celiac disease (allergy to gluten, a protein found in wheat and other related grains).[8]

Drug therapies for osteoporosis

FDA approved drug therapies are antiresorptive agents that prevent further bone loss, with the exception of teriparitide, an anabolic therapy that stimulates new bone protein formation, though to a lesser degree also stimulates osteoclastic bone resorption. The American Academy of Clinical Endocrinologist guidelines on osteoporosis drug therapies include first-line agents alendronate, risedronate, zoledronic acid, and denosumab because all have been shown in clinical trials to reduce vertebral, nonvertebral, and hip fractures (Table 32.2).[9] Alendronate and risedronate are preferred over zoledronic acid and denosumab due to lower cost and oral administration.

Postmenopausal women with family history of breast cancer but without increased risk of thromboembolic disease may find that selective estrogen receptor modulator drug therapy addresses both medical conditions. Estrogen replacement, although effective, has long-term risks of breast cancer and increased risk of cardiovascular disease.

Testosterone replacement for older men poses risks for cardiovascular health and prostate cancer.

Teriparitide has not been shown to reduce fracture risk to a greater extent than antiresorptive drugs, and teriparitide is high cost, requires monitoring for hypercalcemia, and has a black box warning label of osteosarcoma based on rodent toxicology studies. For these reasons, teriparitide is indicated for high fracture risk or when recurrent fractures occur during treatment with antiresorptive drug therapies. Calcitonin is a weak antiresorptive drug that has little clinical utility given the above alternatives.

Prolonged suppression of bone resorption may lead to suppressed bone formation, resulting in fragile bone called osteonecrosis, with clinical consequences of atypical femoral shaft fractures and jaw necrosis following invasive dental procedures. In one United States study of 1.8 million patients aged 45 or older,[10] 142 atypical femoral fractures were identified with a rate of 1.78/100,000 patient-years for those with up to 1.9 years of bisphosphonate use, but 113.1/100,000 patient-years in those with 8 to 9.9 years of use, with the recommendation that bisphosphonate treatment be time limited. Oral bisphosphonate treatment of three to five years, the duration of most clinical trials, has far greater benefit to prevent osteoporotic hip fractures than risk of atypical fractures. Hip fracture incidence in the placebo-treated subjects was as high as 750 hip fractures/100,000/year. Bisphosphonate-treated subjects experienced about 150–375/100,000/year fewer osteoporosis-related hip fractures at a risk of 11/100,000/year of atypical femoral shaft fractures. Osteonecrosis of the jaw was too rare to estimate rates of this adverse experience.

Over time, the withdrawal from oral bisphosphonates, often referred to as "drug holidays," can be associated with bone loss, as measured by serial bone densitometry. Resumption of oral bisphosphonates after several years of drug holiday is appropriate to stop further bone loss. Serial monitoring at intervals of six months to one year of serum markers of bone turnover, such as C telopeptide, Type 1 collagen, is suggested in clinical guidelines,[8] but without clinical trials data to establish a standardized approach.[11] Extrapolation from a European cohort undergoing invasive dental procedures reported no osteonecrosis of the jaw when serum C telopeptide was greater than 150 pg/mL.[12]

Table 32.2 Osteoporosis drug therapies

Drug	Class	Route of administration	Fracture risk reduction		
			Vertebral	Nonvertebral	Hip
Alendronate	Bisphosphonate	Oral weekly	Yes	Yes	Yes
Risedronate	Bisphosphonate	Oral weekly or monthly	Yes	Yes	Yes
Zoledronic acid	Bisphosphonate	Intravenous once yearly	Yes	Yes	Yes
Denosumab	Monoclonal antibody against RANK-L receptor	Subcutaneous every 6 months	Yes	Yes	Yes
Ibandronate	Bisphosphonate	Oral monthly or intravenous every 3 months	Yes	* No effect demonstrated	* No effect demonstrated
Raloxifene	Selective estrogen receptor modulator	Oral daily	Yes	* No effect demonstrated	* No effect demonstrated
Teriparatide	Synthetic parathyroid hormone derivative	Subcutaneous daily	Yes	Yes	* No effect demonstrated
Calcitonin	Synthetic salmon calcitonin	Intranasal daily or subcutaneous daily	Yes	No effect demonstrated	No effect demonstrated

* The lack of demonstrable effect at these sites may be due to insufficient sample size for study.

Nonpharmacologic management of osteoporosis

Smoking cessation, avoidance of phosphate beverages that bind dietary calcium, and alcohol and caffeine intake limited to two servings per day are nonpharmacologic strategies to promote bone health. Weight-bearing exercise stimulates bone formation, and has been estimated in a meta-analysis of clinical trials in postmenopausal women to reduce 20-year relative fracture risks of spine and femoral neck by about 10%. First-line drug therapies reduce fracture risks by 40%–60%, though no trial has combined exercise and drug treatments.[13] Physical activity recommendations for cardiovascular health serve bone health as well. Weight training with improper body mechanics risks nerve entrapment syndromes, soft-tissue injuries, and degenerative spine disease. However, weight-bearing exercise techniques are easy to perform safely in the home setting with proper patient education.

Monitoring of bone metabolism with serial bone density

Serial bone density for monitoring osteoporosis treatment plans is recommended at two-year intervals, although one year is appropriate in high turnover states such as hyperparathyroidism or high-dose steroid use. Bone density monitoring for those with screening studies within normal range or osteopenia and who do not require drug therapies, should be no more frequent than every two years.[14]

Other metabolic bone conditions of older adults

Four common metabolic bone conditions of older adults associated with increased fractures include osteomalacia (inadequately mineralized bone resulting from vitamin D deficiency), hyperparathyroidism (primary, secondary and tertiary), Paget's disease, and renal osteodystrophy (Table 32.3).

Table 32.3 Metabolic bone conditions of older adults

	Bone pathology	Bone turnover state	Diagnostic criteria	Treatment
Osteoporosis	Excess bone resorption	High	Bone densitometry T score $\leq$-2.5	Calcium, vitamin D, and drug therapies
Osteomalacia	Inadequately mineralized bone	Low	Low serum 25-hydroxyvitamin D	Vitamin D
Hyperparathyroidism				
Primary	Excess bone resorption	High	Hypercalcemia and high serum intact PTH	Surgery; cinacalcet
Secondary	Excess bone resorption	High	Low serum 25 vitamin D	Vitamin D; cinacalcet
Tertiary	Excess bone resorption	High		Surgical resection of parathyroid(s)
Paget's disease	Disordered bone resorption and formation	High	Elevated serum markers of bone turnover X-ray	Bisphosphonates
Renal osteodystrophy	Low bone formation	Low	Chronic kidney disease Low serum markers of bone turnover	Vitamin D; phosphate binding agents

Primary hyperparathyroidism is characterized by excessive production of parathyroid hormone, which leads to hypercalcemia via two mechanisms: (a) osteoclast-medicated bone resorption and (b) calcium conservation at the level of the glomerulus. The incidence in men >60 years of age is 1/1,000/year, twice the frequency for older women.[15] Head and neck irradiation in childhood and long-term lithium therapy are risk factors. More than 80% involve a single adenoma, although four-gland hyperplasia can result from either sporadic disease or as a hereditary multiple endocrine neoplasia Type 1 and 2A. The disease course can vary in severity from asymptomatic hypercalcemia to a syndrome of constipation, hypertension, osteoporosis, peptic ulcer disease, pancreatitis, kidney stones, mood disorders, and cognitive impairment. Additional laboratory findings include decreased or low normal serum phosphate, low serum 25-hydroxyvitamin D due to increased conversion to 1,25-dihydroxyvitamin D, possible elevation in serum alkaline phosphatase, urinary calcium excretion <250 mg/g Cr, and serum intact parathyroid hormone >80 pg/mL. Radiographs may show diffuse osteopenia, subperiosteal resorption (a salt-and-pepper appearance

of the phalanges, distal clavicles, or skull), and osteitis fibrosa cystica (deep areas of bone resorption filled by fibrous tissues). Osteopenia on bone density testing may be more severe at the proximal radius, a site with greater cortical bone than the lumbar spine and femoral neck. Definitive therapy for hyperparathyroidism is surgical resection of the adenoma; considered when either of the following are present: serum calcium >1 mg/dL above the upper limit of normal, bone mineral density T score $\leq$2.5, vertebral fracture, creatinine clearance <60 cc/min, nephrocalcinosis, renal calculi, or hypercalciuria > 400 mg/dL.[16] Cinacalcet reduces serum calcium >1 mg/dL and bisphosphonates may reduce bone loss.

Secondary hyperparathyroidism results from prolonged and severe vitamin D deficiency, either from inadequate nutrient intake, chronic kidney disease, or GI malabsorption syndromes including bariatric surgery and inflammatory bowel diseases. Multiple parathyroid gland hyperplasia may occur in chronic states, though early correction of vitamin D deficiency may prevent progression to clinically significant hyperparathyroidism. Tertiary hyperparathyroidism results from prolonged secondary hyperparathyroidism such as end stage renal disease and persists even after renal failure is corrected with organ transplantation.

Otitis deformans, or Paget's disease, is a condition of focal areas of active bone turnover. The prevalence of Paget's disease ranges from 1%–3% in areas of the United States to 10%–15% of older Europeans, with male to female ratio of 3 to 2 and 15% estimated to be familial autosomal dominant inheritance with identified genetic mutations involving osteoclast differentiation and function. The diseased bone is deformed, with thickened cortices and course trabeculations resulting in painful skeletal deformity and fractures. The most commonly affected sites include the femur, spine, pelvis, humerus, tibia, cranium, and sternum, causing hearing loss and nerve compression syndromes of the thoracic and lumbar spine. Osteosarcomas, fibrosarcomas, and benign giant cell tumors develop in 2%–4% of patients with Paget's disease. The pathogenesis of Paget's disease is unknown, but it is hypothesized that the condition is a late manifestation of an earlier paramyxoviral infection such as measles, respiratory syncytial, or canine distemper viruses. Asymptomatic Paget's disease may present as an elevated serum alkaline phosphatase or as incidental radiographic findings.[17] Serum markers of bone turnover such as C telopeptide, and osteocalcin are elevated, particularly when bone formation is markedly increased. Nuclear bone scans using technetium-labeled polyphosphonate or diphosphonate often reveal additional areas of disease not detected on x-ray. The radiographic changes of Paget's disease can be difficult to distinguish from those seen in metastatic prostate or breast cancer. Intravenous zoledronic acid is indicated to treat severe bone pain. Oral bisphosphonate is effective for milder disease. Calcitonin is used when bisphosphonates are contraindicated due to renal insufficiency.

Osteitis fibrosa, or renal osteodystrophy, is inadequately mineralized bone that results from impaired vitamin D metabolism and inadequate calcium absorption due to chronic kidney disease.[19] Simultaneously, cortical bone may experience significant bone resorption due to secondary hyperparathyroidism. Chronic kidney disease is a stronger risk factor for fracture than conventional risk factors such as bone mineral density, sex, race, and age.[20] Bone densitometry may underestimate fracture risk in setting of chronic kidney disease. Renal clearance of serum biomarkers of bone turnover may be impaired in chronic kidney disease. Antiresorptive drug

therapies are contraindicated when chronic kidney disease is associated with low bone formation. In addition, bisphosphonates and denosumab are contraindicated when creatinine clearance falls below 30 mL/min, and parathyroid hormone derivatives are not used when there is secondary hyperparathyroidism associated with vitamin D deficiency. Current treatment strategies are management of vitamin D deficiency, optimization of calcium through calcium phosphate binders, resistance exercise, and fall prevention.

References

1. Siris ES, Adler R, Bilezikian J, et al. The clinical diagnosis of osteoporosis: a position statement from the National Bone Health Alliance Working Group. *Osteoporosis International* 2014;25;1439–1443.

2. US Preventive Services Task Force. Screening for osteoporosis: US Preventive Services Task Force recommendation statement. *Ann Intern Med* 2011;**154**:356–364.

3. Crandall CJ, Larson J, Gourlay ML, et al. Osteoporosis screening in postmenopausal women 50 to 64 years old: comparison of US Preventive Task Force strategy and two traditional strategies in the Women's Health Initiative. *J of Bone and Mineral Research* 2014;**29**:1661–1666.

4. National Osteoporosis Foundation. *Clinician's Guide to Prevention and Treatment of Osteoporosis*. Washington, DC: National Osteoporosis Foundation, 2014.

5. Blake GM, Fogelman I. Role of dual-energy x-ray absorptiometry in the diagnosis and treatment of osteoporosis. *J Clin Densitom* 2007;**10**:102–110.

6. Bolland MJ, Grey A, Avenell A, et al. Calcium supplements with or without vitamin D and risk of cardiovascular events: reanalysis of the Women's Health Initiative limited access dataset and meta-analysis. *BMJ* 2011;**19**:342.

7. Heany RP, Kopecky S, Maki KC, et al. A review of calcium supplements and cardiovascular risk. *Adv Nutr* 2012; **3**(6): 763–771.

8. American Geriatrics Society Workgroup on Vitamin D Supplementation for Older Adults. Recommendations abstracted from the American Geriatrics Society Consensus Statement on vitamin D for prevention of falls and their consequences. *J Am Geriatr Soc* 2014 Jan;**62**(1):147–152.

9. Watts NB, Bilezikian JP, Camacho PM, et al. American Association of Clinical Endocrinologists medical guidelines for clinical practice for the diagnosis and treatment of postmenopausal osteoporosis. *Endocr Pract* 2010 Nov–Dec;**16**(Suppl 3):1–37.

10. Dell RM, Adams AL, Greene DF. Incidence of atypical nontraumatic diaphyseal fractures of the femur. *J Bone Miner Res* 2012;**27**:2544–2550.

11. Bauer D, Krege J, Lane N, et al. National bone health alliance bone turnover marker project: current practices and the need for US harmonization, standardization, and common reference ranges. *Osteoporosis International* 2012;**23**:2425–2433.

12. Kunchur R, Need A, Hughes T, et al. Clinical investigation of C-terminal cross-linking telopeptide test in prevention and management of bisphosphonate-associated osteonecrosis of the jaws. *J Oral Maxiollofac Surg* 2009;**67**:1167–1173.

13. Kelley GA, Kelley KS, Kohrt WM. Effects of ground and joint reaction force exercise on lumbar spine and femoral neck bone mineral density in postmenopausal women: a meta-analysis of randomized controlled trials. *BMC Musculoskeletal Disorders* 2012;**13**:177–196.

14. Cosman F, Jan de Beur S, LeBoff MS, et al. Clinician's guide to prevention and treatment of osteoporosis. *Osteoporosis International* 2014;**10**:2359–2381.

15. Marcocci C, Cetani F. Primary hyperparathyroidism. *New Engl J Med* 2011;**365**:2389–2397.

16. Bilezikian JP, Brandi ML, Eastell R, et al. Guidelines for the management of asymptomatic primary hyperparathyroidism: summary statement from the Fourth International Workshop. *J Clin Endocrinol Metab* 2014;**99**:3561–3569.

17. Ralston SH. Clinical practice. Paget's disease of bone. *N Engl J Med* 2013; **368**:644–650.

18. Hosking D, Lyles K, Brown JP, et al. Long-term control of bone turnover in Paget's disease with zoledronic acid and risedronate. *J Bone Miner Res* 2007;**22**:142–148.

19. Miller PD. Chronic kidney disease and osteoporosis: evaluation and management. *BoneKEy Reports* 2014;**3**: 542–548.

20. Salam SN, Eastell R, Khwaja A. Fragility fractures and osteoporosis in CKD: Pathophysiology and diagnostic methods. *American Journal of Kidney Disease* 2014;**63**:1049–1059.

Chapter 33

Common rheumatologic diseases in the elderly

Jowairiyya Ahmad, MD, and Jennifer Sloane, MD

As the population of the United States ages, rheumatologic disease is quickly becoming one of the more common diagnoses encountered in the geriatric population. According to a recent study, more than 67 million Americans will have arthritis by 2030.[1] In addition to increasing prevalence, disability associated with musculoskeletal disorders is increasing. A recent evaluation of the burden of disease found that worldwide disability associated with musculoskeletal disorders had more than tripled since 2004.[2] With this increased burden of disease, there is a necessity for these diseases to be managed with an interdisciplinary approach. Through appropriate partnership of physical therapists, occupational therapists, physiatrists, orthopedic surgeons, and pain specialists, rheumatologic disease in the elderly can be effectively managed.

Osteoarthritis

Osteoarthritis is the most common type of arthritis. According to 2005 US census data, approximately 27 million Americans suffer from osteoarthritis.[3] Although osteoarthritis was once thought to be a normal consequence of aging, it is now felt to have more of a multifactorial etiology. It results from a complex interplay of a patient's age, genetics, bone mass, hormonal influences, occupation, physical activity, and injuries.[4]

Clinical presentation

Patients with osteoarthritis classically report joint pain that increases at night and with use. They may also have increasing stiffness after prolonged immobility; however, this stiffness should last for 30 minutes or less. Patients may suffer from primary and/or secondary osteoarthritis. Primary osteoarthritis most commonly affects the hands, spine, hips, knees and feet. Secondary osteoarthritis can affect any joint. Secondary osteoarthritis results from an underlying condition such as previous trauma, congenital disorders, endocrinology disorders (diabetes mellitus, acromegaly, hypothyroidism, hemachromatosis), or inflammatory arthritis (calcium pyrophosphate dehydrate deposition disease, rheumatoid arthritis, gout).

The physical examination of a patient with osteoarthritis is likely to reveal tender joints. Patients may also have enlarged joints from bony osteophyte formation or from joint effusions; however, the joints are neither warm nor erythematous. Warmth or erythema should lead to an evaluation for inflammatory causes of the patient's joint pain. Aspiration of joint fluid can sometimes be helpful in making the diagnosis. Synovial fluid from a joint with osteoarthritis will be noninflammatory with less than 2,000 WBC/mm^3. There are no laboratory tests or biomarkers that are helpful in establishing the diagnosis of osteoarthritis. Although osteoarthritis is primarily a clinical diagnosis, radiographs can be helpful to confirm the diagnosis and rule out more serious causes of pain such as fracture or malignancy.

Hand osteoarthritis

Elderly women are at higher risk for development of hand osteoarthritis. Patients with osteoarthritis of the hands commonly have bony enlargement of the joints. The most commonly affected joints are the proximal interphalangeal (PIP) joints, distal interphalangeal (DIP) joints, and first carpometacarpal joints. Patients often report that the symptoms are increased in their dominant hand. Pain may significantly interfere with performance of the activities of daily living. A significant proportion of patients with hand

---

Reichel's Care of the Elderly, 7th Edition, ed. Jan Busby-Whitehead *et al.* Published by Cambridge University Press.
© Cambridge University Press 2016.

osteoarthritis may have erosive disease. These patients may have striking bony proliferation, erythema, or warmth on physical examination. This presentation may often be confused with an inflammatory arthritis but is degenerative in its pathophysiology. Radiographs can sometimes be helpful in differentiating between these diagnoses. Radiographs of patients with hand osteoarthritis classically show joint space narrowing with subchondral sclerosis and marginal osteophytes. Radiographs of erosive osteoarthritis may also show subchondral erosions or a "gull wing" appearance of the distal interphalangeal joints.

Spine and hip osteoarthritis

The cervical and lumbar spine are the most common sites of spine osteoarthritis. Patients may relate pain, stiffness, and difficulty with movement of these areas. They may also have radicular symptoms if nerve root impingement or spinal stenosis exists. Imaging of the spine may show osteophytes resulting in foraminal narrowing, spinal stenosis, or spondylothesis.

Hip osteoarthritis classically presents as referred pain to the groin and thigh but the pain can also radiate to the buttock and knee. Patients usually report that the pain increases with walking but also with prolonged immobility. As the disease progresses, patients may demonstrate decreased range of motion. Radiographs of the hip in osteoarthritis will often show joint space narrowing with osteophyte formation.

Knee osteoarthritis

The knee is the most common site of joint pain in the older adult. Risk factors for osteoarthritis of the knee include increased BMI, previous knee injury, smoking, older age, intensive physical activity, female gender, and presence of hand osteoarthritis.[5] Patients with osteoarthritis of the knee usually report pain that is increased with ambulation, but they can also have stiffness after prolonged immobility. It may also lead to other joint strain secondary to an abnormal gait. Other sources of pain of the knee such as mechanical derangement, anserine bursitis, fracture, or referred pain from the hip or spine should be considered before making a diagnosis of osteoarthritis. Physical examination of a knee affected by osteoarthritis may show crepitus, bony proliferation, and valgus or varus deformity. It may also reveal joint swelling, but the synovial fluid will be noninflammatory with a white blood cell count less than 2,000 WBC/mm^3.

Radiographs may show joint space narrowing that is present more often in the medial joint compartment. They are also likely to show osteophytes.

Foot osteoarthritis

While any joint of the feet can be affected by osteoarthritis, the first metatarsophalangeal (MTP) joint is most commonly involved. Older age and female sex are independent risk factors for developing arthritis of this joint.[6] Patients classically have the physical finding of hallux valgus with lateral deviation at the first MTP joint. Hallux valgus may also result in formation of an inflamed bunion at the site, which may be confused with gout. Radiographs can help differentiate between the two with osteoarthritis of the first MTP showing the classic joint space narrowing and osteophytes.

Treatment

Patients with osteoarthritis are treated with a combination of non-pharmacologic and pharmacologic modalities. Exercise should be encouraged, especially with knee osteoarthritis, as recent studies suggest that exercise, in combination with weight loss, is more effective in pain reduction than weight loss alone.[7] Involvement of occupational and physical therapists is encouraged. Splints, taping, orthotics, and wedged insoles can be helpful adjuncts in treatment.

Pharmacologic treatments for osteoarthritis do not change the natural history of the disease; rather, they focus on management of pain. Acetaminophen is the first-line treatment for osteoarthritis with doses up to 4,000 mg daily showing significant reduction in osteoarthritis pain when compared to placebo.[8] More recent recommendations suggest a maximum of 3,250 mg of acetaminophen daily.[9] The efficacy of this dose in osteoarthritis has not been studied in a large randomized controlled trial. If nonpharmacologic treatments and acetaminophen do not help with the pain, topical nonsteroidal anti-inflammatory medications (NSAIDs) are often preferred in the elderly over oral NSAIDs.[10] Oral NSAIDs can be used in the elderly with careful attention to the possible side effects such as gastrointestinal bleeding and hypercoagulability. Treatment with opioid analgesics may be necessary but should be used sparingly in the elderly due to increased falls and fractures.[11] Supplementation with glucosamine and chondroitin sulfate remains controversial as large-scale studies have shown conflicting results.

Intra-articular injections of corticosteroids or hyaluronic acid often provide relief for patients who have failed nonpharmacologic and pharmacologic treatment. Any joint can be injected with corticosteroid, but the knee is the most common site. Studies have demonstrated that a large majority of patients will have relief with intra-articular steroid injections to their knee.[12] Unfortunately, intra-articular injection with steroids is not curative, and the pain is likely to return. Injection of hyaluronic acid is primarily performed in the knee joint. Results from trials regarding the efficacy of viscosupplementation to the knee with hyaluronic acid have been conflicting with some trials suggesting benefit and others finding it no more effective than intra-articular placebo.[13]

Surgery is an option for some patients who have failed nonoperative treatments. Joint replacement of the knee and the hip are the most common surgical treatments of osteoarthritis. As these are complicated surgeries associated with significant perioperative morbidity, elderly patients must be fully medically evaluated before joint replacement surgery is performed.

Rheumatoid arthritis

Rheumatoid arthritis (RA) affects approximately 1% of the world's population. Recent studies suggest that, in patients older than 60, the overall prevalence may be as high as 2%. It is estimated that there are currently 1.3 million Americans living with RA.[14] Females are affected more often than males.

Clinical presentation

Rheumatoid arthritis is a symmetric inflammatory polyarticular arthritis that classically affects the small joints of the hands and feet. It may also affect medium- and large-size joints; however, this is less typical than the small joint pattern. Patients usually describe stiffness that is increased in the morning, joint pain, and swelling, and, often, constitutional symptoms. Rheumatoid arthritis may present indolently over several months or may present acutely. The majority of patients with RA have a positive rheumatoid factor, but this is neither specific nor sensitive for the diagnosis of RA. Patients may also have a positive antibody to cyclic citrullinated peptide (CCP antibody). CCP antibody has high specificity for the diagnosis of RA but has a lower sensitivity. Radiographs early in RA may be normal. As the disease progresses, one

may see periarticular osteopenia and juxta-articular erosions.

As rheumatoid arthritis often presents in younger people, many elderly with RA have been living with this disease for years. Patients without sustained access to disease modifying antirheumatic drugs may have serious morbidity from their RA. Patients with long-standing RA may have ulnar deviation of their hands, subluxation of numerous joints, swan neck and boutonniere deformities, joint contractures, and rheumatoid nodules. They may have undergone numerous orthopedic surgeries. With long-standing disease, patients may also suffer from extra-articular manifestations of RA such as: uveitis, scleritis, pulmonary fibrosis, and cardiovascular disease.

Elderly-onset RA occurs in patients older than 60 years of age and occurs equally among males and females. Symptoms are more likely to appear abruptly as opposed to insidiously. Large joints such as the shoulder are also more likely to be involved. Patients with elderly-onset RA are less likely to have a positive CCP antibody.[15]

Treatment

The trend in the treatment of RA is to treat the disease early and aggressively. Tight control with disease modifying anti-rheumatic drugs (DMARDs) should be started as soon as possible.

Oral medications are sometimes preferred by the geriatric patient. Nonsteroidal anti-inflammatory medications and corticosteroids may be used to help with pain; however, as these medications are not DMARDs, they should only be used as adjunctive therapy. Initial treatment with hydroxychloroquine or sulfasalazine may be considered for patients with very mild disease or for those with many comorbidities. The majority of patients with a new diagnosis of RA start with weekly oral methotrexate and daily folic acid supplementation. Methotrexate is generally well tolerated by the elderly; however, the weekly dosing schedule may sometimes be confusing to patients. If tight control of the rheumatoid arthritis is not achieved within the first 6 to 12 weeks, additional medications are added to the existing regimen. A recent trial of hydroxychloroquine, sulfasalazine, and methotrexate taken together has proven noninferior to methotrexate and etanercept together.[16] Leflunomide is another oral medication that is often used by itself or in combination with other medications for RA. Tofacitinib was also recently approved for treatment of RA but data in the elderly is limited.

If oral medications do not control the disease or if they cannot be tolerated, biologic medications should be considered. The majority of biologic medications work best when used in combination with oral medications. Vaccinations such as pneumococcal, influenza, hepatitis B, and herpes zoster should be initiated, if possible, before the biologic medications are prescribed. Screening for tuberculosis should also occur before initiation of a biologic medication as these medications are associated with reactivation of latent tuberculosis. Tumor necrosis factor (TNF) alpha inhibitors are the most commonly used biologic medications for RA. Adalimumab, certolizumab, etanercept, golimumab, and infliximab are FDA approved for the treatment of RA. These medications have never been directly compared but seem to have similar efficacy in the treatment of RA. Choice between these medications is usually made based on patient preference and includes issues such as: route of administration, frequency of administration, and cost. Although elderly patients may seem to be at higher risk for adverse events, recent studies have demonstrated that these medications are as safe in the elderly as they are in the general population.[17] Other options for patients who fail or cannot take TNF alpha inhibitors include rituximab, abatacept, and tocilizumab, although none of these medications have been studied specifically in the elderly.

Crystal-induced arthritis

Deposition of monosodium urate crystals (gout) or calcium pyrophosphate crystals (pseudogout) are the most common causes of crystal-induced arthritis. Another cause of crystal-induced arthritis in the elderly, albeit less common, is that induced by calcium phosphate hydroxyapatite crystals.

Gout

Joint pain induced by monosodium urate crystals most commonly affects men and postmenopausal women older than 65 years of age.[18] There is an increasing risk for gout as one grows older due to increased hyperuricemia. Hyperuricemia is defined as a uric acid level greater than 7 mg/dL. Etiologies of hyperuricemia are likely to be multifactorial but may stem from longevity, increased use of diuretics

and aspirin, and a higher prevalence of comorbidities such as hypertension, congestive heart failure, and renal failure. Patients may remain asymptomatic with hyperuricemia for many years before their first attack of gout; however, the degree of the hyperuricemia is directly linked to their risk of gout.[19] As the uric acid rises greater than 7 mg/dL, the uric acid crystals can become insoluble and deposit into the joints or soft tissues, initiating a gout attack.

Clinical presentation

The majority of first gout attacks present with involvement of the metatarsophalangeal joint, foot, or ankle. However, in the elderly, a first attack of gout may be polyarticular or involve the hands. Once the acute attack has resolved, patients enter into the intercritical period where they are asymptomatic from gout. A large majority of patients will eventually experience another acute attack of gout. Over time, if patients remain untreated, the intercritical period shortens and gout can become chronic. Elderly patients with chronic gout may have diffuse tophi, which are sometimes misinterpreted as osteoarthritis.

The definitive diagnosis of acute gout should be established by direct visualization of intracellular monosodium urate crystals under polarized microscopy. Polarized microscopy will demonstrate strongly negative birefringent crystals. In intercritical or chronic gout, the crystals may still be present but not intracellular. Imaging of early acute gout may only show soft tissue swelling or the presence of a joint effusion. Classic radiographic features such as erosions with sclerotic margins and overhanging edges may not be present until many years after the first attack of gout. Visualization of tophi on imaging may also take several years.

Treatment

The treatment of gout in the elderly is essentially the same as that of the general population with the caveat that careful attention must be paid to medication side effects. Colchicine or NSAIDs are most commonly used for the acute episodes. Colchicine is usually prescribed according to renal function and provider discretion. NSAIDs may also help with the inflammation of gout; however, they must be used cautiously in the elderly population as geriatric patients are more likely to experience gastrointestinal, renal, and cardiovascular side effects from NSAIDs.[20] If colchicine or NSAIDs are not tolerated or do not control the symptoms, intra-articular or oral corticosteroids can be used.

Patients who have chronic frequent gout attacks, a severe polyarticular presentation of acute gout, or tophaceous deposits will benefit from medications to lower their uric acid levels. A serum uric acid level below 6 mg/dL is associated with less frequent gout attacks.[21] Allopurinol, febuxostat, probenecid, and pegloticase are FDA-approved treatments for lowering uric acid in gout. These medications should not be initiated nor should dosage be adjusted during an acute episode of gout as this may prolong the acute attack. Allopurinol and febuxostat both inhibit xanthine oxidase. Although rare, allopurinol (and not febuxostat) is associated with a severe hypersensitivity syndrome. This allergic reaction occurs more often in patients with renal insufficiency; however, the drug can still be used cautiously in renal insufficiency.[22, 23] Febuxostat is an option for those who are allergic to allopurinol. It is also approved for use in patients with renal dysfunction as long as the creatinine clearance is greater than 30 mL/min. Probenecid is an uricosuric agent; however, as it is associated with increased nephrolithiasis and cannot be used in patients with renal dysfunction, it is not often prescribed for the elderly. Pegloticase has been recently approved by the FDA. It effectively and rapidly lowers serum uric acid levels, but its use is limited by the development of antibodies to pegloticase and by its high cost.

Elderly patients with gout may also suffer from the effects of polypharmacy. As the use of diuretics may increase serum uric acid, efforts should be made by physicians to try to limit the use of these medications in gout patients. Aspirin can also increase serum uric acid levels; thus, it is important to ensure that patients with gout who are taking aspirin have a definite need for this medication.

Calcium pyrophosphate deposition disease

According to one study, almost 50% of patients older than 84 years of age have evidence of calcium deposition in articular cartilage, or chondrocalcinosis, on radiographs of knees, hands, wrists, and pelvis.[24] There are also metabolic and congenital conditions associated with chondrocalcinosis such as hypothyroidism, hypomagnesemia, hyperparathyroidism, and hemochromatosis. Whereas the majority of patients with radiographic evidence of chrondrocalcinosis will remain asymptomatic, some patients may demonstrate an acute inflammatory arthritis from precipitation of the calcium pyrophosphate crystals. This acute flare of disease is termed pseudogout.

Clinical presentation

An attack of pseudogout may be monoarticular or polyarticular. It may affect any joint but is more common in medium and large joints. It does not affect the first MTP, which may help differentiate it from gout. It may be severe enough to be confused with RA. Trauma, surgery, or severe medical illness can sometimes precipitate an attack. The diagnosis of calcium pyrophosphate deposition disease (CPPD) is made through assessment of synovial fluid under polarized microscopy. One should see weakly positive birefringent rhomboid shaped crystals. An arthrocentesis should show joint fluid that is inflammatory with a WBC greater than 2,000 mm^3. Inflammatory markers are likely to be elevated. Radiographs may show chondrocalcinosis but this is not specific for the diagnosis as it can be found in asymptomatic individuals.

Treatment

There are few randomized controlled trials showing benefit of pharmaceutical treatments for CPPD. NSAIDs are usually the first oral medication to be used. Colchicine is often prescribed in the acute setting and for prophylaxis, but the evidence behind this practice is limited.[25] Other options for treatment of pseudogut include intra-articular or oral steroids.

Basic calcium phosphate hydroxyapatite deposition disease

Deposition of basic calcium phosphate hydroxyapatite crystals often causes a highly destructive arthritis of the shoulders bilaterally. This is seen most often in elderly women and named the Milwaukee shoulder. Synovial fluid may be serosanguinous but, under light microscopy, one may see basic calcium phosphate hydroxyapatite crystals. Radiographs of the shoulder may show severe glenohumeral degeneration with displacement of the humeral head and periarticular calcifications. These patients may be treated with NSAIDs and corticosteroids but the disease may be difficult to control.

Polymyalgia rheumatica/giant cell arteritis

Polymyalgia rheumatica

Polymyalgia rheumatica (PMR) is a disease that is found only in older adults. As one ages, the incidence of PMR also rises with a peak incidence in the eighth decade of life. Women are affected more often than men.[26] People of northern European descent have a significantly higher risk of being affected, but PMR has been seen in all racial and ethnic groups.[27]

Clinical presentation

Patients with PMR classically report pain of the shoulders and pelvic girdle. These symptoms usually occur along with fatigue and morning stiffness. Physical examination usually reveals a patient in severe discomfort at rest; however, besides this finding, the physical examination may be normal.

Although PMR is quite common in the elderly population, as there are no specific diagnostic tests for this condition, there is considerable variation in diagnosis and treatment. The majority of patients with PMR have an erythrocyte sedimentation rate (ESR) greater than 40 and an elevated c-reactive protein (CRP), but some patients may also have normal inflammatory markers.[28] As the diagnosis of PMR may be difficult, imaging has been explored as an adjunct in diagnosis. Magnetic resonance imaging (MRI), ultrasound, and positron emission tomography (PET) may show subacromial bursitis, biceps long head tenosynovitis, trochanteric bursitis, or interspinous bursititis, but these findings are somewhat nonspecific.[29]

Treatment

Responsiveness to treatment with low-dose prednisone has been one of the hallmarks of a diagnosis of PMR. Patients with PMR are usually slowly tapered off the prednisone within one year. Relapses are common and may necessitate increasing the dose and duration of prednisone. No medications have shown success as a steroid-sparing agent for PMR in numerous randomized controlled clinical trials.[30]

Giant cell arteritis

Giant cell arteritis (GCA) is also found exclusively in older adults. Although it may be diagnosed in patients as young as 50 years of age, recent studies have suggested that the mean age of GCA diagnosis is approximately 76 years of age.[31] Similar to PMR, GCA is diagnosed more often in patients of northern European descent.

Clinical presentation

Patients with GCA present with symptoms related to arterial insufficiency. As the temporal artery can often be affected, in the past, GCA was also referred to as temporal arteritis. As it is now clear that GCA can affect numerous other vessels, the disease is more appropriately referred to as GCA. Patients classically present with a combination of headache, jaw claudication, and, possibly, vision loss. Vision loss may occur as a result of ischemia of the retina, choroid, or optic nerve. Patients are also likely to have constitutional symptoms such as fevers and weight loss. They may also have symptoms of PMR. Most clinicians believe that 40%–50% of patients with GCA will also have PMR symptoms. As the aorta is often involved in GCA, patients may have symptoms of lower extremity claudication. A recent study that performed CT angiography on recently diagnosed GCA patients revealed findings suggestive of aortitis in approximately 65% of patients with GCA.[32] Physical examination may be normal or may show artery abnormalities such as enlargement, tenderness, or an absent pulse.

The majority of patients with GCA will have an elevated ESR. It may be as high as 100 mm/hour, but in a small minority of patients, the ESR may be normal.[33] MRI, ultrasound, CT, and PET have also been used in the diagnosis of GCA, but they are not thought to be as specific nor as sensitive as biopsy of the affected artery.[34] Arterial biopsy remains the gold standard for diagnosis.

Treatment

As vision loss can occur rapidly and irreversibly, treatment with 60 mg of prednisone should be initiated quickly if one has a high clinical suspicion. If vision is threatened, high dose pulse intravenous methylprednisolone should be considered. The prednisone needs to be tapered slowly to avoid relapse. Patients may need to take steroids for one to two years.

Remitting seronegative symmetric synovitis with pitting edema

Remitting seronegative symmetrical synovitis with pitting edema (RS3PE) is a disease of people older than 50. Patients typically present with acute pain and subcutaneous swelling of the dorsum of the hands. They may also have a polyarthritis that classically affects the small joints of the hands but may affect any joint. Laboratory tests may reveal elevated inflammatory markers. Imaging may show subcutaneous edema, tenosynovitis, as well as synovitis.[35] Some feel that this syndrome may be a subset of RA or PMR. Low-dose prednisone is very effective in treating this condition.

Sjögren's syndrome

Sjögren's syndrome is the most common medical cause of xerostomia in the elderly. The incidence of Sjögren's syndrome in the elderly is not known; however, estimates of the prevalence range between 1% to 14%.[36]

Clinical presentation

Patients with Sjögren's syndrome usually report dry eyes and dry mouth. There can also be systemic manifestations with neurologic, pulmonary, musculoskeletal, gastrointestinal, hematologic, and renal involvement. Diagnosis can be difficult but usually involves a combination of auto-antibodies (anti-SSA and SSB), ocular staining, and, possibly, labial salivary gland biopsy. A Schirmer test may also be used. This involves placing a piece of paper in the lower lid of the eye. After a specified time, the paper is removed and evaluated for wetness. This test is not specific for Sjögren's syndrome. Other diagnostic tests often used to evaluate patients with sicca include salivary and parotid gland scintigraphy and sialometry. The elderly with Sjögren's syndrome must also be carefully evaluated for the development of lymphoma. The risk of non-Hodgkin's lymphoma – particularly marginal zone lymphoma or mucosa-associated lymphoid tissue (MALT)-type lymphomas – in all patients with Sjögren's syndrome is significantly higher than that of the normal population.[37]

Treatment

Patients with Sjögren's syndrome should try to avoid using antidepressants, antihistamines, anticholinergics, and some neuroleptic medications as these medications can exacerbate symptoms. Salivary and tear substitutes can help with the sicca. Muscarinic agonists such as pilocarpine and cevimeline can also be used to stimulate secretions.

Inclusion body myositis

Inclusion body myositis (IBM) is an idiopathic inflammatory myopathy. It is rare in the general population, with an estimated prevalence of 0.49 to 1.07 per 100,000 in Olmstead County, Minnesota.[38] Although IBM is not frequently encountered in the general population, it is the most common muscle disease of aging. The majority of patients are older than 50 and are more likely to be male.[39] Patients usually present with an insidious onset of muscle weakness, often initially involving the proximal lower extremities first before becoming widespread. The pattern of muscle involvement can be symmetric or asymmetric. Muscle enzymes can be normal or only mildly elevated. Markers of systemic inflammation are normal, and there are no associated autoantibodies. An EMG and MRI can be helpful for diagnosis, but muscle biopsy remains the gold standard. A biopsy should show extensive endomysial inflammation with inflammatory cells surrounding myofibers. Rimmed vacuoles may also be visualized in the myofibers on Gomori trichrome stain. Electron microscopy should show filamentous inclusions and vacuoles. IBM is often resistant to treatment. High-dose prednisone is usually prescribed for several months; however, if the patient does not respond to this treatment, it is discontinued. Methotrexate and azathioprine are also sometimes used, although the data is limited regarding their success.[40]

References

1. Deal CL, Hooker R, Harrington T, et al. The United States rheumatology workforce: supply and demand, 2005–2025. *Arthritis Rheum.* 2007; **56**(3): 722–729.

2. Murray CJL, Vos T, Lozano R, et al. Disability-adjusted life years (DALYs) for 291 diseases and injuries in 21 regions, 1990–2010: a systematic analysis for the Global Burden of Disease Study 2010. *Lancet.* 2012; **380**(9859): 2197–2223.

3. Lawrence RC, Felson DT, Helmick CG, et al. Estimates of the prevalence of arthritis and other rheumatic conditions in the United States: Part II. *Arthritis Rheum.* 2008; **58**(1): 26–35.

4. Neogi T, Zhang Y. Epidemiology of osteoarthritis. *Rheum Dis Clic of N Amer.* 2013; **39**(1): 1–19.

5. Blagojevic, M, Jinks C, Jeffery A, Jordan KP. Risk factors for onset of osteoarthritis of the knee in older adults: a systematic review and meta-analysis. *Osteoarthritis and cartilage.* 2010; **18**(1): 24–33.

6. Roddy E, Zhang W, Doherty M. Prevalence and associations of hallux valgus in a primary care population. *Arthritis Care Res.* 2008; **59**(6): 857–862.

7. Villareal DT, Chode S, Parimi N, et al. Weight loss, exercise, or both and physical function in obese older adults. *N Engl J Med.* 2011; **364**(13):1218–1229.

8. Towheed T, Maxwell L, Judd M, et al. Acetaminophen for osteoarthritis. Available at: http://summaries.coch rane.org/CD004257/acetaminophen-for-osteoarthritis (accessed 19 June 2014).

9. The Acetaminophen Hepatotoxicity Working Group. Recommendations for FDA Interventions to Decrease the Occurrence of Acetaminophen Hepatotoxicity. 2008 Available at: www.fda.gov/downloads/Advisory Committees/CommitteesMeetingMaterials/Drugs/Dr ugSafetyandRiskManagementAdvisoryCommittee/uc m161518.pdf (accessed 20 December 2014).

10. Underwood M, Ashby D, Cross P et al. Advice to use topical or oral ibuprofen for chronic knee pain in older people: randomized controlled trial and patient preference study. *BMJ.* 2008; **336**:138–142.

11. Rolita, L, Spegman, A, Tang, X, Cronstein, BN. Greater number of narcotic analgesic prescriptions for osteoarthritis is associated with falls and fractures in elderly adults. *Jour Am Ger Soc.* 2013; **61**(3): 335–340.

12. Raynauld JP, Buckland-Wright C, Ward R, et al. Safety and efficacy of long-term intraarticular steroid injections in osteoarthritis of the knee: A randomized, double-blind, placebo-controlled trial *Arthritis Rheum.* 2003; **48**(2): 370–377.

13. Bannura RR, Vaysbrot EE, Sullivan MC, et al. Relative efficacy of hyaluronic acid in comparison with NSAIDs for knee osteoarthritis; a systemic review and meta-analysis. *Sem Arthritis and Rheum.* 2014; **43**: 593–599.

14. Rasch EK, Hirsch R, Paulose-Ram R, Hochberg MC. Prevalence of rheumatoid arthritis in persons 60 years of age and older in the United States: effect of different methods of case classification. *Arthritis Rheum.* 2003; **48**(4): 917–926.

15. Innala L, Moller B, Ljung, L, Smedby, T, Södergren, A, Magnusson, S, et al. Age at onset determines severity and choice of treatment in early rheumatoid arthritis. *Arthritis Rheum.* 2012; **64**(10): S908.

16. O'Dell JR, Mikuls TR, Taylor TH, et al. Therapies for active rheumatoid arthritis after methotrexate failure. *N Engl J Med.* (2103); **369**(4): 307–318.

17. Ornetti, P, Chevillotte, H, Zerrak, A, Maillefert, JF. Anti-tumour necrosis factor-α therapy for rheumatoid and other inflammatory arthropathies. *Drugs Aging.* 2006; **23**(11): 855–860.

18. Roddy, F, Mallen CD, Doherty M. Gout. *BMJ* 2013; **1347**: f5648. doi:10.1136/bmj.f5648.

19. Campion EW, Glynn RJ, DeLabry LO. Asymptomatic hyperuricemia: risks and consequences in the Normative Aging Study. *Am J Med.* 1987; **82**: 421–426.

20. Crofford LJ. Use of NSAIDs in treating patients with arthritis. *Arth Res Ther.* 2013; **15** (Supplement 3): S2.

21. Shoji A, Yamanaka H, Kamatani N. A retrospective study of the relationship between serum urate level and recurrent attacks of gouty arthritis: evidence for reduction of recurrent gouty arthritis with antihyperuricemic therapy. *Arthritis Rheum.* 2004; **51**: 321–325.

22. Hande RK, Noone RM, Stone WJ. Severe allopurinol toxicity: description and guidelines for prevention in patients with renal insufficiency. *Am J Med.* 1984; **76**: 47–56.

23. Stamp LK, O'Donnell JL, Zhang M, et al. Using allopurinol above the dose based on creatinine clearance is effective and safe in patients with chronic gout, including those with renal impairment. *Arthritis Rheum.* 2012; **63**(2): 412–421.

24. Wilkins E, Dieppe P, Maddison P, Evison G. Osteoarthritis and articular chondrocalcinosis in the elderly. *Annals Rheum Dis.*1983; **42**(3): 280–284.

25. Terkeltaub RA. Colchicine update: 2008. *Sem arthritis rheum.* 2008; **38**(6): 411–419.

26. Doran MF, Crowson CS, O'Fallon WM, et al. Trends in the incidence of polymyalgia rheumatica over a 30 year period in Olmsted County, Minnesota, USA. *J Rheum.* 2002; **29**(8): 1694–1697.

27. Gonzalez-Gay MA, Vazquez-Rodriguez TR, Lopez-Diaz MJ, et al. Epidemiology of giant cell arteritis and polymyalgia rheumatica. *Arthritis Care Res.* 2009; **61** (10): 1454–1461.

28. Gonzalez-Gay MA, Rodriiguez-Valverde V, Blanco R, et al. Polymyalgia rheumatica without significantly increased erythrocyte sedimentation rate: a more benign syndrome. *Arch Int Med.* 1997; **157**(3): 317–320.

29. Camellino D, Cimmino MA. Imaging of polymyalgia rheumatica: indications on its pathogenesis, diagnosis and prognosis. *Rheumatology* 2012; **51**(1): 77–86.

30. Weyland CM, Goronzy JJ. Giant cell arteritis and polymyalgia rheumatic. *N Engl J Med.* 2014; **371**: 50–57.

31. Kermani TA., Schäfer VS, Crowson CS, et al. Increase in age at onset of giant cell arteritis: a population-based study. *Annals Rheum Dis.* 2010; **69**(4): 780–781.

32. Prieto-González S, Arguis P, García-Martínez A, et al. Large vessel involvement in biopsy-proven giant cell arteritis: prospective study in 40 newly diagnosed patients using CT angiography. *Annals Rheum Dis.* 2012; **71**(7): 1170–1176.

33. Salvarani C, Hunder GG. Giant cell arteritis with low erythrocyte sedimentation rate: Frequency of occurrence in a population-based study. *Arthritis Care Res.* 2010; **45**(2): 140–145.

34. Nesher G. The diagnosis and classification of giant cell arteritis. *J Autoimmunity.* 2014; **48**: 73–75.

35. Klauser A, Frauscher F, Halpern EJ, et al. Remitting seronegative symmetrical synovitis with pitting edema of the hands: ultrasound, color doppler ultrasound, and magnetic resonance imaging findings. *Arthritis Care Res.* 2005; **53**(2): 226–233.

36. Moerman RV, Bootsma H, Kroese, FG, Vissink A. Sjögren's syndrome in older patients. *Drugs & Aging.* 2013; **30**(3): 137–153.

37. Theander E, Henriksson G, Ljungberg O, et al. Lymphoma and other malignancies in primary Sjögren's syndrome: a cohort study on cancer incidence and lymphoma predictors. *Annals Rheum Dis.* 2006; **65**(6): 796–803.

38. Wilson FC, Ytterberg SR, St Sauver JL, Reed AM. Epidemiology of sporadic inclusion body myositis and polymyositis in Olmsted County, Minnesota. *J Rheum.* 2008; **35**(3): 445–447.

39. Greenberg, SA. Inclusion body myositis. *Current Opinion Rheum.* 2011; **23**(6): 574–578.

40. Griggs, RC. The current status of treatment for inclusion body myositis. *Neurology.* 2006; **66**(2 Suppl 1): S30–S32.

Chapter 34

Musculoskeletal injuries in the elderly

Natalie R. Danna, MD, and Joseph D. Zuckerman, MD

Introduction

Orthopedic trauma in the elderly patient presents both a medical and a surgical challenge. This growing population requires injury management tailored to specific patient needs. Injury treatment is based on patient factors, injury factors, and other special considerations in order to optimize outcome. The goal of injury treatment in the elderly patient is enabling return to pre-injury functional status. This chapter will focus on the treatment of some of the more common musculoskeletal injuries encountered in the elderly, including proximal humerus fractures, wrist fractures, hip fractures, ankle fractures, and vertebral compression fractures.

Patient factors

Pre-injury status

The goal of injury treatment in the elderly patient is a return to pre-injury level of function. Therefore, a thorough history that includes pre-injury level of activity and independence is integral to guiding effective orthopedic care. The treatment goals of an independent community ambulator who sustains a hip fracture are different than those of an institutionalized nonambulator. The former requires early operative intervention combined with aggressive postoperative rehabilitation, while the latter requires a less aggressive approach that enables comfortable transfers and the ability to sit. For both, the goal is to return the patient to pre-injury status; however, the approach to each differs significantly.

Systemic disease

Elderly patients often have preexisting medical comorbidities that influence musculoskeletal injury treatment. Cardiopulmonary disease is common in this population and affects the patient's ability to tolerate anesthesia, undergo surgery, and participate in a postoperative rehabilitation program. Cardiopulmonary disease is a major determinant of the American Society of Anesthesiologists preoperative risk assessment.[1]

The presence of neurologic disorders such as Parkinson's disease, Alzheimer's disease, and previous cerebrovascular accident affect injury management. Profound Parkinson's disease that is associated with severe contractures and significant functional incapacity limits the treatment options for both fractures and soft tissue injuries.[2] Patients who have suffered a stroke and resulting neurologic impairment are at an increased risk for fracture as a result of altered gait and balance, coupled with compromised bone quality due to impaired weight bearing and mechanics. Fractures occurring in patients who have suffered a stroke usually occur on the affected side.[3, 4]

Endocrinopathies, such as diabetes and thyroid disorders, are common in the elderly. Diabetic patients are considered to be immunocompromised and have microvascular disease that increases the risk of wound complications and infection following surgery.[5, 6] Independent of other known risk factors, diabetics also have greater risk of sustaining a fracture, longer time to fracture union, and poorer expected outcome of operative fracture fixation as compared to age matched nondiabetic patients.[5–8]

Bone quality

Strong bone should be both appropriately dense and appropriately mineralized. In the elderly, reduction of bone quality – osteopenia – is common and may be

---

Reichel's Care of the Elderly, *7th Edition*, ed. Jan Busby-Whitehead *et al.* Published by Cambridge University Press.
© Cambridge University Press 2016.

caused by either osteoporosis (decreased bone density with normal mineralization) or osteomalacia (deceased mineralization with or without a change in density). Osteopenia is most commonly caused by senile osteoporosis, but also may be caused by other, treatable causes such as nutritional deficiencies, hyperparathyroidism, renal disease, tumors, and Cushing's disease.[9] A thorough medical evaluation should identify any of these treatable causes.

Osteopenia affects fracture management because osteopenic bone is at higher risk for delayed union and nonunion. Additionally, osteopenic bone may affect the ability of the surgeon to achieve stable fixation during operative fracture fixation. Orthopedic implants do not have the same fixation in osteopenic bone as they have in robust, strong bone. Lower forces are required for screw pullout, leading to early failure of fixation. This problem is compounded by the osteopenia that develops, even in normal bone, during periods of immobilization. Several techniques may be employed to mitigate this problem: bone graft, bone graft substitutes, methylmethacrylate cement, and new locked-plating systems.[10]

Several prophylactic and therapeutic medical treatments for osteoporosis are currently available – such as bisphosphonates, parathyroid hormone analogues, calcitonin, and selective estrogen receptor modulators – and should be considered for the elderly patient.[11–13] Osteomalacia in the elderly patient is often the result of nutritional deficiencies, whether due to malabsorption syndromes, aberrant metabolism of calcium, vitamin D, and phosphorus, or excessive use of phosphate-binding medications such as phenytoin or antacids. These conditions are generally treated medically by addressing the cause of the deficiency and providing increased dietary supplementation of the deficient metabolite.

Soft-tissue quality

The most characteristic age-related change in skeletal muscle tissue is a loss of muscle mass secondary to a decrease in the size and/or number of muscle fibers.[14, 15] Functional changes associated with aging are alterations in reaction time, strength, reflex time, coordination, speed, and endurance.[16, 17]

As a result of aging, skin becomes more fragile and less tolerant of handling during surgical intervention. These changes affect the treatment options considered. Age-related attritional changes can compromise soft tissue repair; aggressive surgical management

requiring lengthy rehabilitation may not be warranted in patients with preexisting soft tissue compromise.

Injury factors

Polytrauma

Although patients older than age 65 constitute a minority of the overall population, they represent over 28% of all fatal injuries in the United States.[18, 19] For any operative injury, mortality and morbidity are greater in the geriatric patient. Traditional trauma rating systems used to triage patients and predict outcome are less reliable in the elderly.[20, 21]

Recognition of skeletal injuries in the geriatric trauma patient requires vigilance. The possibility of fractures should be considered in any high-energy trauma. Visceral injuries uncommonly occur without skeletal injury in the elderly trauma patient.[22] Long bone injuries should be immobilized to decrease hemorrhage and minimize the risk of fat embolization. The mortality of acute and delayed complications of pelvic fractures (hemorrhage or sepsis) is 17% in cases of closed pelvic ring fractures, and more than 80% in cases of open fractures.[19] Early stabilization of pelvic ring fractures and long bone fractures facilitates patient mobilization, and improves respiratory function, ultimately resulting in improved outcomes.[23]

Open fractures

Fractures in which the bone is exposed to the outside environment through a defect in the soft tissue cover are known as open fractures. Open fractures in the elderly, particularly those of the lower extremity, should be treated as limb-threatening injuries. Preexisting conditions such as vascular insufficiency, diabetes mellitus, atherosclerosis, osteopenia, and immunocompromise adversely affect the outcome of these injuries and are more common in the geriatric population. The basic tenets of open fracture management must be followed to optimize outcome in this population: timely and meticulous debridement of bone and soft tissue, fracture stabilization, bone grafting, and soft tissue coverage when necessary.[24, 25]

Comminution

Even low-energy fractures in the elderly patient may result in marked comminution, which is more commonly associated with high-energy trauma in the younger patient. This is often the result of relative weakness of osteopenic bone. Comminuted fractures in the geriatric population must be treated with special considerations in mind. The most important determinant of fracture stability is stable bony apposition at the fracture site. This may mean tolerating or intentionally shortening the bone to obtain a stable construct. Patients with evidence of osteoporosis should also be treated medically to improve bone stock and optimize chances of fracture healing.[26]

Intra-articular fractures

Intra-articular fractures require a stable, anatomic reduction to prevent post-traumatic arthrosis and to allow for early range of motion. Early joint motion promotes articular cartilage healing.[27] Intra-articular fractures in an arthritic joint are generally unique to the elderly patient and may require primary prosthetic replacement. This is applicable in displaced intra-articular fractures of the hip and proximal humerus.

Special considerations

Periprosthetic fractures

The treatment of fractures about a total joint replacement is a challenging task. Risk factors include osteopenia and previous revision surgery. Treatment of displaced periprosthetic fractures must be individualized, accounting for early patient mobilization, preservation of limb alignment, and stability of the bone-implant interface.[28, 29] Nonsurgical management may result in limb malalignment and prolonged recumbency with associated pulmonary, genitourinary, and thromboembolic complications. Surgical management is complicated by the presence of the implant, associated osteopenia, and implant instability. This often leads to difficulties with postoperative mobilization of the patient.

Periprosthetic fractures commonly occur at/near the end of an intramedullary portion of an implant (stem) and may result in the loosening of the implant (Figure 34.1). There is a high complication rate of treatment following periprosthetic fractures. Compared to fractures not near implants, there is a higher rate of nonunion, malunion, and infection. These rates are comparable to those of revision joint replacement.[30]

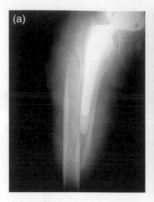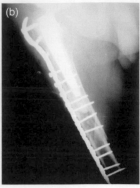

Figure 34.1 (A) Preoperative and (B) postoperative anteroposterior (AP) radiographs of a displaced periprosthetic fracture of the femur distal to a total hip replacement. The implant was stable in the femur and the decision was made to proceed with open reduction and internal fixation of the fracture while retaining the implant in the stable position.

Pathologic fractures

Metastatic disease

The skeleton is the third most common site of metastatic disease. The incidence of bony involvement in patients with a known malignancy is reported to be between 12% and 70%.[31–33] Common primary malignancies that metastasize to the skeleton are lung, breast, renal, thyroid, and brain. Furthermore, primary malignancies and dyscrasias may involve the skeleton, such as lymphoma, myeloma, and chondrosarcoma. The proximal femur is the most common location of pathologic fracture and is involved in over 50% of cases. This is due to the significant mechanical stresses that occur across the hip joint and proximal femur during ambulation.[34]

Treatments are, again, directed at early patient mobilization. Surgical treatment is the standard of care in treatment of neoplastic fractures, especially those of the femur.[35] The goals are to restore function, alleviate pain, facilitate nursing care, decrease hospital stays, and improve patient quality of life. Surgical contraindications are few but may include obtunded mental status, inability to tolerate the operative procedure, and life expectancy less than one or two months.

Atypical fractures of the femur associated with bisphosphonate use

Bisphosphonate treatment is steadily growing in the elderly population. As osteoporosis screening is

464

promoted widely in the lay media, and patients live longer, bisphosphonate use is increasing. With this increasing prevalence have emerged reports of atypical fractures in the metadiaphysis of the femur that are associated with bisphosphonate use.[36] Many patients report prodromal thigh pain. Occasionally, the thigh pain prompts radiographic evaluation before complete fracture occurs (Figure 34.2A).

Investigation of the histology and biomarkers present in the deranged tissue has given rise to the theory that these stem from stress fractures in which bisphosphonate use impairs healing by suppressing bone turnover.[37, 38] In the patient on chronic bisphosphonate treatment, complaints of thigh pain should prompt a radiographic evaluation.

The constellation of cortical thickening, transverse fracture pattern, and a medial spike when the fracture extends through the medial cortex, in the context of a low-energy insult, is the characteristic radiographic presentation (Figure 34.2B).[39] If radiographs are normal but pain persists, a magnetic resonance imaging (MRI) should be performed.[40]

In patients with complete or impending fracture, even those that are nondisplaced, operative treatment is strongly advised to avoid the complications associated with prolonged bed rest.[41, 42] Furthermore, surveillance of the contralateral limb should be performed in these patients with a low threshold for prophylactic treatment, if findings are present,[39] in order to prevent progression and reduce total hospital admission time.[43]

Preoperative considerations

Absolute indications for operative fracture treatment are open fractures, compartment syndrome, and neurovascular compromise. Relative surgical indications include displaced intra-articular fractures in which acceptable reduction and alignment cannot be maintained and fractures that require stabilization in order to mobilize the patient out of bed. Fracture management in the elderly must take into consideration all of the injury factors, patient factors, and special considerations previously described. All aspects must be considered to develop an individualized plan of care.

Timing of surgery in the elderly patient is controversial. Generally, surgery should be performed when comorbid medical conditions have been optimized. Retrospective analayses have offered equivocal assessments on the relationship

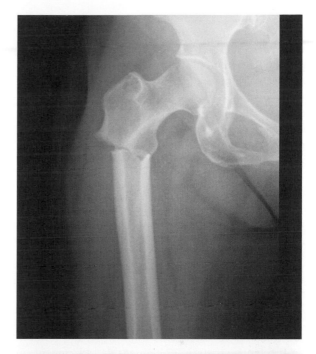

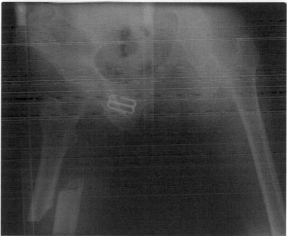

Figure 34.2 (A) AP radiograph of the right hip of a patient on chronic bisphosphonate therapy with a six-month history of thigh pain. There is an incomplete fracture, transversely oriented, from the thickened lateral cortex that does not extend through medial cortex. This patient was taken to the OR for operative stabilization. (B) AP radiograph of the pelvis of patient on chronic bisphosphonate therapy who sustained a fall. Note the hallmarks of atypical femur fractures: subtrochanteric location, transverse fracture line, lateral cortical thickening, and medial cortical spike.

between timing and morbidity.[44, 45] A prospective study from our institution of 367 hip fracture patients demonstrated that surgical delay of more than two days from hospital admission doubled the risk of patient death at one year when age, sex, and number of comorbidities was controlled.[46]

No significant difference has been demonstrated in survival rates in patients undergoing operative treatment of hip fractures with either regional or general anesthetics.[47, 48] There has been demonstrated a reduced incidence of thromboembolic events (DVT, pulmonary embolus) after use of regional anesthesia.[49] Because pulmonary embolism is a significant cause of morbidity and mortality in the geriatric patient, regional anesthesia is preferable when appropriate.

Implant choice should reflect the surgical goal: to achieve a stable fracture construct with anatomic or near anatomic alignment and/or reduction of articular surfaces to allow early mobilization of the patient and range of motion of the affected joint. Fracture impaction restores structural continuity, allows for force transmission across the fracture segment, and decreases the overall forces on the implant, all of which improve outcome and healing potential.

Intramedullary devices are the implant of choice for fractures in osteopenic bone when the location and fracture pattern are amenable. Placement of intramedullary implants is closer to the mechanical axis of the bone; thus, they act as a load-sharing device. Plates, which are placed directly on the bone, are further from the mechanical axis and act as load-bearing devices.

Hip fractures

Principles

Hip fractures in the elderly can be a life threatening injury because of the impact on medical, functional, and psychological status of the patient. More than 250,000 hip fractures occur annually in the United States, which result in over %9 billion in health-care costs. Current age trends predict a doubling of the yearly incidence of hip fractures by the year 2050.[50–52]

The risk of a hip fracture increases with age, doubling every decade after the age of 50. Hip fractures occur most commonly in Caucasian women, followed by Caucasian men, then African-American women and men. This may be due to differences in bone density between these groups. Institutionalized patients are also at an increased risk for hip fracture, often with greater risk of mortality.[53–58]

Hip fractures in the elderly usually occur from low energy trauma. They are categorized by anatomic location into two classes: intra-capsular (femoral neck fractures) or extra-capsular (intertrochanteric and subtrochanteric fractures). Fractures of the femoral neck are intracapsular, extra-articular fractures that occur in the region between the femoral head and the intertrochanteric line. The location of these fractures can compromise the primary blood supply to the femoral head, especially in displaced fractures.

The intertrochanteric region lies outside the hip capsule, in between the greater and lesser trochanters. This area of metaphyseal bone benefits from a rich blood supply and, as a result, carries a lower risk of the healing complications associated with intracapsular fractures. The greater trochanter is a superolateral structure that serves as the insertion point for the hip abductors and short external rotators. The lesser trochanter is located distally at the posteromedial surface of the proximal femur and serves as the attachment site for the iliopsoas. The calcar femorale is a region of bone located along the posteomedial portion of the proximal femur and acts as a cortical strut to transmit the large forces across the intertrochanteric region.

Presentation and initial management

Patients who have sustained a hip fracture present with complaint of hip and groin pain with the inability to bear weight on the affected extremity after a fall. The affected extremity is usually positioned in external rotation and slight hip flexion. This position provides maximal capsular volume and the most comfort from the hematoma that develops in intracapsular fractures; in displaced extracapsular fractures, the displacement of the fracture results in a shortened and externally rotated position of the lower extremity. There will often be a noticeable leg length discrepancy. Evaluation should include a thorough neurovascular exam of the affected extremity as well as examination of all other extremities to exclude concomitant fracture. Neurologic examination should assess mental status and inquire as to loss of consciousness associated with the fall.

Medical consultation should be obtained at the time of presentation to optimize the patient medically for anticipated surgery. Injury radiographs, initial laboratory investigations, chest radiograph, and electrocardiogram should be performed. A baseline arterial blood gas may be warranted since hip fractures carry a risk for thromboembolic phenomena. A Foley catheter should be placed to eliminate the need for positioning on a bedpan or use of a urinal to minimize patient discomfort. Additionally, the Foley catheter allows accurate measurement of urine production, important for volume status assessment in these patients who may not have had adequate fluid intake after their injury due to access or pain. Orthogonal films should include a true anteroposterior (AP) and cross-table lateral (Figure 34.2) of the hip. A cross-table lateral projection is preferable to a frog-leg lateral, as the latter causes the bone fragments to rotate through the fracture site, further displacing fracture fragments causing increased discomfort to the patient and the potential for further injury.

If the diagnosis of a hip fracture is suspected but not confirmed by routine radiographs, further imaging studies are indicated. An AP view with axial traction and internal rotation of the affected limb can improve the visualization of the entire femoral head and neck. If doubt remains, a technetium bone scan or MRI should be obtained. A technetium bone scan requires two to three days after injury to minimize the risk of false-negative, whereas an MRI can accurately diagnose occult fracture within 24 hours after injury.[59] The preferred treatment of hip fractures is operative because it allows early mobilization of the patient, thereby decreasing the risk of cardio-pulmonary events, urinary tract infections, decubitus ulcers, and the rate of mortality in the first year. It also minimizes the period of non–weight bearing, decreases the risk of nonunion/malunion, and increases the ease of transfer. Overall, operative management also decreases the cost of hip fractures, which is becoming increasingly important.[60]

As for any hospitalized patient, the potential for thromboembolic events (DVT or PE) is concerning. In addition to mechanoprophylaxis, chemoprophylaxis should be administered; however, the risk of bleeding in the injured or postoperative patient is an important consideration and must be balanced with the need for prophylaxis. Warfarin, the historic gold standard, requires daily monitoring and carries a significant risk of bleeding. Low molecular weight heparins (LMWH) have been the contemporary choice, effective without the need for laboratory monitoring, although their subcutaneous administration raises compliance concerns post-hospitalization.[61–63] A promising alternative has emerged: rivaroxaban is a direct factor Xa inhibitor, orally administered, with predictable pharmacokinetics and the same efficacy as LWMH.[64] Discussion between the medical and surgical teams should pinpoint the precise starting time postoperatively, but generally chemoprophylaxis should begin 12 hours postoperatively. An inferior vena cava filter may be used when anticoagulation is contraindicated or in patients at a high risk for recurrent thromboembolism.

Outcomes

The goal of surgical treatment of hip fractures is to restore the patient's functional status to the pre-injury level. At one-year follow-up, 41% of patients will regain their pre-injury ambulatory status, 40% will require increased assistance, and 8% will become non-ambulatory.[65]

Mortality rates of hip fracture patients are twice that of age- and sex-matched controls.[44, 66, 67] The highest increase is seen in the first 6 months after injury, and progressively decreases to that of age- and sex-matched controls at one year. However, one-year mortality can be as high as 30%.[67–69]

While the amount of time from injury to surgical treatment has been debated as a predictive factor, a prospective study from our institution in which age, sex, and other comorbidities were controlled, demonstrated that a delay of surgical treatment for more than two days in patients who did not suffer from dementia and were ambulatory prior to injury doubled one-year mortality.[46]

Postoperative rehabilitation should employ a weight bearing as tolerated program. Although some have recommended restricted weight bearing (or even non–weight bearing), in situations when fracture fixation is felt to be suboptimal, we feel that this has a very negative impact on the overall recovery and does not accomplish the intended goal of limiting forces across the hip (and therefore on the fracture fixation). Joint reaction forces across the hip are actually higher with non-weight bearing as opposed to toe-touch weight bearing. When elderly patients are allowed immediate postoperative weight bearing as tolerated, they tend to self-regulate the amount of weight on the injured extremity and will gradually increase the amount of weight bearing as their comfort allows.[70, 71] The approach encourages, rather than limits, their recovery of mobility and ambulation.

Femoral neck fractures

Femoral neck fractures, as previously discussed, are intracapsular fractures. They are generally classified

467

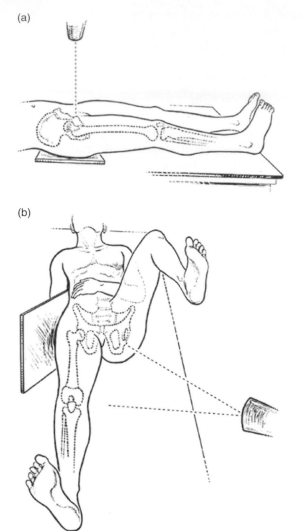

(a)

(b)

Figure 34.3 A sketch depicting the proper method of evaluating suspected hip fractures, demonstrating (A) AP and (B) cross-table lateral radiographs of a displaced fracture of the subcapital femoral neck in a patient with limited ambulatory capability.

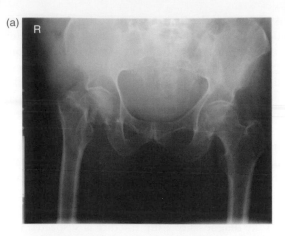

(a)

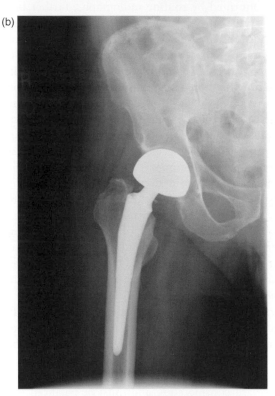

(b)

Figure 34.4 (A), Preoperative and (B) postoperative AP radiographs of a displaced fracture of the subcapital femoral neck in a patient with limited ambulatory capability. This injury is associated with a high incidence of avascular necrosis, compromising healing when the femoral head is retained. Therefore, this fracture was treated with hip hemiarthroplasty.

as nondisplaced or displaced. Nondisplaced fractures may be treated nonoperatively, for the sick or non-ambulatory patient; however, there are reports of increased rates of nonunion. For this reason as well as for earlier mobilization, internal fixation, with cannulated screws or a head screw with side plate (sliding hip screw), is preferable. Displaced fractures are similarly treated for patients under 60 years old. Displaced fractures in patients over 80 years old are treated with arthroplasty, a total hip replacement for healthy, active patients, and hemiarthroplasty for lower-demand patients. For patients between 60 and 80 years old, the decision to fix the fracture versus replacing the joint has to be individualized, taking into account the patient's lifestyle, independence, physiologic age, bone quality, and comorbidities.[72] See Figures 34.3 and 34.4.

468

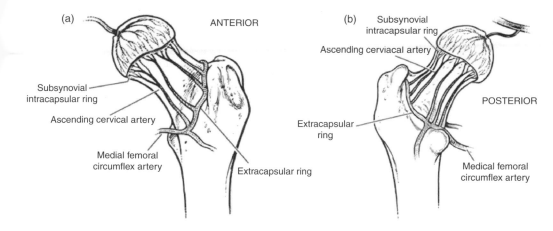

Figure 34.5 Vascular anatomy of the femoral neck.

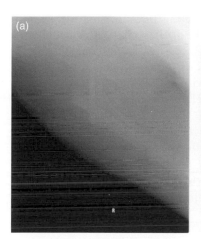
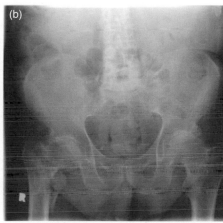

Figure 34.6 (A) Preoperative and (B) postoperative AP radiographs of an unstable intertrochanteric hip fracture. This fracture was fixed with a cephalo-medullary device.

Osteonecrosis of the femoral head and nonunion following femoral neck fractures increase in frequency as the degree of fracture displacement increases. Therefore, nondisplaced fractures have rates of these complications between 5%–10% while these rates are 20%–35% for displaced fractures.[73–79] The presence of these complications is a common indication for revision surgery. See Figure 34.5.

Intertrochanteric hip fractures

Intertrochanteric hip fractures are classified as stable or unstable, based on whether or not the posteriomedial buttress (calcar femorale) is intact or comminuted. This is determined on injury radiographs based upon the position of the lesser trochanter. Stable fractures are characterized by an intact lesser trochanter on the distal fracture fragment, whereas unstable

fractures demonstrate a large, displaced lesser trochanteric fragment. A large, displaced lesser trochanteric fragment is an indication of calcar comminution and an unstable fracture pattern.

Surgery is the treatment of choice for all intertrochanteric hip fractures. Although they have been most commonly treated with extramedullary devices (those that reside outside of the central canal of the femur, such as a sliding hip screw), recently, an increasing number are being treated with cephalomedullary (intramedullary) devices (Figure 34.6). Both methods are accepted forms of operative treatment and have demonstrated similar results and complications in recent prospective, randomized studies.[80–82] The indications and goals for nonoperative treatment are similar to those for femoral neck fractures.

Ankle fractures

The ankle joint is a modified hinge joint consisting of the lateral malleolus (tuberosity on the distal fibula), the medial malleolus (tuberosity on the distal tibia), the plafond (central articular surface of the distal tibia), and the talus. Binding these osseous structures are the lateral collateral ligament, the deltoid ligament, and the tibiofibular syndesmosis. The lateral collateral ligament is composed of three structures: the anterior talofibular ligment, the calcaneofibular ligmament, and the posterior tibiofibular ligament. The deltoid ligament consists of an anterior, superficial portion that attaches to the navicular, sustentaculum tali, and the talus, while the stronger, deeper, posterior portion originates on the posterior colliculus of the medial malleolus and inserts on the medial surface of the talus.

The clinical examination of a patient with a suspected ankle injury should include palpation of the abovementioned osseous and ligamentous structures. Swelling and ecchymoses should be noted. Weight-bearing ability must be determined (patients are rarely able to bear weight on an unstable fracture). A neurovascular exam should be performed, ensuring that ankle dorsi- and plantarflexion are intact, as is great toe flexion and extension. Sensation should be tested over the dorsum of the foot, first web space, medial and lateral edges of the foot, and the plantar surface.

The decision to evaluate an ankle radiographically after injury should be made using the Ottawa Ankle Rules. Only patients with tenderness over the inferior or posterior pole of either malleolus (defined as the distal 6 cm for these guidelines) and the inability to take four steps independently (even if limping) should have x-rays.[83] Radiographic examination should include three views of the ankle: an antero-posterior view, a mortise view (20 degree internal rotation oblique), and a lateral view. Ankle fractures can include isolated lateral malleolus/distal fibula fractures, isolated medial malleolus fractures, fractures of both malleoli (bimalleoloar), or both malleoli and the posterior portion of the tibial plafond (trimalleolar). Isolated fractures of the lateral malleolus should be evaluated with stress views to exclude the presence of a medial soft tissue injury that will lead to ankle instability.[84]

The goal of treatment of ankle fractures in elderly patients is to restore the normal tibiotalar relationship while maintaining a congruous joint surface. Stable injuries, such as isolated lateral malleolus fractures without medial disruption, should be rested in the acute post-injury period with gradual return to weight-bearing as tolerated with the use of a brace or fracture boot.

Bi-malleolar injuries (including their equivalent lateral malleolus fractures combined with medial soft tissue disruption) and fractures associated with talar displacement and joint incongruity are unstable and require operative fixation. Even slight talar incongruity can lead to early post-traumatic arthritis.[85] The primary goal of operative treatment of an elderly patient with an ankle fracture is to obtain or maintain an anatomic relationship of the tibia, fibula, and talus, and thereby joint congruity.

The timing of surgery depends largely on the condition of the soft tissue envelope. Ankle fractures and fracture-dislocations can be associated with significant swelling and the development of fracture blisters. When present, operative treatment should be avoided because of the risk of soft tissue sloughing following the surgical procedure. The return of skin wrinkles about the ankle herald adequate subsidence of swelling. Studies have shown that operative treatment restores anatomic relationships and stability, as well as improving function and pain scores over time.[86, 87] Patients with unstable injuries should remain non–weight bearing until bony union is achieved and soft tissue supporting structures have had the chance to heal.

Proximal humerus fractures

Proximal humerus fractures are common in the elderly population. The proximal humerus is the third most common site of fracture and often occurs as a result of a low energy mechanism, such as a fall from standing position.

The current system used to classify fractures of the proximal humerus fractures was first described by Neer.[88, 89] This classification divides the proximal humerus into four anatomic segments: the head, the shaft, the lesser tuberosity, and the greater tuberosity. A segment is considered independent if it is displaced 1 cm or more, or angulated 45 degrees or more from its anatomic position. Thus, proximal humerus fractures can be defined as one part (minimally displaced), or as two-, three-, or four-part fractures. This system provides treatment guidelines and predicts outcome based upon fracture type.

Minimally displaced fractures account for approximately 85% of all proximal humerus fractures. These fractures have an intact surrounding soft-tissue envelope, and all parts can be expected to move as a single unit. These injuries are treated with an initial period of immobilization in a sling, followed by range of motion exercises beginning about one week post-injury.

Two-part fractures through the surgical neck of the humerus are treated operatively with reduction and internal fixation. Fractures through the anatomic neck are rare and treated with reduction and internal fixation in younger patients and with arthroplasty in older patients. Greater tuberosity fractures are treated operatively if there is greater than 5 mm superior translation, to preserve rotator cuff function. Lesser tuberosity fractures may be treated closed unless there is a block to internal rotation.

Three- and four-part fractures are at increased risk for osteonecrosis of the humeral head and require operative management. Treatment preference – internal fixation versus prosthetic replacement – is determined by patient factors (age, activity level) and fracture factors (bone quality, comminution, and presence of dislocation). Currently, options for prosthetic replacement include hemiarthroplasty or reverse total shoulder arthroplasty (Figure 34.7).

Regardless of treatment approach, elderly patients with displaced proximal humerus fractures require a prolonged, supervised physiotherapy program to optimize functional outcomes. Minimally displaced one-part and adequately reduced two-part fractures can be expected to have good functional outcomes. Poor results may be related to compromise of the rotator cuff, malunion, nonunion, or osteonecrosis. Results of prosthetic replacement are predictable for pain relief, but less consistent for functional recovery.

Distal radius fractures

Distal radius fractures occur more commonly in geriatric patients than any other. The incidence increases dramatically with age, particularly for women, and parallels that seen for fractures of the proximal humerus and proximal femur.[90] Distal radius fractures have been attributed to the presence of osteoporosis, as well as poor eyesight, impaired coordination, and decreased muscular strength.

Unstable fractures are identified by marked comminution, greater than 1 cm of shortening, loss of palmar tilt, greater than 10 degrees of dorsal tilt, and intraarticular displacment (Figure 34.8A, B). Unstable fractures account for 15%–25% of distal radius injuries in the geriatric population and are generally associated with poorer outcome.

Closed reduction and splint/cast application is the treatment of choice for most distal radius fractures in elderly patients and should be attempted initially, even for unstable fractures. If closed reduction is successful, immobilization should continue for six weeks and radiographs should be performed weekly for three to four weeks to ensure that the reduction is maintained.

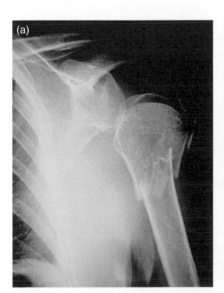
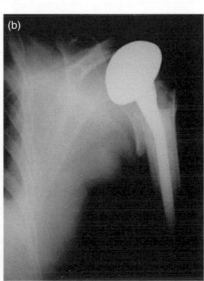

Figure 34.7 (A) Preoperative and (B) postoperative AP radiographs of a displaced three-part fracture of the proximal humerus treated with prosthetic replacement.

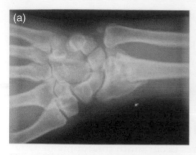 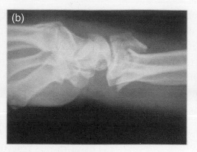 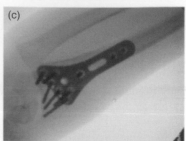

Figure 34.8 (A) AP and (B) lateral radiographs of an unstable distal radius fracture demonstrating significant shortening and comminution as well as loss of radial inclination and palmar tilt. (C) This fracture was indicated for operative fixation, and was repaired using open reduction and internal fixation with a volar plate.

If closed reduction is not successful or not able to be maintained, operative intervention may be necessary, particularly when treating an active-elderly patient with involvement of the dominant extremity. A variety of operative techniques have been described, such as external fixation, percutaneous pin fixation, and internal plate fixation. The choice is often surgeon-dependent, and each option has its own, risk–benefit profile.

Functional outcome after distal radius fracture is often favorable, though dependent on patient factors, treatment method, and quality of reduction. Minimally displaced fractures treated in cast immobilization generally do well with minimal loss of pre-injury function. Surgical fixation of displaced fractures demonstrates good to excellent results in 70%–90% of patients with comminuted, unstable fractures.[91].] However, in low-demand elderly patients, even closed treatment of displaced fractures may yield acceptable functional results despite a cosmetic deformity.[92] Ultimately, the treatment of each patient should be individualized and should be based on fracture type, as well as presence of comorbidities, pre-injury functional status, and hand dominance.

Vertebral compression fractures

In the setting of osteoporotic bone, vertebral compression fractures often result from low-energy trauma (i.e., a simple fall or even just sitting down in an awkward or forceful manner). Jensen et al. have estimated that 44% of women aged 70 or older have vertebral compression fractures.[93] Elderly patients with vertebral compression fractures are at an increased risk for developing other osteoporotic fractures, such as those of the distal radius, proximal femur, and proximal humerus.

Vertebral compression fractures most often occur in the mid-thoracic spine. When vertebral collapse occurs over several adjacent segments, kyphosis (humpback deformity) or scoliosis (lateral compression deformity) may develop.

Vertebral compression fractures may present as an incidental finding; however, most are associated with the acute onset of pain. The location of the pain is typically midline in the thoracolumbar spine, but may be referred to the lumbosacral area. If a neurologic deficit is present, metastatic disease, infection, and Paget's disease must be included in the differential diagnosis.

Physical examination demonstrates decreased spinal range of motion, kyphotic deformity, and midline spinal tenderness to palplation. Radiographic evaluation should include standing AP and lateral views. If the patient is too uncomfortable to stand, then supine radiographs may be obtained. A bone scan can be helpful in differentiating old fractures from acute ones. A CT scan can evaluate the integrity of the posterior elements and to identify more severe injuries, such as burst fractures, that can compromise the spinal canal and cause compression of the neural elements.

Historically, a nonoperative approach has been the mainstay for the treatment of vertebral compression fractures. The protocol should involve appropriate analgesia and a short period of rest followed by mobilization.

Advances in operative techniques have changed the management of compression fractures. Vertebroplasty consists of the percutaneous insertion of a large gauge cannula into the vertebral body. Liquid bone cement is then injected into the vertebra. Vertebral kyphoplasty is similar in principle: percutaneous insertion of a balloon tamp is used to create a cavity within the vertebral body followed by the injection of cement to maintain vertebral height. However, this technique has more potential to correct deformity. Recent studies have demonstrated that as compared to traditional nonoperative treatment of vertebral compression fractures, operative intervention improves pain, restores vertebral height, lessens disability, shortens length of hospital stay, and returns the patient to his or her pre-injury level of function.[94] Meta-analysis comparing vertebroplasty to kyphoplasty suggests that kyphoplasty may be superior to vertebroplasty for patients with pronounced kyphotic deformity or loss of vertebral height, and those with vertebral fissures or fractures compromising the posterior integrity of the vertebrae.[95]

Conclusion

Orthopedic injuries are responsible for significant morbidity and mortality in the geriatric population. As life expectancy continues to increase, the prevalence of these problems will increase as well. The ideal treatment should focus on prevention of predisposing risk factors to these injuries, such as osteoporosis and falls. The primary goals of treatment are to provide analgesia, allow as close to immediate patient mobilization as possible, and return the patient to his/her pre-injury level of function. Treatment should include patient education and rehabilitation to optimize outcome. Each treatment plan should be individualized based on patient factors, injury factors, and the other mitigating variables presented above that are unique to each patient, situation, and injury.

References

1. Owens, W.D., J.A. Felts, and E.L. Spitznagel, Jr., ASA physical status classifications: a study of consistency of ratings. *Anesthesiology*, 1978. **49**(4): 239–43.

2. Bloem, B.R., Y.A. Grimbergen, M. Cramer, et al., Prospective assessment of falls in Parkinson's disease. *J Neurol*, 2001. **248**(11): 950–8.

3. McClure, J. and S. Goldsborough, Fractured neck of femur and contralateral intracerebral lesions. *J Clin Pathol*, 1986. **39**(8): 920–2.

4. Soto-Hall, R., Treatment of transcervical fractures complicated by certain common neurological conditions. In: *Instructional Course Lectures XVII*, Reynolds, F.C., Editor. 1960, St. Louis: CV Mosby; 117–120.

5. Loder, R.T., The influence of diabetes mellitus on the healing of closed fractures. *Clin Orthop Relat Res*, 1988 (**232**): 210–6.

6. Ganesh, SP, R. Pietrobon, W.A. Cecilio, et al., The impact of diabetes on patient outcomes after ankle fracture. *J Bone Joint Surg Am*, 2005. **87**(8): 1712–8.

7. Ahmed, LA, R.M. Joakimsen, G.K. Berntsen, et al., Diabetes mellitus and the risk of non-vertebral fractures: the Tromso study. *Osteoporos Int*, 2006. **17** (4): 495–500.

8. Egol, K.A., N.C. Tejwani, M.G. Walsh, et al., Predictors of short-term functional outcome following ankle fracture surgery. *J Bone Joint Surg Am*, 2006. **88**(5):974–9.

9. Lane, J.M. and V.J. Vigorita, Osteoporosis. *J Bone Joint Surg Am*, 1983. **65**(2):274–8.

10. Fulkerson, E., K.A. Egol, E.N. Kubiak, et al., Fixation of diaphyseal fractures with a segmental defect: a biomechanical comparison of locked and conventional plating techniques. *J Trauma*, 2006. **60**(4):830–5.

11. Bhutani, G. and M.C. Gupta, Emerging therapies for the treatment of osteoporosis. *J Midlife Health*. **4**(3): 147–152.

12. Sammartino, A., D. Cirillo, V.D. Mandato, et al., Osteoporosis and cardiovascular disease: benefit-risk of hormone replacement therapy. *J Endocrinol Invest*, 2005. **28**(10 Suppl):80–4.

13. Gass, M. and B. Dawson-Hughes, Preventing osteoporosis-related fractures: an overview. *Am J Med*, 2006. **119**(4 Suppl 1):S3–S11.

14. Kalu, D.N. and E.J. Masoro, The biology of aging, with particular reference to the musculoskeletal system. *Clin Geriatr Med*, 1988. **1**(2):257–67.

15. Tomonaga, M., Histochemical and ultrastructural changes in senile human skeletal muscle. *J Am Geriatr Soc*, 1977. **25**(3):125–31.

16. McCarter, R., Effects of age on contraction of mammalian skeletal muscle. In: *Aging in muscle*, J. D. G. Kalkor, Editor. 1978, New York: Raven Press; 1–22.

17. Murray, M.P., E.H. Duthie, Jr., S.R. Gmbert, et al., Age-related differences in knee muscle strength in normal women. *J Gerontol*, 1985. **40**(3):275–80.

18. Broos, P.L., K.H. Stappaerts, P.M. Rommens, et al., Polytrauma in patients of 65 and over: injury patterns and outcome. *Int Surg*, 1988. **73**(2): 119–22.

19. Martin, R.E. and G. Teberian, Multiple trauma and the elderly patient. *Emerg Med Clin North Am*, 1990. **8**(2):411–20.

20. DeMaria, E.J., P.R. Kenney, M.A. Merriam, et al., Survival after trauma in geriatric patients. *Ann Surg*, 1987. **206**(6):738–43.

21. Horst, H.M., F.n. Obeid, V.J. Sorensen, and B.A. Biins, Factors influencing survival of elderly trauma patients. *Crit Care Med*, 1986. **14**(8):681–4.

22. Oreskovich, M.R., J.D. Howard, M.K. Copass, and C.J. Carrocp, Geriatric trauma: injury patterns and outcome. *J Trauma*, 1984. **24**(7):565–72.

23. Bone, L. and R. Bucholz, The management of fractures in the patient with multiple trauma. *J Bone Joint Surg Am*, 1986. **68**(6):945–9.

24. Gustilo, R.B. and J.T. Anderson, Prevention of infection in the treatment of one thousand and twenty-five open fractures of long bones: retrospective and prospective analyses. *J Bone Joint Surg Am*, 1976. **58**(4):453–8.

25. Gustilo, R.B., L. Simpson, R. Nixon, et al., Analysis of 511 open fractures. *Clin Orthop Relat Res*, 1969. **66**:148–54.

26. Cornell, C.N., J.M. Lane, and A.R. Poynton, Orthopedic management of vertebral and long bone fractures in patients with osteoporosis. *Clin Geriatr Med*, 2003. **19**(2):433–55.

27. Salter, R.B., D.F. Simmonds, B.W. Malcolm, et al., The biological effect of continuous passive motion on the healing of full-thickness defects in articular cartilage. An experimental investigation in the rabbit. *J Bone Joint Surg Am*, 1980. **62**(8): 1232–51.

28. Scott, R.D., R.H. Turner, S.M. Leitzes, and O.E. Aufranc, Femoral fractures in conjunction with total hip replacement. *J Bone Joint Surg Am*, 1975. **57**(4):494–501.

29. Zickel, R.E., V.G. Fietti, Jr., J.F. Lawsing, and G.V. Cochran, A new intramedullary fixation device for the distal third of the femur. *Clin Orthop Relat Res*, 1977. **125**: 185–91.

30. Johansson, J.E., R. McBroom, T.W. Barrington, and G. A. Hunter, Fracture of the ipsilateral femur in patients wih total hip replacement. *J Bone Joint Surg Am*, 1981. **63**(9):1435–42.

31. Clain, A., Secondary Malignant Disease of Bone. *Br J Cancer*, 1965. **19**:15–29.

32. Jaffe, H., *Tumors and Tumorous Conditions of Bones and Joint*. 1958, Philadelphia: Lea & Febiger.

33. Parrish, F.F. and J.A. Murray, Surgical treatment for secondary neoplastic fractures. A retrospective study of ninety-six patients. *J Bone Joint Surg Am*, 1970. **52**(4): 665–86.

34. Harrington, K., Impending pathologic fractures from metastatic malignancy: Evaluation and management. In: *American Academy of Orthopaedic Surgeons Instructional Course Lectures XXXV*, L. Anderson, Editor. 1986, St. Louis: CV Mosby; 357–381.

35. Harrington, K.D., F.H. Sim, J.E. Enis, et al., Methylmethacrylate as an adjunct in internal fixation of pathological fractures. Experience with three hundred and seventy-five cases. *J Bone Joint Surg Am*, 1976. **58**(8): 1047–55.

36. Papapetrou, P.D., Bisphosphonate-associated adverse events. *Hormones (Athens)*, 2009. **8**(2): 96–110.

37. Neviaser, A.S., J.M. Lane, B.A. Lenart, et al., Low-energy femoral shaft fractures associated with alendronate use. *J Orthop Trauma*, 2008. **22**(5): 346–50.

38. Odvina, C.V., J.E. Zerwekh, D.S. Rao, et al., Severely suppressed bone turnover: a potential complication of alendronate therapy. *J Clin Endocrinol Metab*, 2005. **90**(3): 1294–301.

39. Thompson, R.N., J.R. Phillips, S.H. McCauley, et al., Atypical femoral fractures and bisphosphonate treatment: experience in two large United Kingdom teaching hospitals. *J Bone Joint Surg Br*, 2012. **94**(3): 385–90.

40. Shane, E., D. Burr, P.R. Ebeling, et al., Atypical subtrochanteric and diaphyseal femoral fractures: second report of a task force of the American Society for Bone and Mineral Research. *J Bone Miner Res*, 1987. **29**(1): 1–23.

41. Ha, Y.C., M.R. Cho, K.H. Park, et al., Is surgery necessary for femoral insufficiency fractures after long-term bisphosphonate therapy? *Clin Orthop Relat Res*, 2010. **468**(12): 3393–8.

42. Egol, K.A., J.H. Park, C. Prensky, et al., Surgical treatment improves clinical and functional outcomes for patients who sustain incomplete bisphosphonate-related femur fractures. *J Orthop Trauma*, 2013. **27**(6): 331–5.

43. Banffy, M.B., M.S. Vrahas, J.E. Ready, and J.A. Abraham, Nonoperative versus prophylactic treatment of bisphosphonate-associated femoral stress fractures. *Clin Orthop Relat Res*. **469**(7): 2028–34.

44. Sexson, S.B. and J.T. Lehner, Factors affecting hip fracture mortality. *J Orthop Trauma*, 1987. **1**(4):298–305.

45. Kenzora, J.E., R.E. McCarthy, J.D. Lowell, and C.B. Sledge, Hip fracture mortality. Relation to age, treatment, preoperative illness, time of surgery, and complications. *Clin Orthop Relat Res*, 1984(186): 45–56.

46. Zuckerman, J.D., M.L. Skovron, K.J. Koval, et al., Postoperative complications and mortality associated with operative delay in older patients who have a fracture of the hip. *J Bone Joint Surg Am*, 1995. **77** (10):1551–6.

47. Davis, F.M., D.F. Woolner, C. Frampton, et al., Prospective, multi-centre trial of mortality following general or spinal anaesthesia for hip fracture surgery in the elderly. *Br J Anaesth*, 1987. **59**(9):1080–8.

48. Valentin, N., B. Lomholt, J.S. Jensen, et al., Spinal or general anaesthesia for surgery of the fractured hip? A prospective study of mortality in 578 patients. *Br J Anaesth*, 1986. **58**(3):284–91.

49. Modig, J., T. Borg, G. Karlstrom, et al., Thromboembolism after total hip replacement: role of epidural and general anesthesia. *Anesth Analg*, 1983. **62**(2):174–80.

50. Brody, J.A., Prospects for an ageing population. *Nature*, 1985. **315**(6019):463–6.

51. Frandsen, P.A. and T. Kruse, Hip fractures in the county of Funen, Denmark. Implications of demographic aging and changes in incidence rates. *Acta Orthop Scand*, 1983. **54**(5):681–6.

52. Praemer, A., S. Furner, and D.P. Rice, *Musculoskeletal Conditions in the United States*. 1992, Park Ridge, IL: American Academy of Orthopaedic Surgeons; **vii**, 199.

53. Greenspan, S.L., S.L. Myers, L.A. Maitland, et al., Fall severity and bone mineral density as risk factors for hip fracture in ambulatory elderly. *JAMA*, 1994. **271**(2):128–33.

54. Hinton, R.Y. and G.S. Smith, The association of age, race, and sex with the location of proximal femoral fractures in the elderly. *J Bone Joint Surg Am*, 1993. **75**(5):752–9.

55. Hinton, R.Y., D.W. Lennox, F.R. Ebert, et al., Relative rates of fracture of the hip in the United States. Geographic, sex, and age variations. *J Bone Joint Surg Am*, 1995. **77**(5):695–702.

56. Garraway, W.M., R.N. Stauffer, L.T. Kurland, and W. M. O'Fallon, Limb fractures in a defined population. II. Orthopedic treatment and utilization of health care. *Mayo Clin Proc*, 1979. **54**(11): 708–13.

57. Johnell, O. and I. Sernbo, Health and social status in patients with hip fractures and controls. *Age Ageing*, 1986. **15**(5):285–91.

58. Uden, G. and B. Nilsson, Hip fracture frequent in hospital. *Acta Orthop Scand*, 1986. **57**(5):428–30.

59. Rizzo, P.F., E.S. Gould, J.P. Lynden, and S.E. Asnis, Diagnosis of occult fractures about the hip. Magnetic resonance imaging compared with bone-scanning. *J Bone Joint Surg Am*, 1993. **75**(3): 395–401.

60. Parker, M.J., J.W. Myles, J.K. CAnandramer, and R. Drewett, Cost-benefit analysis of hip fracture treatment. *J Bone Joint Surg Br*, 1992. **74**(2):261–4.

61. Colwell, C.W., Jr., T.E. Spiro, A.A. Trowbridge, et al., Use of enoxaparin, a low-molecular-weight heparin, and unfractionated heparin for the prevention of deep venous thrombosis after elective hip replacement. A clinical trial comparing efficacy and safety. Enoxaparin Clinical Trial Group. *J Bone Joint Surg Am*, 1994. **76**(1):3–14.

62. Geerts, W.H., R.M. Jay, K.I. Code, et al., A comparison of low-dose heparin with low-molecular-weight heparin as prophylaxis against venous thromboembolism after major trauma. *N Engl J Med*, 1996. **335**(10):701–7.

63. Merli, G.J., Update. Deep vein thrombosis and pulmonary embolism prophylaxis in orthopedic surgery. *Med Clin North Am*, 1993. **77**(2): 397–411.

64. Kinov, P., P.P. Tanchev, M. Ellis, and G. Volpin, Antithrombotic prophylaxis in major orthopaedic surgery: an historical overview and update of current recommendations. *Int Orthop*. **38**(1): 169–75.

65. Koval, K.J., M.L. Skovron, G.B. Aharanoff, et al., Ambulatory ability after hip fracture. A prospective study in geriatric patients. *Clin Orthop Relat Res*, 1995. **310**: 150–9.

66. White, B.L., W.D. Fisher, and C.A. Laurin, Rate of mortality for elderly patients after fracture of the hip in the 1980's. *J Bone Joint Surg Am*, 1987. **69**(9):1335–40.

67. Tajeu, G.S., E. Delzell, W. Smith, et al., *Death, debility, and destitution following hip fracture*. J Gerontol A Biol Sci Med Sci, 2014. **69**(3): 346–53.

68. Aharonoff, G.B., K.J. Koval, M.L. Skovron, and J.D. Zuckerman, Hip fractures in the elderly: predictors of one year mortality. *J Orthop Trauma*, 1997. **11**(3):162–5.

69. Seitz, D.P., G.M. Anderson, P.C. Austin, et al., Effects of impairment in activities of daily living on predicting mortality following hip fracture surgery in studies using administrative healthcare databases. *BMC Geriatr*. **14**(1): 9.

70. Koval, K.J., K.D. Friend, G.B. Aharonoff, and J.D. Zuckerman, Weight bearing after hip fracture: a prospective series of 596 geriatric hip fracture patients. *J Orthop Trauma*, 1996. **10**(8):526–30.

71. Koval, K.J., D.A. Sala, F.J. Kummer, and J.D. Zuckerman, Postoperative weight-bearing after a fracture of the femoral neck or an intertrochanteric fracture. *J Bone Joint Surg Am*, 1998. **80**(3):352–6.

72. Probe, R. and R. Ward, Internal fixation of femoral neck fractures. *J Am Acad Orthop Surg*, 2006. **14**(9):565–71.

73. Schmidt, A.H. and M.F. Swiontkowski, Femoral neck fractures. *Orthop Clin North Am*, 2002. **33**(1): 97–111, viii.

74. Cobb, A.G. and P.H. Gibson, Screw fixation of subcapital fractures of the femur – a better method of treatment? *Injury*, 1986. **17**(4): 259–64.

75. Garden, R.S., Malreduction and avascular necrosis in subcapital fractures of the femur. *J Bone Joint Surg Br*, 1971. **53**(2):183–97.

76. Stromqvist, B., L.I. Hansson, L.T. Nilsson, and K.G. Thorngren, Hook-pin fixation in femoral neck fractures. A two-year follow-up study of 300 cases. *Clin Orthop Relat Res*, 1987(218): 58–62.

77. Bentley, G., Treatment of nondisplaced fractures of the femoral neck. *Clin Orthop Relat Res*, 1980(152): 93–101.

78. Calder, S.J., G.H. Anderson, C. Jagger, et al., Unipolar or bipolar prosthesis for displaced intracapsular hip

fracture in octogenarians: a randomised prospective study. *J Bone Joint Surg Br*, 1996. **78**(3):391–4.

79. Keating, J.F., A. Grant, M. Masson, et al., Randomized comparison of reduction and fixation, bipolar hemiarthroplasty, and total hip arthroplasty: treatment of displaced intracapsular hip fractures in healthy older patients. *J Bone Joint Surg Am*, 2006. **88**(2):249–60.

80. Hardy, D.C., P.Y. Descamps, P. Krallis, et al., Use of an intramedullary hip-screw compared with a compression hip-screw with a plate for intertrochanteric femoral fractures. A prospective, randomized study of one hundred patients. *J Bone Joint Surg Am*, 1998. **80**(5):618–30.

81. Adams, C.I., C.M. Robinson, C.M. Court-Brown, and M.M. McQueen, Prospective randomized controlled trial of an intramedullary nail versus dynamic screw and plate for intertrochanteric fractures of the femur. *J Orthop Trauma*, 2001. **15**(6):394–400.

82. Crawford, C.H., A.L. Malkani, S. Cordray, et al., The trochanteric nail versus the sliding hip screw for intertrochanteric hip fractures: a review of 93 cases. *J Trauma*, 2006. **60**(2): 325–8; discussion 328–9.

83. Stiell, I.G., R.D. McKnight, G.H. Greenberg, et al., Implementation of the Ottawa ankle rules. *JAMA*, 1994. **271**(11):827–32.

84. McConnell, T., W. Creevy, and P. Tornetta, 3rd, Stress examination of supination external rotation-type fibular fractures. *J Bone Joint Surg Am*, 2004. **86**-A(10): 2171–8.

85. Ramsey, P.L. and W. Hamilton, Changes in tibiotalar area of contact caused by lateral talar shift. *J Bone Joint Surg Am*, 1976. **58**(3):356–7.

86. Beauchamp, C.G., N.R. Clay, and P.W. Thexton, Displaced ankle fractures in patients over 50 years of age. *J Bone Joint Surg Br*, 1983. **65**(3):329–32.

87. Ali, M.S., C.A.N. McLaren, E. Rouholamin, and B.T. O'Connor, Ankle fractures in the elderly: nonoperative or operative treatment. *J Orthop Trauma*, 1987. **1**(4):275–80.

88. Neer, C.S., 2nd, Displaced proximal humeral fractures. II. Treatment of three-part and four-part displacement. *J Bone Joint Surg Am*, 1970. **52**(6): 1090–103.

89. Neer, C.S., 2nd, Displaced proximal humeral fractures. I. Classification and evaluation. *J Bone Joint Surg Am*, 1970. **52**(6): 1077–89.

90. Alffram, P.A. and G.C. Bauer, Epidemiology of fractures of the forearm: a biomechanical investigation of bone strength. *J Bone Joint Surg Am*, 1962. **44**-A: 105–14.

91. Rozental, T.D. and P.E. Blazar, Functional outcome and complications after volar plating for dorsally displaced, unstable fractures of the distal radius. *J Hand Surg Am*, 2006. **31**(3):359–65.

92. Young, B.T. and G.M. Rayan, Outcome following nonoperative treatment of displaced distal radius fractures in low-demand patients older than 60 years. *J Hand Surg Am*, 2000. **25**(1):19–28.

93. Majd, M.E., S. Farley, and R.T. Holt, Preliminary outcomes and efficacy of the first 360 consecutive kyphoplasties for the treatment of painful osteoporotic vertebral compression fractures. *Spine J*, 2005. **5**(3):244–55.

94. Prather, H., L. Van Dillen, J.P. Metzler, et al., Prospective measurement of function and pain in patients with non-neoplastic compression fractures treated with vertebroplasty. *J Bone Joint Surg Am*, 2006. **88**(2):334–41.

95. Ma, X.L., D. Xing, J.X. Ma, et al., Balloon kyphoplasty versus percutaneous vertebroplasty in treating osteoporotic vertebral compression fracture: grading the evidence through a systematic review and meta-analysis. *Eur Spine J*. **21**(9): 1844–59.

Dermatologic conditions in the elderly

Katherine M. Varman, MD, and Christopher J. Sayed, MD

Introduction

Although the aging process affects every organ system, the physical signs of aging are most apparent on the skin. The skin undergoes many stages of evolution from embryogenesis to young adulthood, and it continues to accrue changes as we age through adulthood. As with any organ, many of the changes are attributable to the normal aging process, but the skin is also burdened with a disproportionate share of environmental exposures that occur through the routine course of our lives. Most notably, ultraviolet radiation (UVR) plays a major role in accelerating the natural aging process of the skin.[1, 2] Many of the stigmata associated with normal aging, such as lentigines, are mostly or entirely due to UVR. This photo-induced skin damage is evident by the stark difference in skin quality between areas exposed to chronic sun exposure such as the face and the double-clothed areas such as the buttocks or female breasts.

The accumulation of natural and UVR-induced changes of the skin results in a radical alteration in both its structure and function. As a result, elderly patients are more susceptible to a number of primary cutaneous inflammatory, infectious, and neoplastic processes than their younger counterparts.[3] Elderly patients are also at risk of developing skin conditions that are related to common systemic diseases such as diabetes, vascular disease, and internal malignancy. It is important that clinicians understand these associations so that the skin conditions are recognized promptly and managed effectively. As the average human lifespan continues to lengthen and the aging population grows, we will continue to see an increase in the amount of skin disease encountered in clinical practice.[4]

In this chapter we will explore the changes in structure and function of the skin that are a result of both natural and UVR-induced aging. The manner in which these changes relate to skin disease in the elderly will be discussed, as well as how to appropriately evaluate and manage skin disease with special consideration for this population.

Structure and function of the skin

Introduction to structure and function

The skin has many important functions in addition to serving as a physical barrier to the environment. It plays a role in vitamin D synthesis, prevention of water loss, and protection from pathogens. It also has a complex immunological microenvironment that interacts with external pathogens and antigens and also provides immune surveillance for cutaneous neoplasms. The skin is composed of distinct layers with overlapping and complimentary roles. Each of these layers undergoes unique changes during the aging process that affect the way they function.

The thinnest and most superficial layer of the skin is the epidermis. The width varies widely, with the thickest epidermis found on the palms and soles and the thinnest on the eyelids. It is composed primarily of keratinocytes, but melanocytes and Langerhans cells are also found in this compartment. The stratum corneum is the outermost layer, comprising mainly lipids and proteins that are crucial for the barrier function of the skin.

Below the epidermis lies the thin basement membrane zone, which divides the epidermis from the dermis. The dermis provides most of the elasticity and durability of the skin. It is composed predominantly of type 3 collagen, which undergoes constant remodeling via production by fibroblasts and degradation by matrix metalloproteinases (MMPs). Unlike the epidermis, the dermis also harbors the nerves, blood vessels, and the adnexal structures of the skin.

Reichel's Care of the Elderly, 7th Edition, ed. Jan Busby-Whitehead *et al.* Published by Cambridge University Press.
© Cambridge University Press 2016.

Table 35.1 Summary of changes in skin structure and function with aging

Change in skin structure or composition	Location	Effect on function
Decreased production of lipid and filaggrin	Epidermis	Xerosis (dry skin), pruritus, decreased physical barrier function
Decreased keratinocyte proliferation	Epidermis	Skin fragility, delayed wound healing
Decreased collagen production and quality	Dermis	Dermal atrophy, skin fragility, easy bruising
Decreased elastin production and quality	Dermis	Decreased skin elasticity, increased fragility
Decreased Langerhans cell numbers and function	Epidermis, dermis	Increased skin infection with candida, dermatophytes, cellulitis Increased risk of cutaneous neoplasm
Fewer melanocytes	Epidermis	Mottled pigmentation, sallow color, increased photosensitivity
Decreased dermal blood vessels	Dermis	Impaired thermoregulation
Decreased subcutaneous fat	Subcutis	Decreased insulation for thermoregulation Decreased cushioning, resulting in increased bruising and risk of pressure ulcers
Decreased eccrine glands	Subcutis	Impaired sweating and thermoregulation
Loss of hair follicles and hair follicle melanocytes	Dermis and subcutis	Decreased hair density Graying of hair

Source: Information from references 1, 3, 5–7, 11.

Deeper still, the subcutaneous fat resides in a plane beneath the dermis and is also present over the entire surface of the body. It is home to medium-sized vessels and nerves and is primarily composed of adipocytes. The functions of the skin described in this section can be attributed to these underlying structures, and alterations in these structures are directly linked to the functional changes summarized in Table 35.1 and discussed in the following paragraphs.[5–7]

Physical barrier function

The epidermis, dermis, and subcutaneous fat all provide physical barrier function, and the epidermis is on the front line. As keratinocytes mature, they fill with proteins and lipids that form the bricks and mortar of the stratum corneum at the surface of the skin. This water-insoluble barrier prevents loss of moisture from the skin and protects it from environmental exposures. The dermis and subcutaneous fat provide both cushion and elasticity that protect the skin from physical trauma as well.[5]

As the epidermis ages, it produces fewer lipids and vital proteins such as filaggrin, which helps prevent epidermal water loss. This results in drier skin that becomes rough and scaly. It also allows for greater exposure to environmental hazards and a predisposition toward eczematous conditions such as asteatotic dermatitis.[8]

Skin tears caused by skin fragility are a frequent finding in photo-aged skin.[8, 9] With time, epidermal proliferation is reduced and leads to atrophy of the epidermis and decreased length of rete ridges, ultimately resulting in less contact with the dermis. Decreased collagen production by fibroblasts and increased matrix metalloproteinase activity, which is enhanced by UVR, result in an average decrease in dermal thickness of up 20% in the elderly compared to younger patients.[10] These changes, coupled with decreased skin elasticity, cause the skin to be a less effective physical barrier to trauma as time passes.[8–11]

Immunologic barrier function

Given its large surface area and constant interaction with the external environment, it is not surprising that the skin is a major hub of immunologic activity. In fact, some estimates suggest that the skin is home to a resident T-cell population that is twice as large as the population of T-cells found in circulation. The skin has the important task of interacting with both harmless and noxious environmental antigens, and must determine how to respond to each appropriately.

Langerhans cells are the primary antigen-presenting cells in the dermis and have a complex interaction with both skin-resident T-cells and those residing in regional lymph nodes. Epidermal Langerhans cells are reduced in number by up to 50% in the elderly and have reduced capacity to stimulate T-cell proliferation,[12] thus making this population more susceptible to cutaneous infections, such as cellulitis, candidiasis, and dermatophytosis.[13] Decreased immune surveillance also leads to increased susceptibility to cutaneous neoplasms.[3]

Delayed-type hypersensitivity responses are also noted to decline in elderly patients. This likely occurs through a combination of impaired ability of skin-resident T-cells to proliferate and respond to antigenic stimulation as well as an increased proportion of regulatory T-cells seen in older patients. The net effect is a decrease in local secretion of inflammatory cytokines – such as TNF-α and IFN-γ – that are responsible for triggering migration of circulating macrophages, neutrophils, and lymphocytes to the skin.[14]

Protection from ultraviolet light

Ultraviolet light is the most ubiquitous and important mutagen that the skin faces. The skin's ability to protect itself through the production and distribution of pigment is an important adaptation for the prevention of both acute and chronic UV-induced changes. Melanin-containing organelles called melanosomes are produced in melanocytes and transferred to keratinocytes, where they are distributed in a fashion that maximally shields the DNA of each cell. As the skin ages, decreases in the number of melanocytes and irregularities in their distribution are manifested as mottled pigmentation and a decrease in number of nevi. Ultimately, this results in increased photosensitivity and susceptibility to UV-induced DNA damage in the epidermis.[11, 15]

Thermoregulation

Maintaining temperature homeostasis is a complicated task, and the skin plays a critical role as the body's primary interface with the external environment. Dilation of the cutaneous vasculature leads to increased shedding of heat, while, conversely, constriction results in conservation of heat. As the number of dermal vessels decreases over time, the ability to regulate temperature homeostasis through this mechanism is diminished.[1, 16–18] The loss and redistribution of subcutaneous fat over time also leads to decreased insulating properties of the skin. The ability to appropriately cool is also challenged by a decrease in the number of eccrine glands responsible for sweating.[1, 18]

Wound healing

The role of the skin as a physical barrier leads to frequent trauma, and when compromised it must regenerate in a fashion that is both rapid and durable. The stages of wound healing are well organized and include the inflammatory phase, proliferative phase, and maturation phase. Although each stage is characterized by a particular set of cytokines and enzymatic activity, their time courses overlap.

The inflammatory phase, which predominates in the first five to seven days of wound healing, starts with coagulation. This is mediated by platelets and the coagulation cascade. As bleeding slows, platelets release important mediators, such as TGF-α, TGF-β, and platelet-derived growth factor. Together these stimulate the first phases of fibroblast and keratinocyte proliferation, chemotaxis of neutrophils and macrophages, and angiogenesis. As neutrophils and macrophages arrive, the cytokine profile is modified through secretion of TNF-α, IL-1, IL-10, and fibroblast growth factor. These inflammatory cytokines help stimulate further epidermal and dermal proliferation, angiogenesis, and prevention of infection.

As these processes accelerate, the proliferative phase begins its five- to seven-day course. Granulation tissue composed of macrophages, fibroblasts, and endothelial cells fill the tissue defect. As an extracellular matrix composed of collagen III, fibrin, and fibronectin is formed, it stimulates the proliferation and migration of keratinocytes that gradually cover the wound.

Following reepithelialization, the wound enters the maturation phase. Proliferation slows, and fibroblasts and matrix metalloproteinases begin the months-long task of forming and remodeling dermal collagen. Collagen III is broken down and replaced by collagen I, and fibroblasts transition to myofibroblasts. As these changes occur, the wound contracts and the tensile strength gradually increases, although it never reaches more than 70% of the tensile strength of normal skin.[20–22]

Despite popular belief, only moderate effects on wound healing seem to occur as part of normal aging. Fibroblast function, which is crucial to wound maturation and scar strength, appears to be preserved during the aging process. Deposition of collagen during wound formation seems to be similar among younger and older patients, though there is likely a small decrease in the rate of keratinocyte proliferation and reepithelialization. On the other hand, there is an increased proportion of elastin formation in wounds in older patients, which may lead to improved appearance of mature scars.[22–24]

Many of the perceived effects of aging on wound healing are due to comorbidities that are far more common in the older population. Venous incompetence increases over time, and the increased venous pressures that result lead to leukocyte trapping in small venules and capillaries. Increased pressure also results in endothelial permeability, which allows leakage of erythrocytes and leukocytes. As these cells accumulate in the dermis, they contribute to an inflammatory profile that often slows the transition from the inflammatory phase to the proliferative phase of wound healing. Diabetes also increases significantly with age and leads to both an arteriolopathy and autonomic instability that causes venous shunting away from the skin. Impaired delivery of oxygen and nutrients to wounds ultimately slows the healing process.[25, 26]

Physical factors such as decreased subcutaneous fat for cushioning and decreased mobility in the elderly lead to a predisposition to develop pressure ulcers. Medications are an additional environmental factor that are more pervasive in older patients and affect wound healing through their effects on coagulation, inflammation, and proliferation. Chronic wounds are a major cause for morbidity in elderly patients as well as a source of significant financial burden to the medical system.[26]

Aesthetic function

The signs of physical aging are a common cause of distress among patients, and they are most easily perceived on the skin. Physical beauty has been shown to have a major influence on socioeconomic success and happiness, and the typical changes seen

with aging are often a major source of patient concern. Lentigines, seborrheic keratoses, rhytides (wrinkles), cherry angiomas, and many other benign and normal skin changes are telltale signs of the normal aging process, many of which are encouraged by sun exposure. Structural changes of the face such as redistribution of subcutaneous fat away from the cheeks, loss of muscle mass, resorption of bone of the forehead and mandible, and loss of elasticity of the dermis all play major roles in the physical manifestations of aging.[1, 11, 27–31] As systemic conditions such as diabetes and venous insufficiency become more common with advancing age, their physical manifestations also become more common and make them part of the physical stigmata of the aging process.[1, 10] Many procedures and products have been developed in attempts to mask the visible signs of aging, and they vary widely in their costs and risks. It is important to realize that many patients undergo these procedures and may present with complications related to them.

Photoaging, or dermatoheliosis, is a major driving factor for many of the changes seen with aging. UVA light (320 nm–400 nm) is responsible for many of the immediate effects seen with sun exposure such as immediate erythema and photosensitivity reactions (i.e., with HCTZ, antibiotics), but is also a major contributor to the process of photoaging. UVB light (290 nm–320 nm) plays a major role in photocarcinogenesis and is a major cause of sunburn and tanning. As both contribute to photoaging, the skin develops telangiectasias, a sallow hue, translucency, dyspigmentation, dryness, and wrinkling. In highly sun-exposed sites, elastic fibers fragment and accumulate, leading to actinic elastosis, which is noted as a pebbly texture frequently seen on the forehead and temples. Lentigines, nevi, and seborrheic keratosis also become more common in sun-exposed locations.[1, 10, 11]

Mitigating the effects of photoaging

Given the inevitability of the aging process, it is not surprising that there is a large market and need for products and strategies to curb its effects on the skin. Although the physical stigmata of aging are common targets of intervention, the need for prevention of skin cancer and other pathologic responses to UV light are major drivers of this trend as well.

Broad spectrum sunscreens that block both UVA and UVB have been proven to reduce the signs of photoaging (grade 2B) as well as the incidence of melanoma and nonmelanoma skin cancer. Inorganic physical blockers such as zinc oxide and titanium dioxide are effective, broad spectrum components of many commercially available sunscreens. Many organic blockers are also available with varying absorption spectra, levels of water resistance, and durations of stability. For this reason, multiple organic ingredients are combined in most commercially available sunscreens to allow for complimentary effects.[33]

Topical retinoids are the most effective and frequently prescribed medications used to address the changes associated with photoaging. Topical retinoic acid, also called tretinoin, is the most commonly used and best researched drug in this class. When used daily over the course of several weeks or months, topical retinoids are moderately effective for the prevention and improvement of roughness, fine wrinkling, and dyspigmentation of the skin. Correlating histologic changes can also be observed, with improved dispersion of melanin, increased collagen, and decreased cellular atypia in sun-damaged skin (grade A).[1, 34–36] Alpha-hydroxy acids found in many over-the-counter cosmeceuticals have been shown to lead to similar improvements, although generally to a lesser extent than topical retinoids (grade B).[37]

There have also been remarkable advances in physical modalities for the treatment of photoaged skin. Neurotoxins such as onabotulinumtoxin-A (Botox) block the release of acetylcholine from motor neurons and are able to reduce the appearance of rhytides that develop with repeated facial movement. Dermal fillers such as hyaluronic acid are also frequently used to treat superficial rhytides and replace volume in locations where it has been lost over time. Various laser procedures, radiofrequency devices, dermabrasion, chemical peels, and surgical procedures have also been developed, and each carries a specific set of potential adverse outcomes. Patients pursuing these treatments should be appropriately counseled on these risks and have access to appropriate follow-up when needed.

Appendages: hair, nails, and glands

Hair has a major cosmetic function for most adults, and its distribution and thickness typically change with time. The majority of patients experience graying of >50% of their hair, and male- and female-pattern alopecia are common causes or hair loss. Hair normally cycles between the active anagen and resting telogen phases, and a larger percentage of hair remains in telogen as patients age. Although hair typically thins on the scalp over time, it often becomes more common on the upper lips and chins of female patients and on the ears, backs, and noses of males.

Similarly, nail growth slows with aging, and the nails become thinner and more brittle. Breakage is more common, and the rate of onychomycosis increases as more patients become infected over time. Complete regrowth of fingernails usually takes about six months, and toenails take up to 18 months. The rate of growth slows by about 35% by the age of 80.[1, 18, 19]

Varying changes are seen in different glands of the skin during the aging process. Decreased numbers of eccrine glands results in decreased sweating and reduced ability for thermoregulation. On the other hand, sebaceous glands required for lipid production on the skin actually increase in number and volume with time. This is sometimes observed as sebaceous hyperplasia, but, despite this increase, the production of lipids decreases by 23%–32% every decade in the aging population. The result is increasing dry, scaly, and pruritic skin.[1, 19, 32]

Benign skin lesions

Acrochordons

Acrochordons, commonly referred to as skin tags, are frequently encountered benign growths in elderly patients. They are typically soft, skin-colored, pedunculated papules found in intertriginous areas such as the neck, axilla, and inguinal folds. The stalk is typically 1 mm–3 mm in diameter, while the attached body can range from 1 mm to over a centimeter. In some instances they are hyperpigmented or have a slightly verrucous surface. Patients who are obese, especially those with acanthosis nigricans, are particularly predisposed to the development of acrochordons. Screening for diabetes mellitis is indicated in these patients, as both acrochordons and acanthosis nigricans are frequent associations.[38]

Although acrochordons are usually asymptomatic and incidental findings in most patients, they are occasionally traumatized by friction in patients who are active or by clothing or jewelry (depending on the location). Cryotherapy of the base or snip removal with forceps and scissors are quick and effective

481

when necessary, but in most cases removal is sought for cosmetic purposes. Larger acrochordons may require local anesthesia and removal with scissors or a blade.

Cherry angiomas

Cherry angiomas (also called cherry hemangiomas) begin to arise in the third and fourth decades of life and are nearly ubiquitous in older patients. These bright red vascular papules can be scattered over any cutaneous surface and are typically 1 mm–5 mm in diameter, although they can occasionally approach a centimeter in size. They are much more common in patients with fair skin and are almost always asymptomatic. Treatment with a vascular laser or electrosurgery can be performed for cosmetic purposes, but intervention is typically unnecessary. Rarely, spontaneous thrombosis results in sudden necrosis and biopsy may be performed due to suspicion of skin cancer, given the abrupt change. Rare reports of multiple eruptive cherry angiomas have been reported in patients with solid and hematologic malignancy, but in the vast majority of cases they are no cause for alarm.[1, 39]

Seborrheic keratosis

Although seborrheic keratoses are extremely common, they are a frequent cause of concern among patients and medical providers. Although these pigmented papules and plaques typically have a classic waxy, "stuck-on" appearance (Figure 35.1), they occasionally raise concern for melanoma due to variations in pigment and growth to sizes greater than what would be expected for a melanocytic nevus. Most are less than a centimeter in diameter, but they can grow to several centimeters in size. They can be few or numerous. These growths arise in the epidermis, are composed of keratinocytes, and, unlike melanocytic proliferations, frequently have a waxy or verrucous texture. Patients often report the ability to partially remove or "pick-off" portions with their fingernails, which can be reproduced in clinic with a tendency of the lesions to crumble slightly with blunt manipulation.

Recognition and reassurance are all that is typically required when counseling patients. Although UV-induced signature mutations have been described in seborrheic keratosis and they have a predilection to

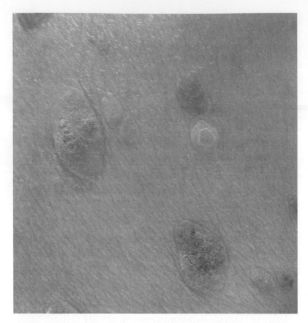

Figure 35.1 Seborrheic keratoses: stuck-on, waxy, crumbling, hyperpigmented papules and plaques. (A black-and-white version of this figure will appear in some formats. For the color version, please refer to the plate section.)

arise in sun-exposed areas, they have no malignant potential. Treatment is sometimes sought when they become inflamed or pruritic. Irritation can occur spontaneously or due to friction from clothing as a result of their predisposition to occur along the waistline or in the inframammary folds in female patients. Inflamed seborrheic keratoses often have a pink or crusted appearance and may be confused for melanoma or non-melanoma skin cancer in sun-exposed areas, which occasionally leads to biopsy. Although no reliably useful topical treatments exist, cryotherapy, curettage, sharp removal, and a number of other destructive methods can be quite effective for lesions that are inflamed or cosmetically displeasing to patients.

Solar lentigines

The solar lentigo, also referred to as an actinic lentigo, is proliferation of melanocytes with increased melanin production limited to the basal layer of the epidermis. As the name implies, it is found with increased incidence in sun-exposed skin.[40] Although they have colloquially been referred to as "liver spots," there is no relationship to hepatic disease. They are usually multiple on the shoulders, face, forearms, and dorsal hands, but can affect any surface with a history of natural or artificial UVR exposure. The pigmentation is typically relatively evenly distributed, and size can range from a few millimeters to 3 cm–4 cm in size. The borders often have a moth-eaten or slightly notched appearance.

Lentigines often darken with exposure to UV light but do not completely fade over time in its absence as is typical of ephilides (freckles). Lentigines are benign; however, the most challenging differential diagnosis is with lentigo maligna, as both can show subtle irregularities of pigment, slightly irregular borders, or sizes that are not typical for most benign melanocytic lesions.[41]

Actinic purpura

Actinic purpura, also referred to as senile or solar purpura, are found in approximately 12% of patients over the age of 50 years, and in up to one-third of elderly patients in long-term care facilities.[42] These asymptomatic, nonpalpable purpura are most common on surfaces routinely exposed to minor trauma, such as the forearms (Figure 35.2). As normal aging and UV light contribute to decreases in collagen and subcutaneous fat, the skin and microvasculature become more susceptible to the routine shearing and mechanical forces that occur with daily activities. More often than not, a specific trigger for a lesion cannot be recalled. The result is the leakage of red blood cells and formation of noninflammatory purpura.

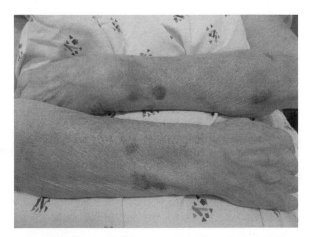

Figure 35.2 Actinic purpura: purpura classically located on the forearm with absence of yellow-green hues. (A black-and-white version of this figure will appear in some formats. For the color version, please refer to the plate section.)

Typical resolution occurs over the course of three weeks without the evolution of yellow and green coloration seen in traumatic purpura. Persistent hyperpigmentation following repeated purpura may result due to hemosiderin deposition over time. Anticoagulants such as aspirin and warfarin can predispose patients to larger and more frequent purpura. Interestingly, decreases in dermal collagen resulting in actinic purpura may correlate to decreased bone collagen and osteoporosis.[43] Palpable purpura, especially on sites beyond the forearms, should raise suspicion of vasculitis. The presence of purpura on the trunk and proximal extremities that evolve with yellow and green coloration should trigger concern for elder abuse.

Other common benign skin lesions

Sebaceous hyperplasia

Sebaceous hyperplasia is commonly noted on the face of elderly patients and occasionally confused with basal cell carcinoma. These symmetric yellow papules typically have a central punctum from which a small droplet of sebum can sometimes be expressed with pressure. They are usually multiple and lack the arborizing vessels seen in basal cell carcinoma. Cosmetic destructive therapies can be pursued.

Epidermal inclusion cysts

Epidermal inclusion cysts (epidermoid cyst, cyst of the follicular infundibulum, sebaceous cyst) are derived of a wall of keratinizing epithelium depositing keratinocytes into a central cavity. They are clinically recognized as dermal or subcutaneous mobile nodules that are usually asymptomatic and do not require treatment. A central pore is sometimes seen, from which the cheesy, foul-smelling contents can be expressed. Manipulation and trauma sometimes lead to rupture of the wall and subsequent inflammatory response. Incision and drainage typically leads to recurrence, thus an excision including the entire wall of the cyst is a more effective method to prevent recurrence. Episodes of acute inflammation can be treated with incision and drainage or intralesional triamcinolone for temporary relief or with antibiotics if superinfection is strongly suspected.[44]

Malignant skin lesions

Skin cancers are the most common malignancies encountered in the United States and are estimated to affect one in five Americans at some point in their lives. Nonmelanoma skin cancer is not required to be reported to cancer registries so incidence estimates vary, but an estimate based on census data and insurance claims in 2006 suggested an incidence of 3.5 million annually with a cost of over $1.5 billion to the medical system. The majority of these will be in the geriatric population.[1, 45–47] Basal cell and squamous cell carcinomas, referred to generally as nonmelanoma skin cancers, make up the large majority of the skin cancers diagnosed. Most are due to sun exposure and are easily treated. Melanoma makes up a smaller percent of skin cancers but leads to the bulk of skin-cancer-related mortality. All types of skin cancers have shown trends toward increasing frequency over the last three decades, likely due to an increasingly aged population. Although strong evidence supporting routine screening skin exams is lacking, it is generally recommended every one to three years after the age of 40, depending on such risk factors as fair skin, family history, and history of UV exposure. For patients at low risk, this can be performed by a primary care physician who is comfortable providing full skin examinations. Patients with a history of skin cancer, multiple atypical pigmented lesions, >50 moles, or long-term immunosuppression should have an ongoing relationship with a dermatologist for routine monitoring.[1, 46] Increasing evidence supports the use of sunscreen and sun avoidance to prevent the incidence of melanoma and nonmelanoma skin cancers, including in patients who have a prior history of skin cancer.[48–50]

Basal cell carcinoma

Of the millions of nonmelanoma skin cancers that develop yearly, 75%–80% of these will be basal cell carcinoma (BCC). Fortunately, BCC has very little metastatic potential and, other than in rare cases, is limited to the skin. Men are affected at a rate of 1.5–2:1 when compared to women, and 75%–80% of BCCs will be found on the head and neck.[45–47] The progenitor cell is likely located in the infundibular section of the pilosebaceous unit; thus BCC does not develop on the palms or soles where pilosebaceous units are absent.[48] The median age of development is 68 years. UVR is the main contributor to the development of BCC, specifically via mutations in the gene *patched* (PTCH1).[51] There is good data demonstrating that regular use of sunscreen and avoidance of tanning (by tanning beds or natural UV exposure)

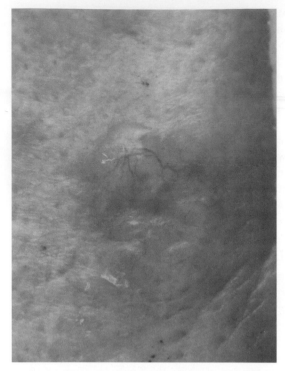

Figure 35.3 Basal cell carcinoma: pearly papule in the retro-auricular area with arborizing telangiectasias. (A black-and-white version of this figure will appear in some formats. For the color version, please refer to the plate section.)

can reduce the lifetime risk of developing this malignancy. Lightly colored hair and eyes, freckles, fair skin, immunosuppression, history of sunburns, radiation exposure, and family history can all contribute to increased risk.[1, 46]

The classic appearance of basal cell carcinoma is a pearly papule or small plaque with arborizing telangiectasias and a rolled border (Figure 35.3). Many subtypes have been described, with the most common being superficial, nodular, and morpheaform (infiltrative, characterized by scarlike features). Ulceration is a finding that is frequently shared among subtypes. Up to 10% of BCCs may have pigment, which may lead to confusion with melanoma. Although mortality is highly unusual, morbidity is frequent. Some BCCs will remain superficial and slow-growing over the course of years, while some will take on aggressive growth patterns and invade into the deep dermis, subcutaneous fat, muscle, or even cartilage and bone. This is especially true on high-risk locations (such as the nose, eyelids, and ears). A small shave biopsy is typically sufficient for diagnosis.[52]

Given the high frequency with which BCC is encountered, it is not surprising that many forms of treatment have been developed. Superficial basal cell carcinoma is contiguous with the epidermis and most easily treated. Electrodessication and curettage allows for rapid treatment in the outpatient setting, little discomfort, and high cure rates. Topical therapy with imiquimod or 5-fluoruracil cream has lower cure rates, but is relatively easy to use unless the patient lacks the physical or mental capacity to apply it regularly. Nodular basal cell carcinoma is treated very effectively with electrodessication and curettage but is less successfully treated with topical therapy in most instances. Standard excisions with 4-mm margins and local anesthesia are reliable in the outpatient setting for most types of basal cell carcinoma and is the treatment of choice for more aggressive subtypes when it is feasible.

For high-risk or cosmetically sensitive locations, tumors with ill-defined borders, recurrent tumors, or tumors >2 cm, Mohs surgery is the ideal method of treatment. Mohs surgeons use frozen section pathology to process tissue and read results within about one hour, and take additional layers of tissue until all margins are clear. Most centers achieve recurrence rates of <1%, and the surgery allows for complex closures to take place on the same day the tumor is excised. See Table 35.2 for a summary of common treatments for nonmelanoma skin cancers.[52–54]

Actinic keratosis and squamous cell carcinoma

Actinic keratoses (AKs) are premalignant precursors to squamous cell carcinoma that develop in sun-damaged skin. Although most will remain in a superficial, precancerous stage, there is an estimated rate of 1% chance per decade for each to evolve to invasive squamous cell carcinoma. Since most patients present with many AKs, the risk quickly accumulates and makes treatment of this early stage essential.

AKs are often described to be "better felt than seen," as they are often subtle visually. They present as erythematous macules or thin papules with sandpaper-like, gritty scale. Palpating high-risk areas such as the forehead, temples, cheeks, and nose is critical for detection. Treating individual lesions with cryotherapy and other destructive techniques is very successful in the office (grade A). Prescription topical treatment is also highly effective for individual lesions

or "field treatments" of widespread actinic damage over larger areas.[52]

In many instances, AKs evolve along a continuum to squamous cell carcinoma in-situ (SCCis), which can then progress to invasive squamous cell carcinoma (SCC). Just as often, however, SCCis and SCC will develop de novo. Like AK, SCCis is limited to the epidermis, but the pathologic features fill the epidermis more fully. The clinical distinction can be difficult, but SCCis tends to be larger and is often resistant to superficial treatment such as cryotherapy that is typically very successful in the treatment of AK.[46, 55] Invasive SCC (Figure 35.4) can also be difficult to distinguish from its more superficial counterparts, but it should be highly suspected of lesions that develop thicker, nodular components, have rapid growth, bleed frequently, or are tender to palpation. At times, invasion of local nerves can cause persistent pain or paresthesia. Any lesion that is present or grows for more than six to eight weeks, recurrently ulcerates or bleeds, and does not heal as expected should be biopsied to rule out nonmelanoma skin cancer. As with BCC, shave biopsy is usually sufficient.

A specific subtype of SCC known as keratoacanthoma typically arises and grows quickly, often reaching sizes of 2 cm or greater over the course of four to six weeks. It tends to have a characteristic central crater that is filled with keratinized debris. In some cases this represents a reactive process, and spontaneous resolution over the course of months is not infrequent. Because it cannot be fully distinguished from well-differentiated invasive SCC, most authors recommend surgical removal following diagnosis.[57]

Although SCCis does not have metastatic potential, invasive SCC can become very aggressive in some instances. Estimates of metastatic disease developing in cutaneous SCC vary, but it is likely in the range of 3%–5%. The lips, ears, genitals, and fingers carry an increased risk. SCCis can be treated similarly to superficial or nodular BCC in most instances, whereas invasive SCC should be treated by standard excision or Mohs surgery, depending on the size and location. [46, 56–58] See Table 35.2 for additional information on the treatment of AKs and nonmelanoma skin cancers.

Following the diagnosis of a first skin cancer, the risk of developing another skin cancer over the next three years increases to more than tenfold that of the

Table 35.2 Common treatments for nonmelanoma skin cancer

	Description	Indications	Advantages	Disadvantages	Cure rates
Mohs micrographic surgery	Surgeon reads frozen section pathology and takes further sections until tumor is cleared	BCC, SCC, SCCis (all grade A). Especially for high-risk locations, large tumors, and recurrent tumors	High clearance rates; single physician can often handle in the office if multiple passes are needed to achieve clear margins	May require several hours	98%–99%
Excision	Excision with local anesthesia, typically 3 mm–4 mm margins with permanent section pathology in the following days	BCC, SCC, SCCis (all grade A)	Short time in the office (30 min–90 min) with local anesthesia	May require larger margins and repairs than Mohs. Requires some restrictions in activities for 7–10 days. Not ideal for some tumors >2 cm or in high-risk locations.	~ 95%–98%
ED&C	Three cycles of curettage followed by electrodessication	Superficial and nodular BCC, SCCis (all grade A)	Fast (~ 10 min); local anesthesia in the office. Minimal wound care.	Likely higher recurrence for ~ 95% more aggressive subtypes and high-risk areas such as face. Circular scar not ideal in some locations.	~ 95%
Imiquimod	Topical immunotherapy activating Toll-like receptor-7. Applied 5× weekly for 6–12 weeks for skin cancer or 2–3× weekly for AKs.	AKs (grade A), superficial (grade A) and nodular BCC (Grade B), SCCis (Grade B)	Patient-controlled, excellent cosmetic outcome	Higher recurrence rate than most physical modalities. May result in significant local inflammation. Chance of patient error.	72%–82% varies with duration and frequency. Lower responses for nodular BCC.
5-Fluorouracil	Pyrimidine analog that blocks DNA synthesis. Twice daily application for 3–6 weeks.	AKs (grade A), superficial (grade B) and nodular (grade D) BCC, SCCis (grade B)	Patient-controlled, excellent cosmetic outcome	Higher recurrence than most physical modalities. May result in significant local inflammation. Chance of patient error.	57%–90%
Photodynamic therapy	Topical precursor of protoporphyrin IX applied and incubated. Red or blue light exposure results in reactive oxygen species production.	AKs (grade A), superficial BCCs (grade A), SCCis	In-office treatment, more physician control than topical pharmacotherapy. Excellent cosmetic outcome.	Higher recurrence than most physical modalities. May result in significant inflammation.	73%–98% clearance reported, protocols vary

Source: Information from references 52–54, 60, 61.

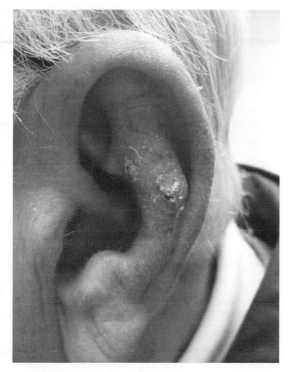

Figure 35.4 Squamous cell carcinoma: crusted nodule on the antihelix, a high-risk location. (A black-and-white version of this figure will appear in some formats. For the color version, please refer to the plate section.)

general population. As more time passes without additional skin cancers developing the risk of subsequent skin cancer gradually falls, but patients remain at increased risk. Although standardized guidelines are lacking, most patients are followed every six months for full skin exams for one to two years following the diagnosis of a nonmelanoma skin cancer and then annually thereafter.[59]

Melanoma

Melanoma makes up less than 5% of skin cancers diagnosed each year, but it accounts for 80% of skin-cancer-related mortality. The rate of melanoma diagnosis is steadily increasing, with an estimated 140,000 melanomas projected to be diagnosed in 2014, which will result in close to 9,700 deaths. Whereas the majority of melanomas are limited to the skin at the time of diagnosis, and survival of those patients approaches 98%, mortality increases significantly in later-stage disease, with <15% of patients surviving at five years after being diagnosed with metastatic disease.[46, 47]

Various factors contribute to the risk of developing melanoma. A number of mutations – including

CDKN2A, melanocortin-1 receptor (linked to fair skin and red hair), and *BRCA 1/2* – are linked to higher rates of melanoma, but environmental risk factors are more common contributors. History of blistering sunburns, cumulative UV exposure, lighter skin types, presence of >50 nevi or atypical nevi, family history, increasing age, and male gender all increase the risk of developing melanoma. Females have higher rates under the age of 40, but the trend reverses, and males over 60 have double the risk of age-matched females.[46, 47]

The clinical diagnosis of melanoma is one of the most challenging aspects of dermatology at any age. Benign nevi (moles) are common benign melanocytic neoplasms that often have overlapping clinical features with melanoma, and 50% of melanomas will develop within nevi. Provider familiarity with the ABCDEs of melanoma (*A*symmetry, *B*order irregularity, multiple *C*olors, *D*iameter >6 mm, and *E*volution) is helpful, but most nevi with one or two of these features, known as atypical nevi, are benign. When patients have many atypical nevi, it is useful to recognize one or two patterns of "signature nevi" in a patient that have a similar appearance so that a lesion that does not match the background pattern will stand out; this is sometimes referred to as the "ugly duckling" rule.[62]

The primary subtypes of melanoma include superficial spreading, nodular, lentigo maligna, and acral lentiginous. Up to 10% of all subtypes may be amelanotic or hypomelanotic. The superficial spreading subtype (Figure 35.5) is the most common subtype at any age, but lentigo maligna becomes increasingly common in elderly, highly sun-damaged skin. It is named for its resemblance to benign lentigines, and distinguishing features are most often the large size and irregular pigmentation of lentigo maligna. Their subtle and prolonged horizontal growth phase often makes detection difficult, but also results in a long lag time before an invasive component develops. Nodular melanoma is less common but has an early vertical growth phase and often presents at more advanced stages. Acral lentiginous melanoma presents on the palms, soles, and nail apparatus. It is the least common type of melanoma overall, but the most common type found in African-American patients.[1, 63]

A biopsy should be performed urgently any time melanoma is suspected. Ideally, excisional biopsy with a scalpel or punch tool is utilized to allow for adequate

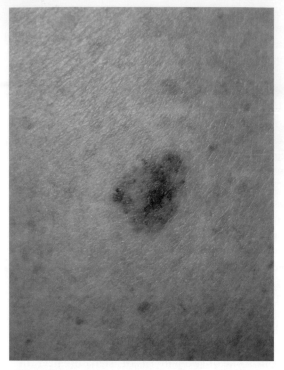

Figure 35.5 Superficial spreading melanoma: irregularly shaped, pigmented plaque with variegated pigment. (A black-and-white version of this figure will appear in some formats. For the color version, please refer to the plate section.)

assessment of the margins and depth of the tumor (grade A). The Breslow depth, measured from the stratum granulosum to the deepest point of invasion, is the most important prognostic factor from biopsy specimens, as it is strongly linked to risk of mortality. Melanoma in-situ, which is limited to the epidermis, carries little to no risk of systemic spread. When ulceration is absent and Breslow depth is <1 mm, 10-year mortality risk is <5% in most instances, whereas tumors >4-mm depth with ulceration have 10-year survival of ~ 50%. Advanced age is associated with more advanced disease at the time of diagnosis and poorer prognosis.[1, 46, 63]

Upon diagnosis of melanoma, excision with margins that increase based on the depth of invasion is indicated (grade A). In most tumors <1 mm without ulceration, local excision is curative and no further workup is indicated. A growing role for Mohs surgery in cosmetically sensitive areas for thin melanomas is being seen as data has generally confirmed high clearance rates and excellent cosmetic and functional outcomes.[64] In tumors with >1 mm Breslow depth, a sentinel lymph node biopsy is generally indicated to provide further prognostic information (grade A). Lymph node dissection is typically performed when a sentinel node is positive, but the benefit is controversial, and it carries risk of substantial morbidity.[65–68]

Metastatic melanoma has a poor prognosis, but, after decades of stagnation, major breakthroughs in treatment have emerged. Standard chemotherapeutic regimens have historically had limited success, but as our knowledge of the immune response to malignancy and the oncogenic pathways that fuel melanoma has grown, so has our ability to manipulate these pathways through the use of very specific drugs. Immunotherapy with new biologics – including ipilimumab that inhibits *CTLA4* and PD-1 inhibitors – are currently in trials and have shown durable responses in a substantial subset of patients.[69] Targeted therapy with *BRAF* inhibitors in patients with melanomas harboring *BRAF* mutations have also led to dramatic responses, although recurrence over several months is seen in >90% of patients.[70] The success of these drugs has been groundbreaking, and it has fueled the ongoing development of many complementary and new agents that are currently in the pipeline.

Similar to nonmelanoma skin cancer surveillance, there are not clear evidence-based guidelines to follow for melanoma screening. Second melanomas develop in 3.5%–4.5% of patients, and local recurrence will occur in more than 4% of patients with the highest risk occurring in the first five years following diagnosis. In most instances, follow-up visits after the diagnosis of melanoma occur every three months for the first year, then every six months in years two through five, and then annually in perpetuity. Visits should include complete skin examination with focus on sites of previous melanoma, lymph node exam, and complete review of systems.[63]

Inflammatory skin diseases

Rosacea

Rosacea is a common, chronic inflammatory condition that predominantly involves the convex surfaces of the central face. It is most common in fair skinned individuals and affects an estimated 1%–10% of this population, with a female predominance.[71–73] Eighty percent of cases will present in adults over 30 years old.[74] There are four morphological subtypes: erythematotelangiectatic (ETR), papulopustular

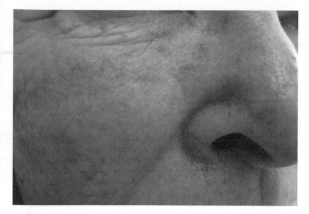

Figure 35.6 Rosacea: erythema, telangiectasias, and scattered papules and pustules. (A black-and-white version of this figure will appear in some formats. For the color version, please refer to the plate section.)

(PPR), phymatous (PhR), and ocular rosacea.[75] It is unknown if the rosacea subtypes represent different stages of a progressive disease, or if they are distinct entities that share common phenotypic features.

Erythematotelangiectatic rosacea is characterized by persistent centrofacial erythema, facial flushing, and scattered telangiectasia on the forehead, nose, and malar cheeks. Flushing is often the primary initial and ongoing symptom of cutaneous rosacea, and it can be accompanied by symptoms of stinging or burning. Exacerbations are often triggered by alcohol, ultraviolet radiation, caffeine, heat, emotion, smoking, and spicy foods. These factors are thought to induce rosacea by dilation of cutaneous vessels.[71] As the name implies, papulopustular rosacea is defined by the development of papules and pustules that typically involve the same distribution in the central face. Lesions can appear acneiform, but unlike acne vulgaris, there are no comedones (Figure 35.6). Phymatous rosacea is easily recognized by marked, nodular tissue hypertrophy that distorts the facial contours. The nose is most commonly involved (rhinophyma), but the chin, cheeks, and ears can also be affected. The fourth subtype, ocular rosacea, must be considered in all patients with cutaneous rosacea. Ocular symptoms are variable and have a range of severity from chronic hyperemia, conjunctivitis, and blepharitis to corneal ulceration and vision-threatening keratitis. Symptoms include redness, burning, watering, dryness, and light sensitivity. Ocular disease has been reported to be present in 33% of patients with skin manifestations and does not necessarily reflect the severity of the skin disease.[76] Eye involvement may precede, occur concurrently, or follow cutaneous disease. It may also occur in the absence of cutaneous disease. Any patient with signs or symptoms of ocular rosacea should be referred for an ophthalmologic evaluation.

Although the precise etiology of rosacea is unclear, research continues to implicate the innate immune system in the pathogenesis of the disease. In affected individuals, exposure to environmental triggers such as ultraviolet light and commensal skin organisms results in an inappropriate activation of the innate immune system. This aberrant activation results in the inflammation and neurovascular hyperreactivity that define the disease. Although there may be a genetic predisposition to developing rosacea, no specific genes have been implicated. The role of the saprophytic mite, *Demodex folliculorum*, is unclear, although mite proteins have been shown to induce innate inflammatory responses.[77] Higher mite density has been found on people with rosacea, and decreasing the mite density is associated with reduced inflammation in recent studies.[78]

All patients with rosacea should be counseled to avoid triggers such as temperature extremes and alcohol, practice sun protection, and use only gentle, hypoallergenic skin products. Cosmetic camouflage with green-tinted facial powder or foundation may be recommended.

Medications classically utilized for papulopustular rosacea include topical metronidazole, azelaic acid, and sulfacetamide-sulfur formulations. For patients who fail topical therapy, either subantimicrobial or fully bacteriocidal doses of oral tetracyclines are the next line therapy. The anti-inflammatory component of tetracyclines, in particular the ability to inhibit proteases, is thought to be responsible for their efficacy. For patients with ETR or persistent erythema, topical brimonidine is a new agent that is available. It is an alpha-2 adrenergic receptor agonist and works immediately to vasoconstrict dilated vessels and diminish redness. Side effects include irritation and risk of rebound erythema and should be discussed with the patient. Topical retinoids are also utilized and are thought to work by inhibiting inappropriate innate immunity activation. Pulsed dye or potassium titanyl phosphate (KTP) lasers are efficacious treatment for both persistent erythema and telangiectasias. They target hemoglobin, resulting in heating and coagulation of the vessels. In severe cases of inflammatory PPR or early phymatous rosacea, oral retinoids such

489

as acitretin or isotretinoin may be beneficial. Adjunctive therapy for phymatous rosacea includes surgical debulking with dermabrasion or laser ablation with a carbon dioxide laser to re-contour the hypertrophic tissue. In all cases, neither oral nor topical steroids are recommended because of the likelihood of inducing dependence and a rebound steroid-induced rosacea.[1, 6, 7, 71]

Seborrheic dermatitis

Seborrheic dermatitis is a chronic inflammatory condition that has a characteristic clinical appearance and distribution. It is recognized as chronic, relapsing erythema that involves the glabella, eyebrows, paranasal region, alar creases, and nasolabial folds. The chest, frontal hairline, and ear canals are also frequently involved (Figure 35.7). There is also a variable degree of skin flaking, from fine dandruff (pityriasis sicca) to thick, greasy adherent scales (pityriasis steatoides).

Although seborrheic dermatitis has a predilection for areas of the body with increased numbers of sebaceous glands, it is not felt to be a disease of sebaceous glands. The etiology is thought to be due to the host response to commensal saprophyte *Malassezia* (formerly *Pityrosporum ovale*).[1, 6, 7, 79] The fungus is not believed to be directly pathogenic; rather, it may incite a host immune response or cause an irritant dermatitis from fungal metabolic byproducts. Patients with Parkinson's disease or HIV may have severe seborrheic dermatitis. The

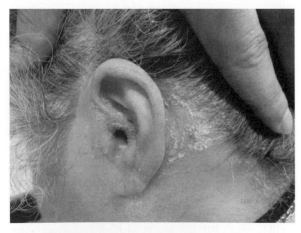

Figure 35.7 Seborrheic dermatitis: erythematous plaques that are flaky, adherent, and slightly greasy affecting the scalp, ear, and retroauricular sulcus. (A black-and-white version of this figure will appear in some formats. For the color version, please refer to the plate section.)

reason for this is unknown, but it improves with treatment of both conditions.

Seborrheic dermatitis can be mild without symptoms or can be quite impressive with erythema and thick scaling (pityriasis amiantacia) of the scalp. There may be itching and, rarely, alopecia. Mild disease is usually controlled with topical antifungals such as ketoconazole 2%, selenium sulfide 2.5%, or ciclopirox 1% shampoo. The shampoo may be used for scalp and/or skin involvement, and the patient is asked to leave the medication on for five to ten minutes before washing it off. It is usually used two to three times a week until control is established, after which it may be used weekly for maintenance. Topical antifungal creams such as ketoconazole 2%, other azole creams, and ciclopirox 1% cream may also be applied directly if preferred. They are also used daily until symptoms are controlled, then decreased to weekly for maintenance. For inflammatory seborrheic dermatitis, topical steroids are beneficial. The strength and formulation chosen are dependent on the location being treated. For the face, low-potency steroids, such as hydrocortisone 2.5% or desonide 0.05% cream, should be used twice a day until improvement. For the scalp and body, mid- to high-potency steroids can be safely used. For the scalp, fluocinolone acetonide 0.01% shampoo is approved by the US Food and Drug Administration, although other formulations (such as solutions or foams) are frequently used off-label, depending on the patient's vehicle preference. Careful consideration must be made if there is a component of rosacea or periorificial dermatitis, because topical corticosteroids are known to cause flares in both of these conditions. Occasionally, short courses or intermittent suppressive doses of oral itraconazole or fluconazole can be beneficial for flares or severe disease.[79]

Whenever seborrheic dermatitis is resistant to therapy, alternative diagnoses should be considered. The primary differential diagnosis of seborrheic dermatitis includes rosacea, psoriasis (particularly for scalp involvement), tinea corporis, systemic lupus erythematosus (SLE), and periorificial dermatitis. History and physical exam are usually sufficient for differentiating these entities.

Psoriasis

Psoriasis is an immune-mediated inflammatory disorder that can have a variety of clinical presentations and can vary greatly in severity. It is most commonly

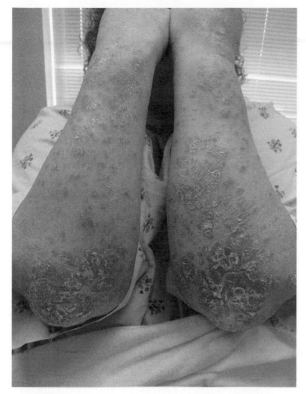

Figure 35.8 Psoriasis: scaly, erythematous plaques with a predilection for extensor surfaces. (A black-and-white version of this figure will appear in some formats. For the color version, please refer to the plate section.)

characterized by erythematous papules and plaques with silvery scale (Figure 35.8) and has several subtypes, including plaque, guttate, inverse, erythrodermic, pustular, and nail psoriasis. It affects 1%–3% of the world's population, and 3.2% of all psoriatic patients have an onset in the geriatric age group over 60 years old.[80] Diagnosis is usually clinical, but a skin biopsy may be required in nonclassical presentations. It is important to approach psoriasis as a systemic disease. It is associated with systemwide inflammation that has deleterious effects on the cardiovascular and hepatic systems. Psoriasis has been shown to be independently associated with an elevated risk of coronary artery disease, type 2 diabetes mellitus,[81] and nonalcoholic fatty liver disease in patients over 55 years old.[82] Other comorbidities that are associated with psoriasis include malignancy, diabetes, metabolic syndrome, depression, inflammatory bowel disease, and serious infections. Psoriatic arthritis (PsA) has been reported to affect from 5% to as high as 30% of patients with

psoriasis,[83] and there is a yearly incidence of newly diagnosed PsA of almost 2% per year.[84, 85] A rheumatologist should evaluate patients with suspected joint involvement.

When evaluating the patient with psoriasis, it is important to consider potential triggers such as infection or medications. *Streptococcus pyogenes* has been associated with new onset of guttate psoriasis as well as flares of existing disease. Medications may also trigger or exacerbate psoriasis. The worst offenders include antimalarial drugs, beta blockers, and lithium. Angiotensin-converting enzyme inhibitors, NSAIDs, and terbinafine have also been reported as inciting agents.[86] Abrupt cessation of corticosteroids is known to provoke erythrodermic and pustular flares, and the TNF-α antagonists have triggered palmoplantar and diffuse pustular psoriasis in patients without a prior history of the disease.

The treatment of psoriasis can be approached in a stepwise manner, and the chosen agents and formulations should be tailored to patient comorbidities as well as preference. The first step in treatment is topical therapy, which includes medium- to high-potency topical steroids (grade A), vitamin D analogs such as calcipotriene and calcitriol (grade B), and tar-based emollients (grade B). For facial or intertriginous areas, low- to mid-potency steroids, calcipotriene, or topical calcineurin inhibitors (such as tacrolimus or pimecrolimus) may be used as alternatives (grade B). For patients who do not have optimal response to topical therapy but are not candidates for systemic therapy, light therapy with nbUVB (311 nm) is a useful adjunct. First-line oral therapies for psoriasis include methotrexate and acitretin (grade A). In severe cases of acute pustular or erythrodermic psoriasis, cyclosporine or infliximab should be instituted due to the rapid onset of action (grade C). For long-term maintenance, methotrexate at 7.5 mg–25 mg weekly is a generally well-tolerated medication that can be tailored to a patient's glomerular filtration rate (GFR). Laboratory monitoring is required, and cumulative methotrexate dose should be followed to determine the need for liver biopsy. Acitretin may be used in the absence of severe renal insufficiency, but it is often harder to tolerate. Side effects include dry skin, photosensitivity, and arthralgia. Acitretin is particularly effective in the treatment of localized palmoplantar pustular psoriasis and is often a first-line agent in such cases. As with methotrexate, laboratory monitoring is required. The biological drugs – including the TNF-α

inhibitors (adalimumab, etanercept, and infliximab) and the anti-IL-17/23 monoclonal antibody, ustekinumab – are also options in the elderly population (grade B). The biologics are associated with a small risk of infection, and the patient should be evaluated for prior exposure to tuberculosis, hepatitis B, and endemic fungal infections prior to initiation. The TNF-α blocking agents have also been associated with demyelinating diseases and hematologic malignancies; however, it is not clear whether the increased risk is due to the underlying disease state or the medication. There is no convincing evidence that relative risk of infection with TNF-α therapy increases with age.[86] Lastly, there are new oral medications on the horizon for the treatment of psoriasis. The janus kinase (JAK) inhibitors have been approved for rheumatoid arthritis, and these – along with phosphodiesterase 4 inhibitors and Th17 pathway inhibitors – are in the final stages of the FDA approval process. Preliminary studies are showing excellent tolerability as well as efficacy.

Atopic dermatitis

Atopic dermatitis (AD) is a common, chronic inflammatory condition of the skin that is estimated to have a lifetime prevalence of about 20%.[87] AD usually has an onset in infancy to early childhood. Adults with AD usually developed the condition as a child; however, there is also a small subset of individuals who present in adulthood. Most studies report 20- to 40-year-olds as the most common age of adult-onset AD, but others have reported an age of onset in patients as old as 79.[88] AD is characterized by erythematous, scaly plaques that range in severity and distribution. In adults, the hands, feet, and the flexural surfaces are frequently involved. Less common, nonflexural morphological variants also occur and include nummular (Figure 35.9), follicular, seborrheic dermatitis-like, and prurigo-like patterns.[88] Affected areas are pruritic, and constant rubbing and inflammation may lead to lichenification of the skin. Complications of AD are often infectious in nature and include bacterial superinfection, dermatophytosis, and eczema herpeticum.

Diagnosis is usually made clinically, although a biopsy may assist in ruling out other diagnoses. Pruritus is always present and can be helpful in distinguishing AD from other common conditions such as psoriasis. Assessing for an allergic contact dermatitis with patch testing is often performed in

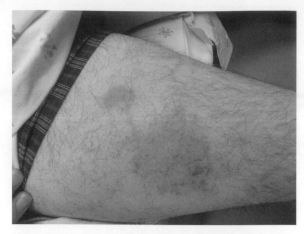

Figure 35.9 Nummular dermatitis: annular, slightly scaly, with pruritic plaques on the extremities. (A black-and-white version of this figure will appear in some formats. For the color version, please refer to the plate section.)

new adult-onset disease or in cases where there is acute worsening. One study showed nearly one-third of 1,022 patients with nummular dermatitis had a reaction to one or more allergens (nickel sulfate was highest at 10.2%).[89] Other conditions on the differential diagnosis that should be considered include pityriasis rosea, lichen simplex chronicus, scabies, tinea corporis, and seborrheic dermatitis.

The etiology of atopic dermatitis is multifactorial. The discovery of the filaggrin mutation in some patients indicates that at least a subset is caused by skin barrier dysfunction. Other subtypes may be predominately due to abnormalities in the immune system. Both of these ultimately result in abnormalities in cutaneous immunity, which is critical for protection against pathogens as well as generating tolerance to benign antigens. These effects account for the clinical findings and complications of AD.

Treatment options range with the severity of disease and degree of impact on the quality of life. All patients should be asked to maintain skin hydration and avoid trigger factors such as heat, low humidity, and any contact allergens that have been identified. Avoidance of aeroallergens and food allergens, although reasonable, has not been shown to be useful for disease control.[90–92] Patients with AD should also be evaluated for superinfections, because they are at an increased risk of bacterial, viral, and fungal skin infections. The mainstay for mild disease is mid- to high-potency topical steroid preparations on the trunk and extremities, and low- to medium-potency topical steroids on the face (grade A). The use of high-potency ointments is frequently employed by dermatologists who prefer short bursts of high-potency steroids to longer treatments with mild- to medium-potency steroids. Aggressive moisturization with thick cream or emollients is important for preserving as much barrier function as possible. Antihistamines can be a useful adjunct for the associated pruritus, particularly for nocturnal itching. For disease that is recalcitrant to topical regimens, narrowband UVB (311 nm) or oral immunomodulating medications are warranted. First-line therapies include methotrexate, azathioprine, and mycophenolate mofetil (grade B). Each has variable efficacy amongst patients, and the first agent is often chosen based on patient comorbidities and the drug side effect profiles. In the case of acute flares, cyclosporine 5 mg/mL/day may be used to establish quick control prior to transitioning to a long-term immunomodulator (grade B).[93]

Pruritus

Pruritus is a common complaint in the elderly population that can be debilitating for patients and challenging to treat. Each year in the United States, more than seven million patients complain of itching at outpatient visits; of these, 1.8 million (25%) are complaints from patients 65 years or older.[94] It is often very frustrating for the patient and can significantly impact the quality of life, causing sleep disturbances and depression. The approach to pruritus involves a thorough history and physical examination and careful exclusion of an infectious etiology, medication side effect, or systemic disease. A complete dermatologic examination should be performed to look for primary or secondary skin lesions.

Pruritus can be grouped into pruritus with skin disease, pruritus without skin disease, and pruritus resulting from secondary skin changes, usually from chronic rubbing or scratching (Table 35.3). If there is skin disease, diagnosis and treatment should be directed at the eruption. This involves careful evaluation of morphological features, distribution, symptoms, and occasionally a skin biopsy. Principal subgroups include primary skin diseases such as atopic dermatitis and Grover's disease, infectious diseases, medications, and physiologic changes of aging skin. Impaired skin barrier function and immunosenescence are two well-described phenomena that occur in aging skin and result in pruritus. Immunosenescence results in impaired cellular immunity, increased risk of

infection, and a cytokine profile that favors inflammation and itch. Skin dryness, or xerosis, worsens over time, and clues that it is causing itch include: temporary relief during bathing, worsening in the winter months, and itching of the extremities more than the trunk. Xerosis should always be treated regardless of whether it is the primary cause of itch. The patient should be asked to avoid soaps, detergents, and astringents, to limit bathing to less than once a day, and to avoid hot water. Application of petrolatum or heavy cream moisturizer should be performed immediately after bathing and throughout the day. Wet wraps may be utilized in severe cases.[95]

Pruritus can also be caused by chronic rubbing or picking of an initial primary lesion or normal skin. The skin's response is to thicken and form well-demarcated, lichenified plaques or papules that we recognize as lichen simplex chronicus (Figure 35.10) and prurigo or "pickers" nodules. Once established, these changes can perpetuate the "itch-scratch" cycle even if the primary cause has resolved. Treatment can be extraordinarily challenging and involves a discussion of the "itch-scratch cycle" with the patient and possibly a psychiatric evaluation. Systemic medications have been used in severe cases.

If there is no rash, this usually indicates a systemic or neurologic cause, and the focus should be directed at patient comorbidities and medications (see Table 35.4).

In some patients, no clear cause will be found on thorough workup. For these patients, a combination of age-related skin changes is often the diagnosis of exclusion. Management is then centered on symptom management and identification of triggers or exacerbating agents.

Lower extremity stasis-related skin changes

Lower extremity chronic venous insufficiency is a common finding in the elderly and is often multifactorial in etiology. There are several dermatoses that are related to chronic venous stasis, the most common of which is stasis dermatitis.

Stasis dermatitis affects a reported 6.2% of patients over the age of 65 and results from chronic venous hypertension.[118] The skin overlying the affected areas can be brightly erythematous or violaceous, or it can appear rusty due to red blood cell extravasation and hemosiderin deposition in the dermis. Eczematous patches or plaques with scaling are typical, and in acute cases the skin can be weeping and

Table 35.3 Differential diagnosis and evaluation of pruritus

Groups	Subgroups	Examples	Possible evaluation
Pruritus with skin disease	Primary dermatologic conditions	Atopic dermatitis Xerosis Urticaria Allergic/irritant dermatitis Lichen planus Cutaneous T-cell lymphoma Grover's disease Bullous pemphigoid	Skin biopsy Patch testing
	Infectious diseases	Scabies Head or pubic lice Dermatophytoses (tinea pedis, capitus, corporis, cruris, versicolor, Majocchi granuloma) Id reaction at distant site	KOH evaluation Mineral oil preparation Skin biopsy with special stains Tissue culture
	Medications	Photosensitizers (thiazides, tetracycline, ACE-inhibitors, CCBs, NSAIDs, quinine, and amiodarone)	Evaluation of medications started within 6 weeks of itch. Skin biopsy
	Physiologic changes of aging skin	Impaired skin barrier function Immunosenescence	Diagnosis of exclusion
Pruritus without skin disease	Systemic disease	Thyroid, liver, and renal disease Hematopoietic disorders (lymphoma, polycythemia vera) Sensory neuropathy due to diabetes	Screening lab work: CBC with differential, fasting plasma glucose, TFTs, LFTs, BUN/Cr, Ca, Phos, TSH, PTH, Ferritin
	Neuropathic	Genital pruritus Forearms (brachioradial pruritus) Midback (nostalgia paresthetica) Herpes zoster (dermatomal)	Nerve impingement, particularly C5–C8 in brachioradial pruritus and T2–T6 in nostalgia paresthetica Examination for lichenification or hyperpigmentation of involved areas
	Medications	ACE inhibitors, salicylates, chloroquine, CCBs	Evaluation of medications started within 6 weeks of itch
Pruritus with secondary skin disease	Due to chronic scratching or rubbing	Lichen simplex chronicus	Psychological evaluation Exclusion of systemic disease Intralesional triamcinolone injections Topical steroids Unna boot wraps Oral antihistamines Systemics: methotrexate, CsA, thalidomide, MMF
		Prurigo nodularis	

CBC – complete blood count, TFT – thyroid function tests, LFT –liver function tests, BUN – blood urea nitrogen, Cr –creatinine, Ca –calcium, Phos – phosphorus, TFTs – thyroid function tests, PTH – parathyroid, CsA – cyclosporine A, MMF – mycophenolate mofetil
Source: Information from references 94–97.

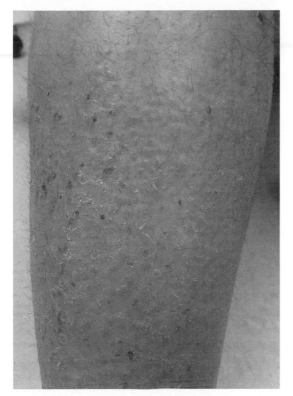

Figure 35.10 Lichen simplex chronicus: thick, excoriated, lichenified plaque on the lower leg at a site of frequent scratching due to contact dermatitis. (A black-and-white version of this figure will appear in some formats. For the color version, please refer to the plate section.)

vesicles may be present. It is not uncommon to have skin breakdown with ulcerations or widespread weeping of serosanguinous transudate.

The treatment for stasis dermatitis is treating the cause of the edema and encouraging fluid redistribution with compression hose, leg elevation, and daily walking. White petroleum jelly is an effective, inexpensive, and non-sensitizing product that may be used to protect and lubricate the skin. Mid- to high-potency corticosteroids such as triamcinolone ointment, with or without occluding leg wraps, are a mainstay of therapy when erythema suggests underlying inflammation. Wet dressings with antiseptic solutions – such as dilute acetic acid, potassium permanganate, or aluminum acetate or subacetate – for two to three hours, two to three times a day followed by application of emollients are useful for weeping or impetiginized areas. In cases of ulceration, barrier creams like zinc oxide are also important to protect the skin from further breakdown and environmental

exposures. Zinc oxide is also available in an impregnated bandage that can be wrapped to create compression (Unna boot). It is important to note that patients with stasis dermatitis are prone to developing contact allergies, and common sensitizers such as neomycin and bacitracin should be avoided.

Areas of stasis dermatitis are also prone to infection. Impetiginized lesions can be treated with antiseptic wraps or topical mupirocin, which is least likely to cause cutaneous sensitization.[119, 120] Secondary cellulitis requires oral antibiotic therapy. Of note, cellulitis can appear similar to stasis dermatitis with warmth, erythema, and edema; a key differentiating feature is the distribution. Stasis dermatitis is almost invariably bilateral, and it is exceedingly rare for cellulitis to be bilateral.

There are several other skin diseases that primarily affect the lower legs and are thought to be associated with chronic venous stasis or other vasculopathy. Acroangiodermatitis is characterized by scaly, red to violaceous papules and plaques located circumferentially on the lower extremities. This condition is characterized by arterio-venous shunts that develop after hyperplasia of the vasculature due to venous hypertension. Schamberg disease is a pigmented purpuric dermatosis that commonly affects the lower extremities and may be caused or potentiated by edema. It appears as small rusty macules with a "cayenne pepper" appearance. The rusty appearance is due to hemosiderin extravasation and deposition caused by superficial capillaritis. It is usually chronic and asymptomatic. Other lower extremity vasculopathies include vasculitis of medium and small vessels, such as leukocytoclastic vasculitis and erythema elevatum diutinum. These vasculitities are often found on the lower extremities, and if they are suspected, the diagnosis is made by skin biopsy. Lastly, lipodermatosclerosis is a lower extremity finding that is related to both diabetes and lower extremity edema. Cutaneous sclerosis with fat degeneration and dermal fibrosis results in hyperpigmented, shiny atrophic appearance of the skin and narrowing of the ankles; often with an "inverted bottle" appearance.

Autoimmune blistering disorders

Autoimmune blistering disorders (ABD) are characterized by the development of autoantibodies against cell-cell adhesion molecules. The distribution and quality of the blisters are defined by the properties of the target antigen. Autoimmune blistering disorders

495

Table 35.4 Treatment of pruritus

Agent	Examples*	Applications
Topical steroids	Desonide Triamcinolone Clobetasol	Primary skin diseases excluding infectious Secondary skin diseases
Topical calcineurin inhibitors	Pimecrolimus Tacrolimus	Alternative to steroid for chronic use or for use on face/genital/intertriginous areas
Topical cooling agents	Menthol Camphor Phenol	For soothing effect; can be kept in the refrigerator for added cooling effect
Topical anesthetics	Pramoxine 1% cream Eutectic mixture of lidocaine 2.5% + prilocaine 2.5% (EMLA) Lidocaine in acid mantle cream Lidocaine patch	Focal pruritus and neuropathic etiologies
Other topicals	Topical Doxepin 5%	Atopic dermatitis Neuropathic itch
	Topical capsaicin 2%–6%	Neuropathic itch
Systemic antihistamines	Diphenhydramine Cetirizine Fexofenadine Loratidine	Focal or systemic pruritus; used frequently despite lack of evidence of efficacy for diseases that are not specifically histamine mediated Use in geriatrics may be limited by anticholinergic effects and confusion
Other systemic medications	Gabapentin 100 mg–300 mg and increased up to 1,800 mg/day.	Neuropathic itch Some primary skin disease Itch associated with systemic disease
	SNRI, esp. mirtazapine	
	SSRI such as paroxetine, sertraline, fluvoxamine	
	Doxepin	Nocturnal pruritus
Adjuvant therapy	nbUVB	ESRD

* Topical steroids are typically applied twice a day to affected areas until improvement or up to two weeks.

SNRIs – selective norepinephrine reuptake inhibitors, SSRIs – selective serotonin reuptake inhibitors
Note: Topical antihistamines generally are not recommended due to the risk of irritant or contact dermatitis and lack of efficacy.
Source: Information from references 98–117.

may be broadly divided into pemphigus and pemphigoid. Pemphigus antigens are located within the epidermis, and the blisters are shallow and clinically flaccid. Pemphigoid antigens are located at the basal layer, and the blisters are therefore deeper and tense when intact (Figure 35.11).[121] Pemphigus and pemphigoid each have subtypes that are clinically distinct; they affect different skin surfaces, have different responses to therapy, and have different natural courses. (See Table 35.5 for a brief review of these disorders.)

Diagnosis of ABDs is usually made using a combination of diagnostic tools, including skin biopsies for traditional hematoxylin and eosin (H&E) as well

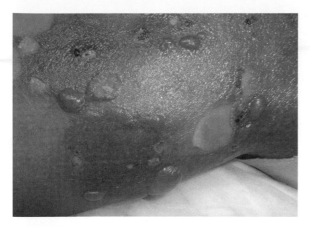

Figure 35.11 Bullous pemphigoid: widespread, tense bullae erupting diffusely on the trunk and extremities. Shallow ulcers are present where bullae have ruptured. (A black-and-white version of this figure will appear in some formats. For the color version, please refer to the plate section.)

as direct immunofluorescence (DIF), which looks for the presence of autoantibodies deposited in the skin. Serum is also collected for enzyme linked immunosorbent assay (ELISA) and indirect IF to detect circulating autoantibodies.

Treatment of the blistering disorders varies slightly depending on the type. The possibility of medication-induced disease should be considered for both pemphigus and pemphigoid appearing lesions. Any offending agent should be discontinued. Early and potentially aggressive therapy may be warranted if mucosal ulcerations are present, because both PV and paraneoplastic pemphigus carry significant morbidity and mortality. Prior to the use of immunosuppressants, 70%–100% of PV patients died within one to five years of disease onset.[122–124] BP is only associated with a slightly increased mortality, and topical steroids are a reasonable first-line therapy, assuming the patient is able to apply the cream twice a day for at least several weeks (grade A).[125] Most of the time, oral glucocorticoids are used to establish control in BP (grade A). This is followed by maintenance immunosuppression with azathioprine, methotrexate, or mycophenolate mofetil (grade C). Tetracycline has also been used beneficially with nicotinamide or dapsone for their anti-inflammatory properties (grade C).[126, 127] Severe, refractory cases are treated with intravenous immunoglobulin and rituximab (grade C). Therapy is usually continued two months after complete remission on minimal therapy.

Treatment of PV is similar to BP. Systemic glucocorticoids are used to establish disease control, and steroid-sparing immunomodulatory agents are employed to maintain remission. (grade A). Azathioprine, mycophenolate mofetil, and dapsone are first-line agents (grade B), followed by rituximab (grade B), cyclophosphamide, and IVIG (grade C) for recalcitrant disease. Topical steroid gels and topical anesthetics like viscous lidocaine are adjuvant therapies. Other additional measures include observation for secondary infection (especially HSV and candida); avoidance of sharp, spicy, or abrasive foods; and good oral hygiene. The goal is long-term remission off therapy, but this can take years to achieve.[125–129]

Infectious skin diseases

Erysipelas and cellulitis

Infections of the skin and soft tissue can be classified by the levels of the skin and structures that are affected by the etiologic pathogen. Erysipelas is an acute infection, usually caused by group A beta-hemolytic streptococcus, that involves both the upper dermis and superficial lymphatics. It typically involves the face or a lower extremity and appears clinically as well-defined, bright red, warm plaques. Pain usually precedes the skin findings, and the patient will often have an acute onset with fever and chills. Progression to lymphangitis and abscess is rare. Mild cases can be treated on an outpatient basis with oral penicillin V or amoxicillin. Alternative parenteral options include intramuscular procaine penicillin, intravenous (IV) ceftriaxone, or IV cefazolin. Cefazolin provides additional coverage against some staphylococcus, which can be useful in cases where the diagnosis is unclear. Treatment for 5–10 days is usually effective. More severe cases require hospitalization for IV therapy.

Cellulitis generally extends deeper into the dermis and subcutaneous tissue than erysipelas. It is differentiated from erysipelas by a less distinct border and a more indolent onset and course. Like erysipelas, there is erythema, tenderness, and pain; however, there is a deeper component that generates an indurated plaque. There may be fluctuance, purulent drainage, or occasionally crepitus (in the case of clostridia or other anaerobic infections). Cellulitis can complicate a surgical wound infection, pressure ulcer, vascular ulcer, or sites of trauma. In the elderly population, sores and fissures between the toes due to tinea pedis and macerated skin are important access portals for

Table 35.5 Classification and presentation of autoimmune blistering disorders

ABD	Subtype	Distribution	Other features
Pemphigoid	Bullous pemphigoid	Generalized or focal May present as itchy urticarial or eczematous plaques Trunk and extremities Rarely involves mucosa	Most common ABD Primarily affects the elderly Chronic, relapsing course, but can have long-term remission Nonscarring
	Mucous membrane pemphigoid (cicatricial pemphigoid)	Any mucosal surface, including oropharyngeal, conjunctiva, nose, esophagus, anal, and genital Cutaneous involvement is less common	Scarring
	Drug-induced pemphigoid*	Trunk and extremities Mucosa not uncommon	Acute and resolves within months after discontinuation of offending drug Nonscarring
Pemphigus	Pemphigus vulgaris	Mucosal only Mucosal and skin	Most common pemphigus Painful oral lesions. Significant morbidity. Long-term remission possible with immunosuppression. May be drug-induced**
	Pemphigus folliaceous	Superficial blisters not usually intact Seborrheic distribution	May mimic Hailey-Hailey or Grover's disease. May be drug-induced**
	Paraneoplastic pemphigus	Characterized by painful, intractable stomatitis. Life-threatening upper airway and pulmonary involvement can occur.	Most commonly associated with non-Hodgkin's lymphoma, chronic lymphocytic leukemia, Castleman's disease, and thymoma
	IgA pemphigus	Grouped vesicles that evolve into pustules, sometimes in annular or circinate patterns Usually trunk and proximal extremities	May be pruritic

* More than 50 different medications have been implicated, including antibiotics, NSAIDs, antiarrhythmics/antihypertensives, diuretics, salicylates, TNF-alpha inhibitors, and diabetes medications among others.[129]

** Penacillamine, captopril, penicillins, cephalosporins, enalapril, rifampin, and NSAIDs.[131–133]

Source: Information from references 121, 122.

pathogens.[134, 135] The lower extremities are a common site of involvement and a population-based study reported the incidence of lower-extremity cellulitis to be 199 per 100,000 person-years. The incidence of cellulitis was found to increase with age.[136]

It is critical to consider the possibility of deeper infection when there are crepitant soft-tissue wounds, central necrosis, or pain that is out of proportion to physical exam findings. These findings suggest a deeper infection such as gangrenous cellulitis, necrotizing fasciitis, synergistic gangrene, or myonecrosis. Soft tissue infections can develop and progress rapidly and are highly lethal, even with quick medical intervention. Identification of the responsible pathogen with wound gram stain and culture is the gold standard in effective antimicrobial therapy in soft tissue infections. Radiographic examination is not indicated and should not delay surgical intervention.

The primary differential diagnosis of cellulitis includes allergic contact or irritant dermatitis, herpes zoster, skin changes secondary to deep vein thrombosis, inflammatory skin conditions such as pyoderma gangrenosum, gout, and stasis dermatitis. Skin abscesses often have surrounding cellulitis. It is important to evaluate for fluctuance or evidence of a cavity, because abscesses require surgical management with incision and drainage.

Treatment of cellulitis is geared toward the most common or suspected pathogens. It is useful to classify cellulitis into purulent versus nonpurulent cellulitis, because purulent cases are often due to methicillin-resistant *S. aureus* (MRSA), whereas nonpurulent cases are usually due to beta-hemolytic streptococci or methicillin-sensitive *S. aureus* (MSSA). Gram-negative aerobic bacilli are identified in a minority of cases. Patient characteristics – such as immunodeficiency, comorbidities, history of hospitalization or surgical procedure, and the location of the infection – should prompt consideration of other etiologic agents. Pressure ulcer cellulitis can be due to both typical skin organisms and facultative and anaerobic microorganisms from the bowel (such as enterococci, Pseudomonas aeruginosa, and Bacteroides fragilis). Other subtypes of cellulitis include periorbital cellulitis, abdominal wall cellulitis, buccal cellulitis (usually *Streptococcus pneumoniae*), and perianal cellulitis (usually group A beta-hemolytic *Streptococcus*). Cultures are not usually useful in the setting of mild infection, and most patients with mild cellulitis may be treated with oral antibiotics.[137] Patients with signs of systemic toxicity should be treated parenterally. Cultures of blood, pus, or bullae are indicated for patients with systemic toxicity, underlying comorbidities, persistent or extensive disease, buccal and periorbital cellulitis, and for special exposures such as animal bites and salt or freshwater.[138]

Herpes zoster

Primary varicella-zoster virus (VZV) infection results in varicella, or chickenpox, which is well recognized as a diffuse vesicular rash. Herpes zoster, commonly known as shingles, is due to the reactivation of latent VZV from the sensory dorsal root ganglia, which results in vesicles occurring in a dermatomal distribution. Herpes zoster is a common cause of morbidity in the United States, particularly for the elderly population. About 1 million people develop zoster each year,

and it is estimated that 32% of the population will experience zoster over their lifetimes.[139, 140] Second attacks of varicella are rare, occurring in only 1%–4% of people, and disseminated lesions usually represent disseminated zoster.[140–142] When breakthrough varicella does occur, it is usually mild and affects people with severe immunodeficiency or those who were immunized with live attenuated varicella vaccine. Unlike varicella, herpes zoster is not seasonal and occurs sporadically throughout the year. Its reactivation is dependent on host risk factors and is not triggered by exposure to another person with varicella or herpes zoster. Intermittent exposure to varicella may in fact confer protection against herpes zoster by boosting host immunity. The elderly population is especially susceptible to zoster due to immune senescence and impaired cellular immunity. Age and conditions resulting in impaired cellular immunity account for the most significant risk of zoster, although female gender, physical trauma in the dermatome, and underlying malignancy have also been reported as risk factors.[143, 144]

In the majority of patients, zoster has a prodrome of neuropathic pain of variable severity and paresthesia in a dermatomal distribution. Patients may present during the prodrome, and shingles should always be on the differential for localized pain out of proportion to clinical exam findings. Vesicles with erythematous bases develop within a few days to weeks after the prodrome (Figure 35.12). Over the next seven to ten days, the vesicles evolve into pustules that dry and crust over. In immunocompromised patients, skin

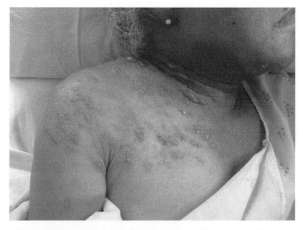

Figure 35.12 Herpes zoster: clustered vesicles on an erythematous base in a dermatomal distribution. Note the sharp demarcation at midline. (A black-and-white version of this figure will appear in some formats. For the color version, please refer to the plate section.)

disease can be severe and cause skin necrosis and scarring. Zoster is contagious, but infectivity has been reported to be about one-third the rate observed after exposure to varicella. In uncomplicated cases, the patient is considered infectious for seven days after the appearance of the rash; however, this can be longer depending on the competency of the immune response. In uncomplicated cases, transmission is thought to be via direct contact with skin lesions. In disseminated cases, the virus can be aerosolized; appropriate airborne precautions should be observed.

The diagnosis of herpes zoster is often clinical; however, several techniques are available in indeterminate cases. A Tzank smear can be performed at the bedside by obtaining a swab from the base of a de-roofed vesicle. Polymerase chain reaction (PCR) or direct immunofluorescence testing of vesicle fluid are other diagnostic options. Enzyme-linked immunosorbent assay (ELISA) may also be available.

Although herpes zoster is self-limited, sequelae can include cutaneous, ocular, neurologic, and visceral complications. Postherpetic neuralgia (PNH) is the most common complication and is defined as pain lasting at least 90 days after resolution of skin lesions. PNH is more common in the elderly and is reported to occur in 20% of patients aged 80 years or older, whereas overall risk of PHN is 10%–15%.[145, 146] Development of PNH correlates with the presence of prodromal pain, initial severity of pain, and patient age. Herpes zoster ophthalmicus (HZO) occurs when VZV reactivates in the ophthalmic division of the trigeminal nerve. Incidence of HZO is reported in 8%–56% of cases.[147, 148] Of those cases, 50%–72% will have eye involvement.[147] Nasociliary branch involvement can lead to neurotrophic keratitis and chronic ulceration of the cornea or acute retinal necrosis. Nasociliary branch involvement is suggested by disease on the nasal tip, referred to as Hutchinson's sign.[149] Involvement of other cranial nerves can affect the associated structures such as the mouth, ears, pharynx, and larynx. Herpes zoster oticus or Ramsay Hunt syndrome occurs with involvement of the facial and auditory nerves and is characterized by ipsilateral facial palsy, ear pain, and vesicles on the external ear canal or tympanic membrane. Tinnitus, vertigo, taste perception, lacrimation, and deafness may also occur. Ramsay Hunt syndrome can also be due to herpes simplex type 2 infection.[150] Immunosuppressed patients are at risk of more severe

complications, including leptomeningitis, meningoencephalitis, segmental or transverse myelitis, and local palsies due to proximal spread of the infection to the meninges and spinal cord. Stroke syndromes due to involvement of the cerebral arteries has also been reported.[151, 152]

Antiviral therapy with acyclovir, famciclovir, or valacyclovir initiated within 72 hours of the onset of the rash can reduce healing time as well as the duration and severity of acute pain.[151–153] It is unclear if antiviral therapy decreases the risk of PHN. There may be a role for oral glucocorticoids for people with severe pain or in cases of cranial polyneuritis or motor neuropathies caused by inflammation and compression of affected nerves. Otherwise, the general consensus has recommended against the use of systemic steroids. Treatment for acute pain and PNH includes lidocaine 5% patches, gabapentin, pregabalin, opioids, and tricyclic antidepressants. Calamine lotion and cool compresses may be applied topically, but occlusive ointments and glucocorticoids should be avoided. Zoster vaccination is indicated in patients who are 60 years of age or older whether or not they have a history of zoster.[154, 155] A large Veterans Affairs Cooperative Study investigated the effects of VZV vaccination and demonstrated that it reduced the risk of zoster by 51.3%, reduced the burden of illness by 61.5%, and reduced the incidence of post-herpetic neuralgia (PHN) by 51.3%.[156] Another study in the elderly showed reduction of PHN by 67%.[157]

Scabies

Scabies is an infestation of the skin by the mite *Sarcoptes scabiei*. The mite is usually transmitted from person to person by direct contact, although it can survive on fomites for 24–36 hours.[158, 159] Scabies are not spread by pets. The female mite burrows along the top layers of the skin where it lays its eggs. An infected person usually harbors about 10–15 female mites. The characteristic intense itch is due to a delayed type-IV hypersensitivity reaction to the mite as well as its feces and eggs.[160] Elderly people living in nursing facilities may be at increased risk of infection due to close contact with other residents and unfortunate suboptimal hygiene conditions.

It is critical to consider scabies in all elderly patients complaining of intense itch that may be out of proportion to skin findings. It is not uncommon for the diagnosis to be overlooked because the patient has another explanation for pruritus. The diagnosis is made by a history of intense itching that often disrupts sleep in conjunction with typical distribution of skin involvement. An important component of the history is whether there are others infected in the household. All areas of the body may be affected, but the exam should focus on the classically involved areas, which include the finger web spaces, axilla, waist, and genitals. There are usually erythematous papules with overlying excoriations in these areas. Linear burrows 2 mm–15 mm long are pathognomonic but not always evident. Some patients will have small vesicles or pustules, and urticaria has also been a presenting symptom. A positive scabies preparation confirms the diagnosis but is not required for treatment.

Patients are treated with either topical permethrin 5% cream or oral ivermectin 200 mcg/kg. For topical treatment, the patient is instructed to massage the cream thoroughly into the skin from the neck to the toes, including the areas under the finger and toenails. The cream is washed off after 8–14 hours. This can be repeated in one to two weeks. Oral treatment may be warranted for patients with persistent or nodular infections or for those who cannot apply the cream appropriately. Two doses of ivermectin 200 mcg/kg, usually given two weeks apart, has been shown to have the same efficacy as a single application of permethrin.[161] The patient's close contacts should also be treated, and the patient is instructed to wash all recently worn clothing and linen in very hot water and to vacuum and clean the home thoroughly. Recently used items can alternatively be placed in a plastic bag for at least three days. It is important to counsel the patient that itching typically persists for a few weeks despite effective treatment because of retained fecal and parasite elements. Medium- or high-potency topical steroids and oral antihistamines can be used to manage pruritus after eradication of the mites.

Onychomycosis

Onychomycosis is infection of the nail bed and plate with a dermatophyte, yeast, or mold. The dermatophyte, *Trichophyton rubrum*, is responsible for the majority of finger and toenail infections. Patients whose hands are frequently in moist conditions also have a similar risk of *Candida* infection due to the environment. Dermatophytic onychomycosis (tinea unguium) is classified as distal subungual, proximal subungual, and white superficial. Distal subungual is the most common subtype. Proximal subungual infections are less common, and may herald underlying immunodeficiency or AIDS. The incidence of onychomycosis increases with age. The risk is likely due to a combination of waning cellular immunity and worsening vascular insufficiency in the elderly population. Diabetes, tinea pedis, psoriasis and genetic predisposition are other risk factors.[162–166]

Onychomycosis is easily recognized as dystrophy of the nail plate with yellow discoloration due to subungual keratinaceous debris. Superficial white onychomycosis has dull, chalky white spots on the surface of the nail plate that spread centrifugally to involve the whole nail plate if left untreated. Onychodystrophy can also be caused by genetic conditions, senile ischemia, chronic trauma, or inflammatory pathologies affecting the nail matrix. Inflammatory conditions like psoriasis or lichen planus will usually involve all of the nails, which would be uncommon for onychomycosis. Onychomycosis is only responsible for 50%–60% of cases of onychodystrophy, so it is important to prove the presence of an infection prior to initiating oral treatment.[167]

Tinea unguium can be diagnosed in the office with potassium hydroxide (KOH) or chlorazol black stains of subungual debris. Nail samples may alternatively be sent to pathology for periodic acid-Schiff (PAS) staining or microbiology for culture. Cultures can be performed for all cases where clinical suspicion is high despite a negative KOH scraping; however, it should be noted that almost one-third of cultures may be falsely negative, and they take four to six weeks for results. Pathologic evaluation with PAS is more costly but is more sensitive than KOH or culture, with one study reporting sensitivities of PAS stain, culture, and KOH at 82%, 53%, and 48%, respectively.[168]

Treatment of dermatophyte onychomycosis with topical agents alone is generally ineffective. Topical agents include terbinafine, azole creams, and ciclopirox. Ciclopirox is available as a nail lacquer, which facilitates penetration into the nail plate. Treatment with ciclopirox lacquer results in resolution in approximately 7% of patients compared to 0.4% using placebo.[169] Adjuvant therapies include topical keratolytic agents, dilute vinegar soaks, antifungal powders, and good foot hygiene. The decision to treat with an oral agent is based on patient comorbidities, discomfort, and preference. Oral treatment is generally recommended for patients who have pain associated with the onychodystrophy and those with a history of, or risk factors for, lower extremity cellulitis. Terbinafine 250 mg daily is the first-line agent for oral therapy and is given for six weeks for fingernails and 12 weeks for toenails. The cure rate is reported to be 76% +/–3%,[170] and overall, long-term recurrence rates are reported as high as 50%.[171–173] It is important to discuss the modest cure rate and risk of recurrence with the patient so that there can be an educated discussion about risks and benefits of treatment. In cases when the decision is made not to treat with oral agents, topical treatments should still be used on a daily to weekly basis for concomitant tinea pedis.

Laser therapy has gained some discussion in the community. The Q-switched and long-pulsed Nd: YAG lasers have been approved for temporary cosmetic improvement of onychomycosis and are widely available at high cost, but studies have not been able to demonstrate an appreciable cure rate or therapeutic benefit beyond temporary improvement in appearance.[174] New lasers that target the organism may yield superior results.

Intertrigo

Intertrigo is a broad term used to describe any inflammatory condition affecting the intertriginous areas. The term is commonly used when referring to candidal intertrigo; however, bacteria and dermatophytes can also cause infections of these areas. In candidal intertrigo, the affected skin is often brightly erythematous and can be weeping and macerated with superficial erosions. It often has characteristic satellite papules or pustular lesions. Erosio interdigitalis blastomycetica is the term for candidal infections involving the interdigital web spaces of the hands or feet. Diagnosis of candidal intertrigo is usually clinical, although a KOH preparation or culture of skin scrapings may be utilized. Diabetes, antibiotic or steroid use, HIV, and other immunosuppressive states are risk factors for developing persistent intertrigo. Treatment of candidal intertrigo involves topical antifungal creams, usually a polyene such as nystatin, or an azole such as miconazole or clotrimazole. It is applied every 12 hours for several weeks, and the patient should also take measures to decrease heat, moisture, and friction. Barrier creams containing zinc oxide can be helpful as can adsorbent powders,

although in some people these can cause more skin irritation. Severe or resistant intertrigo can be treated with a two- to six-week course of an oral azole, usually fluconazole (50 mg–100 mg daily or 150 mg weekly) or itraconazole 200 mg twice a day. In cases of resistant intertrigo, it is important to consider alternative diagnoses such as inverse psoriasis, allergic contact or irritant dermatitis, tinea cruris, seborrheic dermatitis, inverse lichen planus, bacterial intertrigo, and erythrasma.[175] Erythrasma is caused by a corynebacterium infection. A Wood's lamp examination can be performed to look for coral red fluorescence if erythrasma is suspected. Rare conditions that affect the intertriginous areas and that may mimic candidal intertrigo include benign familial pemphigus (Hailey-Hailey) disease, mycosis fungoides, and granular parakeratosis.

Summary

The geriatric population seeks care for a variety of skin conditions. Many of the skin complaints can be attributed to normal physiologic changes of aging, which include benign skin growths, immunosenescence, and generalized xerosis. The accumulation of multiple medical comorbidities and medications can also cause skin disease and discomfort. Additionally, years of sun exposure leads to photoaging and photocarcinogenesis, which may result in a significant burden of cutaneous carcinoma for some individuals. As is the case with many disease processes, the elderly share an increased burden of skin conditions that may present uniquely within their demographic. Being mindful of how to best address these skin conditions and their impact on quality of life is essential to the care of our elderly patients.

References

1. Studdiford J, Salzman B, Tully A. Geriatric Dermatology. In: Arenson C, Busby-Whitehead J, Brummel-Smith K, O'Brien James G, Palmer M, Reichel W, eds. *Reichel's Care of the Elderly: Clinical Aspects of Aging.* 6th ed. New York: Cambridge University Press; 2009; 345–68.

2. Kligman AM, Koblenzer C. Demographics and psychological implications for the aging population. *Dermatol Clin.* 1997 Oct; **15**(4):549–53.

3. Vukmanovic-Stejic M, Rustin MH, Nikolich-Zugich J, Akbar AN. Immune responses in the skin in old age. *Curr Opin Immunol.* 2011 Aug; **23**(4):525–31.

4. Kosmadaki MG, Gilchrest BA. The demographics of aging in the United States: implications for dermatology. *Arch Dermatol.* 2002 Nov; **138**(11):1427–8.

5. Vandergriff T, Bergstresser P. Anatomy and Physiology. In: Bolognia J, Jorrizo J, Schaffer J, eds. *Dermatology.* 3rd ed. Philadelphia: Saunders; 2012; 43–54.

6. Gilchrest BA, Chiu N. Aging and the Skin. In: Beers MH, Berkow R, eds. *The Merck Manual of Geriatrics*, 3rd ed. Whitehouse Station, NJ: Merck and Co, Inc, 2000; 1231–7.

7. Balin AK. Skin Disease, In: Evans JG, Williams TF, Beattie BL, et al., eds. *Oxford Textbook of Geriatric Medicine.* 2nd ed. Oxford: Oxford University Press, 2000; 721–38.

8. Rinnerthaler M, Duschl J, Steinbacher P, et al. Age-related changes in the composition of the cornified envelope in human skin. *Exp Dermatol.* 2013 May; **22**(5):329–35.

9. Stalder JF1, Tennstedt D, Deleuran M, et al. Fragility of epidermis and its consequence in dermatology. *J Eur Acad Dermatol Venereol.* 2014 Jun; **28**(Suppl 4):1–18.

10. Fisher GJ, Varani J, Voorhees JJ. Looking older: fibroblast collapse and therapeutic implications. *Arch Dermatol.* 2008; **144**:666–72.

11. Rabe JH, Mamelak AJ, McElgunn PJ, et al. Photoaging: mechanisms and repair. *J Am Acad Dermatol.* 2006 Jul; **55**(1):1–19.

12. Xu YP, Qi RQ, Chen W, et al. Aging affects epidermal Langerhans cell development and function and alters their miRNA gene expression profile. *Aging (Albany, NY).* 2012 Nov;**4**(11):742–54.

13. Laube S: Skin infections and ageing. *Ageing Res Rev.* 2004; **13**:69–89.

14. Agius E, Lacy KE, Vukmanovic-Stejic M, et al. Decreased TNF-{alpha} synthesis by macrophages restricts cutaneous immunosurveillance by memory CD4+ T cells during aging. *J Exp Med.* 2009; **206**:1929–40.

15. Yaar M, Gilchrest BA. Ageing and photoageing of keratinocytes and melanocytes. *Clin Exp Dermatol.* 2001; **26**:583–91.

16. Waller JM, Maibach HI. Age and skin structure and function, a quantitative approach (I): blood flow, pH, thickness, and ultrasound echogenicity. *Skin Res Technol.* 2005; **11**:221–35.

17. Hughes VA, Roubenoff R, Wood M, et al. Anthropometric assessment of 10-y changes in body composition in the elderly. *Am J Clin Nutr.* 2004; **80**:475–82.

18. Fenske NA, Lober CW. Structural and functional changes of normal aging skin. *J Am Acad Dermatol.* 1986; **15**:571–85.

19. Thomas DR, Burkemper NM. Aging skin and wound healing. *Clin Geriatr Med.* 2013 May; **29**(2):xi–xx.

20. Katz MH, Kirsner RS, Eaglstein WH, et al: Human wound fluid from acute wounds stimulates fibroblast and endothelial cell growth. *J Am Acad Dermatol.* 1991; **25**:1054–8.

21. Kirsner RS, Eaglstein WH: The wound healing process. *Dermatol Clin.* 1993; **11**:629–40.

22. Sandblom PH, Peterson P, Muren A, et al. Determination of the tensile strength of the healing wound as a clinical test. *Acta Chir Scand.* 1953; **105**:252–7.

23. Freedland M, Karmiol S, Rodriguez J, et al. Fibroblast responses to cytokines are maintained during aging. *Ann Plast Surg.* 1995; **35**:290–6.

24. Pienta KJ, Coppey DS. Characterization of the subtypes of cell motility in ageing human skin fibroblasts. *Mech Ageing Dev.* 1990; **56**:99–105.

25. Raffetto JD. Dermal pathology, cellular biology, and inflammation in chronic venous disease. *Thromb Res.* 2009; **123**(Suppl 4):S66–71.

26. Bergan JJ, Schmid-Schonbein GW, Smith PD, et al. Chronic venous disease. *N Engl J Med.* 2006; **355**:488–98.

27. Aharon I, Etcoff N, Ariely D, et al. Beautiful faces have variable reward value: fMRI and behavioral evidence. *Neuron.* 2001; **32**:537–51.

28. Henderson JJA. Facial attractiveness predicts longevity. *Evol Hum Behav.* 2003; **24**:351–6

29. Alam M, Dover JS. On beauty: evolution, psychosocial considerations, and surgical enhancement. *Arch Dermatol.* 2001; **137**:795–807.

30. Rohrich R, Pessa J. The fat compartments of the face: anatomy and clinical implications for cosmetic surgery. *J Plast Reconstr Surg.* 2007; **119**:2219–27.

31. Lambros V. Observations on periorbital and midface aging. *Plast Reconstr Surg.* 2007; **120**:1367–76.

32. Plewig G, Koigman AM. Proliferative activity of the sebaceous glands of the aged. *J Invest Dermatol.* 1978; **70**:314–17.

33. Iannacone MR, Hughes MC, Green AC. Effects of sunscreen on skin cancer and photoaging. *Photodermatol Photoimmunol Photomed.* 2014 Apr–Jun; **30**(2–3):55–61.

34. Creidi P, Vienne M-P, Ochonisky S, et al. Profilometric evaluation of photodamage after topical retinaldehyde and retinoic acid treatment. *J Am Acad Dermatol.* 1998; **39**:960–5.

35. Olsen EA, Katz HI, Levine N, et al. Tretinoin emollient cream for photodamaged skin: results of 48-week, multicenter, double-blind studies. *J Am Acad Dermatol.* 1997 Aug; **37**(2 Pt 1):217–26.

36. Calikoglu E, Sorg O, Tran C, et al. UVA and UVB decrease the expression of CD44 and hyaluronate in mouse epidermis, which is counteracted by topical retinoids. *Photochem Photobiol.* 2006; **82**:1342–7.

37. Dietre CM, Griffin TD, Murphy GF, et al. Effects of alpha-hydroxy acids on photoaged skin. *J Am Acad Dermatol.* 1996; **34**:187–95.

38. Akpinar F, Dervis E. Association between acrochordons and the components of metabolic syndrome. *Eur J Dermatol.* 2012 Jan–Feb; **22**(1):106–10.

39. Fajgenbaum DC, Rosenbach M, van Rhee F, et al. Eruptive cherry hemangiomatosis associated with multicentric Castleman disease: a case report and diagnostic clue. *JAMA Dermatol.* 2013 Feb; **149**(2):204–8.

40. Derancourt C, Bourdon-Lanoy E, Grob JJ, et al. Multiple large solar lentigos on the upper back as clinical markers of past severe sunburn: a case-control study. *Dermatology.* 2007; **214**(1):25–31.

41. Tanaka M, Sawada M, Kobayashi K. Key points in dermoscopic differentiation between lentigo maligna and solar lentigo. *J Dermatol.* Jan 2011; **38**(1):53–8.

42. e Dinato SL, de Oliva R, e Dinato MM, et al. [Prevalence of dermatoses in residents of institutions for the elderly]. *Rev Assoc Med Bras.* Nov–Dec 2008; **54**(6):543–7.

43. Shuster S. Osteoporosis, a unitary hypothesis of collagen loss in skin and bone. *Med Hypotheses.* 2005; **65**(3):426–32.

44. Stone M. Cysts. In: Bolognia J, Jorrizo J, Schaffer J, eds. *Dermatology.* 3rd ed. Philadelphia: Saunders; 2012: 43–54.

45. Rogers, HW, Weinstock, MA, Harris, AR, et al. Incidence estimate of nonmelanoma skin cancer in the United States, 2006. *Arch Dermatol.* 2010; **146**(3):283–7.

46. American Cancer Society. Cancer Facts and Figures 2014. Available at: www.cancer.org/research/cancer factsstatistics/cancerfactsfigures2014/index (accessed July 15, 2014).

47. Stern RS. Prevalence of a history of skin cancer in 2007: results of an incidence-based model. *Arch Dermatol.* 2010 Mar; **146**(3):279–82.

48. Mancebo SE, Hu JY, Wang SQ. Sunscreens: a review of health benefits, regulations, and controversies. *Dermatol Clin.* 2014 Jul; **32**(3):427–38.

49. Green AC, Williams GM, Logan V, Strutton GM. Reduced melanoma after regular sunscreen use: randomized trial follow-up *J Clin Onco.* 2011 Jan 20; **29**(3):257–63; published online on December 6, 2010.

50. Lin JS, Eder M, Weinmann S. Behavioral counseling to prevent skin cancer: a systematic review for the US Preventive Services Task Force. *Ann Intern Med.* 2011 Feb 1; **154**(3):190–201.

51. Youssef KK, Van Keymeulen A, Lapouge G, et al. Identification of the cell lineage at the origin of basal cell carcinoma. *Nat Cell Biol.* 2010; **12**:299–305.

52. Soyer HP, Rigel D, Wurm E. Actinic Keratosis, Basal Cell Carcinoma, and Squamous Cell Carcinoma In: Bolognia J, Jorrizo J, Schaffer J, eds. *Dermatology.* 3rd ed. Philadelphia: Saunders; 2012: 1773–94.

53. Bath FJ, Bong J, Perkins W, Williams HC. Interventions for basal cell carcinoma of the skin. *Cochrane Database Syst Rev.* 2003; **2**:CD003412.

54. Chren MM, Linos E, Torres JS, et al. Tumor recurrence 5 years after treatment of cutaneous basal cell carcinoma and squamous cell carcinoma. *J Invest Dermatol.* 2013 May; **133**(5):1188–96.

55. Röwert-Huber J, Patel MJ, Forschner T, et al. Actinic keratosis is an early in situ squamous cell carcinoma: a proposal for reclassification. *Br J Dermatol.* 2007; **156**:8–12.

56. Brantsch KD, Meisner C, Schonfisch B, et al. Analysis of risk factors determining prognosis of cutaneous squamous-cell carcinoma: a prospective study. *Lancet Oncol.* 2008; **9**:713–20.

57. Schwartz RA. Keratoacanthoma. *J Am Acad Dermatol.* 1994; **30**:1–19.

58. Rowe DE, Carroll RJ, Day CL Jr. Prognostic factors for local recurrence, metastasis, and survival rates in squamous cell carcinoma of the skin, ear, and lip. Implications for treatment modality selection. *J Am Acad Dermatol.* 1992; **26**:976–90.

59. Marcil I, Stern RS. Risk of developing a subsequent nonmelanoma skin cancer in patients with a history of nonmelanoma skin cancer: a critical review of the literature and meta-analysis. *Arch Dermatol.* 2000; **136**:1524–30.

60. Micali G, Lacarrubba F, Nasca MR, et al. Topical pharmacotherapy for skin cancer: part II. Clinical applications. *J Am Acad Dermatol.* 2014 Jun; **70**(6):979.e1–12.

61. Ross K, Cherpelis B, Lien M, Fenske N. Spotlighting the role of photodynamic therapy in cutaneous malignancy: an update and expansion. *Dermatol Surg.* 2013 Dec; **39**(12):1733–44.

62. Scope A, Dusza SW, Halpern AC, et al. The "ugly duckling" sign: agreement between observers. *Arch Dermatol.* 2008 Jan; **144**(1):58–64.

63. Garbe C, Bauer J. Melanoma In: Bolognia J, Jorrizo J, Schaffer J, eds. *Dermatology.* 3rd ed. Philadelphia: Saunders; 2012: 1885–1914.

64. Zitelli JA, Brown C, Hanusa BH. Mohs micrographic surgery for the treatment of primary cutaneous

melanoma. *J Am Acad Dermatol.* 1997 Aug; **37**(2 Pt 1):236–45.

65. Gershenwald JE, Thompson W, Mansfield PF, et al. Multi-institutional melanoma lymphatic mapping experience: the prognostic value of sentinel lymph node status in 612 stage I or II melanoma patients. *J Clin Oncol.* 1999; **17**:976–83.

66. Leiter U, Buettner PG, Bohnenberger K, et al. Sentinel lymph node dissection in primary melanoma reduces subsequent regional lymph node metastasis as well as distant metastasis after nodal involvement. *Ann Surg Oncol.* 2010; **17**:129–37.

67. Kettlewell S, Moyes C, Bray C, et al. Value of sentinel node status as a prognostic factor in melanoma: prospective Observational Study. *BMJ.* 2006; **332**:1423–7.

68. Morton DL, Thompson JF, Cochran AJ, et al. Sentinel-node biopsy or nodal observation in melanoma. *N Engl J Med.* 2006; **355**:1307–17.

69. Sosman JA, Kim KB, Schuchter L, et al. Survival in BRAF V600-mutant advanced melanoma treated with vemurafenib. *N Engl J Med.* 2012 Feb 23; **366**(8):707–14.

70. Chapman PB, Hauschild A, Robert C, et al. Improved survival with vemurafenib in melanoma with BRAF V600E mutation. *N Engl J Med.* 2011; **364**:2507–16.

71. Elewski BE, Draelos Z, Dréno B, et al. Rosacea – global diversity and optimized outcome: proposed international consensus from the Rosacea International Expert Group. *J Eur Acad Dermatol Venereol.* 2011; **25**:188–200.

72. Berg M. Epidemiological studies of the influence of sunlight on the skin. *Photodermatol.* 1989; **6**:80–4.

73. McAleer MA, Fitzpatrick P, Powell FC. Papulopustular rosacea: prevalence and relationship to photodamage. *J Am Acad Dermatol.* 2010; **63**:33–9.

74. Spoendlin J, Voegel JJ, Jick SS, et al. A study on the epidemiology of rosacea in the UK. *Br J Dermatol.* 2012 Sept; **167**(3):598–605.

75. Wilkin J, Dahl M, Detmar M, et al. Standard classification of rosacea: report of the National Rosacea Society Expert Committee on the Classification and Staging of Rosacea. *J Am Acad Dermatol.* 2002; **46**:584–7.

76. Lazararidou E, Clinical and laboratory study of ocular rosacea in northern Greece. *J Eur Acad Dermatol Venereol.* 2011 Dec; **25**(12):1428–31.

77. Lazaridou E, Giannopoulou C, Fotiadou C, et al. The potential role of microorganisms in the development of rosacea. *J Dtsch Dermatol Ges.* 2011; **9**:21–5.

78. Zhao YE, Wu LP, Peng Y, Cheng H. Retrospective analysis of the association between Demodex infestation and rosacea. *Arch Dermatol.* 2010; **146**:896–902.

79. Kastarinen H, Oksanen T, Okokon EO, et al. Topical anti-inflammatory agents for seborrhoeic dermatitis of the face or scalp. *Cochrane Database Syst Rev.* 2014; 5:CD009446.

80. Potts GA, Hurley MY. Psoriasis in the geriatric population. *Clin Geriatr Med.* 2013 May; **29**(2):373–95.

81. Dregan A, Charlton J, et al. Chronic inflammatory disorders and risk of type 2 diabetes mellitus, coronary heart disease, and stroke: a population-based cohort study. *Circulation.* 2014 Sep 2; **130**(10):837–44.

82. Van der Voort EA et al. Psoriasis is independently associated with nonalcoholic fatty liver disease in patients 55 years or older: Results from a population-based study. *J Am Acad Dermatol.* 2014 Mar; **70**(3):517–24.

83. Zachariae H. Prevalence of joint disease in patients with psoriasis: implications for therapy. *Am J Clin Dermatol.* 2003; **4**:441–7.

84. Eder L, Chandran V, Shen H, et al. Incidence of arthritis in a prospective cohort of psoriasis patients. *Arthritis Care Res (Hoboken).* 2011; **63**:619–22.

85. Alamanos Y, Voulgari PV, Drosos AA. Incidence and prevalence of psoriatic arthritis: a systematic review. *J Rheumatol* 2008; **35**:1354–8.

86. Balato N, Managing moderate-to-severe psoriasis in the elderly. *Drugs Aging.* 2014 Apr; **31**(4):233–8.

87. Williams HC, ed. *Atopic Dermatitis: The Epidemiology, Causes and Prevention of Atopic Eczema.* Cambridge: Cambridge University Press, 2000.

88. Ozakaya E. Adult-onset atopic dermatitis. *J Am Acad Dermatol.* 2005 Apr; **52**(4):579–82.

89. Bonamonte D, Foti C, Vestita M, et al. Nummular eczema and contact allergy: a retrospective study. *Dermatitis.* 2012 Jul–Aug; **23**(4):153–7.

90. Garritsen FM, ter Haar NM, Spuls PI. House dust mite reduction in the management of atopic dermatitis: a critically appraised topic. *Br J Dermatol.* 2013; **168**:688–91.

91. Kjaer HF, Eller E, Høst A, et al. The prevalence of allergic diseases in an unselected group of 6-year-old children: the DARC birth cohort study. *Pediatr Allergy Immunol.* 2008; **19**:737–45.

92. Bath-Hextall F, Delamere FM, Williams HC. Dietary exclusions for established atopic eczema. *Cochrane Database Syst Rev.* 2008; **1**:CD005203.

93. Ring J, Alomar A, Bieber T, et al. Guidelines for treatment of atopic eczema (atopic dermatitis) part II: European Dermatology Forum; European Academy of Dermatology and Venereology; European Task Force on Atopic Dermatitis; European Federation of Allergy; European Society of Pediatric Dermatology; Global Allergy and Asthma European Network. *J Eur Acad Dermatol Venereol.* 2012 Sep; **26**(9):1176–93.

94. Berger TG, Shive M, Harper GM. Pruritus in the older patient: a clinical review. *JAMA.* 2013;**310**(22);2443–50.

95. Paul C, Maumus-Robert S, Mazereeuw-Hautier J, et al. Prevalence and risk factors for xerosis in the elderly: a cross-sectional epidermological study in primary care. *Dermatology.* 2011; **223**(3):260–5.

96. Cohen AD, Vander T, Medvendovski E, et al. Neuropathic scrotal pruritus: anogenital pruritus is a symptoms of lumbosacral radiculopathy. *JAAD.* 2005; **52**(1):61–6.

97. Savk O, Savk E. Investigation of spinal pathology in notalgia paresthetica. *J Am Acad Dermatol.* 2005; 52:1085–7.

98. Browning J, Combes B, Mayo MJ. Long-term efficacy of sertraline as a treatment for cholestatic pruritus in patients with primary biliary cirrhosis. *Am J Gastroenterol.* 2003; **98**:2736–41.

99. Klein PA, Clark RA. An evidence-based review of the efficacy of antihistamines in relieving pruritus in atopic dermatitis. *Arch Dermatol.* 1999; **135**:1522–5.

100. Ada S, Seçkin D, Budakoğlu I, Ozdemir FN. Treatment of uremic pruritus with narrowband ultraviolet B phototherapy: an open pilot study. *J Am Acad Dermatol.* 2005; **53**:149–51.

101. Wang H, Yosipovitch G. New insights into the pathophysiology and treatment of chronic itch in patients with end-stage renal disease, chronic liver disease, and lymphoma. *Int J Dermatol.* 2010; **49**:1–11.

102. Davis MP, Frandsen JL, Walsh D, et al. Mirtazapine for pruritus. *J Pain Symptom Manage.* 2003; **25**:288–91.

103. Hundley JL, Yosipovitch G. Mirtazapine for reducing nocturnal itch in patients with chronic pruritus: a pilot study. *J Am Acad Dermatol.* 2004; **50**:889–91.

104. Demierre MF, Taverna J. Mirtazapine and gabapentin for reducing pruritus in cutaneous T-cell lymphoma. *J Am Acad Dermatol.* 2006; **55**:543–4.

105. Sheen MJ, Ho ST, Lee CH, et al. Prophylactic mirtazapine reduces intrathecal morphine-induced pruritus. *Br J Anaesth.* 2008; **101**:711–15.

106. Ständer S, Böckenholt B, Schürmeyer-Horst F, et al. Treatment of chronic pruritus with the selective serotonin re-uptake inhibitors paroxetine and fluvoxamine: results of an open-labelled, two-arm proof-of-concept study. *Acta Derm Venereol.* 2009; **89**:45–51.

107. Mayo MJ, Handem I, Saldana S, et al. Sertraline as a first-line treatment for cholestatic pruritus. *Hepatology.* 2007; **45**:666–74.

108. Wallengren J, Sundler F. Brachioradial pruritus is associated with a reduction in cutaneous innervation

109. Goodkin R, Wingard E, Bernhard JD. Brachioradial pruritus: cervical spine disease and neurogenic/neuropathic [corrected] pruritus. *J Am Acad Dermatol.* 2003; **48**:521–4.

that normalizes during the symptom-free remissions. *J Am Acad Dermatol.* 2005; **52**:142–5.

110. Marziniak M, Phan NQ, Raap U, et al. Brachioradial pruritus as a result of cervical spine pathology: the results of a magnetic resonance tomography study. *J Am Acad Dermatol.* 2011; **65**:756–62.

111. Eschler DC, Klein PA. An evidence-based review of the efficacy of topical antihistamines in the relief of pruritus. *J Drugs Dermatol.* 2010; **9**:992–7.

112. Dawn AG, Yosipovitch G. Butorphanol for treatment of intractable pruritus. *J Am Acad Dermatol.* 2006; **54**:527–31.

113. Kumagai H, Ebata T, Takamori K, et al. Effect of a novel kappa-receptor agonist, nalfurafine hydrochloride, on severe itch in 337 haemodialysis patients: a phase III, randomized, double-blind, placebo-controlled study. *Nephrol Dial Transplant.* 2010; **25**:1251–7.

114. Phan NQ, Bernhard JD, Luger TA, Ständer S. Antipruritic treatment with systemic μ-opioid receptor antagonists: a review. *J Am Acad Dermatol.* 2010; **63**:680–8.

115. Penning JP, Samson B, Baxter AD. Reversal of epidural morphine-induced respiratory depression and pruritus with nalbuphine. *Can J Anaesth.* 1988; **35**:599–604.

116. Gilchrest BA, Rowe JW, Brown RS, et al. Relief of uremic pruritus with ultraviolet phototherapy. *N Engl J Med.* 1977; **297**:136–8.

117. Ko MJ, Yang JY, Wu HY, et al. Narrowband ultraviolet B phototherapy for patients with refractory uraemic pruritus: a randomized controlled trial. *Br J Dermatol.* 2011; **165**:633–9.

118. Yalçin B, Tamer E, Toy GG, et al. The prevalence of skin diseases in the elderly: analysis of 4099 geriatric patients. *Int J Dermatol.* 2006; **45**:672–6.

119. Tomljanović-Veselski M, Lipozencić J, Lugović L. Contact allergy to special and standard allergens in patients with venous ulcers. *Coll Antropol.* 2007; **31**:751–6.

120. Jindal R, Sharma NL, Mahajan VK, Tegta GR. Contact sensitization in venous eczema: preliminary results of patch testing with Indian standard series and topical medicaments. *Indian J Dermatol Venereol Leprol.* 2009; **75**:136–41.

121. Mimouni D. Diagnosis and classification of pemphigus and BP. *Autoimmunity Reviews.* 2014 Apr–May: **13**(4–5):477–81.

122. Bystryn JC, Rudolph JL. Pemphigus. *Lancet.* 2005; **366**:61–73.

123. Grando SA. Pemphigus autoimmunity: hypotheses and realities. *Autoimmunity.* 2012; **45**:7–35.

124. Lever WF. Pemphigus. *Medicine (Baltimore).* 1953; **32**:1–123.

125. Joly P, Roujeau JC, Benichou J, et al. A comparison of oral and topical corticosteroids in patients with bullous pemphigoid. *N Engl J Med.* 2002; **346**:321–7.

126. Goon AT, Tan SH, Khoo LS, Tan T. Tetracycline and nicotinamide for the treatment of bullous pemphigoid: our experience in Singapore. *Singapore Med J.* 2000; **41**:327–30.

127. Gürcan HM, Ahmed AR. Efficacy of dapsone in the treatment of pemphigus and pemphigoid: analysis of current data. *Am J Clin Dermatol.* 2009; **10**:383–96.

128. Singh S. Evidence-based treatments for pemphigus vulgaris, pemphigus foliaceus, and bullous pemphigoid: a systematic review. *Indian J Dermatol Venereol Leprol.* 2011 Jul–Aug; **77**(4):456–69.

129. Mutasim DF. Autoimmune bullous dermatoses in the elderly: diagnosis and management. *Drugs Aging.* 2003; **20**(9):663–81.

130. Stavropoulos PG, Soura E, Antoniou C. Drug-induced pemphigoid: a review of the literature. *J Eur Acad Dermatol Venereol.* 2014 Sep; **28**(9):1133–40.

131. Brenner S, Bialy-Golan A, Ruocco V. Drug-induced pemphigus. *Clin Dermatol.* 1998; **16**:393–7.

132. Brenner S, Goldberg I. Drug-induced pemphigus. *Clin Dermatol.* 2011; **29**:455–7.

133. Feng S, Zhou W, Zhang J, Jin P. Analysis of 6 cases of drug-induced pemphigus. *Eur J Dermatol.* 2011; **21**:696–9.

134. Dupuy A, Benchikhi H, Roujeau JC, et al. Risk factors for erysipelas of the leg (cellulitis): case-control study. *BMJ.* 1999; **318**:1591–4.

135. Semel JD, Goldin H. Association of athlete's foot with cellulitis of the lower extremities: diagnostic value of bacterial cultures of ipsilateral interdigital space samples. *Clin Infect Dis* 1996; **23**:1162–4.

136. McNamara DR, Tleyjeh IM, Berbari EF, et al. Incidence of lower-extremity cellulitis: a population-based study in Olmsted county, Minnesota. *Mayo Clin Proc.* 2007; **82**:817–21.

137. Perl B, Gottehrer NP, Raveh D, et al. Cost-effectiveness of blood cultures for adult patients with cellulitis. *Clin Infect Dis.* 1999; **29**:1483–8.

138. Peralta G, Padrón E, Roiz MP, et al. Risk factors for bacteremia in patients with limb cellulitis. *Eur J Clin Microbiol Infect Dis.* 2006; **25**:619–26.

139. Harpaz R, Ortega-Sanchez IR, Seward JF, Advisory Committee on Immunization Practices (ACIP) Centers for Disease Control and Prevention (CDC). Prevention of herpes zoster: recommendations of the Advisory Committee on Immunization Practices (ACIP). *MMWR Recomm Rep.* 2008; **57**:1–30.

140. Yawn BP, Saddier P, Wollan PC, et al. A population-based study of the incidence and complication rates of herpes zoster before zoster vaccine introduction. *Mayo Clin Proc.* 2007; **82**:1341–9.

141. Straus SE, Ostrove JM, Inchauspé G, et al. NIH conference. Varicella-zoster virus infections: biology, natural history, treatment, and prevention. *Ann Intern Med.* 1988; **108**:221–37.

142. Donahue JG, Choo PW, Manson JE, Platt R. The incidence of herpes zoster. *Arch Intern Med.* 1995; **155**:1605–9.

143. Zhang JX, Joesoef RM, Bialek S, et al. Association of physical trauma with risk of herpes zoster among Medicare beneficiaries in the United States. *J Infect Dis.* 2013; **207**:1007–11.

144. McDonald JR, Zeringue AL, Caplan L, et al. Herpes zoster risk factors in a national cohort of veterans with rheumatoid arthritis. *Clin Infect Dis.* 2009; **48**:1364–71.

145. Bowsher D. Postherpetic neuralgia and its treatment: a retrospective survey of 191 patients. *J Pain Symptom Manage.* 1996; **12**:290–9.

146. Rowbotham M, Harden N, Stacey B, et al. Gabapentin for the treatment of postherpetic neuralgia: a randomized controlled trial. *JAMA.* 1998; **280**:1837–42.

147. Pavan-Langston D. Herpes zoster ophthalmicus. *Neurology* 1995; **45**:S50–1.

148. Ragozzino MW, Melton LJ 3rd, Kurland LT, et al. Population-based study of herpes zoster and its sequelae. *Medicine (Baltimore).* 1982; **61**:310–6.

149. Tomkinson A, Roblin DG, Brown MJ. Hutchinson's sign and its importance in rhinology. *Rhinology.* 1995; **33**:180–2.

150. Diaz GA, Rakita RM, Koelle DM. A case of Ramsay Hunt–like syndrome caused by herpes simplex virus type 2. *Clin Infect Dis.* 2005; **40**:1545–7.

151. Gnann JW Jr. Varicella-zoster virus: atypical presentations and unusual complications. *J Infect Dis.* 2002; **186**(Suppl 1):S91–8.

152. Kost RG, Straus SE. Postherpetic neuralgia–pathogenesis, treatment, and prevention. *N Engl J Med.* 1996; **335**:32–42.

153. Choo PW, Galil K, Donahue JG, et al. Risk factors for postherpetic neuralgia. *Arch Intern Med.* 1997; **157**:1217–24.

154. Adour KK. Otological complications of herpes zoster. *Ann Neurol.* 1994; **35**(Suppl):S62–4.

155. Mishell JH, Applebaum EL. Ramsay-Hunt syndrome in a patient with HIV infection. *Otolaryngol Head Neck Surg.* 1990; **102**:177–9.

156. Levin MJ, Oxman MN, Zang JH, et al. Varicella-zoster virus-specific immune responses in elderly recipients of a herpes zoster vaccine. *J Infect Dis.* 2008 Mar 15; **197**(6):825–35.

157. Oxman MN, Levin MJ, Shingles Prevention Study Group. Vaccination against herpes zoster and postherpetic neuralgia. *J Infect Dis.* 2008; **197**(Suppl 2):S228–36.

158. Fuller LC. Epidemiology of scabies. *Curr Opin Infect Dis.* 2013; **26**:123–6.

159. Arlian LG, Runyan RA, Achar S, Estes SA. Survival and infectivity of Sarcoptes scabiei var. canis and var. hominis. *J Am Acad Dermatol.* 1984; **11**:210–15.

160. Currie BJ, McCarthy JS. Permethrin and ivermectin for scabies. *N Engl J Med.*2010; **362**:717–25.

161. Usha V, Gopalakrishnan Nair TV. A comparative study of oral ivermectin and topical permethrin cream in the treatment of scabies. *J Am Acad Dermatol.* 2000; **42**:236–40.

162. Sigurgeirsson B, Steingrímsson O. Risk factors associated with onychomycosis. *J Eur Acad Dermatol Venereol.* 2004; **18**:48–51.

163. Piérard GE, Piérard-Franchimont C. The nail under fungal siege in patients with type II diabetes mellitus. *Mycoses.* 2005; **48**:339–42.

164. Muñoz-Pérez MA, Rodriguez-Pichardo A, Camacho F, Colmenero MA. Dermatological findings correlated with CD4 lymphocyte counts in a prospective 3 year study of 1161 patients with human immunodeficiency virus disease predominantly acquired through intravenous drug abuse. *Br J Dermatol.* 1998; **139**:33–9.

165. Zaias N, Tosti A, Rebell G, et al. Autosomal dominant pattern of distal subungual onychomycosis caused by Trichophyton rubrum. *J Am Acad Dermatol.* 1996; **34**:302–4.

166. Faergemann J, Correia O, Nowicki R, Ro BI. Genetic predisposition–understanding underlying mechanisms of onychomycosis. *J Eur Acad Dermatol Venereol.* 2005; **19**(Suppl 1):17–19.

167. Gupta AK, Jain HC, Lynde CW, et al. Prevalence and epidemiology of onychomycosis in patients visiting physicians' offices: a multicenter Canadian survey of 15,000 patients. *J Am Acad Dermatol.* 2000; **43**:244–8.

168. Weinberg JM, Koestenblatt EK, Tutrone WD, et al. Comparison of diagnostic methods in the evaluation of onychomycosis. *J Am Acad Dermatol.* 2003 Aug; **49**(2):193–7.

169. Gupta AK, Fleckman P, Baran R. Ciclopirox nail lacquer topical solution 8% in the treatment of toenail onychomycosis. *J Am Acad Dermatol.* 2000; **43**:S70–80.

170. Gupta AK, Ryder JE, Johnson AM. Cumulative meta-analysis of systemic antifungal agents for the treatment of onychomycosis. *Br J Dermatol.* 2004; **150**:537.

171. Sigurgeirsson B, Olafsson JH, Steinsson JB, et al. Long-term effectiveness of treatment with terbinafine vs itraconazole in onychomycosis: a 5-year blinded prospective follow-up study. *Arch Dermatol.* 2002; **138**:353–7.

172. Drake LA, Shear NH, Arlette JP, et al. Oral terbinafine in the treatment of toenail onychomycosis: North American multicenter trial. *J Am Acad Dermatol.* 1997; **37**:740–5.

173. Tosti A, Piraccini BM, Stinchi C, Colombo MD. Relapses of onychomycosis after successful treatment with systemic antifungals: a three-year follow-up. *Dermatology.* 1998; **197**:162–6.

174. Hollmig ST, Rahman Z, Henderson MT, et al. Lack of efficacy with 1064-nm neodymium:yttrium-aluminum-garnet laser for the treatment of onychomycosis: a randomized, controlled trial. *J Am Acad Dermatol.* 2014; **70**:911–7.

175. Yosipovitch G, DeVore A, Dawn A. Obesity and the skin: skin physiology and skin manifestations of obesity. *J Am Acad Dermatol.* 2007 Jun; **56**(6):901–16.

508

Pressure ulcers
Practical considerations in prevention and treatment

Mary H. Palmer, PhD, RN-C, FAAN, ASGF

Introduction

Pressure ulcers have plagued humanity for centuries. A sixteenth-century surgeon, Ambrose Paré, proposed that removing the cause, relieving the pain, and providing nutrition and rest were the first steps in healing.[1, 2] In the mid-twentieth century, Margaret Woodruff, a nurse, echoed this advice by proposing the use of a sheepskin in direct contact with the skin while providing nutritional therapy and measures to improve circulation.[3] Despite intense efforts over the ensuring decades, pressure ulcers continue to affect approximately 7.5 million people globally and are viewed as public health and patient safety issues.[4]

Pressure ulcers cause significant financial burden and human suffering. According to Berlowitz and colleagues in 2009, annual costs in the United States for pressure ulcers were between $9.1 and $11.6 billion. [5] The costs of a hospital-acquired stage IV pressure ulcer during a hospital stay were estimated to be US $129,248.[6] Affected adults describe "endless pain," and one stated, "When they clean it, it is like a needle scraping my nails. It is very painful."[7]

Because of the high incidence and prevalence of pressure ulcers and their complications, costs to the health-care system, pain and suffering for affected adults, and caregiver burden, efforts continue to reduce pressure ulcer rates. One of the goals of Healthy People 2020 is to achieve 10% improvement in pressure-ulcer-related hospitalizations of older adults.[8] Since 2008, the Centers for Medicare and Medicaid Services (CMS) ceased reimbursement to hospitals for pressure ulcers acquired during hospitalization (HAPUs), thus creating an incentive for hospitals to prevent pressure ulcer development.[9]

The purpose of this chapter is to discuss evidence-based literature regarding the prevention and treatment of pressure ulcers in older adults and the need for patient- and family-centered care that supports function, independence, and quality of life.

Background

Skin, the body's largest organ, comprises 10%–15% of body weight and serves to maintain thermoregulation, prevent infection and water loss, and act as a protective covering to underlying tissues and structures of the human body.[10] The skin also mirrors the health of the human organism. The concept of skin failure was proposed, and it was described as an event that occurs during a critical illness in which skin and underlying tissue die.[10] For example, a person not considered at risk for pressure ulcer formation could experience an event such as sepsis, trauma, or myocardial infarction whereby volume depletion results in low blood pressure, which in turn reduces blood flow to the skin. In such events, body parts may also be subjected to prolonged pressure that occludes blood flow to tissue, resulting in localized ischemia and overt changes to the skin.[11]

A consensus conference convened in 2010 concluded that "not all pressure ulcers are avoidable."[12] The panel of experts noted that hemodynamic instability and advanced directives prohibiting artificial hydration and nutrition could create situations when pressure ulcers may be unavoidable.

In addition to changes in a person's medical condition, other factors play a role in pressure ulcer development. A conceptual model identifying key determinants in pressure ulcer development was proposed.[13] Identified direct causal factors included immobility, general skin status, and perfusion.

Reichel's Care of the Elderly, 7th Edition, ed. Jan Busby-Whitehead *et al.* Published by Cambridge University Press.
© Cambridge University Press 2016.

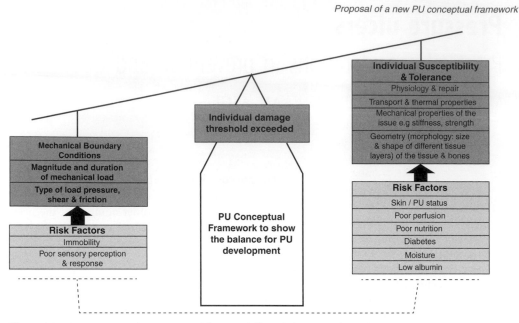

Proposal of a new PU conceptual framework

Figure 36.1 New pressure ulcer conceptual framework (from Coleman et al., 2014).

Indirect factors included moisture, sensory perception, diabetes, low albumin, and poor nutrition (see Figure 36.1). Other factors included in this model were: age, medications, presence of pitting edema, and general health status. Although the model identifies linkages among physiological and biomechanical determinants and patient risk factors for pressure ulcer development, the model requires further development to address varying levels and different combinations of risk factors. Factors not included in the model are those extrinsic to older adults. These include time staff members take to respond to inpatient call lights and nurses' attention to pressure ulcer prevention activities.[14, 15] A systematic literature review concluded that more nursing staff, regardless of the level (i.e., certified nursing assistant, licensed practical nurse, or registered nurse), "led to fewer pressure ulcers."[16] Therefore, factors beyond characteristics of the older adult can influence the development of pressure ulcers.

Because of the significant morbidity and mortality associated with pressure ulcers and because they are considered, for the most part, preventable, effective pressure ulcer prevention has been included in hospital patient safety strategies.[17] Caution should be used when making comparisons across hospitals regarding rates of hospital-acquired pressure ulcers because of the discrepancies in data sources. For

example, authors of one study found little correlation between each hospital's administrative incidence data and point-prevalence surveillance data.[18] An examination of Medicare claims data from fiscal year 2009–2010 found that lower-staged pressure ulcers (such as stage I or stage II) on admission which progressed to stage III or stage IV pressure ulcers were reported as present on admission, thus causing underreporting of hospital-acquired stage III and stage IV pressure ulcers.[19]

Pressure ulcer rates are also of concern in long-term care facilities. These facilities must ensure that "a resident who enters the facility without pressure sores does not develop pressure sores unless the individual's clinical condition demonstrates that they were unavoidable."[20] An updated version of the standardized assessment used in nursing homes, the minimum data set (MDS), was implemented in 2010 to include direct interviews with the nursing home residents and to recognize resident needs.[21] The pressure ulcer section of the MDS version 3.0 differs from MDS version 2.0 by requiring the assessor to provide pressure ulcers counts and stages [using the National Pressure Ulcer Advisory Panel (NPUAP) definitions] and to provide better tracking of pressure ulcers. It also requires reporting of the number and stage of pressure ulcers at admission. In 2011, CMS provided an updated resource for long-term care facilities to use for pressure ulcer prevention and treatment with the aim of helping facilities reduce the rate of high-risk pressure ulcers.[22]

Definitions and stages

Pressure ulcers are an international health concern. The European Pressure Ulcer Advisory Panel (EPUAP) and the NPUAP issued a joint definition of pressure ulcers: "localized injury to the skin and/or underlying tissue usually over a bony prominence, as a result of pressure, or pressure in combination with shear. A number of contributing or confounding factors are also associated with pressure ulcers; the significance of these factors is yet to be elucidated."[23]

The most commonly used category or staging system for pressure ulcers in the United States is the NPUAP classification system, which consists of four pressure ulcer stages and two additional categories: (1) unstageable or unclassified pressure ulcer, and (2) suspected deep tissue injury – depth unknown.[23] The joint EPUAP and NPUAP guidelines began using the term "category" in their classification system for pressure ulcers. Since the term "staging" implies progression from one stage to the next stage, these experts noted that pressure ulcers do not always progress sequentially. The new term "category" was needed to free clinicians from the notion of progression of or reversing stages.[24]

The NPUAP's category for unstageable or unclassified pressure ulcer was defined as "full thickness loss in which actual depth of the ulcer is completely obscured by slough (yellow, tan, gray, green, or brown) and/or eschar (tan, brown, or black) in the wound bed."[23] The actual depth of the pressure ulcer will be either stage III or stage IV after removal of slough and/or eschar in order for the base of the wound to be exposed.[23] Suspected deep tissue injury – depth unknown was defined as "purple or maroon localized area of discolored intact skin or blood-filled blister due to damage of underlying soft tissue from pressure and/or shear." This type of injury can occur after prolonged immobilization and lead to a stage IV pressure ulcer.[10] (See Table 36.1 for a complete description of pressure ulcer stages and categories.)

Epidemiology of pressure ulcers

Secondary analyses of the Medicare Patient Safety Monitoring System database revealed that 4.5% of Medicare beneficiaries who had been discharged from hospitals during a two-year period (January 1, 2006, to December 31, 2007) developed at least one new pressure ulcer.[25] Compared to those who did not develop a pressure ulcer, patients who developed pressure ulcers were more likely to die while in hospital (risk-adjusted OR 2.81, 95% CI 2.44–3.23); had longer hospital stays (risk-adjusted mean length of stay 11.2 days, 95% CI 10.19–11.4, versus 4.8 days, 95% CI 4.7–5.0); and had higher rates of readmission within 30 days (risk-adjusted OR 1.33, 95% CI 1.23–1.45).[25]

Using data from the National Database of Nursing Quality Indicators 2010 Pressure Ulcer Surveys, the rate of hospital-acquired pressure ulcers was determined. Among 710,626 adult patients surveyed in 1,419 hospitals in the United States, the rate of hospital-acquired pressure ulcers was 3.6% in all patients and 7.9% in at-risk patients. Odds of having a hospital-acquired pressure ulcer were lower in Magnet and Magnet-applicant hospitals.[26] (Note: The ANCC's Magnet Recognition Program is "an international organizational credential that recognizes nursing excellence in healthcare organizations."[27]) In 2009, 3.3% of adult patients in intensive care units developed stage III or stage IV pressure ulcers.[28] In older adults who had surgical repair of hip fractures, the cumulative incidence of pressure ulcers stage II or higher at the third day of hospitalization was 6.2% (95% CI 5.4–7.1). The majority of pressure ulcers were classified as stage II and located in the sacral area or the heel.[29] When these patients were followed from hospital admission to 32 days post-hospitalization, the highest adjusted (for multiple factors, including time) acquired pressure ulcer rate, when compared to the home setting, was in the hospital setting (relative rate 2.2, 95% CI 1.3–3.7).[30]

Racial differences in pressure ulcer incidence have been reported. The incidence of stages II, III, and IV pressure ulcers in black nursing home residents was 0.56 per person-year as compared to 0.35 per person-year for whites.[31] Black nursing home residents had fewer stage I pressure ulcers identified than white nursing home residents, perhaps because of the difficulty in detecting nonblanchable erythema in dark pigmented skin.[32] A systematic review, however, indicated that there is limited evidence for the relationship between race and pressure ulcer development.[33] This systematic review also noted that independent predictors for pressure ulcer

Table 36.1 Categories/stages of pressure ulcers

Category/stage I: Nonblanchable erythema	Intact skin with nonblanchable redness of a localized area usually over a bony prominence. Darkly pigmented skin may not have visible blanching; its color may differ from the surrounding area. The area may be painful, firm, soft, warmer or cooler as compared to adjacent tissue. Category I may be difficult to detect in individuals with dark skin tones. May indicate at-risk persons.
Category/stage II: partial thickness	Partial thickness, loss of dermis presenting as a shallow open ulcer with a red pink wound bed, without slough. May also present as an intact or open/ruptured serum-filled or sero-sanginous-filled blister. Presents as a shiny or dry shallow ulcer without slough or bruising.* This category should not be used to describe skin tears, tape burns, incontinence associated dermatitis, maceration, or excoriation.
Category/stage III: full thickness skin loss	Full thickness tissue loss. Subcutaneous fat may be visible, but bone, tendon, or muscle are *not* exposed. Slough may be present but does not obscure the depth of tissue loss. *May* include undermining and tunneling. The depth of a Category/Stage III pressure ulcer varies by anatomical location. The bridge of the nose, ear, occiput, and malleolus do not have (adipose) subcutaneous tissue and category/stage III ulcers can be shallow. In contrast, areas of significant adiposity can develop extremely deep Category/Stage III pressure ulcers. Bone/tendon is not visible or directly palpable.
Category/stage IV: full thickness tissue loss	Full thickness tissue loss with exposed bone, tendon or muscle. Slough or eschar may be present. Often includes undermining and tunneling. The depth of a category/stage IV pressure ulcer varies by anatomical location. The bridge of the nose, ear, occiput, and malleolus do not have (adipose) subcutaneous tissue and these ulcers can be shallow. Category/Stage IV ulcers can extend into muscle and/or supporting structures (e.g., fascia, tendon or joint capsule) making osteomyelitis or osteitis likely to occur. Exposed bone/muscle is visible or directly palpable.
Additional categories/stages for the United States	
Unstageable/unclassified: full thickness skin or tissue loss – depth unknown	Full thickness tissue loss in which actual depth of the ulcer is completely obscured by slough (yellow, tan, gray, green or brown) and/or eschar (tan, brown or black) in the wound bed. Until enough slough and/or eschar are removed to expose the base of the wound, the true depth cannot be determined; but it will be either a Category/Stage III or IV. Stable (dry, adherent, intact without erythema or fluctuance) eschar on the heels serves as "the body's natural (biological) cover" and should not be removed.
Suspected deep tissue injury – depth unknown	Purple or maroon localized area of discolored intact skin or blood-filled blister due to damage of underlying soft tissue from pressure and/or Shear. The area may be preceded by tissue that is painful, firm, mushy, boggy, warmer or cooler as compared to adjacent tissue. Deep tissue injury may be difficult to detect in individuals with dark skin tones. Evolution may include a thin blister over a dark wound bed. The wound may further evolve and become covered by thin eschar. Evolution may be rapid exposing additional layers of tissue even with optimal treatment.

* Bruising indicates deep tissue injury.

Source: National Pressure Ulcer Advisory Panel, www.npuap.org/resources/educational-and-clinical-resources/npuap-pressure-ulcer-stagescategories.

development included mobility/activity, perfusion, and skin/pressure ulcer status.[33]

Few data are available regarding the remission or cure rates of pressure ulcers. Sibbald and colleagues recommended that determining "healability" is important before beginning treatment.[34] These authors also noted that healable wounds should be healed within twelve weeks.[34] An instrument to measure pressure ulcer healing for stages II to IV pressure ulcers – Pressure Ulcer Scale for Healing (PUSH 3.0) – is available at the NPUAP website. This instrument helps to quantify several parameters: surface area (as measured by length multiplied by width of the pressure ulcer), exudate amount, and tissue type. This instrument offers an alternative to a practice known as reverse staging. An international group of experts released a consensus document supporting the NPUAP's position that a healed stage IV ulcer should be classified as a healed stage IV pressure ulcer rather than using a reverse staging technique.[35]

Costs of pressure ulcers prevention and treatment

Available data regarding pressure ulcer surveillance programs in acute care facilities indicate that those programs can lower hospital-acquired pressure ulcer rates and can be cost-saving, with net savings of $127.51 per patient.[36] Costs of treating existing pressure ulcers are high. For example, costs for treating stage I pressure ulcers were reported in 2013 at approximately $2,000, stage II between $3,000 and $10,000, stage III between $5,900 and $14,840, and stage IV between $18,730 and $21,410.[36]

Quality of life

Pressure ulcers cause both acute and chronic pain, are unsightly, and may limit function. Therefore, understanding and measuring patient-reported outcomes is important. Measuring the quality of life of adults living with pressure ulcers has gained importance, and an instrument (PU-QOL) has been developed and tested. It consists of 10 scales: pain, exudate, odor, sleep, movement/mobility, daily activities, vitality, emotional well-being, self-consciousness and appearance, and social participation.[37] This self-reported scale attempts to capture the impact of pressure ulcer prevention and treatment interventions from the affected

adult's perspective. More research about the effects of pressure ulcers on quality of life from the perspectives of the affected adult, family members, and formal caregivers is critically needed.

Pathophysiology of pressure ulcers

Tissue injury can be superficial, deep, or a combination of both. Injury to the skin and deep tissue can occur within four to six hours after sustained loading,[38] and clinically detectable pressure ulcers can develop within two to six hours.[39] Emerging evidence indicates that deep tissue injury may occur under intact skin, but the current staging systems do not sufficiently encompass that type of lesion.[40] Pressure to skin over bony prominences – such as the sacrum, heels, trochanters, femoral condyles, malleoli, or ischial tuberosities – may occlude capillary blood flow and lead to tissue death.[39] Shear forces pull and distort skin, underlying tissues, and blood vessels, leading to tissue damage.[41] This can occur when a supine person is raised to a greater than 30-degree angle or when a patient is pulled up in bed without the use of a pull sheet.

A pathway has been described to explain deep muscle injury as hypoxic reperfusion injury.[42] The compressed area between a bony prominence and pressure point is described as the epicenter of injury. The injury could be from high impact over a short time period or from lower impact over a longer time period. As swelling and edema occur, it leads to further hypoxia at the epicenter and hypoxia spreading to the peri-injured tissue. As microcirculation becomes impaired and further ischemia occurs, irreversible damage takes place. The muscle swells within rigid fascia, leading to compartment syndrome, which requires surgical intervention.[42]

Pressure ulcers are subject to bacterial colonization, which can occur as early as 48 hours.[43] Enzymes released by bacteria break down protein that could otherwise aid wound healing.[44] Fluids from chronic wounds exhibit increased protease levels and proinflammatory cytokine levels as well as decreased levels of growth factors.[43] An impaired healing response in older adults with pressure ulcers may be a result of the interplay among several intrinsic and extrinsic factors, including ischemic and oxidant stress, metabolic disruptions, prolonged application of uneven pressure to tissue, and exposure to shear forces and friction.[43, 45] Some pressure ulcers become infected with multidrug resistant organisms that increase risk of bacteremia and death.[46]

Prevention of pressure ulcers

In 2007 the Institute for Healthcare Improvement included pressure ulcer prevention in its Five Million Lives Campaign.[47] The overall aim of this two-year campaign was to prevent five million incidents of medical harm in participating hospitals. Pressure ulcer prevention includes identifying at-risk individuals and reliably implementing prevention strategies for these individuals. Elements of prevention are (1) assessing for pressure ulcers at admission into a health-care setting, (2) reassessing pressure ulcer risk daily, (3) inspecting skin daily, (4) managing moisture, (5) optimizing nutrition and hydration, and (6) minimizing pressure.[48]

Several screening tools are available, but the Braden Scale is frequently used in health-care facilities in the United States. It consists of six subscales that measure sensory perception level, skin moisture, level of physical activity, mobility, nutrition, and friction/shear.[49] The sensitivity and specificity of this scale are 57.1% and 67.5%, respectively.[50] Scores on the Braden Scale range from 6 to 23, with the lower scores indicating higher risk of pressure ulcer development.[49] Although the tool tends to overpredict pressure ulcer risk (51), the assignment of risks is as follows: 19 to 23, not at risk; 15 to 18, mild risk; 13 to 14, moderate risk; 10 to 12, high risk; and a score of 9 or lower, at very high risk. This tool has high inter-rater reliability for registered nurses (Pearson $r = 0.99$, percent agreement 88%).[49]

In people of color, a score of 18 or below on the Braden Scale was accurate in predicting pressure ulcers.[52] A systematic review indicated that the Braden Scale should not be used for surgical patients; there was low predictive validity for pressure ulcer risk.[49, 53] In the critical care setting, four of the six Braden Scale subscales were associated with increased likelihood of developing a pressure ulcer. These included sensory perception, mobility, moisture, and friction/shear subscales.[54] Both patients who did and did not develop pressure ulcers had been classified at risk using the Braden Scale, indicating that more research is needed to differentiate at-risk adults in critical care units.[54] The ability to differentiate between these groups is essential to effectively implement preventive strategies for at-risk patients as recommended by the joint NPUAP and

EPUAP expert.[55] The EPUAP and NPUAP joint guidelines recommended a structured and systematic approach to risk assessment (24), although no conclusive evidence exists that a systematic and structured risk assessment tool reduces pressure ulcer incidence.[56]

In home health agencies, clinical judgment had been the most commonly used method to assess pressure ulcer risk, especially before the implementation of Outcome and Assessment Information Set (OASIS). When nurses used clinical judgment about pressure ulcers, they considered patients' dependency level and self-care abilities.[57] According to OASIS data from five home health-care agencies in the United States from September 2007 to January 2009, the prevalence of pressure ulcers was 1.3%. Newly developed pressure ulcers were associated with the presence of bowel incontinence, activities of daily living (ADL) dependence, being chairfast or bedfast, and having a pressure ulcer upon admission to home care.[58]

Pressure ulcer prevention interventions

In 2009, the EPUAP and the NPUAP issued joint evidence-based guidelines on pressure ulcer prevention and treatment.[24]

Pressure redistribution and repositioning interventions

There is limited evidence for the use of pressure-redistributing support surfaces (i.e., mattresses, pads, and cushions) to relieve pressure exerted on subcutaneous tissues by body weight when a body part presses against a chair or bed's surface. These support surfaces may be static (such as a mattress) or dynamic (whereby pressure under the body is varied mechanically). When compared to standard hospital mattresses, foam alternatives reduced incidence of pressure ulcers, as did medical sheepskins when compared to standard care.[59] Using dressings prophylactically to mitigate shear on tissue may enhance pressure ulcer prevention and may reduce pressure ulcer incidence.[60, 61] A consensus panel recommended the use of a five-layer soft silicone dressing for high-risk patients (i.e., patients in the emergency department, intensive care unit, or operating room) as part of a strategy to prevent sacral pressure ulcer development.[41] More research is needed to better understand clinical, quality of life, and economic outcomes of the use of dressings in pressure ulcer prevention.[62]

Repositioning has long been considered the cornerstone of pressure ulcer prevention because repositioning relieves or eliminates interface pressure for the maintenance of microcirculation. There is limited research evidence, however, for repositioning to prevent pressure ulcers, especially in regard to repositioning frequency and position (i.e., 30-degree tilt versus 90-degree position).[63] One study in nursing homes found that a repositioning schedule of every three hours using 30-degree tilt was cost-effective when compared to every six hours using 90-degree lateral rotation.[64] Another study in nursing home residents who were placed on high-density foam mattresses did not find a significant reduction in pressure ulcer incidence when two-, three-, or four-hour turning schedules were used.[65] The EPUAP and NPUAP joint guideline recommended repositioning based on the affected person's factors, such as tissue tolerance, activity and mobility levels, health status, skin condition, and patient comfort. The use of support surfaces also influences repositioning frequency.[24] To prevent the effect of shear forces, maintaining the head of bed at 30 degrees or less was recommended.[41]

People who sit for long periods of time may not be able to shift their position, including adults with spinal cord injuries. This population is at increased risk of pressure ulcer development.[24, 66] Evidence exists that pressure-redistributing seat cushions prevent pressure ulcers.[24] Results from one study indicated that air-cell-based cushions provided greater reductions in tissue stresses when compared to foam cushions.[67] Wheelchair users should be taught how to reposition while seated to relieve pressure and increase blood flow to the buttocks.[68]

Nutritional intervention

The EPUAP and NPUAP joint guideline recommends providing high-protein mixed oral or tube feeding supplements to adults at risk of pressure ulcer development. This recommendation is supported by direct evidence from trials conducted in humans.[24]

Topical intervention

Sacral dryness is a risk factor for pressure ulcer development, and moisturizers are relatively inexpensive. Although there is insufficient evidence for prophylactic benefits of topical agents,[62] application of moisturizers to the sacral area has been recommended.[69]

Treatment of pressure ulcers

Maintaining a clean wound base is considered important for healing and closure,[24] but a systematic review found no evidence to support specific cleansing solutions or techniques.[70] The authors of the review noted the limited number and low quality of research studies that were reviewed, making recommendations difficult. The EPUAP and NPUAP joint guideline graded the level of evidence for cleansing and debriding pressure ulcers as being supported by indirect evidence and/or expert opinion. These findings highlight the need for clinicians and researchers to work together to conduct and publish high quality research to provide higher levels of evidence on which to base clinical practice.

Pressure redistribution and repositioning interventions

The NPUAP defined a support surface as "a specialized device for pressure redistribution designed for the management of tissue loads, micro-climate, and/or other therapeutic functions (i.e., any mattresses, integrated bed systems, mattress replacements, overlays, or seat cushions or seat cushion overlays)."[71]

Air-fluidized beds provided moderate-strength evidence of wound improvement when compared to standard hospital beds.[72] In this review, alternating-pressure mattresses and other support surfaces had similar healing rates.[72]

Repositioning to relieve pressure over bony prominences has been a mainstay of pressure ulcer treatment, yet no randomized trials existed to determine its impact on pressure ulcer healing.[73] Keeping the head of the bed at the lowest degree of elevation to avoid shear forces and friction may prevent further pressure ulcer development. The use of a wound electronic medical record that includes photographs of wounds has been recommended as an integral part of treatment.[74]

Wound dressings

Multiple options are available for pressure ulcer dressings. The type of dressing is determined by the tissue in the wound bed, condition of skin surrounding the pressure ulcer, and the condition and treatment goals of the affected adult. Type of dressing may change as wound healing progresses.[24] Presence of exudate, necrotic tissue, and infection also can influence dressing choices.[75] In one systematic review, hydrocolloid dressings, compared to gauze dressings, showed greater reduction in wound size.[72] Overall, there is limited evidence for using specific dressings and topical therapies for wound improvement.[76]

Nutritional intervention

Little systematic evidence exists on the effectiveness of enteral and parenteral nutrition in the prevention of pressure ulcers.[77] Several nutritional guidelines are available, which generally recommend conducting a nutritional assessment including weighing the patient, reviewing food and fluid intake, and investigating unexplained weight loss. Other recommendations include recognizing the effects of malnutrition, correcting an underfed status by designing a diet based on 35 kcal/kg, 1.0 to 1.5 g/kg of protein, and 1mL/kcal of fluids, and evaluating the effects of a nutritional intervention.[78] Protein supplementation was found effective in reducing the size, but not in healing, of pressure ulcers.[72]

Other therapies

Electromagnetic therapy for pressure ulcer treatment has been studied, although two systematic reviews concluded that no evidence exists supporting the benefit of this therapy.[72, 79] The use of therapeutic ultrasound for pressure ulcer healing has also been investigated, and no systematic evidence exists regarding the benefits of this treatment.[80] The authors of the preceding systematic reviews noted that further research is needed.

Results of a meta-analysis on the use of electrical stimulation for chronic wound healing indicated that increased wound healing occurred. The proposed mechanism of electrical stimulation on healing is that it restarts or accelerates wound healing by stimulating fibroblasts and increasing the migration of neutrophils and macrophages.[81] Recent reviews indicate moderate evidence for electrical stimulation as an ancillary intervention for wound healing (82) and improved healing rates.[72] A review of hyperbaric oxygen therapy for chronic wounds noted that no trials that involved pressure ulcers were included in the review.[83]

Surgical interventions for pressure ulcers

In a systematic review, insufficient evidence was available to determine superiority of one approach over another for closure of stage III and stage IV pressure ulcers.[72] Detailed description of surgical interventions is beyond the scope of this chapter.

Pressure ulcer pain management

People with pressure ulcers experience acute and chronic pain from these wounds. A study conducted in nine hospitals in the United Kingdom found that of all patients who had a pressure ulcer, 43.2% reported pain.[84] Words patients use to describe pain from a pressure ulcer include "burning," "shooting," "sharp," "aching," "cutting," and "hot."[85] Pain is caused by irritation of nerve endings in and around the pressure ulcer.[86] Pain is also caused by pressure ulcer treatment such as debridement or pressure applied to the wound from dressings.[86] Many times pain is not addressed as a part of wound care in hospitalized patients, and differences in pain levels are observed in racial groups, with nonwhites reporting more pain.[87] Thus, pain should be assessed using a validated tool such as the McGill Pain Scale (MPS), and it should be treated prior to dressing changes or other treatment interventions, including repositioning and pressure relief.

Results from a mixed-methods systematic literature on pressure ulcer pain indicated need for better communication between the affected adult and health-care provider for effective pain management to occur. Some adults use words such as "misery" or cannot find words to describe pain from pressure ulcers. Gorecki et al. proposed a biopsychosocial model of pain, displayed in Figure 36.2.[88] Because pain from pressure ulcers is chronic and has a significant impact on the lives of affected adults, patient and health-care provider education about promoting health and preventing pain is needed.[88]

Palliative wound care

Despite best care practices, a pear-shaped or horseshoe-shaped pressure ulcer, also called skin changes at life's end (SCALE), may suddenly appear on the sacrum or coccyx when death is near.[89] Because wound healing is not the goal, nor is it feasible, for a person close to death, dressings that alleviate pain and cause little discomfort should be used to cover the wound. The goals of palliative wound care are

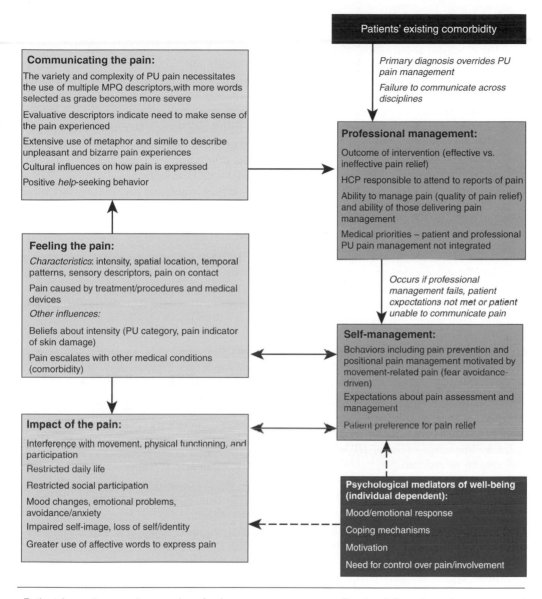

Patients' existing comorbidity

Primary diagnosis overrides PU pain management

Failure to communicate across disciplines

Communicating the pain:

The variety and complexity of PU pain necessitates the use of multiple MPQ descriptors, with more words selected as grade becomes more severe

Evaluative descriptors indicate need to make sense of the pain experienced

Extensive use of metaphor and simile to describe unpleasant and bizarre pain experiences

Cultural influences on how pain is expressed

Positive *help*-seeking behavior

Professional management:

Outcome of intervention (effective vs. ineffective pain relief)

HCP responsible to attend to reports of pain

Ability to manage pain (quality of pain relief) and ability of those delivering pain management

Medical priorities – patient and professional PU pain management not integrated

Feeling the pain:

Characteristics: intensity, spatial location, temporal patterns, sensory descriptors, pain on contact

Pain caused by treatment/procedures and medical devices

Other influences:

Beliefs about intensity (PU category, pain indicator of skin damage)

Pain escalates with other medical conditions (comorbidity)

Occurs if professional management fails, patient expectations not met or patient unable to communicate pain

Self-management:

Behaviors including pain prevention and positional pain management motivated by movement-related pain (fear avoidance-driven)

Expectations about pain assessment and management

Patient preference for pain relief

Impact of the pain:

Interference with movement, physical functioning, and participation

Restricted daily life

Restricted social participation

Mood changes, emotional problems, avoidance/anxiety

Impaired self-image, loss of self/identity

Greater use of affective words to express pain

Psychological mediators of well-being (individual dependent):

Mood/emotional response

Coping mechanisms

Motivation

Need for control over pain/involvement

Patients' experience and expression of pain

Facstors influencing pain management

Figure 36.2 Model of how the nature of pressure ulcer pain influences the impact, communication, and management of that pain (from Gorecki, Closs, Nixon, and Briggs, 2011).

symptom management and improvement of the quality of life.[90] Support of and communication with family caregivers is especially important, as they may believe that pressure ulcers are a sign of neglect. Family members may need assistance to better understand the stages of the dying process and accept that care activities change as death nears. When death is imminent, repositioning to prevent pressure ulcers and supplying food and oral fluids to sustain life may be discontinued.

Measures to maximize dignity and comfort should continue until death occurs.

Interdisciplinary team approach

The prevention and the treatment of pressure ulcers are complex interventions requiring the expertise, collaboration, and involvement of multiple healthcare providers. Central to this activity, however, are the affected older adult and family caregivers. When

517

given an opportunity to participate, adults will share what they know about their health, functioning, desires, and goals, information about their past experiences, and the emotional and physical impact of living with a pressure ulcer. For example, smelling the odor from pressure ulcers left one adult with "an indelible impression," and it created a desire to prevent a pressure ulcer or to participate in healing an existing one.[91] Communication and education are key components to pressure ulcer prevention and treatment. Litigation often starts with families wanting answers about why and how a pressure ulcer started and how it was treated.[92] Thus, staff education about the legal implications of pressure ulcers should also be an ongoing process.[92]

Education of all involved parties is essential to effective teamwork. Multiple stakeholders in the prevention and treatment of pressure ulcers include hospital administration and interprofessional clinical staff of all levels, and educational opportunities should be ongoing.[93] Institutional level quality management of pressure ulcers was found to be positively associated with preventive pressure ulcer quality management at the unit level, indicating pressure ulcer prevention is more than a clinical issue and should be viewed from a systems perspective.[94] Quality improvement initiatives in nursing homes have demonstrated that incidence of stage III and stage IV pressure ulcers can be reduced.[95]

Medical management by physicians, nurse practitioners, or physician assistants of comorbid conditions, such as diabetes mellitus and circulatory diseases, to achieve maximal disease and symptom control is needed to prevent and heal pressure ulcers. Nutritionists, dieticians, geriatricians, wound, ostomy, and continence nurse specialists, and rehabilitation specialists provide key expertise to create and update comprehensive care plans. In addition, surgeons may be needed to perform debridement, and infectious disease specialists may be needed to aggressively treat deep infections.[96]

Communication among clinicians, other healthcare professionals, and family caregivers about the goal and expected outcomes of treatment interventions is essential in the implementation and evaluation of successful interdisciplinary care.

Summary and conclusion

Pressure ulcers are prevalent in health-care delivery settings despite intensive efforts to prevent and treat them. The complex interactions between intrinsic and extrinsic factors that lead to pressure ulcer development are becoming better understood. Knowledge about skin health and skin failure is rapidly increasing, and clinicians need to remain abreast of advances in pressure ulcer prevention, management, and treatment. Organization-wide efforts are needed to reduce incidence of pressure ulcers, facilitate pressure ulcer healing, and promote the dignity and quality of life for affected older adults and their families.

Interprofessional evidence-based interventions to promote good skin health and prevent pressure ulcers remain essential to the well-being of older adults.

References

1. Levine JM. Historical notes on pressure ulcers: the cure of Ambrose Pare. *Decubitus*. 1992 Mar;**5**(2):23–4, 26.

2. Levine JM. Historical perspective on pressure ulcers: the decubitus ominosus of Jean-Martin Charcot. *J Am Geriatr Soc*. 2005 Jul;**53**(7):1248–51.

3. Woodruff MB. To prevent and cure pressure sores. *Am J Nurs*. 1952 May;**52**(5):606.

4. Pieper B, Kirsner RS. Pressure ulcers: even the grading of facilities fails. *Ann Intern Med*. 2013 Oct 15;**159**(8):571–2.

5. Preventing Pressure Ulcers in Hospitals: A Toolkit for Improving Quality of Care [Internet]. Available from: www.ahrq.gov/professionals/systems/long-term-care/resources/pressure-ulcers/pressureulcertoolkit/putool kit.pdf (accessed May 21, 2014).

6. Brem H, Maggi J, Nierman D, et al. High cost of stage IV pressure ulcers. *Am J Surg*. 2010 Oct;**200**(4):473–7.

7. Hopkins A, Dealey C, Bale S, et al. Patient stories of living with a pressure ulcer. *J Adv Nurs*. 2006 Nov;**56**(4):345–53.

8. Healthy People 2020 [Internet]. Available from: www.healthypeople.gov/2020/topicsobjectives2020/over view.aspx?topicid=31 (accessed May 30, 2014).

9. Padula WV, Mishra MK, Makic MB, Sullivan PW. Improving the quality of pressure ulcer care with prevention: a cost-effectiveness analysis. *Med Care*. 2011 Apr;**49**(4):385–92.

10. Langemo DK, Brown G. Skin fails too: acute, chronic, and end-stage skin failure. *Adv Skin Wound Care*. 2006 May;**19**(4):206–11.

11. Bansal C, Scott R, Stewart D, Cockerell CJ. Decubitus ulcers: a review of the literature. *Int J Dermatol*. 2005 Oct;**44**(10):805–10.

12. Black JM, Edsberg LE, Baharestani MM, et al. Pressure ulcers: avoidable or unavoidable? Results of the National Pressure Ulcer Advisory Panel Consensus

Conference. *Ostomy Wound Manage.* 2011 Feb;**57**(2):24–37.

13. Coleman S, Nixon J, Keen J, et al. A new pressure ulcer conceptual framework. *J Adv Nurs.* 2014 Oct;**70**(10):2222–34.

14. Tzeng HM, Grandy GA, Yin CY. Staff response time to call lights and unit-acquired pressure ulcer rates in adult in-patient acute care units. *Contemp Nurse.* 2013 Oct;**45**(2):182–7.

15. Sving E, Gunningberg L, Hogman M, Mamhidir AG. Registered nurses' attention to and perceptions of pressure ulcer prevention in hospital settings. *J Clin Nurs.* 2012 May;**21**(9–10):1293–303.

16. Backhaus R, Verbeek H, van Rossum E, et al. Nurse Staffing Impact on Quality of Care in Nursing Homes: A Systematic Review of Longitudinal Studies. *J Am Med Dir Assoc.* 2014 Jun;**15**(6):383–93.

17. Sullivan N, Schoelles KM. Preventing in-facility pressure ulcers as a patient safety strategy: a systematic review. *Ann Intern Med.* 2013 Mar 5;**158**(5 Pt 2):410–16.

18. Meddings JA, Reichert H, Hofer T, McMahon LF Jr. Hospital report cards for hospital-acquired pressure ulcers: how good are the grades? *Ann Intern Med.* 2013 Oct 15;**159**(8):505–13.

19. Coomer NM, McCall NT. Examination of the accuracy of coding hospital-acquired pressure ulcer stages. *Medicare Medicaid Res Rev.* 2013 Dec 24;**3**(4):10.5600/mmrr.003.04.b03. eCollection 2013.

20. Publication 100–07: State Operations Manual [Internet]. Available from: www.cms.gov/Regulations-and-Guidance/Guidance/Manuals/Internet Only-Manuals-IOMs-Items/CMS1201984.html?DLPage=1&DLSort=0&DLSortDir=ascending (accessed May 30, 2014).

21. Saliba D, Jones M, Streim J, et al. Overview of significant changes in the Minimum Data Set for nursing homes version 3.0. *J Am Med Dir Assoc.* 2012 Sep;**13**(7):595–601.

22. Resource Guide: Pressure Ulcer Prevention and Treatment [10SOW-IIPC NCC-C7-02 110711] [Internet]; 2011. Available from: https://healthinsight.org/Internal/assets/Nursing%20Home/PressureUlcers/PRU_Resource_Guide1_NCC_2012.pdf (accessed May 21, 2014).

23. NPUAP Pressure Ulcer Stages/Categories [Internet]. Available from: www.npuap.org/resources/educational-and-clinical-resources/npuap-pressure-ulcer-stagescategories (accessed May 30, 2014).

24. European Pressure Ulcer Advisory Panel and National Pressure Ulcer Advisory Panel. *Prevention of pressure ulcers: quick reference guide.* Washington, DC: National Pressure Ulcer Advisory Panel; 2009.

25. Lyder CH, Wang Y, Metersky M, et al. Hospital-acquired pressure ulcers: results from the national Medicare Patient Safety Monitoring System study. *J Am Geriatr Soc.* 2012 Sep;**60**(9):1603–8.

26. Bergquist-Beringer S, Dong L, He J, Dunton N. Pressure ulcers and prevention among acute care hospitals in the United States. *Jt Comm J Qual Patient Saf.* 2013 Sep;**39**(9):404–14.

27. Magnet Recognition Program˚ Overview [Internet]; 2014. Available from: www.nursecredentialing.org/Magnet/International/MagnetProgOverview (accessed Apr 22, 2015).

28. Clements L, Moore M, Tribble T, Blake J. Reducing skin breakdown in patients receiving extracorporeal membranous oxygenation. *Nurs Clin North Am.* 2014 Mar;**49**(1):61–8.

29. Baumgarten M, Margolis DJ, Localio AR, et al. Pressure ulcers among elderly patients early in the hospital stay. *J Gerontol A Biol Sci Med Sci.* 2006 Jul;**61**(7):749–54.

30. Baumgarten M, Margolis DJ, Orwig DL, et al. Pressure ulcers in elderly patients with hip fracture across the continuum of care. *J Am Geriatr Soc.* 2009 May;**57**(5):863–70.

31. Baumgarten M, Margolis D, van Doorn C, et al. Black/white differences in pressure ulcer incidence in nursing home residents. *J Am Geriatr Soc.* 2004 Aug;**52**(8):1293–8.

32. Rosen J, Mittal V, Degenholtz H, et al. Pressure ulcer prevention in black and white nursing home residents: a QI initiative of enhanced ability, incentives, and management feedback. *Adv Skin Wound Care.* 2006 Jun;**19**(5):262–8.

33. Coleman S, Gorecki C, Nelson EA, et al. Patient risk factors for pressure ulcer development: systematic review. *Int J Nurs Stud.* 2013 Jul;**50**(7):974–1003.

34. Sibbald RG, Goodman L, Woo KY, et al. Special considerations in wound bed preparation 2011: an update©. *Adv Skin Wound Care.* 2011 Sep;**24**(9):415–36; quiz 437–8.

35. Baharestani MM, Black JM, Carville K, et al. Dilemmas in measuring and using pressure ulcer prevalence and incidence: an international consensus. *Int Wound J.* 2009 Apr;**6**(2):97–104.

36. Spetz J, Brown DS, Aydin C, Donaldson N. The value of reducing hospital-acquired pressure ulcer prevalence: an illustrative analysis. *J Nurs Adm.* 2013 Apr;**43**(4):235–41.

37. Gorecki C, Brown JM, Cano S, et al. Development and validation of a new patient-reported outcome measure for patients with pressure ulcers: the PU-QOL instrument. *Health Qual Life Outcomes.* 2013 Jun 13;**11**:95.

38. Gefen A. How much time does it take to get a pressure ulcer? Integrated evidence from human, animal, and in vitro studies. *Ostomy Wound Manage.* 2008 Oct;**54**(10):26–8, 30–5.

39. Lyder CH. Pressure ulcer prevention and management. *JAMA.* 2003 Jan 8;**289**(2):223–6.

40. Aliano K, Low C, Stavrides S, et al. The correlation between ultrasound findings and clinical assessment of pressure-related ulcers: is the extent of injury greater than what is predicted? *Surg Technol Int.* 2014 Mar;**24**:112–16.

41. Black J, Clark M, Dealey C, et al. Dressings as an adjunct to pressure ulcer prevention: consensus panel recommendations. *Int Wound J.* 2014 Aug;**12**(4):484–8.

42. Smart H. Deep tissue injury: what is it really? *Adv Skin Wound Care.* 2013 Feb;**26**(2):56–8.

43. Mustoe TA, O'Shaughnessy K, Kloeters O. Chronic wound pathogenesis and current treatment strategies: a unifying hypothesis. *Plast Reconstr Surg.* 2006 Jun;**117**(7 Suppl):35S–41S.

44. Gupta S, Baharestani M, Baranoski S, et al. Guidelines for managing pressure ulcers with negative pressure wound therapy. *Adv Skin Wound Care.* 2004 Nov-Dec;**17**(Suppl 2):1–16.

45. Scott EM, Buckland R. Pressure ulcer risk in the peri-operative environment. *Nurs Stand.* 2005 Oct 26_Nov 1;**20**(7):74, 76, 78 passim.

46. Braga IA, Pirett CC, Ribas RM, et al. Bacterial colonization of pressure ulcers: assessment of risk for bloodstream infection and impact on patient outcomes. *J Hosp Infect.* 2013 Apr;**83**(4):314–20.

47. 5 Million Lives Campaign: Overview [Internet]; 2015. Available from: www.ihi.org/Engage/Initiatives/Comp leted/5MillionLivesCampaign/Pages/default.aspx (accessed Apr 22, 2015).

48. Duncan KD. Preventing pressure ulcers: the goal is zero. *Jt Comm J Qual Patient Saf.* 2007 Oct;**33**(10):605–10.

49. Braden BJ, Maklebust J. Preventing pressure ulcers with the Braden scale: an update on this easy-to-use tool that assesses a patient's risk. *Am J Nurs.* 2005 Jun;**105**(6):70–2.

50. Pancorbo-Hidalgo PL, Garcia-Fernandez FP, Lopez-Medina IM, Alvarez-Nieto C. Risk assessment scales for pressure ulcer prevention: a systematic review. *J Adv Nurs.* 2006 Apr;**54**(1):94–110.

51. Brown SJ. The Braden Scale: a review of the research evidence. *Orthop Nurs.* 2004 Jan–Feb;**23**(1):30–8.

52. Maklebust J, Sieggreen MY, Sidor D, et al. Computer-based testing of the Braden Scale for Predicting Pressure Sore Risk. *Ostomy Wound Manage.* 2005 Apr;**51**(4):40–2, 44, 46 passim.

53. He W, Liu P, Chen HL. The Braden Scale cannot be used alone for assessing pressure ulcer risk in surgical patients: a meta-analysis. *Ostomy Wound Manage.* 2012 Feb;**58**(2):34–40.

54. Cox J. Predictive power of the Braden scale for pressure sore risk in adult critical care patients: a comprehensive review. *J Wound Ostomy Continence Nurs.* 2012 Nov–Dec;**39**(6):613–21; quiz 622–3.

55. Stausberg J. The Braden Scale and Care Dependency Scale each demonstrate at least 70% sensitivity and specificity for identifying inpatients at risk of pressure ulcer. *Evid Based Nurs.* 2011 Jan;**14**(1):20–1.

56. Moore ZE, Cowman S. Risk assessment tools for the prevention of pressure ulcers. *Cochrane Database Syst Rev.* 2014 Feb 5;**2**:CD006471.

57. Balzer K, Kremer L, Junghans A, et al. What patient characteristics guide nurses' clinical judgement on pressure ulcer risk? A mixed methods study. *Int J Nurs Stud.* 2014 May;**51**(5):703–16.

58. Bergquist-Beringer S, Gajewski BJ. Outcome and assessment information set data that predict pressure ulcer development in older adult home health patients. *Adv Skin Wound Care.* 2011 Sep;**24**(9):404–14.

59. McInnes E, Jammali-Blasi A, Bell-Syer S, et al. Preventing pressure ulcers–Are pressure-redistributing support surfaces effective? A Cochrane systematic review and meta-analysis. *Int J Nurs Stud.* 2012 Mar;**49**(3):345–59.

60. Call E, Pedersen J, Bill B, et al. Enhancing pressure ulcer prevention using wound dressings: what are the modes of action? *Int Wound J.* 2015;**12**(4):408–13.

61. Clark M, Black J, Alves P, et al. Systematic review of the use of prophylactic dressings in the prevention of pressure ulcers. *Int Wound J.* 2014;**11**(5):460–71.

62. Moore ZE, Webster J. Dressings and topical agents for preventing pressure ulcers. *Cochrane Database Syst Rev.* 2013 Aug 18;**8**:CD009362.

63. Gillespie BM, Chaboyer WP, McInnes E, et al. Repositioning for pressure ulcer prevention in adults. *Cochrane Database Syst Rev.* 2014 Apr 3;**4**:CD009958.

64. Moore Z, Cowman S, Posnett J. An economic analysis of repositioning for the prevention of pressure ulcers. *J Clin Nurs.* 2013 Aug;**22**(15–16):2354–60.

65. Bergstrom N, Horn SD, Rapp MP, et al. Turning for ulcer reduction: a multisite randomized clinical trial in nursing homes. *J Am Geriatr Soc.* 2013 Oct;**61**(10):1705–13.

66. Anton L. Pressure ulcer prevention in older people who sit for long periods. *Nurs Older People.* 2006 May;**18**(4):29–35.

67. Levy A, Kopplin K, Gefen A. An air-cell-based cushion for pressure ulcer protection remarkably reduces tissue stresses in the seated buttocks with respect to foams:

finite element studies. *J Tissue Viability*. 2014 Feb;**23**(1):13–23.

68. Sonenblum SE, Vonk TE, Janssen TW, Sprigle SH. Effects of wheelchair cushions and pressure relief maneuvers on ischial interface pressure and blood flow in people with spinal cord injury. *Arch Phys Med Rehabil*. 2014 Jul;**95**(7):1350–7.

69. Reddy M, Gill SS, Rochon PA. Preventing pressure ulcers: a systematic review. *JAMA*. 2006 Aug 23;**296**(8):974–84.

70. Moore ZE, Cowman S. Wound cleansing for pressure ulcers. *Cochrane Database Syst Rev*. 2013 Mar 28;**3**: CD004983.

71. National Pressure Ulcer Advisory Panel Support Surface Standards Initiative: Terms and Definitions Related to Support Surfaces [Internet]; 2007. Available from: www.npuap.org/wp-content/uploads/2012/03/ NPUAP_S3I_TD.pdf (accessed Apr 22, 2015).

72. Smith ME, Totten A, Hickam DH, et al. Pressure ulcer treatment strategies: a systematic comparative effectiveness review. *Ann Intern Med*. 2013 Jul 2;**159** (1):39–50.

73. Moore ZE, Cowman S. Repositioning for treating pressure ulcers. *Cochrane Database Syst Rev*. 2012 Sep 12;**9**:CD006898.

74. Rennert R, Golinko M, Kaplan D, et al. Standardization of wound photography using the wound electronic medical record. *Adv Skin Wound Care*. 2009 Jan;**22**(1):32–8.

75. Canadian Agency for Drug Health and Technologies Health. *Dressing Materials for the Treatment of Pressure Ulcers in Patients in Long-Term Care Facilities: A Review of the Comparative Clinical Effectiveness and Guidelines*. Ottawa, Canada: Canadian Agency for Drugs and Technologies in Health; 2013. CADTH Rapid Response Reports.

76. Saha S, Smith MEB, Totten A, et al. Pressure Ulcer Treatment Strategies: Comparative Effectiveness. Comparative Effectiveness Review No. 90. (Prepared by the Oregon Evidence-based Practice Center under Contract No. 290–2007-10057-I.) AHRQ Publication No. 13-EHC003-EF. Rockville, MD: Agency for Healthcare Research and Quality; 2013. Available at: www.effectivehealthcare.ahrq.gov/reports/final.cfm (accessed May 27, 2014).

77. Langer G, Schloemer G, Knerr A, et al. Nutritional interventions for preventing and treating pressure ulcers. *Cochrane Database Syst Rev*. 2003;(4)(4):CD003216.

78. Schols JM, de Jager-v d Ende MA. Nutritional intervention in pressure ulcer guidelines: an inventory. *Nutrition*. 2004 Jun;**20**(6):548–53.

79. Aziz Z, Flemming K. Electromagnetic therapy for treating pressure ulcers. *Cochrane Database Syst Rev*. 2012 Dec 12;**12**:CD002930.

80. Baba-Akbari Sari A, Flemming K, Cullum NA, Wollina U. Therapeutic ultrasound for pressure ulcers. *Cochrane Database Syst Rev*. 2006 Jul 19;(**3**)(3): CD001275.

81. Gardner SE, Frantz RA, Schmidt FL. Effect of electrical stimulation on chronic wound healing: a meta-analysis. *Wound Repair Regen*. 1999 Nov–Dec;7(6):495–503.

82. Kawasaki L, Mushahwar VK, Ho C, et al. The mechanisms and evidence of efficacy of electrical stimulation for healing of pressure ulcer: a systematic review. *Wound Repair Regen*. 2014 Mar–Apr;**22**(2):161–73.

83. Kranke P, Bennett MH, Martyn-St James M, et al. Hyperbaric oxygen therapy for chronic wounds. *Cochrane Database Syst Rev*. 2012 Apr 18;**4**:CD004123.

84. Briggs M, Collinson M, Wilson L, et al. The prevalence of pain at pressure areas and pressure ulcers in hospitalised patients. *BMC Nurs*. 2013 Jul 31; **12**(1):19.

85. Rastinehad D. Pressure ulcer pain. *J Wound Ostomy Continence Nurs*. 2006 May–Jun;**33**(3):252–7.

86. de Laat EH, Scholte op Reimer WJ, van Achterberg T. Pressure ulcers: diagnostics and interventions aimed at wound-related complaints: a review of the literature. *J Clin Nurs*. 2005 Apr;**14**(4):464–72.

87. Stotts NA, Puntillo K, Bonham Morris A, et al. Wound care pain in hospitalized adult patients. *Heart Lung*. 2004 Sep–Oct;**33**(5):321–32.

88. Gorecki C, Closs SJ, Nixon J, Briggs M. Patient-reported pressure ulcer pain: a mixed-methods systematic review. *J Pain Symptom Manage*. 2011 Sep;**42**(3):443–59.

89. Sibbald RG, Krasner DL, Lutz J. SCALE: skin changes at life's end: final consensus statement: October 1, 2009. *Adv Skin Wound Care*. 2010 May;**23**(5):225–36; quiz 237–8.

90. Schim SM, Cullen B. Wound care at end of life. *Nurs Clin North Am*. 2005 Jun;**40**(2):281–94.

91. Latimer S, Chaboyer W, Gillespie B. Patient participation in pressure injury prevention: giving patient's a voice. *Scand J Caring Sci*. 2014;**28**(4):648–56.

92. Fife CE, Yankowsky KW, Ayello EA, et al. Legal issues in the care of pressure ulcer patients: key concepts for healthcare providers–a consensus paper from the International Expert Wound Care Advisory Panel©. *Adv Skin Wound Care*. 2010 Nov;**23**(11):493–507.

93. Armstrong DG, Ayello EA, Capitulo KL, et al. New opportunities to improve pressure ulcer prevention and treatment: implications of the CMS inpatient hospital care Present on Admission (POA) indicators/hospital-acquired conditions (HAC) policy. A consensus paper from the International Expert Wound Care Advisory Panel. *J Wound Ostomy Continence Nurs*. 2008 Sep–Oct;**35**(5):485–92.

94. Bosch M, Halfens RJ, van der Weijden T, et al. Organizational culture, team climate, and quality management in an important patient safety issue: nosocomial pressure ulcers. *Worldviews Evid Based Nurs.* 2011 Mar;**8**(1):4–14.

95. Lynn J, West J, Hausmann S, et al. Collaborative clinical quality improvement for pressure ulcers in nursing homes. *J Am Geriatr Soc.* 2007 Oct;**55**(10):1663–9.

96. Niezgoda JA, Mendez-Eastman S. The effective management of pressure ulcers. *Adv Skin Wound Care.* 2006 Jan–Feb;**19**(Suppl 1):3–15.

37

Anemia and other hematological problems in the elderly

Satish Shanbhag, MBBS, MPH, and Rakhi Naik, MD, MHS

Anemia in the elderly

Definition of anemia and prevalence

Anemia is defined by the World Health Organization (WHO) criteria as a hemoglobin concentration of less than 12 grams/deciliter (g/dL) in adult women and less than 13 g/dL in men.[1] Based on recent large population cohort studies, nearly 10% of adults over the age of 65 years are anemic,[2, 3] with prevalence estimates as high as 20%–30% in adults over 80 years of age.[3, 4]

Common etiologies of anemia

The most common identifiable causes of anemia in older persons include iron deficiency, chronic kidney disease (CKD), myelodyplastic syndrome (MDS), and anemia of inflammation.[3, 5] However, despite thorough investigation, in nearly 20%–40% of elderly individuals, the underlying etiology of anemia may never be identified.[3, 5] This entity, known as unexplained anemia of the elderly (UAE), may be due to the underlying biology of aging and may encompass elements from the known forms of anemia such as erythropoietin deficiency,[6] inflammation,[7] or poor marrow reserve.[8, 9]

Clinical consequences of anemia

Regardless of the underlying etiology of anemia, low hemoglobin is clearly associated with an increased risk of hospitalization and overall mortality in elderly individuals.[2, 10–13] In addition, anemia in older adults appears to be associated with poor physical functioning,[13, 14] including an increased risk of falls and increased frailty.[15, 16] Neurologic dysfunction is also more prevalent among older individuals with anemia and is associated with an increased risk of cognitive decline, poor cognition, and dementia.[17–19] As a result, diagnosis of the etiology of anemia and targeted strategies to improve low hemoglobin has become an essential component of the care of geriatric populations.

Approach to anemia

Classification of anemia

Traditional classification of anemia involves use of the mean corpuscular volume (MCV), which characterizes anemia based on the predominant red blood cell size. MCV categorization was initially developed to (1) identify probable differential diagnoses for the underlying etiology of the anemia, and (2) provide a guide for targeted workup for anemia. Although tremendous overlap exists between MCV categories and the underlying cause for anemia, especially in the elderly population where the etiology may be multifactorial, MCV still remains a useful paradigm to guide workup and diagnosis of anemia in older individuals. A general scheme using MCV includes:

- Microcytic anemia, defined as MCV <80 fL, which generally points to underlying etiologies such as iron deficiency, thalassemia trait, or anemia of inflammation.
- Normocytic anemia, defined as MCV 80 fL–100 fL, which is associated with anemia of inflammation, CKD-associated anemia, or unexplained anemia.
- Macrocytic anemia, defined as MCV >100 fL, which can be related to vitamin B12 deficiency, alcoholism, medications, or MDS.

In addition to MCV, reticulocyte percentage and absolute reticulocyte count are important laboratory parameters for the workup of any anemia, as a

---

Reichel's Care of the Elderly, 7th Edition, ed. Jan Busby-Whitehead *et al.* Published by Cambridge University Press.
© Cambridge University Press 2016.

decreased reticulocyte count suggests a hypoprolifera-tive anemia and increased count may suggest periph-eral destruction. The reticulocyte count is often used in conjunction with additional laboratory tests to make a final diagnosis. Specific laboratory tests will be outlined further in each relevant subsection.

Initial evaluation of anemia

Anemia in the elderly is often detected on routine laboratory examination, since a complete blood count (CBC) is an essential part of routine follow-up of geriatric patients. Anemia may be transient, as can be observed with acute illness, or may be long-stand-ing, as in individuals with underlying comorbidities. The need for additional workup or referral to hema-tology requires an assessment of the (1) trajectory of hemoglobin values, (2) severity of anemia, and (3) presence of additional cytopenias.

The stability of anemia can be an important clue about the etiology of low hemoglobin in older indivi-duals. For patients with a long history of laboratory records, persistent and stable hemoglobin values often point to anemia of inflammation, CKD, or unex-plained anemia of the elderly. Thorough evaluation of underlying comorbidities is warranted for those with stable anemia, as low hemoglobin may be the first clue to subclinical disease, especially renal dys-function. Other causes such as nutritional deficiencies or bone marrow disorders are usually associated with a clear downtrend in hemoglobin, since they are generally caused by a progressive decline in red cell production. These disorders are also associated with a progressive trend in MCV, such as the new develop-ment of microcytosis with iron deficiency or the new development of macrocytosis with MDS.

Assessment of the severity of anemia is also important to guide the need for further workup, refer-ral, or urgent management. Although there is no clear cut-off for the definition of significant anemia, gen-erally a new anemia of <10–11 g/dL warrants further investigation. Abrupt severe anemia may indicate acute bleed, infection, or acute illness. Progressive severe anemia may occur in the context of underlying bone marrow disorders such as MDS or multiple myeloma, nutritional deficiency, or worsening CKD. Anemia that becomes transfusion-dependent always warrants thorough workup and treatment. Although it is not unusual for severe anemia to develop during a hospitalization secondary to inflammation, daily phlebotomy, medications, and hemoglobin values

should be expected to rebound to baseline values within several weeks post-discharge.

The evaluation of anemia must also involve an assessment for abnormalities in the white blood cell count (WBC) and platelet count. The presence of one or more additional cytopenias may point toward an underlying bone marrow process and warrants inves-tigation. Obtaining a WBC differential is particularly useful in the setting of leukopenia or leukocytosis, as it can often direct the diagnostic workup. A further discussion of WBC and platelet disorders is detailed later in the text.

Microcytic anemias

Iron deficiency anemia

The workup of any degree of anemia in the elderly should involve evaluation for iron deficiency anemia, given its high prevalence, association with underlying gastrointestinal malignancy or disease,[20] and ease of management. Although iron deficiency anemia is one of the most common reasons for low hemoglobin in the elderly population, it is notoriously one of the most difficult etiologies to diagnose.[21] Classically, iron deficiency is associated with microcytosis; how-ever, it may also occur in the absence of anemia or may manifest as normocytic anemia.[22] Additional parameters in the CBC that may point to a diagnosis of iron deficiency include an elevated red cell distri-bution width (RDW) and/or thrombocytosis, although these are not always present.

In addition to a CBC, the relevant laboratory stu-dies that should be sent in the evaluation of iron deficiency include serum iron, total iron binding capacity (TIBC), transferrin saturation, and ferritin. Iron deficiency occurs in discrete stages starting with the depletion of iron stores (ferritin), followed by decrease in available iron (iron, percent transferrin saturation), and finally by the development of anemia and microcytosis. The definitional cut-offs for iron deficiency vary; however, a serum iron <60 mcg/dL, transferrin saturation <16%–20%, and ferritin <40 ng/mL is usually indicative of absolute iron deficiency. Concurrent chronic inflammation, which is present in a significant proportion of older individuals, may result in false increases in the ferritin level,[23] such that empiric iron therapy may be the only reliable way to diagnose deficiency.[21] Functional iron deficiency in the setting of chronic inflammation also presents a diagnostic conundrum, as inflammation may cause an iron-deficient state secondary to iron sequestration and inability to utilize available iron stores.[6]

Because anemia occurs in the late stages of iron deficiency, patients may describe symptoms preceding the development of hematologic abnormalities. Symptoms that should be elicited during a targeted history for iron deficiency should include fatigue, pica (especially pagophagia, that is, ice chewing), and evidence of bleeding. Fatigue and pica symptoms may occur in a majority of individuals with absolute iron deficiency related to blood loss or malabsorption;[24] however, patients may not recognize their decreased energy or craving behaviors until these symptoms improve with iron therapy. Bleeding assessment should include history of hematochezia, melena, symptoms of peptic ulcer disease, or other abnormal mucosal blood loss.

Gastrointestinal (GI) blood loss due to chronic gastritis, arteriovenous malformation (AVM), and colorectal cancer remains a common cause of iron deficiency in the elderly population, with nearly half of anemic individuals demonstrating an identifiable GI lesion on endoscopic evaluation.[20] Baseline screening with upper endoscopy and colonoscopy is, therefore, recommended for evaluation of iron deficiency in all older individuals.

Management of iron deficiency involves oral or IV iron supplementation. Because iron deficiency may be difficult to diagnose in the presence of other comorbidities in elderly individuals, empiric iron therapy for isolated anemia can often be trialed and may result in discernible hemoglobin response.[21] IV iron formulations may be needed in those with severe iron deficiency, oral iron intolerance, or ongoing blood loss. In patients with chronic kidney disease, especially those requiring erythropoietin stimulating agents (ESAs), iron supplementation is often recommended for individuals with a transferrin saturation <20%–30% and ferritin <100 ng/mL–500 ng/mL to allow for maximal ESA response.[25]

Thalassemia

The thalassemias are a clinically heterogeneous group of disorders caused by reduced or absent production of either the α- or β-chain of hemoglobin. Clinically significant thalassemia syndromes are usually diagnosed in childhood or adolescence; therefore, geriatricians are unlikely to encounter a patient with anemia due to thalassemia who will require intervention or treatment. However, clinically silent α- and

β-thalassemia syndromes known as thalassemia trait or minor, are common in certain populations, especially those of Mediterranean, African, Middle Eastern, Indian, and Southeast Asian backgrounds. [26] Although it does not require specific management, thalassemia trait results in microcytosis, which may confuse the diagnosis of iron deficiency. A careful review of historical lab values can often help in distinguishing thalassemia trait from iron deficiency, since microcytosis in thalassemia is lifelong and is associated with mild or no anemia, normal RDW, and MCVs that are generally <75 fL.[27] Hemoglobin electrophoresis may be useful in detecting β-thalassemia trait, as hemoglobin A2 levels will be increased; however, a similar test does not exist to diagnose α-thalassemia trait. In those cases, a trial of empiric iron therapy with normalization of iron studies but persistence of microcytosis may suggest thalassemia trait.

Normocytic anemias

Anemia of inflammation

Anemia of inflammation (AI), also known as anemia of chronic disease, is a term used to describe the low hemoglobin that has been observed with acute and chronic illness. Although initially thought to be associated with conditions with overt inflammation such as infectious, rheumatologic, and neoplastic disease, it is now clear that AI occurs in many circumstances, including aging itself. In fact, it is thought that unexplained anemia of the elderly may be a subset of AI with a similar underlying pathophysiology.[5, 28] The mechanism of this type of anemia is thought to be multifactorial and may involve relative erythropoietin deficiency, decreased erythropoietin responsiveness, impaired iron utilization, and shortened red cell survival.[6, 29, 30] The pathophysiology also likely involves impaired bone marrow response secondary to the suppressive effect of pro-inflammatory cytokines, which appear to be upregulated with aging.[28, 31]

By recent estimates, AI is thought to be the underlying reason for low hemoglobin in approximately one-third of persons older than 65.[3] Laboratory evaluation usually reveals a normocytic anemia, although microcytosis with AI can also be observed in severe cases. Functional iron deficiency may coexist with AI; therefore, features of iron deficiency anemia such as increased RDW are also common.[32] Iron studies may reveal a low serum iron, low transferrin saturation, and normal or elevated ferritin. Hepcidin, a peptide hormone produced by hepatocytes, is a major regulator of iron metabolism in AI. Upregulation of hepcidin in response to inflammation results in impaired iron absorption and iron sequestration, leading to the observed changes in iron studies.[33] However, commercially available hepcidin assays are not yet routinely used in clinical practice. Direct measurement of inflammatory markers such as C-reactive protein (CRP) and erythrocyte sedimentation rate (ESR) is not usually indicated, given the variability of these cytokines in AI;[34] however, they may be useful for older individuals suspected of having rheumatologic disease or chronic infection. In patients suspected of having AI, a thorough evaluation for chronic disease (such as diabetes mellitus, congestive heart failure, and CKD) is warranted, as anemia is common in these conditions and may demonstrate pathophysiologic and morphologic features typical of AI.[33]

The mainstay of treatment for AI is management of the underlying condition; however, anemia secondary to ongoing inflammation or to changes secondary to aging itself may persist despite optimal therapy. Blood transfusion may be required in severe cases, although consensus transfusion goals in the elderly have not been established. Restrictive transfusion for hemoglobin <7 g/dL in asymptomatic individuals appears to be safe.[35] However, older persons – especially those with underlying cardiovascular disease – may become symptomatic at a high hemoglobin threshold. Generally, transfusion is reserved for patients who are thought to have symptomatic anemia characterized by increased fatigue, dyspnea on exertion, or palpitations, which usually does not occur until hemoglobin levels drop below 9 g/dL–10 g/dL.[36]

Given the high prevalence of functional iron deficiency in AI, empiric iron therapy may be warranted in a majority of affected individuals. Treatment with ESAs may also be used in AI to decrease transfusion requirements and improve symptoms, especially in those with underlying CKD or malignancy.

Anemia of chronic kidney disease

CKD is defined as a reduced estimated glomerular filtration rate (eGFR) of <60 mL/min per 1.73 m^2 and is associated with anemia even in early stage disease. The prevalence and degree of anemia is directly correlated to the severity of CKD, with nearly 90% of individuals with an eGFR <25 mL/min–30 mL/min demonstrating low hemoglobin levels.[37] The mechanism of anemia related to CKD involves components of chronic inflammation, functional iron deficiency, and erythropoietin deficiency. Erythropoietin is a glycoprotein growth factor produced by the kidney in response to hypoxemia. The primary role of erythropoietin is to stimulate maturation of erythrocytes, thereby increasing red blood cell production and promoting oxygen delivery.[38] Impaired erythropoietin synthesis in the setting of CKD is, therefore, an important cause of anemia in kidney disease.

Laboratory values often reveal a normocytic anemia that is virtually indistinguishable from AI, given the overlap in pathophysiology. Similar to AI, iron studies may reveal functional iron deficiency with reduced serum iron and percent saturation and normal ferritin levels. Serum erythropoietin levels are not generally required for diagnosis of anemia in kidney disease, since absolute deficiency may not be present despite a relative decrease in production.[39]

Treatment of anemia in patients with CKD involves iron supplementation and ESA support with the goal of decreasing transfusion requirements, alleviating symptoms, and improving patient outcomes.[40] Absolute iron deficiency is likely to be present in individuals with CKD at a transferrin saturation <20% and ferritin levels <100 ng/mL;[41] therefore, iron supplementation and workup for underlying cause is required in those patients. In addition, functional iron deficiency may result in ESA nonresponsiveness, especially in dialysis-dependent kidney disease; therefore, higher goals of transferrin saturation of <30% and ferritin <500 ng/mL may be appropriate.[25] ESA support is recommended for those on dialysis for a hemoglobin <10 g/dL after adequate iron repletion. However, because high hemoglobin goals are associated with adverse outcomes including death,[42] ESA support should be withheld for hemoglobin >11 g/dL. For CKD patients not on dialysis, ESA support can be initiated on an individual basis to improve symptoms that are related to the underlying anemia.

Macrocytic anemias

Vitamin B12 deficiency

Cobalamin (vitamin B12) deficiency is associated with macrocytic anemia due to impaired DNA synthesis and ineffective erythropoiesis. Deficiency of vitamin B12 is common in individuals older than 65 and may be associated with dementia, although the etiologic link is not yet clear.[43] Reduced vitamin B12 levels in older populations are often due to malabsorption in the setting of hypochlorhydria, gastric or intestinal surgery, or pernicious anemia. Dietary deficiency is rare, except in the case of strict vegetarianism or chronic malnutrition.

Laboratory evaluation in individuals with vitamin B12 deficiency reveals isolated macrocytic anemia, although pancytopenia may be present in severe cases and may be indistinguishable from MDS. In true deficiency, serum vitamin B12 levels are generally lower than 200 pg/mL; however, levels between 200 pg/mL and 300 pg/mL may also be associated with true vitamin B12 deficiency, and elevated levels of methylmalonic acid (MMA) and homocysteine are required to verify the diagnosis.[44] Antibodies to intrinsic factor (IF) should be checked in patients with verified vitamin B12 deficiency, as they are highly specific for pernicious anemia.[45] Evaluation of the peripheral blood smear may reveal macro-ovalocytes and hypersegmented neutrophils, which are a hallmark of this condition.

In individuals with pernicious anemia or an anatomic cause for vitamin B12 deficiency such as gastric bypass surgery, treatment with cobalamin supplementation is required lifelong. The most commonly prescribed regimen includes intramuscular injection of vitamin B12 at 1,000 mcg daily for one week, followed by 1,000 mcg weekly for four weeks, then 1,000 mcg monthly. Alternative regimens using oral cobalamin supplementation at supra-normal doses of 1,000 mcg–2,000 mcg daily may also be considered and can overcome deficiency due to malabsorption.[46] Full hematologic responses usually do not occur for approximately two months, although a reticulocyte response and normalization of MMA and homocysteine levels should be noted within the first week of therapy.[44]

Myelodysplastic syndrome

MDS is a clonal disorder of hematopoetic stem cells resulting in impaired production and maturation of bone marrow elements. The median age at diagnosis of MDS is 65–70 years, with less than 10% of cases occurring in individuals younger than 50 years of age. [47] The pathophysiology of MDS is due to a host of acquired genetic, epigenetic, and chromosomal alterations, and as a result, there is significant clinical heterogeneity in presentation and disease course.[48]

Initial presentation of MDS can vary widely from asymptomatic isolated anemia on routine testing to debilitating disease. Symptoms, when present, are secondary to the degree and type of cytopenias, although constitutional symptoms such as anorexia and weight loss may also occur in severe cases. Anemia may result in significant fatigue, weakness, and dyspnea. Thrombocytopenia may lead to petechiae, easy bruisability, and mucosal bleeding. Neutropenia may result in recurrent bacterial or fungal infection such as pneumonia and sinusitis. Because MDS is often associated with functional impairment of platelets and neutrophils, symptoms can occur with even modest levels of thrombocytopenia and leukopenia.

Macrocytic anemia may be the first manifestation of MDS in the elderly. Macrocytosis in older individuals without any obvious underlying cause such as nutritional deficiency or excessive alcohol intake should be considered suspicious for MDS.[49] Elevated RDW is usually present due to heterogeneity of red cell production, and reticulocyte count is usually inappropriately low, reflecting ineffective erythropoiesis. Whereas anemia is found in nearly all patients with MDS, thrombocytopenia and neutropenia is present in only about a third of individuals at diagnosis.[47] Peripheral blood smear examination may reveal features suggestive of MDS such as hypogranular neutrophils and abnormal nuclear segmentation; however, definitive diagnosis always requires bone marrow examination. Typical features of the bone marrow include hypercellularity, dysplasia, increase in blast percentage, and karyotypic abnormalities. However, in early or mild disease, bone marrow examination may be equivocal, especially if dysplasia is not prominent and chromosomal mutations cannot be identified.

Prognosis in MDS is generally dictated by the risk of progression to acute leukemia. Median survival can range from less than one year to greater than five years, depending on the stage of disease at presentation. Cytopenias, cytogenetic abnormalities, and blast percentage are generally used to determine severity of MDS at diagnosis and have been found to predict survival in MDS.[50]

Treatment for MDS in older individuals depends on the risk category of disease and baseline performance status. Management may include the use of growth factors such as ESAs, chemotherapy, hypo-methylating agents, or allogeneic stem cell transplantation. Generally, aggressive therapy is reserved for high-risk MDS, with the overall goal of modifying disease course by decreasing the risk to progression to acute leukemia and improving overall survival. Low-risk disease, on the other hand, can often be treated with supportive care alone to improve quality of life and reduce transfusion requirements.[51]

Autoimmune hemolytic anemias

Warm autoimmune hemolytic anemia (AIHA) is characterized by IgG antibodies that react with red cells antigens at room temperature and cause hemolysis. Reticulocytosis, microspherocytes on peripheral blood smear, a positive direct Coomb's test, elevated lactate dehydrogenase (LDH) levels, and reduced to absent serum haptoglobin are all lab abnormalities typical for this disorder. Patients with ongoing hemolysis can compensate for weeks to months before presenting to medical care and usually have spleno-megaly (red cell destruction occurs mainly in the spleen in warm AIHA) along with the sequelae of anemia.[52] AIHA is often associated with underlying lymphoproliferative disorders such as CLL and auto-immune disease; therefore, a workup for underlying etiology is warranted.

Cold agglutinin disease is a type of autoimmune hemolytic anemia characterized by predominantly IgM antibodies binding to the red cell surface and causing complement-mediated red cell destruction at below normal body temperatures. This is a disease of the elderly with a median age at diagnosis of 67 years. Similar to AIHA, cold agglutinin disease is often associated with underlying malignancy. Non-Hodgkin lymphomas, monoclonal gammopathies, and CLL are present in a large majority of patients diagnosed with cold aggutinins, thereby making the recognition of a background inciting factor important when this diagnosis is made.[53–55]

Characteristic features of cold agglutinin disease are symptoms related to anemia along with acrocya-nosis and livedo reticularis, both phenomena related to cold exposure in the peripheries. The blood smear has a characteristic look of clumped red cells, and the automated cell counter is often unable to give an accurate read on the hemogram until the sample is warmed to room temperature. There is limited evidence on therapeutic efficacy in this disorder, but the monoclonal anti-CD20 antibody rituximab seems to

have the best initial response rates in cases that require treatment.[53, 55]

Thrombocytopenia

Overview

Platelets are the dominant cells involved in the primary hemostatic process that occurs in response to vascular injury. The major functions of platelets include adherence, activation, aggregation, and initiation of coagulation; therefore, an overall reduction in platelet number may result in bleeding, especially at sites of frequent vascular injury such as mucosal surfaces.[56] However, although absolute platelet count is clearly a major determinant of hemostatic function, the rate of production and function of platelets also plays a role in determining bleeding risk.

Thrombocytopenia is defined by a platelet count below 150,000/μL. The severity of thrombocytopenia is often categorized by absolute platelet count, with values between 100,000/μL and 150,000/μL defined as mild, 50,000/μL–99,000/μL defined as moderate, and <50,000/μL defined as severe.[57] The underlying mechanisms of thrombocytopenia most commonly include impaired platelet production, peripheral platelet destruction, and splenic sequestration; however, rarely platelet consumption may occur in micro-thrombotic diseases such as thrombotic thrombocytopenia purpura (TTP) or disseminated intravascular coagulation (DIC). Processes that result in impaired platelet production or function, such as MDS, generally lead to bleeding at moderate counts, whereas those that cause thrombocytopenia primarily by peripheral destruction, such as immune thrombocytopenic purpura (ITP), result in bleeding only at severely low counts, since platelet production is preserved.

The evaluation of thrombocytopenia in older individuals should involve an assessment of the trend in platelet count, severity of disease, and associated cytopenias. Stable mild to moderate thrombocytopenia often points to systemic disease (such as liver disease) or medications, whereas progressive, severe thrombocytopenia may suggest a more acute process such as ITP. The presence of additional cytopenias may suggest an underlying bone marrow disorder and should prompt a thorough evaluation. Symptoms, if present, may include mucosal bleeding such as recurrent epistaxis, gum bleeding, GI bleeding, or hematuria. Skin findings include petechiae and spontaneous bruising.

Wet purpura (blood blisters on the mucosal surfaces of the mouth) are a marker of severe thrombocytopenia or severely impaired platelet function and, therefore, require immediate evaluation and management.

Isolated thrombocytopenia may be the first manifestation of chronic liver disease or cirrhosis – including virus-associated hepatitis, alcoholic liver disease, or nonalcoholic fatty liver.[58, 59] The pathophysiology of thrombocytopenia in liver disease appears to be related primarily to hypersplenism in the setting of portal hypertension, as the spleen can sequester up to 90% of platelet mass;[60] however, decreased thrombopoietin synthesis may also play a role in severe disease.[61]

Immune thrombocytopenic purpura

ITP is an acquired disorder caused by the development of autoantibodies against platelet antigens, leading to the premature destruction of platelets in the peripheral circulation by splenic macrophages.[62] ITP is quite common in older individuals, and the incidence appears to increase steadily with age. The average incidence rate for ITP among adults is about two cases per 100,000 person-years, increasing to nearly five cases per 100,000 person-years in people over the age of 60.[63]

ITP should be suspected in any elderly patient with isolated thrombocytopenia and relatively minimal bleeding symptoms compared to the platelet count. Clinically apparent symptoms of thrombocytopenia usually do not occur until the platelet count is lower than approximately 20,000/μL, given the robust bone marrow response that often accompanies this condition. The degree and course of low platelets, especially in the elderly, may vary from chronic moderate thrombocytopenia to a severe acute drop in platelet count.

An underlying etiology of ITP cannot be found in many cases; however, secondary ITP may occur in the setting of viral infection – especially hepatitis C and human immunodeficiency virus (HIV) – and lymphoproliferative disorders such as chronic lymphocytic leukemia (CLL). All adult patients suspected to have ITP should undergo testing for hepatitis C and HIV, given the strong association with ITP.[64] Antiplatelet antibody testing has limited utility in ITP, since its predictive value is generally poor.[65] Peripheral flow cytometry should usually be reserved for patients who have an absolute lymphocytosis or

suspicion of CLL based on physical examination or blood smear. In addition, bone marrow biopsy is usually not routinely warranted even in older individuals unless additional cytopenias are present or symptoms are concerning for a bone marrow process.[64] Evaluation of the peripheral smear in ITP usually reveals normal erythrocyte and WBC morphology with occasional large (young) platelets. Unlike in children, ITP tends to be chronic in adult patients; therefore, treatment is often aimed at stabilizing the platelet count and preventing symptoms, rather than curing the disease itself. Because bleeding risk does not usually increase until severe thrombocytopenia develops, treatment is generally initiated only if the platelet count is below 30,000/μL. First-line therapy usually involves the use of prednisone at a dose of 1 mg/kg that is tapered slowly over a course of weeks to months. Intravenous immunoglobulin (IVIg) may also be used in severe cases. If clinically significant thrombocytopenia recurs after this initial course, second-line therapy with immunosuppressive agents such as rituximab may be considered.[66]

Hematologic malignancies in the elderly

Multiple myeloma

Myeloma, a plasma cell neoplasm, is one of the most common hematologic malignancies in the elderly, responsible for an estimated 24,000 new cases and 11,000 deaths per year in the United States. Despite the five-year survival in myeloma improving dramatically in the last two decades (from 30.7% in 1994 to 45.1% in 2006), myeloma remains a major cause of morbidity in the elderly, with an estimated 83,367 people living with myeloma in the United States.[67] Myeloma is a disease of the elderly, and the incidence of the malignancy increases significantly with age; in fact the median age of patients diagnosed with myeloma is 69 years.[68] The prevalence of myeloma is also much higher in African Americans, who have about twice the incidence rates as Caucasians across all age-groups. (See Figure 37.1.)

Multiple myeloma commonly presents with a hypoproliferative anemia, which is present in about 75% of patients at the time of diagnosis. The anemia is typically normocytic, but macrocytosis may be observed in about 10% of patients.[69] The

Table 37.1 Light chain ratio showing improvement with institution of therapy in a patient with lambda light-chain secretory myeloma with response in quantitative serum-free lambda light chain levels and improvement of the kappa/lambda ratio

	Normal range	Diagnosis	1 month into therapy	2 months into therapy	6 months into therapy
Serum-free kappa chains	3.3–19.4 mg/L	7.2	1.6	2.5	10.8
Serum-free lambda chain	5.7–26.3 mg/L	2890	564	260	148
Kappa/lambda ratio	0.26–1.65	0	0	0.01	0.07

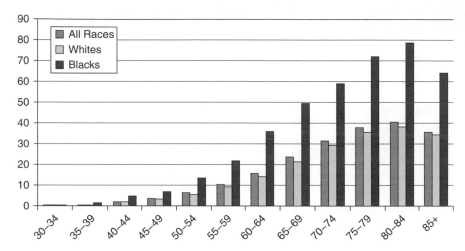

Figure 37.1 Age-specific SEER incidence rates, 2007–2011. Data is from the SEER (Surveillance, Epidemiology, and End Results) program.

mechanism of anemia can be multifactorial, including impaired hematopoiesis secondary to marrow infiltration by clonal plasma cells and impaired renal function due to direct effects of the monoclonal protein. In addition to anemia, patients with myeloma may develop bony lytic lesions, hypercalcemia, and renal damage from the monoclonal protein.

Given the high prevalence of myeloma in the elderly, a workup for anemia should include an evaluation for monoclonal gammopathy. About 80% of patients with multiple myeloma have clonal plasma cells that secrete the entire immunoglobulin molecule, which consists of both a heavy and light chain, while 20% of patients have cells that produce only the light chain fragment of the immunoglobulin molecule.[69] This can make the diagnosis of myeloma somewhat challenging, as patients with light-chain only secretory myeloma do not present with increased gamma globulins (gamma gap) and cannot be diagnosed easily with serum protein electrophoresis alone.

Although serum protein electrophoresis and immunofixation (SPEP and SIFE) can be used to detect clonal immunoglobulins, they are not sensitive for detecting light-chain only disease, because light chains are rapidly cleared in the urine. In the past, urine studies (urine protein electrophoresis and immunofixation) were required to detect urinary light chains, also known as Bence-Jones proteinuria. The advent of the serum-free kappa and lambda light chain assay, however, has considerably improved the diagnostic ease in detecting patients with light-chain only secretory myeloma and assessing response to therapy.[70] Because myeloma is a clonal disease, the plasma cells secrete only either kappa or lambda restricted immunoglobulin molecules, and an abnormal ratio of kappa to lambda light chains can be seen in the serum at diagnosis. The light chain assay is also a very useful tool to assess burden of disease, as improvement in the kappa/lambda ratio denotes response to therapy.

Another important plasma-cell dyscrasia that is frequently found in the elderly is monoclonal gammopathy of undetermined significance (MGUS). MGUS is an asymptomatic, premalignant clonal plasma cell or lymphoproliferative disorder defined by the presence of a serum M-protein <3 g/dL, bone marrow biopsy demonstrating <10% clonal plasma cells, and the absence of end organ damage. MGUS is not considered a cancer; however, it is a premalignant state. MGUS always precedes the development of multiple myeloma, initially in the form of smoldering myeloma and ultimately in the development of symptomatic myeloma with end-organ damage. However, a majority of elderly patients will never progress to multiple myeloma in their lifetime and will remain in the category of MGUS.

In a predominantly Caucasian population in Olmsted County, Minnesota, the prevalence of MGUS was about 4.6% in those between the ages of 70 and 79 years and rose to 6.6% in those over 80.[71] This prevalence is about two to three times higher in African Americans. Risk stratification is based on quantification of the monoclonal protein, the free light chain ratio, and characteristics of the clonal immunoglobulin molecule. These factors can help define the risk of progression to a symptomatic multiple myeloma. The risk of progression at 20 years can be as high as 58% in high-risk MGUS, 37% in high-intermediate-risk MGUS, 21% in low-intermediate-risk MGUS, and 5% in low-risk MGUS.[72]

A discussion of therapies for myeloma is out of the scope of this chapter, but suffice it to say that myeloma therapy has evolved to include novel agents such as lenalidomide and bortezomib, which in combination can result in >95% response rates in patients with newly diagnosed myeloma.[73] A majority of elderly patients with myeloma are not considered eligible for high-dose chemotherapy and autologous stem-cell transplantation due to their age and comorbidities.

The leukemias

Chronic lymphocytic leukemia (CLL) is one of the most commonly encountered leukemias in clinical practice in the elderly. Of an estimated 52,380 cases of leukemia diagnosed annually in the United States, approximately 30% of cases are CLL and 11% are chronic myeloid leukemia (CML).[74] CLL is a B-cell chronic lymphoproliferative neoplasm characterized by progressive accumulation of mature, clonal lymphocytes in the bone marrow and peripheral blood. The natural history of the disease, as defined in the 1970s by Rai and colleagues, can vary widely, with median survival times from diagnosis ranging from >150 months in patients presenting with stage 0 disease (defined by lymphocytosis alone) to only 19 months in patients with stage III and stage IV disease

(characterized by the presence of anemia and thrombocytopenia, respectively).[75] The incidence of CLL increases dramatically with age from seven cases per 100,000 person-years in those between 50 and 64 years of age to 20 cases per 100,000 person-years in those between 65 and 74, and 30 cases per 100,000 person-years in those 75 or older.[76]

Anemia itself is not the usual presentation in patients with newly diagnosed CLL, as it can take several years to get to the level of marrow infiltration required to cause disruption of normal hematopoiesis. Thus, hypoproliferative anemia, marked by a low reticulocyte count, is usually seen years after diagnosis. Other mechanisms of anemia include autoimmune hemolysis, which can occur in about 4% of patients with CLL and is commonly seen as a presenting sign of CLL.[77] Autoimmune hemolysis detected in patients with CLL is generally characterized by an elevated reticulocyte count (indicative of a bone marrow responsive to anemia) and the presence of an IgG warm autoantibody, which can often be detected on a direct Coombs test. Other immune phenomena associated with CLL include ITP and pure red cell aplasia (PRCA), which are thought to be the result of immune dysregulation.[78]

The distinction between a hypoproliferative anemia and hemolysis is important, as the treatment can be very different; steroids and the anti-CD20 monocolonal antibody rituximab form the backbone of therapy for autoimmune hemolysis, while targeted or combination chemotherapy aimed at the CLL clone forms the mainstay of treatment for anemia related to dense marrow infiltration by the leukemia. The introduction of new oral agents such as the Bruton's tyrosine kinase inhibitor ibrutinib have the potential to dramatically alter the natural history of even patients with high-risk CLL who relapse after chemotherapy.[79]

CML is a myeloproliferative neoplasm characterized by unregulated growth of cells in the granulocytic lineage (Table 37.2) and is commonly accompanied by thrombocytosis. Hypoproliferative anemia can be seen in advanced cases of patients presenting in accelerated or blast phase. In contrast to CLL, CML is treated rather than observed, even in asymptomatic patients, with highly effective targeted molecules (tyrosine kinase inhibitors) like imatinib.

Acute myelogenous leukemia (AML) is characterized by accumulation of undifferentiated myeloid precursors (blasts) in the bone marrow and blood

531

Table 37.2 Contrasting hemograms in the leukemias

	Normal range	Stage 0 CLL	CML	AML
White blood count	4.5–11 k/cu mm	33	82	60
Hemoglobin	13.9–16.3 g/dL	15.7	14.4	8
Platelets	150–350 k/cu mm	195	895	30
Neutrophils	40%–70%	18%	63%	20%
Lymphocytes	24%–44%	70%	5%	5%
Bands, myelocytes, and metamyelocytes	0%–1%	0%	22%	5%
Atypical lymphs	0%–1%	8%	0%	0%
Basophils	0%–2%	0%	7%	0%
Blasts	0%–1%	0%	1%	70%

with rapidly progressive anemia and thrombocytopenia. It is responsible for about 36% of newly diagnosed leukemias in the United States.[74] Incidence of AML increases with age, with incidence rates of 10 cases per 100,000 person-years in those aged 65–69, 15 cases per 100,000 person-years in those aged 70–74, and 20 per 100,000 person-years in those aged 75–79.[80] AML is a highly aggressive malignancy that is rapidly fatal when untreated. Treating AML in the elderly is very challenging, as the course of therapy required to "cure" this cancer is very poorly tolerated in the older adult. Biologic rather than chronological age comes into play to select those few elderly able to tolerate the rigors of months of intensive chemotherapy regimens required to induce a remission. AML is incurable with chemotherapy alone in the majority of patients; recent advances in stem-cell transplant technology have made allogeneic transplants accessible to the select fit elderly with minimal comorbidities.[81]

Myeloproliferative neoplasms

Polycythemia vera (PV), essential thrombocytosis (ET), and primary myelofibrosis (PMF) are all myeloproliferative neoplasms (MPN) that exhibit clonal proliferation and differentiation of mature terminal myeloid cells. PV is unique in its epo-independent expansion of the red cell mass with incidence rates that rise with age – in fact, the highest incidence rate of PV is for men aged 70–79 (24 cases/100,000 persons/year).[82]

Virtually all patients with PV have the *V617F* mutation (a change of valine to phenylalanine at the 617 position) in the Janus kinase 2 (*JAK2*) gene.[83] This mutation leads to constitutive tyrosine phosphorylation activity that promotes hypersensitivity to cytokines/growth factors and induces epo-independant erythrocytosis. Approximately half of the patients with ET and PMF also have the *JAK2 V617F* mutation.

Classic clinical findings in these patients with PV include thrombocytosis, erythrocytosis, leukocytosis/neutrophilia, and thrombocytosis with palpable splenomegaly and symptoms of itching and flushing. They have a significant thrombotic risk that can be reduced by phlebotomy (hematocrit goal of 45% in men and 42% in women), anti-platelet agents, and cytoreductive therapy.[84–86]

ET presents with chronic unexplained thrombocytosis; young patients with ET may be asymptomatic and not require therapy, but patients over the age of 60 are considered high-risk for thrombotic events. The incidence of ET rises with age, with the median age of presentation at 72 years.[87] Patients at high risk of thrombosis may benefit from cytoreductive therapy with hydroxyurea or anagrelide in addition to antiplatelet agents.[88–91]

PMF is the rarest of the three *JAK2* mutations associated MPNs; it remains a disease of the elderly, with a median age at presentation of about 67 years.[87] Common signs at presentation include leukocytosis with a neutrophil predominance, tear drop cells on the peripheral blood smear due to marrow fibrosis, and extramedullary hematopoiesis, splenomegaly, pruritus, and macrocytic anemia. Ruxolitinib, a *JAK1/JAK2* inhibitor, has shown activity in patients with PMF and can be beneficial in reducing splenomegaly and symptomatology.[92, 93]

Summary

In summary, we have outlined here the approach to anemia and hematological disorders in the elderly, with an emphasis on common causes of anemia and general guidelines for initial therapy.

References

1. Blanc B, Finch C, Hallberg L, et al. Nutritional anaemia: report of a WHO scientific group. *WHO Tech Report Series* 1968;**405**:5–37.

2. Zakai NA, Katz R, Hirsch C, et al. A prospective study of anemia status, hemoglobin concentration, and mortality in an elderly cohort: the Cardiovascular Health Study. *Arch Intern Med* 2005;**165**:2214–20.

3. Guralnik JM, Eisenstaedt RS, Ferrucci L, et al. Prevalence of anemia in persons 65 years and older in the United States: evidence for a high rate of unexplained anemia. *Blood* 2004;**104**:2263–8.

4. Izaks GJ, Westendorp RG, Knook DL. The definition of anemia in older persons. *JAMA* 1999;**281**:1714–7.

5. Artz AS, Thirman MJ. Unexplained anemia predominates despite an intensive evaluation in a racially diverse cohort of older adults from a referral anemia clinic. *J Gerontol A Biol Sci Med Sci* 2011;**66**:925–32.

6. Ferrucci L, Semba RD, Guralnik JM, et al. Proinflammatory state, hepcidin, and anemia in older persons. *Blood* 2010;**115**:3810–6.

7. Adler AS, Kawahara TL, Segal E, Chang HY. Reversal of aging by NFkappaB blockade. *Cell Cycle* 2008;**7**:556–9.

8. Chambers SM, Shaw CA, Gatza C, et al. Aging hematopoietic stem cells decline in function and exhibit epigenetic dysregulation. *PLoS Biol* 2007;**5**:e201.

9. Chambers SM, Goodell MA. Hematopoietic stem cell aging: wrinkles in stem cell potential. *Stem Cell Rev* 2007;**3**:201–11.

10. Culleton BF, Manns BJ, Zhang J, et al. Impact of anemia on hospitalization and mortality in older adults. *Blood* 2006;**107**:3841–6.

11. Zakai NA, French B, Arnold AM, et al. Hemoglobin decline, function, and mortality in the elderly: the cardiovascular health study. *Am J Hematol* 2013;**88**:5–9.

12. Dong X, Mendes de Leon C, Artz A, et al. A population-based study of hemoglobin, race, and mortality in elderly persons. *J Gerontol A Biol Sci Med Sci* 2008;**63**:873–8.

13. Denny SD, Kuchibhatla MN, Cohen HJ. Impact of anemia on mortality, cognition, and function in community-dwelling elderly. *Am J Med* 2006;**119**:327–34.

14. Penninx BW, Guralnik JM, Onder G, et al. Anemia and decline in physical performance among older persons. *Am J Med* 2003;**115**:104–10.

15. Penninx BW, Pluijm SM, Lips P, et al. Late-life anemia is associated with increased risk of recurrent falls. *J Am Geriatr Soc* 2005;**53**:2106–11.

16. Chaves PH, Semba RD, Leng SX, et al. Impact of anemia and cardiovascular disease on frailty status of community-dwelling older women: the Women's Health and Aging Studies I and II. *J Gerontol A Biol Sci Med Sci* 2005;**60**:729–35.

17. Deal JA, Carlson MC, Xue QL, et al. Anemia and 9-year domain-specific cognitive decline in community-dwelling older women: The Women's Health and Aging Study II. *J Am Geriatr Soc* 2009;**57**:1604–11.

18. Zilinski J, Zillmann R, Becker I, et al. Prevalence of anemia among elderly inpatients and its association with multidimensional loss of function. *Ann Hematol* 2014;**93**(10):1645–54.

19. Hong CH, Falvey C, Harris TB, et al. Anemia and risk of dementia in older adults: findings from the Health ABC study. *Neurology* 2013;**81**:528–33.

20. Joosten E, Ghesquiere B, Linthoudt H, et al. Upper and lower gastrointestinal evaluation of elderly inpatients who are iron deficient. *Am J Med* 1999;**107**:24–9.

21. Pang WW, Schrier SL. Anemia in the elderly. *Curr Opin Hematol* 2012;**19**:133–40.

22. Cook JD, Flowers CH, Skikne BS. The quantitative assessment of body iron. *Blood* 2003;**101**:3359–64.

23. Keel SB, Abkowitz JL. The microcytic red cell and the anemia of inflammation. *N Engl J Med* 2009;**361**:1904–6.

24. Rector WG Jr. Pica: its frequency and significance in patients with iron-deficiency anemia due to chronic gastrointestinal blood loss. *J Gen Intern Med* 1989;**4**:512–3.

25. Moist LM, Troyanov S, White CT, et al. Canadian Society of Nephrology commentary on the 2012 KDIGO Clinical Practice Guideline for Anemia in CKD. *Am J Kidney Dis* 2013;**62**:860–73.

26. Martin A, Thompson AA. Thalassemias. *Pediatr Clin North Am* 2013;**60**:1383–91.

27. Muncie HL Jr, Campbell J. Alpha and beta thalassemia. *Am Fam Physician* 2009;**80**:339–44.

28. Price EA, Mehra R, Holmes TH, Schrier SL. Anemia in older persons: etiology and evaluation. *Blood Cells Mol Dis* 2011;**46**:159–65.

29. Corazza F, Beguin Y, Bergmann P, et al. Anemia in children with cancer is associated with decreased erythropoietic activity and not with inadequate erythropoietin production. *Blood* 1998;**92**:1793–8.

30. Weiss G, Goodnough LT. Anemia of chronic disease. *N Engl J Med* 2005;**352**:1011–23.

31. Artz AS, Xue QL, Wickrema A, et al. Unexplained anaemia in the elderly is characterised by features of low grade inflammation. *Br J Haematol* 2014;**167** (2):286–9.

32. Allen LA, Felker GM, Mehra MR, et al. Validation and potential mechanisms of red cell distribution width as a prognostic marker in heart failure. *J Card Fail* 2010;**16**:230–8.

33. Roy CN. Anemia of inflammation. *Hematology Am Soc Hematol Educ Program* 2010;**2010**:276–80.

34. Merchant AA, Roy CN. Not so benign haematology: anaemia of the elderly. *Br J Haematol* 2012;**156**:173–85.

35. Goodnough LT, Levy JH, Murphy MF. Concepts of blood transfusion in adults. *Lancet* 2013;**381**:1845–54.

36. Finch CA, Lenfant C. Oxygen transport in man. *N Engl J Med* 1972;**286**:407–15.

37. Kazmi WH, Kausz AT, Khan S, et al. Anemia: an early complication of chronic renal insufficiency. *Am J Kidney Dis* 2001;**38**:803–12.

38. Erslev AJ. Erythropoietin. *N Engl J Med* 1991;**324**:1339–44.

39. Donnelly S, Shah BR. Erythropoietin deficiency in hyporeninemia. *Am J Kidney Dis* 1999;**33**:947–53.

40. Ma JZ, Ebben J, Xia H, Collins AJ. Hematocrit level and associated mortality in hemodialysis patients. *J Am Soc Nephrol* 1999;**10**:610–19.

41. Fernandez-Rodriguez AM, Guindeo-Casasus MC, Molero-Labarta T, et al. Diagnosis of iron deficiency in chronic renal failure. *Am J Kidney Dis* 1999;**34**:508–13.

42. Phrommintikul A, Haas SJ, Elsik M, Krum H. Mortality and target haemoglobin concentrations in anaemic patients with chronic kidney disease treated with erythropoietin: a meta-analysis. *Lancet* 2007;**369**:381–8.

43. Andres E, Loukili NH, Noel E, et al. Vitamin B12 (cobalamin) deficiency in elderly patients. *CMAJ* 2004;**171**:251–9.

44. Carmel R. How I treat cobalamin (vitamin B12) deficiency. *Blood* 2008;**112**:2214–21.

45. Nimo RE, Carmel R. Increased sensitivity of detection of the blocking (type I) anti-intrinsic factor antibody. *Am J Clin Pathol* 1987;**88**:729–33.

46. Eussen SJ, de Groot LC, Clarke R, et al. Oral cyanocobalamin supplementation in older people with vitamin B12 deficiency: a dose-finding trial. *Arch Intern Med* 2005;**165**:1167–72.

47. Ades L, Itzykson R, Fenaux P. Myelodysplastic syndromes. *Lancet* 2014;**383**:2239–52.

48. Will B, Zhou L, Vogler TO, et al. Stem and progenitor cells in myelodysplastic syndromes show aberrant stage-specific expansion and harbor genetic and epigenetic alterations. *Blood* 2012;**120**:2076–86.

49. Anttila P, Ihalainen J, Salo A, et al. Idiopathic macrocytic anaemia in the aged: molecular and cytogenetic findings. *Br J Haematol* 1995;**90**:797–803.

50. Greenberg PL, Tuechler H, Schanz J, et al. Revised international prognostic scoring system for myelodysplastic syndromes. *Blood* 2012;**120**:2454–65.

51. Zeidan AM, Linhares Y, Gore SD. Current therapy of myelodysplastic syndromes. *Blood Rev* 2013;**27**:243–59.

52. Gehrs BC, Friedberg RC. Autoimmune hemolytic anemia. *Am J Hematol* 2002;**69**:258–71.

53. Crisp D, Pruzanski W. B-cell neoplasms with homogeneous cold-reacting antibodies (cold agglutinins). *Am J Med* 1982;**72**:915–22.

54. Berentsen S. Cold agglutinin-mediated autoimmune hemolytic anemia in Waldenstrom's macroglobulinemia. *Clin Lymphoma Myeloma* 2009;**9**:110–12.

55. Berentsen S, Ulvestad E, Langholm R, et al. Primary chronic cold agglutinin disease: a population based clinical study of 86 patients. *Haematologica* 2006;**91**:460–6.

56. Smyth SS, McEver RP, Weyrich AS, et al. Platelet functions beyond hemostasis. *J Thromb Haemost* 2009;**7**:1759–66.

57. Williamson DR, Albert M, Heels-Ansdell D, et al. Thrombocytopenia in critically ill patients receiving thromboprophylaxis: frequency, risk factors, and outcomes. *Chest* 2013;**144**:1207–15.

58. Mendes FD, Suzuki A, Sanderson SO, et al. Prevalence and indicators of portal hypertension in patients with nonalcoholic fatty liver disease. *Clin Gastroenterol Hepatol* 2012;**10**(9):1028–33.

59. Sheikh MY, Raoufi R, Atla PR, et al. Prevalence of cirrhosis in patients with thrombocytopenia who receive bone marrow biopsy. *Saudi J Gastroenterol* 2012;**18**:257–62.

60. Aster RH. Pooling of platelets in the spleen: role in the pathogenesis of "hypersplenic" thrombocytopenia. *J Clin Invest* 1966;**45**:645–57.

61. Peck-Radosavljevic M, Zacherl J, Meng YG, et al. Is inadequate thrombopoietin production a major cause of thrombocytopenia in cirrhosis of the liver? *J Hepatol* 1997;**27**:127–31.

62. Kuwana M, Okazaki Y, Ikeda Y. Splenic macrophages maintain the anti-platelet autoimmune response via uptake of opsonized platelets in patients with immune thrombocytopenic purpura. *J Thromb Haemost* 2009;**7**:322–9.

63. Frederiksen H, Schmidt K. The incidence of idiopathic thrombocytopenic purpura in adults increases with age. *Blood* 1999;**94**:909–13.

64. Neunert C, Lim W, Crowther M, et al. The American Society of Hematology 2011 evidence-based practice guideline for immune thrombocytopenia. *Blood* 2011;**117**:4190–207.

65. Cines DB, Blanchette VS. Immune thrombocytopenic purpura. *N Engl J Med* 2002;**346**:995–1008.

66. Provan D, Stasi R, Newland AC, et al. International consensus report on the investigation and management of primary immune thrombocytopenia. *Blood* 2010;**115**:168–86.

67. Surveillance, Epidemiology, and End Results Program (SEER) Stat Fact Sheet: Myeloma. National Cancer Institute. Available at: http://seer.cancer.gov/statfacts/html/mulmy.html (accessed June 30, 2014).

68. DeSantis CE, Lin CC, Mariotto AB, et al. Cancer treatment and survivorship statistics, 2014. *CA Cancer J Clin* 2014;**64**:252–71.

69. Kyle RA, Gertz MA, Witzig TE, et al. Review of 1027 patients with newly diagnosed multiple myeloma. *Mayo Clin Proc* 2003;**78**:21–33.

70. Katzmann JA, Clark RJ, Abraham RS, et al. Serum reference intervals and diagnostic ranges for free kappa and free lambda immunoglobulin light chains: relative sensitivity for detection of monoclonal light chains. *Clin Chem* 2002;**48**:1437–44.

71. Kyle RA, Therneau TM, Rajkumar SV, et al. Prevalence of monoclonal gammopathy of undetermined significance. *N Engl J Med* 2006;**354**:1362–9.

72. Rajkumar SV, Kyle RA, Therneau TM, et al. Serum free light chain ratio is an independent risk factor for progression in monoclonal gammopathy of undetermined significance. *Blood* 2005;**106**:812–17.

73. Richardson PG, Weller E, Lonial S, et al. Lenalidomide, bortezomib, and dexamethasone combination therapy in patients with newly diagnosed multiple myeloma. *Blood* 2010;**116**:679–86.

74. Cancer Facts and Figures. American Cancer Society. Available at: www.cancer.org/research/cancerfactsstatistics/allcancerfactsfigures/index (accessed July 30, 2014).

75. Rai KR, Sawitsky A, Cronkite EP, et al. Clinical staging of chronic lymphocytic leukemia. *Blood* 1975;**46**:219–34.

76. Surveillance, Epidemiology, and End Results Program (SEER) Fast Stats 2014. National Cancer Institute. Available at: http://seer.cancer.gov/faststats/selections.php (accessed July 30, 2014).

77. Mauro FR, Foa R, Cerretti R, et al. Autoimmune hemolytic anemia in chronic lymphocytic leukemia: clinical, therapeutic, and prognostic features. *Blood* 2000;**95**:2786–92.

78. Diehl LF, Ketchum LH. Autoimmune disease and chronic lymphocytic leukemia: autoimmune hemolytic anemia, pure red cell aplasia, and autoimmune thrombocytopenia. *Semin Oncol* 1998;**25**:80–97.

79. Byrd JC, Furman RR, Coutre SE, et al. Targeting BTK with ibrutinib in relapsed chronic lymphocytic leukemia. *N Engl J Med* 2013;**369**:32–42.

80. Surveillance, Epidemiology, and End Results Program (SEER) Cancer Statistics Reviews (CSR) 1975–2011. National Cancer Institute. Available at: http://seer.cancer.gov/csr/1975_2011 (accessed July 30, 2014).

81. Sorror ML, Sandmaier BM, Storer BE, et al. Long-term outcomes among older patients following nonmyeloablative conditioning and allogeneic hematopoietic cell transplantation for advanced hematologic malignancies. *JAMA* 2011;**306**:1874–83.

82. Ania BJ, Suman VJ, Sobell JL, et al. Trends in the incidence of polycythemia vera among Olmsted County, Minnesota residents, 1935–1989. *Am J Hematol* 1994;**47**:89–93.

83. Baxter EJ, Scott LM, Campbell PJ, et al. Acquired mutation of the tyrosine kinase JAK2 in human myeloproliferative disorders. *Lancet* 2005;**365**:1054–61.

84. Marchioli R, Finazzi G, Specchia G, et al. Cardiovascular events and intensity of treatment in polycythemia vera. *N Engl J Med* 2013;**368**:22–33.

85. Landolfi R, Marchioli R, Kutti J, et al. Efficacy and safety of low-dose aspirin in polycythemia vera. *N Engl J Med* 2004;**350**:114–24.

86. Passamonti F. How I treat polycythemia vera. *Blood* 2012;**120**:275–84.

87. Mesa RA, Silverstein MN, Jacobsen SJ, et al. Population-based incidence and survival figures in essential thrombocythemia and agnogenic myeloid metaplasia: an Olmsted County Study, 1976–1995. *Am J Hematol* 1999;**61**:10–15.

88. Beer PA, Erber WN, Campbell PJ, Green AR. How I treat essential thrombocythemia. *Blood* 2011;**117**:1472–82.

89. Cortelazzo S, Finazzi G, Ruggeri M, et al. Hydroxyurea for patients with essential thrombocythemia and a high risk of thrombosis. *N Engl J Med* 1995;**332**:1132–6.

90. Harrison CN, Campbell PJ, Buck G, et al. Hydroxyurea compared with anagrelide in high-risk essential thrombocythemia. *N Engl J Med* 2005;**353**:33–45.

91. Gisslinger H, Gotic M, Holowiecki J, et al. Anagrelide compared with hydroxyurea in WHO-classified essential thrombocythemia: the ANAHYDRET Study, a randomized controlled trial. *Blood* 2013;**121**:1720–8.

92. Harrison C, Kiladjian JJ, Al-Ali HK, et al. JAK inhibition with ruxolitinib versus best available therapy for myelofibrosis. *N Engl J Med* 2012;**366**:787–98.

93. Verstovsek S, Mesa RA, Gotlib J, et al. A double-blind, placebo-controlled trial of ruxolitinib for myelofibrosis. *N Engl J Med* 2012;**366**:799–807.

Chapter

38 Cancer in the elderly

Caroline Mariano, MD, FRCPC, and Hyman Muss, MD

Introduction

Cancer represents one of the most common clinical problems encountered in the everyday care of older adults. Cancer is currently the second leading cause of death in North America. Currently about 50% of cancer diagnoses occur in patients over 65, but this number is expected to increase to 70% by 2030. This increase is driven in part by the shifting demographics, increasing life expectancy, and improved mortality from cardiovascular disease.[1]

The association of cancer with aging also has biologic foundations. The cellular and genetic changes that occur in cancer development parallel those associated with the aging process. Accumulation of genetic instability, telomere shortening, and epigenetic alterations all contribute to cancer risk. Chronic inflammation is also increasingly understood as an important contributor to cancer risk in the elderly.[2]

The aging cancer population as impact across the treatment spectrum from screening decisions, multimodality treatment options, survivorship, and end-of-life care. The older patients are increasing recognized as victims of health-care disparities during each stage of care.

The management in the older adult cancer population is further compounded by the rapidly evolving treatment landscape in oncology. Treatment is becoming increasingly complex, involving newer technologies in surgery and radiation and novel targeted chemotherapeutic options. Although many of these treatments have improved toxicity profiles, they are inevitably more costly. In the United States, the cost of cancer care is expected to increase from $125 billion in 2010 to $158 billion in 2020.[3] Thus, value in cancer care is becoming an important focus moving forward and is one of the major priorities of the American Society of Clinical Oncology (ASCO).

This chapter will review the approach to the principles of geriatric oncology and how these are applied in the most commonly encountered tumor types. Principles of supportive care in the older cancer patients will also be discussed.

Principles of geriatric oncology

Life expectancy, geriatric assessment, and defining goals of treatment

Older cancer patients are different than younger cancer patients as they frequently have other comorbid illnesses that compete with cancer as a cause for mortality. Frequently the effect on survival of comorbid illness far exceeds the risk of dying of cancer. The goals of treatment of older cancer patients also differ from their younger counterparts; older patients with serious illness are much less likely to accept treatment that would result in loss of independence or cognition.[4] When evaluating the older cancer patient, the first issue to address is life expectancy exclusive of the cancer diagnosis. Life expectancy varies greatly among older patients of similar age and must be factored in to any treatment decision. A series of user-friendly models are available on the Internet (www.eprognosis.org) that can estimate life expectancy in a variety of settings based on clinical and geriatric assessment parameters. An example using two patients of similar age but with markedly different clinical and geriatric assessment variables shows the value of up to one of these models in predicting survival (Table 38.1).

A formal comprehensive geriatric assessment (CGA) is time-consuming and frequently not readily

---

Reichel's Care of the Elderly, 7th Edition, ed. Jan Busby-Whitehead *et al.* Published by Cambridge University Press.
© Cambridge University Press 2016.

Table 38.1 Five- and ten-year all-cause mortality risk for two male patients (one well and one sick) using the combined Schonberg-Lee calculator

Variable	Well	Sick
Age	75–79 years	75–79 years
Gender	Male	Male
BMI	≥ 25	<25
Patient's self-reported health	Good	Fair
Chronic lung disease	No	Yes
Prior cancer	No	No
Congestive heart failure	No	No
Diabetes or high blood sugar	No	No
Describe cigarette use	Former smoker	Current smoker
Difficulty walking a 1/4 mile without help	No	Yes
Overnight hospitalization in last 12 months	No	One
Help in routine daily activities	No	No
Memory problems interfering with managing finances	No	No
Memory problem interfering with bathing or showering	No	No
Difficulty pushing or pulling large objects	No	Yes
Risk of 5-year mortality	**23%**	**69%**
Risk of 10-year mortality	**34%–43%**	**93%**

Source: Modified from www.eprognosis.org.

available. To help overcome this barrier, several screening instruments have been developed that identify vulnerable or frail patients who should be referred for formal geriatric assessment.[5,6] To further expedite cancer management in older patients, care providers are probably best advised to learn how to do a geriatric assessment using minimal resources. Brief geriatric assessment tools that include evaluation of activities of daily living (washing, dressing, etc.), instrumental activities of daily living (such as using the telephone, shopping, etc.), falls, psychosocial status – including anxiety and depression, social support, nutritional status, and medication use – have been developed for use in the oncology setting and have been shown to be feasible in academic and community settings.[7–9] In addition, a detailed list of comorbid illnesses and their effects on function is obtained. This brief geriatric assessment requires

only about 10 minutes of professional time and 20–30 minutes for patients to complete the other scales; in geriatric oncology programs about 25% of patients need assistance with this.[9] Such a brief geriatric assessment can identify problems that when addressed can be improved by prudently utilizing proven interventions (e.g., identifying a fall and then referring the patient for evaluation and management). Multiple studies have shown that geriatric assessment (GA) variables combined with clinical information can predict severe chemotherapy toxicity in elders,[10–12] and that these measures are superior to standard assessment of performance status.[10] Furthermore, GA variables, particularly physical function, have been shown to be predictive of mortality in older cancer patients.[13] Studies are ongoing to evaluate if GA directed interventions can improve outcomes.

After estimating life expectancy and completing a geriatric assessment, the goals and options of cancer treatment can be better defined. For patients with potentially curable cancers who have long estimated life expectancy but whose cancers are likely to recur or need immediate treatment, standard therapies would be considered. The goal here would be to cure or improve the chances of cure. When cure is not an option, the goals of therapy are palliation of symptoms (if any) and control of the cancer for as long as possible. Depending on the results of the geriatric assessment and the potential effects of cancer treatment on function, optimal treatment decisions can be offered. Final decision making should be patient-centered, with the patient's (and his or her family's, if appropriate) choice taking precedent. The goals of treatment for older patients with serious illness may be markedly different from younger patients with the same stage and extent of cancer. One classic study of older patients noted that approximately 75% of patients would decline therapy that improved their survival if it resulted in severe functional impairment, and almost 90% would decline if it affected their cognitive function.[4]

Clinical trials

In spite of the fact that older patients represent the majority of those with cancer, they are woefully underrepresented in clinical trials.[14, 15] Although there is now an expanding literature on outcomes for older patients with cancer treated with surgery, radiation therapy, and chemotherapy, the poor accrual of older patients to newer large phase III practice-changing trials limits the generalizability of these results for optimizing care in older patients. Older cancer patients who have life expectancies exceeding five years and who are fit should be offered participation in state-of-the-art clinical trials. Although there are several well-defined barriers to trial participation among older patients, an inherent age bias among oncologists is probably the major reason for not offering older patients clinical trial involvement;[16] when offered, older and younger patients have similar participation rates.[16] A paucity of trials exists for patents with poor performance status and/or frailty. Specific trials need to be devised for these groups as findings from mainstream phase III trials are not generalizable to this population. In addition, different endpoints may be more relevant for older patients than standard outcome variable such as response rates, progression-free status, and overall survival. Such trials might focus on the effects of treatment on function, quality of life, and other endpoints that are of major concern for elders.

Breast cancer

Epidemiology

Breast cancer is the second most commonly diagnosed cancer in the world, and the most common cancer in women. In 2012, 1.67 million breast cancers were diagnosed. The highest rates are in North America and Western Europe, with age standardized incidence rates of 85 per 100,000.[17] The average age of breast cancer diagnosis is 61, and 41% of breast cancers are diagnosed in women over 65.[18]

Risk factors

A number of risk factors have been identified for breast cancer and are summarized in Table 38.2. Traditional reproductive factors are less relevant in

Table 38.2 Risk factors for breast cancer in women aged >65 [19])

	Approximate relative risk increase
Nonmodifiable risk factors	
Age >70 vs. <30	18
White vs. black race	1.04
Hereditary breast cancer mutation (*BRCA1/2*)	3–7
First-degree relative with breast cancer	1.2–1.6
Factors related to estrogen	
Nulliparity	1.1–1.3
Early menopause, late menarche	1.1–1.7
Use of hormone replacement therapy	1.2–1.4
Lifestyle/environmental factors	
High body mass index	1.4–1.8
Alcohol: >3 drinks per day	1.5
Radiation to chest under age 30	3–8

539

older women, as increasing age becomes the dominant risk factor for developing new cancers.[19] Although 1 in 28 women aged 40–59 will be diagnosed with breast cancer, that number increases to 1 in 15 for women over the age of 70.[18]

It is common for older women to have a family history of breast cancer; however, a specific mutation is identified in only a small number of patients. Higher number and lower age at diagnosis of relatives confers higher risk. About 5%–6% of breast cancers are caused by inherited germ-line mutations in genes such as *BRCA1* and *BRCA2*. Although cancers owing to these mutations are typically diagnosed at a younger age, the risk in carriers is lifelong.[20] The Gail prediction model (available online) is a useful tool that incorporates many of these factors, but it is less reliable in older women.[21]

The relationship of hormone replacement therapy (HRT) to breast cancer risk has been clearly established. Longer duration of HRT use, higher dose, and use of combination estrogen-progestin products are associated with the highest risk. [22] In postmenopausal women, increased body mass index (BMI) is associated with an increased risk of breast cancer.[23] Conversely physical activity has been shown to lower the risk by as much as 25%.[24] Alcohol increases the risk of breast cancer in a dose-dependent manner, whereas cigarette smoking confers only a modest increase in risk.[25] Exposure to radiation, such as in treatment for Hodgkin's lymphoma, increases breast cancer risk, particularly when the exposure is at a young age.[26, 27]

Characteristics of breast cancers in older women

Breast cancers in older women are more likely to be estrogen receptor (ER) positive, progesterone receptor positive, human epidermal growth factor receptor 2 (HER-2) negative, and of lower grade compared to younger women. These factors are typically associated with a less aggressive phenotype. However, older women are more likely to present with larger tumors and tumors that have spread to regional lymph nodes. These observations are partially explained by later presentation and detection, although older women tend to develop axillary lymph node spread with relative small primary tumors.[28]

Screening and prevention

The use of screening mammography in older women is extremely controversial. Only one major screening trial included women aged 70–74 and failed to show a statistically significant improvement in breast cancer mortality in the screened group. Mammographic false positive rates decrease with increasing age.[29] However, for women with decreasing life expectancy, the number needed to screen to prevent a breast cancer death increases exponentially. Modeling studies suggest that extending mammography to include women between 70 and 80 years of age may prevent between one and four breast cancer–related deaths per 1,000 women screened. There was no difference in effect between annual and biannual screening.[19]

Currently the US Preventive Services Task Force (USPSTF) recommends mammography every two years for women aged 50–74.[29] The American Geriatric Society (AGS) recommends continued screening every one to two years for women up to age 85 who have five or more years of remaining life expectancy.[30] A reasonable approach is for women 75 and older with estimated survival greater than 5–10 years to discuss the pros and cons of mammography with their primary care physician and that a recommendation be made on an individual basis.

For postmenopausal women with a high risk of breast cancer, chemoprevention has been shown to decrease new cases of breast cancer by as much as 50%. Tamoxifen, raloxifene, examestane, and anastrazole have all proven effective in randomized controlled trials. However, the modest impact on mortality and potential adverse effects have prevented widespread use.[31, 32] Thus, chemopreventive strategies should only be offered for very high-risk women with long life expectancy.

Clinical presentation and diagnosis

The vast majority of breast cancer patients will present as a result of screening or with a palpable mass. A breast mass in an older woman is more likely to be malignant than in a younger woman. Although additional imaging with targeted mammography, magnetic resonance imaging (MRI), or ultrasound may be helpful, core needle biopsy is the optimal method to establish the diagnosis. About 5%–10% of women in developed countries will present with metastatic disease at the time of their initial diagnosis. Common sites of metastases include bone, lung, liver, and brain.

Table 38.3 Breast cancer staging and prognosis [62]

T stage		N stage	
Tis	Carcinoma in situ (DCIS or LCIS)	N0	No lymph node (LN) involvement
T1	Tumor ≤ 2 cm	N1mic	Micrometastatases to axillary LN 0.2 mm to 2 mm
T2	Tumor 2 cm–5 cm	N1	Metastases in 1–3 axillary LN
T3	Tumor ≥ 5 cm	N2	Metastases in 4–9 axillary LN
T4	Tumor involves chest wall or skin, inflammatory breast cancer	N3	Metastases ≥ 10 axillary LN, infraclavicular or supraclavicular LN
M stage			
M1	Any distant metastases		
Stage grouping		**5-year relative survival**	
Stage 0	TisN0	100%	
Stage 1	T1N0, T1N1mic	100%	
Stage 2	T2N0, T3N0, T2N1, T1N1	93%	
Stage 3	T3N1, T4 any N, any T N2, any T N3	72%	
Stage 4	any T, any N M1	22%	

Staging

Breast cancer is staged using the TNM, which describes the primary tumor, affected lymph nodes, and distant metastasis (Table 38.3). For most women newly diagnosed with breast cancer, extensive staging investigations are not required. All women should have a detailed history and physical examination (with careful assessment of breast, skin, and lymph nodes), bilateral mammography, CBC, liver function tests, and alkaline phosphatase (ALP). For women with locally advanced disease, imaging of the chest and liver and a bone scan are recommended.[33]

Prognosis

Overall the prognosis for breast cancer is excellent, with close to 90% of patients alive five years after diagnosis (Table 38.3).[34] When assessing prognosis for elderly patients, competing causes of mortality must also be considered. Several online tools have been developed to help assess the relative benefit of various treatment strategies. Adjuvant! Online® allows users to enter breast cancer stage, grade, and hormone status as well as an estimate of comorbidities relative

to age.[35] Adjuvant! Online then estimates the benefit of various treatment modalities. Predict UK is a similar tool that allows users to enter more information about the breast cancer and estimates 5- and 10-year survival.[28]

Management

Early stage disease
Ductal carcinoma in situ

Ductal carcinoma in situ (DCIS) is a precursor to invasive ductal carcinoma. DCIS is most commonly treated with breast-conserving surgery (BCS) and radiation. There is little data about management of older women with DCIS. Older women with DCIS are less likely to have recurrence and more likely to die of non–breast cancer causes compared to younger women.[36] Therefore, many women, particularly those with small amounts of low-grade disease, can be adequately treated with surgery alone. In women with ER positive disease, adjuvant therapy with tamoxifen can reduce the risk of ipsilateral and contralateral DCIS and breast cancer, although absolute survival benefit is minimal.

Local therapy: surgery and radiation

The standard of care for early stage operable breast cancer is mastectomy or BCS followed by radiation therapy. For clinically node negative patients, axillary lymph node dissection (ALND) has largely been replaced by less invasive sentinel lymph node biopsy (SLNB). However, the optimal management of the axilla is controversial – particularly in older women with early stage disease – and axillary dissection is not warranted in all patients with positive SLNB.

Both BCS and mastectomy have very low operative mortality rates, with morbidity and mortality driven by the presence of comorbidities and not age. For women with limited life expectancy (i.e., less than five years) or extreme surgical risk or women who refuse surgery, treatment with primary endocrine therapy for women with hormone-receptor positive tumors is an option that can provide disease control.[37]

Radiation therapy to the breast after BCS is generally safe and well tolerated in older women. Several trials have questioned the benefit of radiation in older women with low risk hormone-receptor positive tumors. The CALGB 9343 trial randomized women aged 70 and older with stage 1, ER positive breast cancer treated with BCS plus tamoxifen versus tamoxifen plus radiation. In long-term follow-up, patients treated with radiation had a 2% risk of local-regional recurrence compared to 10% in those treated with tamoxifen alone; however, there was no difference in survival.[38] A similar trial in the United Kingdom showed that treatment with radiation improved the risk of ipsilateral breast cancer recurrence (4.1% vs 1.3%), but other outcomes were similar.[39]

Systemic adjuvant therapy

Systemic adjuvant treatment with endocrine therapy, chemotherapy, or both is frequently recommended in addition to surgery in potentially curable patients to lower the risk of recurrence and improve survival. Endocrine therapy is the mainstay of therapy in women with hormone-receptor positive tumors. The addition of chemotherapy is appropriate for some older women with hormone-receptor positive tumors, and many older women with hormone-receptor negative or HER-2 positive tumors.[40]

Endocrine therapy

Adjuvant endocrine therapy has been consistently shown to improve outcomes in women with ER positive breast cancers regardless of age. Tamoxifen has been used for this purpose for decades. Although generally well tolerated, it carries a small risk of endometrial carcinoma (less than 2% over 10 years of use) and venous thromboembolic disease, and has drug interactions with some selective serotonin reupdate inhibitors (SSRIs). In postmenopausal women, aromatase inhibitors (examestane, letrozole, and anastrazole) have shown improvement in disease-free survival compared to tamoxifen alone. However, aromatase inhibitors carry a risk of arthralgias and loss of bone density. Some studies have also suggested increased cardiovascular events with these agents.[41]

Careful discussion, assessment of cancer recurrence risk, life expectancy, and comorbidities are necessary when selecting endocrine therapy in older women. All women treated with aromatase inhibitors should be counseled about bone health and bone density and closely monitored. Endocrine therapy is recommended for at least five years after diagnosis, but recent data suggest that longer durations of tamoxifen may lead to lower risks of relapse.[41, 42]

Chemotherapy and targeted therapy

Adjuvant chemotherapy has been shown to improve survival in women with high-risk breast cancer. The most effective regimens are multiagent, including an anthracycline and a taxane, but they are also the most toxic.[43] Although fear of toxicity in older women is widespread, the decision to offer chemotherapy should not be based on age. The pivotal CALGB 49907 study randomized women over 65 to capecitabine versus multiagent chemotherapy and found that women randomized to the capecitabine arm had inferior overall survival.[44] Trastuzumab in combination with chemotherapy dramatically improves outcomes for HER-2 positive breast cancer patients, and the effect appears independent of age.[45]

Both anthracyclines and trastuzumab are associated with a small risk of heart failure. Older age and preexisting heart disease increases this risk.[46] For women at high risk for heart failure, anthracyclines may be omitted in favor of taxane-based regimens. All women treated with trastuzumab require a baseline cardiac evaluation and routine monitoring during treatment. "Chemo brain" is a common concern among breast cancer patients. Although data has been mixed, patients may experience cognitive changes with chemotherapy that persist in long-term follow-up, and this is an active area of ongoing research.[47, 48]

Locally advanced disease

Women who present with locally advanced or inoperable cancer require careful multidisciplinary evaluation. The best outcomes are achieved using neoadjuvant systemic therapy, surgery, and radiation. However, this approach may not be feasible in frail elderly patients. Neoadjuvant endocrine therapy for those with ER positive tumors may be effective in this situation as would primary radiation therapy.[49]

Metastatic disease

The median overall survival for metastatic breast cancer is two to three years; however, the course is extremely variable among patients. For all women, previous therapy, comorbid disease, functional status, and goals of care must be considered when making treatment decisions.[40]

For women with ER positive disease, hormonal therapy can provide disease control with minimal toxicity for months to years. In patients with ER negative or organ-threatening disease, chemotherapy including anthracyclines, taxanes, vinca alkyloids, and capecitabine can be used. Typically sequential single agents are used to minimize toxicity. Trastuzumab and other anti-HER-2 therapies are also extremely effective in women with HER-2 positive metastatic disease. For women with bone metastases, bisphosphonates and denosumab prevent skeletal related events including hypercalcemia and bony pain.

Survivorship

After curative treatment, breast cancer survivors should be followed with regular history, physical examination, and mammography. Monitoring for recurrence with blood work, tumor markers, and other imaging studies is not recommended.[50] Women should be encouraged to participate in regular physical activity, maintain a healthy weight, and consume a diet low in fat. There is evidence that these lifestyle interventions improve treatment related side effects and may decrease risk of recurrence.[24, 51, 52]

Prostate cancer

Epidemiology

Prostate cancer is the fourth most common cancer globally, with an estimated 1.1 million cases diagnosed in 2012.[17] Incidence rates vary widely across regions depending on the use of prostate specific antigen (PSA) testing. In North America, it is the most common cancer diagnosed in men, with an age standardized incidence rate of 97 per 100,000, and it is the second leading cause of male cancer–related deaths.[17]

Prostate cancer is a disease of older men. In autopsy series, up to 73% of men over 80 have prostate cancer.[53] The average age at diagnosis in the United States is 66 years old, and 70% of prostate cancer deaths occur in men aged 75 and older.[18]

Risk factors

African Americans have higher prostate cancer incidence, lower age at diagnosis, and more aggressive disease compared to Caucasians, findings that are independent of socioeconomic factors.[54] Having a first-degree relative with the disease doubles baseline risk. *BRCA2* carriers have a fourfold increase in prostate cancer risk, and the role of other genes is being investigated.[55]

Cigarette smoking has a minor impact on development of prostate cancer, but worsens outcomes after diagnosis.[56] Some studies have found that lycopene (found in tomatoes) and soy products decrease the risk of prostate cancer.[57] Unfortunately results have not been conclusive.

Screening and prevention

PSA is a glycoprotein produced exclusively by prostate epithelial cells. It can be elevated in benign and malignant conditions. Unfortunately, its use as a screening test has been plagued by lead-time bias and length-time bias (Figure 38.1).

The two largest PSA screening trials, enrolling more than 200,000 men, have now reported long-term outcomes with conflicting results. The European trial found a decrease in prostate cancer mortality of 20% in the screened group aged 55–59 with a number needed to invite to screen of 1,055.[58] In the American trial, which used a combination of PSA screening and digital rectal exam (DRE), no difference in prostate cancer mortality was found. However, 52% of patients in the control group received at least one PSA test.[59]

Neither trial enrolled men aged 75 and older, and most consensus groups do not endorse PSA screening in this age group. However, PSA testing remains common practice in the United States, even among patients with limited life expectancy.[60, 61] In our opinion, the potential harms, including complications from biopsy

543

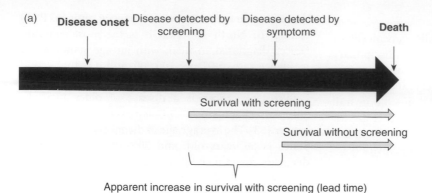

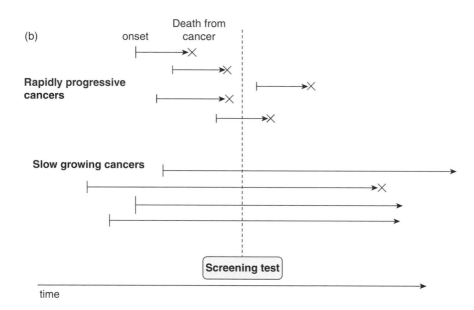

Figure 38.1 Lead-time and length-time bias. (A) Lead-time bias: early detection of slow growing cancers artificially increases cancer-specific survival. (B) Length-time bias: a screening test performed at one point in time in a population is more likely to detect indolent, slow growing cancers compared to quickly growing cancers.

and long-term side effects from unnecessary prostate cancer treatment, outweigh any potential benefits of PSA screening in patients 70 and older.

Clinical presentation and diagnosis

Most men presenting with prostate cancer are asymptomatic. Urinary symptoms are more likely to be caused by concurrent benign prostatic hyperplasia (BPH). Finding cancer tissue in transurethral prostate resection (TUPR) specimens is another common presentation; 5%–10% of patients present with metastatic disease. Prostate cancer usually spreads to regional lymph nodes, bladder, bone, and lung.

Staging

Workup for prostate cancer should include history, physical examination, DRE, and PSA. Abnormal PSA

or DRE are typically followed up with transrectal ultrasound guided biopsy. Although prostate cancer can be staged using the TNM system,[62] a more useful classification creates prognostic groups based on PSA, Gleason score, and T stage (Table 38.4). Additional staging with bone scan and computed tomography (CT) scan of the pelvis is only necessary for patients with intermediate or higher risk disease.

Prognosis

Overall the prognosis for prostate cancer is excellent, with a relative 10-year survival of 99%.[34] Men over 70 tend to present with more aggressive cancers and have worse survival.[63] Long-term side effects from prostate cancer treatment are also more common in older patients.[64, 65] The challenge is to identify patients who are likely to die from prostate cancer rather than other causes. Assessment of tumor biology and geriatric assessment is helpful in this regard.

Management

Localized disease

For patients with early prostate cancer, a number of treatment options are available, which can be daunting for both clinicians and patients (Table 38.5). Few head-to-head trials exist to compare strategies.

Watchful waiting

In watchful waiting patients are treated with palliative therapy only if their disease becomes symptomatic.

This is a strategy typically reserved for patients with limited life expectancy who are not felt to be candidates for curative treatment.

Active surveillance

Active surveillance is an increasingly utilized option in patients with low risk prostate cancer. It involves a fixed schedule of PSA monitoring and prostate biopsies. Cancer is treated if there is clear evidence of progression. About half of patients end up receiving treatment, and outcomes do not appear to be compromised by the delay in treatment.[66]

Radical prostatectomy

Radical prostatectomy (RP) involves removal of all prostate tissue and seminal vesicles. Open, laparoscopic and robotic techniques have similar rates of complications. Surgeon experience most consistently predicts rate of surgical complications and cancer recurrence.[67] Impotence is the most common side effect; rates vary depending on preoperative sexual function and tumor location. Urinary incontinence is common postoperatively, but most patients recover within two years.

Radiation therapy

External beam radiation therapy (EBRT) delivers a therapeutic dose of radiation to the prostate bed,

Table 38.4 Prognostic grouping for prostate cancer [33]

Risk group	PSA	Gleason score	Stage
Low risk	<10	≤6	T1, T2a
Intermediate risk	10–20	7	T2b, T2c
High risk	≥20	8–10	T3a
Very high risk	Any	Any	T3b, T4
Metastatic	Any	Any	N1 or M1

Table 38.5 Strategies to treat localized prostate cancer

Strategy	Patient selection	Advantages	Disadvantages
Watchful waiting	Frail; limited life expectancy	Avoids treatment in patients likely to die from noncancer causes	Risk of undertreating elderly patients
Active surveillance	Low risk disease Educated about disease process	Spares treatment for many patients	Risk of biopsy-related complications Anxiety of living with cancer
Radical prostatectomy	Acceptable surgical risk; tumor not fixed to surrounding tissue	Excellent long-term cancer control Bowel dysfunction rare	Surgical risks Impotence common
Radiation therapy	Able to lie flat and tolerate daily treatments	Excellent long-term cancer control No operative risk Can treat disease beyond prostate bed	Gastrointestinal side effects High symptom burden during treatment Impotence common
Brachytherapy	Low or intermediate risk Prostate volume <50 cc Able to tolerate anesthesia	Excellent long-term cancer control Single treatment	Risk of long-term urinary dysfunction Impotence common

typically given in daily fractions over six weeks. Fields can be extended to cover extra-prostatic disease. Sexual dysfunction is a common side effect, but rates are generally lower compared to RP.[68, 69] About 50% of patients will experience urinary symptoms during treatment, but most resolve. Radiation proctitis occurs in about 20% of men, with a small risk of long-term gastrointestinal side effects.

Brachytherapy

In brachytherapy, a radioactive source is implanted into the prostate to deliver a high dose of radiation directly to the tumor. With appropriate patient selection and operator experience, it offers similar cancer control outcomes to EBRT and RP.[64] Sexual dysfunction is common, again with rates lower than surgery. Gastrointestinal side effects are less common than with EBRT, but about 15% of patients report urinary dysfunction in long-term follow-up.[68, 69]

Advanced or recurrent prostate cancer

Advanced prostate cancer is a heterogeneous disease. Many patients have only biochemical evidence of cancer, detected by rising PSA after curative treatment, and will die from other causes. Other patients have diffusely metastatic disease leading to a high burden of morbidity and mortality.

Hormone sensitive disease

The first-line treatment of advanced prostate cancer is androgen deprivation therapy (ADT), most commonly accomplished with gonadotropin-releasing hormone agonists. Long-term ADT is associated with loss of libido, fatigue, decreased bone mineral density, decreased muscle mass, reduced insulin sensitivity, increased cholesterol, and subtle changes in cognition. [70] The PR7 trial compared intermittent versus continuous ADT in patients with biochemical recurrence only. Overall survival was similar between arms, but intermittent therapy was associated with lower costs and a small improvement in quality of life (QOL). Only 45% of deaths in the trial were due to prostate cancer. A similar trial in men with documented metastatic disease also showed some improvement in QOL with intermittent ADT, but median overall survival was shorter (5.1 years versus 5.8 years).[71, 72]

Castrate resistant prostate cancer

When patients fail ADT, anti-androgens such as bicalutamide can provide disease stabilization, but patients eventually progress to a hormone resistant state.

Until 2011, docetaxel was the only drug shown to improve survival in castrate resistant prostate cancer (CRPC). With the development of newer agents, the median overall survival is now more than two years. Docetaxel has been consistently shown to benefit older men, and fit elderly patients were represented in clinical trials of most novel agents (Table 38.6).[73] Since many of these therapies are less toxic than traditional chemotherapy, a wider spectrum of patients can be offered treatment.[74] These therapies are also being actively investigated in earlier stage disease. Because of the rapidly changing therapeutic landscape, patients with reasonable functional status should be referred to a medical oncologist for a discussion about their options.

Colorectal cancer

Epidemiology

Colorectal cancer (CRC) is the fourth most common cancer worldwide. It is the third most common cause of cancer-related deaths in the United States,[18] with 70% of deaths occurring in patients over 70.[75] In North America, the age standardized incidence rate is 30 per 100,000.[17] The average age at diagnosis is 69.

Risk factors

A number of risk factors for CRC have been identified. Age remains the most common risk factor, with incidence increasing in each decade of life.[18] Rates are about 25% higher in men versus women. African Americans have higher rates of CRC, lower age at diagnosis, and higher mortality rates – for reasons that are unclear.

A personal history of polyps, particularly large adenomatous polyps with tubulovillous or villous histology, increases CRC risk by 3.5–6.5 times. A family history of CRC or high-risk polyps will also increase risk.[76] Hereditary CRC syndromes such as Lynch syndrome, account for about 5%–10% of cases and cancers usually diagnosed in younger patients. Inflammatory bowel disease, particularly ulcerative colitis, greatly increases CRC risk.

Obesity and moderate alcohol use both confer a 1.5-fold increase in CRC risk.[77] Diabetes also increases the risk of CRC, independent of lifestyle factors.

Table 38.6 Agents used in treatment of advanced CRPC

Drug	Mechanism of action	Elderly patients in registration trial	Benefits/advantages	Side effects/disadvantages
Docetaxel	Taxane-type chemotherapy	20% age $\geq$75	Improved survival by 2.4 months Improved QOL	Fatigue, neuropathy, myelosuppression
Abiraterone	Oral androgen biosynthesis inhibitor	28% age $\geq$75	Improved survival by 4.8 months Well tolerated, improved QOL	Fluid retention, hypokalemia
Enzalutamide	Oral anti-androgen	25% age $\geq$75	Improved survival by 4.8 months Well tolerated, improved QOL	Seizures (rarely), fatigue, hot flashes
Radium-223	Alpha-emitting radiopharmaceutical targeting bone	Median age 71	Improved survival by 3.6 months Decreased pain, QOL	Mild diarrhea, thrombocytopenia
Cabazitaxel	Taxane-type chemotherapy	9% age $\geq$75; max age 80	Improved survival by 2.4 months	Neutropenia common; 6% treatment-related deaths in elderly
Sipileucel -T	Immunotherapy	73% age $\geq$65	Improved survival by 4.1 months	Infusion reactions; very costly

Source: Adapted from reference 74.

Physical activity decreases the risk of CRC by up to 27%.[78] The links to diet are less clear, but lower consumption of red meat and a high consumption of fruit and fiber have been shown to be protective in some studies.

Screening and prevention

CRC screening recommendations have evolved considerably, and differ between major consensus groups.[79, 80] Most screening tests have not been extensively validated in the elderly. Because of lag time and the long natural history of CRC, models suggest that it takes 10 years for patients to ultimately derive benefit from CRC screening.[81] Therefore, fit older patients may benefit from screening, if life expectancy is greater than 10 years.[82]

Both the endoscopic screening and stool-based tests are used for CRC screening. Sensitive fecal occult blood testing (FOBT) annually or biennially decreases CRC mortality by 15%–25%.[83] Fecal immunochemical-based testing (FIT) offers improved sensitivity and specificity compared to guaiac-based FOBT. Endoscopic screening offers both diagnostic and therapeutic opportunities. Flexible sigmoidoscopy every five years or colonoscopy every 10 years are both options. Although colonoscopy has the advantage of evaluating the whole colon, older patients are more likely to suffer from complications of colonoscopy.[84, 85]

We recommend that clinicians offer CRC screening to patients aged 50–75, either with FIT testing (or FOBT if not available) yearly or endoscopic screening, if estimated life expectancy is greater than 10 years. For patients older than 75 with a long life expectancy, the decision to screen must be individualized.[81, 86]

Meta-analysis of chemoprevention trials have shown that aspirin use is associated with 6%–7% absolute decrease in the risk of developing CRC or adenomas. However, this must be weighed against potential adverse events and does not replace screening.[87]

547

Table 38.7 Colorectal cancer staging and prognosis

T stage		N stage	
Tis	In situ: intraepithelial or invasion of lamina propria	N0	No lymph node (LN) involvement
T1	invades submucosa	N1	Metastases in 1–3 regional LN
T2	invades muscularis propria	N2	Metastases in ≥ 4 regional LN
T3	invades through muscularis propria		
T4	Tumor penetrates visceral peritoneum or adherent to other organs		
M stage			
M1	Distant metastases		
Staging group		**5-year relative survival**	
Stage 1	T1-2 N0	90%	
Stage 2	T3-4 N0	70%	
Stage 3	Any T, N1 or N2	36%	
Stage 4	Any T, any N, M1	20%	

Source: Information from references 18, 62.

Clinical presentation

Only about 30% of CRCs are diagnosed through screening in North America. Common presenting symptoms include iron deficiency anemia, change in bowel habits, abdominal, and weight loss; 5%–10% of patients will present with an acute obstruction. Patients with rectal cancers are more likely to present with hematochezia, tenesmus, and pain, a small percentage will be palpated on DRE.[88] In symptomatic patients, the next step should be referral for colonoscopy. Using screening tests such as FOBT is not appropriate for diagnostic evaluation.

About 20% of patients in developed countries will present with metastatic disease. Common sites of CRC spread are intra-abdominal lymph nodes, liver, lung, and peritoneum.

Staging

CRC is staged using the TNM system (Table 38.7). All patients with suspected CRC should have a complete colonoscopy and biopsy of suspicious lesions. Rectal cancers are defined as tumors arising below the peritoneal reflection, which is usually 12 cm–15 cm from the anal verge.

Preoperatively all patients with CRC stage 2 and above should have a CT scan of the abdomen and pelvis, CBC, and carcinoembryonic antigen (CEA) level. The role of chest imaging is controversial as it often picks up indeterminate lesions, particularly in older patients. A PET scanning offers increased sensitivity but is less reliable in lesions under 1 cm, and should not be routinely preformed.[33]

Surgical planning for rectal cancers is more complicated, so additional local-regional staging including pelvic MRI and endorectal ultrasound is often required.

Prognosis

Overall, the five-year relative survival for CRC is 65% (Table 38.7). In early stage disease, other factors such as grade, genetic features of the tumor, and comorbidities are important determinants of outcome. Adjuvant! Online* is a useful web-based tool that allows users to enter cancer stage and grade as well as an estimate of comorbidities.[89] The benefit of various treatment modalities can then be estimated.

Management

Stage 1–3 (early stage) disease

Local therapy: surgery and radiation

The goal of oncologic surgery is complete removal of the tumor and regional lymph nodes, typically with partial colectomy. Although operative mortality is low, frail elderly patients have a higher risk. A preoperative geriatric assessment is helpful to counsel patients and optimize comorbid conditions. Unfortunately elderly patients remain undertreated and are more likely to undergo noncurative or emergency surgery.[85]

Local management of rectal cancer is complex and requires multidisciplinary evaluation. The surgical procedure of choice is a total mesorectal excision (TME). In cancers stage T3 and above, the addition of pelvic radiation (often with concurrent chemotherapy) improves outcomes.

In frail elderly patients with symptomatic CRC, surgical consultation is still warranted as minimally invasive procedures can sometimes be performed to relieve bleeding or obstruction.

Adjuvant chemotherapy

The use of adjuvant 5-flurouracil (5-FU) based chemotherapy is well tolerated, and this treatment has been shown to decrease recurrence rates and improve survival from colon cancer for several decades (Table 38.8). However, the use of adjuvant chemotherapy in rectal cancer is less well established.

The vast majority of stage 2 colon cancers are cured with surgery alone, and adjuvant chemotherapy provides little benefit. However, in selected patients with high-risk disease, it may be considered.[90]

For stage 3 colon cancer, the standard of care is six months of adjuvant chemotherapy with a combination of 5-FU/leucovorin and oxaliplatin (FOLFOX). The relative risk reduction of cancer relapse with the use of 5-FU alone is 35% compared with placebo. In a landmark clinical trial, the addition of oxaliplatin in stage 3 colon cancer improved overall survival at five years to 73% compared to 69% with 5-FU alone.[91] There is ongoing debate about the benefit of oxaliplatin in older patients. In subgroup analyses of two randomized control trials, patients older than 70 did not derive any benefit from oxaliplatin.[92] However, in large cohort analyses, older patients have similar outcomes to younger patients treated with FOLFOX.[93] Neuropathy occurs in 90% of patients during treatment with oxaliplatin and persists at one year in about one-third of patients. This can ultimately result in functional limitations in elderly persons.[94]

Regardless, older patients as a group remain undertreated with adjuvant chemotherapy.[94]

Table 38.8 Chemotherapy agents used in treatment of colorectal cancer

Agent	Mechanism of action	Common toxicities
Infusional 5-FU	Cytotoxic antimetabolite	Diarrhea, mucositis
Capecitabine	Oral 5-FU derivative, renally cleared	Hand-foot syndrome, diarrhea
Oxaliplatin	Cytotoxic platinum derivative	Neuropathy, myelosuppression
Irinotecan	Cytotoxic DNA topoisomerase inhibitor	Diarrhea, myelosuppression
Cetuximab	Monoclonal antibody against epidermal growth factor receptor	Infusion reactions, rash, hypomagnisemia
Panitumumab		
Bevacizumab	Monoclonal antibody targeting vascular endothelial growth factor (VEGF)	Hypertension, proteinuria, impaired wound healing; rare arterial thromboembolism but higher risk in elderly
Aflibercept	Decoy VEGF receptor	Hypertension, proteinuria, venous and arterial thrombosis
Regorafenib	Tyrosine kinase inhibitor with multiple targets	>50% of risk of grade 3–4 toxicity; rash, diarrhea, fatigue

Table 38.9 NSCLC cancer staging per 2010 update [18, 62]

T stage		N stage	
T1	Tumor ≤3 cm	N0	No lymph node (LN) involvement
T2a	Tumor 3 cm–5 cm	N1	Ipsilateral peribronchial, intrapulmonary or hilar LN
T2b	Tumor 5 cm–7 cm		
T3	Tumor >7 cm *or* invading chest wall, diaphragm, mediastinal pleura, main bronchus, parietal pericardium, phrenic nerve. Atelectasis, tumor nodule in same lobe.	N2	Ipsilateral mediastinal or subcarinal LN
N3	Contralateral *or* supraclavicular LN		
T4	Invasion of surrounding organs, great vessels or mediastinum. Separate nodules in different ipsilateral lobe.		
M stage			
M1a	Malignant effusion, contralateral nodule		
M1b	Distant metastases		
Stage grouping		**Approximate 5-year survival**	
Stage 1	T1-2a N0	45–50%	
Stage 2	T1-2N1, T2b-T3N0	30%	
Stage 3	Any T4, any N2-N3, T3N1	5–14%	
Stage 4	Any T, any N, M1	1%	

Treatment decisions should be based on life expectancy, tumor biology, functional statu and patient preference, not age alone.[75]

Follow-up

For the first five years after curative treatment, patients should be routinely followed with clinical evaluation, colonoscopy, CEA levels, and imaging of the liver and chest. This allows for early detection of recurrent disease, which could be amenable to resection. For patients who would not be candidates for further surgery or chemotherapy, active surveillance should not be pursued.[95]

Stage 4 (advanced stage) disease

The median survival of advanced CRC is approximately two years, and many patients maintain good QOL.

A subset of patients with isolated liver or lung metastases may be cured with surgical resection or high-dose radiation therapy to the metastatic site. Careful multidisciplinary evaluation is necessary to plan and sequence treatment. Surgical approaches can also be helpful in palliation of symptoms such as obstruction or bleeding in advanced disease.

Chemotherapy remains the mainstay of treatment for most patients with metastatic CRC. Several targeted biologic agents have been developed that improve outcomes (Table 38.9). Typically agents are used sequentially with 5-FU remaining the backbone. Chemotherapy "breaks" can be used safely to preserve QOL and lesson toxicity.[96] Frail older patients may also benefit from dose modifications to avoid serious toxicity.[97] Unfortunately older patients have been underrepresented in metastatic CRC trials, but the existing evidence suggests that fit older patients derive similar benefit as their younger counterparts.[75]

Lung cancer

Epidemiology

Lung cancer is the most common cancer diagnosed worldwide with 1.8 million new cases in 2012.[17] It is also the leading cause of cancer-related deaths. In developed countries, overall rates are decreasing; lung cancer is more common in men, but rates in women are increasing. In the United States, the average age of lung cancer diagnosis is 70;[18] 85% of lung cancer cases are classified as non-small cell lung cancer (NSCLC), which can be further subdivided into subtypes including adenocarcinoma, squamous cell carcinoma, and large cell carcinoma. Small cell lung cancer (SCLC) accounts for the majority of remaining cases.

Risk factors

Tobacco accounts for 90% of lung cancer cases and will increase lung cancer risk 10–30 times depending on amount of exposure. Overall heavy smokers (at least one pack per day) have a 30% lifetime risk of lung cancer.[98] Exposure to second-hand smoke will also increase risk, with a relative risk increase of 1.2.[99]

Other risk factors include therapeutic thoracic radiation for other malignancies and exposure to toxins including arsenic, nickel, and radon. Air pollution likely contributes to 1%–2% of lung cancer cases.[100] Patients with chronic lung disease – including chronic obstructive pulmonary disease (COPD), pulmonary fibrosis, and tuberculosis – carry an increased risk for cancer; the effect appears to be mediated by inflammation.[100]

Interestingly a chemoprevention trial of beta-carotene found that supplementation increased lung cancer rates.[101] The role of genetic factors in lung cancer predisposition is poorly understood, but research is ongoing.

Screening and prevention

The best and most cost-effective preventive measure for lung cancer is smoking cessation. In North America, approximately 9% of people aged 65 and older are current smokers.[99] Worldwide, tobacco use continues to increase, particularly in developing countries, where there are fewer limits on advertising and lower rates of taxation on tobacco products.[102] Smoking cessation will gradually decrease lung cancer risk over 15 years, which then plateaus at approximately two times baseline risk. Even in patients diagnosed with lung cancer, smoking cessation improves mortality.[103]

For many years screening for lung cancer was not thought to be effective, until the publication of the National Lung Cancer Screening Trial (NLST). This trial enrolled 53,000 people aged 55–74 at high risk for lung cancer. Patients were deemed at high risk if they had at least a 30-pack year history of smoking, were current smokers, or had quit within 15 years. Participants were randomized to low-dose CT chest versus chest x-ray annually for three years. The study found a 20% decrease in lung cancer mortality in the CT scanned group, with a number needed to screen of 320. In the CT group, 24% of patients had an abnormal result, 96% of which were false positives. Biopsies were performed in high volume expert centers, and the risk of complications was 4.5 per 10,000 people screened.[104] In addition 25% of surgeries performed were for lesions that were benign. More recently models have been developed to predict probability of cancer in nodules identified on CT screening.[105]

Several organizations, including the US Preventive Services Task Force (USPSTF), have recommended screening for patients who fit NLST criteria.[106] We recommend that lung cancer screening be discussed with these high-risk patients who have a life expectancy greater than five years and would be able to tolerate lung cancer treatment. Patients who elect to be screened should be referred to a center with expertise in interpretation and evaluation of lung nodules. Smokers should be counseled about cessation, regardless of age or comorbidities.

Clinical presentation

Many patients with early lung cancer are asymptomatic. Local symptoms can include cough, hemoptysis, chest pain, and dyspnea.[107] More than 50% of patients will present with advanced lung cancer; metastases to liver, bone, brain, and adrenal glands are most common. Weight loss at presentation is associated with adverse prognosis. A variety of paraneoplastic phenomena are associated with lung cancer. Hypercalcemia and hypertrophic osteoarthopathy are commonly associated with NCLCL. Small cell lung cancer is associated with SIADH (syndrome of inappropriate antidiuretic hormone) and a variety of neurologic and endocrine paraneoplastic syndromes.

Staging and diagnosis

NSCLC is staged using the TNM system, updated in 2010 (Table 38.9). Clinically SCLC is divided into limited stage disease, cancer limited to the lung that can be encompassed in one radiation port, and extensive stage disease.

All patients with suspected lung cancer should have a detailed history and physical examination. Initial imaging should include a CT scan of the chest and upper abdomen. This can usually identify a site for biopsy. A core biopsy, rather than FNA, should be obtained whenever possible. Brain imaging should be performed in all patients with SCLC, and patients with stage 3 or 4 NSCLC.[33]

Patients with potentially resectable NSCLC should be referred for multidisciplinary evaluation. Further staging investigations include positron emission tomography (PET) scan, mediastinal lymph node evaluation (either with endobronchial ultrasound or mediastinoscopy), and full pulmonary function tests.[108]

Management of non-small cell lung cancer

Early stage

Surgery is the standard of care in patients with stage 1 and 2 NSCLC and offers the potential for cure in 60%–70% of patients. Careful preoperative assessment is crucial, including mediastinal staging and detailed assessment of lung function and functional capacity. Fit patients should be considered for partial or complete pnemonectomy, depending on tumor location. For patients not eligible for surgery, treatment with stereotactic radiation therapy is another potentially curative modality.[109, 110]

In patients with stage 2 and some patients with stage 1B NSCLC, the addition of four cycles of cisplatin-based adjuvant chemotherapy has been shown to improve five-year overall survival by up to 15%.[111] Subset analyses of clinical trials showed that although older patients often received lower doses or fewer cycles of chemotherapy, they still derived survival benefit, without compromising long-term QOL.[112]

Locally advanced

The management of locally advanced lung cancer is complex, and practices vary widely between centers. In general, multimodality therapy including surgery, radiation, and chemotherapy offers the best outcomes. Unfortunately, few elderly patients were enrolled in clinical trials for stage 3 lung cancer. The existing evidence suggests that fit older patients still benefit from aggressive therapy, but they may be at higher risk for pneumonitis, myelosuppression, and cardiac complications.[113, 114]

Metastatic NCLC

The outcomes for advanced NSCLC are poor with a median overall survival of 6–12 months. The mainstay of treatment for most patients is platin-based chemotherapy. In large reviews, treatment with chemotherapy offers improvement in both survival and QOL.[115] Several trials have now proven that patients older than 70 also benefit from chemotherapy.[116, 117] The addition of bevacizumab, an anti-angiogenesis agent, to chemotherapy improves outcomes in some patients, but it is associated with a higher rate of serious toxicities in older people.[118]

Fortunately, recent advances have allowed for identification of "driver mutations" in some NSCLC patients. One example is the epidermal growth factor receptor (EGFR) mutation, which occurs in about 15% of patients with adenocarcinoma. In these patients, treatment with oral tyrosine kinase inhibitors targeting EGFR has proven more effective and far less toxic compared to cytotoxic chemotherapy.[119] Similarly a small percentage of adenocarcinoma patients will have anaplastic lymphoma kinase (ALK) fusion oncogene driver mutation, which can be effectively treated with oral therapy. Therefore even elderly patients who refuse chemotherapy should be referred to medical oncology to discuss other therapeutic options.

Patients with metastatic lung cancer often have a high symptom burden. Many interventions are available to address symptoms including radiation therapy and indwelling pleural catheters. In a pivotal study, early referral to specialist palliative care was shown to improve both QOL and survival in patients with stage 4 NSCLC, despite lower utilization of chemotherapy in the intervention group.[120]

Management of SCLC

SCLC is a very aggressive disease, with a tumor doubling time of approximately 60 days. Standard treatment of limited stage disease is a concurrent radiation and platin-based chemotherapy. This offers a response rate of 80%–90%, but only 10%–15% of patients will ultimately be cured.[121]

The mainstay of treatment for extensive stage disease is platinum-based chemotherapy. With treatment, the median survival is approximately 9 months. As in NSCLC, elderly patients are often undertreated, but evidence suggests that they derive similar benefits to their younger counterparts. Patients with limited stage SCLC and extensive stage SCLC without brain metastases have improved survival when treated with prophylactic cranial radiation. The benefit is consistent in older patients;[122] however, whole brain irradiation is associated with neurocognitive side effects, which may have a more significant impact in the frail elderly.[123]

Principles of symptom management and palliative care in cancer patients

Systems of care

Palliative care is a discipline that includes principles of medicine, nursing, and other allied health professions to care for patients with serious illness. Palliative care focuses on symptom control, optimization of function, and clear communication about goals of care. These skills are necessary in the everyday care of cancer patients by all providers. Specialty palliative care teams are available in many centers and can address complex patient needs. Specialty palliative care does not preclude use of cancer-directed or potentially life-prolonging treatment. In the oncology population, integration of palliative care has been consistently shown to improve QOL and reduce health-care costs. Furthermore one study showed improved survival in lung cancer patients referred for early palliative care.[120, 124]

Hospice is also an interdisciplinary model, but it focuses specifically on maximizing QOL in the face of terminal illness. In the United States, hospice is a comprehensive care system funded by Medicare and Medicaid. Eligibility includes an estimated life expectancy of less than six months and selection of a treatment plan with comfort as the primary focus.[125]

Symptom management of geriatric oncology

Pain

Assessment

Cancer-related pain remains a common problem among elderly cancer patients, and advanced age is associated with undertreatment. Assessment of pain can be challenging, particularly when a patient presents with cognitive impairment and multiple comorbidities. Most older patients, even those with moderate severity dementia, can self-report the presence and severity of pain. For patients with more severe cognitive impairment, providers can use nonverbal pain cues. Validated scales have been developed such as the Checklist of Nonverbal Pain Indicators, which includes vocal complaints, facial grimaces, bracing, restlessness, and rubbing.[126] The Pain Assessment in Advanced Dementia Scale (PAINAD) is a similar scale which is specific for patients with advanced dementia.[127] Neuropathic pain differs from nociceptive pain and often described as burning or shock like, and can be associated with paresthesias. All patients should also be assessed for depression, which can impact perception and management of pain.

Treatment

Nonpharmacologic interventions can be effective in lowering pain scores. Patient and caregiver education about pain is crucial, and models have shown that collaborative care can improve pain outcomes. Cognitive behavioral therapy has been shown to be an effective adjunct for cancer-related pain, although it has not been studied specifically in the geriatric oncology population.[128] Exercise is effective in management of several pain syndromes. In the oncology setting, regular exercise can prevent or decrease arthalgias in breast cancer patients treated with aromatase inhibitors.[129]

Many pharmacologic therapies can be used in management of cancer-related pain (Table 38.10). Opioids are often underutilized in the geriatric population due to concerns of toxicity and addiction. However, when initiated at low doses with slow titration, they are usually well tolerated. All opioids cause constipation and should be prescribed with a bowel regimen. Combination analgesics such as oxycodone-acetaminophen (Percocet®) can decrease pill burden, but difficulty in titration limits their use in the oncology setting. Multiple agents have been promoted to treat neuropathic pain, including anticonvulsants and antidepressants. However, the majority of evidence for these agents is in noncancer patients.

The goal of therapy should be reducing pain severity while preserving functional status and minimizing adverse effects. This can be achieved in the majority of older cancer patients. Those with persistent pain or

Table 38.10 Pharmacologic agents used in cancer-related pain [30]

Medication	Advantages/uses	Considerations in the elderly
Nonopioids		
Acetaminophen	Well tolerated; wide spectrum of use	Reduce dose if severe hepatic impairment
NSAIDs	Useful in bone pain, inflammatory lesions	Use with caution: risk of renal impairment, delirium, cardiac toxicity
Opioids		
Tramadol	Mixed opioid and central neurotransmitter effect; may help neuropathic pain	Lowers seizure threshold; caution with seritonergic agents
Morphine	Multiple preparations; inexpensive	Active metabolites; caution in renal failure
Hydromorphone	Fewer active metabolites; high potency	Caution in renal failure, liver failure
Oxycodone	Few toxic metabolites	Only oral formulation; caution in liver failure
Fentanyl	Transdermal; safe in renal failure	Lowest dose patch (12 mcg) equivalent to ~50 mg morphine/24 h, peak effect in 18–24 h; caution in liver failure; variable absorption if patient is malnourished
Methadone	Inexpensive; safe in renal failure; effective in neuropathic pain	Requires experienced prescriber; complex pharmacokinetics; prolongs QTc; caution in liver failure
Other adjuvant agents		
Gabapentin/pregabalin	Modest effect in neuropathic pain	Can cause sedation; titrate slowly
Serotonin–norepinephrine reuptake inhibitors (duloxetine, venlafaxine)	Effective in painful chemotherapy induced neuropathy, treatment of depression; some effect in neuropathic pain	Monitor cognitive effects; drug interactions; withdrawal effects
Tricyclic antidepressants	Used in neuropathic pain	Avoid in elderly due to anticholinergic effects
Bisphosphonates	Prevent pain from bony metastases	Caution in renal failure; risk of osteonecrosis
Glucocorticoids	Wide spectrum of use; anti-inflammatory;safe in renal failure	Use with caution: risk of delirium, hyperglycemia, multiple long-term complications

unmanageable side effects should be referred to a palliative care or pain specialist.

Nausea and vomiting

Chemotherapy-induced nausea and vomiting (CINV) is a common concern among cancer patients. Interestingly the risk of CINV is lower in older patients, but the same treatment strategies should be employed across age groups. A combination of pharmacologic therapy remains the mainstay for both

treatment and prevention of CINV (Table 38.11); different strategies can be employed for acute (within 24 hours) or delayed emesis.[130] These regimens are extremely effective in preventing vomiting, but nausea can be a more difficult problem.

In the absence of emetogenic chemotherapy nausea and vomiting is often multifactorial. Patients should be assessed for medication side effects, constipation, hypercalcemia, and CNS metastases. If pharmacologic therapy is warranted, agents that target

Table 38.11 Pharmacologic agents used in management of CINV

Class	Utility	Considerations in the elderly
NKI receptor antagonists (aprepitant, fosaprepitant)	Prevents acute and delayed CINV for moderate-highly emetogenic regimens; may be steroid sparing	Drug interactions common
5HT-3 antagonists (ondansentron)	Prevents acute CINV; some effect in delayed CINV	Causes constipation; QTc prolongation
Dexamethasone	Prevents acute and delayed CINV; enhances effect of 5HT-3 antagonists	Multiple side effects; avoid chronic use
D2 antagonists (prochlorperazine metoclopramide)	Uses PRN for acute and delayed emesis	QT prolongation; risk of extrapyramidal symptoms with prolonged use

dopaminergic pathways such as metoclopramide, prochlorperazine, and haloperidol are effective. Ondansetron is the agent of choice in radiation-therapy induced nausea and vomiting.[131]

Bowel dysfunction

Up to 80% of older cancer patients experience constipation. It contributes to nausea, delirium, and pain, particularly in frail elders.[132] Again the causes are multifactorial and it can be related to medications (particularly opioids), disease burden, bowel obstruction, and dietary changes. Nonpharmacologic measures including increasing fluid, increasing mobility, and increasing fiber intake can sometimes be helpful. All patients with persistent constipation should be prescribed a regular laxative. Both stimulant type and osmotic laxatives are effective. Polyethylene glycol-based products (PEG, Miralax*) are often the best tolerated in older patients. Stool softeners are not recommended in the palliative care population due to lack of effect.[133, 131, 130, 123] Methylnaltrexone is a peripheral opioid antagonist, administered subcutaneously, that is effective in relief of severe constipation associated with opioids.[131]

Diarrhea in an older cancer patient requires careful evaluation, particularly to assess for infection, degree of dehydration, and the possibility of overflow diarrhea. Patients with new onset fecal incontinence should be evaluated for spinal cord compression. Underlying causes should be treated and volume status optimized. If diarrhea remains a problem, particularly when associated with chemotherapy, loperamide can be prescribed.[131]

Neuropathy

Neuropathy is a common side effect of multiple chemotherapeutic agents including platinums, vinca alkyloids, taxanes, and bortezemib. The most common syndrome is a peripheral sensory neuropathy, characterized by anesthesia and dysesthesia, which can sometimes be painful. Age does not appear to be a risk factor for chemotherapy-induced neuropathy (CIN); however, neuropathy will have a more profound functional impact in frail elderly patients and those with underlying neurologic or motor problems.

After treatment, CIN can be very slow to improve, and some patients are left with permanent deficits. For this reason, clinicians must carefully evaluate patients during treatment and make appropriate dose adjustments. There are no effective agents to improve neuropathy once it has developed. Duloxetine is the only agent shown in a randomized control trial to improve pain related to CIN.[134]

Dyspnea

Dyspnea is a common symptom at the end of life and can have a significant impact on QOL and function. All patients should have an evaluation and appropriate diagnostic testing to evaluate underlying causes such as heart failure, pulmonary emboli, COPD, pleural effusions, infection, and so on. Objective measures such as oxygen saturation and respiratory rate may not correlate with the subjective sensation of dyspnea. Oxygen provides symptomatic improvement for hypoxic patients with dyspnea, but not for those with nonhypoxic causes. A fan directed to the face may provide relief in patients with normal saturation.[135]

555

Opioids are a mainstay of pharmacologic therapy for dyspnea. Their effectiveness has been shown in multiple clinical trials, many of which included older patients.[136] Morphine is the most well studied agent and can be effective at low doses. In older patients, caution should be taken to manage potential side effects. Treatment with opioids in the palliative care setting rarely causes respiratory depression and is not associated with increased or hastened mortality.[137] Treatment with low-dose, rapid-acting benzodiazepines such as lorazepam can also be effective, particularly when an anxiety component of the symptoms exists.

Cancer-related fatigue

Fatigue is a common symptom throughout the spectrum of illness. In older persons, this is compounded by age-related decreases in muscle strength and sarcopenia. No single strategy has been proven to alleviate cancer-related fatigue; therefore, clinicians should first focus on assessment and management of contributing factors. Clinicians should evaluate for anemia, depression, sleep disturbance, endocrine dysfunction, electrolyte imbalances, and nutritional deficiencies. [131] Management of concurrent symptoms such as pain, constipation, and nausea will often improve fatigue. Nearly all cancer therapies are associated with fatigue. It is not clear whether age increases this risk. When treatment-related fatigue consistently interferes with function or QOL, dose modification or treatment breaks should be considered.

For patients during and after curative cancer treatment, an exercise program can help restore energy, sleep patterns, physical function, and QOL. In advanced disease, incorporation of moderate physical activity can also be beneficial. Occasionally a trial of psychostimulants, steroids, or megastrol can be useful, but these strategies have not been specifically evaluated in the older patients and all carry significant risk of adverse reactions.

Conclusions

The management of cancer in the older patient remains a challenge, which has been complicated by gaps in education and resource availability. There is a major gap in geriatric knowledge and training among oncologists; likewise, primary care physicians, including geriatricians, are unaware of the potential benefits of modern cancer treatments. Coupled with the projected shortage of oncologists and geriatricians in the years to come, this lack of training in geriatrics will further compound the challenges for a health-care system currently in crisis.[138] Education of cancer care providers is a pressing need and is currently being addressed by many organizations. Ideally, such training in geriatrics should begin in medical school, continue throughout residency, and be part of maintenance of certification. Outstanding resources exist to train practitioners about key issues related to the care of older patients and several are listed in Table 38.12.

Geriatric oncology is a rapidly growing field, and new research will undoubtedly lead to more rational assessment and management of older cancer patients. We believe that interdisciplinary care and education are the keys to better outcomes in this population.

Key references

Geriatric assessment

- Puts, et al. An update on a systematic review of the use of geriatric assessment for older adults in oncology. *Annals of Oncology* 2013;25(2):1–9.
- Hurria, et al. Predicting Chemotherapy Toxicity in Older Adults with Cancer: A Prospective Multicenter Study. *J Clin Oncol* 2011;29:3457–3465.

Breast cancer

- Biganzoli, et al. Management of elderly patients with breast cancer: updated recommendations of the International Society of Geriatric Oncology (SIOG) and European Society of Breast Cancer Specialists (EUSOMA). *Lancet Oncology* 2012;13:e148–e160.
- Walter and Schonberg. Screening mammography in older women: a review. *JAMA* 2014;311 (13):1336–1347.

Prostate cancer

- Resnick, et al. Long-term functional outcomes after treatment for localized prostate cancer. *N Engl J Med* 2013;368:436–445.
- Mukherji, et al. New treatment developments applied to elderly patients with advanced prostate cancer. *Cancer Treatment Reviews* 2013;39:578–583.

Table 38.12 Internet resources helpful in the management of older cancer patients

Name	Description
ASCO University http://university.asco.org/geriatric-oncology	Online modules that explore different care options for older patients with various malignancies. Also has Maintenance of Certification (MOC) module on geriatric oncology.
International Society of Geriatric Oncology (SIOG) www.siog.org	Website provides useful links to geriatric oncology guidelines and other educational materials.
Adjuvant! (adjvuvantonline.com) www.adjuvantonline.com/index.jsp	Calculate benefits of adjuvant therapy for patients with colon, lung, and breast cancer. Effect of comorbidity on treatment benefit can be calculated.
ePrognosis http://eprognosis.ucsf.edu/default.php	A series of calculators for estimation of life expectancy based on studies of older adults in different health-care settings. Includes smartphone application which can be applied to screening decisions.
CARG (Cancer and Aging Research Group) www.mycarg.org	A group of researchers with major interest in geriatric oncology research. Opportunities for mentoring. Also online chemotherapy toxicity calculator and geriatric assessment tools.
Moffitt Cancer Center Senior Adult Oncology Program Tools http://moffitt.org/cancer-types–treatment/cancers-we-treat/senior-adult-oncology-program-tools	The CRASH score – online tool for estimating the toxicity of chemotherapy. Site also has other geriatric calculators.
Lineberger Comprehensive Cancer Center Geriatric Oncology http://unclineberger.org/geriatric	Free PowerPoint slide sets of core lectures in geriatrics as well as other resources.

Colorectal cancer

- McCleary, et al. Refining the chemotherapy approach for older patients with colon cancer. *J Clin Oncol*. 2014 Aug 20;32(24):2570–2580
- Papamichael, et al. Treatment of the elderly colorectal cancer patient: SIOG expert recommendations. *Ann Oncol* 2009;20(1):5–16.
- Day, et al. Colorectal cancer screening and surveillance in the elderly patient. *Am J Gastroenterol* 2011;106(7):1197–1206.

Lung cancer

- Gajra and Jatoi. Non–small-cell lung cancer in elderly patients: a discussion of treatment options. *J Clin Oncol*. 2014 Aug 20;32(24):2562–2569.
- Meoni, et al. Medical treatment of advanced non-small cell lung cancer in elderly patients: a review of the role of chemotherapy and targeted agents. *J Geriatr Oncol* 2013 l;4:282–290.

Symptom management

- Naeim, et al. Supportive care considerations for older adults with cancer. *J Clin Oncol*. 2014 Aug 20;32(24):2627–2634.
- Cancer Care Ontario: www.cancercare.on.ca/toolbox/symptools. Evidence based symptom management guidelines available online and algorithms or as a smartphone application.

References

1. Shih YC, Hurria A. Preparing for an epidemic: cancer care in an aging population. *Am Soc Clin Oncol Educ Book* 2014;**34**:133–137.
2. Lopez-Otin C, Blasco MA, Partridge L, et al. The hallmarks of aging. *Cell* 2013 Jun 6;**153**(6):1194–1217.
3. Mariotto AB, Yabroff KR, Shao Y, et al. Projections of the cost of cancer care in the United States: 2010–2020. *J Natl Cancer Inst* 2011 Jan 19;**103**(2):117–128.
4. Fried TR, Bradley EH, Towle VR, Allore H. Understanding the treatment preferences of seriously ill patients. *N Engl J Med* 2002 Apr 4;**346**(14):1061–1066.

5. Ramsdale E, Polite B, Hemmerich J, et al. The Vulnerable Elders Survey-13 predicts mortality in older adults with later-stage colorectal cancer receiving chemotherapy: a prospective pilot study. *J Am Geriatr Soc* 2013 Nov;**61**(11):2043–2044.

6. Min LC, Elliott MN, Wenger NS, Saliba D. Higher vulnerable elders survey scores predict death and functional decline in vulnerable older people. *J Am Geriatr Soc* 2006 Mar;**54**(3):507–511.

7. Hurria A, Cirrincione CT, Muss HB, et al. Implementing a geriatric assessment in cooperative group clinical cancer trials: CALGB 360401. *J Clin Oncol* 2011 Apr 1;**29**(10):1290–1296.

8. Hurria A, Gupta S, Zauderer M, et al. Developing a cancer-specific geriatric assessment: a feasibility study. *Cancer* 2005 Nov 1;**104**(9):1998–2005.

9. Williams GR, Deal AM, Jolly TA, et al. Feasibility of geriatric assessment in community oncology clinics. *J Geriatr Oncol* 2014 Jul;**5**(3):245–251.

10. Hurria A, Togawa K, Mohile SG, et al. Predicting chemotherapy toxicity in older adults with cancer: a prospective multicenter study. *J Clin Oncol* 2011 Sep 1;**29**(25):3457–3465.

11. Extermann M, Boler I, Reich RR, et al. Predicting the risk of chemotherapy toxicity in older patients: the Chemotherapy Risk Assessment Scale for High-Age Patients (CRASH) score. *Cancer* 2012 Jul 1;**118**(13):3377–3386.

12. Puts MT, Santos B, Hardt J, et al. An update on a systematic review of the use of geriatric assessment for older adults in oncology. *Ann Oncol* 2014 Feb;**25**(2):307–315.

13. Soubeyran P, Fonck M, Blanc-Bisson C, et al. Predictors of early death risk in older patients treated with first-line chemotherapy for cancer. *J Clin Oncol* 2012 May 20;**30**(15):1829–1834.

14. Hutchins LF, Unger JM, Crowley JJ, et al. Underrepresentation of patients 65 years of age or older in cancer-treatment trials. *N Engl J Med* 1999 Dec 30;**341**(27):2061–2067.

15. Sacher AG, Le LW, Leighl NB, Coate LE. Elderly patients with advanced NSCLC in phase III clinical trials: are the elderly excluded from practice-changing trials in advanced NSCLC? *J Thorac Oncol* 2013 Mar;**8**(3):366–368.

16. Kemeny MM, Peterson BL, Kornblith AB, et al. Barriers to clinical trial participation by older women with breast cancer. *J Clin Oncol* 2003 Jun 15;**21**(12):2268–2275.

17. Ferlay J, Soerjomataram I, Ervik M, et al. GLOBOCAN 2012 v1.0, Cancer Incidence and Mortality Worldwide. 2012;11. Available at: http://globocan.iarc.fr (accessed Jan 15, 2014).

18. Howlader N, Noone A, Krapcho M, et al. SEER Cancer Statistics Review, 1975–2010, based on November 2012 SEER data. Available at: http://seer.cancer.gov/csr/19 75_2010 (accessed Jan 15, 2014).

19. Walter LC, Schonberg MA. Screening mammography in older women: a review. *JAMA* 2014 Apr 2;**311** (13):1336–1347.

20. Van der Kolk DM, de Bock GH, Leegte BK, et al. Penetrance of breast cancer, ovarian cancer and contralateral breast cancer in *BRCA1* and *BRCA2* families: high cancer incidence at older age. *Breast Cancer Res Treat* 2010 Dec;**124**(3):643–651.

21. Cummings SR, Lee JS, Lui LY, et al. Sex hormones, risk factors, and risk of estrogen receptor-positive breast cancer in older women: a long-term prospective study. *Cancer Epidemiol Biomarkers Prev* 2005 May;**14** (5):1047–1051.

22. Rossouw JE, Anderson GL, Prentice RL, et al. Risks and benefits of estrogen plus progestin in healthy postmenopausal women: principal results from the Women's Health Initiative randomized controlled trial. *JAMA* 2002 Jul 17;**288**(3):321–333.

23. Van den Brandt PA, Spiegelman D, Yaun SS, et al. Pooled analysis of prospective cohort studies on height, weight, and breast cancer risk. *Am J Epidemiol* 2000 Sep 15;**152**(6):514–527.

24. Lynch B, Neilson H, Friedenreich C. Physical activity and breast cancer prevention. *Recent Results Cancer Res* 2011;**186**:13–42.

25. Chen WY, Rosner B, Hankinson SE, et al. Moderate alcohol consumption during adult life, drinking patterns, and breast cancer risk. *JAMA* 2011 Nov 2;**306**(17):1884–1890.

26. Travis LB, Hill DA, Dores GM, et al. Breast cancer following radiotherapy and chemotherapy among young women with Hodgkin disease. *JAMA* 2003 Jul 23;**290**(4):465–475.

27. Pukkala E, Kesminiene A, Poliakov S, et al. Breast cancer in Belarus and Ukraine after the Chernobyl accident. *Int J Cancer* 2006 Aug 1;**119**(3):651–658.

28. Wishart GC, Bajdik CD, Dicks E, et al. PREDICT Plus: development and validation of a prognostic model for early breast cancer that includes HER2. *Br J Cancer* 2012 Aug 21;**107**(5):800–807.

29. Nelson HD, Tyne K, Naik A, et al. Screening for breast cancer: an update for the US Preventive Services Task Force. *Ann Intern Med* 2009 Nov 17;**151**(10):727–737, W237–W242.

30. Durso S, Sullivan G editors. *Geriatrics Review Syllabus*, 8th ed. New York: American Geriatric Society; 2013.

31. Visvanathan K, Hurley P, Bantug E, et al. Use of pharmacologic interventions for breast cancer risk reduction: American Society of Clinical Oncology

clinical practice guideline. *J Clin Oncol* 2013 Aug 10;**31**(23):2942–2962.

32. Moyer VA, US Preventive Services Task Force. Medications to decrease the risk for breast cancer in women: recommendations from the US Preventive Services Task Force recommendation statement. *Ann Intern Med* 2013 Nov 19;**159**(10):698–708.

33. National Comprehensive Cancer Network (NCCN) guidelines. Available at: www.nccn.org (accessed Nov 1, 2013).

34. Siegel R, Ma J, Zou Z, Jemal A. Cancer statistics, 2014. *CA Cancer J Clin* 2014 Jan;**64**(1):9–29.

35. Ravdin PM, Siminoff LA, Davis GJ, et al. Computer program to assist in making decisions about adjuvant therapy for women with early breast cancer. *J Clin Oncol* 2001 Feb 15;**19**(4):980–991.

36. Kong I, Narod SA, Taylor C, et al. Age at diagnosis predicts local recurrence in women treated with breast-conserving surgery and postoperative radiation therapy for ductal carcinoma in situ: a population-based outcomes analysis. *Curr Oncol* 2014 Feb;**21**(1): e96–e104.

37. Hind D, Wyld L, Beverley CB, Reed MW. Surgery versus primary endocrine therapy for operable primary breast cancer in elderly women (70 years plus). *Cochrane Database Syst Rev* 2006 Jan 25;**1**: CD004272.

38. Hughes KS, Schnaper LA, Bellon JR, et al. Lumpectomy plus tamoxifen with or without irradiation in women age 70 years or older with early breast cancer: long-term follow-up of CALGB 9343. *J Clin Oncol* 2013 Jul 1;**31**(19):2382–2387.

39. The PRIME II trial: Wide local excision and adjuvant hormonal therapy ± postoperative whole breast irradiation in women ≥ 65 years with early breast cancer managed by breast conservation. Abstract S2-01. 36th Annual San Antonio Breast Cancer Symposium; December 2013.

40. Biganzoli L, Wildiers H, Oakman C, et al. Management of elderly patients with breast cancer: updated recommendations of the International Society of Geriatric Oncology (SIOG) and European Society of Breast Cancer Specialists (EUSOMA). *Lancet Oncol* 2012 Apr;**13**(4):e148–e160.

41. Burstein HJ, Prestrud AA, Seidenfeld J, et al. American Society of Clinical Oncology clinical practice guideline: update on adjuvant endocrine therapy for women with hormone receptor-positive breast cancer. *J Clin Oncol* 2010 Aug 10;**28**(23):3784–3796.

42. Davies C, Pan H, Godwin J, et al. Long-term effects of continuing adjuvant tamoxifen to 10 years versus stopping at 5 years after diagnosis of oestrogen receptor-positive breast cancer: ATLAS, a randomised trial. *Lancet* 2013 Mar 9;**381**(9869):805–816.

43. Early Breast Cancer Trialists' Collaborative Group (EBCTCG), Peto R, Davies C, et al. Comparisons between different polychemotherapy regimens for early breast cancer: meta-analyses of long-term outcome among 100,000 women in 123 randomised trials. *Lancet* 2012 Feb 4;**379**(9814):432–444.

44. Muss HB, Woolf S, Berry D, et al. Adjuvant chemotherapy in older and younger women with lymph node-positive breast cancer. *JAMA* 2005 Mar 2;**293**(9):1073–1081.

45. Albanell J, Ciruelos EM, Lluch A, et al. Trastuzumab in small tumours and in elderly women. *Cancer Treat Rev* 2014 Feb;**40**(1):41–47.

46. Chavez-MacGregor M, Zhang N, Buchholz TA, et al. Trastuzumab-related cardiotoxicity among older patients with breast cancer. *J Clin Oncol* 2013 Nov 20;**31**(33):4222–4228.

47. Hutchinson AD, Hosking JR, Kichenadasse G, et al. Objective and subjective cognitive impairment following chemotherapy for cancer: a systematic review. *Cancer Treat Rev* 2012 Nov;**38**(7):926–934.

48. Mandelblatt JS, Jacobsen PB, Ahles T. Cognitive effects of cancer systemic therapy: implications for the care of older patients and survivors. *J Clin Oncol* 2014 Aug 20;**32**(24):2617–2626.

49. Macaskill EJ, Renshaw L, Dixon JM. Neoadjuvant use of hormonal therapy in elderly patients with early or locally advanced hormone receptor-positive breast cancer. *Oncologist* 2006 Nov–Dec;**11**(10).1081–1088.

50. Khatcheressian JL, Hurley P, Bantug E, et al. Breast cancer follow-up and management after primary treatment: American Society of Clinical Oncology clinical practice guideline update. *J Clin Oncol* 2013 Mar 1;**31**(7):961–965.

51. Rock CL, Demark-Wahnefried W. Nutrition and survival after the diagnosis of breast cancer: a review of the evidence. *J Clin Oncol* 2002 Aug 1;**20**(15):3302–3316.

52. Rock CL, Doyle C, Demark-Wahnefried W, et al. Nutrition and physical activity guidelines for cancer survivors. *CA Cancer J Clin* 2012 Jul–Aug;**62**(4):243–274.

53. Delongchamps NB, Singh A, Haas GP. The role of prevalence in the diagnosis of prostate cancer. *Cancer Control* 2006 Jul;**13**(3):158–168.

54. Hoffman RM, Gilliland FD, Eley JW, et al. Racial and ethnic differences in advanced-stage prostate cancer: the Prostate Cancer Outcomes Study. *J Natl Cancer Inst* 2001 Mar 7;**93**(5):388–395.

55. Zheng SL, Sun J, Wiklund F, et al. Cumulative association of five genetic variants with prostate cancer. *N Engl J Med* 2008 Feb 28;**358**(9):910–919.

56. Kenfield SA, Stampfer MJ, Chan JM, Giovannucci E. Smoking and prostate cancer survival and recurrence. *JAMA* 2011 Jun 22;**305**(24):2548–2555.

57. Yan L, Spitznagel EL. Soy consumption and prostate cancer risk in men: a revisit of a meta-analysis. *Am J Clin Nutr* 2009 Apr;**89**(4):1155–1163.

58. Schroder FH, Hugosson J, Roobol MJ, et al. Prostate-cancer mortality at 11 years of follow-up. *N Engl J Med* 2012 Mar 15;**366**(11):981–990.

59. Andriole GL, Crawford ED, Grubb RL 3rd, et al. Prostate cancer screening in the randomized Prostate, Lung, Colorectal, and Ovarian Cancer Screening Trial: mortality results after 13 years of follow-up. *J Natl Cancer Inst* 2012 Jan 18;**104**(2):125–132.

60. Drazer MW, Prasad SM, Huo D, et al. National trends in prostate cancer screening among older American men with limited 9-year life expectancies: evidence of an increased need for shared decision making. *Cancer* 2014 May 15;**120**(10):1491–1498.

61. Moyer VA, US Preventive Services Task Force. Screening for prostate cancer: US Preventive Services Task Force recommendation statement. *Ann Intern Med* 2012 Jul 17;**157**(2):120–134.

62. AJCC (American Joint Committee on Cancer). *Cancer Staging Manual*. 7th ed. New York: Springer-Verlag; 2010.

63. Sun L, Caire AA, Robertson CN, et al. Men older than 70 years have higher risk prostate cancer and poorer survival in the early and late prostate specific antigen eras. *J Urol* 2009 Nov;**182**(5):2242–2248.

64. Keyes M, Crook J, Morton G, et al. Treatment options for localized prostate cancer. *Can Fam Physician* 2013 Dec;**59**(12):1269–1274.

65. Alemozaffar M, Regan MM, Cooperberg MR, et al. Prediction of erectile function following treatment for prostate cancer. *JAMA* 2011 Sep 21;**306**(11):1205–1214.

66. Shappley WV 3rd, Kenfield SA, Kasperzyk JL, et al. Prospective study of determinants and outcomes of deferred treatment or watchful waiting among men with prostate cancer in a nationwide cohort. *J Clin Oncol* 2009 Oct 20;**27**(30):4980–4985.

67. Trinh QD, Bjartell A, Freedland SJ, et al. A systematic review of the volume-outcome relationship for radical prostatectomy. *Eur Urol* 2013 Nov;**64**(5):786–798.

68. Vordermark D. Quality of life and satisfaction with outcome among prostate-cancer survivors. *N Engl J Med* 2008 Jul 10;**359**(2):201; author reply 201–2.

69. Resnick MJ, Koyama T, Fan KH, et al. Long-term functional outcomes after treatment for localized prostate cancer. *N Engl J Med* 2013 Jan 31;**368**(5):436–445.

70. Schulman C, Irani J, Aapro M. Improving the management of patients with prostate cancer receiving long-term androgen deprivation therapy. *BJU Int* 2012 Jun;**109**(Suppl 6):13–21.

71. Hussain M, Tangen CM, Berry DL, et al. Intermittent versus continuous androgen deprivation in prostate cancer. *N Engl J Med* 2013 Apr 4;**368**(14):1314–1325.

72. Crook JM, O'Callaghan CJ, Duncan G, et al. Intermittent androgen suppression for rising PSA level after radiotherapy. *N Engl J Med* 2012 Sep 6;**367**(10):895–903.

73. Italiano A, Ortholan C, Oudard S, et al. Docetaxel-based chemotherapy in elderly patients (age 75 and older) with castration-resistant prostate cancer. *Eur Urol* 2009 Jun;**55**(6):1368–1375.

74. Mukherji D, Pezaro CJ, Shamseddine A, De Bono JS. New treatment developments applied to elderly patients with advanced prostate cancer. *Cancer Treat Rev* 2013 Oct;**39**(6):578–583.

75. Papamichael D, Audisio R, Horiot JC, et al. Treatment of the elderly colorectal cancer patient: SIOG expert recommendations. *Ann Oncol* 2009 Jan;**20**(1):5–16.

76. Atkin WS, Morson BC, Cuzick J. Long-term risk of colorectal cancer after excision of rectosigmoid adenomas. *N Engl J Med* 1992 Mar 5;**326**(10):658–662.

77. Kitahara CM, Berndt SI, de Gonzalez AB, et al. Prospective investigation of body mass index, colorectal adenoma, and colorectal cancer in the prostate, lung, colorectal, and ovarian cancer screening trial. *J Clin Oncol* 2013 Jul 1;**31**(19):2450–2459.

78. Boyle T, Keegel T, Bull F, et al. Physical activity and risks of proximal and distal colon cancers: a systematic review and meta-analysis. *J Natl Cancer Inst* 2012 Oct 17;**104**(20):1548–1561.

79. Rex DK, Johnson DA, Anderson JC, et al. American College of Gastroenterology guidelines for colorectal cancer screening 2009 [corrected]. *Am J Gastroenterol* 2009 Mar;**104**(3):739–750.

80. US Preventive Services Task Force. Screening for colorectal cancer: US Preventive Services Task Force recommendation statement. *Ann Intern Med* 2008 Nov 4;**149**(9):627–637.

81. Lee SJ, Leipzig RM, Walter LC. Incorporating lag time to benefit into prevention decisions for older adults. *JAMA* 2013 Dec 25;**310**(24):2609–2610.

82. Gross CP, Soulos PR, Ross JS, et al. Assessing the impact of screening colonoscopy on mortality in the medicare population. *J Gen Intern Med* 2011 Dec;**26**(12):1441–1449.

83. Hewitson P, Glasziou P, Watson E, et al. Cochrane systematic review of colorectal cancer screening using the fecal occult blood test (hemoccult): an update. *Am J Gastroenterol* 2008 Jun;**103**(6):1541–1549.

84. Lieberman DA, Weiss DG, Bond JH, et al. Use of colonoscopy to screen asymptomatic adults for colorectal cancer. Veterans Affairs Cooperative Study Group 380. *N Engl J Med* 2000 Jul 20;**343**(3):162–168.

560

85. Colorectal Cancer Collaborative Group. Surgery for colorectal cancer in elderly patients: a systematic review. *Lancet* 2000 Sep 16;**356**(9234):968–974.

86. Hoffman RM, Walter LC. Colorectal cancer screening in the elderly: the need for informed decision making. *J Gen Intern Med* 2009 Dec;**24**(12):1336–1337.

87. Rothwell PM, Wilson M, Elwin CE, et al. Long-term effect of aspirin on colorectal cancer incidence and mortality: 20-year follow-up of five randomised trials. *Lancet* 2010 Nov 20;**376**(9754):1741–1750.

88. Majumdar SR, Fletcher RH, Evans AT. How does colorectal cancer present? Symptoms, duration, and clues to location. *Am J Gastroenterol* 1999 Oct;**94** (10):3039–3045.

89. Gill S, Loprinzi C, Kennecke H, et al. Prognostic web-based models for stage II and III colon cancer: A population and clinical trials-based validation of numeracy and adjuvant! online. *Cancer* 2011 Sep 15;**117**(18):4155–4165.

90. Benson AB 3rd, Schrag D, Somerfield MR, et al. American Society of Clinical Oncology recommendations on adjuvant chemotherapy for stage II colon cancer. *J Clin Oncol* 2004 Aug 15;**22**(16):3408–3419.

91. Andre T, Boni C, Mounedji-Boudiaf L, et al. Oxaliplatin, fluorouracil, and leucovorin as adjuvant treatment for colon cancer. *N Engl J Med* 2004 Jun 3;**350**(23):2343–2351.

92. Tournigand C, Andre T, Bonnetain F, et al. Adjuvant therapy with fluorouracil and oxaliplatin in stage II and elderly patients (between ages 70 and 75 years) with colon cancer: subgroup analyses of the Multicenter International Study of Oxaliplatin, Fluorouracil, and Leucovorin in the Adjuvant Treatment of Colon Cancer trial. *J Clin Oncol* 2012 Sep 20;**30**(27):3353–3360.

93. Sanoff HK, Carpenter WR, Martin CF, et al. Comparative effectiveness of oxaliplatin vs non-oxaliplatin-containing adjuvant chemotherapy for stage III colon cancer. *J Natl Cancer Inst* 2012 Feb 8;**104**(3):211–227.

94. Muss HB, Bynum DL. Adjuvant chemotherapy in older patients with stage III colon cancer: an underused lifesaving treatment. *J Clin Oncol* 2012 Jul 20;**30**(21):2576–2578.

95. Meyerhardt JA, Mangu PB, Flynn PJ, et al. Follow-up care, surveillance protocol, and secondary prevention measures for survivors of colorectal cancer: American Society of Clinical Oncology clinical practice guideline endorsement. *J Clin Oncol* 2013 Dec 10;**31**(35):4465–4470.

96. Chibaudel B, Tournigand C, Andre T, de Gramont A. Therapeutic strategy in unresectable metastatic colorectal cancer. *Ther Adv Med Oncol* 2012 Mar;**4**(2):75–89.

97. Seymour MT, Thompson LC, Wasan HS, et al. Chemotherapy options in elderly and frail patients with metastatic colorectal cancer (MRC FOCUS2): an open-label, randomised factorial trial. *Lancet* 2011 May 21;**377**(9779):1749–1759.

98. Samet JM, Wiggins CL, Humble CG, Pathak DR. Cigarette smoking and lung cancer in New Mexico. *Am Rev Respir Dis* 1988 May;**137**(5):1110–1113.

99. Centers for Disease Control and Prevention (CDC). State-specific prevalence of current cigarette smoking among adults, and policies and attitudes about secondhand smoke – United States, 2000. *MMWR Morb Mortal Wkly Rep* 2001 Dec 14;**50**(49):1101–1106.

100. Brenner DR, Boffetta P, Duell EJ, et al. Previous lung diseases and lung cancer risk: a pooled analysis from the International Lung Cancer Consortium. *Am J Epidemiol* 2012 Oct 1;**176**(7):573–585.

101. Omenn GS, Goodman GE, Thornquist MD, et al. Effects of a combination of beta carotene and vitamin A on lung cancer and cardiovascular disease. *N Engl J Med* 1996 May 2;**334**(18):1150–1155.

102. World Health Organization. WHO report on the global tobacco epidemic, 2013: enforcing bans on tobacco advertising, promotion and sponsorship; 2013. Available at: www.who.int/toba cco/global_report/2013/en.

103. Parsons A, Daley A, Begh R, Aveyard P. Influence of smoking cessation after diagnosis of early stage lung cancer on prognosis: systematic review of observational studies with meta-analysis. *BMJ* 2010 Jan 21;**340**:b5569.

104. National Lung Screening Trial Research Team, Aberle DR, Adams AM, et al. Reduced lung-cancer mortality with low-dose computed tomographic screening. *N Engl J Med* 2011 Aug 4;**365**(5):395–409.

105. McWilliams A, Tammemagi MC, Mayo JR, et al. Probability of cancer in pulmonary nodules detected on first screening CT. *N Engl J Med* 2013 Sep 5;**369**(10):910–919.

106. Moyer VA. Screening for Lung Cancer: US Preventive Services Task Force Recommendation Statement. *Ann Intern Med* 2013 Dec 31;**160**(5):330–338.

107. Chute CG, Greenberg ER, Baron J, et al. Presenting conditions of 1539 population-based lung cancer patients by cell type and stage in New Hampshire and Vermont. *Cancer* 1985 Oct 15;**56**(8):2107–2111.

108. Detterbeck FC, Postmus PE, Tanoue LT. The stage classification of lung cancer: *Diagnosis and Management of Lung Cancer, 3rd ed*: American College of Chest Physicians evidence-based clinical practice guidelines. *Chest* 2013 May;**143**(5 Suppl):e191S–210S.

109. Grills IS, Mangona VS, Welsh R, et al. Outcomes after stereotactic lung radiotherapy or wedge resection for

stage I non-small-cell lung cancer. *J Clin Oncol* 2010 Feb 20;**28**(6):928–935.

110. Senthi S, Lagerwaard FJ, Haasbeek CJ, et al. Patterns of disease recurrence after stereotactic ablative radiotherapy for early stage non-small-cell lung cancer: a retrospective analysis. *Lancet Oncol* 2012 Aug;**13**(8):802–809.

111. Butts CA, Ding K, Seymour L, et al. Randomized phase III trial of vinorelbine plus cisplatin compared with observation in completely resected stage IB and II non-small-cell lung cancer: updated survival analysis of JBR-10. *J Clin Oncol* 2010 Jan 1;**28**(1):29–34.

112. Fruh M, Rolland E, Pignon JP, et al. Pooled analysis of the effect of age on adjuvant cisplatin-based chemotherapy for completely resected non-small-cell lung cancer. *J Clin Oncol* 2008 Jul 20;**26**(21):3573–3581.

113. Hardy D, Cormier JN, Xing Y, et al. Chemotherapy-associated toxicity in a large cohort of elderly patients with non-small cell lung cancer. *J Thorac Oncol* 2010 Jan;**5**(1):90–98.

114. Schild SE, Mandrekar SJ, Jatoi A, et al. The value of combined-modality therapy in elderly patients with stage III nonsmall cell lung cancer. *Cancer* 2007 Jul 15;**110**(2):363–368.

115. NSCLC Meta-Analyses Collaborative Group. Chemotherapy in addition to supportive care improves survival in advanced non-small-cell lung cancer: a systematic review and meta-analysis of individual patient data from 16 randomized controlled trials. *J Clin Oncol* 2008 Oct 1;**26**(28):4617–4625.

116. Quoix E, Zalcman G, Oster JP, et al. Carboplatin and weekly paclitaxel doublet chemotherapy compared with monotherapy in elderly patients with advanced non-small-cell lung cancer: IFCT-0501 randomised, phase 3 trial. *Lancet* 2011 Sep 17;**378**(9796):1079–1088.

117. Effects of vinorelbine on quality of life and survival of elderly patients with advanced non-small-cell lung cancer: the Elderly Lung Cancer Vinorelbine Italian Study Group. *J Natl Cancer Inst* 1999 Jan 6;**91**(1):66–72.

118. Ramalingam SS, Dahlberg SE, Langer CJ, et al. Outcomes for elderly, advanced-stage non small-cell lung cancer patients treated with bevacizumab in combination with carboplatin and paclitaxel: analysis of Eastern Cooperative Oncology Group Trial 4599. *J Clin Oncol* 2008 Jan 1;**26**(1):60–65.

119. Mok T, Wu Y, Thongprasert S, et al. Phase III, randomised, open-label, first-line study of gefitinib vs carboplatin/paclitaxel in clinically selected patients with advanced nonsmall-cell lung cancer (IPASS). *Ann Oncol* 2010;**21** (Suppl 8): 1.

120. Temel JS, Greer JA, Muzikansky A, et al. Early palliative care for patients with metastatic non-

small-cell lung cancer. *N Engl J Med* 2010 Aug 19;**363**(8):733–742.

121. Gaspar LE, Gay EG, Crawford J, et al. Limited-stage small-cell lung cancer (stages I–III): observations from the National Cancer Data Base. *Clin Lung Cancer* 2005 May;**6**(6):355–360.

122. Eaton BR, Kim S, Marcus DM, et al. Effect of prophylactic cranial irradiation on survival in elderly patients with limited-stage small cell lung cancer. *Cancer* 2013 Nov 1;**119**(21):3753–3760.

123. Dietrich J, Monje M, Wefel J, Meyers C. Clinical patterns and biological correlates of cognitive dysfunction associated with cancer therapy. *Oncologist* 2008 Dec;**13**(12):1285–1295.

124. Parikh RB, Temel JS. Early specialty palliative care. *N Engl J Med* 2014 Mar 13;**370**(11):1075–1076.

125. Medicare hospice benefits. 2013 August 2013;02154. Available at: www.medicare.gov.

126. Feldt KS. The checklist of nonverbal pain indicators (CNPI). *Pain Manag Nurs* 2000 Mar;**1**(1):13–21.

127. Schuler MS, Becker S, Kaspar R, et al. Psychometric properties of the German "Pain Assessment in Advanced Dementia Scale" (PAINAD-G) in nursing home residents. *J Am Med Dir Assoc* 2007 Jul;**8**(6):388–395.

128. Integration of behavioral and relaxation approaches into the treatment of chronic pain and insomnia: NIH Technology Assessment Panel on Integration of Behavioral and Relaxation Approaches into the Treatment of Chronic Pain and Insomnia. *JAMA* 1996 Jul 24–31;**276**(4):313–318.

129. Randomized trial of exercise vs usual care on aromatase inhibitor-associated arthralgias in women with breast cancer. Abstract S3-03. San Antonio Breast Cancer Symposium 2013; December 2013.

130. Basch E, Prestrud A, Hesketh P, et al. Antiemetics: American Society of Clinical Oncology clinical practice guideline update. *J Clin Oncol* 2011 November 1 2011;**29**(31):4189–4198.

131. Cancer Care Ontario Symptom Assessment and Management Tools. 2014; Available at: www.cancer care.on.ca/toolbox/symptools (accessed on Jan 15, 2014).

132. Barford K, D'Olimpio J. Symptom management in geriatriconcology: practical treatment considerations and current challenges. *Curr Treat Options Oncol* 2008 June 2008;**9**(2):204–214.

133. Librach SL, Bouvette M, De Angelis C, et al. Consensus recommendations for the management of constipation in patients with advanced, progressive illness. *J Pain Symptom Manage* 2010 Nov;**40**(5):761–773.

134. Smith EM, Pang H, Cirrincione C, et al. Effect of duloxetine on pain, function, and quality of life

among patients with chemotherapy-induced painful peripheral neuropathy: a randomized clinical trial. *JAMA* 2013 Apr 3;**309**(13):1359–1367.

135. Galbraith S, Fagan P, Perkins P, et al. Does the use of a handheld fan improve chronic dyspnea? A randomized, controlled, crossover trial. *J Pain Symptom Manage* 2010 May;**39**(5):831–838.

136. Ben-Aharon I, Gafter-Gvili A, Paul M, et al. Interventions for alleviating cancer-related dyspnea: a systematic review. *J Clin Oncol* 2008 May 10;**26**(14):2396–2404.

137. Hallenbeck J. Pathophysiologies of dyspnea explained: why might opioids relieve dyspnea and not hasten death? *J Palliat Med* 2012 Aug;**15**(8):848–853.

138. Hurria A, Naylor M, Cohen HJ. Improving the quality of cancer care in an aging population: recommendations from an IOM report. *JAMA* 2013 Nov 6;**310**(17):1795–1796.

Chapter 39

Eye problems of the aged

Jessica L. Kalender-Rich, MD, Michelle R. Boyce, MD, and Jason A. Sokol, MD

Ocular disorders of aging

The management of ocular health in the rapidly aging US population presents an ever-expanding challenge to primary care providers, geriatricians, and ophthalmologists alike. The United States defines visual impairment as vision with corrective lenses of worse than 20/40 but better than 20/200 in the better seeing eye. Vision worse than 20/200 with corrective lens is the definition of legal blindness.[1] Approximately, 4.1 million Americans are visually impaired, and 1.2 million Americans 40 years and older are legally blind according to the most recent census data.[2] In a population-based study, the rate of visual impairment in individuals 80 years and older was 15–30 times greater than individuals 40–50 years old.[3] In addition, because many eye diseases can be insidious in onset, the American Academy of Ophthalmology recommends a comprehensive eye exam every one to two years in otherwise healthy individuals over the age of 65.[4] (See Box 39.1.)

Preventing blindness is an important factor in assisting the elderly to function autonomously and to lead a productive life. Blinding disorders can cause significant personal, familial, and societal burdens. The total annual economic impact of visual impairment in adult Americans reaches approximately $51.4 billion.[5] Timely ophthalmological evaluation allows for preventative diagnoses and treatment of potentially blinding eye diseases.

Eyelids and lacrimal system

The eyelid can be anatomically divided into an anterior and posterior lamella by the tarsal plate. The anterior lamella is composed of cilia or lashes, dermis, orbicularis oculi muscle, and lid retractors (Figure 39.1A). The posterior lamella is composed of the tarsal plate and the palpebral conjunctiva (Figure 39.1B).

The major function of the eyelid is to protect the surface of the globe. Additionally, it serves to distribute the tear film across the optically clear cornea. The tear film is integral in protecting the cornea and ensuring vision. The tear film serves multiple functions to the underlying cornea including providing (1) lubrication and protection, (2) a smooth optical surface, (3) antimicrobial properties, and (4) necessary nutrients. The tear film is composed of three layers: lipid, aqueous, and mucin. The meibomian glands, sebaceous glands, and apocrine glands produce the lipid layer of the tear film that serves to slow evaporation of the aqueous tears. The aqueous portion is produced by the lacrimal and accessory lacrimal glands. Conjunctival goblet cells produce the mucinous layer, which assists in the adherence of the tear film to the ocular surface. The tears drain via the upper and lower lid puncta, canalicular system, nasolacrimal sac and nasolacrimal duct to exit beneath the inferior turbinate of the nose.

Abnormalities of the eyelid are particularly important to recognize in the setting of conditions that may cause the eyelid not to close completely. In those cases,

---

BOX 39.1 Ocular disorders of aging

1. The rate of visual impairment in individuals 80 years and older is 15–30 times greater than individuals 40–50 years old.[3]
2. Because many eye diseases can be insidious in onset, the American Academy of Ophthalmology recommends a comprehensive eye exam every one to two years in otherwise healthy individuals over the age of 65.

Reichel's Care of the Elderly, *7th Edition*, ed. Jan Busby-Whitehead *et al*. Published by Cambridge University Press. © Cambridge University Press 2016.

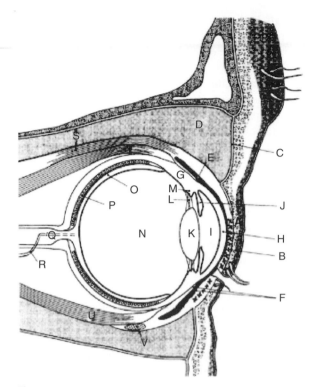

Figure 39.1 Cross-section anatomy of the eye, orbit, and eyelids: (A, B) posterior lamellae of eyelid, (C) orbital septum, (D) orbital fat, (E) superior fornix and conjunctiva, (F) inferior fornix and conjunctiva, (G) sclera, (H) cornea, (I) anterior chamber, (J) iris, (K) lens, (L) zonular fibers, (M) ciliary body and muscle, (N) vitreous body, (O) retina, (P) choroid, (Q) optic nerve, (R) central retinal artery, (S) levator muscle, (T) superior rectus muscle, (U) inferior rectus, and (V) inferior oblique muscle.

special attention is needed to ensure all functions of the eyelid are met using other means, such as artificial tears.

Eyelid structural changes associated with aging

Structural changes of the eyelid can affect an older adult's vision both by physically obstructing the visual fields and preventing the eyelid from performing its vital protective functions. These eyelid malpositions may produce tearing and ocular discomfort secondary to mechanical irritation of the cornea or failure of the eyelids to protect and lubricate the cornea leading to exposure keratopathy. Medical therapies with aggressive lubrication may be a temporizing measure, but the definitive treatment of these structural changes is generally surgical.

Dermatochalasis is the most common eyelid change observed in the elderly. It is characterized by a progressive laxity and resulting redundancy of eyelid skin, which can obstruct the superior visual field. This condition may be associated with blepharoptosis or ptosis, both commonly due to stretching or dehiscence of the lavatory aponeurotic. Blepharoptosis is abnormal low-lying upper eyelid margin obstructing the superior portion of the cornea. Ptosis is the drooping of the upper eyelid.

Horizontal eyelid laxity can cause lagophthalmos, or the inability to close the lids completely. Entropion, or the inward rotation of the eyelid margin, may result from involutional changes or chronic scarring processes of the conjunctiva, such as Stevens-Johnson syndrome or ocular cicatricial pemphigoid. This may be accompanied by trichiasis, or malpositioned eyelashes. Ectropion, the outward rotation of the lid margin, may be a consequence of involutional, cicatricial, paralytic, or inflammatory processes of the skin, orbicularis oculi muscle, or lid retractors. Structural changes can also be a common cause of chronic tearing, or epiphora. Obstruction of any portion of the lacrimal drainage system can cause epiphora. Involutional stenosis of the nasolacrimal duct is the most common type of nasolacrimal duct obstruction in elderly persons.[6] The treatment of the obstruction is dependent on the location. If the lacrimal "pump" (lid laxity) is the etiology for tearing, treatment is a lid tightening or ectropion repair. Punctal stenosis can typically be treated by a short in office procedure (punctoplasty). A lacrimal sac and nasolacrimal duct obstruction require silicone intubation and dacryocystorhinostomy (DCR). The DCR procedure requires the creation of a bony ostium between the lacrimal sac and the nasal cavity. A complete workup for epiphora would involve investigations into dry eye and blepharitis, both of which are discussed in this chapter.

Eyelid neoplasms

Basal cell carcinoma (BCC) is the most common malignancy of the eyelids, accounting for more than 90% of eyelid neoplasms. Risk factors for BCC include fair skin, ultraviolet exposure and cigarette smoking. BCC most frequently affects the upper eyelids and involvement of the medial canthus is associated with a worse prognosis. These lesions are typically painless and very slow growing and may not be noticed by patients, especially those with poor vision. The lesions appear as a nodular ulcer with raised rolled borders (rodent ulcer). Lesions can be associated with surrounding skin changes including ectropion, entropion, dimpling of skin, and loss of eyelashes or madarosis. Due to the slow progression of these lesions, metastasis is rare. The diagnosis is made by excisional biopsy. The technique of Mohs' micrographic surgery, the careful stepwise excision and microscopic monitoring of the surgical margins, produces a lower recurrence rate in addition to preserving the maximal amount of tissue.[7]

Squamous cell carcinoma (SCC) of the eyelid is 40 times less common than BCC, but it is much more aggressive. SCC most commonly occurs in the lower lid and can rapidly spread with local extension. Metastasis occurs in only 0.5% of SCCs that arise from sun-damaged skin, although metastasis may be more common in tumors that arise from chronically inflamed areas.[8] Lesions appear flat with overlying telangiectasia and scaling. As with BCC changes of the associated skin can be seen including ectropion, entropion, and madarosis. Surgical excision with wide margins and frozen sections is the treatment of choice due to the potentially deadly nature of this neoplasm.

Sebaceous cell carcinoma a highly malignant neoplasm arising from the eyelid lid sebaceous glands. Sebaceous cell carcinoma is found more often in the elderly and in women. It occurs two times more often in the upper lid as compared to the lower.[9] This lesion can masquerade as common benign lesions, so a high index of suspicion is critical. Chronic, unilateral blepharitis, recurrent chalazia and associated madarosis are highly suspicious signs of this disorder. A full-thickness eyelid biopsy with permanent sections is required for a correct diagnosis. These neoplasms can exhibit skip lesions and pagetoid spread making Mohs' surgery risky. The prognosis of sebaceous cell carcinoma is worse than that of BCC or SCC, with a mortality rate of 20% secondary to metastasis.[10] Treatment includes wide excision with sentinel lymph node biopsy in patients with high-risk features.

Secorrheic keratosis, actinic keratosis, and keratoacanthoma are examples of some common nonmalignant tumors on the eyelid. These require close follow-up and, frequently, excisional biopsy.

Blepharitis

Blepharitis is an extremely common condition characterized by anterior eyelid inflammation and posterior eyelid meibomian gland dysfunction. Clinically these entities lead to symptoms of burning, foreign body sensation, redness, mild itching, and tearing. These symptoms are frequently worse in the evening and are exacerbated by prolonged reading or wind exposure.

Blepharitis may be secondary to infectious or noninfectious causes. Organisms that inhabit the eyelids can also produce inflammation of the lids and cornea. The most common infectious cause of blepharitis is staphylococcus. Symptoms of staphylococcal blepharitis include collarettes, or material deposited at the base of the eyelashes, madarosis (lash loss), mild mucopurulent discharge, chronic conjunctivitis, and corneal changes. Treatment for staphylococcal blepharitis includes daily lid hygiene and topical antibiotics. Lid hygiene consists of scrubbing the eyelid margins with dilute baby shampoo or an over the counter commercial preparation. Warm compresses may then be applied to the lids with a clean washcloth. An antibiotic ointment, such as erythromycin or bacitracin, should be applied to the lids before bedtime for at least six weeks.

Noninfectious types of blepharitis include seborrheic blepharitis and meibomian gland dysfunction. Seborrheic blepharitis is characterized by oily lid margins, crusting of the lashes, conjunctivitis, and seborrheic dermatitis. Meibomian gland dysfunction is characterized by thickened irregular lid margins with inflammation around the orifices of the glands on the posterior eyelid surface. When expressed, the material within the glands may have a thick consistency. Acne rosacea has been associated. The treatment for noninfectious blepharitis includes lid hygiene, warm compresses, and systemic doxycycline.

Aqueous tear deficiency can additionally contribute to symptoms of dry eye in patients with blepharitis. These patients may be evaluated by examining the tear meniscus, tear breakup time, or a shortened interval between the blink and the separation of the tear film, and Schirmer testing, or a measure of tear production over a given period of time. Treatment of aqueous tear deficiency includes over the counter artificial tears, lubricating ointment at bedtime, and punctal occlusion.

Conjunctiva

Conjunctivitis affects all age groups; it is classified into acute or chronic and infectious or noninfectious subtypes. It does not cause structural damage to the eye except very rarely and with specific bacterial infections. Conjunctivitis typically presents with non-specific symptoms such as irritation, discharge, photophobia, and itching. The conjunctiva is typically diffusely erythematous, and a slit-lamp examination may reveal follicular or papillary response.

Bacterial conjunctivitis is less common than viral conjunctivitis in adults and is characterized by copious mucopurulent discharge. Although bacterial, the disease is generally self-limited and symptoms resolve in two to seven days without treatment. Treatment may be started at presentation or at day three or four if symptoms are failing to resolve or worsening. Treatment includes topical broad-spectrum antibiotic agent such as a fluoroquinolone drop for five to seven days. The antibiotic regimen should be modified according to culture results. Any patient with neisseria infection should be followed daily and treated systemically with intravenous antibiotic therapy because of the potential rapid destructive clinical course.

Viral conjunctivitis is most commonly caused by adenovirus. Patients may have associated systemic symptoms of an upper respiratory tract infection. In contrast to bacterial infections, the discharge is more watery, but patients can have severe crusting of lashes in the morning. The disease is self-limited, lasting up to 10 days. Epidemic keratoconjunctivitis is a more virulent strain of adenoviral conjunctivitis. This syndrome is characterized by a highly contagious, rapidly spreading conjunctivitis commonly with preauricular lymphadenopathy, photophobia, and blurry vision. Viral conjunctivitis does not require and should not be treated with antibiotics. Therapies include aggressive use of lubricants and symptomatic relief with cool compresses. Severe cases may require topical steroids under the care of an ophthalmologist.

Allergic conjunctivitis is most often associated with symptoms of seasonal allergies and it is characterized by itching and a stringy, white discharge. The most effective treatment is environmental control of the offending allergen. As this not always possible, symptomatic treatment includes cold compresses and combined mast-cell stabilizer-antihistamine topical preparations. In severe cases, topical steroids can also be used under the care of an ophthalmologist.

Chronic conjunctivitis is defined as symptoms for greater than three weeks. The differential includes the systemic diseases of Chlamydia, molluscum contagiosum, conjunctival malignancy, ocular cicatricial pemphigoid, sebaceous cell carcinoma, eyelid malpositions, and irritation from medication drops such as glaucoma medications. If a neoplastic or cicatricial systemic process is suspected, a conjunctival biopsy should be performed.

Cornea

The cornea (Figure 39.1H) is the major refracting or focusing surface of the eye allowing transmission of light to the retina. The cornea consists of five layers: epithelium, Bowman's layer, stroma, Descemet's membrane, and endothelium. The endothelium functions as a metabolic pump containing Na + –K + ATPase transporting fluid out of the cornea to keep the optical system dehydrated and clear. The number of endothelial cells decreases with age but is unlikely to decrease to level at which corneal edema results. Corneal edema can occur with corneal dystrophies or secondary to trauma to endothelial cells during intraocular surgery.

Fuchs endothelial corneal dystrophy is a common cause of corneal edema in the elderly. Fuchs is characterized by corneal epithelial and stromal edema due to endothelial cell dysfunction and loss. This leads to the formation of guttata, or thickened areas of Descemet's membrane due to stromal edema. These guttata can become pigmented and have a beaten bronze appearance. This condition is commonly bilateral, although it may be asymmetric. Patients are frequently asymptomatic until a significant amount of corneal edema accumulates causing symptoms of blurry vision that is worse in the morning and that clears throughout the day. This phenomenon is thought to be secondary to corneal dehydration associated with evaporation from the ocular surface throughout the day. As the condition progresses and more endothelial cell function is lost, epithelial edema or bullae may occur, causing pain. Early treatment strategies involve dehydrating the cornea with topical hyperosmotic agents. If corneal decomposition continues, these patients can go onto require corneal transplantation.

Trauma to the endothelial cells during intraocular surgery can cause a similar appearing pathology of corneal edema. Patients with low endothelial cell counts or corneal dystrophies are at a higher risk for this complication. Cataract surgery is the most commonly performed intraocular surgery in the United

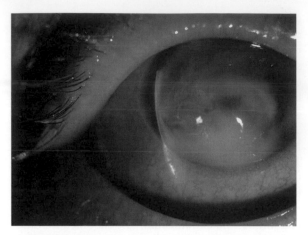

Figure 39.2 Infectious keratitis; noted features include mattering of the eyelashes, injected conjunctiva, corneal haze, and hypopyon (anterior chamber collection of white blood cells). (A black-and-white version of this figure will appear in some formats. For the color version, please refer to the plate section.)

States. Corneal stromal edema following cataract surgery is termed pseudophakic bullous keratopathy. This condition can also be initially managed with hyperosmotic agents but often progresses to require a corneal transplantation.

Decreased vision and pain along with acute onset red eye, pain, photophobia, and tearing can also signify infectious processes of the cornea (Figure 39.2). Contact lens wearers experience corneal infections at a much higher rate than the general population. Additionally, these patients are at risk for infection by highly virulent microbes including Pseudomonas and Acanthamoeba. Acanthamoeba is found in soil, swimming pools, hot tubs, and lake water and is resistant to freezing and the levels of chlorine routinely used. These patients commonly present with eye pain that is out of proportion to the appearance of the infectious process. Acanthamoeba infections can be devastating to the cornea, especially when diagnosis and treatment are delayed. Contact lens wearers with suspected infection should be urgently referred to an ophthalmologist. Infectious keratitis in non–contact lens wearers can be caused by a wide range of organisms. Staphylococcal infections can be associated with blepharitis as reviewed above and may lead to slowly progressive peripheral corneal infiltrates. In contrast, gram-negative bacterial infections such as neisseria progress rapidly and may lead to corneal perforation. Fungal keratitis is most common in southern climates and immunocompromised persons. Herpes simplex and varicella zoster infections can be mild and self-limited or may cause severe corneal infections with corneal anesthesia and scarring. Varicella zoster infections also produce pain and vesicular skin lesions in a dermatomal distribution.

The management of most corneal infections includes gram and giemsa stains of material obtained by scraping the bed of the ulcer, if present, as well as culture and sensitivity testing. Initial treatment may include frequent topical application of fortified broad-spectrum antibiotics and/or topical fluoroquinolone antibiotics. Modification of the treatment regimen is based on culture results and clinical response. Additional tests, such as confocal scanning, may be necessary to diagnose fungal or Acanthamoeba infections. Prolonged topical therapy is usually successful in clearing the infection, but surgical treatment may be necessary in cases with residual corneal scaring. Herpes simplex keratitis is generally treated with topical antiviral agents. Oral acyclovir may be helpful in treating and preventing recurrent keratitis. Acute varicella zoster infections are treated for 7–10 days with oral antivirals acyclovir 800 mg five times daily, famciclovir 500 mg three times daily, or valacyclovir 1 g three times daily to minimize ocular complications.[11] Steroids can rapidly exacerbate herpetic infections; thus, topical steroids should only be administered under the care of an ophthalmologist.

Presbyopia

Presbyopia is the most common ocular condition affecting the aging population. At approximately 40 years of age, people progressively lose the ability to accommodate, or focus on a near target. Normal accommodation is produced by ciliary muscle contraction, allowing relaxation of the zonules that hold the intraocular crystalline lens in place. This causes the crystalline lens to change shape and focusing power. Without the ability of the lens to adapt appropriately, patients need visual aids, usually in the form reading glasses or bifocals, to assist them in focusing on near targets.

Cataracts

An estimated 20.5 million Americans over the age of 40 have cataracts.[12] The prevalence increases to nearly 70% in Americans older than 75.[13] The natural crystalline lens is positioned behind the iris and supported by zonular fibers that arise from the

BOX 39.2 Cataracts and presbyopia

1. An estimated 70% of Americans over the age 75 have cataracts. Once the vision is unable to be corrected with a change in lens prescription, the patient may be offered cataract surgery based on an ophthalmologist's evaluation.

2. Visual acuity following cataract surgery is 20/40 or better in 97% of patients without coexisting ocular pathology. Patients have significant improvement in their quality of life and overall visual function.

internal layers of the eye (Figures 39.1K and 39.1L). It is composed of three layers. The zonular fibers are connected to a lens capsule and beneath the lens capsule is outer cortical layer of fibers and an inner nuclear layer. A cataract is an opacity in any of the three layers of the natural lens that that normally develops with aging. At present there are no therapies to prevent the formation of cataracts. (See Box 39.2.)

Cataracts can vary in appearance dependent on which layer of lens the opacity is located. Opacity in the nuclear layer is known as nuclear sclerosis. Nuclear sclerosis occurs as the number and density of lens fibers increases over time. Initially this thickening of the natural lens may cause a shift in the focusing power of the eye allowing the patient to read without glasses. Vision continues to decline as the lens progressively thickens and yellows eventually requiring surgical removal to restore vision. Cortical cataracts are opacities in the cortical layer of the natural lens. They often appear spoke-shaped and impair vision to varying degrees. Posterior subcapsular cataracts are opacities just anterior to the posterior capsule of the natural lens. Visual impairment and glare symptoms are found in bright light with both cortical and posterior subcapsular cataracts.

There are systemic conditions that have been found to increase and accelerate the presentation of cataracts. In particular, diabetes mellitus is associated with early onset and a higher incidence of cataracts. Large osmotic shifts, such as those occurring in hyperglycemic episodes, lead to the formation of cataracts due to swelling of the lens fibers. Blunt trauma, electrical shock or ionizing radiation has also been found to cause cataract formation. Lastly many drugs have been linked to cataract progression including long-term topical or systemic corticosteroids, chlorpromazine, amiodarone, and phenothiazides.

Nonsurgical management of cataracts entails accurate refraction and eyeglass correction. Eventually, the vision does not improve significantly with a change in lens prescription and the patient may be offered cataract surgery based on an ophthalmologist's evaluation.

Cataract surgery

Recent technological advances in cataract surgery have been extraordinary. Extracapsular cataract extraction and phacoemulsification are microsurgical techniques that remove the cataract and leave the posterior lens capsule intact so that an intraocular lens may be implanted in the native lens capsule. Most recently, ophthalmic lasers have been introduced into the market to assist in cataract extraction. Intraocular lens implants are small disc-shaped pieces of polymethylmethacrylate, acrylic, silicone, or hydrogel that are manufactured with differing powers. The power of the implant is determined by the optical properties of each patient's eye, which is measured pre-operatively. Cataract surgery is an outpatient procedure, the majority being done under local anesthetic and mild intravenous sedation. Ideally, following cataract surgery distance glasses are not required because refractive error is taken into account with intraocular lens power selection. However, most patients will require reading glasses for near vision following cataract surgery; multifocal and accommodative intraocular lens are gaining favor to allow patients to see clearly at all distances without glasses. Visual acuity following cataract surgery is 20/40 or better in 97% of patients without coexisting ocular pathology. Patients have significant improvement in their quality of life and overall visual function, such as nighttime and daytime driving, community and home activities, mental health, and life satisfaction.[14]

The most common complication is opacification of the posterior lens capsule occurring in approximately 20%–30% of patients. The posterior capsular opacification can be cleared with an in-office laser procedure. Retinal detachment is one of the more serious sequelae following cataract surgery with a lifetime incidence of 0.7%. Cystoid macular edema following cataract surgery may cause temporary and sometimes permanent visual impairment. Cystoid macular edema is characterized by intraretinal edema. Patients present with a gradual loss in central vision most commonly occurring 6–10 weeks postoperatively. Approximately, 75% cases improve without intervention. Topical steroids and NSAIDS may be useful in cases that do not spontaneously improve. More rare, but sight threatening complications of cataract surgery include intraocular lens dislocation, endophthalmitis, and expulsive choroidal hemorrhage.

Bacterial endophthalmitis is a true emergency and one of the most feared complications of intraocular surgery. This most commonly occurs within two weeks of the surgery. Less than 1 in 1,000 surgeries are complicated by acute bacterial endophthalmitis. [15] The most common organism implicated is staphylococcus epidermis. Patients typically present with acute eye pain and loss of vision. Anterior chamber inflammation may be associated with a hypopyon, or layered leukocytes. Emergent referral to an ophthalmologist is necessary if this condition is suspected. Surgical removal of the infected vitreous body with instillation of intravitreal antibiotics and steroids has been reported to be successful in treating this condition.

Glaucoma

Glaucoma is a group of diseases with characteristic optic nerve fiber layer atrophy and corresponding visual field loss. Glaucoma is the second most common cause of blindness in the United States. The incidence is highest in African Americans and Hispanics. Glaucoma is a very slowly progressive disease. It is estimated that of the 2.2 million people who develop glaucoma, approximately half are unaware of their disease.[16] Glaucoma is characterized into open-angle and closed-angle depending on the etiology of the restriction of aqueous outflow. The known risk factors for primary open-angle glaucoma include high intraocular pressure, age, race, and family history. Once the damage occurs in adults, it is irreversible. Early detection and treatment are essential to prevent permanent loss of visual function.

Intraocular pressure is the function of three features of the eye: the rate of aqueous fluid production by the ciliary body (Figure 39.lM), the resistance to aqueous outflow through the trabecular meshwork, and the venous pressure of the episcleral veins. Glaucoma therapies target one or more of these pathophysiological mechanisms. Intraocular pressure between 21 mmHg and 8 mmHg is considered to be normal; however, glaucoma may develop with intraocular pressure in the normal range, so called

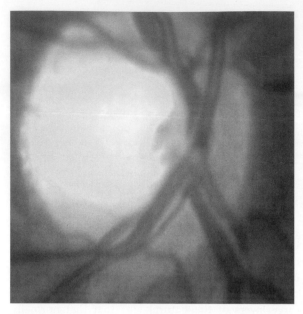

Figure 39.3 Glaucomatous cupping of the optic nerve; a loss of the nerve fiber layer is noted temporally. (A black-and-white version of this figure will appear in some formats. For the color version, please refer to the plate section.)

normal-tension glaucoma. Intraocular pressure can be measured easily in the office by a primary care provider with a handheld tonometer.

Also, routine direct ophthalmoscopy of the optic disc in all adult patients by the primary care provider can help identify glaucoma. Optic nerve atrophy is characterized by an increased size or asymmetry of the central cupped out portion of the optic nerve in comparison to the remaining neural rim, the so called "cup/disc ratio." The cup/disc ratio varies – usually 0.3 (the central cup occupies 30% of the optic nerve head) in Caucasians and 0.5 in African Americans is considered normal. Larger cups or asymmetric cups should raise the suspicion of glaucoma (Figure 39.3). Additionally, the disc rim should have uniform thickness without notches or hemorrhages.

Open-angle glaucoma

Primary open-angle glaucoma (POAG) has no obvious macroscopic mechanical restriction to outflow. Primary open-angle glaucoma is the most common form of glaucoma in the United States, constituting 70% of glaucoma in adults. POAG is asymptomatic as elevated intraocular pressure is chronic and often does not produce any sensation of pain or discomfort. Known as the thief of sight, glaucomatous visual field loss develops insidiously initially affecting the peripheral visual fields and sparing the central visual acuity until very late in the disease. The diagnosis of POAG is made by finding characteristic optic cupping and typical visual field changes in the presence of an open, normal-appearing angle.

Steroid-induced glaucoma is a type of secondary open-angle glaucoma. Patients who are taking systemic or topical steroids may develop high intraocular pressure and glaucomatous damage. The steroids modify the intracellular structure of the trabecular meshwork cells and increase the resistance to outflow. This effect may or may not be reversible following discontinuation of the steroids.

Angle-closure glaucoma

Acute angle-closure glaucoma has visible impediment to aqueous outflow, most commonly because of mechanical blockage by the peripheral iris. Acute angle-closure glaucoma occurs in only 0.1% of people older than age 40 in the United States, but it is considered an ophthalmic emergency. Anatomically narrow anterior chamber angle predisposes a patient to acute angle-closure glaucoma. Risk factors include hyperopia, Asian ancestry, and female sex. The peak prevalence is between 55 and 70 years of age.[17] The anterior chamber depth decreases normally with age because of the growth of the lens.

In patients who already have a narrow chamber angle, the iris becomes opposed to the anterior surface of the lens. The attack often occurs in the evening during periods of dim illumination when the pupil becomes moderately dilated and has the greatest surface contact with the anterior lens. The iris lens contact impedes the normal flow of aqueous fluid from its production site behind the iris to its drainage site in the trabecular meshwork. Intraocular pressure builds up behind the iris, causing the peripheral iris to bow forward and further obstruct the outflow of aqueous. During this time the aqueous fluid production continues. The result is a very rapid rise in intraocular pressure that causes severe pain, corneal edema, iris ischemia and thus a mid-dilated and poorly reactive pupil. Additional symptoms of blurred vision especially with haloes around lights are in relation the corneal edema.

Medications can predispose patients with anatomically narrow angles to develop angle closure glaucoma. Patients who have undergone pharmacological dilation may develop angle-closure glaucoma as the dilation slowly wanes and the iris becomes arrested in mid-dilation. Medications with anticholinergic side effects, such as decongestants, tricyclic antidepressants, and antispasmodics can also precipitate and angle-closure attack. Patients with a suspicious clinical appearance and elevated intraocular pressure should be referred to an ophthalmologist for immediate management.

The acute goal of treatment for angle closure glaucoma is to lower the intraocular pressure as rapidly as possible with medical treatment. The angle obstruction is then definitively treated by with a laser iridectomy. Laser iridectomy creates a hole in the iris to provide an alternative channel for aqueous flow into the anterior chamber. Additionally, laser iridectomy is performed in the fellow eye to protect against further attacks of angle-closure glaucoma.

Glaucoma management

The goal of glaucoma treatment is to lower intraocular pressure to a low enough level to prevent further damage to the optic nerve and visual field. Medical management is the initial treatment in the United States. Glaucoma medications drain through the nasolacrimal duct system and are absorbed by the nasal mucosa, thus leading to potential systemic side effects of these topical medications. Primary care physicians should question their patients about ophthalmic medications.

Beta blockers (Timolol) are an older generation of medications that were considered first line for many years and still are by many practicing ophthalmologists. They lower intraocular pressure by reducing aqueous fluid production. Beta blockers are generally well tolerated but are contraindicated in patients with bradycardia and pulmonary disease. Systemic side effects of beta blockers include bradycardia, heart block, bronchospasm, impotence, lethargy, masking of hypoglycemia, and exacerbation of myasthenia gravis.

Adrenergic alpha2-agonists (Brimonidine) have minimal systemic side effects and are potent inhibitors of aqueous fluid production. Side effects include ocular irritation and dry mouth. They may be safer than beta blockers in the geriatric population.

Prostaglandin analogs (Latanoprost, Bimatoprost, Travoprost) lower intraocular pressure by increasing uveoscleral outflow and have minimal systemic side effects. Ocular side effects include increased

BOX 39.3 Vitreous and retina

Rhegmatogenous retinal detachment
1. Retinal detachment is seen in persons older than 50 with risk factors including a history of intraocular surgery and myopia.
2. Symptoms of retinal detachment include flashes of light, floaters in the vision, and a peripheral visual field defect described as a curtain or shade over part of the visual field.
3. Rapid referral to an ophthalmologist is indicated if a retinal detachment is suspected.
Age-related macular degeneration
1. Age-related macular degeneration (AMD) is the leading cause of legal blindness in the United States in people over 50 years of age.
2. Anti-VEGF treatments have dramatically changed the visual prognosis of this disease offering stabilization and even improvement in vision.
3. Low-vision aids can be helpful for persons with loss of central vision associated with AMD.

pigmentation of the iris and periocular skin as well as increased growth of the eye lashes or hypertrichosis. This once-a-day drop is becoming a common first line therapy for glaucoma patients of any age.

Topical carbonic anhydrase inhibitors (Dorzolamide, Brinzolamide) have fewer systemic side effects than the oral medications but are less potent. The oral carbonic anhydrase inhibitors (Acetazolamide) lower intraocular pressure by reducing aqueous fluid production. The systemic side effects of the oral drugs can be more serious in older individual and often limit their use in the elderly. The systemic side effects include metallic taste, paresthesias, malaise, weight loss, metabolic acidosis, renal lithiasis, diarrhea, and pancytopenia.

Laser is another treatment option in the arsenal against glaucoma. Laser trabeculoplasty is applied by directing a small, focused argon or diode laser at the trabecular meshwork. The desired result is an improvement in outflow facility and reduction in intraocular pressure. Studies in patients with POAG have shown laser trabeculoplasty to be safe and effective, although there is a decline in success rate from year one (60%) to year four (44%).[18] Practice patterns in the United States vary as to whether patients are offered laser trabeculoplasty prior to glaucoma filtration surgery.

Glaucoma filtration surgery is offered after more conservative therapies have failed to provide adequate control of the glaucoma. One surgical technique for POAG entails the creation of a fistula from the anterior chamber of the eye to the subconjunctival space. Lastly, another technique involves the implantation of an artificial drainage device in the subconjunctival space with a tube placed into the anterior chamber to allow drainage of aqueous fluid.

Vitreous and retina

The neurosensory retina is composed of 10 layers with millions of photoreceptors to capture light rays and convert them into electrical impulses (Figure 39.1O). As the eye ages, a host of conditions can affect the vitreoretinal interface, the retinal circulation, the retinal pigment epithelial choroidal complex, and the optic nerve. (See Box 39.3.)

Posterior vitreous detachment

Posterior vitreous detachment (PVD) is a very common condition that occurs in approximately 75% of patients older than 65 years of age. The vitreous is a jellylike substance that occupies 80% of the volume of the eye (Figure 39.1N). With increasing age, portions of the vitreous body begin to liquefy. This process remains asymptomatic until a PVD occurs. A PVD occurs when liquefaction of the vitreous body occurs to the point that it separates from the retina. Patients will often describe flashes of light and floaters. Photopsias, or flashes of light, are often described as arc-shaped, "lightning bolts" in the peripheral visual field. Flashes are caused by traction of the partially detached vitreous base tugging on the retina, which creates an electrical stimulus. Floaters are also a common symptom with multiple etiologies as they are caused by opacities in the vitreous body forming shadows on the underlying retina. Floaters may represent aggregation of the vitreous gel, blood, or pigment from the retina.

The most obvious and bothersome floater is the separation of the vitreous body from the optic nerve. Known as a Weiss ring, it may appear to the patient to be an insect or cobweb moving around in the vision.[19]

Approximately 15% of patients with acute symptomatic PVD have a retinal tear placing them at risk for a retinal detachment. If a blood vessel is torn during vitreous separation, the vitreous cavity can fill with blood and result in a dramatic decrease in vision. A vitreous hemorrhage can be an indicator for an increased risk of a retinal tear. Approximately 50%–70% of patients with a PVD-associated vitreous hemorrhage have retinal tears, whereas only 10%–12% patients without vitreous hemorrhage have associated retinal tears.[19]

Rhegmatogenous retinal detachment

Retinal detachment secondary to a tear or hole (rhegma) in the retina is typically seen in persons older than 50. Risks include a history of intraocular surgery, such as cataract extraction, or those who have myopia. Symptoms of retinal detachment include flashes of light and floaters in the vision. Patients will report a decline in central vision if the macula is involved. A patient may report a curtain or shade over part of the visual field. Examination of the retina by binocular indirect ophthalmoscopy is the most important way to identify retinal tears and detachments. Rapid referral to an ophthalmologist is indicated if a retinal detachment is suspected.

Epiretinal membrane

Epiretinal membrane (ERM) is typically seen in patients older than age 50 and occurs in both eyes in 20% of cases. ERM most commonly occurs secondary to a vitreous detachment due to proliferation of glial cells on the retinal surface. Contraction of the ERM on the surface of the retina causes retinal distortion and visual symptoms of distorted images (i.e., perception of a squiggly line). ERMs may also cause loss of retinal capillary integrity that may lead to cystoid macular edema. Most cases of ERM are closely observed. Rarely vision is severely affected and surgical removal of the ERM can be performed. There is an increased risk of retinal detachment following ERM surgery.

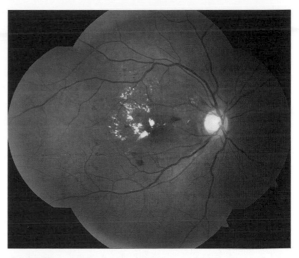

Figure 39.4 Nonproliferative diabetic retinopathy; noted features include dot and flame hemorrhages, microaneurysms, and hard exudates throughout the fundus. (A black-and-white version of this figure will appear in some formats. For the color version, please refer to the plate section.)

Retinal vascular disorders

Diabetic retinopathy

Diabetic retinopathy is the leading cause of blindness in individuals aged 20–64 in the United States. After 20 years of diabetes, approximately 99% type 1 diabetics and 60% of type 2 diabetics will have some retinopathy.[20] Type II diabetics should be examined yearly by an ophthalmologist for evidence of retinopathy starting at the time of diagnosis. Type I diabetics should be examined within five years of diagnosis or after age 10, whichever comes first. The earliest signs of diabetic retinopathy include microaneurysms, dot and blot hemorrhages, cotton wool spots, and venous beading (Figure 39.4). Proliferative diabetic retinopathy is evidenced by the formation of new retinal blood vessels on the surface of the retina and in the vitreous cavity. These fragile abnormal blood vessels cause vitreous hemorrhages and exert traction on the retina causing retinal detachments. Additionally, abnormal retinal capillaries can leak serous fluid causing macular edema. Macular edema can severely reduce central vision is type II diabetics.

Laser photocoagulation has proved beneficial for the treatment of proliferative diabetic retinopathy and maculopathy.[21] The goal of laser photocoagulation in proliferative diabetic retinopathy is to halt the progression of new blood vessels by reducing the ischemic stimulus. Pars plana vitrectomy (PPV), or surgical removal of the vitreous, can also be an important technique for clearing the vitreous cavity of blood and removing the fibrovascular scaffold that results in retinal detachment by traction from new blood vessels. Recently, anti-vascular endothelial growth factor (anti-VEGF) intravitreal injections have been shown to be clinically useful in the treatment proliferative diabetic retinopathy, although these medications are not yet FDA approved for this indication.

Retinal vein occlusion

Retinal vein occlusion can affect the central retinal vein or more distal branch. Symptoms include loss of central vision and/or peripheral visual field defects. Associated systemic conditions include hypertension, diabetes, cardiovascular disease, and arteriosclerosis. Acute findings on fundus examination are the classic "blood and thunder" appearance including venous tortuosity, retinal hemorrhages, retinal edema, and cotton wool spots. In central retinal vein occlusion (CRVO), these changes are observed throughout the fundus, but only the regions of the occluded branch veins (BRVO) are affected in those cases. In BRVO the site of occlusion is at an arteriovenous crossing site. This is thought to be related to arterial wall thickening due to systemic factors of hypertension, atherosclerosis and hyperlipidemia eventually resulting in complete occlusion of the vein. Laser photocoagulation offers proven benefit for the two major complications, macular edema and retinal neovascularization.[22] Additionally, anti-VEGF therapies have clinically shown to be beneficial for the treatment of the complications of retinal vein occlusions. Retinal vein occlusions result in massive retinal ischemia. Retinal ischemia stimulates neovascularization of the retina and other structures of the eye that can lead to complications such as vitreous hemorrhage and neovascular glaucoma.

Retinal artery occlusion

Acute retinal artery occlusion results in infarction of the inner retina secondary to an embolus or an intraluminal thrombus. Patients typically present with sudden, painless loss of vision and visual field defects. The retina becomes white, edematous, and a cherry red spot may be present in cases of central retinal artery occlusion. Evaluation and management of patients is focused on the embolic workup. A complete stroke workup including Carotid Doppler testing and cardiac echocardiogram are important tests in this evaluation. Giant cell

arteritis (GCA) is a rare cause of retinal artery occlusion but should be considered in patients in their sixties or older, since failure to recognize and treat this etiology can lead to rapid loss of vision bilaterally. This condition is discussed later in the chapter.

Choroidal disorders

Age-related macular degeneration

Age-related macular degeneration (AMD) is the leading cause of legal blindness in the United States in people over 50 years of age. Persons older than 60 are at greatest risk and the prevalence of this disorder increases with age. Its hallmark is the loss of central vision with deterioration of the macula, the highly sensitive portion of the retina responsible for central vision.

Two forms of AMD occur, the dry type (non-neovascular) in 85% of eyes and the wet type (neovascular) in 15%. Additionally, a sudden drop in vision can occur on rare occasions when the dry form of AMD converts to the wet form. The dry form is characterized by drusen deposits under the retina and atrophy of the central macula. The majority of patients with dry AMD have milder visual impairment. Choroidal neovascularization, or abnormal vessel growth under the retina, is the characteristic finding in wet AMD (Figure 39.5). The neovascularization results in hemorrhage and lipid exudates in

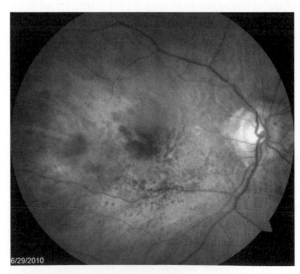

Figure 39.5 Wet age-related macular degeneration; subretinal hemorrhage denotes the choroidal neovascularization. (A black-and-white version of this figure will appear in some formats. For the color version, please refer to the plate section.)

the macula. These entities cause severe damage and vision loss.

For many years, laser photocoagulation was the only treatment with proven benefit for the choroidal neovascularization.[23] Anti-VEGF treatments have been shown to be beneficial and superior in the treatment of choroidal neovascularization. The anti-VEGF medications ranibizumab and aflibercept have recently been FDA approved for the treatment of neovascular AMD. The anti-VEGF medication bevacizumab is commonly used off label for this indication by many vitreoretinal specialists. This revolution in treatment has dramatically changed the visual prognosis of patients with AMD. Some of the anti-VEGF treatments have demonstrated stabilization or even improvement in visual acuity.[24] Low-vision aids can be helpful for persons with loss of central vision.

Optic nerve disorders

Giant cell arteritis/temporal arteritis/ arteritic ischemic optic neuropathy

GCA is a systemic disease with many names that most commonly presents with weight loss, headache, scalp tenderness, jaw claudication, malaise, and proximal muscle weakness. GCA is a primary vision-threatening disorder that affects the optic nerve and causes an optic neuropathy. Patient may present transient vision loss prior to a complete occlusive event that leads to severe vision loss. Tenderness or an enlarged temporal artery may be a sign of temporal arteritis. An elevated ESR and C-reactive protein as well as a low platelet count can support the suspicion of GCA, but the diagnosis is made based on history and clinical examination. Biopsy should also be performed if the diagnosis of GCA is entertained as nearly 10% of patients with this condition have a normal ESR. If the diagnosis is suspected, high-dose intravenous steroids should be administered immediately, without waiting for the biopsy. The role of steroids is to protect against vision loss in the unaffected eye, which can occur within hours or days after the first. Temporal artery biopsy should be performed within two weeks of initiating steroid therapy because pathological features can change with duration of treatment, making the definitive diagnosis more challenging.

Nonarteritic ischemic optic neuropathy

Nonarteritic ischemic optic neuropathy is an infarction of the optic nerve. It is associated with hypertension, diabetes mellitus, obstructive sleep apnea, and conditions that cause hypoperfusion of the optic nerve such as hypotension. Patient presents with acute, painless loss of vision, commonly noticed upon waking from sleep. Vision may vary from normal with loss of a portion of the visual field to no light perception (NLP). NLP vision should prompt the examiner to consider GCA. Patients may present with partial edema of the optic nerve head and hemorrhages within the nerve fiber layer. Treatment is focused on minimizing the risk factors for a repeat event.

Low vision

When treatment to prevent vision loss fails, patients are left with very poor vision and may struggle with simple activities of daily living. Part of the continuum of care is to aid these patients in making the most of their remaining vision. There are ophthalmologists and organizations available in many communities that specialize in low vision rehabilitation. Visual acuity of less than 20/40 with corrective lenses, a central loss of vision, a large peripheral loss of vision or a loss in contrast sensitivity would all be indications to refer a patient for low vision rehabilitation. The goal of low vision rehabilitation is to help people learn new strategies to complete daily tasks. A wide range of low vision aids are available including handheld magnifiers, digital desktop magnifiers, magnifying spectacles, large-print books, talking watches, and computers that magnify printed materials. As an addition to these physical aids, control of the environment is very important. Some simple recommendations include using bright lights while reading, lighting dim areas such as stairs and closets, controlling glare in outdoor situations with a wide brim hat or dark tinted sunglasses that wrap around the side of face, and increasing contrast between colors whenever possible. Additional information distributed by the American Academy of Ophthalmology as well as a handout for low vision patients can be found at one. aao.org.

References

1. Centers for Disease Control and Prevention. Why is vision loss a public health problem? 2009. www.cdc.gov/ visionhealth/basic_information/vision_loss.htm (accessed June 29, 2014).

2. National Eye Institute. Vision Problems in the US: Prevalence of Adult Vision Impairment and Age-Related Eye Disease in America. 2012. http://vision problemsus.org/index.html (accessed June 29, 2014).

3. Tielsch JM, Sommer A, Witt K, et al. Blindness and visual impairment in an American urban population. *The Baltimore Eye Survey. Arch Ophthalmol.* 1990; **108**: 286–290.

4. American Academy of Ophthalmology Preferred Practice Committee. *Comprehensive Adult Eye Examination.* San Francisco: American Academy of Ophthalmology; 2010.

5. Rein DB, Zhang P, Wirth KE, et al. The economic burden of major adult visual disorders in the United States. *Arch Ophthalmol.* 2006; **124**: 1754–1760.

6. Tantenbaum MMC. Lacrimal drainage system. In: Tasman WJE, ed. *Duane's Clinical Ophthalmology.* Philadelphia: Lippincott; 2006: vol **4**, chap 13.

7. Rubin AI, Chen EH, Ratner D. Basal-cell carcinoma. *N Engl J Med.* 2005; **353**: 2262–2269.

8. Vaughn GI DR, Gayre GS. Eyelid malignancies. In: Yanoff M DJ, Aggsburger JJ, eds. *Ophthalmology.* Philadelphia: Mosby; 2004: chap 93.

9. Shields JA, Demirci H, Marr BP, et al. Sebaceous carcinoma of the eyelids: personal experience with 60 cases. *Ophthalmology.* 2004; **111**: 2151–2157.

10. Jacobiec FA. Sebaceous tumors of the ocular adnexa. In: Albert DA, Jacobiec FA, eds. *Principles and Practice of Ophthalmology.* Philadelphia: Saunders; 1994.

11. Pepose JS. The potential impact of the varicella vaccine and new antivirals on ocular disease related to varicella-zoster virus. *Am J Ophthalmol.* 1997; **123**: 243–251.

12. The Eye Disease Prevalence Research Group. Prevalence of cataract and pseudophakia/aphakia among adults in the United States. *Arch Ophthalmol.* 2004; **122**: 487–494.

13. Klein BE, Klein R, Lee KE. Incidence of age-related cataract: the Beaver Dam Eye Study. *Arch Ophthalmol.* 1998; **116**: 219–225.

14. Brenner MH, Curbow B, Javitt IC, et al. Vision change and quality of life in the elderly: response to cataract surgery and treatment of other chronic ocular conditions. *Arch Ophthalmol.* 1993; **111**: 680–685.

15. Javitt JC, Yitale S, Canner JK, et al. National outcomes of cataract extraction: Endophthalmitis following inpatient surgery. *Arch Ophthalmol.* 1991; **109**: 1085–1089.

16. American Academy of Ophthalmology Preferred Practice Committee. *Primary Open Angle Glaucoma.* San Francisco: American Academy of Ophthalmology; 2010.

17. Coleman AL, Brigatti L. The glaucomas. *Minerva Med.* 2001; **92**: 365–379.

18. Weinand FS, Althen F. Long-term clinical results of selective laser trabeculoplasty in the treatment of primary open angle glaucoma. *Eur J Ophthalmol.* 2006; **16**: 100–104.

19. Van Overdam KA, Bettink-Remeijer MW, Klaver CC, et al. Symptoms and finding predictive for the development of new retinal breaks. *Arch Ophthalmol.* 2005; **123**: 479–484.

20. Klein R, Klein BE, Moss SE, et al. The Wisconsin Epidemiologic Study of Diabetic Retinopathy II. *Arch Ophthalmol.* 1984; **102**: 520–526.

21. Early photocoagulation for diabetic retinopathy. ETDRS report number 9. Early Treatment Diabetic Retinopathy Study research group. *Ophthalmology.* 1991; **98**: 766–785.

22. Branch Vein Occlusion Study Group. Argon laser photocoagulation for macular edema in branch vein occlusion. *Am I Ophthalmol.* 1984; **98**: 271–282.

23. Macular Photocoagulation Study Group. Argon laser photocoagulation for neovascular maculopathy: five-year results from randomized clinical trials. *Arch Ophthalmol.* 1991; **109**: 1109–1114.

24. Abraham P, Yue H, Wilson L. Randomized, double-masked, sham-controlled trial of ranibizumab for neovascular age-related macular degeneration: PIER study year 2. *Am J Ophthalmol.* 2010; **150**: 315–324.

Chapter 40

Geriatric otolaryngology

Rebecca J. Kamil, BS, Carrie Nieman, MD, MPH, and Frank R. Lin, MD, PhD

Introduction

Many otolaryngologic conditions, including age-related hearing loss, vertigo, dysphagia, and voice changes, become increasingly prevalent with aging and substantially affect the functioning of older adults. This chapter discusses the expected anatomical and physiological age-related changes as well as the etiology, presentation, and treatment of common head and neck conditions that geriatricians will encounter.

Ear

Outer ear

Age-related changes

The external auditory canal changes with age. The lateral cartilaginous ear canal weakens with age, reducing structural rigidity, and outgrowths in the medial bony ear canal (e.g., benign exostoses) can further narrow the canal, leading to cerumen impaction and difficulty fitting a hearing aid.[1, 2] Atrophy of the surface epithelium and decreased apocrine gland function of the ear canal predisposes to dryness, scaling, and trauma.

Common pathologies

Cerumen impaction is a frequent consequence of age-related changes in the external auditory canal.[3, 4] Cerumen protects the ear with antimicrobial properties and by capturing foreign particles and is normally eliminated from the ear canal with epithelial migration. In older adults, apocrine glands atrophy, decreasing the watery component of cerumen, producing cerumen that is drier, harder, and less likely to be expelled.[2, 5] Hearing aids and the thicker, fuller tragal hairs associated with normal aging can further impede the canal's normal "self cleaning" mechanism.[5] Every patient should be regularly evaluated for impaction at clinic visits.[3] Cerumen can be removed with curettage (ideally done with an operative otoscope head, such as a Welch Allyn Operating Otoscope #21700), suction, topical cerumenolytics, or irrigation with warm water. However, irrigation should be avoided in patients who are diabetic, immunocompromised, or those with perforated tympanic membranes due to the risk of precipitating an acute otitis externa or media.[3, 6, 7] Preventive measures include counseling against cotton swab use and encouraging the regular use of emollients like mineral oil or glycerin.[3]

Squamous cell carcinoma, basal cell carcinoma, and actinic keratoses can affect the pinna.[8] With age, skin becomes atrophic due to dermal thinning, disorganized collagen deposition, and decreased elastic tissues and mitotic divisions. Free radicals produced secondary to ultraviolet light exposure promote cross-linking of fibrous proteins and DNA. Risk factors for skin cancer include age, sun exposure, Type I–II skin types on the Fitzpatrick scale, and history of multiple sunburns.[9, 10] Squamous cell carcinoma may present as a red patch, often preceded by actinic keratosis.[9] Basal cell carcinoma presents as an elevated, pink, waxy nodular lesion with a clearly demarcated capillary bed. Maintain a high level of suspicion for malignancy and refer for biopsy when accompanied by persistent otalgia, recurrent otitis externa, bleeding, hearing loss, facial nerve weakness/paralysis, or granulation tissue.[11]

Acute otitis externa (AOE) is a bacterial infection of the external auditory canal often precipitated by a break in the skin secondary to water exposure or manipulation, such as cotton swab use.[12] The

Reichel's Care of the Elderly, *7th Edition*, ed. Jan Busby-Whitehead *et al.* Published by Cambridge University Press.
© Cambridge University Press 2016.

setting of a warm, moist ear canal encourages bacterial growth of common pathogens such as *Pseudomonas aeruginosa* and *Staphylococcus aureus*. The patient presents with pruritus, purulent discharge, pain, and, at times, conductive hearing loss due to canal narrowing.[12, 13] On physical exam, pulling the pinna elicits significant pain, distinguishing AOE from otitis media.[12] Topical treatment with antiseptic or antibiotic eardrops, with or without steroids, is first-line treatment. Although several meta-analyses of randomized controlled trials have not demonstrated clinically significant differences between topical treatments, ciprofloxacin, and steroid preparation (Cipro HC with hydrocortisone or Ciprodex with dexamethasone) twice a day for 7–10 days is a common, albeit expensive, treatment.[13, 14] Cheaper options include a neomycin, polymyxin, and hydrocortisone preparation (Cortisporin Otic Suspension), which can be given three to four times a day, or antiseptic treatment with acetic acid 2.0%, with or without hydrocortisone 1.0%.[13, 14] If soft tissue swelling limits drug delivery, eardrops may be administered with a wick, along with pain medication and frequent debridement by the physician if needed.[12, 14] Systemic antibiotic treatment, with coverage of *Pseudomonas aeruginosa* and *Staphylococcus aureus*, is reserved as adjunctive treatment if the patient is diabetic or immune deficient, if the infection has spread beyond the ear canal, or if topical therapy is unable to be delivered effectively.[14] If significant debris, impaction, or failure of initial antibiotic course occurs, referral to an otolaryngologist is needed.

Malignant otitis externa is a feared complication of AOE and is a rare, potentially lethal infection of the soft tissue and bone of the external auditory canal and skull base by *Pseudomonas aeruginosa*.[12, 15] Classically, this complication occurs in older, diabetic, and immunocompromised patients. Symptoms include severe otalgia for ≥ 4 weeks, purulent otorrhea, and, occasionally, cranial neuropathies, particularly facial paralysis.[12] On physical exam, granulation tissue is seen along the ear canal floor. Long-term intravenous antibiotics and correction of immunosuppression (e.g., glucose control in diabetics) are the primary treatment, whereas surgery is reserved for debridement. Suspicion for malignant otitis externa requires emergent referral to an otolaryngologist.

Herpes zoster oticus is a vesicular rash of the external ear canal accompanied by severe pain and hearing loss and, when accompanied by facial paralysis, is called Ramsay Hunt syndrome.[15] Caused by reactivation of latent herpes virus, the incidence increases with age due to the decline of cellular immunity.[16] With a worse prognosis than Bell's palsy, early treatment with steroids and antiviral medication and an urgent appointment with an otolaryngologist are essential.[17] Treatment for Ramsay Hunt syndrome includes 500 mg famciclovir three times a day for seven days or 800 mg acyclovir five times a day for 7 to 10 days.[18] Oral prednisone of 60 mg daily for 3 to 5 days should also be prescribed.[17] Close monitoring, early audiometric testing, and documentation of the degree of facial paralysis are important in following disease progression and establishing prognosis.

Middle and inner ear

Age-related changes

The middle and inner ear undergo changes with age, including stiffening and thinning of the tympanic membrane and middle ear ossicles, death of inner and outer cochlear hair cells, atherosclerotic changes of inner-ear vessels, and devascularization of the spiral ligament, which impact a patient's auditory and vestibular systems.[1, 2, 19]

Common pathologies

Although otitis media is a common pediatric problem, it may also occur in older adults, often coinciding with upper respiratory tract infections or allergic rhinitis.[20] Acute otitis media presents with rapid onset of pain and possibly fever, accompanied by fullness and erythema of the tympanic membrane and an effusion. Treatment includes amoxicillin 500 mg three times a day for 7–10 days for uncomplicated otitis media, and amoxicillin/clavulanate 875 mg twice a day or 500 mg three times a day for 10–14 days for diabetic or immunocompromised patients.[21] In complicated cases, myringotomy may be performed in the office by an otolaryngologist to provide immediate symptomatic relief.[20] Referral to an otolaryngologist is needed if middle ear effusions are persistent for ≥ 8 weeks, particularly if unilateral, to rule out a nasopharyngeal lesion.[22, 23]

In older adults, acquired cholesteatomas may present as a chronically draining ear with purulent otorrhea, hearing loss, tinnitus, vertigo, and/or facial nerve palsy.[24, 25] On otoscopic exam, there can be tympanic membrane retraction, white debris, granulation tissue, and ossicular erosion. Cholesteatomas are due to squamous epithelium in the middle ear, mastoid, or epitympanium. It is unknown how cholesteatomas form, but hypotheses involve epithelial migration or implantation secondary to instrumentation. Cholesteatomas are benign but can lead to significant morbidity secondary to erosive expansion and damage to surrounding structures. A computed tomography (CT) temporal bone scan without contrast and audiogram are essential to early workup and can be ordered before referral to an otolaryngologist. Treatment by an otolaryngologist generally involves surgical removal. Untreated cholesteatomas can lead to serious complications, including CSF otorrhea, labyrinthine fistulas, ossicular erosion, facial nerve paralysis, mastoiditis, and meningitis.

Auditory

Age-related hearing loss

Treatment of age-related hearing loss generally involves evaluation by an audiologist (a clinician with a master's or doctoral degree in audiology) or hearing instrument specialist/hearing aid dispenser (a technician licensed by the state to dispense and fit hearing aids). Nearly all insurance programs will cover the cost of audiologic testing by an audiologist with a physician's referral, but they will not cover hearing aids, which range from $3,000 to $10,000 for bilateral fitting and follow-up care by an audiologist or hearing aid dispenser. Several need-based outreach programs provide access to discount or free hearing aids through an application process that can be coordinated by the referring audiologist. Over-the-counter assistive listening devices (e.g., Pocket Talker, Comfort Duett) and personal sound amplifiers (devices worn on/in the ear similar to a hearing aid but sold as a consumer electronic device not explicitly for the treatment of hearing loss) can also provide amplification and may be a good option, particularly when hearing aids are not possible due to limited time or financial resources.

For older adults with severe to profound hearing loss who no longer obtain significant benefit from hearing aids, cochlear implantation is an option. Cochlear implantation among older adults is a routine outpatient procedure with a safety profile comparable to implantation in younger adults and children and associated with significant gains in speech perception and quality of life.[26, 27] A cochlear implant directly stimulates the cochlear nerve, bypassing the impaired cochlea, and can restore access to sound and language for many adults with severe hearing loss. Cochlear implantation is covered by Medicare and most other private insurance programs. If there is concern for a severe hearing loss, referral to an otolaryngologist who performs cochlear implants, generally at larger academic centers, is warranted.

Sudden sensorineural hearing loss

Sudden sensorineural hearing loss can be distinguished from an acute conductive hearing loss by history, otoscopy, and the Weber and Rinne tests.[28–30] Sudden sensorineural hearing loss involves at least a 30-decibel hearing loss over three contiguous frequencies that generally occurs acutely and less commonly over one to three days. [28, 31] Patients may notice pressure in the affected ear and transient dizziness.[28, 31] A history and physical should include information about trauma, ear pain, drainage, fever, and other associated illnesses to distinguish between an acute otitis media, which simply requires observation or oral antibiotics/decongestants, and a true sensorineural loss.[28, 32] Sensorineural loss is caused by pathology to the inner ear or auditory nerve from viral infection, tumor, or other etiologies and requires immediate referral to an otolaryngologist for audiologic confirmation, workup, and treatment. Treatment within the first several days is critical for the efficacy of oral corticosteroids (generally 14–21 days of prednisone 1 mg/kg/day with taper) and/or intratympanic steroids (injected directly into the middle ear) in helping to aid hearing recovery.[28]

Tinnitus

Tinnitus is the perception of sound in the absence of external noise.[33] The physical exam and history can differentiate between pulsatile and nonpulsatile tinnitus. Pulsatile tinnitus presents with a rhythmic whooshing sound corresponding to the heartbeat, whereas nonpulsatile tinnitus is described as a ringing or buzzing sound. Persistent pulsatile tinnitus could reflect vascular or other pathologic etiologies (e.g., vascular tumor, benign intracranial hypertension, carotid stenosis) and should be further worked up. Initial workup may include listening for carotid bruits, obtaining a carotid ultrasound, and brain MRI with contrast to evaluate for intracranial masses.

Referral to an otolaryngologist is indicated if pulsatile tinnitus is persistent. Nonpulsatile tinnitus is more common and often seen in the setting of hearing loss and can be exacerbated by neck or back strain, stress, or temporomandibular joint problems. If nonpulsatile tinnitus is sporadic and not bothersome, generally no further evaluation is needed. If it is occasionally bothersome, ambient stimulation, which includes using a sound generator when sleeping or having a radio on in the background, is a simple, low-cost approach to decrease attention directed at tinnitus. Tinnitus is commonly associated with hearing loss, and amplification can assist with symptom management. Tinnitus retraining therapies (e.g., neuromonics) are an option for patients whose daily function is severely impacted, but must be used daily for weeks to months with the aim of decreasing loudness and annoyance. If tinnitus worsens, is very bothersome, or is accompanied by vertigo or change in hearing, evaluation by an otolaryngologist is warranted with further referrals for specialized tinnitus management, including tinnitus retraining, biofeedback, and cognitive behavioral therapy.

Balance

Age-related changes

Presbytasis is the loss of balance due to aging and is caused by changes in mobility, vision, proprioception, and vestibular function.[2] Balance disorders are worsened by polypharmacy and decreased muscle tone of older adults, which increases the risk of falls and worsens health outcomes.[8]

Common pathologies

Vertigo is the sensation of movement in the absence of movement. Benign paroxysmal positional vertigo (BPPV) is the most common cause of vertigo among older adults and is caused by the displacement of otoconia into the semicircular canals.[34] The displacement leads to brief, episodic vertigo lasting one minute or less precipitated by head movements, most commonly turning over in bed. Performing the Dix-Hallpike maneuver and observing for nystagmus can diagnose posterior semicircular canal BPPV.[34–36] Treatment involves maneuvers that shift the otoconia back into place, such as the Epley manuever.[34, 37] If refractory to treatment, referral to an otolaryngologist is necessary.[35]

Another common peripheral cause of vertigo, Ménière's disease, is characterized by spontaneous episodes of vertigo accompanied by fluctuating, low-frequency hearing loss, tinnitus, and a sense of aural fullness.[38] The natural history of Ménière's disease can range from rare episodes to extended periods of vertigo.[34] An individual episode generally lasts for less than one hour.[38] The disorder is thought to originate from excess endolymph within the inner ear that leaks into perilymph, which excites, then inhibits, cranial nerve VIII and basal hair cells.[34, 39] If Ménière's is suspected, referral to an otolaryngologist is needed. Initial treatment involves a low-salt diet (<1,500 mg of sodium per day) and triameterene/hydrochlorothiazide with intratympanic steroids reserved for more refractory cases.[8, 34, 40]

Migrainous vertigo occurs in roughly 25% of migraine patients and is the second most common cause of episodic vertigo.[34, 38, 41] Vertigo can range from seconds to days and occurs in the absence of or prior to a migraine. Pharmacologic treatment consists of migraine treatment with triptans, calcium channel blockers, and beta blockers. Lifestyle measures such as exercise and cutting back on caffeine, sugar, fat, alcohol, and tobacco are also important.

Throat
Swallowing

Age-related changes

Swallowing is a synchronized series of muscle contractions that allows a food bolus to safely enter the stomach.[2, 42] With aging, this process can become problematic due to weakness of masticatory, tongue, and facial muscles. Older patients experience longer swallowing phases that lead to an increased risk of aspiration. This is compounded by the high prevalence of neurologic disorders and polypharmacy in older adults.

Common pathologies

Dysphagia is common in the older population and can be secondary to gastroesophageal reflux disease (GERD), Zenker's diverticulum, autoimmune disease, and neurologic diseases like cerebrovascular accidents.[8, 42] Further functional tests include the modified barium swallow and flexible endoscopy while swallowing.[2] Referral to a speech-language pathologist is often warranted when dysphagia persists, with further evaluation by an otolaryngologist as needed. Treatment of the underlying pathological process is necessary along with rehabilitation. For instance, Zenker's diverticulum is commonly treated with surgery by otolaryngologists.[43] Moreover, simple measures like a soft diet and head-of-bed elevation can help tremendously.

Voice

Age-related changes

The voice undergoes age-related changes including calcification of the laryngeal cartilage, decreased muscular tone, joint stiffening, and bowing of the vocal folds.[2, 44] These changes are compounded by age-related decreases in secretions, nerve conduction speed, and pulmonary function.

Common pathologies

There are numerous etiologies of voice disorders, including GERD, COPD, vocal cord paralysis, and neurologic disorders.[2, 44] Treating the underlying cause and rehabilitation of the voice often involves a multidisciplinary approach with speech pathologists, otolaryngologists, neurologists, and pulmonologists. Treatment of vocal cord paralysis and presbylaryngis with injectables can be done in an office setting or the operating room. Furthermore, hydration and avoidance of tobacco are essential, and sialogogues may be helpful. Warning signs for neoplasm include progressive hoarseness, dysphagia, and a palpable mass, particularly in a smoker.[44]

Nasal cavity and sinus

Age-related changes

Aging of the nasal cavity and sinuses involves decreased smell and taste secondary to loss of olfactory epithelium.[2, 8] Drugs, radiation, trauma, and infections can compound this loss. Loss of moisture due to atrophy of glandular tissue can lead to excessive nasal dryness and increase the risk of epistaxis.[45] This dryness is exacerbated by common medications prescribed to older adults, especially anticoagulants. Lower mucociliary clearance and immunosenescence increase the risk of infection and inflammation.[45–47]

Common pathologies

Rhinitis is common among older adults and can be classified into allergic and nonallergic types.[45] Due to the phenomenon of immunosenescence, nonallergic rhinitis has a higher prevalence in older adults. These two entities are differentiated by skin or blood allergen testing but may coexist in certain patients. Vasomotor rhinitis, a type of nonallergic rhinitis, is thought to be caused by a dysregulated autonomic nervous system, leading to overstimulation of the parasympathetic system.[45, 48] Drug-induced rhinitis is commonly caused by aspirin, NSAIDs, and phosphodiesterase-5 inhibitors, all of which are commonly prescribed to older adults.[45] Rhinitis medicamentosa stems from overuse of intranasal decongestants. Atrophic rhinitis involves degenerative changes of the mucosa, excessive cholinergic activity, and architectural changes of the nasal cavity's blood vessels and connective tissue. Gustatory rhinitis involves copious rhinorrhea during meals. General rhinitis symptoms include rhinorrhea, sneezing, coughing, nasal drainage, difficulty smelling, and postnasal drip. Initial treatment modalities can include intranasal steroids (e.g., fluticasone nasal), antihistamines, and anticholinergics as well as second-generation antihistamines.[45, 49]

Sinusitis is inflammation or infection of the sinus cavities; it may occur independently of or concurrent with rhinitis.[8, 50] Bacteria, viruses, and other noninfectious etiologies can cause acute sinusitis. Suspect a bacterial cause when symptoms are present for 10 or more days or worsen after a period of initial improvement. Symptoms can last up to four weeks and involve congestion, sneezing, purulent nasal discharge, epistaxis, and facial pain and fullness. For acute uncomplicated cases, imaging is not recommended. Amoxicillin is the treatment of choice for acute bacterial sinusitis and trimethoprim-sulfamethoxazole or macrolides for penicillin allergics, while symptomatic relief is given for viral causes.[51] Treatment can also include intranasal steroids and hypertonic (3%–5%) saline nasal irrigation. Limited evidence, which demonstrates modest benefit in symptom relief, supports adjunctive systemic corticosteroids.[52] Antihistamines, decongestants, anticholinergics, leukotriene inhibitors, and mucolytics can also be employed.[51]

Chronic sinusitis is common among older adults due to decreased effectiveness of the aging immune system.[8] Chronic sinusitis results from allergies or viral infections that lead to increased secretions, poor mucocilary function, and obstruction with possible superimposed bacterial infection. If obstruction continues, the sinus mucus membranes can undergo fibrosis, which further impairs the ability to clear pathogens. Chronic rhinosinusitis is defined as 12 weeks or longer of two or more of the following: mucopurulent drainage, congestion, facial pain/pressure/fullness, decreased smell, as well as documentation of purulence or edema in the nasal cavity, polyps, or radiographic imaging of sinus inflammation.[50] When symptoms of headache and facial pain predominate, physicians must differentiate chronic sinusitis from migraine, which is challenging given overlap in symptoms and patient demographics.[53] Referral to an otolaryngologist is needed if symptoms persist for more than four weeks.

Invasive fungal sinusitis is potentially life threatening but generally only needs to be considered in diabetic and immunocompromised patients.[54, 55] Mucormycosis is a rare, potentially fatal infection that occurs in the setting of ketoacidosis, hematologic malignancy, and neutropenia. Mucosal gangrene results from infiltration of vasculature with fungi. Symptoms include congestion, fever, sinus pain, rhinorrhea, cranial nerve palsies, abrupt change in vision, and alterations in consciousness. The infection can erode through adjacent bone, spread along blood vessels and nerves, and lead to intracranial involvement and death. A CT and nasal endoscopy are needed to classify spread, and treatment is intravenous antibiotics and urgent surgery.

Epistaxis has a bimodal distribution with peaks in children and older adults.[56] With aging, the nasal cavity experiences loss of fat and sclerosing of small vasculature.[45] Older adults also experience increased nasal dryness, atrophic rhinitis, neoplasms, and drugs that predispose to bleeding.[56] Secondary causes of epistaxis include trauma, iatrogenic injury, and liver disease. Most bleeds occur from the anterior septum and can be easily treated by having the patient put his/her chin to the chest (which avoids blood going into the nasopharynx), liberal application of topical decongestant, and firmly pinching the lower lateral cartilages of the nose to fully obstruct the nostrils for 5–10 minutes (10–15 minutes if the patient is taking an anticoagulant). Prevention of epistaxis with nasal moisture is essential and includes regular nasal saline sprays with daily application of petroleum-based jelly to the nares.

Lastly, anosmia is a common complaint in older adults and can be due to rhinitis, loss of olfactory neuroepithelial cells, drugs, neoplasms, and Alzheimer's disease.[57] If symptoms worsen, are particularly bothersome, or do not appear to be secondary to rhinitis, referral to an otolaryngologist may be warranted.

Oral cavity

Age-related changes

The oral cavity tends to become drier with age due to decreased glandular acinar tissue, making dry mouth a common complaint.[2, 45] Older adults are at risk for dental caries and gum disease because of decreased yet thicker saliva and lower IgA levels. There is also noted mandibular and maxillary bone resorption, which can worsen the fit of dentures. Ill-fitting dentures can cause paresthesia and a burning sensation from persistent contact with the mental nerve. Sensory abilities decline with decreased olfactory cells and taste buds, which can result in malnutrition.

Common pathologies

White lesions are often found in the oral cavity of older adults and have a wide differential diagnosis (Table 40.1).[54] Oral candidiasis is most commonly due to a fungal infection by *Candida albicans* and frequently seen in the elderly because of the high prevalence of immunocompromised states and diabetes. Candidiasis can also be secondary to

Table 40.1 Characteristics of common oral lesions [54, 58, 61]

Lesion	Characteristics	Management
Candidiasis	White plaques with an erythematous foundation that can be removed; angular chelitis may be present	Topical nystatin or azole class antifungals
Leukoplakia	White patch that cannot be removed	Refer for biopsy and removal
Erythroplakia	Red velvety lesion	Refer for biopsy and removal
Neoplasm	Persistent ulcer or protruding mass	Refer for biopsy, removal, and management

inhalational steroid use, dentures, or antibiotic treatment. On oral exam, there are white plaques with erythematous foundations. Cytology or culture can be performed but are not necessary for diagnosis. Treatment is with topical antifungals in the form of lozenges, liquids, or creams.[54, 58] Oral leukoplakia is a white patch that cannot be rubbed away and generally results from persistent irritation leading to hyperkeratosis.[59, 60] Oral leukoplakia is a diagnosis of exclusion, and malignant transformation is uncommon. Similarly, erythroplakia is an oral red, velvety lesion that is a diagnosis of exclusion. However, it is less common but with higher malignant potential.[60] Referral for biopsy by an otolaryngologist or oral surgeon can rule out malignancy, and subsequent management involves removal of the lesion with surgical or laser treatments and avoidance of risk factors.[61]

The parotid gland can be bilaterally enlarged secondary to viral infections or autoimmune disorders like Sjögren's syndrome.[62, 63] Bacterial parotitis is common among older adults and can be secondary to dehydration or obstruction of Stensen's duct by a sialolith. Presentation involves sudden onset of unilateral warmth, erythema, pain, and edema over the cheek and can be accompanied by fever, purulent exudate, and, often, trismus. With milking of the parotid (i.e., firmly stroking the parotid from the anterior tragus to the corner of the mouth), cultures can be obtained from the Stensen's duct for suspected bacterial parotitis to aid in antibiotic selection. Treatment involves intravenous hydration, antibiotics, regular use of sialogogues (hard, sour candies), aggressive external and bimanual cheek massage two to three times daily to "milk" the gland, application of heat, and, if needed, surgical drainage of an abscess or stone removal.[64] Empiric treatment for *Staphylococcus aureus* with vancomycin 15 mg/kg IV q12 and clindamycin 600 mg IV q8h may be warranted, particularly given the prevalence of MRSA among nursing home residents.[64, 65] Acute bacterial parotitis in frail, elderly adults has a poor prognosis, so early intervention is vital.[62, 66]

Facial nerve palsy

Bell's palsy is a sudden-onset, idiopathic facial paralysis and is thought to be secondary to reactivation of latent herpes simplex virus.[17] Incidence increases with age, and facial palsy can also be secondary to cholesteatomas, trauma, and parotid gland and skull base tumors.[17, 67] The degree of facial paralysis is an important prognostic indicator, where total paralysis is less likely to regain full function. Loss of facial sensation in the affected area, otalgia, hyperacusis, taste changes, and decreased lacrimation are common. Evaluation includes thorough head and neck examination involving palpation of the parotid gland and neurologic testing focusing on cranial nerves and cerebellar function. Treatment consists of 60 mg of prednisone daily for seven to fourteen days with 5-day taper, or 50 mg prednisolone for 10 days within 72 hours of symptom onset.[68] Although the efficacy of antivirals is controversial, early treatment with 1,000 mg valacyclovir three times a day for one week is a treatment option.[68–71] To prevent corneal damage, it is essential to use moisturizing eye drops frequently and protect the involved eye at night.[17] Referral to an otolaryngologist or neurologist is warranted unless the history and physical are strongly consistent with a simple Bell's palsy.[68]

Head and neck cancer

The risk of head and neck cancer increases with age due to the cumulative exposure of carcinogens and immunosenescence.[2] Thyroid cancer tends to be more aggressive in older adults, so midline neck masses should be treated with high suspicion. Presentation of head and neck cancer varies widely depending on the site of lesion. Nasopharyngeal cancers can present with a variety of symptoms, including nasal obstruction, epistaxis, Eustachian tube dysfunction, otalgia, and cranial neuropathies.[72] Oral cavity carcinoma presents with a persistent, ulcerative lesion, while swollen lymph nodes can be the presentation of lymphoma or a nonspecific finding of many head and neck cancers.[59] Referral to an otolaryngologist is necessary in any cases concerning possible head and neck cancer.

Further reading

Key references include:

- *Bailey's Head and Neck Surgery – Otolaryngology*, 5th Edition. Baltimore, MD: Lippincott Williams & Wilkens, 2014.
- *Cummings Otolaryngology – Head and Neck Surgery*, 5th Edition. Philadelphia, PA: Mosby Elsevier, 2010.

- American Academy of Otolaryngology – Head and Neck Surgery Guidelines. Available at: www.entnet.org/guidelines.

References

1. Weinstein BE. Aging of the outer, middle and inner ear and neural pathways. In: *Geriatric Audiology*. 2nd ed. New York, NY: Thieme; 2000:55–80.

2. Seshamani M, Kashima ML. Special considerations in managing geriatric patients. In: Flint PW, Haughey BH, Lund VJ, et al., eds. *Cummings Otolaryngology Head & Neck Surgery*. 5th ed. Philadelphia, PA: Mosby Elsevier; 2010:230–238.

3. Roland PS, Smith TL, Schwartz SR, et al. Clinical practice guideline: cerumen impaction. *Otolaryngol Head Neck Surg.* 2008;**139**:S1–S21.

4. Lum CL, Jeyanthi S, Prepageran N, et al. Antibacterial and antifungal properties of human cerumen. *J Laryngol Otol.* 2009;**123**:375–378.

5. Kutz JW, Isaacson B, Roland PS. Aging and the auditory and vestibular system. In: Johnson JT, Rosen CA, eds. *Bailey's Head and Neck Surgery: Otolaryngology*. Vol **2**. 5th ed. Philadelphia, PA: Lippincott Williams & Wilkins; 2014:2615–2623.

6. Rubin J, Yu VL, Kamerer DB, Wagener M. Aural irrigation with water: a potential pathogenic mechanism for inducing malignant external otitis? *Ann Otol Rhinol Laryngol.* 1990;**99**:117–119.

7. Weinroth SE, Schessel D, Tuazon CU. Malignant otitis externa in AIDS patients: case report and review of the literature. *Ear Nose Throat J.* 1994;**73**:772–774, 777–778.

8. Bailey BJ. Geriatric otolaryngology. In: Bailey BJ, Johnson JT, eds. *Head and Neck Surgery – Otolaryngology*. Vol **1**. 4th ed. Philadelphia, PA: Lippincott Williams & Wilkins; 2006:235–245.

9. Nathan CO, Lian TS. Cutaneous malignancy. In: Johnson JT, Rosen CA, eds. *Bailey's Head and Neck Surgery: Otolaryngology*. 5th ed. Philadelphia, PA: Lippincott Williams & Wilkins; 2014:1723–1738.

10. Fitzpatrick TB. Soleil et peau [Sun and skin]. *Journal de Médecine Esthétique.* 1975;**2**:33–34.

11. Ussmuller J, Hartwein J, Rauchfuss A, Sanchez-Hanke M. Primary carcinoma of the ear canal. Clinical aspects, intratemporal growth behavior and surgical strategy. *HNO.* 2001;**49**:256–263.

12. Linstrom CJ, Lucente FE. Diseases of the external ear. In: Johnson JT, Rosen CA, eds. *Bailey's Head and Neck Surgery: Otolaryngology*. 5th ed. Philadelphia, PA: Lippincott Williams & Wilkins; 2014:2333–2357.

13. Handzel O, Auwaerter PG. Otitis externa. Available at: www.hopkinsguides.com/hopkins/ub/view/Johns_Ho pkins_ABX_Guide/540407/all/Otitis_Externa?q=acut e%20otitis%20externa. Accessed May 8, 2014.

14. Rosenfeld RM, Schwartz SR, Cannon CR, et al. Clinical practice guideline: acute otitis externa. *Otolaryngol Head Neck Surg.* 2014;**150**:S1–S24.

15. Guss J, Ruckenstein MJ. Infections of the exernal ear. In: Flint PW, Haughey BH, Lund VJ, et al., eds. *Cummings Otolaryngology Head and Neck Surgery*. 5th ed. Philadelphia, PA: Mosby Elsevier; 2010:1944–1949.

16. Burke BL, Steele RW, Beard OW, et al. Immune responses to varicella-zoster in the aged. *Arch Intern Med.* 1982;**142**:291–293.

17. Vrabec JT, Lin JW. Acute paralysis of the facial nerve. In: Johnson JT, Rosen CA, eds. *Bailey's Head and Neck Surgery: Otolaryngology*. 5th ed. Philadelphia, PA: Lippincott Williams & Wilkins; 2014:2503–2518.

18. Uscategui T, Doree C, Chamberlain IJ, Burton MJ. Antiviral therapy for Ramsay Hunt syndrome (herpes zoster oticus with facial palsy) in adults. *Cochrane Database Syst Rev.* 2008;**4**:CD006851.

19. Etholm B, Belal A Jr. Senile changes in the middle ear joints. *Ann Otol Rhinol Laryngol.* 1974;**83**:49–54.

20. Casselbrant ML, Mandel EM. Otitis media in the age of antimicrobial resistance. In: Johnson JT, Rosen CA, eds. *Bailey's Head and Neck Surgery: Otolaryngology*. 5th ed. Philadelphia, PA: Lippincott Williams & Wilkins; 2014:1479–1506.

21. Handzel O, Auwaerter PG. Acute Otitis Media, Adult. Available at: www.hopkinsguides.com/hopkins/ub/view/ Johns_Hopkins_ABX_Guide/540408/3/Acute_Otitis_M edia_Adult_?q=otitis%20media. Accessed May 8, 2014.

22. Ramakrishnan K, Sparks RA, Berryhill WE. Diagnosis and treatment of otitis media. *Am Fam Physician.* 2007;**76**:1650–1658.

23. O'Reilly RC, Sando I. Anatomy and physiology of the eustachian tube. In: Flint PW, Haughey BH, Lund VJ, et al., eds. *Cummings Otolaryngology Head and Neck Surgery*. 5th ed. Philadelphia, PA: Mobsy Elsevier; 2010:1866–1875.

24. Meyer TA, Strunk CL, Lambert PR. Cholesteatoma. In: Johnson JT, Rosen CA, eds. *Bailey's Head and Neck Surgery: Otolaryngology*. Vol **2**. 5th ed. Philadelphia, PA: Lippincott Williams & Wilkins; 2014:2433–2446.

25. Chang CYJ. Cholesteatoma. In: Lalwani AK, ed. *Current Diagnosis and Treatment in Otolaryngology – Head and Neck Surgery*. 3rd ed. New York, NY: McGraw-Hill; 2012.

26. Sprinzl GM, Riechelmann H. Current trends in treating hearing loss in elderly people: a review of the technology and treatment options – a mini-review. *Gerontology.* 2010;**56**:351–358.

27. Chen DS, Clarrett DM, Li L, et al. Cochlear implantation in older adults: long-term analysis of complications and device survival in a consecutive series. *Otol Neurotol.* 2013;**34**:1272–1277.

28. Stachler RJ, Chandrasekhar SS, Archer SM, et al. Clinical practice guideline: sudden hearing loss. *Otolaryngol Head Neck Surg.* 2012;**146**:S1–S35.

29. Bagai A, Thavendiranathan P, Detsky AS. Does this patient have hearing impairment? *JAMA.* 2006;**295**:416–428.

30. Thijs C, Leffers P. Sensitivity and specificity of Rinne tuning fork test. *BMJ.* 1989;**298**:255.

31. Oliver ER, Hashisaki GT. Sudden sensory hearing loss. In: Johnson JT, Rosen CA, eds. *Bailey's Head and Neck Surgery: Otolaryngology.* Vol **2**. 5th ed. Philadelphia, PA: Lippincott Williams & Wilkins; 2014:2589–2595.

32. Conlin AE, Parnes LS. Treatment of sudden sensorineural hearing loss: I. A systematic review. *Arch Otolaryngol Head Neck Surg.* 2007;**133**:573–581.

33. Cosetti MK, Roehm PC. Tinnitus and hyperacusis. In: Johnson JT, Rosen CA, eds. *Bailey's Head and Neck Surgery: Otolaryngology.* 5th ed. Philadelphia, PA: Lippincott Williams & Wilkins; 2014:2597–2614.

34. Agrawal Y, Minor LB, Carey JP. Peripheral vestibular disorders. In: Johnson JT, Rosen CA, eds. *Bailey's Head and Neck Surgery: Otolaryngology.* 5th ed. Philadelphia, PA: Lippincott Williams & Wilkins; 2014:2701–2716.

35. Bhattacharyya N, Baugh RF, Orvidas L, et al. Clinical practice guideline: benign paroxysmal positional vertigo. *Otolaryngol Head Neck Surg.* 2008;**139**:S47–S81.

36. Dix MR, Hallpike CS. The pathology symptomatology and diagnosis of certain common disorders of the vestibular system. *Proc R Soc Med.* 1952;**45**:341–354.

37. Hilton M, Pinder D. The Epley (canalith repositioning) manoeuvre for benign paroxysmal positional vertigo. *Cochrane Database Syst Rev.* 2004;**2**:CD003162.

38. Ishiyama G, Ishiyama A. Central vestibular disorders. In: Johnson JT, Rosen CA, eds. *Bailey's Head and Neck Surgery: Otolaryngology.* 5th ed. Philadelphia, PA: Lippincott Williams & Wilkins; 2014:2717–2732.

39. Schuknecht HF. Meniere's disease: a correlation of symptomatology and pathology. *Laryngoscope.* 1963;**73**:651–665.

40. Phillips JS, Westerberg B. Intratympanic steroids for Meniere's disease or syndrome. *Cochrane Database Syst Rev.* 2011;**7**:CD008514.

41. Kayan A, Hood JD. Neuro-otological manifestations of migraine. *Brain.* 1984;**107**(Pt 4):1123–1142.

42. Lundy DS. Swallowing – patient safety and medicinal therapy for ear, nose, and throat disorders. In: *Geriatric Care Otolaryngology.* Alexandria, VA: American Academy of Otolaryngology – Head and Neck Surgery Foundation; 2006:86–101.

43. Eibling DE. Management of intractable aspiration. In: Johnson JT, Rosen CA, eds. *Bailey's Head and Neck Surgery: Otolaryngology.* Vol **1**. 5th ed. Philadelphia, PA: Lippincott Williams & Wilkins; 2014:859–867.

44. Benninger MS, Abitbol J. Voice – dysphonia and the aging voice. In: *Geriatric Care Otolaryngology.* Alexandria, VA: American Academy of Otolaryngology – Head and Neck Surgery; 2006:66–85.

45. Varga-Huettner VE, Pinto J. Physiology of the aging nose and geriatric rhinitis. In: Onerci TM, ed. *Nasal Physiology and Pathophysiology of Nasal Disorders.* Heidelberg: Springer; 2013:165–181.

46. Kim SW, Mo JH, Kim JW, et al. Change of nasal function with aging in Korean. *Acta Otolaryngol Suppl.* 2007;(558):90–94.

47. Alford RH. Effects of chronic bronchopulmonary disease and aging on human nasal secretion IgA concentrations. *J Immunol.* 1968;**101**:984–988.

48. Lal D, Corey JP. Vasomotor rhinitis update. *Curr Opin Otolaryngol Head Neck Surg.* 2004;**12**:243–247.

49. Sur DK, Scandale S. Treatment of allergic rhinitis. *Am Fam Physician.* 2010;**81**:1440–1446.

50. Rosenfeld RM, Andes D, Bhattacharyya N, et al. Clinical practice guideline: adult sinusitis. *Otolaryngol Head Neck Surg.* 2007;**137**:S1–S31.

51. Suh JD, Chiu AG. Medical management of chronic sinusitis. In: Johnson JT, Rosen CA, eds. *Bailey's Head and Neck Surgery: Otolaryngology.* 5th ed. Philadelphia, PA: Lippincott Williams & Wilkins; 2014:586–594.

52. Venekamp RP, Thompson MJ, Hayward G, et al. Systemic corticosteroids for acute sinusitis. *Cochrane Database Syst Rev.* 2014;**3**:CD008115.

53. Deconde AS, Mace JC, Smith TL. The impact of comorbid migraine on quality of life outcomes after endoscopic sinus surgery. *Laryngoscope.* 2014;**124**(8):1750–1755.

54. Wein RO, O'Leary M. Stomatitis. In: Johnson JT, Rosen CA, eds. *Bailey's Head and Neck Surgery: Otolaryngology.* 5th ed. Philadelphia, PA: Lippincott Williams & Wilkins; 2014:736–756.

55. Adelson RT, Marple BF, Ryan MW. Fungal rhinosinusitis. In: Johnson JT, Rosen CA, eds. *Bailey's Head and Neck Surgery: Otolaryngology.* 5th ed. Philadelphia, PA: Lippincott Williams & Wilkins; 2014:557–572.

56. Bleier BS, Schlosser RJ. Epistaxis. In: Johnson JT, Rosen CA, eds. *Bailey's Head and Neck Surgery: Otolaryngology.* 5th ed. Philadelphia, PA: Lippincott Williams & Wilkins; 2014:501–508.

57. Holbrook EH, Leopold DA. Olfaction. In: Johnson JT, Rosen CA, eds. *Bailey's Head and Neck Surgery: Otolaryngology.* 5th ed. Philadelphia, PA: Lippincott Williams & Wilkins; 2014:371–378.

58. Gonsalves WC, Chi AC, Neville BW. Common oral lesions: Part I. Superficial mucosal lesions. *Am Fam Physician*. 2007;75:501–507.

59. Deschler DG, Erman AB. Oral cavity cancer. In: Johnson JT, Rosen CA, eds. *Bailey's Head and Neck Surgery: Otolaryngology*. 5th ed. Philadelphia, PA: Lippincott Williams & Wilkins; 2014:1849–1874.

60. Vaezi A, Grandis JR. Head and neck tumor biology. In: Johnson JT, Rosen CA, eds. *Bailey's Head and Neck Surgery: Otolaryngology*. 5th ed. Philadelphia, PA: Lippincott Williams & Wilkins; 2014:1645–1671.

61. Gonsalves WC, Chi AC, Neville BW. Common oral lesions: Part II. Masses and neoplasia. *Am Fam Physician*. 2007;75:509–512.

62. Coutaz M, Morisod J. The acute bacterial parotitis of the elderly. *Rev Med Suisse*. 2009;5:1942–1945.

63. Butt FY. Benign diseases of the salivary glands. In: Lalwani AK, ed. *Current Diagnosis and Treatment in Otolaryngology-Head and Neck Surgery*. 3rd ed. New York, NY: McGraw-Hill; 2012:chap 18.

64. Rogers J, McCaffrey TV. Inflammatory disorders of the salivary glands. In: Flint PW, Haughey BH, Lund VJ, et al., eds. *Cummings Otolaryngology Head & Neck Surgery*. 5th ed. Philadelphia, PA: Mosby Elsevier; 2010:1151–1161.

65. Bartlett JG. Parotitis. Available at: www.hopkinsguides.com/hopkins/ub/view/Johns_Hopkins_ABX_Guide/540418/3/Parotitis?q=facial%20palsy (accessed May 8, 2014).

66. Coutaz M. Acute bacterial parotitis in the frail elderly subject: a harbinger of death? *J Am Med Dir Assoc*. 2014;15(5):269–270.

67. Rowlands S, Hooper R, Hughes R, Burney P. The epidemiology and treatment of Bell's palsy in the UK. *Eur J Neurol*. 2002;9:63–67.

68. Baugh RF, Basura GJ, Ishii LE, et al. Clinical practice guideline: Bell's palsy. *Otolaryngol Head Neck Surg*. 2013;149:S1–S27.

69. Engstrom M, Berg T, Stjernquist-Desatnik A, et al. Prednisolone and valaciclovir in Bell's palsy: a randomised, double-blind, placebo-controlled, multicentre trial. *Lancet Neurol*. 2008;7:993–1000.

70. Gronseth GS, Paduga R, American Academy of Neurology. Evidence-based guideline update: steroids and antivirals for Bell palsy: report of the Guideline Development Subcommittee of the American Academy of Neurology. *Neurology*. 2012;79:2209–2213.

71. Schwartz SR, Jones SL, Getchius TS, Gronseth GS. Reconciling the clinical practice guidelines on Bell's palsy from the AAO-HNSF and the AAN. *Otolaryngol Head Neck Surg*. 2014;150:709–711.

72. Wei WI, Chua DTT. Nasopharyngeal carcinoma. In: Johnson JT, Rosen CA, eds. *Bailey's Head and Neck Surgery: Otolaryngology*. Vol 2. 5th ed. Philadelphia, PA: Lippincott Williams & Wilkins; 2014:1875–1897.

Dental care for the elderly patient

Allen D. Samuelson, DDS

Preface

The goal of an ethical dental professional is to provide patient-centered and preventive-directed care for patients. The American Dental Association (ADA) defines dentistry as "evaluation, diagnosis, prevention and/or treatment (nonsurgical, surgical or related procedures) of diseases, disorders and/or conditions of the oral cavity, maxillofacial area and/or the adjacent and associated structures and their impact on the human body; provided by a dentist, within the scope of his/her education, training and experience, in accordance with the ethics of the profession and applicable law."[1] The standard levels of prevention that apply to medicine are applicable to dentistry. Primary prevention "forestalls the onset, reverses the progression of and arrests the disease process before treatment becomes necessary." Secondary prevention involves "routine treatment methods to terminate a disease process and restore tissues to as near normal as possible." Tertiary prevention "employs measures to replace lost tissues and to rehabilitate patients to the point that physical capabilities and/or mental attitudes are as near normal as possible after the failure of primary prevention."[2]

The practicing physician must have a basic knowledge of the oral and maxillofacial region as well as the pathological changes likely to occur, as these changes may reflect systemic health. Recent research has shown a correlation between oral health and systemic health, such that the relationship can no longer be ignored. Specifically, periodontitis has been linked to cardiovascular disease and diabetes as well as to pre-term low-birth-weight infants.[3–15] Oral disease such as periodontitis and dental caries, specifically root surface caries, is particularly prevalent in the elderly population.

The baby boomer generation will present challenges to the medical health-care system and to those delivering dental care. The rate of edentulism for those over age 65 has dropped from 40% in the 1980s to around 20% in the beginning of the twenty-first century. Furthermore, there will be a large increase in older adults retaining their natural teeth over the next few decades. Therefore, dental caries and periodontitis will be present in many geriatric patients due to the increase in retention of teeth.[16–19]

Introduction

As the initial portion of the aero-digestive tract, the maxillofacial structures form an important, interrelated complex of skin, mucosa, joints, bones, glandular tissues, vessels, ligaments, tendons, nerves, and teeth. Many diseases can affect one or more of these structures, and therefore effect change or loss of function, which can result in decreased quality of life. Discomfort, dysfunction, or malformations in this region can severely affect an individual's ability to thrive.[20]

Oral prosthetic devices are often used to improve comfort, function, health, and esthetics. These devices can be fixed or removable prostheses, such as dental implants, fixed partial dentures, crowns, dentures (full and partial), jaw positioning and protective devices, orthodontic hardware, as well as obturators to repair deformations. Elderly patients are more likely to have one or more of these devices in their mouths. Oral prostheses may fit and function very well or very poorly. Over time, they can fatigue and fail, requiring repair or replacement.

Since an oral prosthesis can fail over time, the general or geriatric medicine physician is in a good position to screen for problems by including a brief

---

Reichel's Care of the Elderly, 7th Edition, ed. Jan Busby-Whitehead *et al.* Published by Cambridge University Press.
© Cambridge University Press 2016.

dental history as well as an oral and maxillofacial examination within the framework of the routine general physical examination. The time-honored history and techniques of inspection, palpation, percussion, and auscultation are certainly valid when examining the maxillofacial structures and oral cavity. This chapter serves as an introduction to the general characteristics, basic anatomy, and age-related changes that can be expected in the oral cavity and maxillofacial region.[21–32]

Oral mucosa

General characteristics and anatomy

Mucosa is the lining epithelium and connective tissue of the oral cavity and has similar functions to that of the skin in that it serves as a barrier for protection of underlying structures. There are differing levels of mucosal thickness and keratinization depending on location. There are three distinct types of mucosa present in the oral cavity: masticatory, lining, and specialized. The gingiva and hard palate are lined with masticatory mucosa that is keratinized. Masticatory mucosa does not stretch and serves to bear the forces and friction of mastication. The soft palate, ventral tongue, floor of mouth, and the alveolar and buccal mucosa are all nonkeratinized and designed to stretch and allow for movement of the underlying muscular and bony tissues. The mucosa on the dorsum of the tongue and vermillion border of the lips is known as specialized mucosa. The tongue is coated with taste buds and papillae of various types (foliate, fungiform, filiform, circumvallate) and the vermillion border, only present in humans, serves as a transitional zone between skin and mucosa on the lips. All mucosal tissues should be moist and pink or red in color without ulcerations, masses, inflammation, cleft, or defect. Depending on the skin tones of the individual, racial pigmentation may be present in various areas of the mucosal surfaces, including the tongue. The tongue should be clean and pink without staining or hyperplastic papillae. The mucosal tissues present over the alveolar ridges should be smooth, pink, firm, and without ulcerations.

Age-related changes

Although there is conflicting data as to exactly how aging affects the oral mucosa, it is generally agreed that change does occur. The lining mucosal tissues in older adults are thinner, smoother, and drier than those of younger cohorts. There are studies that indicate nutritional factors such as iron or B-vitamin deficiencies, and not age per se, may be the cause of these changes. The floor of the mouth and ventral tongue can exhibit varicosities. Additionally, the tongue mucosa may likewise become thinner with loss of filiform papillae. Moreover, sun exposure can cause changes in the vermillion border – specifically, a loss of distinct delineation.

The most worrisome mucosal lesion is that of oral cancer. (See Box 41.1.)

There are many types of cancerous lesions that may occur in the oral cavity, including melanoma, squamous cell carcinoma, and various sarcomas. The most common oral cancer is squamous cell carcinoma. Squamous cell carcinoma can appear as a white, red, or mixed lesion, generally firm and painless. Common regions of occurrence are the floor of the mouth, ventral tongue, and palatal tissues.

Several mucosal changes can be manifestations of oral side effects of medications. These can include xerostomia, lichenoid drug reaction (resembling lichen planus), mucositis, gingival hyperplasia, and allergic reactions. Xerostomia is particularly worrisome as it causes oral discomfort. Without saliva there is a lack of the buffering capacity and lubrication, and teeth are at high risk for dental caries. This will be discussed later in the text. Additionally, there are several systemic diseases that may manifest in the oral structures, such as diabetes mellitus, Crohn's disease, leukemia, and lymphoma.

Examination techniques

The oral mucosa should be inspected with good lighting. Make certain that all removable prosthetic devices have been removed from the mouth prior to the examination. The lips and buccal and labial mucosa should be inspected for macules, papules, ulcerations, or other abnormalities. The hard and soft palate can likewise be inspected. These structures can also be palpated using the bimanual technique or with a single digit in order to detect intramucosal masses or tenderness over any region. Residual ridges bearing a prosthetic device such as a denture should be inspected and palpated for irritation, reactive lesions, or other pathological entity. In patients who use tobacco and alcohol, the risk for oral cancerous lesions is elevated.

BOX 41.1 Cancer: oral/neck radiation/chemotherapy consideration

Chemotherapeutic agents and radiation (particularly radiation to the head and neck) pose risks of several oral complications, including:

1. Mucositis causing pain, risk of infection, and difficulty with nutrition and hydration.
2. Xerostomia and salivary gland dysfunction – leading to oral discomfort, dysguesia, and difficulty swallowing, speaking, and chewing. The risk of dental caries increases greatly.
3. Taste alterations
4. Neurotoxicity
5. Bleeding (generally – platelets should be 50 k–65 k before dental extraction)
6. Radiation caries – can be very rapidly progressing
7. Trismus/tissue fibrosis – can limit access to the oral cavity greatly
8. Osteoradionecrosis – may require hyperbaric oxygen prior to any surgical work (e.g., dental extraction)

It is CRITICAL for a physician who is caring for a patient who is planned to have radiation (particularly to the head and neck), chemotherapy, or immune suppressive agents (e.g., post-transplant) to refer to a dentist for a full evaluation of the patient to optimize treatment and prevention and quality of life long term.

Source: National Cancer Institute – PDQ Cancer Information Summaries. Oral Complications of Chemotherapy and Head/Neck Radiation (PDQ®) Health Professional Version. Last update April 10, 2014. www.cancer.gov/cancertopics/pdq/supportivecare/oralcomplications/HealthProfessional (accessed May 11, 2014.)

Joints and osteology

General characteristics and anatomy

The maxilla and mandible articulate via the temporomandibular joint (TMJ). This bilateral, complex structure defined as a ginglymoid diarthroidial joint allows for many of the functions listed in the introductory paragraph. This joint is unique in that it allows for translation and rotation in two axes. A fibrocartilaginous disk is interposed between the condyler head of the mandible and the fossa in the skull base. The TMJ should display a good range of motion laterally and in protrusion without limitations, deviations, pain, dysfunction, or noise. The average maximum voluntary opening for the human mouth is about 50 mm–55 mm and for lateral movements approximately 10 mm–11 mm. The teeth, known as gomphoses or immobile joints, will be discussed later in the chapter. (See Box 41.2.)

The maxillofacial osteology is complex. There are many bones working in concert for the survival, protection, and function of the person. There are several foramina where nerves, blood vessels, and lymphatics exit. The mandible and maxilla are the primary bony structures of concern in this chapter. Both the mandible and maxilla are intramembranous bones in that they are formed by ossification of the mesenchymal tissues in the developing fetus and newborn. There should be facial symmetry, and these bones, along with others, should provide for good support of the facial soft tissues. Several muscles of mastication have their origin and insertion on the maxilla and mandible to allow for the motor functions listed in the introductory paragraph. Located within several bones of the maxillofacial region are sinus cavities of various sizes. The maxillary sinus is located within the maxillary bones and should be healthy and pain free. Intraorally, all bony tissue should be covered with nonulcerated lining or masticatory mucosa unless a recent dental extraction has occurred. There may be protuberances of bone on the buccal or lingual of the alveolus. These rock hard, immobile structures are generally normal and are termed "exostoses" or "tori."

Age-related changes

The TMJ may develop pain related to arthritis or other functional disturbances. Arthritic changes can cause pain, deviations, and limitations of motion. Noises such as clicking, popping, or crepitations within the joint can signal displacement or distortion of the articular disc mentioned previously.[33]

Many of the changes that occur in the peripheral skeleton and joints occur in the maxillofacial region. Periosteal expansion, thinning of cortical bone, and gradual loss of trabecular bone can cause fragility and loss of support for the dental structures. If teeth are lost,

589

BOX 41.2 Antiresorptive and other medications and osteonecrosis of the jaws

There are several medications used for a variety of reasons ranging from osteoporosis to metastatic bone disease that can adversely affect bone healing, particularly in the jaws. The physician considering placing a patient on one of these medications, particularly via the intravenous route, should refer the patient to a dentist for a comprehensive dental examination. During the comprehensive examination it should be determined if restorative and surgical treatment is needed, and preventive education should be stressed. Examples of medication classes that may affect bone/soft tissue healing in the mouth include:

1. IV and oral bisphosphonates
2. receptor activator of nuclear factor kappa-B (RANK) ligand inhibitors
3. antiangiogenic medications
4. tyrosine kinase inhibitors

The ideal time frame for referral is *prior to* the initiation of these treatments. It is *critical* for a physician who is caring for a patient for whom these classes of medications are to be prescribed to refer the patient to a dentist for a full evaluation to optimize prevention and treatment.

Source: Ruggiero SL, Dodson TD, et al. Medication-Related Osteonecrosis of the Jaw – 2014 – Update. American Association of Oral and Maxillofacial Surgeons: Special Committee on Medication-Related Osteonecrosis of the Jaws. Available at: www.aaoms.org.

this can result in loss of alveolar bone, which will continue throughout life. When alveolar bone loss becomes severe, prosthetic reconstruction can become difficult. Additionally, osteoporosis may be a risk factor for the development of periodontal disease, which can result in loss of alveolar bone and teeth.[34–35]

Examination techniques

The bones of the maxillofacial region should be inspected for symmetry and masses. They can be palpated to note masses, tenderness, or fracture. The sinus cavities, particularly the maxillary sinus, can be percussed to evaluate pain and transilluminated to evaluate for mucosal changes indicative of sinusitis. The TMJ can be inspected for range of motion, deviations, or other dysfunction. It can also be palpated for tenderness and clicks, pops, or crepitations. The TMJ can be auscultated directly anterior to the tragus of the ear to evaluate for joint sounds. Intraorally, the bony structures of the maxilla and mandible can be inspected and palpated to note any pathological entities.

Muscles of mastication and facial expression

General characteristics and anatomy

There are two major muscle groups in the maxillofacial region: the muscles of facial expression innervated by cranial nerve VII (facial nerve with five branches) and the muscles of mastication innervated by cranial nerve V (trigeminal nerve with three main divisions and several branches). These structures work together to accomplish the functions listed in the introductory paragraph. Also, there are numerous muscles of facial expression that should work symmetrically to provide for facial animation. The muscles of mastication act to depress, elevate, rotate, and translate the mandible to allow for a full range of mobility free of limitations, deviations, or pain. The major depressors of the mandible are the lateral (external) pterygoid, digastrics, and the temporalis muscles. The major elevators of the mandible are the medial (internal) pterygoid, masseter, and temporalis muscles.

Age-related changes

Certainly, generalized weakness may occur as a patient ages. Specifically, myofacial pain is manifested as muscle pain in the maxillofacial region. The patient often states that the "side of my face is sore or tender," and does not necessarily point directly to the joint itself. Bell's palsy is another disorder that affects the muscles of facial expression and will manifest as palsy or as an asymmetrical disfigurement.

Examination techniques

The muscles of facial expression can be inspected for symmetry during facial animation or in a static pose. The muscles of mastication can be inspected for symmetry and palpated for masses or to examine for tenderness. The muscles of mastication can be palpated extraorally and intraorally. Masticatory strength can be tested by having the individual bite on a tongue depressor. Range of motion can be evaluated as well.

Nerves

General characteristics and anatomy

The maxillofacial complex is richly innervated via the 12 pairs of cranial nerves as well as the cervical nerves. These nerves should provide for motor, sensory, proprioceptive, and autonomic functions without pain, dysesthesia, parasthesia, or dysfunction. The major nerve providing sensory and motor input in the maxillofacial region is the trigeminal. The trigeminal nerve has three divisions: ophthalmic, maxillary, and mandibular. As previously discussed, the facial nerve provides for facial expression and contributes to the taste response. The facial nerve also supplies secretory fibers to both the submandibular and sublingual salivary glands. Taste response is completed by contributions from the vagus and glossopharyngeal nerves. Branches of the glossopharyngeal nerve also supply the secretory fibers to the parotid gland.

Age-related changes

Trigeminal neuralgia (TN) is a relatively common cause of facial pain in the elderly. The symptom complex is characterized by a trigger point, generally intraorally, with subsequent severe, lancinating pain of a few seconds to minutes duration. TN may be an early sign of multiple sclerosis.[36] Moreover, TN resulting from previous infection with the herpes zoster virus is a severely debilitating illness that is difficult to treat.

Examination techniques

The neurological examination portion of the dental physical examination includes the 12 pairs of cranial nerves. Motor, sensory, and autonomic function can be examined with relative ease. The muscles of facial expression can be examined by inspecting the face for symmetry during facial animation and in static pose. The muscle of mastication can be tested by having the patient bite on a tongue depressor while the physician attempts to remove it from the mouth. Sensation can be assessed by swiping a wisp of cotton in the region of each division of the trigeminal nerve. Autonomic function can be assessed subjectively by a query about mouth dryness and objectively by examining the mouth directly.

Glandular tissue

The primary glandular tissues of note are the major and minor salivary glands and lymphatic tissues. The salivary glands serve to produce sufficient amounts of saliva for food bolus preparation, assist in taste, provide initial enzymatic breakdown of food, provide immunological protection against microorganisms, and lubricate the oral mucosa. Salivary glands contain mucous cells, serous cells, or a combination. Serous cells produce watery saliva, whereas mucous cells produce saliva thicker in quality. Major salivary glands include the parotid, submandibular, and sublingual. There are also many minor or accessory salivary glands. The parotid glands are located laterally in the face near the anterior aspect of the tragus and below the lobe of the ear. The submandibular and sublingual glands are located in the floor of the mouth. The minor salivary glands are located in the labial mucosa and palate. Lymphatic tissues such as the tonsils, adenoids, and accessory tissues are present in the mouth. There are also lymphoid tissues present within the salivary glands.

Age-related changes

Age-related changes include xerostomia from a variety of causes, including medications, Sjögren's syndrome, and radiation to the head and neck. In addition to these causes, there are typically more ductal cells than acinar cells in the older adult, which can result in less salivary production. Additionally, calcifications within the gland called sialoliths can block salivary flow, leading to swelling, pain, stasis, and infection. Xerostomia can lead to difficulty with eating, speaking, prosthetic retention, glossodynia, oral pain and discomfort. Lacking the buffering capacity of saliva when xerostomic, the teeth are at high risk for caries. (See Box 41.3.)

Examination techniques

Salivary glands can be inspected for symmetry and swelling by examining the face from the anterior. The tissues in the mouth can be inspected for swellings and asymmetry. The glands can be palpated extraorally for masses or tenderness. Intraorally, if the

591

BOX 41.3 Xerostomia (dry mouth) may have devastating effects on oral health

Saliva can be thought of, figuratively speaking, as the blood supply of the mouth. Salivary hypofunction can lead to xerostomia that can introduce a constellation of side effects, adversely affecting the quality of life of the patient. The three main reasons why xerostomia occurs are medications, radiation therapy, and disease. Over 400 medications, including chemotherapeutic agents, may contribute to xerostomia. Diseases that may contribute to a dry mouth include Sjögren's syndrome, diabetes, and autoimmune disorders.

Symptoms indicative of dry mouth may include:

1. generalized caries (sometimes rapidly progressive)
2. difficulty swallowing
3. taste alteration
4. oral discomfort, burning, pain
5. speech disturbances
6. mucosal and gingival irritation

Physicians should be sensitive to the fact that well over 400 medications may cause dry mouth. Xerostomia can have rapid and devastating effects on the teeth and the health of the masticatory system. It is *critical* for the physician to refer patients to a dentist if the patient complains of dry mouth.

Sources: Turner MD, Ship JA. Dry mouth and its effects on the oral health of elderly people. Journal of the American Dental Association. September 2007;138:15S–20S.
Folke S, Fridlund B. The subjective meaning of xerostomia – an aggravating misery. *International Journal of Qualitative Studies on Health and Well-Being.* 2009; 4:245–255.

mirror or tongue depressor being used adheres to the mucosa, this may indicate dryness or xerostomia. Also, if you suspect xerostomia, you can administer the cracker test. Obtain a saltine cracker to investigate whether the patient can adequately chew and swallow it. If not, xerostomia may be a problem. The clinician may also attempt to "milk" the glands to assess patency and flow from the parotid duct located in the buccal mucosa bilaterally opposite the upper molar teeth or the submandibular duct, located in the anterior floor of the mouth. Likewise, the anterior lip can be everted, dried with a 2 × 2 gauze, and inspected for flow from the minor salivary glands evident as discrete beads of saliva. Additionally, bimanual palpation of the floor of the mouth can be performed to assess symmetry and locate masses or tenderness.

Vessels

The oral and maxillofacial region is rich in blood supply provided mainly from branches of the external carotid and basilar arteries. The arteries of the head and neck should display a normal pulse without bruits.

Age-related changes

Changes that occur in the vascular system include skin, mucosal, and, rarely, intraosseous. Telangiectasia and

angiomas may occur on the skin of the face and neck. Intraorally, the most frequent finding is caviar tongue or lingual varicosities. Intraosseous lesions such as arterio-venous (A-V) malformation may be present. Although rare, tooth removal in the area of an A-V malformation may cause life-threatening blood loss. Temporal (giant cell) arteritis and headaches of various causes are relatively common and may be the result of congestive heart failure, transient ischemia, and increased intracranial pressure.

Examination techniques

Inspection extraorally, intraorally, and radiographically may reveal lesions indicative of vascular pathology. Palpation may reveal mucosal lesions involving the vascular system.

Periodontium

Three important structures comprise the periodontium: alveolar bone, periodontal ligament, and gingival tissues. Alveolar bone is present in both the mandible and maxilla and forms the housing for the teeth. It contains both cortical and cancellous bone. Alveolar bone provides firm support for the teeth, the interface being designated a gomphosis or immobile joint. Surrounding each tooth at the root area is the periodontal ligament, which provides a cushioning effect for the teeth upon occlusion (biting). The ligament runs in several different orientations, counterbalancing vertical and lateral forces placed on the teeth. The gingiva surrounding the teeth is comprised of masticatory and lining musoca and serves to protect the underlying bony and dental structures. The tissues immediately adjacent to the teeth are masticatory and keratinized, and the gingiva below this tissue is lining mucosa and non-keratinized.

Age-related changes

Gingivitis and periodontitis are the two most prominent diseases of the periodontium. These are inflammatory in nature, and the extreme result is tooth mobility or loss. Gingivitis manifests the cardinal signs of inflammation in the gingiva. Periodontitis is an inflammatory-mediated destruction of the periodontium and manifests as bone loss, loose teeth, and generally inflamed gingival tissues. Other presentations of gingival or periodontal disease may occur, such as acute necrotizing ulcerative gingivitis, aggressive periodontitis, and periodontal abscess. There may indeed be substantial bone loss in the apparent absence of local factors (plaque, calculus). Poor control of diabetes and immune deficits also can be contributing factors to the exacerbation of periodontal disease. Systemic illnesses such as leukemia can affect the appearance of the gingival tissues, generally manifesting as hyperplasia, friability, and hemorrhage. Poor oral health and hygiene is a risk for aspiration pneumonia in debilitated patients.[37, 38]

Examination techniques

The periodontium can be inspected for loss, abscesses, purulence, bleeding, and general inflammation. The periodontium can be palpated as well for masses or tenderness. Oral cancerous lesions can also occur on the gingival tissues.

Teeth

There are 20 primary or milk teeth and 32 adult or permanent teeth. There can be additional teeth known as supernumerary. One or more primary teeth can occasionally be retained into adulthood, especially if there is no permanent successor. Teeth are designated as central incisors, lateral incisors, cuspids (canines), 1st and 2nd bicuspids (premolars), and 1st, 2nd, and 3rd molars. There are several methods for numbering teeth, with the military designation being the most common in the United States. The teeth are numbered 1–32 beginning in the upper right, proceeding to the upper left, continuing to the lower posterior left, and proceeding to the lower posterior right. Anterior and posterior are general positional designations for teeth such as the 1st molar, which is the most posterior tooth present. Positional designations for individual teeth are mesial (toward the dental midline), distal (away from the dental midline), lingual (toward the tongue), and facial or buccal (toward the cheek). There are four separate layers of various mineral compositions in dental structure: enamel (90% mineral and the hardest substance in the human body), dentin (70% mineral), cementum (50% mineral), and pulpal tissue (0% mineral; comprised of nerves, blood vessels, and lymphatics). Teeth generally exhibit a white, yellow, or light gray hue of varying chromas. Teeth may also take on the color of the restorative material used to repair lost tooth structure. The teeth should all be present and occlude or fit together smoothly upon closing with no interferences. The upper teeth are generally slightly facial to the lower teeth. Teeth should be clean with minimal plaque, tartar (calculus), or food debris.

Age-related changes

Although poor oral hygiene may be present at any age, an elderly individual may be more prone to this due to loss of manual dexterity, visual deficit, or cognitive decline. Teeth may be lost due to caries, periodontitis, or fracture. As a result of loss of teeth, a poor occlusal or interdigitating relationship may occur, leading to tipped, rotated, or increased spacing between teeth. Besides dental caries and periodontal disease, a variety of factors can lead to tooth structure loss, including attrition, abrasion, erosion, and abfraction. Attrition is loss of tooth structure due to tooth-to-tooth contact. Abrasion is loss of tooth structure due to dietary or environmental materials (e.g., sand or dust, coarse dietary components, tobacco, etc.).

Examination techniques

The teeth should be inspected for the presence of calculus, plaque, and food debris. Plaque only requires about 24 hours to form, and tartar (calculus) can form in as few as three days. The teeth can be inspected for caries, wear, and fractured cusps or other tooth components. The teeth can be palpated for tenderness or looseness. A tongue blade may be used to push on the teeth from several directions for this assessment. The teeth can be percussed to assess for tenderness as well. To assess for tooth fracture, a tongue blade may be applied over the tooth in question, and a bite force can be applied to elicit any tenderness. The general occlusion of the teeth can be assessed by having the patient bite the teeth together. Normally there is an overjet (maxillary teeth project out over the mandibular teeth) and overbite (maxillary teeth overlap the mandibular teeth), and the teeth fit together evenly and symmetrically.

Prosthetics

A variety of prosthetic devices may be present in the mouth. These devices may be permanently affixed to the mouth or removable. Appliances may be worn to aid in mastication and for aesthetics. These appliances should be well adapted and not painful. Appliances may be worn to aid in protecting the dentition due to grinding or bruxism, to position the jaw in a certain way, or to straighten the teeth. Dental implants affixed to the jaw should be immobile and well functioning. Any prosthetic devices should allow for smooth, symmetrical, and pain-free closure and functioning. All prosthetic devices used for whatever purpose should be clean and free of plaque, calculus, or food debris.

Age-related changes

There are myriad prosthetic devices that may be present in the mouth for a variety of reasons. It is critical for patients to be followed closely by their dental professional if they wear a prosthetic device. However, if there is minimal follow-up the device may become ill-fitting due to changes and loss of oral structures.[39] Fixed prosthetics, if preventive measures are not in place, can gather plaque, calculus, and infectious organisms. Patients may then suffer from recurrent or new caries around the device at the margins between the prosthesis and the natural tooth.

Furthermore, nutritional deficiencies can affect the tissues' response to trauma from prosthetic devices. Moreover, poor oral and prosthesis hygiene may be present. Oral mucosal lesions (epulis and papillary hyperplasia) can be associated with removable prosthetic devices. Fungal infections appearing as either beefy red areas or as curdlike plaques that wipe off easily are relatively common under removable appliances. A potassium hydroxide staincan confirm this diagnosis. If there are lesions associated with the prosthetics, both the prosthesis and the attendant tissue must be treated for full resolution. Individuals wearing removable prosthesis should keep the prosthesis out of their mouth for at least six hours a day to allow the tissues to breathe and minimize infection (such as fungal).

Examination techniques

Removable prosthetic devices should be removed upon examination of the mouth. They should be inspected for cleanliness and integrity. Once placed in the mouth, they should be inspected for proper general fit and function. Of course, a subjective history from the patient may also alert the practitioner to potential problems with the prosthesis. Fixed devices (crowns, bridges, implants, etc.) should be inspected for cleanliness, as well as the condition of the periodontium surrounding them.

Prevention and special patient considerations

Ideally, the maintenance of oral and systemic health involves co-therapy between the patient and the medical and dental care team. Patients should be engaged in their own health in such a way as to minimize the need for dental and medical intervention. Prevention involves sensitivity to genetic tendencies (family history), control of habits (tobacco cessation), dietary considerations (carbohydrate discipline), oral hygiene (conscious application of brushing and flossing), and maintenance of good systemic health, as this may limit medication use and facilitate maintenance of salivary, oral mucosal, and dental integrity.

However, when patients become disabled for whatever reason (physical or cognitive impairment), caregivers must be engaged in the process of education and administration of preventive measures to the degree that they have the ability. The dental team should assist the caregiver and medical team in this endeavor to preserve and protect the dentition for as long as possible. Conservative and compassionate dental care – keeping comfort, function, health, and esthetics in mind – are excellent guiding principles.

Summary and recommendations

Oral health is intimately related to systemic health and directly related to quality of life. Frail, home-bound, and institutionalized older adults are particularly susceptible to oral health problems and should be screened carefully at the initial medical visit. Nursing homes are required by law to have a contract with a dentist or assist in locating a dentist for their clients. [31] Oral treatment planned for all older adults, particularly frail elders, should take into account psychosocial, medical, and functional abilities and circumstances to fashion a plan that is realistic, given the preceding parameters. However, all older adults should be reminded that proper nutrition, oral hygiene, and cessation of habits such as tobacco use, are critical to maintaining oral health. As in all medical specialties, prevention and patient education are paramount. Therefore, all adult patients should be screened or evaluated by an oral health professional so that optimal health can be achieved and maintained.

References

1. www.ada.org/en (accessed May 9, 2014).

2. Harris NO, Godoy G. *Primary Preventive Dentistry.* 5th ed. New York: Appleton and Lange; 1999.

3. Glick, M DMD (ed.). The Oral-Systemic Disease Connection: An Update for the Practicing Dentist. *JADA.* 2006; 137(special supplement):1S–40S.

4. Paquette DW, Nichols T, Williams RC. Oral Inflammation, CVD, and Systemic Disease. Connections: *Oral and Systemic Health Review.* July 2005; 1(1): 1–8.

5. Paquette DW. Periodontal Disease and the Risk for Adverse Pregnancy Outcomes. *Grand Rounds in Oral and Systemic Medicine.* Nov 2006; 1(4): 14–24.

6. Moritz AJ, Mealey, BL. Periodontal Disease, Insulin Resistance, and Diabetes Mellitus: A Review and Clinical Implications. *Grand Rounds in Oral and Systemic Medicine.* May 2006; 1(2): 13–20.

7. DePaola, DP (guest ed.). Proceedings and Consensus Opinion from the Global Oral and Systemic Health Summit. *Grand Rounds Supplement.* Feb 2007; 1–20.

8. Beck JD, Slade G, Offenbacher S. Oral Disease, Cardiovascular Disease and Systemic Inflammation. *Periodontology.* June 2000; 23: 110–120.

9. The American Journal of Cardiology and Journal of Periodontology Editor's Consensus: Periodontitis and Atherosclerotic Cardiovascular Disease. *J Periodontology.* 2009; 80: 1021–1032.

10. Babu, NC, Gomes AJ. Systemic Manifestations of Oral Diseases. *J Oral Maxillofac Pathol.* May–Aug 2011; 15(2): 144–147.

11. Parks ET, Lancaster H. Oral Manifestations of Systemic Disease. *Dermatol Clin.* Jan 2003; 21(1): 171–182.

12. Islam NM, Bhattacharyya I et.al. Common Oral Manifestations of Systemic Disease. *Otolaryngol Clin North Am.* Feb 2011; 44(1): 161–182.

13. Swinson B, Witherow H et al. Oral Manifestations of Systemic Diseases. *Hosp Med.* Feb 2004; 65(2): 92–99.

14. Parameters on Systemic Conditions Affected by Periodontal diseases. *J Periodontol.* 2000; 71: 880–883.

15. Parameters on Periodontitis Associated with Systemic Conditions, *J Periodontol.* 2000; 71: 876–879.

16. www.cdc.gov/aging/help/dph-aging/state-aging-health.html (accessed May 11, 2014).

17. US Department of Health and Human Services. *Oral Health in America: A Report of the Surgeon General.* Rockville, MD: US Department of Health and Human Services, National Institute of Dental and Craniofacial Research, National Institutes of Health; 2000.

18. Beltrán-Aguilar ED, Barker LK, Canto MT, et al. Surveillance for Dental Caries, Dental Sealants, Tooth Retention, Edentulism, and Enamel Fluorosis – United States, 1988–1994 and 1999–2002. *MMWR* 2005; 54(3): 1–44.

19. Vargas CM, Kramarow EA, Yellowitz JA. *The Oral Health of Older Americans. Aging Trends; No. 3.* Hyattsville, MD: National Center for Health Statistics; 2001: 1–8.

20. MacEntee M, Hole R, Stoler E. The Significance of the Mouth in Old Age. *Soc Sci Med.* 1997; 45: 1449–1458.

21. Holm-Pederson P, Löe H (eds.). *Textbook of Geriatric Dentistry.* 4th ed. New York: McGraw Hill; 1999.

22. Hazzard WR, Blass JP. *Principles of Geriatric Medicine and Gerontology.* New York: McGraw-Hill Professional; 2003.

23. Wade, ML, Suzuki, JB. Issues Related to Diagnosis and Treatment of Bisphosphonate-induced Osteonecrosis of the Jaws. *Grand Rounds in Oral and Systemic Medicine* May 2007; 2(2): 46–53.

24. Bhaskar, SN. *Orban's Oral Histology and Embryology.* 10th ed. Philadelphia: C.V. Mosby; 1986.

25. Ten Cate, AR. *Oral Histology Development, Structure, and Function.* 2nd ed. Philadelphia: C.V. Mosby; 1985.

26. Regezi JA, Sciubba JJ. *Oral Pathology Clinical-Pathologic Correlations.* Philadelphia: W.B. Saunders; 1989.

27. Montgomery RL. *Head and Neck Anatomy with Clinical Correlations.* New York: McGraw-Hill; 1981.

28. Hollinshead, HW. *Anatomy for Surgeons: The Head and Neck.* Baltimore: Lippincott Williams & Wilkins; 1982.

29. Okeson JP. *Management of Temporomandibular Disorders and Occlusion.* 4th ed. Philadelphia: C.V. Mosby; 1998.

30. Sheiham A. Oral Health, General Health, and Quality of Life (Editorial). *Bulletin of the World Health Organization* Sep 2005; **83**(9): 644–645.

31. Matear DW. Demonstrating the Need for Oral Health Education in Geriatric Institutions. *Probe* Mar–Apr 1999; **33**(2): 66–71.

32. Federal Nursing Home Reform Act from the Omnibus Budget Reconciliation Act of 1987 (OBRA 1987).

33. Widmalm SE, Westesson PL, Brooks SL, et al. Temporomandibular Joint Sounds: Correlation to Joint Structure in Fresh Autopsy Specimens. *Am J Orthod Dentofacial Orthop.* Jan 1992; **101**(1): 60–69.

34. Al Habashneh R, Alchalabi H, Khader YS, et al. Association between Periodontal Disease and Osteoporosis in Postmenopausal Women in Jordan. *J Periodontol.* Nov 2010; **81**(11): 1613–1621.

35. Pelelassi E, Nocopoulou-Karayianni K, Archontopoulou AD, et al. The Relationship Between Osteoporosis and Periodontitis in Women Aged 45–70 Years. *Oral Dis.* May 2012; **18**(4): 353–359.

36. Danesh-Sani SA, Rahimdoost A, Soltani M, et al. Clinical Assessment of Orofacial Manifestation in 500 Patients with Multiple Sclerosis. *J Oral Maxillofac Surg.* Feb 2013; **71**(2): 290–294.

37. Ueda K. Preventing Aspiration Pneumonia by Oral Health Care. *JMAJ.* 2011; **54**(1): 39–43.

38. Liantonio J, Salzman B, Snyderman D. Preventing Aspiration Pneumonia by Addressing Three Key Risk Factors: Dysphagia, Poor Oral Hygiene, and Medication Use. *Annals of Long Term Care* Oct 2014; **22**(10).

39. Wolfart S, Weyer N, Kern M. Patient Attendance in a Recall Program After Prosthodontic Rehabilitation: A 5-Year Follow-up. *Int J Prosthodont.* Sept–Oct 2012; **25**(5): 491–496.

Chapter 42

Foot health in the elderly

Diana Homeier, MD, and Louise Ye, DO, LAc

Introduction

Foot health is important to the overall well-being of the older adult. Maintaining healthy and pain-free feet can assist in maintaining mobility and functional independence. A large percentage of older adults have foot pain that alters their ability to function independently.[1] Foot conditions can be a major cause of pain, discomfort, and disability.[2] They are also associated with an increased risk of falls.[3] Foot problems may be the result of a primary foot disorder or a manifestation of systemic disease.

The care of feet is often neglected during the routine office visit and physical examination. Because the foot can impact overall function, the podiatric exam for either preventive or problem-related issues is an important part of geriatric care [4] Once problems are identified, management may involve definitive treatment, proper footwear, or a referral to an appropriate specialist.

Foot examination

Health-care practitioners should regularly examine their geriatric patients' feet. Older adults may not be vigilant about their feet and may lack the vision, sensation, or flexibility to adequately check their own feet.[5] The foot examination may begin with the evaluation of the patient's shoes. The type of shoe worn and ability to ambulate in the shoe can give clues to underlying foot problems.[6] The foot exam then includes a dermatologic, orthopedic, vascular, neurologic, and functional assessment.[1] The dermatologic exam is an evaluation of the condition of the skin and the presence of discoloration, hyperkeratotic lesions, ulcerations, infection, and nail abnormalities. The orthopedic assessment includes an evaluation of any foot deformities (hallux valgus,

digiti flexus) as well as arthritic changes. A vascular assessment includes the palpation of the posterior tibial and dorsalis pedis pulses and inspection of skin and temperature for signs of vascular disease. The neurologic exam comprises an evaluation of motor and sensory function, including a monofilament test when indicated.[1] The functional exam is an assessment of the patient's gait and mobility.

Skin and nail conditions

Skin changes that occur with aging and skin pathologies that occur elsewhere on the body can also occur on the foot (see Figure 42.1). Xerosis (excessively dry

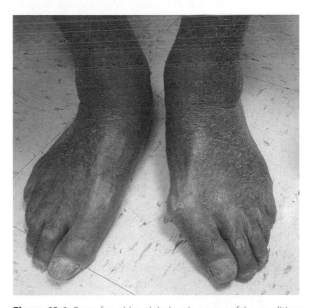

Figure 42.1 Feet of an older adult showing many of the conditions that can happen with aging. Xerosis is present on both legs and feet. Onychomycosis is present bilaterally. Hallux valgus (bunion) is noted on the left foot. Digiti flexus (hammertoe) is present in the right second toe. (A black-and-white version of this figure will appear in some formats. For the color version, please refer to the plate section.)

Reichel's Care of the Elderly, 7th Edition, ed. Jan Busby-Whitehead *et al.* Published by Cambridge University Press.
© Cambridge University Press 2016.

skin) is a very common problem for older adults. Xerosis is due to a lack of hydration and lubrication. The skin may form fissures or cracks (common on the heel) that increase the risk of possible ulceration and infection. Emollients applied after bathing can be helpful. Urea cream or solution can be used as a keratolytic. A heel pad or cup can also be used to minimize trauma to the heel.[5]

Pruritis is common in older patients and may be related to dry skin and cold weather. The patient may complain of itching and scratching, and the foot examination may reveal excoriations. An examination should be done to rule out tinea, urticarial, or other skin lesions.[7] Treatment of pruritis consists of skin lubricants and topical steroids if warranted. If needed, antihistamines can be helpful, but they have side effects that can be dangerous in older patients.

Venous stasis dermatitis is caused by venous insufficiency and can manifest as edema, induration, discoloration, and ulcerations of the skin. It starts most commonly in the medial aspect of the ankle. Management includes elevation and compression stockings to improve venous return and manage edema. Emollients and topical corticosteroids can help to manage the dermatitis. Antibiotics may be indicated when infection is present.[8]

Hyperkeratotic lesions

Hyperkeratotic lesions such as tyloma (callus) and heloma (corn) are thickened and hardened areas of the skin that have developed over time due to constant friction or pressure or over bony prominences.[9] Ill-fitting shoes may be a factor in the development of these lesions. Other factors include contractures, gait changes, deformities, loss of skin tone and elasticity, loss of soft tissue with age, and atrophy of the plantar fat pad.[10] Generally, these are not harmful, but patients often present with pain, ulceration, or infection that can limit their ambulation.[11] Patients with vascular or neurologic disorders will need to examine their feet frequently to check for signs of skin irritation, ulceration, and bone infection.[9]

It is often hard to differentiate corns and calluses. Corns are usually smaller than calluses and have a central core that is surrounded by irritated skin. Corns are often painful with pressure. On the other hand, calluses are rarely painful and often larger. These usually develop on the stratum corneum, the outermost layer, on the soles of the feet, under the heels or balls.[12] It is important to differentiate corns and calluses from verruca (warts) or other similar appearing lesions.[10]

Treatment for hyperkeratotic lesions is dependent upon the patient and the effect on function. The primary focus should be placed on removing pressure and preventing ulceration or further injury. Considerations for treatment include padding, shoe modification, emollients, debridement, and orthoses. When the lesion is on the plantar aspect of the foot, treatment should be aimed at dispersing the weight. [9] The lesions can be treated with salicylic acid plasters and debulking.[12] Surgical revision may be indicated in some cases. The problem may be recurrent or persist because of the residual deformity and underlying conditions such as diabetes.[11]

Ulceration

An ulceration is a soft tissue injury that leads to an open wound or sore that is difficult to heal. It can result in complete loss of the epidermis and may go as deep as the dermis and subcutaneous fat. There are several different stages of ulcers. Risk factors for ulcer development include lack of mobility and prolonged stress on the tissue.[13] Ulcers can lead to poor quality of life, high mortality due to sepsis, and increased hospitalization.

There are three types of ulcerations that need to be taken into consideration: arterial, neurotrophic, and venous stasis ulcers. The ulcers are defined by their appearance, location, and the surrounding tissue.

Arterial (ischemic) ulcers are often on the heels, tips of the toes, between toes, or anywhere there are bony prominences. Patients complain of severe pain worsening at night. Patients often feel better after hanging the leg over the side of the bed.[14] There is usually very poor circulation causing poor tissue granulation and color changes (pale white/yellow, gray color when the leg is elevated, and redness reappears when the leg is dangling).[9]

Neurotrophic ulcers are usually located on the bottom of the feet beneath pressure points or hyperkeratoic lesions. There is often no pain associated with this type of ulcer. There is an increased incidence with elderly who have diabetes due to a loss of foot sensation and changes in the sweat-producing glands. Patients often complain of tingling, numbness, or burning sensation. The ulcers appear punched-out with a calloused, white fibrotic rim.[9]

Venous stasis ulcers occur in patients with poor venous circulation in the leg. They primarily occur below the knee, just above the ankle. Due to the poor circulation, risk of infection and prolonged healing often occur.[13]

Treatment should be focused on reducing pressure to the area and preventing infection. Pressure reduction can be obtained with dressings, orthoses, shoe modifications, and special depth shoes. In order to prevent infection of the ulcerated area, wound care is essential. The wound must be kept clean, and the wound base must be healthy to permit healing. Appropriate wound care may include debridement and/or antibiotics (when indicated). Vascular ulcers may warrant further evaluation with a vascular specialist. It is essential to improve vascular supply to the area and minimize worsening of conditions.[10]

Onychomycosis

Onychomycosis is one of the most prevalent nonbacterial diseases of the toenail. It is usually caused by dermatophytes (*Trichophytum rubrum* or *T. mentagrophytes*).[15] Other causes include yeasts and nondermatophyte fungi. Factors that contribute to this disease can include occlusive footwear, repeated trauma, sports participation, comorbid diseases such as diabetes, peripheral vascular disease, genetic predisposition, and foot hygiene.

The incidence of onychomycosis increases with age.[16] As the population ages, the nails also change. The nail calcium concentration decreases along with iron. Blood circulation diminishes and nail growth becomes retarded, increasing the susceptibility to infection.[15]

The patient often presents with discoloration and increased thickness in the toenail (see Figure 42.1). The infection may cause distal subungual, white superficial, proximal subungual, or total dystrophic changes. The superficial variety does not involve the nail plate, whereas the distal and proximal kind affect both the nail bed and the nail plate. When the nail plate is involved, hypertrophy and deformity is the result, and external pressure to the nail may cause pain.[10] It is important to rule out any other diseases that may mimic onychomycosis such as trauma, lichen planus, and psoriasis. Only approximately half of the suspected onychomycosis is truly due to a fungal infection and the other half is due to other causes that may lead to variation of nail morphology.[17] Therefore, confirmation of a fungal infection is imperative.

Diagnosis can be made based on laboratory confirmation with potassium hydroxide smear, culture, nail biopsy and less frequently immunohistochemistry, restriction fragment length polymorphisms, and polymerase chain reaction assays. It is important to get the correct specimen sampling and to use proper technique to prevent false negatives.[16]

After diagnosis is confirmed, management includes systemic and topical antifungals, keratolytic agents, debridement, photodynamic therapy, and surgical removal. Elders often do well with serial nail debridement as this decreases chances of infection, ingrown toenails, corns, and ulceration.[9] Treatment is often challenging because treatment is lengthy as the infection is usually embedded within the nail and difficult to reach. Factors that can indicate poor prognosis include the amount of nail involvement, nail dystrophy, mold, dermatophytoma, immunosuppression, and poor circulation.[16]

Tinea pedis

Tinea pedis, otherwise known as athlete's foot, is also caused by contagious dermatophytic fungal infection, such as *T. rubrum* or *T. mentagrophytes*. It affects the skin and causes scaling, flaking, and itching. It can be an extension of onychomycosis. In most cases, the disease is transmitted in warmer and moist communal areas where people walk barefoot, such as locker rooms and showers.[7]

Tinea pedis can occur in the interdigital spaces and on the sole of the foot. The diagnosis can usually be made clinically through thorough history and physical. Treatment consists of conservative measures such as allowing the feet to ventilate and remain dry with good hygiene. Topical antifungal medication is usually the treatment of choice such as clotrimazole, miconazole nitrate, and terbinafine hydrochloride. For severe or refractory infections, oral terbinafine is most effective, but it is important to be aware of the side effects that may occur with any oral medications.[15]

Other nail disorders

Ingrown toenail (onychocryptosis) is an incurvation of the edge of the nail into the nail groove. This is usually due to poor self-care (nail cutting) or narrow fitting shoes.[15] When this occurs, an abscess or an infection may result. If treatment is not initiated, periungual granulation tissue forms and complications such as deformity and involution may be the outcome. Treatment may include excision, partial avulsion, fulgeration, desiccation or caustics, and astringents.[11]

Paronychia is a localized infection involving the lateral or medial nail wall, most often caused by a spike of ingrown nail. This requires incision and drainage of the abscess with removal of the nail tissue. Antibiotics may also be necessary if there is surrounding cellulitis or if the patient is diabetic. Nonhealing granulation tissue in the nail groove may be an indication for a biopsy as Kaposi sarcoma, melanoma, and squamous cell carcinoma can present in this manner.[9]

There are many nail dystrophies that can occur in the older adult. They are usually the result of repeated trauma, underlying diseases, or degenerative changes. These nail conditions can be a source of pain, ulceration, and infection. Treatment should be individualized and may include specialized shoes, orthoses, debridement, and possible excision.

Subungal hematomas are common in the elderly secondary to microtrauma. However, when pigmented lesions are noted under the nail, it is important to rule out melanoma.[9]

Common foot disorders in elderly

Forefoot

Hallux valgus

Hallux valgus, commonly known as bunion, affects one-third of people over age 65. It is characterized by subluxation of the first metatarsal phalangeal joint and lateral deviation, greater than 15 degrees, of the great toe toward the lesser toes (see Figure 42.1).[18] The tissues around the joint may become swollen and sore. It may lead to restricted movement and thickening of the skin. Patients often complain that it is difficult to wear shoes or find shoes that are comfortable. Bunions may eventually lead to bursitis, which is inflammation of small fluid-filled pads (bursae); hammertoe, a bend in the middle joint of the toe, usually the one next to the big toe; and metatarsalgia, which is inflammation of the ball of the foot. Conservative management may include adaptive shoes (wider shoes or shoes with wider toe), proper padding and taping, anti-inflammatory medication,

and applying ice. In some cases, the patient remains symptomatic and may require surgical management. Bunion surgery has been found to reduce symptoms and improve patient ability to comfortably wear shoes.[19]

Digiti flexus

A digiti flexus (hammertoe) or contracted toe is a deformity arising from increased extension at the metatarsophalangeal joint (MPJ), flexion of the proximal interphalangeal joint (PIPJ), and hyperextension of the distal interphalangeal joint (DIPJ) of the lesser toes causing it to be permanently bent, resembling a hammer (see Figure 42.1).[15] Two other types of toe deformities are claw toe and mallet toe. Claw toe deformity is an extension contracture of the MPJ and flexion of both PIPJ and DIPJ. Mallet toe consists of flexion at the DIPJ only. A "crossover" second toe deformity occurs when the hallux valgus deformity crosses over the second MPJ causing subluxation.[20] Hammertoes are often painful and may be associated with hyperkeratotic lesions from abnormally shaped toes rubbing on shoes.

Treatments should be focused on alleviating pain and caring for keratotic lesions. Management may be nonsurgical or surgical. The conservative approach includes physical therapy, proper-sized shoes (wider and deeper), padding, and orthotic devices. Debridement of hyperkeratotic lesions can also be beneficial along with corticosteroid injections to decrease inflammation or bursitis. Taping and splinting mild crossovers to prevent further worsening of conditions may be helpful. Surgical correction may be necessary for more severe cases.[20]

A hammertoe deformity may progress to metatarsal-phalangeal dislocation. This is a dislocation of the phalanx on top of the metatarsal head. This can result in chronic pain and possibly a source of callus or ulceration. Treatment usually consists of shoe accommodation (wide toe shoes) or surgical correction of the joint.[5]

Sesamoiditis

Sesamoiditis is inflammation of the sesamoid bones and usually affects those that are under the first metatarsal joint of the hallux. There are normally two sesamoid bones and may be comprised of two separate pieces. The function of the sesamoid bones is to act as a hinge for the flexor tendons, which allows the big toe to bend downward.[21]

Sesamoiditis is caused by repetitive motions, sudden bending upward of the big toe, direct trauma, osteoporosis, or osteoarthritis. Treatment involves rest, proper-fitting shoes, and padding with proper arches to prevent continual impact to the sesamoid bones. Anti-inflammatory medications, corticosteroid injections, and immobilization may also be used.[21]

Fracture of phalanx/stress fracture

Stress fracture can develop from overuse and occurs in the weight-bearing bones of the foot. It is more common in patients with chronic inflammatory arthropathies, severe osteoporosis, joint deformities, or chronic corticosteroid injections.[20] This happens when overused muscles are unable to minimize the shock of repeated impacts and thus transfer the stress to the bones, leading to small fractures. The most common sites of stress fractures are the second and third metatarsals of the foot.[20] The patient may complain of gradually increasing pain and swelling on top of the foot. The patient may also notice bruising. A stress fracture is often difficult to see on an x-ray and may require a bone scan, magnetic resonance imaging (MRI), or computed tomography (CT) scan.

A conservative approach is to wear proper footwear and orthoses. It is important to immobilize and modify activities. Normal activities can be resumed after adequate healing which may take six to eight weeks.[20] Strength training and physical therapy will be of great benefit for these patients after recovery.

Other fractures may occur from falls or trauma in older adults. This may be due to instability or neuropathy. When there are fractures of the phalanges, this can affect the balance and ambulation of the patient. [22] Referral to a specialist may be necessary, depending on complications such as osteomyelitis and displacement. If the fractures are nondisplaced, often buddy taping and immobilization with boot or cast are appropriate. A displaced fracture may be reducible or irreducible. If reducible, a cast will be placed to prevent movement. If irreducible or open fracture, open reduction may be required.

Morton's neuroma

Morton's neuroma is a benign lesion that involves the compression of the common digital nerve occurring in the third intermetatarsal space. The patient will complain of numbness and tingling, and/or radiating,

shooting, or burning pain on weight bearing. Occasionally the pain may be described as "walking on a lump."[23] It may be relieved by removing or changing the footwear. The symptoms may be replicated with direct pressure at the intermetatarsal space. A click may be felt or heard with compression to the forefoot and applying plantar pressure, known as Mulder's sign. Other maneuvers that can be used are Grauthier's test (applying medial to lateral pressure of the forefoot) and Bratkowski test (hyperextending the toes, rolling the thumb over the symptomatic area and feeling a mass).[20]

It is important to differentiate Morton's neuroma from other diseases such as stress fracture, osteoarthritis, neoplasm, bursitis, or capsulitis. An x-ray, ultrasound, or MRI may be helpful to rule out other musculoskeletal pathology.[24] Initial treatment should be focused on orthoses and corticosteroid injections to decrease pressure and irritation of the nerve. For some patients, this may not be enough, and surgical neurectomy or nerve decompression could be considered. Cryogenic neuroablation is an option to preserve structures, but is less effective on large neuromas.[23]

Midfoot

Pes planus

Pes planus (also known as flatfoot) is a postural deformity in which the arch of the foot is touching or nearly touching the ground. This can be congenital or acquired. When the patient is standing, the longitudinal arch collapses, causing a subluxation of joints. [5] Many patients with pes planus are asymptomatic and untreated. However, as they age the deformity can become more rigid and cause pain and stress on foot and ankle joints. The primary goal of management is the reduction of pressure through weight loss and arch support orthoses. Surgery is reserved for serious cases when other measures have failed.[25]

Posterior tibial tendon dysfunction

Posterior tibial tendon dysfunction is the most common cause of acquired flatfoot in the older adult.[26] It is defined as the gradual tearing of the tibialis posterior tendon. The tibialis posterior tendon lies directly behind the medial malleolus and passes to the plantar surface of the foot to insert primarily onto the navicular bone. Its function is to invert and plantar flex the foot. As the tendon is serially

601

damaged, there is collapse of the longitudinal arch. This can lead to subluxation of the tarsal joints and even the ankle.[5]

Most patients present with an insidious onset of unilateral flatfoot deformity. Patients complain of pain and swelling along the medial foot and ankle, pain in the arch that can radiate to the medial calf muscle. The arch can progressively collapse. There are four stages described. Stage 1 is tendinitis and degeneration of the tibialis posterior tendon. Stage 2 describes a ruptured tendon that is functionally incompetent. In stage 3 the deformity becomes rigid and fixed. In stage 4 there is a valgus ankle deformity.[27]

Treatment is dependent on the stage of the disease at the time of presentation. Stage 1 deformity may be treated with orthoses, casting, or a brace. Stage 2 may involve tendon transfer or arthrodesis. Stages 3 and 4 usually require arthrodesis.[27]

Heel

Plantar fasciitis

Heel pain is a common complaint among older adults. Plantar fasciitis is the most common cause of heel pain. It is caused most frequently by an overuse injury at the origin of the plantar fascia due to excessive stress or pronation. The classic history is sharp pain localized to the insertion of the fascia that is most severe when the patient arises, eases somewhat after walking, but increases again with increased weight bearing. If the condition becomes chronic, the pain may be dull and constant.[28] Radiographs may reveal a plantar calcaneal spur. However, these have also been reported to be present in 27% of people without any symptoms.[28]

The differential diagnosis includes calcaneal stress fracture, plantar fascial tear, tarsal tunnel syndrome, plantar calcaneal bursitis, and bone contusion. Initial management may include stretching of the Achilles tendon and plantar fascia as well as proper footwear. A heel lift or cushion, orthoses, anti-inflammatory medication, physical therapy, and steroid injections can also be helpful. Difficult cases may require night splints, extracorporeal shock wave therapy or possibly surgery (open plantar fasciotomy).[28]

Fat pad atrophy

The heel fat pad may undergo atrophy with aging. This can cause heel pain while walking which is noticeably worse when the patient is walking barefoot and somewhat relieved by shoes. On examination, these patients will have little to no fat pad present on palpation over the heel, and there may be hyperkeratotic lesions overlying the heel. Treatment is with proper shoe support and shoe inserts.[5]

Achilles tendonitis

The Achilles tendon inserts on the posterior aspect of the calcaneus. Inflammation and degeneration of the tendon can cause posterior heel pain that may run along the course of the tendon. On examination, the patient may have tenderness with palpation or squeezing of the tendon. Treatment may consist of anti-inflammatory medication, warm compresses, orthoses or heel lifts, and physical therapy exercises. [2] Achilles tendon tear or rupture should be considered if the patient had trauma or sudden onset of pain with push-off of the foot.

Tarsal tunnel syndrome

The tarsal tunnel is located posterior and inferior to the medial malleolus. Within the tarsal tunnel lies the tibialis posterior tendon, flexor digitorum longus tendon, flexor hallicus longus tendon, and the posterior tibial nerve.[29] Tarsal tunnel syndrome (TTS) is a compressive entrapment neuropathy of the posterior tibial nerve or one of its branches.[30] It is an uncommon condition that occurs more often in patients with a history of trauma or rheumatoid arthritis. The patient with TTS complains of pain in the heel, sole, and/or toes, often described as burning. The pain may radiate proximally and may worsen at night. The differential diagnosis includes plantar fasciitis, Morton's neuroma, and systemic diseases that can cause a neuropathy. On examination, there may be tenderness over the nerve, decreased sensation, and some muscle wasting and weakness in the region of the nerves affected.[30] The diagnosis is difficult, and electrodiagnostic testing may be useful. Treatment includes orthoses, anti-inflammatory medications, steroid injections, and surgical release.

Systemic diseases in the foot

Diabetes

Diabetes is the number one systemic condition affecting foot health in the elderly.[5] It is estimated that 15% of diabetics will develop foot ulceration and 20% of ulcers will lead to amputation.[31] The National

Diabetes Advisory Board has stated that 50%–75% of amputations could be prevented with proper surveillance, education, and early intervention.[31] It is imperative for the geriatric practitioner to have a high level of surveillance and care for the feet of their diabetic patients. Older diabetics may suffer from neuropathy, vascular disease, and skin changes due to their diabetes. Due to sensory, vision, and mobility changes, it may be more difficult for an older diabetic to note changes to their feet.

Prevention of foot ulcers in older diabetics is the most important strategy. Routine (at least annual) foot examination and patient education as well as proper footwear and reduction of pressure points are facets of this care. The diabetic foot assessment should include a skin assessment, neuropathic assessment (pressure sense with 10-gm monofilament test, vibration sense using 128 Hz tuning fork, position, pain, and temperature), structural assessment for abnormalities, and vascular assessment.[32] Additional keys to prevention of foot ulcers include glycemic control, treatment of foot deformities and hyperkeratotic lesions, smoking cessation, and monitoring for/treatment of arterial disease.[5]

Once a diabetic foot ulcer develops, a comprehensive assessment and proper management are key to reduce the potential for amputation.[31] Documentation of the wound and its progress should be carefully undertaken. The presence of infection must be considered and treated appropriately. Recognizing underlying osteomyelitis can be a challenge. Radiographs can be helpful (usually takes two weeks to see infectious changes on plain radiographs), but MRI or leucocyte scans may be necessary in some patients.[32]

In patients with poorly controlled diabetes and peripheral neuropathy, a swollen, warm, red foot without ulceration could indicate Charcot neuroarthropathy.[33] Charcot neuroarthropathy (or Charcot foot) begins with inflammation, bone resorption and fragmentation, and joint dislocation. It can progress to bony consolidation and fusion as well as new bone formation. The end result is a deformed foot that is less functional. Because the patient has neuropathy, they are unaware of the stresses or injuries to the foot that occur over time. The diagnosis may be made by radiograph or by clinical presentation of an erythematous, warm, neuropathic foot with a change in shape, but without an open wound. The goals of treatment are foot stability and prevention of skin injury. Treatment may involve immobilization, bisphosphonates, and surgery. If treatment is initiated early in the course of the disease process, there is better probability of preserving function.[33]

Gout

Gout, also known as podagra, is another common foot pain complaint. This was once known as the "disease of kings" because it was attributed to overindulgence of food and wine. This medical condition is characterized by a painful and often disabling form of arthritis in joints, most often in the big toe.[34] In gout there is an excess of uric acid that collects in the blood and tissues and sodium urate crystals deposit in the joints and elsewhere. This may happen when there is an increase in uric acid production or when the kidneys are unable to remove the uric acid from the body adequately. Acute gouty attacks occur when tophi, an accumulation of the crystalline and amorphous urate, are formed.[34]

There are two types of gout: primary and secondary. Primary gout is due to an inherited metabolic abnormality whereas secondary gout is a result of an acquired disease or environmental factor specifically food, alcohol, and medications.[34] Certain foods such as shellfish and red meats have high purine and calorie content, as do fructose-sweetened drinks and food. Diuretic medications, aspirin, and immunosuppressants such as cyclosporine also increase uric acid content in the body.

Classic presentation of a gouty attack is an erythematous, swollen joint – often the big toe or foot with severe pain with weight bearing. The most common location is the MPJ of the great toe. Elderly people, particularly women who are taking diuretics, may present with urate deposits in preexisting Heberden's nodes that may or may not be painful.[34, 35] Some other types of arthritis can mimic gout, so a thorough history and physical is imperative.

The diagnosis of gout is primarily clinical. Uric acid level is usually elevated, but medication and the timing of an acute attack can alter this. Confirmation is made by visualization of urate crystals via needle aspiration of the affected joint. Strong, negative birefringent needle-shaped crystals are seen under the microscope.

Treatment with nonsteroidal anti-inflammatory drugs (NSAIDs), steroids, and/or colchicine are usually the first step to treatment of an acute attack. However, caution must be used in prescribing NSAIDs to elderly patients. Colchicine may also interact with other prescribed medications (e.g., a statin may slow liver metabolism causing accumulation).[36] It is also important to emphasize diet and lifestyle changes. Medications (such as allopurinol and probenecid) can provide long-term prophylaxis for those with recurrent attacks along with concurrent well-managed comorbidities.

Care of the geriatric foot

Foot care is an important part of overall health care for older adults. Healthy feet are fundamental to mobility, comfort, and independence in function. All older patients should have a foot examination performed at least annually. Geriatric practitioners are in an ideal position to perform this examination, provide basic education and treatment, and refer the patient to a specialist when needed.

Patient education includes a discussion about self-examination (using a mirror if needed), foot hygiene, skin care, foot safety, and proper footwear. In discussing foot safety, the older adult may be reminded to wear shoes or slippers even when at home to prevent injury. Socks made of cotton or wool are preferred because they can provide a barrier against wetness. Some sources recommend white socks because they can show drainage.[37]

Proper footwear is important for foot health. Patients should be warned to break in new shoes slowly to prevent injury.[2] There have been multiple studies evaluating the ideal footwear type for older adults at risk of falls. What is known thus far is that older adults should wear shoes both inside and outside the house that fit appropriately because walking barefoot or in socks alone increases the risk of falls. [38] Older patients should wear low-heel shoes with a thin, firm sole to optimize foot position. A tread sole and a treaded beveled heel might help to prevent falls on slippery surfaces.[38] Breathable materials that can stretch such as leather and canvas are preferable to plastic.[37]

Shoe modifications and orthoses can be used for patients at higher risk for foot injury or with foot deformities. For example, extra depth shoes can provide more space for deformed toes. Orthoses can be used to support a joint, accommodate, or correct a deformity, and to redistribute weight.[39] There are multiple forms of orthoses available, and they can be made to specifically fit the patient's foot and needs. There are sophisticated technologies (such as computerized gait analysis) for difficult or complex cases.

References

1. Helfand AE. Primary considerations in managing the older patient with foot problems, chap 122. In: Halter JB, Ouslander JG, Tinetti ME, et al., editors. *Hazzard's Geriatric Medicine and Gerontology*. 6th ed. New York: McGraw Hill Medical; 2009.

2. Kosinski M, Ramcharitar S. In-office management of common geriatric foot problems. *Geriatrics*. 1994;**49**(5):43.

3. Stubbs B, Binnekade T, Eggermont L, et al. Pain and risk for falls in Community dwelling older adults: systematic review and meta-analysis. *Archives of Physical Medicine and Rehabilitation*. 2014;**95**:175–187.

4. Stults BM. Preventive health care for the elderly in personal health maintenance. *West J Med.* 1984;**141**:832–845.

5. Albreski DA. Diseases and disorders of the foot. In: Durso SC, Sullivan GM, editors in chief. *Geriatrics Review Syllabus: A Core Curriculum in Geriatric Medicine*, 8th ed. New York: American Geriatrics Society; 2013.

6. Alexander IJ. *The Foot Examination and Diagnosis*. 2nd ed. New York: Churchill Livingstone; 1997.

7. Helfand AE. Foot health in the elderly: podogeriatric overview. In: Arenson C, Busby-Whitehead J, Brummel-Smith K, et al., editors. *Reichel's Care of the Elderly, Clinical Aspects of Aging*. 6th ed. New York: Cambridge; 2009.

8. Grant-Kels JM. Dermatologic diseases and disorders. In: Durso SC, Sullivan GM, editors in chief. *Geriatrics Review Syllabus: A Core Curriculum in Geriatric Medicine*. 8th ed. New York: American Geriatrics Society; 2013.

9. Ward K, Kosinski MA, et al. Podiatry. In: Fillit H, Rockwood K, editors. *Brocklehurst's Textbook of Geriatric Medicine and Gerontology*. 7th ed. Philadelphia: Saunders, an imprint of Elsevier; 2010.

10. Helfand AE. Foot problems. In: Evans J, Williams T., editors. *Oxford Textbook of Geriatric Medicine*. 2nd ed. Oxford: Oxford University Press; 2000.

11. Helfand AE, Robbins JM. Foot problems. In: Ham R, Sloane P., editors. *Ham's Primary Care Geriatrics: A Case-Based Approach*. 6th ed. Philadelphia: Saunders, an imprint of Elsevier; 2014.

12. Goldstein BG, Goldstein AO, et al. Overview of benign lesions of the skin. 2014 Jun [cited 2014 Jul 8]. Available from: www.uptodate.com/contents/overview-of-benign-lesions-of-the-skin?source=search_result&search=corns+and+callus+goldstein&selectedTitle=1%7E150.

13. Alguire PC, Scovell S. Overview and management of lower extremity chronic venous disease. *UpToDate.* June 2014 [updated 2014 May 5]. Available from: www.uptodate.com/contents/overview-and-manage ment-of-lower-extremity-chronic-venous-disease?sou rce=search_result&search=overview+and+manage ment+of+lower+extremity+chronic+venous+diseas e&selectedTitle=1%7E150.

14. Neschis, DG, Golden, MA. Clinical features and diagnosis of lower extremity peripheral artery disease. *UpToDate.* June 2014 [updated 2014 Jun 12]. Available from: www.uptodate.com/contents/clinical-features-a nd-diagnosis-of-lower-extremity-peripheral-artery-di sease?source=search_result&search=Clinical+features +and+diagnosis+of+lower+extremity+peripheral&sel ectedTitle=1%7E150.

15. Baran R. The nail in the elderly. *Clin in Derm.* 2011; **29**: 54–60.

16. Welsh O, Ver-Cabrera L, Welsh E. Onychomycosis. *Clin in Derm.* 2010; **28**: 151–159.

17. Allevato MAJ. Diseases mimicking onychomycosis. *Clin in Derm.* 2010; **28**: 164–177.

18. Dufour AB, Casey VA, Golightlu YM, Hannan MT. Characteristics associated with hallux valgus in a population-based study of older adults: the Framingham foot study. *Arthr Care & Research.* In Press. Accepted 2014 Jun 17.

19. Ferrari J. Hallux valgus deformity. *UpToDate.* 2014 Jun [updated 2013 May 15]. Available from: www.upto date.com/contents/hallux-valgus-deformity-bunion?s ource=search_result&search=hallux+valgus&selected Title=1%7E20.

20. Thomas JL, Blitch EL, Chaney DM, et al. Diagnosis and treatment of forefoot disorders. Section 1: Digital deformities. *Journal of Foot and Ankle Surgery.* 2009; **48**: 230–272.

21. American Health Network. Indiana: American Health Network-Central Services Organization; 2014. Available from: www.ahni.com/Specialties/Foot+and+Ankle/Arti cles/Common+Disorders/Sesamoiditis.html.

22. Gravlee JR, Hatch RL, et al. Toe fractures in adults. *UpToDate.* 2014 Jun [updated 2013 Jun 13]. Available from: www.uptodate.com/contents/toe-fractures-in-adults.

23. Adams II WR. Morton's neuroma. *Clin Podiatr Med Surg.* 2010; **27**: 535–545.

24. Jain S, Mannan K. The diagnosis and management of Morton's neuroma: a literature review. *Foot Ankle Spec.* 2013; **6**: 307–317.

25. Caselli MA, George DH. Foot deformities: biomechanical and pathomechanical changes associated with aging, part I. *Clin Podiatr Med Surg.* 2003; **20**: 487–509.

26. Katchis SD. Posterior tibial tendon dysfunction. In: Ranawat CS, Positano RG, editors. *Disorders of the Heel, Rearfoot and Ankle.* Philadelphia: Churchill Livingstone; 1999.

27. Geideman WM, Johnson JE. Posterior tibial tendon dysfunction. *Orthop Sports Phys Ther.* 2000; **30**: 68–77.

28. Healey K, Chen K. Plantar fasciitis: current diagnostic modalities and treatments. *Clin Podiatr Med Surg.* 2010; **27**: 369–380.

29. Ahn JM, El-Khoury GY. Radiologic evaluation of chronic foot pain. *Am Fam Physician.* 2007; **76**: 975–983.

30. Wallach DM, Katchis SD. Tarsal tunnel syndrome. In: Ranawat CS, Positano RG, editors. *Disorders of the Heel, Rearfoot and Ankle.* Philadelphia: Churchill Livingstone; 1999.

31. Helfand AE. Assessing and preventing foot problems in older patients who have diabetes mellitus. *Clin Podiatr Med Surg.* 2003; **20**: 573–582

32. Khanolkar MP, Bain SC, Stephens JW. The diabetic foot. *Q J Med.* 2008; **101**: 685–695.

33. Botek G, Anderson MS, Taylor R. Charcot neuroarthropathy: an often overlooked complication of diabetes. *Clev Clinic J Med.* 2010; **77**(9): 593–599.

34. Scott JT. Gout and other crystal arthropathies. In: Evans J, Williams T., editors. *Oxford Textbook of Geriatric Medicine.* 2nd ed. Oxford: Oxford University Press; 2000.

35. Dieppe PA. Investigation and management of gout in the young and the elderly. *Annals of Rheumatic Diseases.* 1991; **50**: 263–266.

36. Crittenden DB. New therapies for gout. *Annu Rev Med.* 2013; **64**: 325–337.

37. Bryant JL, Beinlich, NR. Foot care: focus on the elderly. *Orthop Nursing.* 1999; **18**(6): 53–60.

38. Menant JC, Steele JR, Menz HB et al. Optimizing footwear for older people at risk of falls. *J Rehab Research and Development* 2008; **45**: 1167–1182.

39. Esquenazi A, Thompson E. Management of Foot Disorders in the Elderly. In: Felsenthal G, Garrison SJ, Steinberg FU, editors. *Rehabilitation of the Aging and Elderly Patient.* Baltimore: Williams & Wilkins; 1994.

Surgical care of the elderly

Deepika Koganti, MD, David W. Rittenhouse, MD, and Michael S. Weinstein, MD, FACS, FCCM

Although the elderly make up approximately 13% of the US population, they represent 30%–50% of patients requiring elective and emergent surgical care (including trauma care).[1–3] The geriatric population is increasing, and although age remains an independent risk factor for mortality, more surgeons are operating on the elderly than ever before. Between 2000 and 2020, it is projected that a surgeon's caseload will grow by 14%–47% solely because of the increase in the geriatric population.[2] Of potential interest, almost 10% of Medicare patients have surgery during their last week of life, which raises concerns about the appropriateness and benefits of such procedures.[4, 5] The purpose of this chapter is to highlight key issues in geriatric surgery, focusing on perioperative risk assessment, medication assessment, communication issues, and postoperative care.

Preoperative care: risk assessment

One of the central tenets of perioperative planning for the patient is to weigh the potential harm against the benefit of the operation in terms of return to acceptable function and/or alleviation of suffering. This tenets holds in the elective as well as the acute setting. Risk assessment involves a thorough evaluation of the patient's functional and physical status, as well as elicitation of patient centered goals of therapy, ideally in partnership with the patient's primary care provider.

Traditional risk assessment has focused on cardiac risk and mortality outcomes. For instance, the Revised Cardiac Index, published in 1999 by Lee et al. in *Circulation*, is part of the American Heart Association and American College of Cardiology guidelines and is used to predict perioperative cardiac complications.[6] Such risk assessment has

also assisted with potential risk modification, for instance with the use of perioperative blockade. The American College of Surgeons National Surgery Quality Improvement Program developed a risk calculator to estimate morbidity and mortality for a patient undergoing surgery. This calculator takes into account many relevant factors regarding the geriatric population such as functional and nutritional status. This online tool is available at http://riskcalculator.facs.org/PatientInfo/Patient Info. No one calculator has been clearly deemed superior; therefore, most physicians utilize these different tools to obtain an overall idea of the patient's perioperative risk.

Refined preoperative assessment tools and the use of frailty measures have led to better insight into the difference between chronologic and physiologic age. Along with this shift has come focus not only on mortality and complications as outcomes, but also on functional status, discharge disposition, rehospitalization, and other quality-of-life measures. Some newly identified risk predictors are relatively simple. For example, a positive history of falls in the past six months in elderly patients undergoing colorectal surgery predicts increased complications and readmissions, as well as increased rates of discharge to a care facility instead of home.[7] The evaluation of sarcopenia based on computed tomography imaging of the psoas muscle is another novel method of assessment of frailty and risk. Sarcopenia, or loss of muscle mass, appears to be a predictor of increased physiologic age, frailty, loss of independence following surgery or injury, and increased mortality.[8, 9]

In addition to these uncomplicated approaches, a multidimensional comprehensive geriatric assessment (CGA) performed by a multi-disciplinary geriatric team is recommended. Such a program has

Reichel's Care of the Elderly, 7th Edition, ed. Jan Busby-Whitehead *et al.* Published by Cambridge University Press.
© Cambridge University Press 2016.

been demonstrated to predict adverse outcomes post-operatively in the geriatric population undergoing elective procedures.[10] The CGA includes: cognitive assessment, depression screening, consideration of risk factors for delirium, alcohol and drug use, cardiopulmonary evaluation, burden of comorbidity, polypharmacy assessment, physical function and history of falls, frailty, nutritional assessment, social support and goals of therapy.[10–12] Ideally, this work in preoperative assessment will allow not only appropriate selection of patients but will also lead to proactive risk modification and improved outcomes for all geriatric patients in need of surgical care.[13]

Medications assessment

Certainly medication assessment in the surgical geriatric patient is critical. Evaluation of the need for anticoagulation in the perioperative period is an essential part of medication assessment. Vitamin K antagonists such as warfarin are usually held five days preoperatively. However, in patients who are at high risk for thromboembolism, anticoagulation should be bridged instead of completely stopped.[14] Urgent procedures require reversal of these agents with the administration of vitamin K if a 12-hour delay is acceptable, or with fresh frozen plasma or a prothrombin concentrate if more urgent intervention is required. Other oral anticoagulants such as dabigatran, rivaroxaban, and apixaban, have shorter half-lives but may not be easily reversed in cases of emergency. Antiplatelet therapies such as clopidogrel are held seven days prior to surgery. Continuation of aspirin has been controversial. However, holding aspirin preoperatively has been associated with withdrawal syndrome and increased risk of thromboembolism.[15] It is advised that aspirin be continued perioperatively. Similarly, for some patients in the period of high risk for cardiac stent thrombosis, continuation of all antiplatelet therapy through the perioperative period may be warranted.

The patient will often be NPO at midnight for surgery the next day, therefore it is crucial to know which medications to continue and which to withhold on the day of surgery. Medications that should be continued include beta blockers, anti-arrhythmics, asthma medications, gastroesophageal reflux therapies, and statins. It appears quite important to continue beta blockers since their withdrawal perioperatively has been shown to increase morbidity and mortality.[16] Continuation of angiotensin converting enzyme (ACE) inhibitors is controversial as their continuation has been associated with improved outcomes in cardiac surgery patients, but their use has also been associated with severe intraoperative refractory hypotension. Medications that should be held the day of surgery include insulin, oral hypoglycemic agents, and diuretics unless prescribed for congestive heart failure.

Preoperative communication

An in-depth discussion of goals of care is paramount to ensure the surgeon, the patient, and his or her family are in agreement. At times, communication with the patient themselves may be complicated because of dementia or delirium, reinforcing the critical importance of involving family early on in the decision-making process.[17] A goal-oriented approach may be recommended over the usual disease/procedure-oriented method, especially for elderly patients with multiple medical problems facing the end of life. The patient and her social support figures are the experts in the patient's goals, values, expectations, and hopes. The surgeon caring for this population needs to be well versed in the variety of options to help choose the best treatment plans that maximize the likelihood of meeting those goals. In certain situations, more conservative treatments may be associated with a better quality of life.[18]

Older patients naturally are more likely to have do not resuscitate (DNR) orders and other limitations placed on burdensome treatments, often outlined in advanced directives. Literature exists concerning the effect of DNR orders on outcomes as well as the surgical care. For example Saager, et al. found that preexisting DNR orders are not associated with increased postoperative morbidity at 30 days in a cohort of surgical patients from the American College of Surgeons National Surgery Quality Improvement Program database.[19] However, Kazaure and colleagues found that DNR orders were an independent risk factor for 30-day mortality in a cohort of patients from the same database.[20] Unfortunately, at times a DNR order is conflated with less care and patients with such orders may be afforded less opportunities for certain types of interventions. It is important to review such orders explicitly in the preoperative planning. DNR orders or other limitations to life-prolonging therapies need not be a barrier to consideration of operative intervention especially for procedures aimed for symptom relief. Most societies, including the American College of Surgeons, recommend a practice of required reconsideration, in which exploration of the goals and values associated with a DNR order inform a careful discussion to evaluate whether to rescind or leave in effect the DNR order. If the order is rescinded at the time of the operation, a clearly defined perioperative time period should be established.[21]

Postoperative care: prevention and management of complications, disposition

Postoperative complications in the elderly population are responsible for significant morbidity, mortality, and functional derangements. The most common complications that occur postoperatively in geriatric surgery are neurologic, cardiac, and pulmonary. Postoperative delirium is the number one neurologic complication, with rates reported between 15% and 53% of general patients and up to 80% for patients in the intensive care unit.[22] Importantly, the development of delirium is independently associated with poor outcomes. Some risk factors associated with delirium include cognitive impairment, sleep deprivation, immobility, visual impairment, hearing impairment, and dehydration. Implementing certain protocols such as orienting the patient throughout the day, using noise reduction strategies at night, encouraging early physical therapy and ambulation, reinstituting visual and hearing aids immediately postoperatively, and ensuring adequate oral intake have been shown to decrease the incidence of delirium.[22] Other factors associated with increased risk of delirium include inadequate pain control, electrolyte abnormalities, and opioid use.[23] Adequate pain control can be complicated in the elderly secondary to decreased renal and hepatic function, drug–drug interactions, and cognitive impairment. Medications without significant effects on mental status such as NSAIDs and IV acetaminophen are preferred. However, opiates should be used if necessary for pain control. Clinical status should be carefully monitored for any signs of sedation that could signal respiratory depression. To avoid adverse side effects, the rule "start low and go slow" should be employed for narcotic dosing.[24] Regional blocks preoperatively can decrease postoperative pain medication use and should be done if appropriate. Neuraxial

blockades have also been shown to improve survival and decrease complications such as venous thromboembolism and respiratory depression.[25]

Although age has not been shown to be an independent risk factor in cardiac postoperative care, acute myocardial infarction has a higher mortality in the elderly population. As previously discussed, patients who were on beta blockers preoperatively for ACCF/AHA guideline indications should be continued on them postoperatively.[16] Careful attention to fluid balance is critical in avoiding both cardiac and pulmonary insufficiency in the perioperative period. It is often too easy to tip the scale in either direction in patients, for example, with aortic stenosis or diastolic dysfunction. Unfortunately, tools for assessing intravascular volume remain inadequate, and attention to weight, intakes and outputs, and physical assessment remain important tools.

Pulmonary complications have been shown to strongly correlate with age. Patients 60–69 years of age experience twice the number of pulmonary complications of those less than 60 years, whereas patients aged 70–79 have three times as many complications. Risk factors include the use of long-acting neuromuscular blockage, decreased lung expansion, surgery close to the diaphragm, and aspiration. To ensure lung expansion and avoid shallow breathing, early mobilization, adequate pain control, and incentive spirometry should be employed. Elderly patients are also at a higher risk of aspiration due to weakened oropharyngeal reflexes, which can be compounded by swallowing disorders. Appropriate aspiration precautions should be practiced and sedation avoided.

Hypothermia has been associated with many postoperative events such as cardiovascular complications and surgical site infection. The elderly are more prone to developing hypothermia due to physiologic changes including impaired central thermoregulation, vasoconstriction, and decreased metabolic activity.[23] Therefore, aggressive thermoregulation with the use of warming devices should be carried out perioperatively.

Polypharmacy is also a significant cause of postsurgical complications in the elderly with over 25% of hospitalized geriatric patients receiving an inappropriate medication.[26] The START and STOPP criteria or Beer's criteria can be used to determine appropriateness of a patient's medical regimen.[27, 28] These criteria have been utilized to assess for medications that may increase the risk of postoperative complications as well as medications that may result in the increased risk of falls and traumatic injuries.

Unlike the younger population, elderly patients are less likely to be discharged home after surgery. Both preoperative risk factors and post-surgical complications play a role in disposition. For example, the incidence of being discharged to a facility after a minor surgery was 0.8% in nonfrail and 17.4% in the frail. The incidence after major surgery was 2.9% in nonfrail versus 42.11% in frail patients.[29] Interdisciplinary team efforts to facilitate early mobilization may improve functional independence in this population.

Emergency surgery and trauma

Patients who present with surgical emergencies and traumatic injuries pose the challenge of an unexpected, often radical change in health status. Risk prediction and outcomes following emergency surgical care is challenging. Similar to elective cases, elderly patients undergoing emergent abdominal surgery experience higher postoperative complications and mortality rates than younger patients. Emergency abdominal surgeries are among the most common cases performed in patients over 80 years old.[30] Risk factors that were found to correlate with poor outcomes in older emergent patients include higher ASA class, preoperative shock, malignancy, increased time between presentation and OR, and preoperative steroids. Knowledge of the mortality rates and risk factors can be used by the surgeon to better inform the patient in discussing his or her expectations regarding postoperative outcome. Collaboration among geriatricians and surgeons in emergency surgery has not been studied but may help reduce postoperative mortality and improve outcomes such as has been seen in the trauma literature discussed in the following paragraphs.

Currently, the elderly comprise 20%–30% of all trauma patients. However, by 2050, this number is estimated to significantly increase so that at least 40% of injured patients admitted for surgical care will be over 65 years old.[31] Falls, motor vehicle accidents, and pedestrian–versus–motor vehicle collisions are the major culprits of trauma in this population. Elderly patients experience complications at a higher rate with one in three geriatric patients having an in-hospital adverse event versus one in five younger adults.[32] Preexisting comorbidities along with decreased physiologic reserve play a significant role

in the worse outcomes. However, clinical mismanagement can contribute to adverse events. In-hospital care of the elderly with issues such as medications and management of new and existing comorbidities has been improved when a geriatric team is consulted within 24 hours of the trauma.[33] The integration of the geriatric service consult with the trauma team allows for a comprehensive evaluation for the overall plan of care, prevention of complications from existing comorbidities or the onset of new issues, medication management, and discharge planning.[34]

Postoperative communication challenges

Some of the greatest challenges in communication and decision making occur when the postoperative course does not meet the hopes and expectations of patients, families, surgeons, and other health-care providers. When complications ensue, prognosis for recovery and more importantly, functional recovery, diminishes. In the ideal setting, such outcomes and possible courses of action would have been discussed in the preoperative conversation and continued postoperatively. Although understanding the patient- and family-centered goals and expectations remains paramount, consideration of the surgeon's perspective may shed light on the complicated dynamic. Intensivists, geriatricians, and other non-surgical providers have observed that surgeons may be reluctant to limit or forego life-prolonging therapies in postoperative patients. Schwarze and colleagues have coined the term surgical "buy-in" to help understand this phenomenon. [35] They describe a complex process in which surgeons may expect a commitment to aggressive postoperative interventions aimed at rescue following high-risk surgical procedures. The process appears to stem from a strong sense of responsibility both for the patient and for complications that ensue. Unfortunately the request for withdrawal or limitation of life-sustaining therapies may be an unwelcome conversation, and responsibility for an unfavorable outcome might be shifted to the patient or family. Understanding this unique surgical perspectives may help nonsurgeons better negotiate challenging end-of-life decision making in the postoperative period.

Furthermore, it is important to consider how such conflicts may result from practices and policies that focus on mortality outcomes alone.[36] More investigation will be required to better define meaningful outcome measures in the geriatric population that are patient-centered and stem from the full range of possible outcomes that may be seen as favorable in the eyes of the patient.

Conclusion

As our population ages, the surgical care of the elderly will continue to challenge the surgical workforce. With increased focus and understanding of the unique aspects of the geriatric population, we hope to improve the delivery of surgical care both by enhancing safety and ensuring care aligned with patient goals and preferences. Communication and collaboration among surgeons, geriatricians, patients, and families will allow for optimal management and improved outcomes.

References

1. Elixhauser A, Andrews RM. Profile of inpatient operating room procedures in US Hospitals in 2007. *Archives of Surgery*. 2010; **145** (12): 1201–1208.

2. Etzioni DA, Liu JH, O'Connell JB, et al. Elderly patients in surgical workloads: a population-based analysis. *American Surgeon* 2003; **69**: 961–965.

3. Bonne, S, Schuerer, DJ. Trauma in the older adult: epidemiology and evolving geriatric trauma principles. *Clinics in Geriatric Medicine* 2013; **29**(1): 137–150.

4. Teno JM, Gozalo PL, Bynum JPW, et al. Change in end-of-life care for Medicare beneficiaries: site of death, place of care, and health care transitions in 2000, 2005, and 2009. *JAMA*. 2013; **309**: 470–477.

5. Kwok AC, Semel ME, Lipsitz SR, et al. The intensity and variation of surgical care at end of life: a retrospective cohort study. *Lancet*. 2011; **378**: 1408–1413.

6. Ford MK, Beattie WS, Wijeysundera DN. Systematic review: prediction of perioperative cardiac complications and mortality by the revised cardiac risk index. *Annals of Internal Medicine* 2010; **152**(1): 26–35.

7. Jones TS, Dunn C., Wu DS, et al. Relationship between asking an older adult about falls and surgical outcomes. *JAMA Surgery* 2013; **148**(12): 1132–1138.

8. Fairchild B, Webb TP, Xiang Q, et al. Sarcopenia and frailty in elderly trauma patients. *World Journal of Surgery* 2014; **39**(2): 373–379.

9. Englesbe MJ, Patel SP, He K, et al. Sarcopenia and mortality after liver transplantation. *Journal of the American College of Surgeons* 2010; **211**(2): 271–278.

10. Kim KI, Park KH, Koo KH, et al. Comprehensive geriatric assessment can predict postoperative morbidity and mortality in elderly patients undergoing elective surgery. *Archives of Gerontology and Geriatrics* 2013; **56**(3): 507–512.

11. Partridge JSL, Harari D, Martin FC, Dhesi JK. The impact of pre-operative comprehensive geriatric assessment on postoperative outcomes in older patients undergoing scheduled surgery: a systematic review. *Anaesthesia* 2014; **69**(s1): 8–16.

12. Chow W, Rosenthal RA, Merkow RP, et al. Optimal preoperative assessment of the geriatric surgical patient: a best practices guideline from the American College of Surgeons National Surgical Quality Improvement Program and the American Geriatrics Society. *Journal of the American College of Surgeons* 2012; **215**: 453–466.

13. Harari D, Hopper A, Dhesi J, et al. Proactive care of older people undergoing surgery ('POPS'): designing, embedding, evaluating and funding a comprehensive geriatric assessment service for older elective surgical patients. *Age and Ageing* 2007; **36**(2): 190–196.

14. Douketis JD, Spyropoulos AC, Spencer FA, et al. Perioperative management of antithrombotic therapy: antithrombotic therapy and prevention of thrombosis: American College of Chest Physicians evidence-based clinical practice guidelines. *Chest Journal* 2012; **141**(2 suppl): e326S–e350S.

15. Gerstein NS, Schulman PM, Gerstein WH, et al. Should more patients continue aspirin therapy perioperatively?: clinical impact of aspirin withdrawal syndrome. *Annals of Surgery* 2012; **255**(5): 811–819.

16. Fleischmann KE, Beckman JA, Buller CE, et al. 2009 ACCF/AHA focused update on perioperative beta blockade: a report of the American College of Cardiology Foundation/American Heart Association Task Force on Practice Guidelines. *Circulation* 2009; **120**(21): 2123–2151.

17. Oresanya LB, Lyons WL, Finlayson E. Preoperative assessment of the older patient: a narrative review. *JAMA* 2014; **311**(20): 2110–2120.

18. Mack JW, Weeks JC, Wright AA, et al. End-of-life discussions, goal attainment, and distress at end of life: predictors and outcomes of receipt of care consistent with preferences. *J Clin Oncol*. 2010; **28**: 1203–1208.

19. Saager L, Kurz A, Deogaonkar A, et al. Pre-existing do-not-resuscitate orders are not associated with increased postoperative morbidity at 30 days in surgical patients. *Crit Care Med*. 2011: **39**(5): 1036–1041.

20. Kazaure H, Roman S, Sosa JA. High mortality in surgical patients with do-not-resuscitate orders: analysis of 8256 patients. *Archives of Surgery* 2011; **146**(8): 922–928.

21. www.facs.org/about-acs/statements/19-advance-directives (accessed Nov. 9, 2015).

22. Inouye SK. Delirium in older persons. *N Engl J Med* 2006; **354**(11): 1157–1165.

23. Sieber FE, Barnett SR. Preventing postoperative complications in the elderly. *Anesthesiology Clinics* 2011; **29**(1): 83–97.

24. Falzone E, Hoffmann C, Keita H. Postoperative analgesia in elderly patients. *Drugs Aging.* 2013; **30**(2): 81–90.

25. Rodgers A, Walker N, Schug S, et al. Reduction of postoperative mortality and morbidity with epidural or spinal anaesthesia: results from overview of randomised trials. *BMJ* 2000; **321**(7275): 1493.

26. Finlayson E, Maselli J, Steinman MA, et al. Inappropriate medication use in older adults undergoing surgery: a national study. *J American Geriatric Society* 2011; **59**(11): 2139–2144.

27. Gallagher P, Ryan C, Byrne S, et al. STOPP (Screening Tool of Older Person's Prescriptions) and START (Screening Tool to Alert doctors to Right Treatment): consensus validation. *International Journal of Clinical Pharmacology and Therapeutics* 2008; **46**(2): 72–83.

28. American Geriatrics Society 2012 Beers Criteria Update Expert Panel. American Geriatrics Society updated Beers Criteria for potentially inappropriate medication use in older adults. *J American Geriatric Society* 2012; **60**(4): 616–631.

29. Makary MA, Segev DL, Pronovost PJ, et al. Frailty as a predictor of surgical outcomes in older patients. *Journal of the American College of Surgeons* 2010; **210**(6): 901–908.

30. Deiner S, Westlake B, Dutton RP. Patterns of surgical care and complications in elderly adults. *J American Geriatric Society* 2014 May; **62**(5): 829–835.

31. MacKenzie EJ, Morris JA Jr, Smith GS, Fahey M. Acute hospital costs of trauma in the United States: Implications for regionalized systems of care. *J Trauma* 1990; **30**: 1096–1101.

32. Knudson MM, Lieberman J, Morris JA, et al. Mortality factors in geriatric blunt trauma patients. *Arch Surg* 1994; **129**(4): 448–453.

33. Fallon WF Jr, Rader, E, Zyzanski S, et al. Geriatric outcomes are improved by a geriatric trauma consultation service. *Journal of Trauma-Injury, Infection, and Critical Care* 2006; **61**(5): 1040–1046.

34. DeGolia PA, Rader EL, Peerless JR, et al. Geriatric trauma care: integrating geriatric medicine consultation within a trauma service. *Clin Geriatr.* 2009; **17** (1): 38, 42.

35. Schwarze ML, Bradley CT, Brasel KJ. Surgical buy-in: the contractual relationship between surgeons and patients that influences decisions regarding life-supporting therapy. *Crit Care Med.* 2010; **27**: 157–161.

36. Schwarze ML, Brasel KJ, Mosenthal, AC. Beyond 30-day mortality: aligning surgical quality with outcomes that patients value. *JAMA Surgery* 2014; **149**(7): 631–632.

Chapter 44

Rehabilitation in the elderly

Paul Thananopavarn, MD, Angela Lipscomb-Hudson, MD, and Tanya Zinner, MD

Introduction

One of the most challenging and important aspects of geriatrics is maintaining an elderly person's function and quality of life. Functional independence is certainly one of the top priorities of people as they age. In a survey conducted by the National Council on Aging, Americans' greatest concerns about growing older were "not being able to take care of myself" and "being a burden."[1] Unfortunately, a multitude of physiologic changes that come with age lower a person's functional reserve capacity to withstand and recover from insults due to illness or accidents. However, the resulting impairments may be amenable to rehabilitation in an effort to restore function and independence.

Age and function

Functional aging may follow one of four models or paths.[2] The first model represents a person of good health and a large functional reserve who never becomes dependent with age, but then has a sudden catastrophic event or illness that leads to a quick demise (Figure 44.1). The second model describes a person who suffers from a series of debilitating events, but is temporarily able to recover most, but not all, function through healing and rehabilitation (Figure 44.2). The third model is of a person with a low functional reserve due to aging and disease who slips easily into a state of dependence (Figure 44.3). These models emphasize (1) the importance of maintaining a large functional reserve through preventive care, exercise, nutrition, and good fortune, and (2) that rehabilitation can be useful whenever there is a loss of function, but has the greatest potential in those with a high baseline functional status. The fourth model (Figure 44.4) relates to persons aging with a developmental disability. Rehabilitation medicine

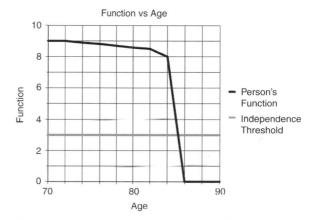

Figure 44.1 Older person with a high functional reserve who suffers a catastrophic illness.

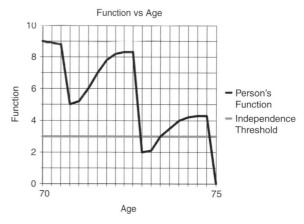

Figure 44.2 Person with a high functional reserve who suffers debilitating events but is able to recover through rehabilitation.

helps maximize a disabled person's potential early in development and may also be necessary later in life to recover function and quality of life. As more people survive and live longer with developmental or

---

Reichel's Care of the Elderly, 7th Edition, ed. Jan Busby-Whitehead *et al.* Published by Cambridge University Press.
© Cambridge University Press 2016.

Table 44.1 Definitions of impairment, activity, and participation

Term	Definition	Example
Impairment	Loss of body part or function	Broken hip from a fall
Activity (disability)	Loss of ability to perform an activity	Inability to walk and perform basic self-care
Participation (handicap)	Loss of ability to participate in a life situation	Unable to live independently at home

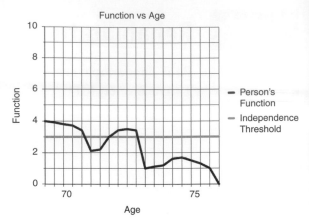

Figure 44.3 Older person with low functional reserve who declines into a state of dependence.

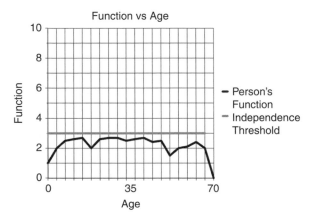

Figure 44.4 Person with a significant developmental disability who requires rehabilitation interventions early in life, then periodically during the aging process.

early-acquired disabilities, there will be more challenges in maintaining their function and the function of their caregivers in the face of aging.

Rehabilitation medicine physicians (physiatrists), geriatricians, and others caring for the elderly often find that there may be no perfect treatment for a disease or functional impairment that comes with aging. Rather, a compensatory mechanism must be found to help restore function. A simple example would be a hearing aid for presbycusis, which does not completely restore hearing but aids the elder in day-to-day interactions. More serious impairments, such as spastic hemiparesis from a stroke, have no simple restorative device and will have profound effects on the person's function, psychological state, social role, and relationships. The rehabilitation of this individual will therefore be a complex process that will require using a broader biopsychosocial model of medicine.

Impairment, activity, and participation

The World Health Organization provides a contextual framework through the terms "impairment," "activity," and "participation" to understand how the loss of a body function affects a person's ability to care for him- or herself and fulfill a role in society (Table 44.1).[3] The terms "activity" and "participation" have replaced the older terms "disability" and "handicap," respectively.

A person suffering from a hip fracture from a fall provides an excellent example of how to apply our understanding of the impairment, activity, and participation model as a framework for the rehabilitation process. First, the fracture must be fixed and direct medical consequences of surgery addressed. Second, skilled physical and occupational therapy is employed to improve the activities of mobility and self-care. Lastly, consideration of the person's motivation, pre-fall and post-surgery functional status, home environment, and caregiver support will determine whether the patient may recover at home or in a short-term rehabilitation facility. Ideally, with successful rehabilitation, the patient may regain full participation in life and return to independent living.

The functional assessment

A physician or practitioner leading the rehabilitation efforts of an elder must first assess and optimize the treatment of any medical problem that may act as a barrier to rehabilitation. For example, cognitive impairments from delirium, dementia, or depression

Table 44.2 Descriptors of functional ability and FIM* scoring

FIM score	Term	Definition
0		Activity does not exist
1	Dependent	Person needs 100% help to perform activity
2	Maximum assist	Person needs 75% help to perform activity
3	Moderate assist	Person needs 50% help to perform activity
4	Minimum assist	Person needs 25% help to perform activity
5	Contact guard stand-by assist	Person can perform activity with someone nearby to prevent fall or to provide verbal cues
6	Modified independent	Person can complete activity independently with an assistive device (e.g., walker)
7	Independent	Person completes activity independently

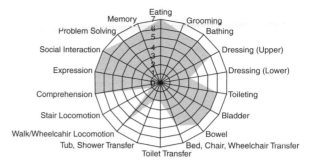

Figure 44.5 Graphical representation of the FIM instrument for a cognitively intact elder who has mobility and self-care impairments after a hip fracture.

may retard the participation in mobility training and the relearning of self-care skills. Poor cardiac or pulmonary status will reduce endurance and tolerance to therapy. Arthritic joint pain may limit range of joint motion and weight-bearing ability. Other complications of immobility, including pressure ulcers, venous thromboembolism, constipation, urinary incontinence, and disuse myopathy need to be prevented or addressed, as they can limit progress toward functional independence. Once the geriatric medical evaluation has been completed, the rehabilitation practitioner can focus on specific components of the geriatric assessment related to function and rehabilitation potential.

Premorbid functional status

A person's functional status prior to the onset of an illness or impairment is one of the most important factors in determining rehabilitation potential.[4] If an elder suffers an injury causing a loss of function, rehabilitation can hope to improve the person's function close to his baseline premorbid functional status. Consider the example of an elder able to walk community distances without an assistive device versus a person confined to a wheelchair due to severe spinal stenosis. If both suffer a unilateral amputation below the knee, the first elder's prognosis for walking with a prosthetic is good, whereas the debilitated elder's prognosis for ambulation is poor and would not be a reasonable goal for rehabilitation.[5]

Current functional status

A person's functional status with a new impairment is the determinant of how much and what type of rehabilitation is necessary. There are many instruments to measure and communicate function, including the Barthel Index and the FIM® Instrument (FIM).[6, 7] The FIM scale is the instrument used by inpatient rehabilitation facilities (IRFs) to measure the amount of assistance a person needs across 18 functional domains. These domains can be divided into five mobility categories, eight activities of daily living (ADL) categories, and five cognitive/communication categories (Figure 44.5).

Each functional domain is scored from 0 to 7, with 0 signifying that the activity does not exist and 7 indicating that the person is fully independent. The terms and definitions that correspond to the numerical scores are part of the normal functional vocabulary of rehabilitation and are useful in describing a patient's ability to perform any type of activity (Table 44.2).[8]

The FIM instrument can be scored by any trained professional who is working with and observing the patient. For example, a nursing assistant trained in the

FIM can score a patient's toilet transfer activity when assisting the patient, not requiring scoring by an occupational therapist. Typically, the FIM score is the sum of all the measured domains and is measured at the beginning and end of the inpatient rehabilitation stay to quantify functional progress.

Living environment and equipment

A person's home living environment, including accessibility, is important to establish early in the rehabilitation process. Is the abode one or two story? If it is a two-story house, is there a possibility for a first floor set-up? How many stairs are there to get into the house? Are there handrails? These are just some of the questions that are necessary to determine the functional goals that are achievable to enable a person to return and thrive at home. For a person who is expected to be wheelchair level, plans for a ramp and measurements of door widths need to be done early, in case construction or modifications are necessary. An elder's current stock of equipment and assistive devices, such as walkers, wheelchairs, commodes, and braces, needs to be assessed with the assistance of therapists for condition, fit, and appropriateness.

Social and caregiver support

The presence of a willing and able caregiver or supportive community of helpers is vital in the rehabilitation process, particularly for elders with major functional impairments. Often, there are limits to what can be achieved during the initial rehabilitation process, so caregivers must be identified early as part of the rehabilitation team, trained, and supported as they care for the elder through extended rehabilitation efforts at home. In the post-acute system, caregivers are important in the following ways: (1) a patient with a caregiver is more likely to be admitted to an inpatient facility for intensive rehabilitation, as the potential for home discharge is greater; (2) in the subacute rehabilitation setting, a person with a caregiver is more likely to return home than be relegated to long-term nursing home care.[9]

The elder's perception of impairment and rehabilitation goals

Asking elders' perceptions of why they think they have a functional problem may reveal underlying problems and barriers to the rehabilitation process. For example, a practitioner may assume that a hospitalized elder is not able to walk due to generalized weakness from extended bed rest. Yet when the practitioner asks, "Why do you think it is hard for you get up and walk?" the patient may reveal that he has knee pain from gout. Treatment of the gout will then relieve the pain, which was the major barrier to the mobilization process.

Another important component of the rehabilitation assessment is inquiring about a person's functional goals. This will assist with assessing motivation and with rehabilitation planning. An example would be asking a traumatic trans-tibial amputee his ultimate rehabilitation goal. If his goal is to be able to jog like he did before he lost his leg, a practitioner will plan for higher-level prosthetic components and intensive physical therapy for gait training. On the other hand, if the same patient feels that he is depressed and has no interest in walking, a referral to a psychologist or psychiatrist and an amputee support group may be a priority.

The rehabilitation physical exam

A comprehensive general geriatric physical exam should be completed; however, in the rehabilitation setting, more focus is placed on the neurologic and musculoskeletal aspects of the exam, as these two systems have the most effect on mobility, self-care skills, and cognitive function.

The rehabilitation team

The rehabilitation of an elderly person can be a complex process, requiring the expertise of multiple therapists and medical professionals. It is incumbent on a practitioner to understand the unique skills of each professional to be able to call on appropriate members to form an effective rehabilitation team. The patient and family are always the focus of our efforts and are considered active members of the team (Table 44.3).

Rehabilitation settings

Multidisciplinary versus interdisciplinary rehabilitation

Rehabilitation of an elderly person can potentially succeed in several different settings, including the hospital, inpatient rehabilitation facility (IRF), skilled nursing facility (SNF), outpatient rehabilitation center, assisted-living facility, or in the home. In higher-level rehabilitation settings, including IRFs and some

Table 44.3 The rehabilitation team

Physical therapist	Specializes in improving a person's mobility, including balance and gait. May recommend assistive devices such as canes and walkers. May use manual therapy and administer physical modalities such as heat and therapeutic ultrasound.
Occupational therapist	Specializes in improving basic self-care skills (ADL), such as bathing and dressing, and higher level IADL, including cooking and driving. May recommend home modifications and adaptive equipment, such as reachers or commodes. OTs can manufacture functional splints and can improve function in persons with vision impairment or neglect using compensatory techniques.
Speech therapist	Focuses on evaluating and treating speech, voice, language, and cognitive impairments. Can evaluate and treat dysphagia.
Rehabilitation nurse	Monitors vital signs, administers medications, performs wound care, manages bowel and bladder problems, assists with patient education and safety.
Recreational therapist	Specializes in the reintegration of the patient back into the community. Works on reducing stress and pain through relaxation techniques and diversion.
Neuropsychologist	Evaluates and treats cognitive, behavioral, and psychological impairments.
Orthotist/prosthetist	Manufactures and fits assistive devices such as ankle foot orthoses or prosthetic limbs to be worn by the patient.
Social worker	Identifies and coordinates resources to help the elder receive necessary services and equipment.
Primary physician/physiatrist	Evaluates the elder, manages medical issues, coordinates services, and orders equipment. A physiatrist is a physician with specialized training in rehabilitation medicine and the care of individuals with disabilities.

SNFs, the rehabilitation process is carefully coordinated and planned among therapy, medical, and social support services, making the experience an interdisciplinary effort. The group activity of this interdisciplinary team is synergistic, producing more than what the team members could produce separately.[10] In the outpatient or home setting, multiple therapy and medical services are available but usually not closely coordinated, making the experience multidisciplinary rather than interdisciplinary.[11]

Inpatient rehabilitation facilities

IRFs are suitable for patients with complex rehabilitation, nursing, *and* medical needs, such as a person with a spinal cord injury, amputation, burn, major multiple trauma, traumatic brain injury, or neurologic disorder (such as stroke, multiple sclerosis, or Parkinson's disease). Elders who have suffered hip fractures can qualify for inpatient rehabilitation if there is sufficient medical need to remain in a hospital setting. Patients must be able to participate in three hours of therapy a day, five days a week, in at least two

disciplines of physical therapy (PT), occupational therapy (OT), or speech therapy (ST). Severely debilitated medical patients with complex medical problems – such as renal failure, recent organ transplant, cancer, or left ventricular assist devices (LVAD) for heart failure – may also qualify if they have sufficient therapy needs to justify intensive rehabilitation. An IRF can be attached to a hospital or be a freestanding facility. Hospital-based facilities have better access to radiology, specialists, and associated procedures such as dialysis. The rehabilitation team is headed by a physiatrist who formulates a detailed treatment plan, visits the patient at least three times a week to address medical and therapy issues, and leads weekly interdisciplinary team meetings that proactively address any barriers to rehabilitation. A typical length of stay is 14 days, with the expectation that the patient's goal is to return to the community, not to an SNF. Medicare Part A covers inpatient rehabilitation as part of the elder's inpatient hospitalization days, with an average cost to Medicare of $1,500 a day.[12]

Subacute rehabilitation

Many nursing facilities have beds designated for skilled nursing and rehabilitation, along with long-term care beds for elders needing custodial care. SNFs are suitable for patients with more straightforward or less medically complex conditions, such as hip fractures, elective joint replacements, or debility due to a common illness such as pneumonia or a urinary tract infection with sepsis. In most cases, to qualify for Medicare-covered skilled services, a patient must have a three-day qualifying inpatient hospital stay and skilled nursing needs (IV antibiotics, enteral tube feeds, wound care) *or* rehabilitation needs in either PT, OT, *or* ST. Patients typically get one to two and a half hours of therapy a day. A physician must visit the patient upon admission and at least once every 30 days; however, a patient undergoing rehabilitation is often seen one or more times a week by a physician or physician extender. The typical cost of an SNF rehabilitation stay approaches $500 a day. [13] Medicare will cover 100% of an elder's stay at an SNF for the first 20 days and 80% of the cost thereafter for a total of 100 days, as long as there is a skilled nursing or therapy need. More often than not, a person will improve, plateau with therapy gains, and no longer qualify for Medicare-covered skilled nursing or therapy services before the 100-day mark. At that point, the elder returns to the community or is responsible for covering the cost of custodial care in the nursing home, unless the person has Medicaid or long-term-care insurance coverage.

Home health and outpatient rehabilitation

Intermittent multidisciplinary therapy and skilled nursing can be provided in the home or assisted-living facility if the patient is homebound and has sufficient caregiver support. Each type of therapy or nursing service can visit the patient two to three times per week at home. Once the elder is not homebound, outpatient therapy can provide longer, more intensive therapy, often with equipment not found in the home. Cost to Medicare is in the range of $100–$200 per visit and is subject to Medicare payment caps.

Selecting the rehabilitation setting for the elder

Studies that have attempted to compare rehabilitation outcomes for stroke,[14–16] hip fracture,[17–18] and joint replacement [19, 20] patients in various settings – IRF, SNF, or home health (HH) – do not definitely favor one setting over another. IRFs tended to demonstrate better functional outcomes than SNFs.[14–20] However, the results are confounded by selection bias and lack of uniform functional measurements, and by the fact that many patients will progress through multiple rehabilitation settings. In these studies and in practice, IRF patients have more complex medical and rehabilitation diagnoses, yet are able to tolerate three hours of therapy. SNF patients tend to be older and have cognitive deficits. HH patients are more likely to be younger, healthier, and have good home support. [16, 18]

Fee-for-service Medicare expenditures for post-acute care have risen, reaching $61.2 billion a year in 2011,[12] partly because Medicare reimburses each rehabilitation setting separately each time an elder accesses this service. In an effort to save on costs, Medicare complicates rehabilitation disposition decisions by putting artificial barriers to access – for example, the three-hour daily (15 hours per week) therapy rule for IRFs, three-day qualifying stay for SNFs, and homebound status for HH. Major changes appear to be underway as Medicare is exploring converting to a "bundle" payment system,[21] allowing only one payment for all post-acute and rehabilitation services per qualifying episode. Quality metrics would be in place to prevent patients from receiving inadequate care in the effort to save on costs. A bundled payment system would create financial incentives for providers and health-care systems to find the most cost-effective mix of post-acute medical and rehabilitation care that can produce good outcomes for patients and prevent hospital readmissions.

Geriatric assistive devices

Practitioners often order assistive devices for an elderly person to enhance safety with mobility or independence with self-care. Each device has the potential to help, but its use comes at an increased financial and energy cost. Improper or ill-fitted equipment can also pose a safety hazard that promotes a fall. A practitioner must know the potential benefits and risks of a piece of equipment and seek the assistance of a therapist who can help properly fit the device and train the elder on proper use.

Canes provide an extra point of contact with the ground, adding stability and tactile information about

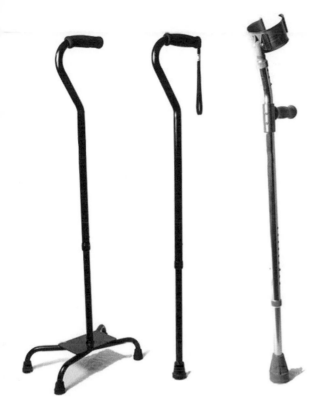

Figure 44.6 Four-point and single-point cane with offset handles. Forearm crutch.

the ground with walking.[23] A simple hook cane is useful for improving walking balance and proprioception, but it can be unstable as the force placed on the handle is not directly over the point of ground contact. A cane with an off-set handle places the handle's center of gravity directly over the ground contact point, allowing more stable weight bearing. No more than 15% of body weight should be placed through a cane. The cane should be fitted so that the top of the handle comes to about the wrist crease with the elbow flexed to about 15–20 degrees when holding the cane.[23] To off-load a painful lower extremity joint, the cane should be held by the contralateral hand and advanced with the painful limb. Canes can come with foot attachments with three or four points of contact, increasing the cane's stability, but at the cost of more weight, less natural gait pattern, and potential difficulty with stairs.

Axillary crutches are rarely used in the geriatric population, as they are difficult to handle, inherently unstable, and may cause axillary nerve compression if improperly used. Forearm or Lofstrand crutches have a cuff around the proximal forearm that allows hands to be free without dropping the crutch. They are easier to maneuver than axillary crutches and are often used for gait training after joint replacement surgery.[24]

Walkers provide a large base of support that can assist in walking stability. With the use of both upper extremities, a walker can help off-load a lower extremity. The disadvantages of walkers are that they can be difficult to maneuver (especially with stairs), promote poor back posture, and decrease arm swing.[25] Standard walkers with no wheels are very stable but require picking up to move forward, which slows down gait and requires significant upper body strength. They may be helpful for people after lower extremity surgery with weight-bearing restrictions or for people with cerebellar ataxia.[25] More commonly, elders use two-wheeled walkers or four-wheeled "rollator" type walkers (Figure 44.7). Two-wheeled walkers maintain a more normal gait pattern compared to standard walkers and can still be used for weight bearing. Rollators may be too easily moved to prevent a fall and therefore cannot be used for significant weight bearing. Rollators are well suited to help elders who need frequent rest breaks or use oxygen, as they often have fold-down seats or baskets to carry oxygen or other personal items.[25]

A manual wheelchair can be used by an elderly person if she is unable or unsafe to walk, or it can be used to help a caregiver transport a patient. A wheelchair needs to be carefully fitted to the patient by a therapist or wheelchair vendor to maximize its functional utility. Some considerations may include selecting: the proper seat height to allow propulsion with feet along with hands, elevating foot rests for comfort or edema control, detachable arm rest for slide board transfers, specialized seat cushion to prevent pressure ulcers, customized seat back to compensate for postural deformities, and lightweight design to reduce work to manually propel the chair or to lift the wheelchair for transport.[26]

Elders with severe weakness may require the assistance of a power-operated mobility device (Figure 44.8). A powered wheelchair's benefit of enhanced longer-range mobility at home and in the community must be balanced against the risk of worsening weakness, balance, and endurance from muscle disuse. Motorized systems are costly, potentially difficult to transport, and require extensive documentation for Medicare payment approval. Powered

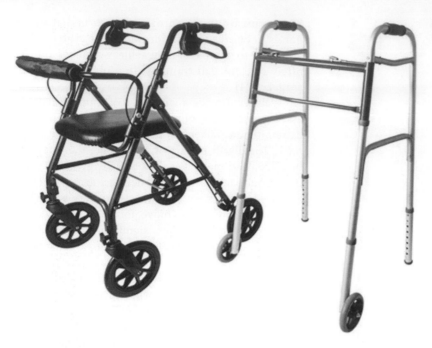

Figure 44.7 Two-wheeled and four-wheeled walkers.

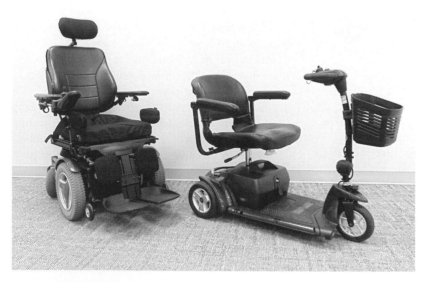

Figure 44.8 Motorized wheelchair and scooter.

scooters can be a less costly alternative that may be lighter and easier to disassemble/transport, but they have a wider turning radius and fewer seating customization possibilities as compared to powered wheelchairs. Scooters may be difficult to transfer into and cannot accommodate changes that come with progressive functional decline, such as those encountered in patients with multiple sclerosis or amyotropic lateral sclerosis. All powered mobility requires intact cognitive faculties and "behind the wheel" testing and training to ensure safe use.[26]

An assortment of aids to help the elderly with self-care activities can be prescribed, usually with the assistance of an occupational therapist. These include simple devices, such as mechanical "reachers" to pick up objects, dressing hooks to pull up pants, tub benches for safer bathing, and raised commodes to help with toilet transfers (Figure 44.9). For some patients with upper extremity hemiparesis, advanced rehabilitation centers are using more complex mechanical devices. One example is the Myopro™ myoelectric upper arm orthosis, which is a battery-

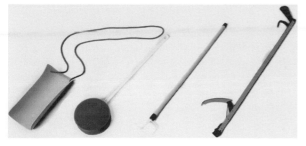

Figure 44.9 Sock aid, long-handle sponge, dressing hook, reacher.

powered arm brace that augments weak elbow flexor and/or extensor muscles to assist in such activities as eating, grooming, and picking up objects (Figure 44.10). Other centers are exploring ways to regenerate organs, muscles, and nerves to restore movement and vital functions. Despite our technological advances, we are many years away from being able to replace the most valuable and versatile aid of all: a human caregiver.

Rehabilitation of common geriatric problems

Stroke

With over 795,000 Americans experiencing a stroke each year, stroke has become the leading cause of long-term disability.[27] Unfortunately, despite procedural and pharmaceutical improvement in the treatment of stroke, 40% of stroke patients are left with moderate functional impairment and 15%–30% with severe disability.[28] The most common impairments after a stroke include motor weakness, sensory deficits, and problems with speech, language, cognition, swallowing, and vision. Spontaneous neurological recovery mostly occurs within the first three months post-stroke, with the most rapid functional recovery occurring in the first 30 days. Usually, there is very little functional motor recovery after six months post-stroke, but swallowing, speech, and sensory dysfunction may gradually improve over a longer period of time.[29] Some poor prognostic signs include no recovery in the first three to four weeks after a stroke, flaccid paralysis at four weeks post-stroke, severe neurological neglect, severe cognitive deficits, and advanced age.[28] Older stroke survivors may have a poorer stroke recovery prognosis given their increased likelihood of comorbid medical

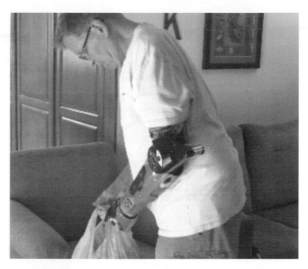

Figure 44.10 Myopro™ myoelectric upper arm orthosis. Photo courtesy of Myomo Corporation.

conditions and prior strokes.[30] Units specialized in organized stroke care and rehabilitation provide better patient outcomes for stroke patients.[31] Compared to general wards, these stroke units have demonstrated reduced mortality, improved recovery of mobility and self-care skills, and a greater likelihood of patients being able to return home. These advantages have been found to extend to stroke patients over the age of 75.[32]

A stroke resulting in significant impairments requires an interdisciplinary team for successful rehabilitation. Consider the example of a 70-year-old man with a history of atrial fibrillation who suffers a large right middle cerebral artery embolic stroke resulting in left spastic hemiplegia, hemianesthesia, hemianopsia, neglect, aprosody, dysphagia, and uninhibited neurogenic bladder. The patient has undergone all appropriate testing and lab work, has been initiated on appropriate secondary stroke prevention, and has avoided complications of immobility. A rehabilitation physician or physiatrist performs a medical and functional assessment of the patient and formulates a rehabilitation plan, which would need to include physical therapy, occupational therapy, speech therapy, nursing, recreational therapy, orthotics, and social case management. Early in the process, the patient's and family's needs and functional goals are explored. This aids in setting appropriate expectations, motivates and engages the patient, and results in improved outcomes.[33]

Motor recovery in hemiplegic stroke progresses in phases.[34, 35] Initially, there is flaccid paralysis and areflexia. Neurologic recovery may be heralded by return of deep tendon reflexes, increased tone, and spasticity. Early voluntary movement may then return in uncoordinated "synergistic" patterns where entire groups of extensor or flexor muscles across multiple joints of a limb co-contract upon initiation of movement. Fortunate hemiplegics may progress to regain functional control of individual muscles and return to normal tone, often in a proximal to distal manner.

Traditional rehabilitation therapies attempt to enhance natural motor recovery and control using physical sensory and motor stimulation, with considerable controversy on whether to promote or suppress synergisms. Rehabilitation also now includes more task-oriented therapy where rehabilitation is focused on acquisition of skills for performance of meaningful and relevant tasks. Programs aim to be challenging, progressive, and optimally adapted to the patient's capabilities and environment, and invoke active participation to prevent learned disuse.[33] An example of this is constraint-induced movement therapy (CIMT), a technique in which a hemiparetic patient uses her weak limb while her strong, unaffected limb is constrained by wearing a mitt. CIMT has been shown to promote cortical reorganization and motor recovery.[35] A practiced form of gait therapy for hemiplegia is body-weight-supported treadmill training (BWSTT), which involves suspending the patient over a treadmill with the therapist assisting in leg movement through the gait cycle (Figure 44.11). BWSTT has shown superior effectiveness over traditional gait training, but requires specialized equipment and significant effort from a therapist moving the paretic leg.[36] Other interventions under study that may prove helpful in enhancing recovery include robotic-assisted motor retraining,[37] functional electrical stimulation,[38] use of neurostimulant medications that augment norepinephrine,[39] and noninvasive brain stimulation using magnetic fields or direct transcranial current to activate dormant brain tissue.[40]

Spasticity is an upper motor neuron condition in which muscles are continuously contracting due to damage of the central nervous system involved in movement. The associated stiffness or tightness may cause difficulty with performing ADL or walking, but may assist gait in some circumstances by preventing knee buckling. Therapy for spasticity is designed to

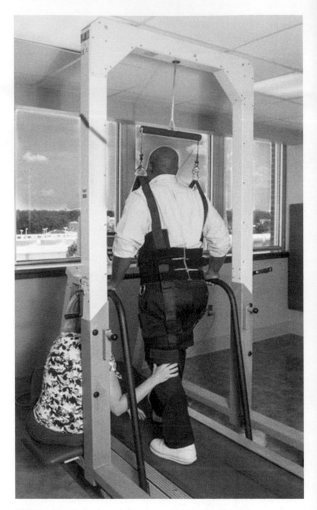

Figure 44.11 Body-weight-supported treadmill training.

reduce muscle tone, maintain or improve range of motion and mobility, increase strength and coordination, and improve comfort.[41, 42] Therapy may include stretching and strengthening exercises, limb positioning, application of cold packs, and electrical stimulation. Oral centrally acting medications such as baclofen, tizanidine, and valium can be used to treat spasticity but must be used with caution in the elderly, as they can cause sedation or confusion. Alternatives include phenol nerve blocks and botulinum toxin injections that reduce muscle tone without causing sedating side effects.

Orthotics are often prescribed to reduce or control spasticity while preserving range of motion and enhancing joint stability in paretic limbs.[43] A common upper extremity orthosis fashioned by occupational therapists is the resting hand split. This orthotic

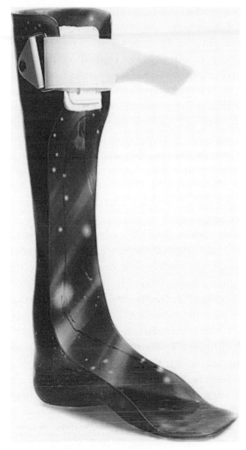

Figure 44.12 Ankle foot orthosis.

prevents contractures and reduces spasticity by keeping the wrist and fingers in relative extension, thereby breaking up the flexion synergy pattern. For a paretic or spastic lower extremity, an orthotist is commonly asked to manufacture ankle foot orthosis (AFO). AFOs come in many forms and have the potential to reduce foot drop by limiting plantar flexion in the swing phase of gait (Figure 44.12). In stance phase, an AFO limits dorsiflexion of the ankle, which in turn enhances knee extension and reduces knee buckling. Elongating the footplate to prevent toes from curling under can interrupt plantar flexion synergism, reducing spasticity and the incidence of ankle contractures.

Pain after stroke most commonly occurs in the hemiparetic shoulder and must be addressed for elder comfort and to allow progress with therapy. The incidence of shoulder pain ranges from 34%–84%, and it correlates with the severity of motor impairment.[44] The etiologic cause of post-stroke shoulder pain can be challenging to ascertain and requires a proper shoulder exam and, at times, radiographic imaging. The differential diagnosis includes glenohumeral subluxation due to muscle weakness, bursitis/tendonitis/rotator cuff tear from improper pulling or positioning of the arm, adhesive capsulitis due to spasticity and immobility, heterotopic ossification, and complex regional pain syndrome.[45]

To reduce shoulder subluxation, it is important to support the arm while the patient is seated or standing, using a vertical cuff sling or wheelchair lap tray. However, classic arm slings that promote adduction and internal rotation of the arm can increase the risk for developing adhesive capsulitis or frozen shoulder. Early hemiplegic shoulder rehabilitation goals include pain prevention using gentle range of motion, proper positioning, spasticity control, and caregiver education. However, once pain begins, a practitioner may need to consider physical modalities, massage, shoulder taping, topical and oral pain medications, neuromuscular electrical stimulation,[46] or corticosteroid injections,[47] depending on the pain etiology.

Dysphagia is a common sequelae of a stroke, occurring in approximately 40% of stroke patients. [48] A speech language pathologist (SLP) screens for swallowing dysfunction by identifying signs such as impaired cough or gag, drooling, coughing or choking with meals, pocketing of food, and dysphonia. High-risk patients will need to undergo a modified barium swallow or fiberoptic endoscopic evaluation of swallowing (FEES) to assess the severity of dysphagia and to determine fluid and meal consistency recommendations. Techniques taught by SLPs to reduce aspiration risk include elevating the bed to at least 30 degrees, turning the head to the paretic side, and performing a chin tuck when eating. Severe dysphagia may require alternative routes of nutrition intake, including consideration of a gastrostomy tube.[49]

Cognitive and communication impairments are influenced by the location of the stroke and are evaluated and treated by an SLP. Aphasias can be broadly categorized into Broca's or productive aphasia, in which a patient has difficulty with speaking but has intact comprehension, or Wernicke's or receptive aphasia, in which comprehension is impaired but speech is intact. Patients with impaired comprehension are a challenge to rehabilitate, given their limited ability to understand and follow commands. Another factor affecting cognitive performance may be depression, which can affect 25%–79% of patients after stroke.[50] Risk factors for post-stroke depression include prior psychiatric history, significant impairment in ADL, high severity of deficits, female gender, nonfluent aphasia, cognitive impairment, and lack of social support. Treatment of depression with an antidepressant medication like an SSRI (selective serotonin reuptake inhibitor) has been shown to be beneficial in aiding in post-stroke recovery.[50]

Most stroke patients with significant impairments will benefit from inpatient rehabilitation provided they are able to tolerate and actively participate in intensive therapy. The effectiveness of an interdisciplinary team approach can be demonstrated in the management of post-stroke urinary incontinence in a 70-year-old woman due to a disinhibited and spastic bladder. During the weekly interdisciplinary team meeting, factors such as UTI, left neglect, hemianopsia, weakness with transfers, and decreased motivation due to depression are identified as barriers to urinary continence. The physiatrist prescribes antibiotics for the UTI, and an antidepressant for depression. Physical therapy works on strengthening and transfers, while occupational therapy works on toileting and visual scanning training for neglect. Nursing begins a timed toileting routine with a commode placed on the right side of the bed. A psychologist implements cognitive-behavioral treatment for depression, and case management contacts the family to order home equipment and therapy and to set up family training. This type of coordinated effort is rarely found in less intensive rehabilitation settings.

Parkinson's disease

The most common movement disorder encountered among geriatric rehabilitation patients is Parkinson's disease. The incidence of Parkinson's disease increases with age, affecting 1%–2% of the population over 65 and more than 4% of those over 85.[51] In spite of optimal pharmacological treatment, functions such as gait, transfers, posture, balance, and speech can progressively deteriorate, leading to impaired self-care, mobility, stability, communication, and quality of life. Newer treatments such as deep brain stimulation procedures may extend the period of functional stability but may not be an option for all patients nor be entirely successful in restoring normal movement.

One of the most studied rehabilitation strategies in Parkinson's disease is the use of external sensory cues. This is based on the hypothesis that people with Parkinson's disease have less central delivery of proprioceptive input but can compensate by using visual cues to activate alternative neural networks in the cerebellum to promote movement. Visual cues – including the use of floor stripes, timing lights, and mirrors – have been frequently found to increase stride length.[52] Auditory cues are hypothesized to replace the "internal timekeeping" function of the degenerated basal ganglia to help initiate movement. Auditory cues, including the use of metronomes and music, may be effective in increasing gait cadence.[53] Treadmill training and gait training with external rhythmic or intermittent auditory, visual, proprioceptive, or cognitive cueing have demonstrated short-term improvement in gait speed, step length, freezing, and balance in the Parkinson's patient; however, sustained improvement has not been demonstrated.[54, 55]

More traditional PT focusing on interventions to improve postural control, balance, and gait have shown immediate and short-term benefit in Parkinson's patients.[56–59] Physical therapy may help train patients with assistive devices, including the use of modified ski poles to walk in a pattern similar to cross country skiing to improve gait velocity[60] or the use of four-wheeled walkers, which can reduce freezing of gait, festination, and retropulsion (falling backward).[61]

In Parkinson's disease, speech volume and articulation may be low or reduced, and dysphagia may be an issue; both problems can be addressed by a speech therapist. The best-studied treatment for hypokinetic dysarthria that has shown clinical effectiveness is the Lee Silverman Voice Treatment (LSVT®).[62] In essence, the patient is trained to "think loud and think shout" in order to increase the strength of the respiratory muscles to move air and to enhance vocal cord adduction to produce voice. Other studied voice treatments include Pitch Limiting Voice Treatment (PLVT®), in which the emphasis is to "speak loud and low," a treatment that addresses the strained, high-pitched voice that may result from LSVT but still has comparable efficacy.[63]

Hip fracture

Hip fractures are common within the geriatric population, ranking as one of the top causes of hospitalization among the elderly.[64] More than 95% of hip fractures are caused by falls, with 258,000 hip fractures in 2010.[65, 66] Approximately 50% of patients sustaining a hip fracture are unable to regain an independent level of functioning.[67] In addition to a significant increase in the risk of death and morbidity following hip fracture, the economic impact is enormous, with an estimated cost of over $20 billion in the United States in 1997.[68–70]

The majority of hip fractures require surgery, and early repair (within 24–48 hours) is recommended as long as the patient is medically stable.[71, 72] The type of repair is determined in large part by the location of the fracture. The vascularity of the intertrochanteric region (extracapsular) typically allows good healing with proper reduction and fixation. Conversely, the relatively poor blood supply of the femoral neck (intracapsular) leads to a higher rate of complications after fracture.

The goal after hip fracture repair is early mobilization, both to optimize functional status and to prevent common complications from immobility, such as pneumonia, muscle weakness, delirium, and pressure sores. Early ambulation, starting within 48 hours of surgery, has been shown to accelerate functional recovery.[73] Particularly in the elderly, the ability to bear weight on the injured extremity is crucial for ambulation. It appears that for certain fracture patterns, patients with normal protective sensation can safely bear weight sooner than is allowed by most protocols.[74] It is important to educate patients on appropriate hip precautions in order to avoid hip dislocation after surgery. For a patient who underwent a posterior approach total or hemi hip arthroplasty, this includes no hip flexion greater than 90 degrees, no hip adduction past neutral (i.e., no crossing the legs), and no internal rotation of the affected extremity. This can be difficult in patients with memory impairment, but studies show that the presence of mild or moderate dementia should not preclude inclusion in a rehabilitation program.[75, 76]

Unfortunately, establishing evidence-based strategies for improving mobility after hip fracture surgery remains difficult due to insufficient and contradicting evidence.[77] However, there is some support for early in-hospital multidisciplinary geriatric intervention,[78] as well as for an intensive upper body exercise program with its positive effect on mobility and balance.[79] Functionally oriented exercise after hip fracture has been shown to be beneficial longer term as well, continuing in the home setting for up to nine months following discharge from traditional rehabilitation services.[80]

Another important area to consider in the rehabilitation of the elderly hip fracture patient is proper nutrition, with particular attention to vitamin D and protein deficiency. Both can have an impact on bone mass and falls.[81, 82] Checking a vitamin D level as well as looking at the protein status in at-risk patients is relatively inexpensive and should be addressed prior to discharge. Oral supplements and patient and family education, with planned follow-up with the primary care physician post discharge, are prudent. In addition, looking at the need for additional medication for osteoporosis and performing a falls risk assessment are important to consider in this population.

Lower extremity amputation

In the elderly population, complications of diabetes and peripheral vascular disease account for the majority of lower extremity amputations. The primary surgical goal is to save as much limb length as possible while allowing adequate healing. However, function and cosmesis of the prosthesis need to be taken into account as well when choosing the length of the residual limb. Mortality rates are high with both above and below knee amputations, and appear to be related to serious comorbidities such as kidney and heart disease, dementia, and reduced preoperative functional status.[83] Preoperative mobility, independence in activities of daily living, ability to stand on one leg, fitness, and intact cognition are all predictors of good walking ability after lower limb amputation. [84] The energy expenditure required to walk with an above-knee prosthesis is increased 100% compared to normal walking, making independent ambulation with an above-knee amputation in older individuals difficult. This compares to an approximately 40% increase over normal walking with a below-knee prosthesis (Figure 44.13), which many elderly patients are able to tolerate.[85] The physical therapist can help assess the K-level of a given patient to determine which prosthetic components are covered by Medicare. K-levels are a rating system (0–4) used by Medicare to indicate an individual's rehabilitation potential with a prosthesis, based on the potential of the patient to ambulate and navigate her environment. A K-level 0 amputee is nonambulatory, a K-level 2 amputee is a community ambulator, whereas a

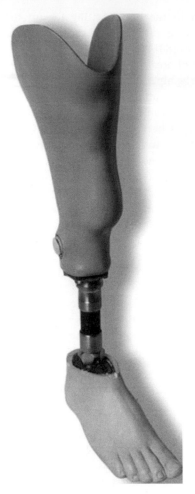

Figure 44.13 Basic trans-tibial prosthesis.

K-level 4 amputee is an active adult performing high-impact athletic activities.

Range of motion and strengthening exercises as well as pre-prosthetic education focus on avoiding flexion contractures at the hip and knee, which can interfere with future prosthetic function. In addition, issues such as depression over the lost limb, stump pain and phantom limb pain management, hygiene and skin issues, prosthetic fitting and managing stump volume variations, safe use of the prosthetic, and fall prevention should be addressed by the rehabilitation team.[86]

Conclusion

Restoring or maintaining an elder's function and independence through rehabilitation can be one of the most challenging and rewarding aspects of a geriatric practice. It involves not just evaluating elders' medical and functional issues, but also assessing their motivation, goals, caregiver support, and environment for recovery. More complex rehabilitation issues require a multidisciplinary team approach that may involve physical modalities, specialized medications, adaptive equipment, multiple therapies, and professionals specialized in rehabilitation. By understanding how to overcome the multiple impairments that can come with age, we can promote full participation in society and enhance an elder's quality of life.

References

1. The United States of Aging Survey 2013. Available at: www.ncoa.org/assets/files/pdf/united-states-of-aging/2013-survey/USA13-Full-Report.pdf (accessed March 27, 2014).

2. Lunney JR, Lynn J, Hogan C. Profiles of older Medicare decedents. *J Am Geriatr Soc.* 2002;**50**:1108–1112.

3. World Health Organization Health Topics on Disabilities. Available at: www.who.int/topics/disabilities/en (accessed March 29, 2014).

4. Mosqueda LA. Assessment of rehabilitation potential. *Clin in Geriatr Med.* 1993;**9**:689–703.

5. Harris KA, van Schie L, Carroll SE, et al. Rehabilitation potential of elderly patients with major amputations. *J Cardiovasc Surg.* 1991;**32**:463–467.

6. Mahoney FI, Barthel D. Functional evaluation: the Barthel Index. *Maryland State Medical J.* 1965;**14**:56–61.

7. Granger CV, Hamilton BB, Linacre JM, et al. Performance profiles of the functional independence measure. *Am J of Phys Med Rehab.* 1993; **72**(2):84–89.

8. Hamilton BB, Laughlin JA, Fiedler RC, Granger CV. Interrater reliability of the 7-level functional independence measure (FIM). *Scandinavian J of Rehabil Med.* 1994;**26**:115–119.

9. Forester AJ, Murff HJ, Peterson JF, et al. The incidence and severity of adverse events affecting patients after discharge from the hospital. *Ann Intern Med.* 2003;**138**:161–167.

10. Melvin JL. Interdisciplinary and multidisciplinary activities and the ACRM. *Arch Phys Med Rehab.* 1980;**61**:379–380.

11. Norrefalk JR. How do we define multidisciplinary rehabilitation? *J Rehabil Med.* 2003;**35**:100–101.

12. Medicare Payment Advisory Commission. Health care spending and the Medicare program. Available at www.medpac.gov/documents/Jun13DataBookEntireReport.pdf (accessed May 10, 2014).

13. Office of the Inspector General, Department of Health and Human Services. Changes in skilled

nursing facilities billing in fiscal year 2011. Available at http://oig.hhs.gov/oei/reports/oei-02-09-00204.pdf (accessed May 10, 2014).

14. Deutsch A, Granger CV, Heinemann AW, et al. Poststroke rehabilitation: outcomes and reimbursement of inpatient rehabilitation facilities and subacute rehabilitation programs. *Stroke.* 2006;**37**:1477–1482.

15. Chan L, Sandel ME, Jette AM, et al. Does postacute care site matter? A longitudinal study assessing functional recovery after a stroke. *Arch Phys Med Rehab.* 2013;**94**:622–629.

16. Kramer AM, Steiner JF, Schlenker RE, et al. Outcomes and costs after hip fracture and stroke: a comparison of rehabilitation settings. *JAMA.* 1997;**277**:396–404.

17. Munin MC, Seligman K, Dew MA, Effect of rehabilitation site on functional recovery after hip fracture. *Arch Phys Med Rehabil.* 2005;**86**:367–372.

18. Mallison T, Deutsch A, Bateman J, Comparison of discharge functional status after rehabilitation in skilled nursing, home health, and medical rehabilitation settings for patients after hip fracture repair. *Arch Phys Med Rehab.* 2014;**95**:209–217.

19. Dejong G, Horn SD, Smout RJ, et al. Joint replacement rehabilitation outcomes on discharge from skilled nursing facilities and inpatient rehabilitation facilities. *Arch Phys Med Rehabil.* 2009;**90**:1284–1296.

20. DeJong G, Tian W, Smout RJ, et al. Long-term outcomes of joint replacement rehabilitation patients discharged from skilled nursing and inpatient rehabilitation facilities. *Arch Phys Med Rehabil.* 2009;**90**:1306–1316.

21. Centers for Medicare and Medicaid Services. Bundled Payments for Care Improvement (BPCI) Initiative: general information. Available at: http://innovation.cms .gov/initiatives/bundled-payments (accessed May 10, 2014).

22. Kaye HS, Hang T, LaPlante MP. *Mobility Device Use in the United States.* Disability Statistics Report No. 14. Washington, DC: National Institute on Disability and Rehabilitation Research, US Department of Education; 2000.

23. Kumar R, Roe MC, Scremin OU. Methods for estimating the proper length of a cane. *Arch Phys Med Rehabil.* 1995;**76**:1173–1175.

24. Faruqui SR, Jaeblon T. Ambulatory assistive devices in orthopaedics: uses and modifications. *J Am Acad Orthop Surg.* 2010;**18**:41–50.

25. Bradley SM, Hernandez CR. Geriatric assistive devices. *Am Fam Phys.* 2011;**84**:405–411.

26. Koontz AM, Karmarkar AM, Spaeth DM, et al. Wheelchairs and seating systems. In: Braddom RL, Chan L, Harrast MA (eds.). *Physical Medicine and Rehabilitation.* Philadelphia: Elsevier, Philadelphia, 2011: 373–401.

27. American Stroke Association. Impact of Stroke. Available at: www.strokeassociation.org/STROKEO RG/AboutStroke/Impact-of-Stroke-Stroke-statistics_ UCM_310728_Article.jsp (accessed May 27, 2014).

28. Duncan P. AHA/ASA-endorsed practice guidelines management of adult stroke rehabilitation care, a clinical practice guideline. *Stroke.* 2005; **36**:e100–e143.

29. Jorgensen HS, Nakayama H, Raaschou HO, Olsen TS. Neurological and functional recovery: the Copenhagen stroke study. *Phys Med Rehabil Clin N Am.* 1999;**10**(4):887–906.

30. Kammersgaard LP, Jørgensen HS, Reith J, et al. Short- and long-term prognosis for very old stroke patients: the Copenhagen stroke study. *Age Ageing.* 2004;**33**(2):149.

31. Stroke Unit Trialists Collaboration. Organised inpatient (stroke unit) care for stroke. *Cochrane Database Syst Rev* 2007; **4**: CD000197.

32. Gresham GE, Duncan PW, Stason WB, et al. *Post Stroke Rehabilitation.* Clinical Practice Guideline No.16. Rockville, MD: US Department of Health and Human Services. Public Health Service, Agency for Health Care Policy and Research. AHCPR Publication No. 1995:95–0662.

33. Langhorne, P, Bernhardt J, Kwakkel G. Stroke rehabilitation. *Lancet.* 2011,**377**:1693–1702.

34. Brunnstrom S. Associated reactions of the upper extremity in adult patients with hemiplegia; an approach to training. *Phys Ther Rev.* 1956;**36**:225–236.

35. Wolf SL, Winstein CJ, Miller JP, et al. Effect of constraint-induced movement therapy on upper extremity function 3 to 9 months after stroke: The EXCITE randomized clinical trial. *JAMA.* 2006;**296** (17):2095–2104.

36. Hesse S, Bertelt C, Jahnke MT, et al. Treadmill training with partial body weight support compared with physiotherapy in nonambulatory hemiparetic patients. *Stroke.* 1995;**26**(6):976–981.

37. Ferraro M, Palazzolo JJ, Krol J, et al. Robot-aided sensorimotor arm training improves outcome in patients with chronic stroke. *Neurology.* 2003;**61**:1604–1607.

38. Yan T, Hui-Chan C, Li L. Functional electrical stimulation improves motor recovery of the lower extremity and walking ability in subjects with first acute stroke. *Stroke.* 2005;**36**:80–85.

39. Gladstone DJ, Danells CJ, Armesto A, et al. Physiotherapy coupled with dextroamphetamine for motor rehabilitation after hemiparetic stroke: a randomized, double-blind, placebo-controlled trial. *Stroke.* 2006;**37**:179–185.

40. Harvey RL, Nudo RJ. Cortical brain stimulation: a potential therapeutic agent for upper limb motor recovery following stroke. *Top Stroke Rehabil.* 2007;**14**:54–67.

41. McGuire J, Harvey RL. The prevention and management of complications after stroke. *Phys Med Rehabil Clin N Am.* 1999;**10**:857–874.

42. Scanlan S, McGuire J. Effective collaboration between physician and occupational therapist in the management of upper limb spasticity after stroke. *Top Stroke Rehabil.* 1998;**4**:1–13.

43. Good D, Supan T. Basic principles of orthotics in neurological disorders. In: Aisen M (ed.). *Orthotics in Neurological Rehabilitation.* New York, NY: Demos Publications, 1992:1–23.

44. Najenson T, Yacubovich E, Pikielni SS. Rotator cuff injury in shoulder joints of hemiplegic patients. *Scandinavian J Rehabil Med.* 1971;**3**:131–137.

45. Barlak A, Unsal S, Kaya K, et al. Poststroke shoulder pain in Turkish stroke patients: relationship with clinical factors and functional outcomes. *Int J Rehabil Res.* 2009;**32**:309–315.

46. Chantraine A, Banbeault A, Uebelhart D, Gremion G. Shoulder pain and dysfunction in hemiplegia: effects of functional electrical stimulation. *Arch Phys Med Rehabil.* 1999;**80**:328–331.

47. Viana R, Pereira S, Mehta S, et al. Evidence for therapeutic interventions for hemiplegic shoulder pain during the chronic stage of stroke: a review. *Top Stroke Rehabil.* 2012;**19**:514–522.

48. Martino R, Foley N, Bhogal S, et al. Dysphagia after stroke: incidence, diagnosis, and pulmonary complications. *Stroke.* 2005;**36**:2756–2763.

49. Foley N, Teasell R, Martino R, et al. Dysphagia treatment post stroke: a systematic review of randomised controlled trials. *Age Ageing.* 2008;**37**:258–264.

50. Spalletta G, Caltagirone C Stein J, et al. Depression and other neuropsychiatric disorders. In: Harvey R, Stein J, Winstein C, et al. (eds.). *Stroke Recovery and Rehabilitation*, 2nd ed. New York, NY: Demos Publications; 2009: 455.

51. DeRijk MC, Breteler MB, Graveland GA, et al. Prevalence of Parkinson's disease in the elderly: the Rotterdam Study. *Neurology.* 1995;**45**:2143–2146.

52. Rubinstein TC, Giladi N, Hausdorff JM. The power of cueing to circumvent dopamine deficits: a review of physical therapy treatment of gait disturbances in Parkinson's disease. *Move Disord.* 2002;**70**:289–297.

53. Moroz A, Edgley SR, Lew HL, Chae J. Rehabilitation interventions in Parkinson disease. *PMR.* 2009;**1**:S42–48.

54. Ransmayr G. Physical, occupational, speech and swallowing therapies and physical exercise in Parkinson's disease. *J Neural Transm.* 2011;**118**:773–781.

55. Petzinger GM, Walsh JP, Akopian G, et al. Effects of treadmill exercise on dopaminergic transmission in the 1-methyl-4-phenyl-1, 2, 3, 6-tetrahydropyridine-lesioned mouse model of basal ganglia injury. *J Neurosci.* 2007;**27**:5291–5300.

56. Toole T, Hirsch MA, Forkink A, et al. The effects of a balance and strength training program on equilibrium in Parkinsonism: a preliminary study. *NeuroRehabilitation.* 2000;**14**:165–174.

57. Hirsch MA, Toole T, Maitland CG, et al. The effects of balance training and high-intensity resistance training on persons with idiopathic Parkinson's disease. *Arch Phys Med Rehabil.* 2003;**84**:1109–1117.

58. Jobges M, Heuschkel G, Pretzel C, et al. Repetitive training of compensatory steps: a therapeutic approach for postural instability in Parkinson's disease. *J Neurol Neurosurg Psychiatry.* 2004;**75**:1682–1687.

59. Stankovic I. The effect of physical therapy on balance of patients with Parkinson's disease. *Int J Rehabil Res.* 2004;**27**:53–57.

60. Baastile J, Langbein WE, Weaver F, et al. Effect of exercise on perceived quality of life of individuals with Parkinson's disease. *J Rehabil Res Devel.* 2003;**37**:529–534.

61. Kegelmeyer DA, Parthasarathy S, Kostyk SK, et al. Assistive devices alter gait patterns in Parkinson disease: advantages of the four-wheeled walker. *Gait Posture.* 2013;**38**:20–24.

62. Ramig LO, Sapir S, Countryman S, et al. Intensive voice treatment (LSVT) for patients with Parkinson's disease: a 2-year follow up. *J Neurol Neurosurg Psychiatry.* 2001;**71**:493–498.

63. deSwart BJM, Wilemse SC, Maassen BAM, et al. Improvement of voicing in patients with Parkinson's disease by speech therapy. *Neurology.* 2003;**60**:498–500.

64. Agency for Healthcare Research and Quality. Statistical Brief #6: Hospitalizations in the Elderly Population, 2003. Available at: www.hcup-us.ahrq.go v/reports/statbriefs/sb6.jsp (accessed June 28, 2014).

65. Hayes WC, Myers ER, Morris JN, et al. Impact near the hip dominates fracture risk in elderly nursing home residents who fall. *Calcified Tissue Internat.* 1993;**52**:192–198.

66. National Center for Health Statistics. National Hospital Discharge Survey (NHDS), Available at: www.cdc.gov/nchs/hdi.htm (accessed September 14, 2011).

67. Morrison RS, Chassin MR, Siu AL. The medical consultant's role in caring for patients with hip fracture. *Ann Intern Med.* 1998;**128**:1010.

68. Wolinsky FD, Fitzgerald JF, Stump TE. The effect of hip fracture on mortality, hospitalization, and functional status: a prospective study. *Am J Public Health.* 1997;**87**:398.

69. Bentler SE, Liu L, Obrizan M, et al. The aftermath of hip fracture: discharge placement, functional status change, and mortality. *Am J Epidemiol.* 2009;**170**:1290.

70. Braithwaite RS, Col NF, Wong JB. Estimating hip fracture morbidity, mortality and costs. *J Am Geriatric Soc.* 2003;**51**:364–370.

71. Shiga T, Wajima Z, Ohe Y. Is operative delay associated with increased mortality of hip fracture patients? Systematic review, meta-analysis and meta-regression. *Can J Anaesth.* 2008;**55**:146–154.

72. Orosz GM, Magaziner J, Hannan EL, et al. Association of timing of surgery for hip fracture and patient outcomes. *JAMA.* 2004;**291**:1738–1743.

73. Oldmeadow LB, Edward ER, Kimmell LA, et al. No rest for the wounded: early ambulation after hip surgery accelerates recovery. *ANZ J Surg.* 2006;**76**:607–611.

74. Kubiak EN, Beebe MJ, North K, et al. Early weight bearing after lower extremity fractures in adults. *J Am Acad Orthop Surg.* 2003;**21**:727–738.

75. Huusko TM, Karppi P, Avikainen V, et al. Randomised, clinically controlled trial of intensive geriatric rehabilitation in patients with hip fracture: subgroup analysis of patients with dementia. *BMJ.* 2000;**321**:1107–1111.

76. Rolland Y, Pillard F, Lauwers-Cances V, et al. Rehabilitation outcome of elderly patients with hip fracture and cognitive impairment. *Disabil Rehabil.* 2004;**26**:425–31.

77. Handoll HHG, Sherrington C, Mak JCS. Interventions for improving mobility after hip fracture surgery in adults. *Cochrane Database Syst Rev.* 2011 Mar 16;**3**: CD001704. doi. 10.1002/14651858.CD001704, pub4.

78. Vidan M, Serra JA, Moreno C, et al. Efficacy of a comprehensive geriatric intervention in older patients hospitalized for hip fracture: a randomized, controlled trial. *J Am Geriatr Soc.* 2005;**53**:1476–1482.

79. Mendelsohn ME, Overend TJ, Connelly DM, et al. Improvement in aerobic fitness during rehabilitation after hip fracture. *Arch Phys Med Rehabil.* 2008;**89**:609–617.

80. Latham NK, Harris BA, Bean JF, et al. Effect of a home-based exercise program on functional recovery following rehabilitation after hip fracture. A randomized clinical trial. *JAMA.* 2014;**311**:707–709.

81. Garoon M, FitzGerald O. Vitamin D deficiency; subclinical and clinical consequences on musculoskeletal health. *Cur Rheum Rep.* 2012;**14**:286–293.

82. Bischoff HA, Stahelin HB, Dick W, et al. Effects of vitamin D and calcium supplementation on falls: a randomised controlled trial. *J Bone Mineral Res.* 2003;**18**:343–351.

83. Rosen N, Gigi R, Haim A, et al. Mortality and reoperations following lower limb amputations. *IMAJ.* 2014;**16**:83–87.

84. Sansam K, Neumann V, O'Connor R, Bhakta B. Predicting walking ability following lower limb amputation: a systematic review of the literature. *J Rehabil Med.* 2009;**41**:593–603.

85. Waters RL, Perry D, Antonelli D, Hislop H. Energy cost of walking of amputees: the influence of level of amputation. *J Bone Joint Surg Am.* 1976;**58**:42–46.

86. Patnera E, Pourtier-Piotte C, Bensoussan L, Coudeyre E. Patient education after amputation: systematic review and experts' opinions. *Ann Phys Rehabil Med.* 2014;**57**:143–212.

Chapter **45**

Geriatric sexuality

Lisa Granville, MD

Introduction

Sexuality is an important part of health and quality of life at all ages and thus is an important area for healthcare providers to address. As the baby boom generation ages, different attitudes and mores regarding sexuality are coming forward as a result of growing up in the "free love" generation. In time, discussion of sexuality with older adults is anticipated to be more direct, open, and often initiated by well-informed patients. Now, however, a number of fallacies regarding sexuality later in life prevail. Many prefer to believe that sexuality in older adults simply does not exist. Brogan notes that "there is a general societal belief that old people are, or should be, asexual and a false assumption exists that physical attractiveness depends on youth and beauty."[1] Alternatively, sexuality in older adults is considered a laughing matter. Comical cards and ones on old age often give messages about physical weakness and failures in sexual performance.[2] Misinformation and misperceptions about sexuality and older adults are held by both patients and clinicians. Failure to adequately address sexuality and diagnose and treat sexual problems can lead to depression and social withdrawal,[3] self-discontinuation of those medications with adverse side effects to sexual satisfaction,[4] and increased risk for sexually transmitted infections including HIV/AIDS.[5]

Sexual activity

The number of years of potential sexual activity in later life is increasing.[6] The demographic trends of Americans living longer, with increasing active life expectancy, and smaller families, allows many older adults greater privacy to engage in sexual activity. Data on sexual activity of older Americans, available

from three studies, reveals and reinforces some consistent trends. In 2009 the AARP surveyed 1,670 people 45 years and older.[7] The National Survey of Sexual Health and Behavior, conducted in 2009, included 14- to 94-year-olds with 1,008 people over age 50.[8] From 2005–2006, the National Social Life, Health and Aging Project (NSHAP) surveyed 3,005 Americans 57–85 years old.[9] In all three studies, across all age groups, sexuality was more important to men than women. Men had more frequent sexual thoughts, feelings of sexual desire, and engagement in self-stimulation than women.[7–9] Adults with partners were much more likely than those without partners to engage in interpersonal sexual activities such as kissing, hugging, oral sex, and intercourse.[7, 9, 10] Adults with partners expressed more importance to having a satisfying sexual relationship, more frequent sexual intercourse, and more sexual satisfaction overall.[7, 9, 11]

Although they represent 5%–10% of the older adult population, there is very little known about the sexuality of the lesbian, gay, bisexual, and transgender (LGBT) population. In 2011, the Institute of Medicine issued a report calling for more research on the LGBT population with an increased focus on LGBT elders, racial and ethnic subpopulations, and bisexual and transgender people.[12] Today's older adults grew up in an environment much less supportive of diversity. Examples include creation of an official diagnosis in 1952 of homosexuality as a sociopathic personality disturbance and Senator McCarthy including gay men and lesbians on his blacklist. In 1973 the American Psychiatric Association removed homosexuality from the *Diagnostic and Statistical Manual of Mental Disorders*.[12] The Still Out, Still Aging MetLife Study conducted in 2010 surveyed 1,201 LGBT people aged 45–64 and found the extent of disclosure of

Reichel's Care of the Elderly, 7th Edition, ed. Jan Busby-Whitehead *et al.* Published by Cambridge University Press. © Cambridge University Press 2016.

sexual orientation and/or gender identity varied significantly. Whereas 74% of gay men and 79% of lesbians were completely or mostly out, this applied to only 39% of transgender and 16% of bisexual people. Moreover, LGBT respondents indicated that healthcare providers are among the groups to whom they have not come out.[13]

Both physical and emotional aspects to sexuality and the desire for intimacy continue throughout life.[11] Physical closeness can be expressed in many ways including holding hands, hugging, kissing, mutual stroking, masturbating, oral sex, and intercourse. Studies have shown that for older adults the current level of activity correlates with past sexual frequency, and most older adults desire more activity than what they have.[14] Lack of partners and lack of privacy are significant obstacles for sexual expression. Adults living in age-segregated environments, such as retirement communities, express more interest in sexual activity and engage in sexual activity more often than their cohorts who are not age-segregated.[10] Some older adults report that sex became more pleasurable and of greater importance with age.[11]

In the National Survey of Behavior and Health, the incidence of vaginal intercourse declined from 51% of women aged 50–59 to 22% of women over 70 years primarily as a result of the loss of a male partner.[8] Avis examined the impact of age and gender on sexual function and found that older women reported a cessation of sexual relations due to the death of a spouse (36%), illness of a spouse (20%), or a spouse's inability to perform sexually (18%). Only 10% of the older women reported a cessation of sexual activity due to their own illness, loss of interest, or inability to perform.[15] Szwabo noted that as roles change within a relationship, so can the sexual behaviors of the couple. If the wife has assumed the caregiver "nursing" role, it may make sexual feelings and expressions less intense as the spouse may be seen as a patient rather than a sexual partner.[16] Adults of both genders without partners appear to adjust their sexual expectations and priorities. In one study it was noted that most people reporting no importance of sex were found to have no current partner and no anticipation of a partner in their lifetime.[11]

NSHAP revealed that the decline in sexual activity with age is largely mitigated by partner availability. The prevalence of sexual activity declined with age from 73% among those 57–64 years old, to 26%

among those 75–85 years old. However, for older adults who still had a partner, sexual activity remained prevalent with 65% of those aged 57–64 and 54% of those aged 75–85 having sexual activity at least two to three times per month. Among those who were sexually active, about half of both women and men reported at least one bothersome sexual problem. Yet only 22% of women and 38% of men reported having discussed sex with a physician since the age of 50.[9]

Barriers to treatment

Several barriers to seeking treatment for sexual problems were revealed in an interview study of 45 adults aged 50–92 years old.[17] Patients expressed a preference to consult a general practitioner of similar age and gender with the goal of minimizing embarrassment by discussing concerns with someone likely to have had similar experiences. Patient perceptions of providers' attitudes limited interactions if perceptions existed that older people are or should be asexual or access to treatments involve age-based rationing. In this study, 97% said they would discuss sexuality if the provider brought it up, and 80% stated a willingness to return for a designated sexual concerns appointment.

Both providers and patients may mistakenly attribute sexual problems to "normal aging," and both may lack knowledge about services and resources. As with many potentially sensitive issues it appears that patients are waiting for their physicians to raise the topic.

> Among those who were sexually active, about half of both women and men reported at least one bothersome sexual problem, yet only 22% of women and 38% of men reported having discussed sex with a physician since the age of 50. *This emphasizes that sexuality is still not adequately discussed in health-care settings.*

Sexual response cycle and common disorders

The traditional model of the human sexual response cycle has four phases described in a linear progression.[18] The first phase, desire, involves the brain and one's interest in or urge for sexual activity. The second phase, arousal, involves the vascular system and the body's response to stimulation. In men this is primarily recognized by penile erection, and in women by vaginal lubrication and genital engorgement. The peak of arousal is referred to as plateau. The third phase, orgasm, involves the spinal cord and perineal musculature. In this phase the body experiences involuntary contractions of the pelvic muscles and reproductive organs, and men experience ejaculation of seminal fluid. In the fourth phase, resolution, the body recovers from orgasm with a physiological rest period. Recent studies reveal greater variability, flexibility, and a more circular nature to sexual response. In both genders the relationship between desire and arousal is complex with variable order and overlap; the motivations for sex are multiple.[18] The *Diagnostic and Statistical Manual of Mental Disorders, Fifth Edition* (DSM-5) has adjusted criteria for diagnosing sexual dysfunctions. It has combined desire and arousal disorders in women into one classification, and created separate diagnostic classifications for men and women.[19]

In 1966 Masters and Johnson's landmark study of older sexuality noted that natural aging leads to a need for more time to engage in sexual activities. Advancing age is associated with delayed arousal and a greater need for genital stimulation, reduced penile rigidity and vaginal lubrication, loss of the sensation of ejaculatory inevitability, and increasing anorgasmia.[20]

Tables 45.1 and 45.2 outline gender-specific sexual response cycle markers, changes with aging, and common disorders for men and women.[6, 9, 18] Whereas women experience menopause and its impact on sexuality over a relatively short period of time, men's physiologic changes are thought to occur over a longer period of time with less awareness as change is occurring. The physiological changes associated with age alone are an insufficient cause to cease sexual activity, and for some these changes are felt to enhance sexual activity.

Misconceptions regarding sexually transmitted infections

Since sexually transmitted infections (STIs) are primarily a health issue of young people, there is very limited information on this topic in the older population. Lacking research, it is unclear if STIs are increasing in the older population or if the increased numbers merely reflect the rapidly expanding

population in general. There are several issues that increase the potential for older adults to acquire STIs. Longer, more active living combined with increased rates of divorce augments the number of new sexual partners.[21] Age-related changes in the immune system may increase susceptibility to HIV infection.[22] Postmenopausal women are more susceptible to the transmission of the HIV virus because of atrophic changes in the vaginal mucosa leading to microabrasions as a result of intercourse.[21, 22] For older adults, negotiating safer sex may be unfamiliar and challenging, they lack knowledge to identify HIV/AIDS risk factors, and they are less likely to use condoms.[5, 21, 22] Public health promotion materials regarding STIs fail to adequately target older adults.[5, 21] Health-care providers lack awareness of seniors' sexuality, fail to engage in conversations about risks, and are less likely to test for the virus.[5, 21, 23]

Until recently, many national health agencies provided stratified STI and HIV data only up to ages 45 to 49.[21] In 2005, people over age 50 accounted for 15% of new HIV/AIDS diagnoses, 24% of those living with HIV/AIDS, and 35% of AIDS deaths.[24] It is estimated that by 2015, 50% of the HIV population in America will be 50+ years old.[21, 22] In the 1980s, the primary route of HIV transmission in older adults was contaminated blood because older adults have higher rates of medical procedures. With routine testing of the blood supply, sexual intercourse and needle sharing are now the main sources of HIV infection.[5] In recognition of the increasing prevalence of HIV, the Center for Disease Control and Prevention issued a guideline in September 2006 advocating that "in all health-care settings, screening for HIV infection should be performed routinely for all patients aged 13–64 years. Older adults who are at increased risk should also be screened."[25] The US Preventive Services Task Force April 2013 guideline concurs with this screening as a grade A recommendation, indicating there is high certainty that the net benefit is substantial.[26]

> In 2005, people over age 50 accounted for 15% of new HIV/AIDS diagnoses, 24% of those living with HIV/AIDS, and 35% of AIDS deaths.[24] It is estimated that by 2015, 50% of the HIV population in America will be 50+ years old.[21, 22]
> *This emphasizes that STIs are increasing and that HIV is especially prevalent among "older" adults.*

Table 45.1 Men

Sexual response cycle: men	Markers	Changes with aging	Disorders**
Desire: brain	Desire/urge for sexual activity	Testosterone decrease in 55+ may affect libido	Hypoactive sexual desire disorder (affected by illness, performance anxiety, relationship problems) NSHAP data:* Lack of interest – 28.2%; 28.5%; 24.2% Performance anxiety – 25.1%; 28.9%; 29.3%
Arousal: vascular system	Penile erection Genital engorgement Testes Scrotum	Longer time for arousal (often need physical stimulation), erections less firm, sperm production declines	Erectile disorder (most common male dysfunction); sexual arousal disorder; sexual pain disorder NSHAP data:* Difficulty achieving, maintaining erection – 30.7%; 44.6%; 43.5% Sex not pleasurable – 3.8%; 7.0%; 5.1% Intercourse pain – 3.0%; 3.2%; 1.0%
Plateau (peak of arousal)	Full penile erection Testicular elevation and swelling Pre-ejaculatory fluid		Premature ejaculation NSHAP data:* Climax too quickly 29.5%; 28.1%; 21.3%
Orgasmic: spinal cord and perineal musculature	Involuntary rhythmic contractions of the pelvic muscles, reproductive organs Ejaculation of seminal fluid	Ejaculatory control improves, fewer contractions per orgasm, volume of ejaculate decreased	Orgasmic disorder NSHAP data:* Inability to climax – 16.2%; 22.7%; 33.2%
Resolution	Subjective sense of relaxation "Refractory period"	Physiologically extended refractory period	

* NSHAP respondents were asked about presence of a problem for "several months or more" during the previous 12 months; data is divided into three age groups: 57–64 years, 65–74 years, and 75–85 years, respectively.

** The disorders listed are based on DSM-IV-TR classification in use at the time of the NSHAP study data collection.

HIV in the elderly population

Misdiagnosis and delayed diagnosis of HIV in the older population occurs because HIV symptoms can be similar to other conditions associated with aging: weakened immune system, weight loss, fatigue, swollen lymph nodes, skin rashes, respiratory problems, depression, and decreased cognition or physical abilities. Delay in diagnosis is concerning because it is associated with an increased risk of both AIDS and death. Increasing age is also an independent predictor of AIDS and death among those with HIV.[21] HIV-infected elders are frequently isolated due to the dual stigma of being old and living with a sexually transmitted infection. Both of these factors make it difficult for seniors to disclose their disease state to family and friends, thereby forfeiting the social support needed to assist with their psychosocial requirements and treatment plans.[23]

Effective antiretroviral therapy (ART) for HIV has allowed many infected people to live to 50+ years and is making AIDS-defining illnesses increasingly rare in those with ART-suppressed HIV.[22] Initiating ART at age 50+ is associated with an overall mortality risk 32% higher than those initiating ART at ages 25–49.[21]

Table 45.2 Women

Sexual response cycle: women	Markers	Changes with aging	Disorders**
Desire: brain	Desire/urge for sexual activity	Unclear: theory of low estrogen causing decreased libido is being reconsidered	Hypoactive sexual desire disorder (most common female dysfunction; affected by illness, performance anxiety, relationship problems) NSHAP data:* Lack of interest – 44.2%; 38.4%; 49.3% Performance anxiety – 10.4%; 12.5%; 9.9%
Arousal: vascular system	Vaginal lubrication Clitoral erection Genital engorgement Vulva Vagina Uterus Breast changes	Less increase in breast size, reduced elasticity of vaginal walls, decreased vaginal lubrication, less muscle tension Often related to estrogen deficiency	Sexual arousal disorder; sexual pain disorder NSHAP data:* Lubrication difficulty – 35.9%; 43.2%; 43.6% Sex not pleasurable – 24.0%; 22.0%; 24.9% Intercourse pain – 17.8%; 18.6%; 11.8%
Plateau (peak of arousal)	Vasocongestion of outer third of uterus, vagina Elevation of uterus		
Orgasmic: spinal cord and perineal musculature	Involuntary rhythmic contractions of the pelvic muscles, reproductive organs	Fewer contractions per orgasm, ability for multiple orgasms may decrease	Orgasmic disorder NSHAP data:* Inability to climax – 34.0%; 32.8%; 38.2%
Resolution	Subjective sense of relaxation	May have refractory period	

* NSHAP respondents were asked about presence of a problem for "several months or more" during the previous 12 months; data is divided into three age groups: 57–64 years, 65–74 years, and 75–85 years, respectively.

** The disorders listed are based on DSM-IV-TR classification in use at the time of the NSHAP study data collection.

HIV-associated non-AIDS (HANA) conditions are increasing and are associated with advancing age and chronic inflammation. HANA conditions include cardiovascular disease, infectious and noninfectious cancers, osteopenia/osteoporosis, liver disease, renal disease, and neurocognitive decline. There is an emerging consensus that HIV and/or its treatment affects the process of aging and/or development of disease; people with HIV experience increased morbidity and mortality.[22] In 2012, the National Institute of Health identified HIV and aging as an area of critical need for research and outlined specific knowledge gaps.[22]

In older people with HIV, multimorbidity is becoming the norm. Individuals are surviving long enough to experience HIV as a chronic disease, and increased survival results in social supports of family and friends falling away, thus increasing the challenge of coordinating their care.[27] Recognizing the importance of geriatric concepts to the aging HIV population, a special meeting convened at the White House on HIV and Aging in 2010. This collaboration between the American Geriatrics Society and the American Academy of HIV Medicine focused on developing clinical treatment strategies and created a frequently updated online site in recognition of the rapidly evolving developments in HIV and aging (www.AAHIVM.org/hivandagingforum).[27]

Impact of common medical conditions and surgical procedures

A number of medical conditions contribute to sexual dysfunction and raise patient concerns regarding health consequences of sexual activity. Medical conditions and their treatments may negatively alter one's perception of body image, create preoccupation with concern of symptom exacerbation, reduce exercise tolerance, and limit flexibility and positions of comfort. Tables 45.3 and 45.4 outline patient advice for common medical conditions and common surgical procedures.[28–32]

Gender-specific conditions

Erectile dysfunction (ED) is the most common disorder of men's sexual health. ED is defined as the recurrent inability to attain or maintain a penile erection sufficient for sexual performance. ED shares risk factors with cardiovascular disease and is now also recognized as an independent marker for increased risk for cardiovascular disease.[31] Management of ED provides an opportunity for cardiovascular risk reduction. The prevalence of ED increases with age. In the Massachusetts Male Aging Study of 1,290 men aged 40–70 years, the probability of severe ED tripled from 5.1% to 15%; the probability of moderate ED doubled from 17% to 34%, and the probability of mild ED remained constant at 17%.[33] Many medical conditions and their treatments contribute to the development of ED. Common etiologies include diabetes mellitus, hypertension, cardiac disease, chronic kidney disease, depression, anxiety, and prostate cancer surgery and radiation.[18, 34]

Treatment options are varied and include lifestyle modification, medications, penile implants, and vacuum devices. Lifestyle modification is aimed at increasing exercise, weight loss to lower BMI below 30 kg per m^2, and smoking cessation [SOE=C]. For most men, PDE5 inhibitors, such as sildenafil citrate, are the first-line treatment option for ED, including those men with diabetes mellitus and spinal cord injury and use of antidepressants [SOE=A].[35] PDE5 inhibitors are considered equally efficacious [SOE=A], and in the presence of sexual stimulation they are 55%–80% effective. Side effects of these medications include headache, flushing, and dyspepsia. PDE5 inhibitors should not be used by men taking nitrates.[35] Intracavernosal injection of vasoactive agents, such as alprostadil, are also effective [SOE=B].

The most commonly reported side effect is penile pain; some men are averse to needle use. Intracavernosal therapy has a success rate of 70%–90%.[36] Intraurethral insertion of vasoactive agents is an alternative. This approach is termed medicated urethral system for erection (MUSE) and is successful 43%–60% of the time.[36] Side effects include urethral irritation in patients and some partners. Vacuum pump with constrictive bands is a common alternative to medications; it is contraindicated in men with sickle cell anemia or blood dyscrasias, and those taking anticoagulants. This method often achieves an erection; however, patient satisfaction varies between 27% and 74%.[37] The vacuum device requires some skill and an understanding partner. Men receiving adequate training report better device satisfaction.[29] Penile implants are generally reserved for those in whom alternatives were unsuccessful. The operation requires destruction of the corpus cavernosus, thus eliminating any future pharmacologic treatments.[29]

> ED is now recognized as an independent marker for increased risk for cardiovascular disease.[31] Management of ED provides an opportunity for cardiovascular risk reduction.
>
> *This emphasizes that recognition of sexual dysfunction may have more impact than just quality of life; for some providers it may be a motivator to explore sexuality.*
>
> Highlighted references:
>
> DeLamater J. Sexual expression in later life: a review and synthesis. *Journal of Sex Research* 2012; 49(2–3): 125–141.
>
> *Provides a detailed review of sexuality and sexual dysfunction in the geriatric population.*
>
> Lindau ST, Schumm LP, Laumann EO, Levinson W, O'Muircheartaigh CA, Waite L. A study of sexuality and health among older adults in the United States. *N Engl J Med* 2014; 357:762–774.
>
> *Provides the results from the National Social Life, Health and Aging Project survey of 3,005 people aged 57–85 years.*
>
> Work Group for the HIV and Aging Consensus Project. Summary report from the Human Immunodeficiency Virus and Aging Consensus Project: treatment strategies for clinicians managing older individuals with the human immunodeficiency virus. *J Am Geriatr Soc* 2012; 60:974–979.
>
> *Provides clinical treatment strategies for the growing 50+ population with HIV/AIDS and raises awareness of online site where information is frequently updated.*

Table 45.3 Common medical conditions

Condition	Advice and information
Cardiovascular disease (CVD)	• Male erectile dysfunction (ED) affects 44%–65% with CVD, 80% with heart failure • ED is a marker for CVD; often precedes CVD event by 2–5 years
Arrhythmia with implantable cardioverter defibrillator (ICD)	• Worry of causing an arrhythmia or shock may exist, especially among those who have experienced ICD shocks during sex • For some, the ICD will be seen as a "rescuer," and sexual interest and activity may increase
Myocardial infarction	• Abstinence often advised for 8–14 weeks, although there is limited data to support this practice • Duration of abstinence depends primarily on patient desire, general fitness, and conditioning • Ability to climb 1–2 flights of stairs is generally considered adequate fitness for sexual activity
Angina	• Late morning activity after a full night's rest • Use of supine position to reduce exertion level • Creation of a relaxed atmosphere for sexual encounters
Heart failure exacerbation with pulmonary edema	• Abstain from sexual activity 2–3 weeks or until ability to climb 1–2 flights of stairs is restored
Hypertension	• No need to limit sexual activity • Be aware that antihypertensive medication and untreated hypertension lead to erectile dysfunction in men; effects in women not well studied
Stroke	• Sexual function may be impaired; desire is usually unaffected • If loss of desire is present, screen for depression • Physical stimulation can be focused on the unaffected side of the body • Pillows and headboards can be used for support
Emphysema and other causes of shortness of breath	• Use intervals of rest • Select positions requiring limited exertion • Use oxygen as needed
Arthritis	• Use general pain reduction approaches: exercise, rest, warm baths, and analgesics prior to exertion • Try different sexual positions to minimize joint pain • Use time of day when pain and stiffness are least severe
Diabetes mellitus (DM)	• Male ED is 2–5 times more common than in general population; 49% of men 65+ with type 2 DM • For some men, establishing good control of diabetes reestablishes potency. • If diabetes is already well controlled, ED is likely irreversible; consider ED management (PDE5 inhibitors effective).
Dementia	• Inappropriate sexual behaviors (ISB) lack universal definition; some are labeled inappropriate only because performed publicly • Lack of privacy, attitudes of family/caregivers have influence • ISB prevalence 1.8%–25%; more common in hospital than community setting
Depression	• Sexual desire is affected • Treatment of depression restores sexual interest

Note: Selective serotonin reuptake inhibitors (SSRIs) are associated with orgasmic dysfunction, decreased sexual desire, and decreased arousal

Table 45.4 Common surgical procedures

Condition	Advice and information
Hysterectomy	• Abstinence advised 6–8 weeks to allow adequate wound healing • Women sensitive to cervical and uterine contractions during orgasm may notice the loss of these sensations • Depression is common and may impair desire
Oophorectomy	• Effects of decreased androgen, estrogen, progesterone not well studied • Sexual frequency is sometimes increased with removed fear of pregnancy
Mastectomy	• Loss of desire occurs with embarrassment, perceived loss of femininity, fear of being unattractive • Periodic depression common for 1–2 years post procedure • Rehabilitation programs encouraged for patients and partners to deal with physical/psychological concerns and enhanced communication
Prostatectomy	• Abstinence advised for 6 weeks to allow wound healing • Transurethral resection of prostate, used for benign prostatic hypertrophy, leads to retrograde ejaculation and erectile dysfunction • Complete prostatectomy, used for prostate cancer, leads to erectile dysfunction in 60% or more
Orchiectomy	• Psychological impact substantial; physical impairment of function limited • Counseling before and after surgery is highly advocated

Sexual encounter enhancements

Sex toys

Health-care providers should develop a general awareness of the types of sex toys that are commonly used as well as related health-care considerations. There are several reasons why a patient may develop an interest in toys, including lack of a partner, returning to the dating scene, and interest in adding variety. The patient may look to the health-care provider for guidance in how to use toys, validation that toy use is an acceptable practice, and health risk education. In addition to these roles, the physician may need to assist in retrieval of misplaced or out-of-reach equipment.

The following guidelines facilitate the safe use of toys. When putting something in a body opening, be aware that sharp, breakable, and hard-to-hold-on-to objects can be problematic and are discouraged from use. One should listen to his or her body; pain is a good indicator to slow down, pull out, or explore other options. Toys should be cleansed thoroughly between use with soap and water and allowed to dry completely. When cleaning porous materials (silicone, latex), a little bleach can be added. Battery or electronically operated equipment should not be

completely submerged. A condom can be used on many toys and will significantly facilitate cleanliness. Condoms should always be changed between partners and when moving from anus to vagina. Using a toy with only one individual, termed dedicated use, is another effective strategy for safer sex practices.

Lubricants

There are many different lubricants available. Lubricants are used with condoms, with toys, for masturbation, for anal sex, and frequently in postmenopausal women for vaginal dryness. When selecting a lubricant there are three main considerations: the ingredients; the purpose; and the reactions between the chemicals and the person, toys, and safer sex supplies. The three main types of lubricants are water-based, silicone-based, and oil-based. Water-based lubricants are popular because they are safe to use with latex condoms and rubber toys. Advantages include ease of cleaning, stain free unless color has been added, nongreasy feel, and reactivation with water or saliva. Silicone-based lubricants last a long time, don't dry out, and small amounts are very effective. Limitations include difficulty in cleaning, damage to silicone toys, and vaginal irritation and infections. Oil-based lubricants are most often used

637

for male masturbation. Limitations include difficulty in cleaning, they are not recommended for vaginal use, and they may damage rubber toys and latex condoms.

Lubricants may have additives. Anal lubricants may contain benzocaine as a desensitizing agent. Although this may assist initiation of anal sex, caution is advised that decreased sensation may increase injuries. Additives may also include flavors and scents. Plain lubricants taste mildly chemical and slightly bitter. Edible lubricants are water based and often contain glycerin. Patients should be advised that in warm, moist environments, such as the vagina, sugar promotes yeast and bacterial infections.

Lubricants also vary in consistency from light liquids to heavy gels. Heavier lubricants are recommended for anal sex. Patients are encouraged to test a small quantity of lubricant for adverse reactions, especially if using it for vaginal intercourse.

Coital positions

With advancing age a number of factors may influence a patient's preference for coital positions. Considerations include limited exercise tolerance, pain aggravated by certain positions, and embarrassment related to medical devices (ostomy pouch) or procedures (mastectomy, orchiectomy). The man on top (missionary) position facilitates intimacy, including talking, hugging, kissing, eye contact, and close body contact. Touching by the man is limited because he must hold himself up, and prolonged activity may be physically challenging. Women may find this position uncomfortable if the man is heavy. The woman on top position facilitates intimacy for similar reasons. With the woman in control of depth, speed, and rhythm of penetration, a woman's orgasm may be facilitated and pain with penetration can be minimized. This position works well for partners of different heights. Prolonged activity may be physically challenging for the woman. The sitting/kneeling position may be a desired alternative for patients with abdominal bloating, discomfort, or medical devices. Although some consider lack of eye contact impersonal, this may be an advantage for those embarrassed by altered body image. If this position is hard on the knees, use of a chair may facilitate comfort. The rear entry (doggie-style) position also facilitates touching, is easy on the muscles, and requires less energy than those positions previously mentioned. This position facilitates deep penile penetration and has limited eye

contact. The side-by-side (spoons) position requires the least amount of energy and is therefore useful for patients with limited mobility or stamina. This position facilitates touching, close body contact, and slower encounters. With increased time and less deep penile penetration, this position is especially useful for patients with premature ejaculation.

Conclusion

Patients of all ages have concerns about sexuality. Many providers, however, may not feel comfortable talking about sexual issues or even taking a sexual history, especially with their older patient population. Gaining a comfort level in this area comes with practice and with personal knowledge of the potential changes and concerns associated with sexuality in the aging population.

References

1. Brogan M. The sexual needs of elderly people: addressing the issue. *Nursing Standard* 1996; **10**:42–45.

2. Bytheway B. *Ageism*. Buckingham, UK: Open University Press, 1995.

3. Nicolosi A, Moreira ED Jr, Villa M, Glasser DB. A population study of the association between sexual function, sexual satisfaction and depressive symptoms in men. *J Affect Disord* 2004; **82**:235–43.

4. Finger WW, Lund M, Slagle MA. Medications that may contribute to sexual disorders: a guide to assessment and treatment in family practice. *J Fam Pract* 1997; **44**:33–43.

5. Milaszewski D, Greto E, Klochkov T, Fuller-Thompson E. A systematic review of education for the prevention of HIV/AIDS among older adults. *Journal of Evidence-Based Social Work* 2012; **9**(3):213–30.

6. DeLameter J. Sexual expression in later life: a review and synthesis. *Journal of Sex Research* 2012; **49**(2–3):125–41.

7. American Association of Retired Persons. *Sex, Romance and Relationships: AARP Survey of Midlife and Older Adults* (Pub. No. D19234). Washington DC: AARP; 2010.

8. Herbenick D, Reece M, Schick V, et al. Sexual behavior in the United States: results from a national probability sample of men and women ages 14–94. *J Sex Med* 2010; **7** (suppl 5):255–65.

9. Lindau ST, Schumm LP, Laumann EO, et al. A study of sexuality and health among older adults in the United States. *N Engl J Med* 2014; **357**:762–74.

10. Weinstein S, Rosen E. Senior adult sexuality in age segregated and age integrated communities. *Int J Aging Hum Devel* 1988; **27**:261–70.

11. Gott M, Hinchcliff S. How important is sex in later life? The views of older people. *Social Science and Medicine* 2003; **56**:1617–28.

12. IOM (Institute of Medicine). *The Health of Lesbian, Gay, Bisexual, and Transgender People: Building a Foundation for Better Understanding.* Washington, DC: National Academies Press; 2011.

13. MetLife. *Still Out, Still Aging: The MetLife Study of Lesbian, Gay, Bisexual, and Transgender Baby Boomers.* Westport, CT: MetLife Mature Market Institute; 2010.

14. Ginsberg TB, Pomerantz SC, Kramer-Feeley V. Sexuality in older adults: behaviours and preferences. *Age and Ageing* 2005; **34**:475–80.

15. Avis NE. Sexual functioning and aging in men and women: community and population-based studies. *Journal of Gender-Specific Medicine* 2000; **2**(2):37–41.

16. Swabo P. Counseling about sexuality in the older person. *Clin Geriatr Med* 2003; **19**:595–604.

17. Gott M, Hinchcliff S. Barriers to seeking treatment for sexual problems in primary care: a qualitative study with older people. *Family Practice* 2003; **20**(6):690–95.

18. Bhasin S, Basson R. Sexual dysfunction in men and women. In Melmed S, Polonsky K, Larsen P, Kronenberg H. (eds.) *Williams Textbook of Endocrinology,* 12th edition. Philadelphia: Elsevier Saunders, 2011.

19. Sungur MZ, Gunduz A. A comparison of DSM-IV-TR and DSM-5 definitions for sexual dysfunctions: critiques and challenges. *J Sex Med* 2014; **11**:364–73.

20. Masters WH, Johnson VE. *Human Sexual Response.* Boston: Little, Brown, and Co; 1966.

21. Poynten IM, Grulich AE, Templeton DJ. Sexually transmitted infections in older populations. *Curr Opin Infect Dis* 2013; **26**:80–85.

22. High KP, Brennan-Ing M, Clifford DB, et al. HIV and aging: state of knowledge and areas of critical need for research: a report to the NIH Office of AIDS Research by the HIV and Aging Working Group. *J Acquir Immune Defic Syndr* 2012; **60**:S1–S18.

23. Karpiak SE, Shipley RA, Cantor MH. *Research on Older Adults with HIV.* New York: AIDS Community Research of America, 2006.

24. HIV/AIDS among persons aged 50 and older, [online]. Available at www.cdc.gov/hiv/pdf/library_factsheet_HIV_among_PersonsAged50andOlder.pdf (accessed July 13, 2014).

25. Branson BM, Handsfield HH, et al. Revised recommendations for HIV testing of adults, adolescents, and pregnant women in health-care settings. *MMWR* 2006 Sep 22; **55**(RR14):1–17.

26. US Preventive Services Task Force. Screening for HIV, Topic Page [online]. Available at www.uspreventive servicestaskforce.org/uspstf/uspshivi.htm (accessed July 13, 2014).

27. Work Group for the HIV and Aging Consensus Project. Summary report from the Human Immunodeficiency Virus and Aging Consensus Project: treatment strategies for clinicians managing older individuals with the human immunodeficiency virus. *J Am Geriatr Soc* 2012; **60**:974–79.

28. Morley JE, Tariq SH. Sexuality and disease. *Clin Geriatr Med* 2003; **19**:563–73.

29. Morales A. Erectile dysfunction: an overview. *Clin Geriatr Med* 2003; **19**:529–38.

30. Palacio-Cena D, Losa-Iglesias ME, Alvarez-Lopez C, et al. Patients, intimate partners and family experiences of implantable cardioverter defibrillators: qualitative systematic review. *J Advanced Nursing* 2011; **67**(12):2537–50. [PMID: 21615459]

31. Nehra A, Jackson G, Miner M, et al. The Princeton III Consensus recommendations for the management of erectile dysfunction and cardiovascular disease. *Mayo Clin Proc* 2012, **87**(8).766–78. [PMCID: PMC3498341]

32. Abdo CHN. Sexuality and couple intimacy in dementia. *Curr Opin Psychiatry* 2013; **26**:593–98.

33. Johannes CB, Araujo AB, Feldman HA, et al. Incidence of erectile dysfunction in men 40 to 69 years old: longitudinal results from the Massachusetts Male Aging Study. *J Urol* 2000; **163**:460–63.

34. Tapscott AH, Hakim LS. Office-based management of impotence and Peyronie's disease. *Urol Clin N Am* 2013; **40**:521–43.

35. Heidelbaugh JJ. Management of erectile dysfunction. *Am Fam Physician* 2010; **81**:305–12.

36. McVary KT. Clinical practice: erectile dysfunction. *N Engl J Med* 2007; **357**:2472–81.

37. Mulligan T, Reddy S, Gulur PV, et al. Disorders of male sexual function. *Clin Geriatr Med* 2003; **19**:473–81.

Chapter

46

Aging in adults with intellectual disabilities and severe and persistent mental illness

Jan S. Greenberg, PhD, Marsha R. Mailick, PhD, and Eun Ha Namkung, MSW

Introduction

This chapter examines the health and social status of older persons with intellectual disabilities (ID) and older persons with severe and persistent mental illness (SPMI). Although they are distinct populations, they share a variety of characteristics that affect their clinical needs and, hence, their interactions with community-based health-care practitioners. First, for both groups, community-based living and services are now the norm. This is a sharp contrast to several decades ago, when residential, social, and health services were provided largely in isolated state-supported institutional settings. Second, their historic segregation from the general public has resulted in lack of knowledge about these populations by health practitioners, many of whom have little understanding of their special needs. Third, both groups rely heavily on the care and assistance provided by family members. Although the social stigma associated with SPMI and to a lesser extent ID has masked the prevalence of family-based care, greater awareness of and support for family caregivers has resulted in increased demands for basic social and health services for relatives with disabilities. Furthermore, since few adults with ID or SPMI marry and most outlive their parents, their siblings often inherit some measure of responsibility during old age.

In this chapter we discuss the populations with ID and SPMI sequentially. We present relevant information for practitioners regarding health, cognitive, functioning, and social challenges associated with the aging process, and available evidence-based treatments developed to meet these challenges.

Intellectual disabilities

Definition

The American Association on Intellectual and Developmental Disabilities (AAIDD) defines ID as a disability characterized by significant limitations both in intellectual functioning (an IQ score of approximately 75 or below) and adaptive behavior, as well as the collection of conceptual, social, and practical adaptive skills.[1] This disability originates before the age of 18 years. Although the cause of an ID is not known in many cases, some of the more common known causes include Down syndrome (DS), fetal alcohol syndrome, fragile X syndrome, and genetic conditions and birth defects.[2] Many aging individuals with autism also have ID.

Population characteristics and demographic trends

Prevalence

The true size of the older population with ID is not known. The estimates by the AAIDD for older adults aged 60 and over with ID range between 600,000 and 1.6 million.[3] It is estimated that there were 641,860 older people with ID aged 60 or older in the year 2000, and the number is expected to roughly double to 1.2 million by 2030, when the youngest members of the baby boom generation reach age 60.[4]

Life expectancy and mortality

Although persons with ID often die at an earlier age than do adults without a disability, there has been a marked increase in the life expectancy of persons with

Reichel's Care of the Elderly, 7th Edition, ed. Jan Busby-Whitehead *et al.* Published by Cambridge University Press. © Cambridge University Press 2016.

ID, primarily as a result of improved health care and community-based services. Mortality is closely related to severity of ID as the median life expectancies for people with mild, moderate, and severe levels of disability have been estimated to be 74.0, 67.6, and 58.6 years, respectively.[5] Persons with DS have an elevated risk of premature death, reflecting their general earlier onset of aging, including Alzheimer's disease (AD).[6,7] However, as a result of contemporary service delivery models and better medical care, life expectancy approaches that of the general population for many adutls with ID.[8] Consequently, the population of older persons with ID is considerably larger than in the past and will continue to grow rapidly.

Demographic and social characteristics

Although persons with ID are more likely to be male (due to the many X-linked causes of ID), the gender profile shifts as populations age with a higher percentage of females (51%) in those 65 years or older.[9] It is estimated that the percentage of adults with ID of all ages who live with families is as high as 75%.[10] However, according the National Core Indicators Adult Consumer Survey 2009–2010 on people with ID served by state systems, most adults aged 65 or older live in group homes (39%) or institutional settings (30%), while 9% live independently, 5% live in a parent's or relative's home, and 17% live in a range of other settings such as agency-operated apartments and foster care homes.[9] Older adults are more likely to live in provider-based settings (e.g., group homes) than their younger counterparts.[9] This phenomenon is partly due to the mortality of the parents and siblings.

Age-related changes

Older people with ID show a greater risk of obesity, metabolic syndrome, respiratory infections (in those with severe ID), low bone mass density, and other age-related health risks compared to the general population.[4, 11] This is due to biological factors related to disabilities, limited access to adequate health care, lack of physical activity, and poor nutrition.[4, 12]

Research on the relationship between dementia and ID has been dominated by studies of aging individuals with DS because by age 35 to 40, a majority of adults with DS display the key neuropathological changes characteristic of AD. Although the formation of plaques and neurofibrilllary tangles associated with dementia may occur during the thirties and forties, the clinical onset of AD tends to be in the fifties.[13, 14] Higher-order functional abilities are typically first affected, and it is only as the disease progresses that more basic activities of daily living are affected, which mirrors the progression of AD in the general population.[15] There are several studies that have investigated the risks for dementia in individuals with DS, but few definitive risk factors other than age have been identified.[15] Coppus studied a cohort of 506 individuals with DS aged 45 and older and found that the cumulative risk for AD doubled every five years, from 8.9% among those 45–49 years of age to 32.1% at ages 55–59.[16] After age 60, Coppus found that the cumulative incidence decreased to 25.6%, explaining the decrease as potentially due to the increased mortality of adults with comorbid DS and dementia. Future cohorts of individuals with DS will be very different than today's aging cohort as they have had far better access to medical care and to educational and rehabilitative services.[15] It is unknown how these cohort differences will affect the risk of future generations of aging adults with DS for developing AD.

Other research has examined the risk of dementia in adults with ID over the age of 65 who do not have DS.[17,18] Whereas Zigman and colleagues found no evidence of increased risk,[18] Strydom and colleagues found an increased standardized morbidity ratio of 2.8 associated with ID.[17] These differences might be explained by taxonomic considerations concerning whether persons with mild cognitive impairments (MCI) are classified together with dementia or as a separate entity.[19] Individuals with ID may have a similar risk for dementia to individuals without ID when dementia cases are limited to those with probable or definite dementia, but are at an increased risk when the definition is expanded to include those with MCI. [20] In consideration of the difficulty in differentiating between MCI and mild dementia for adults with ID, clinicians should focus on assessing the level of support aging individuals need in order to live in the community, irrespective of their diagnosis.

The pattern for age-related changes in functional performances mirrors that of cognitive declines, with those with DS showing the fastest rates of decline.[21] A nine-year longitudinal study of 150 midlife adults with DS found that during the early years of adulthood and early midlife, persons with DS showed a similar pattern of change and stability in functional abilities and behavior problems compared to those with ID due to other causes.[13] However, relative disadvantages in cognitive and functional abilities among adults with DS increased markedly as they entered late-midlife and the aging years.[14] Older persons with DS were less proficient in daily living skills than either younger persons with DS or age-matched persons with other forms of ID.[21, 22]

In addition, older adults with ID are more likely than those under the age of 65 with ID to have a physical disability (21% vs. 15%) and hearing loss (9% vs. 5%) and be legally blind (11% vs. 8%).[9] Although reports indicate a reduction of problematic behaviors (e.g., withdrawal, aggression) with aging, older adults with ID have approximately twice the risk of developing depression as their age peers without ID.[23] Older adults with ID also are more likely to have a diagnosis of a mental illness (44%) than those younger than age 65 (35%).[9]

Due to the long-term use of psychoactive and neuroleptic medications, the ID population is notable for the prevalence of polypharmacy and for frequent complications associated with the long-term use of multiple medications. National Core Indicator Data indicate that 35% of older adults with ID aged 65 or older take medications indicated for mood disorder, 25% for anxiety disorders, 19% for psychotic disorders, and 18% for behavior problems.[9] Thus, "medication-related problems, including polypharmacy, adverse drug effects, drug interactions, and risks associated with longer-term use, may be a particular concern for many adults with DD."[22, p.213]

Evidence-based interventions

Promising results from health promotion programs for the younger population suggest that adults with ID can benefit from structured efforts to reduce chronic disease risk through lifestyle changes.[12, 24] In a review of interventions to promote healthy aging in adults with ID, Heller and Sorensen classified health interventions into three broad categories: fitness/exercise only; interventions that used mixed approaches or focused on health education; and interventions aimed at health-care screening services, which typically involved either a comprehensive medical exam by a physician or nurse practitioner or screening for specific medical conditions such as high blood pressure, cancer, or heart disease.[12] In general, these three broad groups of interventions have been shown to have beneficial effects and can play a role in reducing health disparities for aging adults with ID. However, for the most part, these studies were designed as small-scale pilot efforts to evaluate the feasibility and efficacy of a newly developed intervention. Also, only a few focused exclusively on adults in middle age and old age. Thus, future research is needed evaluating these interventions using randomized control group designs.

Although several promising health promotion interventions designed for older adults with ID are in the development stage, there are several obstacles to successfully engaging individuals with ID as active participants in treatment. Communication difficulties among older persons with ID are a major barrier to providing health screening and other health services.[12] Physicians often rely on caregivers and family members as sources of medical histories. Clinical reports indicate that a major issue in the provision of health services is the extended time needed for obtaining relevant information, diagnostic testing, and explanation of treatments. Furthermore, some adults with ID have to be desensitized before invasive procedures can be performed.[22]

Older adults with autism spectrum disorders

Autism spectrum disorders (ASDs) are complex, lifelong, neurodevelopmental conditions with complex genetic etiology that can cause significant social, communication, and behavioral challenges.[25] Autism was first identified by Kanner in 1943; hence, the first persons to be diagnosed with autism are now in their seventies. ASD was historically thought to be rare, but it is estimated that about 1 in 68 children had ASD in 2010, which is more than double the rate in 2000.[26] It has been estimated that approximately 25% of the increase in the prevalence rates for ASD are due to changes in diagnostic practices rather than due to putative etiologic factors.[27] Owing to a combination of population aging, the increasing prevalence of ASD, and the demand for services by persons with ASD across the lifespan, improving knowledge about aging and autism has become a very high priority.

Autism is a "lifelong disorder whose features change with development,"[28, p. 527] and the details of these changes over midlife and old age are just now being explored.[29] Mailick and colleagues have conducted a 12-year longitudinal study of 406 families of individuals with autism.[30] At the beginning of the study, 38% of the sample was between the ages of 22 and 52. Over this time period, there was an age-related decline in health, with a more rapid decline after age 45. Medication use tended to increase around age 45, but there was a steady decline in behavior problems across all age groups.[31] There also was a general decline in social activities but not in functional abilities.[32, 33] These findings suggest that there is considerable variability in how individuals with ASD age.

In recognition of the difficulties that older persons with ASD may face, interventions for ASDs may include specific behavioral and speech therapy, as well as pharmacotherapies to treat associated features such as anxiety and depression. However, the evidence on effectiveness and safety of interventions for adults with ASD has not been well established at any age.[29] No medications are currently available to treat the core symptoms of ASD. Only one medication, risperidone, has been approved by the Food and Drug Administration (FDA) specifically for use among individuals with ASD who have serious behavior problems, and there are few clinical studies addressing the effectiveness of other medications in this population.[34]

Severe and persistent mental illness

Definition

Severe and persistent mental illness (SPMI) in adults aged 18 or older refers to disorders commonly accompanied by psychotic symptoms, including schizophrenia, schizoaffective disorder, bipolar disorder, and severe forms of major depression that typically develop in late adolescence or early adulthood and are lifelong conditions, resulting in significant impairment in daily living activities and in social, vocational, and educational functioning.[35]

Older adults with SPMI are a diverse and heterogeneous group with respect to their level of social, occupational, and psychological functioning. The largest subgroup of the population with SPMI consists of persons with schizophrenia, and longitudinal research suggests that the life course of schizophrenia is not one of necessarily progressive decline.[36] Rather, some persons experience fluctuations in symptoms in old age, others have long periods when they are relatively asymptomatic, and still others appear to recover.[37, 38] In a review of the research on older adults with schizophrenia, Jeste and Maglione concluded that "positive symptoms of schizophrenia become less severe, substance abuse becomes less common, and mental health functioning often improves."[39, p.966] However, many individuals with schizophrenia experience debilitating symptoms into their later life. Even elders who show few residual signs of having suffered a long-term mental illness face many challenges because of the secondary effects associated with social isolation and financial impoverishment as well as the emergence of health problems related to the long-term side effects of psychotropic medication use.

Population characteristics and demographic trends

Prevalence

In 2012, there were an estimated 9.6 million adults with SPMI, representing 4.1 percent of all US adults. However, the data suggest that there was a lower rate of SPMI among those aged 50 and older (3.0%) compared with those aged 25 or younger (4.1%) or those aged 26 to 49 (5.2%).[40] The lower prevalence of SPMI in the older population is likely due to the remission of psychotic symptoms, premature mortality of the population, and the lack of aging-appropriate diagnostic criteria.[41, 42] Nevertheless, we have witnessed an unprecedented increase in the population of older adults with SPMI in the past decade, and the increase in the number and proportion of the population will continue, in part because of the aging of the baby boomer generation.

Life expectancy and mortality

The life expectancy for persons with an SPMI is shorter than that for the general population by 8–32 years.[43, 44] A review of 37 articles drawn from 25 countries found that people with schizophrenia have a 2.5 times higher risk of dying compared with the general population, and this substantial gap has widened over time. [45] The higher mortality in schizophrenia is due to both suicide and medical problems: 30%–40% of the excess deaths in schizophrenia are due to suicide and injuries, and about 60% are due to medical conditions such as cardiovascular diseases.[46]

Demographic and social characteristics

Although SPMI is more prevalent in women (3.6%) than men (2.4%) aged 50 or older, the gender difference in this age group is much smaller than that in younger age groups.[40] The average age of onset of schizophrenia is 2 to 10 years later in women than in men, and for women a second peak occurs between the ages of 40–45.[47] Women with schizophrenia tend to have milder symptoms initially, and progress to more severe symptoms as they age.[48] Although the reasons for the later onset of schizophrenia in women than in men as well as gender differences in disease course are unknown, one potential explanation involves the role of estrogen, which may serve a protective role to delay illness onset and lead to some new cases during menopause.[48, 49]

People with SPMI are likely to live in poverty and be less educated.[50] These adults are less likely to marry and have children than the general population, leading to smaller social networks than their age peers.[40, 51] Unlike earlier years when institutionalization was common, about 85% of older persons with SPMI reside in the community, and one-third to one-half live with family members.[52]

Age-related changes

Medical comorbidity is the rule for older adults with SPMI, with increasing risk also noted for this population. Studies on middle-aged and older persons with SPMI report that they are at increased risk for cardiovascular diseases, respiratory diseases, and diabetes relative to the age-matched general population.[53–55] Research suggests that similar biological mechanisms that are associated with age-related health problems such as shorter telomere length and increased inflammation are also associated with an increased risk of mental illness.[56]

One of the possible explanations for rapid physical aging in SPMI is the cumulative long-term effect of poor health behaviors and their general lack of access to adequate and appropriate health care.[57] Older people with schizophrenia are more likely to smoke,[58] use substances,[59] and maintain a sedentary lifestyle compared to those without a mental illness.[41, 60] Older age also is a risk factor for many long-term side effects of antipyschotics, including metabolic syndrome and movement disorders,[39] which may contribute to the poor health outcomes of persons with SPMI.[41] Compared with their counterparts without psychiatric disorders, older adults

with schizophrenia or bipolar disorder show a higher risk of cognitive deficits and poorer neurological performance.[61–63] However, the degree of cognitive decline may vary by diagnosis. In individuals with bipolar, an accelerated decline of cognitive functioning in older age was found.[64] Some cross-sectional studies on schizophrenia also found sharper age-associated declines in cognitive functioning among older adults with schizophrenia than those without the illness,[65, 66] whereas a longitudinal study suggests that the overall pattern and rate of cognitive changes with aging appear parallel between the two groups of individuals.[67]

Evidence-based treatments for older adults with SPMI

Over the past decade, there has been a rapid growth in the number of carefully designed studies to evaluate newly developed nonpharmacological treatments to improve the cognitive, social, and physical functioning of older adults with serious mental illness.[68–75] Bartels and his colleagues have been at the forefront of an effort to develop treatments to improve the physical health of older adults. They adapted the Illness, Management and Recovery (IMR) program, which is an evidence-based practice designed to help patients with serious mental illness self-manage their illness, by extending it to age-related medical conditions commonly experienced by older adults with SPMI.[68] Known as the Integrated Illness, Management and Recovery (I-IMR) program, it contains both a general medical illness component that consists of an individually tailored curriculum for the self-management of general medical illness as well as the standard psychiatric component. In a study comparing I-IMR to the usual standard of care, Bartels and his colleagues found that I-IMR was associated with greater overall improvement in the patient's self-management skills, improvement in self-management of diabetes, and a reduction in hospitalizations.

Bartels and his group also developed a combined skills training and health management (ST+HM) intervention for older adults with severe mental illness.[69] The intervention targets independent living skills, social skills, and effective management of medical health care needs. In a study comparing ST+HM to the HM intervention alone, individuals who received the ST intervention in addition to HM had better functional outcomes with respect to independent living skills, social skills, and health management skills at a one-year follow-up compared to those who received HM alone.

Finally, Bartels and his colleagues developed a peer collaborative training to improve the access of older persons with serious mental illness at risk for cardiovascular disease.[70] The training consists of nine weekly peer co-led patient education and skills training sessions and a 45-minute video-based training for primary care providers. In a study of 17 older adults aged 50 and older with mental illness, participants assumed a more active role in their health care and showed significant improvement in their health care–related communication skills.

In addition to Bartels' group, several other teams have evaluated new treatments to improve the health of older adults with SPMI. The Helping Older People Experience Success (HOPES) program was developed to improve both the psychosocial functioning and reduce the long-term medical burden of older adults living in the community.[71] In a randomized trial of 183 older adults with SMI aged 50 or older, HOPES participants showed significant improvements in social skills, psychosocial and community functioning, negative symptoms, and self-efficacy compared to those in the treatment as usual group.

McKibbin and colleagues developed a lifestyle intervention for middle-aged and older patients with schizophrenia and type 2 diabetes mellitus.[72] The program, Diabetes Awareness and Rehabilitation Training (DART), consisted of 24 weekly, 90-minute sessions addressing diabetes education, nutrition, and lifestyle exercise. Sixty-four persons with schizophrenia who were 40 years or older were randomly assigned to DART or standard care. Results showed significant reductions in BMI and plasma trigylcerides for DART participants compared to those receiving standard care.[72]

Van Citters and colleagues examined whether participation in an individualized, community-integrated In SHAPE health promotion program would result in improved physical health behaviors.[73] In SHAPE promotes healthy eating and exercise behaviors and is provided in mainstream community settings. In a pilot study of 76 persons with SMI, participation over a nine-month period was associated with increased exercise, vigorous activity, and leisurely walking. Participants demonstrated a reduction in waist circumference and a decrease in the severity of negative symptoms.

There is a much smaller but growing evidence-based practice aimed at improving the cognitive, social, and daily functioning of older adults with serious mental illness. Granholm and his colleagues developed a 24-session weekly group therapy intervention that combined cognitive-behavioral therapy with social skills and problem-solving training to improve the functioning of mid-life and aging persons with schizophrenia.[74] In a randomized control trial, patients aged 42–74 receiving the cognitive behavior social skills training demonstrated significantly greater skill acquisition and self-reported higher levels of community living skills compared to those receiving the standard of care.

Multiple studies have demonstrated the benefits of cognitive training for patients with SMI, but these studies have focused mainly on younger patients with few targeting older adults with SPMI. McGurk and Mueser found that older adults showed few improvements in cognitive functioning from cognitive training, although they did demonstrate a significant reduction in negative symptoms. [75] This study suggests that cognitive rehabilitation methods may need to be tailored to address the special needs of older patients with severe mental illness.

All of the preceding interventions assume that the patient is receiving standard medications for the treatment of SPMI. However, the long-term safety and effectiveness of antipsychotic medications in older adults with SPMI has not been adequately studied. Older adults with SPMI appear at increased risk for experiencing side effects associated with psychiatric medications. In a study of four commonly prescribed atypical antipsychotics (aripiprazole, olanzapine, quetiapine, and risperidone) in a group of 332 middle-aged and older outpatients with psychotic symptoms, 36% had metabolic syndrome, and approximately 24% had serious side effects.[76] Since a large number of age-related changes may affect the metabolism and absorption of antipsychotic medications, it is generally recommended that older patients be started on a low initial dose (25%–50% provided to a younger adult) and slowly increase it until a therapeutic effect is realized.[76] Family and friends need to vigilantly monitor side effects to help determine whether the medications having their intended effect.

Family caregiving for older adults with ID and SPMI

The family is the primary provider of informal support to persons with ID and SPMI throughout their lives, showing continued high involvement even after the adult with disabilities moves from the family home.[77] In studies on older adults with SPMI and their caregivers, about one-eighth to one-third of the older adults lived with their family caregivers.[78] Regardless of residential arrangement, the caregivers provided high levels of support for their older family member with ID or SPMI, such as personal care, shopping, transportation, money management, and the management of behavioral problems and psychiatric symptoms.[77, 78]

Due to lifelong caregiving responsibility coupled with their own aging, family caregivers are likely to face physical and psychological challenges. Of concern, one out of four family caregivers of adults with ID is older than the age of 60.[10] Family caregivers of aging adults with ID and SPMI experience significant levels of caregiver burden, and higher levels of psychological stress and poorer physical health than their age peers without caregiving responsibilities.[79–81] Esbensen and Seltzer found that the behavior problems and health declines associated with DS were associated with higher levels of caregiver burden among family caregivers of adults with DS.[82] The long-term effects of lifelong caregiving may not become apparent until later life. Using population data, Seltzer and colleagues found that midlife parents of individuals with ID were similar to their age peers with respect to health and mental health.[80] However, by early old age, these parents had poorer health and mental health than the comparison group.[79]

Although research on families caring for adults with ID has primarily focused on the long-term effects on the family, there is evidence that the effects are bidirectional, with the family environment shaping life course outcomes of adults with ID. In a longitudinal study over a 22-year time span of 75 aging adults with DS, Esbensen and colleagues found that parental psychological functioning and the quality of the relationship between the parent and the adult with DS were significant predictors of adult outcomes approximately 12 years later.[83] These findings indicate that the influence of the family environment persists over the life course and highlight the need

for researchers to focus on the reciprocal effects between the adult with ID and the family context. Interventions aimed at strengthening the family could potentially make an impact on further reducing disability and promoting aging-in-place among older persons with ID.

One of the major concerns for aging families of adults with ID is the fear of who will provide care after the parent's death. Heller and Caldwell developed a peer support intervention to support aging caregivers and adults with ID in planning for the future.[84] The intervention consists of a legal/financial training session followed by five additional small group workshops. A one-year follow-up survey found that the intervention reduced caregiver burden and increased the likelihood that families would engage in future planning activities such as completing a letter of intent or a special needs trust. The success of this intervention suggests the need to adapt it for aging families of adults with SMPI.

Final considerations

Several specific issues are often confronted by health-care practitioners serving these populations. First, guardianship status may have to be clarified. Many persons with mental disabilities have legal guardians with either full or limited powers who therefore must participate in clinical and treatment decision making. However, guardianship and competency often are not clearly established, leading to confusion among health-care professionals as they seek to care for these populations. Second, although most persons with ID and/or SPMI are poor and may be covered by Medicaid, state-specific differences in covered benefits limit access to services in many locales, and thus must be considered. Third, there are few specialists experienced in the provision of health services to people with ID and/or SPMI. If possible, practitioners should locate such specialists for consultation and assistance. This is particularly important for the management of problematic behaviors (a condition characteristic of both populations), for which the propensity to overuse medication should be balanced with the activation of behavioral intervention programs and community supports.

The lack of knowledge about the aging process for these groups is complicated by the common absence of detailed medical histories and the reliance on family caregivers as health surveillance reporters, who themselves are aging. With current projections for increases in the size of both populations, access to high-quality health care is critical. To this end, health-care practitioners can be both active participants in increasing the quality of life of persons with ID and SPMl and contributors to a growing literature on their health-care needs.

References

1. American Association on Intellectual and Developmental Disabilities (AAIDD) [Internet]. Washington DC: Definition of Intellectual Disability; 2013 [cited 2014 Jun 5]. Available from: http://aaidhttp://aaidd.org/intellectual-disability/definition#.U7RwDaNPPTod.

2. Centers for Disease Control and Prevention (CDC) [Internet]. Atlanta: Developmental Disabilities; 2013 [cited 2014 Jun 5]. Available from: www.cdc.gov/ncbddd/developmentaldisabilities/facts.html.

3. AAIDD [Internet]. Washington DC: Fact Sheet: Aging – Older Adults and Their Aging Caregivers; 2005 [cited 2014 Jun 5]. Available from: www.ddas.vermont.gov/ddas-publications/publications-dementia/publications-dementia-documents/fs-aging.

4. Heller K. People with intellectual and developmental disabilities growing old: an overview. Impact [Internet]. 2010 winter; [cited 2014 Jun 5]; 23(1). Available from: http://ici.umn.edu/products/impact/231/2.html.

5. Bittles AH, Petterson BA, Sullivan SG, et al. The influence of intellectual disability on life expectancy. *J Gerontol A Biol Sci Med Sci.* 2002 Jul; **57**:M470–2.

6. Perkins EA, Moran JA. Aging adults with intellectual disabilities. *JAMA.* 2010;**304**:91–2.

7. McCarron M, McCallion P, Reilly E, Mulryan N. A prospective 14-year longitudinal follow-up of dementia in persons with Down syndrome. *J Intellect Disabil Res.* 2014;**58**:61–70.

8. Coppus AM. People with intellectual disability: what do we know about adulthood and life expectancy? *Dev Disabil Res Rev.* 2013 Aug;**18**(1):6–16.

9. Taub S, Bershadsky J, Moseley C. Using National Core Indicators Data to understand the experiences of older adults with intellectual disabilities. Presented at the AAIDD Annual Meeting. Minnesota. 2011; [cited 2014 Jun 5]. Available from: www.nationalcoreindicators.org/upload/presentation/Experiences_of_Older_Adults.pdf.

10. Braddock D, Hemp R, Rizzolo MC. *The State of the States in Developmental Disabilities.* Boulder (CO): University of Colorado, Coleman Institute for Cognitive Disabilities and Department of Psychiatry; 2008.

11. de Winter CF, Bastiaanse LP, Hilgenkamp TI, et al. Overweight and obesity in older people with intellectual disability. *Res Dev Disabil.* 2012 Mar–Apr;**33**(2):398–405.

12. Heller T, Sorensen A. Promoting healthy aging in adults with developmental disabilities. *Dev Disabil Res Rev.* 2013 Aug;**18**(1):22–30.

13. Esbensen AJ, Seltzer MM, Krauss MW. Stability and change in health, functional abilities and behavior problems among adults with and without Down syndrome. *Am J Ment Retard.* 2008,**113**:263–77.

14. Zigman WB, Schupf N, Haveman M, Silverman V. The epidemiology of Alzheimer disease in intellectual disability: results and recommendations from an international conference. *J Intellct Disabil Res.* 1997;**41**:76–80.

15. Zigman WB. Atypical aging in Down syndrome. *Dev Disabil Res Rev,* 2013;**18**:51–67.

16. Coppus A, Evnhuis GJ, Verbenrne F, et al. Dementia and mortality in persons with Down's syndrome. *J Intellct Disabil Res.* 2006,**50**:768–77.

17. Strydom A, Hassiotis A, King M, Livingston G. The relationship of dementia prevalence in older adults with intellectual disability (ID) to age and severity of ID. *Psycholl Med.* 2009 Jan;**39**(1):13–21.

18. Zigman WB, Schupf N, Devenny DA, et al. Incidence and prevalence of dementia in elderly adults with mental retardation without down syndrome. *Am J Ment Retard.* 2004 Mar;**109**(2):126–41.

19. Krinsky-McHale SJ, Silverman W. Dementia and mild cognitive impairment in adults with intellectual disability: Issues of diagnosis. *Dev Disabil Res Rev.* 2013;**18**(1):31–42.

20. Silverman W, Zigman W, Krinsky-McHale S, et al. Intellectual disability, mild cognitive impairment, and risk for dementia. *J Policy Pract Intellect Disabil.* 2013 Sep;**10**(3):245–51.

21. Evenhuis HM, Hermans H, Hilgenkamp TI, et al. Frailty and disability in older adults with intellectual disabilities: results from the healthy ageing and intellectual disability study. *J Am Geriatr Soc.* 2012 May;**60**(5):934–8.

22. Minhan PM. Aging in adults with developmental disabilities. In: Arenson C, Busby-Whitehead J, Brummel-Smith K, et al., eds. *Reichel's Care of the Elderly: Clinical Aspects of Aging.* New York: Cambridge University Press; 2009: 210–20.

23. Shooshtari S, Martens P, Burchill C, et al. Prevalence of depression and dementia among adults with developmental disabilities in Manitoba, Canada. Int J Family Med [Internet]. 2011 [cited 2014 Jun 5]: [about 9 p.]. Available from: www.hindawi.com/journals/ijfm/2011/319574.

24. Marks B, Sisirak J, Heller T. *Exercise and Nutrition Health Education Curriculum for Adults with Developmental Disabilities.* Philadelphia: Brookes Publishing; 2010.

25. Newschaffer CJ, Croen LA, Daniels J, et al. The epidemiology of autism spectrum disorders. *Annu Rev Public Health.* 2007;**28**:235–58.

26. CDC [Internet]. Washington DC: Autism Spectrum Disorder; 2013 [cited 2014 Jun 5]. Available from: www.cdc.gov/ncbddd/autism/index.html.

27. King M, Bearman P. Diagnostic change and the increased prevalence of autism. *Int J Epidemiol.* 2009;**38**(5):1224–34.

28. Piven J, Harper J, Palmer P, Arndt S. Course of behavioral change in autism: a retrospective study of high-IQ adolescents and adults. *J Am Acad Child Adolesc Psychiatry.* 1996 Apr;**35**(4):523–9.

29. Piven J, Rabins, P. and on behalf of the Autism-in-Older Adults Working Group. Autism Spectrum Disorders in older adults: toward defining a research agenda. *J Am Geriatr Soc.* 2011;**59**:2151–5.

30. Smith LE, Greenberg JS, Mailick MR. The family context of autism spectrum disorders: Influence on the behavioral phenotype and quality of life. *Child Adolesc Psychiatr Clin N Am,* 2014; **23**(1):143–55.

31. Esbensen AJ, Greenberg JS, Seltzer MM, Aman, MG. A longitudinal investigation of psychotropic and non-psychotropic medication use among adolescents and adults with autism spectrum disorders. *J Autism Devl Disord.* 2009;**39**(3),1339–49.

32. Smith LE, Maenner M, Seltzer MM. Developmental trajectories in adolescents and adults with autism: the case of daily living skills. *J Am Acad Child Adolesc Psychiatry.* 2012;**51**(6), 622–31.

33. Taylor JL, Mailick MR. A longitudinal examination of 10-year change in vocational and educational activities for adults with autism spectrum disorders. *Dev Psychol.* 2014 Mar;**50**(3):699–708.

34. Williams, SK, Scahill L, Vitiello B, et al. Risperidone and adaptive behavior in children with autism. *J Am Acad Child Adolesc Psychiatry.* 2006; **45**(4):431–9

35. National Advisory Council. Health care reform for Americans with severe mental illnesses: report of the National Advisory Mental Health Council. *Am J of Psychiatry.* 1993 Oct;**150**(10):1447–65.

36. Zipursky RB, Reilly TJ, Murray RM. The myth of schizophrenia as a progressive brain disease. *Schizophr Bull.* 2013 Nov;**39**(6):1363–72.

37. Cohen CI, Iqbal M. Longitudinal study of remission among older adults with schizophrenia spectrum disorder. *Am J Geriatr Psychiatry.* 2014;**22**(5):450–8.

38. Auslander LA, Jeste DV. Sustained remission of schizophrenia among community dwelling older outpatients. *Am J of Psychiatry.* 2004 Aug;**161**(8):1490–3.

39. Jeste DV, Maglione JE. Treating older adults with schizophrenia: challenges and opportunities. *Schizophr Bull.* 2013 Sep;**39**(5):966–8.

40. Substance Abuse and Mental Health Services Administration (SAMSHA). Results from the 2012 *National Survey on Drug Use and Health: Mental Health Findings,* NSDUH Series H-47, HHS Publication No. (SMA) 13–4805. Rockville, MD: Substance Abuse and Mental Health Services Administration; 2013.

41. Bartels SJ. Caring for the whole person: integrated health care for older adults with severe mental illness and medical comorbidity. *J Am Geriatr Soc.* 2004 Dec;**52**(12 Suppl):S249–57.

42. Jeste DV, Blazer DG, First M. Aging-related diagnostic variations: need for diagnostic criteria appropriate for elderly psychiatric patients. *Biol Psychiatry.* 2005 Aug;**58**(4):265–71.

43. Druss BG, Zhao L, Von Esenwein S, et al. Understanding excess mortality in persons with mental illness: 17-year follow up of a nationally representative US survey. *Med Care.* 2011 Jun;**49**(6):599–604.

44. Colton CW, Manderscheid RW. Congruencies in increased mortality rates, years of potential life lost, and causes of death among public mental health clients in eight states. *Prev Chronic Dis.* 2006 Apr;**3**(2):A42.

45. Saha S, Chant D, McGrath J. A systematic review of mortality in schizophrenia: is the differential mortality gap worsening over time? *Arch Gen Psychiatry.* 2007 Oct;**64**(10):1123–31.

46. Parks J, Svedsen D, Singer P, Foti ME. *Morbidity and Mortality in People with Serious Mental Illness.* Alexandria, VA: National Association of State Mental Health Program Directors; 2006.

47. Lindamer LA, Lohr JB, Harris MJ, et al. Gender-related clinical differences in older patients with schizophrenia. *J Clin Psychiatry.* 1999 Jan;**60**(1):61–7.

48. Riecher-Rössler A, Häfner H. Gender aspects in schizophrenia: bridging the border between social and biological psychiatry. *Acta Psychiatr Scand Suppl.* 2000;(407):58–62.

49. Dickerson FB. Women, aging, and schizophrenia. *J Women Aging.* 2007;**19** (1/2):49–61.

50. Saraceno B, Levan I, Kohn R. The public mental health significance of research on socio-economic factors in schizophrenia and major depression. *World Psychiatry.* 2005;**4**(3):181–5.

51. Kessler RC, Chiu WT, Demler O, Walters EE. Prevalence, severity, and comorbidity of 12-month DSM-IV disorders in the National Comorbidity Survey Replication. *Arch of Gen Psychiatry.* 2005;**62**(6):617–27.

52. Mechanic D, McAlpine DD. Use of nursing homes in the care of persons with severe mental illness: 1985 to 1995. *Psychiatr Serv.* 2000 Mar;**51**(3):354–8.

53. Jin H, Folsom D, Sasaki A, et al. Increased Framingham 10-year risk of coronary heart disease in

middle-aged and older patients with psychotic symptoms. *Schizophr Res.* 2011 Feb;**125**(2–3):295–9.

54. Hennekens CH, Hennekens AR, Hollar D, Casey DE. Schizophrenia and increased risks of cardiovascular disease. *Am Heart J.* 2005;**150**:1115–21.

55. Sokal J, Messias E, Dickerson FB, et al. Comorbidity of medical illnesses among adults with serious mental illness who are receiving community psychiatric services. *J Nerv Ment Dis.* 2004 Jun;**192**(6):421–7.

56. Kirkpatrick B, Messias E, Harvey PD, et al. Is schizophrenia a syndrome of accelerated aging? *Schizophr Bull.* 2008 Nov;**34**(6):1024–32.

57. Wang PS, Demler O, Kessler RC. Adequacy of treatment for serious mental illness in the United States. *Am J Public Health.* 2002 Jan;**92**(1):92–8.

58. Dickerson FB, Pater A, Origoni AE. Health behaviors and health status of older women with schizophrenia. *Psychiatr Serv.* 2002 Jul; **53**(7):882–4.

59. Hendrie HC, Lindgren D, Hay DP, et al. Comorbidity profile and healthcare utilization in elderly patients with serious mental illnesses. *Am J Geriatr Psychiatry.* 2013 Dec;**21**(12):1267–76.

60. Scott D, Happell B. The high prevalence of poor physical health and unhealthy lifestyle behaviours in individuals with severe mental illness. *Issues Ment Health Nurs.* 2011;**32**(9): 589–97.

61. Moore DJ, Savla GN, Woods SP, et al. Verbal fluency impairments among middle-aged and older outpatients with schizophrenia are characterized by deficient switching. *Schizophr Res.* 2006 Oct;**87**(1–3):254–60.

62. Weisenbach SL, Marshall D, Weldon AL, et al. The double burden of age and disease on cognition and quality of life in bipolar disorder. *Int J Geriatr Psychiatry* [Internet]. 2014 Feb [Epub ahead of print]. Available from Willey Online Library: http://onlineli brary.wiley.com/doi/10.1002/gps.4084/full.

63. Depp CA, Moore DJ, Sitzer D, et al. Neurocognitive impairment in middle-aged and older adults with bipolar disorder: comparison to schizophrenia and normal comparison subjects. *J Affect Disord.* 2007;**101**(1–3):201–9.

64. Gildengers AG, Mulsant BH, Begley A, et al. The longitudinal course of cognition in older adults with bipolar disorder. *Bipolar Disord.* 2009 Nov;**11**(7):744–52.

65. Loewenstein DA, Czaja SJ, Bowie CR, Harvey PD. Age-associated differences in cognitive performance in older patients with schizophrenia: a comparison with healthy older adults. *Am J Geriatr Psychiatry.* 2012;**20**(1):29–40.

66. Fucetola R, Seidman LJ, Kremen WS, et al. Age and neuropsychologic function in schizophrenia: a decline in executive abilities beyond that observed in healthy volunteers. *Biol Psychiatry.* 2000;**48**(2):137–46.

67. Heaton RK, Gladsjo JA, Palmer BW, et al. Stability and course of neuropsychological deficits in schizophrenia. *Arch Gen Psychiatry.* 2001;**58**(1):24–32.

68. Bartels SJ, Pratt SI, Mueser KT, et al. Integrated IMR for psychiatric and general medical illness for adults aged 50 or older with serious mental illness. *Psychiatr Serv*; 2014 Mar;**65**(3):330–7.

69. Bartels SJ, Forester B, Mueser KT. Enhanced skills training and health care management for older persons with severe mental illness. *Community Ment Health J.* 2004 Feb;**40**(1):75–90.

70. Bartels SJ, Aschbrenner KA, Rolin SA, et al. Activating older adults with serious mental illness for collaborative primary care visits. *Psychiatr Rehabil J.* 2013 Dec;**36**(4):278–88.

71. Mueser KT, Pratt SI, Bartels SJ, et al. Randomized trial of social rehabilitation and integrated health care for older people with severe mental illness. *J Consult Clin Psychol.* 2010 Aug;**78**(4):561–73.

72. McKibbin CL, Patterson TL, Norman G, et al. A lifestyle intervention for older schizophrenia patients with diabetes mellitus: a randomized controlled trial. *Schizophr Res.* 2006 Sep;**86**(1–3):36–44.

73. Van Citters AD, Pratt SI, Jue K, et al. A pilot evaluation of the In SHAPE individualized health promotion intervention for adults with mental illness. *Community Ment Health J.* 2010 Dec;**46**(6):540–52.

74. Granholm E, McQuaid JR, McClure FS, et al. A randomized, controlled trial of cognitive behavioral social skills training for middle-aged and older outpatients with chronic schizophrenia. *Am J Psychiatry.* 2005 Mar;**162**(3):520–9.

75. McGurk SR, Mueser KT. Response to cognitive rehabilitation in older versus younger persons with severe mental illness. *Am J Psychiatr Rehabil.* 2008;**11**(1):90–105.

76. Jin H, Shih PA, Golshan S, et al. Comparison of longer-term safety and effectiveness of 4 atypical antipsychotics in patients over age 40: a trial using equipoise-stratified randomization. *J Clin Psychiatry.* 2013 Jan;**74**(1):10–8.

77. Seltzer MM, Krauss MW, Hong J, Orsmond GI. Continuity or discontinuity of family involvement following residential transitions of adults who have mental retardation. *Mental Retardation.* 2001;**39**(3):181–94.

78. Cummings SM, Kropf NP. Formal and informal support for older adults with severe mental illness. *Aging Ment Health.* 2009;**13**(4):619–27.

79. Seltzer MM, Floyd FJ, Song J, et al. Midlife and aging parents of adults with intellectual and developmental disabilities: impacts of lifelong parenting. *Am J Intellect Dev Disabil.* 2011;**116**(6):479–99.

80. Seltzer MM, Greenberg JS, Floyd FJ, et al. Life course impacts of parenting a child with a disability. *Am J Ment Retard*, 2001;**106**(3):265–86.

81. Cummings S, MacNeil G. Caregivers of older clients with severe mental illness: perceptions of burdens and rewards. *Fam Soc*, 2008;**89**:51–60.

82. Esbensen AJ, Seltzer MM. Accounting for the "Down syndrome advantage." *Am J Intellect Dev Disabil.* 2011;**116**(1):3–15.

83. Esbensen AJ, Mailick MR, Silverman W. Long-term impact of parental well-being on adult outcomes and dementia status in individuals with Down syndrome. *Am J Intellect Dev Disabil.* 2013;**118**(4):294–309.

84. Heller T, Caldwell J. Supporting aging caregivers and adults with developmental disabilities in future planning. *Ment Retard.* 2006 Jun;**44**(3):189–202.

Chapter 7

Community-based long-term care for the elderly

Déon Cox Hayley, DO, Myra Hyatt, LSCSW, and Mindy J. Fain, MD

Introduction

Community-based long-term care encompasses a wide array of medical and nonmedical diagnostic, preventive, therapeutic, rehabilitative, personal, social, supportive, and palliative services in a variety of settings for individuals who have lost some capacity for self-care because of a chronic illness or physical, cognitive, or emotional impairment. Some support services allow the patient to remain at home (including adult day care, home health services, home medical care, and telemedicine), whereas other services require a change of residence (such as assisted-living, adult-care homes, and continuing-care retirement communities). The goal of care is to build on interprofessional expertise and teamwork to promote the optimally independent level of physical, social, and psychological functioning in the least restrictive environment.

Older adults are high users of health care. In 2012, 23% of those aged 75 and older had 10 or more medical visits in the last year as compared to 14% of those aged 45–64.[1] Most older adults with chronic health problems prefer to remain at home or in a homelike setting.[2] A minority of older adults (3.5% of all 65+ and 10% of those 85+) live in nursing homes, and there has been a trend toward community-based services to provide support.

Community-based long-term care services focus on the older adult's medical and psychosocial needs and aim to maintain function, prevent acute exacerbations of chronic illness, and avoid unnecessary and costly emergency room visits and hospitalizations. Services include assistance with activities of daily living (ADLs) and instrumental activities of daily living (IADLs). In addition, this care seeks to maintain the patient's safety and provide comfort and assurance. It may entail hands-on or supervisory human assistance, assistive devices, and technology such as computerized medication reminders and emergency alert systems.[3]

Comprehensive geriatric assessment, a multidimensional and interdisciplinary process, embodies a formal approach to match the patient's needs with available resources to provide safe, effective, and high-quality care.[4, 5] Case/care managers are often the point of entry to in-home and community-based services; they are responsible for the determination of the patient's needs. Case management is often provided by a nurse, social worker, or private consultant. A key component of such management involves a review of an individual's socioeconomic, environmental, psychological, and physical health challenges, and the development of a care plan for services or treatment.

The role of the physician in long-term care is vital because, by definition, these patients are often medically complex with restricted ability to manage their own care, and are therefore very vulnerable to further insults to their health. The primary care physician caring for patients who need long-term care will most likely be responsible for authorizing and supervising complex medical plans of care, advocating for the patient, and promoting a collaborative interdisciplinary team effort. Physicians certify patient eligibility for Medicare-funded home health care (HHC), including nursing care, rehabilitative therapies, and hospice care. Medicare has assigned billing codes specifically for physicians who coordinate long-term-care services under Medicare. Physicians also provide a critical consultative function for community-based services funded by other sources.

Community-based care enables the older adult with disabilities to live more independently and may

Reichel's Care of the Elderly, 7th Edition, ed. Jan Busby-Whitehead *et al.* Published by Cambridge University Press.
© Cambridge University Press 2016.

reduce the probability of institutionalization; however, sometimes the challenges posed by limited availability, access, and affordability of services prohibit continued care in the community.

Home care

Home care is defined by the American Medical Association (AMA) as "the provision of equipment and services to the patient in the home for the purpose of restoring and maintaining his or her maximal level of comfort, function and health ... and is a collaborative effort of the patient, family, and professionals."[6] Home care includes a wide array of services: home health care, medical house calls, special programs, home hospice, and long-term supportive care, such as caregiving and home-delivered meals.[7]

Home health care

Medicare skilled home health care (HHC) was designed to provide acute and post-acute care following hospitalization, but it is also useful for the provision of episodic skilled care for the older patient who has difficulty coming to office appointments. HHC includes skilled nursing care, health monitoring, dispensing of medications, psychiatric care, physical and other rehabilitative therapies, personal care, homemaker services, and health education of patients, family members, and caregivers. With technological advances, HHC diagnostic and therapeutic procedures may include intravenous antibiotics, transfusions, chemotherapy, dialysis, enteral and parenteral nutrition, and mechanical ventilation. The use of tele-monitoring systems offers the options of telehome care and "electronic house calls" to assist with chronic disease management programs.

The older patient in need of HHC often has complex medical problems and functional impairments. In order to receive HHC through Medicare, assessments are required to determine medical necessity, including the acuity of the problem, underlying comorbidities, the severity of the patient's functional disability and homebound status, and potential interventions. This process includes a determination of the appropriate level of care and services, and the patient and/or caregiver's ability to implement the plan of care. Most primary care physicians will be involved in ordering, certifying, and overseeing complex home-care plans for their homebound patients, including documentation of a face-to-face evaluation. The details of the care plan are often generated by nurses and therapists who then implement them. This process should be collaborative and include the expertise of all interdisciplinary team members.[8]

Medicare and Medicaid pay for most of HHC, though other reimbursement programs include private insurance, managed care, the Older Americans Act, and self-pay. In 2010, there were over 10,000 Medicare-certified home health agencies, and an additional unknown number of agencies not certified.[9] Medicare-covered services are part-time, intermittent, skilled services that are limited to homebound patients. This care must be ordered by a physician; administered by a core provider such as a nurse, physical therapist, or speech therapist; and must be appropriate to the patient's illness and/or injury. As skilled care is provided only temporarily, it is critical that the patient and caregiver learn and carry out tasks such as the use and maintenance of tubes and catheters and the changing of dressings. Other services, such as those provided by a social worker or home health aide, may be reimbursed but only when the patient is receiving care from one of the three core skilled services. Reimbursement models other than Medicare may include considerations of cost-effectiveness, patient prognosis, and the opportunity to achieve certain outcomes of care. This may include care for patients who are not homebound, but who require services such as infusion therapy.

The website Home Health Compare, sponsored by the Centers for Medicare and Medicaid Services (CMS), an agency of the US Department of Health and Human Services (DHHS) – www.medicare.gov/homehealthcompare/search.html – can help providers, patients, and families assess quality measures of Medicare-certified home health agencies.

Medical house calls

There are a significant number of homebound older adults who have difficulty accessing primary medical care, and their care is disproportionately managed in the emergency room or the acute care setting.[10] In fact, it has been suggested that with focus on acute inpatient care, we are actually neglecting the care of those at home.[11] The vulnerable, elderly, homebound patients may receive care at home through home visits or "house calls." House calls are now more financially feasible for clinicians through modestly higher reimbursement from Medicare, as well as innovative business models based on potential cost savings for health plans, commercial insurers, and other payors from reductions in unnecessary utilization. As a result, the number of house calls performed has grown significantly. However, there are still many office-based primary care providers who – owing to perceived poor reimbursement; time-inefficiencies; concerns about safety, liability, and legal issues; lack of equipment; and perhaps lack of training do – not see patients at home.

Medical house calls are provided by physicians, physician's assistants, and nurse practitioners in the home as part of an ongoing office-based practice, a hospital-based program, a free-standing practice, special programs such as the Veteran's Administration (VA), or specialty programs through academic medical centers. Models range from single providers to team-based care that can include social workers, nurses, and others. House calls can provide longitudinal primary care as well as assessment and management of acute/sub-acute care. Programs frequently coordinate with home health agencies and community-based organizations, such as home-delivered meals, to support patients in their homes. The growth and positive published outcomes of many specialized house call/home-care programs are encouraging. Positive outcomes of these programs include optimization of home safety, enhancement of patient and family education, identification of common geriatric issues that would otherwise go unrecognized,[12] increased likelihood of dying in a location of choice,[13] decreased hospital admissions,[14] and reduced health-care costs.[15]

The VA's Home Based Primary Care (HBPC) program for frail veterans has led the country as a model for comprehensive, interdisciplinary home care. The HBPC program targets patients for whom clinic-based care is not effective, and covers clinician visits, skilled nursing care, and nonskilled care as well as case management. The VA's HBPC program has demonstrated significantly lower total costs (without shifting costs to Medicare) and reduced hospital and nursing home use.[16, 17]

Another established model of care, the Care Transitions Intervention (www.caretransitons.org), developed by Eric Coleman, focuses on the critical transition of medical care of the patient from hospital to home. The model is operationalized by transition coaches (usually nurse practitioners), and has

repeatedly shown that it can decrease hospital readmissions and decrease costs.[18, 19]

Other programs across the country caring for large numbers of chronically ill patients have demonstrated very remarkable reductions in emergency room visits, hospitalizations, length of stay in hospital, and cost savings through a primary care, home-based team approach.[20] In addition, there are specialty home-care programs designed for targeted care of specific medical problems, such as heart failure.

Independence at Home, a Medicare demonstration program supported by the Affordable Care Act and modeled on the demonstrated successes of the VA's HBPC program, began in 2012 and aims to enroll 10,000 home-limited Medicare patients with multiple chronic medical problems. In this three-year, shared-savings program, patients are provided longitudinal primary care and care coordination services in the home for medical and social service needs by teams headed by physicians or nurse practitioners. Quality, patient satisfaction, and cost savings will be measured.[21]

Importantly, a comprehensive set of evidence-based process quality indicators for homebound seniors developed by the Home-based Primary Care Quality Initiative provides a quality framework to evaluate home-based primary medical care.[22]

Residential care facilities

The landscape is changing in regards to the array of residential facilities available for the older adult. The variety of facilities and what they offer can be daunting. Independent-living and assisted-living (AL) facilities, as well as residential or personal care homes, adult board and care, domiciliary care, and congregate living homes are examples of residential care facilities (RCFs). RCFs were designed as less expensive, and often more appropriate, alternatives to nursing home placement for older persons with chronic care needs. There is still much variability ranging from the definition of facilities, to services provided, to regulation. Consequently, RCFs blur the line between community and institutionally based long-term care.

In addition, continuing care retirement communities (CCRCs) are designed to cross the spectrum for individuals with increasing care needs over time.

653

In 2010, the National Survey of Residential Care Facilities reported 31,100 RCFs with a capacity for 971,900 residents. About 50% of RCFs were small facilities (4–10 residents), 16% had 11–25 residents, 28% had 26–100 residents, and 7% had capacity for more than 100. Larger RCFs are more likely to be affiliated with a chain and offer services such as physical and occupational therapy and case management.

Although both nursing homes and RCFs provide housing and care to elders with disabilities, a number of important characteristics differentiate them, including the foundation of how care is provided, what care is provided, regulation, and payment.

Whereas nursing homes were developed on a medical model where physicians direct and order care and nurses are the primary providers of care, RCFs were developed more on a residential model where medical care is not central. In fact, most RCFs do not have physicians on site and there are fewer nursing staff.

Just as RCFs were designed to be different from nursing homes, their regulation was also designed differently. Unlike nursing homes, where the CMS sets the standards that qualify a facility for federal Medicare/Medicaid funding, states are the primary regulators of RCFs. Across states, there are no generally agreed upon standards for care and no consensus about which RCFs should be licensed. States establish their own requirements and may provide little oversight or protection for residents. This has resulted in large numbers of disabled older adults receiving care in what is a largely unregulated industry.

Generally, RCF costs are not covered by Medicare, Medicaid, or private insurance; however, resources vary from state to state, and more facilities have been receiving Medicaid support in recent years.[23] Residency can be costly, and the average monthly rate in 2010 was $3,165 for AL facilities.[24]

Assisted living is one example of an RCF. AL facilities originally were designed to serve those who needed intermediate care – between independent living and a nursing home. ALs may offer individual houses, townhouses, condominiums, or apartments that often incorporate disability features and assistive technology. They can be located in freestanding facilities or on a campus with other facilities.

Assisted living traditionally has provided meals; housekeeping; recreational, social, and educational activities; transportation; emergency help; and only limited assistance with ADLs and personal care.

However, more and more ALs are offering many levels of care as individuals decline in function and are reluctant to move to a nursing home. Services offered vary from facility to facility, including assistance with medication administration, ADLs, and other nursing care. The National Center for Assisted Living (NCAL) has been leading a quality initiative and encouraging standards and evaluation in assisted living.[25]

Dependencies and comorbidities vary among residents. More than half (54%) of residents in AL are over 85 years old. In 2010, 72% of residents received assistance with bathing, 52% received assistance with dressing, 36% received assistance with toileting, 25% received assistance with transferring, and 22% received assistance with eating. Dementia is common among residents (42%), and 17% of facilities have dementia special care units. These units include special features for the care of residents with dementia, such as dementia-specific activities and programming (91%), doors with alarms (90%), specially trained staff (88%), and locked exit doors (76%).[26]

Other RCFs such as adult board and care, or personal care homes, may not be exclusive to older adults; they may also serve those who require supervision and some personal care with few onsite medical services. They are privately operated and are often converted single-family homes. State law and local zoning regulations determine the exact number of residents allowed (approximately 2–20).

Facilities such as board and care homes typically provide a basic room (may be shared), meals, some assistance with daily activities, custodial help (including reminders to take medications, laundry, housekeeping, transportation), and supervision. Depending on licensing, the home may provide assistance with ADLs (such as bathing and grooming), dispensing of medications, dementia care, basic nursing care, and social, recreational, and spiritual activities. Many board and care homes are unlicensed, and states may only infrequently monitor the licensed homes.

Other supportive services

There are other services that support functionally impaired older adults in their ADLs and IADLs to allow them to remain safely at home.

Informal caregiving, the most common form of long-term care in the United States, is unpaid care in the home provided by family or friends. Most community-dwelling older adults with long-term care needs (61.3%) get care from paid and unpaid caregivers – an average of 177 hours per month.[27] Estimates of the percentage of family or informal caregivers who are women range from 59% to 75%.[28] The fact that 30% of persons caring for elderly long-term care users were themselves aged 65 or older brings additional concerns.[29] Informal long-term care often demands intense effort, and affects the physical and psychological health of the caregiver. Use of caregiver support services has been shown to have positive effects; available services include the National Family Caregiver Support Program, support groups, and respite care.

The federally administered Older Americans Act funds local area agencies on aging to support community social and nutrition services, especially for low-income elders and Native Americans. This program also supports information and referral sources. Home- and community-based services (HCBS) money comes through Medicaid and supports nonmedical community services.[30]

There are many other community-based supportive services for the older adult at home, or in local nutrition or senior centers, and often are provided by volunteers for low cost. Benefits may include transportation, social activities, mentoring, meals, and assistance with housekeeping and personal care.

Other programs

Adult day care

Adult day-care programs serve those who need assistance or supervision during the day. These programs offer respite to family members and caregivers, and provide them with the opportunity to go to work and handle personal business. More than 3,500 adult day centers are operating in the United States. Half of participants have some cognitive impairment, and 59% require assistance with two or more ADLs.[31] There are three types of day-care models: social, medical, and special purpose that serve the need of a particular comorbid illness (e.g., dementia). Medical models focus on skilled health care and rehabilitative services; some have workshops for memory improvement and incontinence.

Adult day-care programs generally provide supervision, a meal and snacks, recreation, and health care/monitoring for physical, mental, or social impairments. Participants do not require 24-hour institutional care, yet they are not capable of full-time, independent living.

The majority of states require licensing or certification of programs through licensing, certification, and definition of programs. Regulations regarding types and number of staff and funding vary from state to state. Programs may be funded at least in part by Medicaid, the Older Americans Act, and various state sources. Programs can only receive funding from Medicare or Medicaid if medical services are provided. Therefore, the out-of-pocket fees for patients can be costly.

Studies support several positive effects of adult day care, including decreased behavioral problems in patients with dementia who attend programs, and day-care services may substitute for specific types of home-based formal services.[32, 33]

Hospice care

Hospice is a palliative and supportive care program for terminally ill patients and their families, with the goal of providing a comfortable and dignified death at home. The hospice movement began in response to the belief that burgeoning technology and pursuit of a cure were interfering with the humanitarian care of the dying patient. The Medicare hospice benefit (MHB) was funded as a capitated system with rules for eligibility and covered services; it serves as a guideline for hospice services provided by other payers.

More than 90% of hospice days are provided for patients in their residence (which may be their house or other residential facility) by an interdisciplinary team with expertise in the physical, psychological, social, and spiritual needs of the dying patient and family. Interdisciplinary team members include skilled nurses, hospice physician, nurse practitioner, home health aides, social workers, chaplains, volunteers, and bereavement counselors. Other levels of hospice care include continuous home care for brief periods for symptom management, temporary respite, or inpatient hospice care if the patient is not able to be maintained at home.

On admission to the hospice program, the patient, doctor, and interdisciplinary team develop a plan of care that focuses on palliation and optimization of quality of life, and identifies the patient's goals of care and services. Importantly, no Medicare regulation specifies which interventions are "palliative"; as a result, each hospice has its own guidelines, a decision determined by both philosophical and financial considerations.

The MHB requires that the patient have an anticipated survival of less than six months. However, prognostication is difficult. Cancer is the most common referring diagnosis, and patients with dementia are markedly underrepresented in hospice care. The National Hospice Organization has developed general criteria for referral for hospice, and guidelines for prognosis in chronic disease such as heart disease, pulmonary disease, stroke, dementia, renal disease, and liver disease.[34] For patients with advanced chronic disease, difficulties with prognostication often result in late referrals by the physician.

The use of hospice services has grown, and it is estimated that in 2007, 30% of patients with Medicare who died had accessed at least three days of hospice care. However, average length of stay in hospice in 2012 was 18.7 days, less than three weeks. Eighty-four percent of hospice patients in 2012 were aged 65 and over.[35]

The National Hospice and Palliative Care Organization (NHPCO) has been a leader in setting and monitoring quality standards for end-of-life care. It has been shown that hospice enrollment improves care quality for Medicare patients. Hospice enrollment is associated with fewer 30-day hospital readmissions and in-hospital deaths, and significantly fewer hospital and ICU days. Moreover, hospice care reduced Medicare expenditures per patient by thousands of dollars.[36, 37] But importantly, hospice care is associated with quality of life, with a focus on symptom control, interaction with family, and function as well as emotional and spiritual needs at the end of life.[38, 39]

The program of all-inclusive care for the elderly

Many states have requested "waivers" to pay for normally uncovered home- and community-based services for Medicaid-eligible persons who might otherwise be institutionalized. One state option is known as the Program of All-Inclusive Care for the Elderly (PACE) a capitated benefit that features a comprehensive service delivery system and integrated Medicare and Medicaid financing.[40]

Participants must be at least 55 years old, live in the PACE service area, and be certified as eligible for nursing home care by the appropriate state agency. While enrolled, the participant must receive Medicare and Medicaid benefits solely through the PACE organization. PACE benefits for all participants include a comprehensive package of services, such as medical care, personal care and support, meals, transportation, restorative therapies, prosthetics and other durable medical equipment, medications, laboratory tests, x-rays and other diagnostic procedures, acute inpatient care, nursing facility care, and other services determined necessary by an interdisciplinary team. PACE care is provided in adult day health centers, homes, hospitals, and nursing homes. Each PACE center must have a comprehensive interdisciplinary team that is responsible for initial and periodic assessments, care planning, and coordination of 24-hour care delivery.

There has been recent growth in the development of PACE sites and data to support how PACE programs can reduce hospitalizations, hospital readmissions, and potentially avoidable hospitalizations.[41]

The Veterans Health Administration

The Veterans Health Administration (VHA) offers a spectrum of geriatric and extended care services to enrolled veterans through its 159 VHA medical centers, more than 700 ambulatory care and community-based clinics, 134 nursing homes, and 42 domiciliaries. Recognized as a national leader in geriatric models of care, more than 90% of the VHA medical centers provide comprehensive home and community-based outpatient long-term care programs. Among the continuum of services are the Home-Based Primary Care Program, contract home health care, adult day health care, homemaker and home health aide (H/HHA), community residential and domic iliary care, respite care, home hospice care, and telehealth programs.

References

1. Department of Health and Human Services, Administration of Aging. Health and Health Care [cited 2014 Oct 16]. Available at: www.aoa.gov/aoaroot/aging_statistics/Profile/2013/14.aspx.

2. Kirby JB, Lau DT. Special Committee on Aging. *Development in Aging: 1997 and 1998*, Volume 1, Report 106–229. Washington, DC: United States Senate, 2000.

3. Community and individual race-ethnicity and home health care use among elderly persons in the United States, *Health Serv Res.* 2010;45(5 pt1):1251–67.

4. Martin DC, Marycz RK, McDowell BJ, et al. Community-based geriatric assessment. *J Am Geriatr Soc.* 1985;33(9):602–6.

5. Stuck AE, Siu AL, Wieland GD, et al. Comprehensive geriatric assessment: A meta-analysis of controlled trials. *Lancet.* 1993;**342**:1032–6.

6. American Medical Association, Council on Scientific Affairs. Home Care in the 1990's. *JAMA.* 1990;**263**(9):1241–4.

7. Levine SA, Boal J, Boling PA. Home Care. *JAMA.* 2003;**290**(9):1203–7.

8. Caffry C, Sengupta M, Moss A, et al. Home Health Care and Hospice Care Discharged Patients: United States 2000 and 2007. *National Health Statistics Report.* 2011;38.

9. National Association for Home Care & Hospice. Basic Statistics about Home Care. Washington, DC. 2010 [cited 2014 Oct 16]. Available at: www.nahc.org/assets/1/7/10HC__Stats.pdf.

10. Brickner PW, Duque ST, Kaufman A, et al. The homebound aged: a medically unreached group. *Ann Intern Med.* 1975;**82**(1):1–6.

11. Landers SH. Bringing Home the "Medical Home" for Older Adults. *Cleve Clin J Med.* 2010;**77**(10):661–75.

12. Ramsdell JW, Swart JA, Jackson JE, Renvall M. The yield of a home visit in the assessment of Geriatric Patients. *J Am Geriatr Soc.* 1989;**37**(1):17–24.

13. Holley APH, Gorawara-Bhat R, Dale W, Hayley D. Palliative access through care at home: Experiences with an urban, geriatric home palliative care program. *J Am Geriatr Soc.* 2009;**57**(10):1925–31.

14. Mims RB, Thomas LL, Conroy LV. Physician housecalls: A complement to hospital based medical care. *J Am Geriatr Soc.* 1977;**25**(1):25–34.

15. Pearson S, Inglis SC, McLennan SN, et al. Prolonged effects of a home-based intervention in patients with chronic illness. *Arch Intern Med.* 2006;**166**(6):645–50.

16. Edes T, Kinosian B, Davis D, et al. Financial savings of home based primary care for frail veterans with chronic disabling disease. Abstract presentation, American Geriatrics Society Annual Scientific Meeting, 2010.

17. Edes T, Tompkins H. Quality measure of reduction of inpatient days during home based primary care (HBPC). *J Am Geriatr Soc.* 2007;**55**(4, Suppl):S7.

18. Coleman EA, Min S, Chomiak A, Kramer AM. Post-hospital care transitions: Patterns, complications, and risk identification. *Health Serv Res.* 2004;**39**:1449–65.

19. Coleman EA, Parry C, Chalmers S, Min SJ. The care transitions intervention: Results of a randomized controlled trial. *Arch Intern Med.* 2006;**166**:1822–8.

20. DeJonge KE, Jamshed N, Gilden D, et al. Effects of home-based primary care of Medicare costs in high-risk elders. *J Am Geriatr Soc.* 2014; doi:10.1111/jgs.12974.

21. Independence at Home Demonstration, Section 3024 of the Affordable Care Act [cited 2014 Oct 16]. Available at: www.cms.gov/Medicare/Demonstration-Projects/DemoProjectsEvalRpts/Medicare-Demonstrations-Items/CMS1240082.html.

22. Smith KL, Soriano TA, Boal J. Brief communication. National quality-of-care standards in home-based primary care. *Ann Intern Med.* 2007;**146**:188–92.

23. Mollica RL. State Medicaid reimbursement policies and practices in assisted living. *Prepared for National Center for Assisted Living, American Health Care Association.* Washington, DC. 2009.

24. Caffrey C, Sengupta N, Park-Lee E, et al. Residents Living in Residential Care Facilities United States 2010. *NCHS Data Brief,* No. 91. Hyattsville, MD: National Center for Health Statistics; 2012.

25. American Health Care Association. Available at: www.ahcancal.org/ncal/quality/qualityinitiative/Pages/default.aspx.

26. Park-Lee E, Sengupta M, Harris-Kojetin LD. Dementia Special Care Units in Residential Care Communities: United States, 2010. *NCHS Data Brief.* 2013 Nov;**134**:1–8.

27. Johnson R, Weiner J. *A profile of frail older Americans and their caregivers. The Retirement Project. Occasional Paper Number 8.* Washington, DC: Urban Institute; February 2006.

28. Arno PS, Levine C, Memmott MM. The economics of informal caregiving. *Health Aff (Millwood).* 1999;**18**(2):182–8.

29. US Department of Health and Human Services. *The Characteristics of Long-term Care Users.* Rockville: Agency for Healthcare Research and Quality, 2001, and Thompson L. Long-term care: Support for family caregivers. Washington, DC: Georgetown University, 2004. Long-Term Care Financing Project.

30. US Department of Health and Human Services [Internet]. Washington DC: Administration for Community Living [cited 2014 Oct 16]. Available at: www.aoa.gov.

31. Siebenaler K, O'Keeffe J, O'Keeffe C, et al. Regulatory Review of Adult Day Services: Final Report. U.S. Department of Health and Human Services. 2005 [cited 2014 Oct 16]. Available at: http://aspe.hhs.gov/daltcp/reports/adultday.htm#acknow.

32. Zarit SH. Effects of adult day care on daily stress of caregivers: A within-person approach. *J Gerontol B Psychol Sci Soc Sci.* 2011; **66**(5):538–46.

33. Skarupski KA. Use of home-based formal services by adult day care clients with Alzheimer's disease. *Home Health Care Serv Q.* 2008; **27**(3):217–39.

34. National Hospice Organization Medical Guidelines Task Force, *Medical guidelines for determining prognosis in selected non-cancer diseases.* Arlington, VA: National Hospice Organization, 1996.

35. National Hospice and Palliative Care Organization. NHPCO's Facts and Figures: Hospice Care in America

657

2013 Edition [cited 2014 Oct 16] Available at: http://www.nhpco.org/sites/default/files/public/Statistics_Research/2013_Facts_Figures.pdf.

36. Kelley AS, Deb P, Du Q, et al. Hospice enrollment saves money for Medicare and improves care quality across a number of different lengths-of-stay. *Health Aff (Millwood).* 2013 Mar;32(3):552–61. doi: 10.1377/hlthaff.2012.0851.

37. Taylor DC, Osterman J, VanHoutvan CH, et al. What length of hospice use maximizes reduction in medical expenditures near death in the US Medicare program? *Soc Sci Med.* 2007;65(7):1466–78.

38. Wallston K, Burger C, Smith R, Baugher R. Comparing the quality of death for hospice and non-hospice patients. *Med Care.* 1988;26(2):177–82.

39. Black B, Herr K, Fine P, et al. The relationships among pain, nonpain symptoms, and quality of life measures in older adults with cancer receiving hospice care. *Pain Med.* 2011;12(6): 880–9.

40. Centers for Medicare and Medicaid Services. Quick Facts about Programs for All-Inclusive Care for the Elderly (PACE). CMS Publication No. 11341 2008 [cited 2014 Oct 16]. Available at: www.npaonline.org/website/download.asp?id=2378&title=Quick_Facts_about_PACE_(CMS_Publication).

41. Segelman M, Szydlowski J, Kinosian B, et al. Hospitalizations in the program of all-inclusive care for the elderly. *J Am Geriatr Soc.* 2014;62:320–4.

Chapter

48

Post-acute care and institutional long-term care for the elderly

Rebecca D. Elon, MD, MPH, Marshall B. Kapp, JD, MPH, and Fatima Sheikh, MD, MPH

Historical considerations: the evolution of institutional long-term care

American hospitals and nursing facilities have a common progenitor: the colonial period almshouse. The eighteenth-century almshouses received dependent persons who lacked the financial or family resources to maintain themselves in the general community, including the aged, orphaned, debilitated, and mentally or physically ill. The almshouses served a general welfare function by providing substitute households for the poor and infirmed.[1]

The Philadelphia Almshouse was founded in 1732 and provided the first government-sponsored care of the poor in the colonies. It subsequently evolved into Philadelphia General Hospital.[2] The first American public hospital started as a six-bed infirmary ward in the New York City Almshouse, founded in 1736. It subsequently evolved into Bellevue Hospital.[3] The Baltimore City Almshouse, founded in 1774, evolved into the Baltimore City Hospitals.[4]

In 1751, the Pennsylvania Hospital in Philadelphia opened its doors as the first voluntary hospital in America, built with private donations specifically to care for the sick.[5] Other early voluntary hospitals included New York Hospital opening in 1791 and the Massachusetts General Hospital opening in Boston in 1821.[6] Although these institutions were built with private donations for the purpose of taking care of the sick, there was little that medicine had to offer in that era. Hospitals took care of the ill and dying who had no home and family to care for them. Hospitals were viewed as "houses of death" and were considered "unhappy necessities."[1] The preferred site of medical care, including any surgery and childbirth, was in

the family home. It was not until the late nineteenth century, with the adoption of principles of antisepsis, use of anesthesia for surgery, availability of x-rays to improve diagnosis, and the emergence of professionally trained nurses, that hospitals evolved into places to care for people of all socio-economic classes suffering from acute illness.[1]

In the early nineteenth century, women's and church groups began to establish shelters for "worthy individuals of their own ethnic or religious background," to keep formerly respectable individuals from being relegated to the almshouse.[7] The Philadelphia Indigent Widows' and Single Women's Society founded one of the earliest "old age homes" in 1823, but an applicant had to provide a "certificate of good character."[7] Many similar institutions had entrance fees, so impoverished individuals still found the almshouse as their last refuge in old age.[7]

As American hospitals began curing episodes of illness, rather than caring for indigent people who were infirm or dying, the average length of stay in the hospitals dropped from the pre-1880 level of more than 4 weeks to 18 days by 1900. By 1923, the average length of stay per hospital episode was 12.5 days.[1] Those who were chronically debilitated were sent to the almshouses, if they lacked family or resources to continue their care at home. During this period, private voluntary charitable institutions arose to care for the convalescing and "the incurable."[8, 9]

The Social Security Act of 1935 had a provision that persons residing in public institutions were ineligible to receive benefits. This provision, though later rescinded, is credited with the rise of the for-profit nursing home industry. Those aged persons who required daily assistance, but lacked family to care for them at home, could use their Social Security income to pay for domiciliary care in a private setting.

Reichel's Care of the Elderly, 7th Edition, ed. Jan Busby-Whitehead *et al.* Published by Cambridge University Press.
© Cambridge University Press 2016.

659

Passed in 1946, the Hill-Burton Act promoted the expansion of institutional health care in the United States in the post–World War II era. Federal grants and loans helped hospitals and nursing facilities with new construction and modernization. In return, the health-care institutions agreed to provide a reasonable volume of services to those unable to pay. Although the Hill-Burton Act funds were no longer available after 1997, there are 170 health-care institutions in the United States that remain obligated, as recipients of Hill-Burton funding, to provide free or reduced-cost care.[10]

The health-care landscape changed dramatically with the passage of the Medicare and Medicaid legislation in 1965. Medicare fueled the growth and dominance of hospital medicine. The growth of the nursing home industry in the 1970s was fueled by the Medicaid program, since Medicaid covered the cost of nursing care in the institutional setting for disabled persons who were unable to pay privately.

In the late 1970s, containment of hospital costs became a priority for the Medicare program. The prospective payment system (PPS) based upon diagnosis-related groups (DGRs) was introduced in 1980 as a novel approach to paying hospitals. This system incentivized hospitals financially to discharge patients at or below the average length of stay for their diagnostic group. Hospitals were noted to discharge patients "quicker and sicker." Nursing facilities stepped up to assist in this transition by admitting patients under the institutional Medicare Part A skilled nursing benefit for short-term post-acute care.[11] Post-acute care has become the major focus of many nursing facilities because it generates higher revenue than the traditional long-term care (LTC) programs, which have decreased in census due to the increasing numbers of community-based options now available.

The governmental funding bias toward institutional care can be traced back to the early nineteenth century, when in 1828 it was noted that "the government hoped to restrict expenditures for public assistance by making the almshouse the only source of government assistance to the poor."[1] Today, the modern nursing facility has replaced some functions of the almshouse, as the refuge of last resort for those whose care needs exceed the capacity of their families and communities. Despite the fact that most nursing facilities are owned and operated by private corporations, most of their revenue comes from governmental sources, such as Medicaid, Medicare, and individuals' Social Security checks.

In the 1970s, advocacy groups began grass roots campaigns to try to expand community-based options for disabled persons of all ages. The 1999 Supreme Court *Olmstead* decision required states to create more community options for Medicaid recipients. Many states offered "Medicaid wavier" slots to help move lower-acuity indigent residents out of the nursing facilities into assisted-living facilities (ALFs). Medicaid waiver programs also provided funds for expanded services in the person's own home, at times paying family caregivers, to allow nursing home residents to move back into the community. The private market expansion of ALFs starting in the 1990s allowed those older persons with financial resources and ADL dependencies to find care outside of nursing facilities. The nursing facilities were then left with the highest medical acuity, most behaviorally disturbed, and most dependent indigent residents.

In summary, both modern American hospitals and nursing facilities can trace their origins to the colonial period almshouses. As hospitals evolved in their ability to diagnose, treat, and cure acute illness, medical and surgical care left the private family home and moved into the hospital. Nursing facilities assumed the residential care of chronically ill and dependent persons, whose long-term needs exceeded the capacity of their families. As more chronic care now is moving back into community settings, nursing facilities are focusing on post-acute, short-term care. Although programs such as the Eden Alternative and the Pioneer Network continue to try to assist nursing facilities in developing more homelike LTC environments,[12, 13] the emphasis on post-acute care and preventing hospitalization demands ongoing evolution of nursing facilities into more sophisticated medical facilities.

Current post-acute and long-term care programs

Short-stay residents/patients in the nursing facility

Post-acute care

Although the American nursing facility is considered a site for "institutional long-term care," short-stay, short-term care programs continue to grow and are increasingly dominant within nursing facilities. Most nursing facilities provide rehabilitation services for patients after stroke, joint replacement, and fracture repair, as well as for reconditioning and strengthening after an acute medical illness or surgery. Medicare Part A includes a benefit that pays 100% for the first 20 days of skilled nursing facility care, if indicated by the patient's needs and progress. This benefit is only activated if the patient has a three-night qualifying stay in an acute care hospital prior to nursing facility admission. With the increased use of "observation status" rather than actual hospital admission, some Medicare enrollees may not be eligible for the skilled nursing benefit. After the first 20 days, there is a daily co-payment for the care provided on days 21–100. Some, but not all, Medi-gap, secondary insurance policies will pay this copayment. After 100 days total, the Medicare benefit is exhausted and the patient converts to private pay if ongoing institutional skilled care or long-term care is required.[11] People who are enrolled in Medicare managed care programs will have different rules and requirements governing their eligibility for skilled nursing facility rehabilitation and post-acute services. The three-night hospital stay is typically waived for skilled benefit eligibility.

A major focus in the care of the post-acute population has been on the readmission rate back to the acute care setting within the first 30 days after nursing facility admission. Since the Medicare program penalizes the hospital through nonpayment for selected readmissions, hospitals and post-acute facilities have started to work together to analyze and improve the process of transitions of care. Improvements in the clinical capacities of the nursing facility staff, the care rendered by the medical staff, and improved hand-offs from the hospital team have helped decrease the rate of readmission nationwide. Programs such as INERACT have helped facilities focus on improving the care and reducing the readmissions.[14] The emphasis on reducing unnecessary readmissions has pushed the nursing facility into an increasingly medical model, trying to provide acute medical care in addition to the traditional residential long-term and short-term rehabilitative care.

In order to monitor the post-acute care patients adequately, medical visits typically need to be made at least weekly, or more often if patients are experiencing medical complications or setbacks in their rehabilitation progress. Some medical practices are experiencing Medicare audits claiming that this frequency of visits is medically unnecessary, since the historic requirement for Medicare payment for nursing facility visits was once every 30 days for the first 90 days, followed by once every 60 days thereafter. Although good documentation of the medical necessity of the visit should stand up against an audit, this added threat and burden is making some physicians question their ongoing participation in this arena of care. Although Centers for Medicare and Medicaid Services (CMS) is penalizing hospitals for excessive readmissions, it may be simultaneously challenging the work of the nursing facility medical staff to help realize the lower readmission rate through the provision of more frequent, attentive, and expert medical care.

Respite care residents/patients

Another group of people who may be short-term residents/patients of nursing facilities are those who are admitted for respite care. These people generally pay the daily rate out of pocket, unless they have a respite care benefit with a long-term care insurance policy or a Veterans Administration benefit, or they are enrolled in Medicare Home Hospice. A typical respite care scenario would be the short-term admission of a person with dementia who requires 24-hour supervision at home, so that the family caregiver could take a trip, attend to his or her own personal health issues such as the need for elective surgery, or just have a rest. Respite care residents/patients are expected to return to their homes in a matter of days or weeks.

Terminal care/hospice care in the nursing facility

End-of-life care has become part of the scope of practice of US nursing facilities. A decade or more ago, many nursing facilities transferred back to the hospital any resident/patient who was dying, for fear that a death in the facility might lead to a charge of negligence. With greater acceptance of advance directives and advance care planning, residents and their families may have greater autonomy in deciding how they want the end of life to be approached. For those who recognize that repeated hospitalizations as death approaches and attempts at cardiopulmonary resuscitation for people with end-stage conditions are rarely useful and often traumatic to the dying person, hospice-type care in the nursing facility is increasingly accepted. With the strong emphasis on avoiding

661

unnecessary hospital readmissions from nursing facilities, determining prognosis and transitioning dying patients to a palliative care plan has become a critically important aspect of nursing facility medicine.

Although the Medicare Hospice benefit may be applied within the nursing facility, it cannot be implemented along with the Medicare Part A skilled nursing benefit. Because the Medicare Hospice benefit does not pay for the room-and-board aspect of nursing home care, those who qualify for the Medicare Part A skilled nursing benefit would have an increase in their out-of-pocket expenses by signing on to Medicare Hospice. Under these circumstances, hospice-type care may be employed without invoking the Medicare Hospice benefit per se. The Medicare payment for a nursing facility resident enrolled in hospice goes to the hospice organization, and the nursing facility must bill the hospice for its daily rate. This bureaucratic detail inhibits many nursing facilities from enthusiastically referring their end-of-life residents to hospice organizations. Hospice benefits and services for nursing facility residents have also been an active area of Medicare fraud and abuse investigations, inhibiting many hospice organizations from enthusiastically pursuing service in such settings. Despite these concerns, the hospice team often makes a huge difference in helping the nursing facility staff control a resident's end-of-life symptoms. The hospice benefit also provides additional support to families struggling with a loved one's death in a nursing facility. Moreover, the hospice benefit provides bereavement care for the surviving family member after the loved one's death.

Long-stay residents in the nursing facility

Typically, more than half of the long-term care residents in a nursing facility suffer from dementia. Over the last decade, in response to the market demand for higher-amenity, more homelike environments, the assisted-living industry has built thousands of facilities that provide care in the community for frail elders who have dementia. This trend has left the more medically complex, functionally and behaviorally impaired residents with dementia in the nursing facility. It has also made lack of resources a distinguishing feature between those persons with dementia who can afford to enter assisted-living facilities versus those who cannot and are admitted to a nursing facility with Medicaid payment.

Disabled younger persons must resort to living within a nursing facility, when community options are inadequate for their care needs. The social needs of younger, physically impaired persons are dramatically different from the needs of frail elders with dementia, and often the nursing facility struggles with meeting those needs. Although the preadmission screening and referral process (PASAR) is mandated by federal law and requires nursing facilities to identify persons with developmental disabilities and chronic mental illness to promote community placement, it is rare that the preadmission screening and referral process actually results in an alternative site of care for these specialized populations. Specialized facilities and better community options are necessary to meet the needs of younger persons with functional deficits, including those with developmental disabilities and chronic mental illness. Despite the *Olmstead* decision, it has been challenging to overturn centuries of institutional bias. The nursing facility often remains the community resource and refuge of last resort.

Structure of nursing facility medical practice

Primary care practitioner, continuity of care model

It may be desirable from a continuity of care perspective for a primary care physician to continue to care for his or her own patients once they enter a nursing facility. The long-established doctor–patient relationship can help the nursing home staff understand the new resident within a historical context. The physician can help the patient and family adjust to the strange, new environment and serve as a patient advocate within the facility. It was not long ago that primary care physicians followed their patients across any site of care in which they found themselves. Today, however, emergency room visits are usually managed by the emergency medicine physician, hospital admissions are managed by the hospital-based inpatient team hospitalist physician, and when intensive care is required, the ICU attending is often an intensivist. Likewise, when nursing facility care is needed, the care is often provided by a physician and nurse practitioner team devoting all of their time to nursing facility practice.

The ideal of continuity of care that was taught to twentieth-century medical students as a hallmark and pillar of quality primary care has fallen victim to the demand for efficiency, productivity, and the industrialization of medical care delivery in twenty-first-century America. Physicians today are more likely to define their practice by a particular site of care, rather than by wherever the physician's patient may be located.

Post-acute/LTC practitioner, unassigned admissions

Some physicians in private practice will accept patients under their care within the nursing facility when the patients' own attending physicians do not attend there. These patients are termed "unassigned admissions," as opposed to the patients who are assigned to their community physicians who are on staff at the facility. The physicians accepting unassigned admissions typically make visits on site at the nursing home several days each week and are responsive to the nursing staff calls when they are not on site. Often new physicians in a community will find it advantageous to work with the local nursing facility early in their career to build a caseload while the office-based practice is growing. Once the office practice has grown and is demanding more time, the physician may take him- or herself off of the unassigned admissions roster or may leave the nursing facility practice entirely.

Medical practices employing physicians, nurse practitioners (NPs), and physician assistant (PAs) to work exclusively in nursing facilities are increasingly common. Some of these practices are multistate in scope. Some of these large practices are forcing the independent practitioners out of business, when the nursing facility decides to preferentially give all of the unassigned patients and residents to one group. Sub-specialists who previously were never seen within a nursing facility, are now rounding regularly in many settings to assist facilities with congestive heart failure programs, infection control, post-operative follow-up, physiatry-guided rehabilitation, and others. The landscape of medical practice in nursing facilities is rapidly changing as nursing facilities continue to evolve into a more medically focused site of care.

Full-time facility-based physician

Some physicians work full time within a nursing facility. Settings employing full-time nursing home physicians include: academic facilities such as those affiliated with medical schools or teaching hospitals; governmental facilities such as Veterans Administration or state-owned nursing facilities; large religious or nonsectarian not-for-profit nursing facilities; and some large for-profit nursing facility chains.

Nurse practitioner and physician assistant care of nursing facility residents

Although the scope of practice and licensing requirements for NPs and PAs vary state to state, federal Medicare policy has had a major impact on the ability of these professionals to function within nursing facilities. In the late 1990s, Medicare's decision to allow NPs and PAs to have their own provider numbers and bill the Medicare system as independent practitioners allowed the expansion of NPs and PAs practice within nursing facilities. The NP or PA visits are billed under the same current procedural terminology codes used by the physicians, but Medicare reimburses their work at a discounted rate relative to physician reimbursement. Authorization of prescriptive privileges for NPs and PAs that occurred in many states in the 1990s also promoted their ability to play a major role in nursing facility care.

Improving quality of care through legal regulation of nursing facilities

Regulatory environment overview

Nursing facilities in the United States today are extensively regulated legally in a broad variety of ways.[15] The regulatory environment, both as it exists and is perceived by providers, their risk managers, and insurers exerts a powerful influence on the access to, and quality of, services experienced by nursing facility residents.

First, nursing facilities are subject to regulatory penalties being imposed as part of the required annual state licensure renewal and Medicare/Medicaid survey and certification processes. Applicable standards for nursing facilities are contained in state licensure statutes and the federal Nursing Home Quality Reform Act (NHRA) (part of the Omnibus Budget Reconciliation Act of 1987, Public Law 100–203) and its implementing administrative regulations (codified at 42 Code of Federal Regulations Part 483). Under the NHRA, each nursing facility is required to "care for its residents in such a manner and in such an environment as will promote maintenance or enhancement of the quality of life of each resident" and to "provide services and activities to attain or maintain, for each resident, the highest practicable physical, mental and psychological well-being." For each admitted resident, a facility must collect information according to a defined minimum data set (MDS), using a resident sssessment instrument (RAI), about an individual's physical, mental, and emotional condition. Using this information, facilities must develop and implement an individualized plan of care for each resident.

The federal government contracts with the states to assess, through their survey agencies, whether nursing facilities meet federal standards as determined by annual surveys and complaint investigations. Through its State Operations Manual (SOM) (containing interpretive guidelines and survey protocols), the CMS establishes specific investigative procedures for state surveyors to use. In contrast, complaint investigations, also conducted by state surveyors but following the individual state's procedures (set within federal guidelines and time frames), usually target a single alleged problem in response to a complaint filed against a facility by a resident, a resident's family or friends, or disgruntled facility employees. Quality-of-care problems identified during either annual surveys or complaint investigations are classified into 1 of 12 categories according to their scope (i.e., the number of residents potentially or actually affected) and their severity (i.e., extent of possible harm).

Sanctions for deviation from required regulatory standards range from the draconian to the relatively mild. These may include the following: suspension or revocation of the facility's license to operate; termination of the Medicare and/or Medicaid provider agreement that is necessary for the facility's financial survival, temporary receivership, denial of payment for all admissions or for new admissions, civil money penalties, state monitoring, transfer of residents, a directed plan of correction, or directed in-service training.

In addition to being subject to mandatory federal and state government–established standards, many nursing facilities voluntarily agree to comply with the standards set by private accrediting bodies, most notably the Joint Commission (JC). Hospitals obtain a "deemed status" when accredited by the Joint Commission. "Deemed status" means that through JC accreditation, hospitals are thereby assumed to be in compliance with all governmental requirements. This makes a separate government inspection for JC-accredited hospitals unnecessary. Although nursing facilities are prohibited from claiming "deemed status" when JC accredited, a number of nursing facilities pursue private accreditation as a marketing and quality assurance tool.

Specific aspects of the regulatory environment
Criminal prosecutions

Criminal prosecutions may be initiated by local prosecutors and states' attorneys general charging nursing facilities and/or individual staff members with abuse and neglect of residents and, in the case of deceased residents, even homicide. Also, federal prosecutors working in collaboration with the Department of Health and Human Services' Office of the Inspector General have brought several criminal indictments against nursing facilities. These are based on the theory that a nursing facility that bills the Medicare or Medicaid programs for payments, when the care provided was of substandard quality, is guilty of defrauding the government in violation of the False Claims Act (FCA). The submission of allegedly fraudulent claims through the mail or electronic transfers allows the government to additionally invoke the Mail and Wire Fraud Acts, which are considered predicate offenses (i.e., offenses that may create criminal liability) under the federal Racketeer Influenced and Corrupt Organizations (RICO) Act. Moreover, most states have enacted their own counterparts to the federal FCA, making it unlawful to fraudulently bill their respective state Medicaid programs.

Criminal prosecutions initiated against nursing facilities are relatively infrequent, but extensively publicized when they do occur and carry the possibility of substantial penalties upon conviction or guilty plea. In addition to criminal penalties, conviction under the civil version of the FCA exposes nursing facilities to significant monetary fines. The threat of legal action being brought against a nursing facility is exacerbated by the right of private individuals to act as "private attorneys general" or "relators" and bring their own civil FCA *qui tam* (whistleblower) actions against nursing facilities. If the government chooses to bring a criminal prosecution based on the relator's evidence, then the relator receives between 15% and 25% of the ultimate recovery.

Civil litigation

Historically, nursing facility residents have been statistically underrepresented as plaintiffs in private civil lawsuits brought by or on behalf of particular residents against specific facilities and/or their staff members claiming professional malpractice. Attorneys working under contingency fee arrangements generally have not been eager to represent old, frail, unemployed individuals with short life expectancies because such individuals have a limited ability to command substantial compensatory damages under the American civil justice system. Nursing facility residents whose care is paid for by Medicaid have lacked a financial incentive to sue because most of their financial recovery would ordinarily be diverted either to repay the state for providing care or to resident spend down until a new period of Medicaid eligibility became effective. Furthermore, proving that the nursing facility's negligent conduct proximately or directly caused the injury often is difficult for a plaintiff who already had multiple, serious underlying medical problems. Finally, the majority of older nursing facility residents just do not have the physical and mental stamina, and the availability of adequate support by family or friends, needed to initiate, prosecute, and (literally) outlive the demands of complex civil litigation.

For a variety of reasons, including the enactment of legislation in multiple jurisdictions facilitating (and even encouraging) the filing of personal injury claims against nursing facilities, the increased availability of a cadre of willing plaintiff expert witnesses, and a growing propensity of trial juries to award large judgments (often including punitive or exemplary damages) in nursing facility malpractice cases, the legal picture has changed markedly. The plaintiffs' personal injury bar has discovered and now cultivated this potentially lucrative sphere of practice, as widespread advertising for nursing facility clients by plaintiffs' attorneys abundantly illustrates. As plaintiffs' attorneys representing allegedly injured residents and/or their families often work collaboratively with nursing facility residents' advocates, long-term care ombudsmen offices, consumer groups, and government and private regulators, the volume of civil malpractice actions brought against nursing facilities and staff has escalated dramatically. Most civil claims initiated against nursing facilities stem factually from alleged medical care problems (such as the development of pressure ulcers and the occurrence of medication errors), falls, resident-to-resident assaults, resident abuse, elopements, and violations of residents' rights.[16, 17]

Many nursing facilities are beginning to include in their admission agreements a clause in which the resident (or surrogate) agrees to submit any future claim against the facility to an arbitration process as either a substitute for or a precondition of filing a civil tort claim in the courts. These clauses have been challenged in several cases, with different courts taking differing positions on nursing facility arbitration clause enforceability.

Informed consent

The common law doctrine of informed consent, as embodied in OBRA 1987 and the Medicare/Medicaid Conditions of Participation, prohibits nursing facilities, through their personnel, from doing any sort of diagnostic, therapeutic, or research intervention to a resident without the informed, decisionally capable, and voluntary permission of that resident or his or her surrogate decision maker. An individual may not even be admitted to a nursing facility in the first place without the informed, voluntary authorization of a legally empowered decision maker (either the resident personally or the resident's surrogate). The informed consent doctrine embodies the ethical principle of autonomy or self-determination, which protects the bodily and mental integrity of the resident. The doctrine is built on the premise, supported by evidence, that coercive treatment is detrimental to the resident's overall quality of life.

In addition to judge-made informed consent precedents, constraints are placed on the right of nursing facility providers to intervene in a resident's life without appropriate authorization by federal and state resident rights statutes and regulations. For example, 42 CFR §483.10(b) specifies, among other provisions:

(3) The resident has the right to be fully informed in language that he or she can understand of his or her total health status, including but not limited to, his or her medical condition;

(4) The resident has the right to refuse treatment, to refuse to participate in experimental research, and to formulate an advance directive.

This resident informed choice right is echoed in every state nursing facility licensure statute.

Restraints

The use of both physical or mechanical restraints and psychotropic drugs in nursing facilities is a subject addressed extensively in the OBRA 1987 legislation

665

and implementing regulations. The *Guidance to Surveyors for Long Term Care Facilities* published by CMS defines physical restraints as "any manual method or physical or mechanical device, material, or equipment attached or adjacent to the resident's body that the individual cannot remove easily which restricts freedom of movement or normal access to one's body."[18] Examples might include side rails on a resident's bed, fabric that restricts a resident's movement, and a tray or belt used to confine a resident to a chair, or mittens on one's hands. As an alternative to physical restraints, a nursing facility may include in a resident's care plan devices that monitor a resident's attempts to stand, graphic and verbal reminders to ask for assistance, and physical exercise to improve balance and correct body positioning. Additionally, there are a number of behavioral intervention programs that have been successfully implemented to reduce restraint use.

The same *Guidance* defines chemical restraints as "any drug that is used for discipline or convenience and not required to treat medical symptoms." In turn, discipline "is defined as any action taken by the facility for the purpose of punishing or penalizing residents." Punishment is not treatment. Convenience "is defined as any action taken by the facility to control a resident's behavior or manage a resident's behavior with a lesser amount of effort by the facility and not in the resident's best interest."[18]

Applicable legal provisions clearly convey policymakers' intentions to eliminate the unnecessary and inappropriate utilization of these previously prevalent behavior control modalities. 42 CFR §483.13(a) dictates: "The resident has the right to be free from any physical or chemical restraints imposed for purposes of discipline or convenience, and not required to treat the resident's medical symptoms." The American Geriatrics Society (AGS) cautions providers to avoid relying on the use of physical restraints to manage behavioral symptoms of older adults with delirium: "The use of physical restraints for [NF] residents is now widely accepted as a sign of poor quality of care."

Nonetheless, according to the CMS *Guidance to Surveyors*:

[I]f the resident needs emergency care, restraints may be used for brief periods to permit medical treatment to proceed unless the facility has a notice indicating that the resident has previously made a valid refusal of the treatment in question. If a resident's unanticipated violent or aggressive behavior places him/her or others in imminent danger, the resident does not have the right to refuse the use of restraints. In this situation, the use of restraints is a measure of last resort to protect the safety of the resident or others and must not extend beyond the immediate episode.

In the realm of chemical restraints, resident rights are protected by 42 CFR §483.25(l)(2), which states:

[b] ased on a comprehensive assessment of a resident, the facility must ensure that –

(i) Residents who have not used antipsychotic drugs are not given these drugs unless antipsychotic drug therapy is necessary to treat a specific condition as diagnosed and documented in the clinical record; and

(ii) Residents who use antipsychotic drugs receive gradual dose reductions, and behavioral interventions, unless clinically contraindicated, in an effort to discontinue these drugs.

The antipsychotic medications referenced are both the conventional, or first-generation medications (such as haloperidol, fluphenazine, perphenazine, thiothixene, thioridazine, chlorpromazine, and others) and the second-generation or atypical antipsychotics (such as risperidone, olanazepine, quetiapine, ziprasidone, aripiprazole, clozapine, and others).

In addition to the conditions of participation for Medicare and Medicaid, every state guarantees nursing home residents the right to be free from excessive physical and chemical restraints as part of the respective state's resident bill of rights. These state provisions are completely consistent with both the spirit and letter of the federal prohibitions.

In July 2012, the CMS started posting data on the nursing home compare website regarding the percentage of both long-stay and short-stay residents receiving antipsychotic medications. CMS stated a goal of having a 15% reduction of antipsychotic medication use for behavioral management of residents with dementia that would bring the national average down to approximately 20%.[19] Various behavioral interventions have been associated with a 12%–20% reduction in the use of anti-psychotic medications in nursing facility residents with dementia.[20] Nursing facility pharmacists (many of whom are employed on a consultant basis) must review the appropriateness of all residents' medications on a monthly basis and recommend changes when appropriate. They are often the ones who are recommending gradual dose reductions (GDRs) for antipsychotic medications. A Cochrane Review of the topic of gradual dose reductions for antipsychotic medication for behavioral symptoms concluded that although GDRs are generally well tolerated, those whose neuropsychiatric symptoms were most severe would likely benefit clinical from continued antipsychotic treatment without GDR.[21]

Although it is generally accepted that use of both conventional and atypical antipsychotic medications is associated with an increased risk of death when used to treat neuropsychiatric symptoms (NPS) of dementia, there are studies that challenge the causal link, stating that the severity of the NPS that most closely correlates with the mortality risk.[22]

Drug prescription and management

Even when drugs are prescribed for the proper clinical indications, they may be associated with possible toxicities and dangerous interactions. Liability might be imposed for negligence in monitoring and/or inadequately responding even when the resident assessment and initial prescription were defensible. (Common medications in this category include the vitamin K antagonist anticoagulants.) The absence of a strong evidence base underlying a prescription makes it less defensible, particularly for off-label prescribing. Moreover, when a particular medication is discontinued for a resident, adequate monitoring to detect any adverse reactions is a reasonably expected part of the standard of care.

In 2009, the Drug Enforcement Administration (DEA) determined that the common practice of off-site institutional pharmacies dispensing controlled substances on the basis of chart orders in nursing facilities was in violation of their licensing under the Controlled Substances Act. Since the pharmacies serving most community nursing facilities are licensed as retail pharmacies, they must obtain a valid prescription prior to dispensing any controlled medication to nursing facilities. Accommodation for emergency dispensing was made through allowance of up to a three day supply of Schedule 2 medications to be dispensed via a phone call to the pharmacy by the prescriber, with a prescription subsequently returned to the pharmacy within a seven-day window. This requirement has consumed many hours of extra work for the clinicians practicing in nursing facilities.[23] The DEA regulations allowing electronic prescribing of controlled substances within certain guidelines has eased this burden to some degree.

Elopement

Another sphere of concern is the risk of a resident being injured during an elopement. Wandering refers to a resident with cognitive impairments moving aimlessly about inside a facility, without an appreciation of personal safety needs, while elopement is when a resident leaves a safe area unsupervised and unnoticed and enters into harm's way. Residents who elope are differentiated from wanderers because they make purposeful, overt, and often repeated attempts to leave the nursing facility and its premises. High risk factors for wandering and elopement include dementia, delusions, hallucinations, and schizophrenia.

The problem of elopement risk among mentally compromised nursing facility residents is high on the professional radar screen of the American plaintiffs' personal injury bar. Key to risk management to control elopement-related dangers is thorough, timely (on both an initial and an ongoing basis) assessment of the resident's likelihood of engaging in wandering or elopement behavior and the development, implementation, and monitoring of an individualized treatment plan based on that assessment.

Other aspects of regulation

Nursing facilities also may be subject to suit for discriminating in their provision of services. Requirements of the Americans with Disabilities Act (ADA) and the Rehabilitation Act, as well as their state counterparts, regarding affirmative obligations to accommodate disabled persons apply with full force to nursing facilities both as places of public accommodation and recipients of government payments. Moreover, a nursing facility encounters the possibility of legal claims based on allegations that, by providing inadequate services, it violated express or implied promises made to the resident in the admission agreement or contract.

Opportunities for improvement

Despite the useful functions it serves, the prevailing regime of command and control regulation coupled with private malpractice litigation is inadequate, and may actually undermine the task of maximizing resident quality of care and quality of life in nursing facilities.[16, 17]

The public certainly has a proper interest in monitoring how public funds are spent. But government simply is not capable of specifying in advance in prescriptive regulatory language all the conditions it does, or should, want the providers of publicly funded services to meet nor of enunciating foolproof standards by which to evaluate and enforce the quality of services provided. Moreover, counterproductive effects of the current regulatory schema are undeniable when overly defensive, risk-averse provider behavior results and predominates. The failure of malpractice tort litigation, one additional form of regulation, to meaningfully elicit more desirable provider behavior has also been documented.[24]

The prevailing regulatory atmosphere can smother salutary innovation in nursing facility behavior. This is especially troubling when a culture change movement seems to be taking hold and showing promise to revolutionize nursing home life so much for the better.[25] Unfortunately, however, regulation that is perceived by service providers as unduly intrusive and inflexible, inspires legal anxiety rather than support. This acts as a powerful disincentive to nursing facility adoption of resident-centered practices that are believed to place the facility and its staff collectively and individually at risk of litigation or regulatory citations.

A number of government initiatives, however, seem to be moving in a culture change direction, as an alternative to traditional command-and-control regulation and after-the-fact litigation for damages. For example, Medicare Quality Improvement Organizations (QIOs) are working collaboratively with nursing homes to try to improve resident care by reducing pressure ulcers and minimizing the use of physical restraints.[26] The QIO program also played a significant role in recruiting nursing facilities to participate in the National Nursing Home Quality Care Collaborative (NNHQCC).[27]

Under Section 6102 of the Affordable Care Act (ACA), each nursing facility (including those in corporate chains) is required to participate in a Quality Assurance and Performance Improvement (QAPI) program. On June 7, 2013, CMS made available the initial set of introductory materials to help nursing facilities to establish a foundation to implement and sustain QAPI. This exercise represents an opportunity

for the government, industry, and consumers and their representatives to work together as collaborators pursuing common objectives, rather than as adversaries working at cross-purposes.[27, 28]

Another section of the ACA presents a further chance to explore options to strict command-and-control regulation of nursing facilities. Recognizing the potential of a robust competitive marketplace to encourage nursing facilities who are eager to recruit and retain residents by performing better, nursing facilities now must provide additional information to be included in the Nursing Home Compare feature that appears on Medicare's website. The additional information concerns facility ownership and affiliated parties, governing boards and organizational structure, staffing data, summary information about substantiated complaints, adjudicated criminal violations by facilities and employees, and any civil monetary penalties levied against a facility or its staff. This information will be considered by those selecting a nursing facility for themselves or a loved one. The intention of its inclusion is to positively motivate nursing facility owners, administrators, and trustees to reduce the negative aspects through detailed public disclosure.

Many states have developed their own "technical assistance programs" that provide on-site consultation and training for nursing facility staff.[29] Compared to existing state nursing home enforcement-oriented regulatory regimes, these programs represent a more cooperative, corrective approach to quality.

Quality improvement in nursing facilities: The role of the medical practitioners

AMDA – the Society for Post-Acute and Long-Term Care Medicine – is the professional organization whose major focus is improving medical care in nursing facilities. It originally was comprised of physicians working as nursing facility medical directors, but has broadened its mission to support attending physicians, nurse practitioners and physician assistants working in nursing facilities. AMDA recently published a list of competencies for attending physicians in nursing facilities.[30]

AMDA has developed a certification program for nursing facility medical directors and is the major source of educational programs to train physicians in the nursing facility medical director role. The nursing facility medical director should have a major role in the facility's quality improvement process. This includes a duty to oversee the process of quality assurance and performance improvement in collaboration with other leadership of the facility. The medical director helps to assure that effective medical care is provided to the residents of a nursing facility. The medical director evaluates the performance of physicians and nurse practitioners within a facility, including professionalism and medical care, and provides timely feedback to the providers about their performance. The medical director also participates in the dissemination of current and changing guidelines about medical care, as well as state and nationwide standards for nursing home care. He or she also ensures that the facility meets acceptable standards of care, and evaluates the efficacy of the policies and procedures of a facility, while helping to update and revise policies as needed.

AMDA has created clinical practice guidelines that are useful to help guide the facility medical director and attending physicians in the treatment of commonly occurring conditions in nursing facility residents and patients. Another organization that has guidelines relevant to the nursing facility is APIC, the Association for Professionals in Infection Control and Epidemiology. It publishes infection control guidelines that are specific to the nursing facility setting.[31]

The nursing facility medical director and clinical staff should be aware of the facility's CMS five-star rating and federal quality indicators and work with the facility leadership toward improvement of the indicators and ratings.[32, 33] Some states assess family satisfaction with nursing facility care and post the findings on line. Physicians wishing to keep their board certifications active will be assessing patient or family satisfaction and practice actions toward improving patient safety as part of their personal quality assessment activities for maintenance of board certification.

Quality medical care in nursing facilities requires physicians, NPs, and PAs who are knowledgeable and up to date in the technical aspects of care, who are able to work effectively with the nursing staff and interdisciplinary team, who can work to improve transitions between sites of care, who are committed to take the time to communicate honestly and compassionately, who are committed to care that is truly focused on the resident/patient and family's well-being, and

who have the courage and tenacity to challenge the status quo. Quality medical care emanates from the understanding that it is truly an honor and privilege to serve those persons entrusted to our care in our ever-evolving nursing facilities.

References

1. Starr P. *The Social Transformation of American Medicine: The rise of a sovereign profession and the making of a vast industry*. New York: Basic Books; 1982.

2. www.philadelphia-reflections.com/blog/1015.htm (last accessed Jan. 27, 2015).

3. www.nyc.gov/html/hhc/bellevue/html/about/about.shtml (last accessed Jan. 27, 2015).

4. Sewell JE. *Medicine in Maryland: The practice and the profession 1799–1999*. Baltimore, MD: Johns Hopkins University Press; 1999.

5. www.pennmedicine.org/pahosp/about (last accessed Jan. 27, 2015).

6. Rosenberg, CE. *The Care of Strangers: The rise of America's hospital system*. New York: Basic Books; 1987.

7. www.4fate.org/history.html (last accessed Jan. 27, 2015).

8. The Keswick Home for Incurables, founded in 1883: www.keswick-multicare.org/about (last accessed Jan. 27, 2015).

9. The Washington Home for Incurables, founded in 1888: www.thewashingtonhome.org/#!history/c1z60 (last accessed 1/27/2015).

10. www.hrsa.gov/gethealthcare/affordable/hillburton (last accessed Jan. 27, 2015).

11. *Medicare and You Handbook*: www.medicare.gov/Publications/Search/Results.asp?PubID=10050&Type=PubID (last accessed Jan. 27, 2015).

12. The Eden Alternative: www.edenalt.org (last accessed Jan. 27, 2015).

13. The Pioneer Network: www.pioneernetwork.net (last accessed Jan. 27, 2015).

14. Interventions to Reduce Acute Care Transfers: http://interact2.net (last accessed Jan. 27, 2015).

15. Aka PC, Deason LM, Hammond A. Political factors and enforcement of the nursing home regulatory regime. *J Law & Health* 2011;24(1):1–42.

16. Konetzka RT, Park J, Abbo E. Malpractice litigation and nursing home quality of care. *Health Services Research* 2013;48:1920–1938. doi:10.1111/1475-6773.12072

17. Mukamel DB, Weimer DL, Harrington C, et al The effect of state regulatory stringency on nursing home quality. *Health Services Research* 2012;47:1791–1813. doi:10.1111/j.1475-6773.2012.01459.x

18. www.cms.gov/Regulations-and-Guidance/Guidance/Manuals/downloads/som107ap_pp_guidelines_ltcf.pdf; page 71 (last accessed Nov. 14, 2015).

19. www.cms.gov/Medicare/Provider-Enrollment-and-Certification/CertificationandComplianc/Downloads/AntipsychoticMedicationQM.pdf (last accessed Jan. 27, 2015).

20. Thompson Coon J, Abbott R, Rogers M, et al. Interventions to reduce inappropriate prescribing of antipsychotic medications in people with dementia resident in care homes: A systematic review. *J Am Med Direc Assoc.* 2014 Oct;**15**(10):706–711. doi:10.1016/j.jama.2014.06012

21. Declercq T, Petrovic M, Agerwal M, et al. Withdrawal versus continuation of chronic antipsychotic drugs for behavioral and psychological symptoms in older people with dementia. *Cochrane Database Syst Rev* 2013 March 28;**3**:CD007726. doi 10.1002/14651858.CD007722.pub2

22. Lopez OL, Becker JT, Chang YF, et al. The long term effects of conventional and atypical antipsychotics in patients with probable Alzheimers Disease. *Am J Psychiatry* 2013 Sept;**170**(9):1051–5105. doi 10.1176/appi.ajp.203.12081046

23. Elon R, Schlosberg C. Levenson S, Brandt N. DEA enforcement in Long-Term Care: Is a collaborative correction feasible? *J Am Med Direc Assoc.* 2011;**12**:263–269.

24. Stevenson DG, Spittal MJ, Studdert DM. Does litigation increase or decrease health care quality? A national study of negligence claims against nursing homes. *Medical Care* 2013;**51**:430–436. doi:10.1097/MLR.0b013e3182881ccc

25. Zimmerman, S., Shier, V., & Saliba, D. Transforming nursing home culture: Evidence for practice and policy. *The Gerontologist* 2014;*54*:S1–S5. doi:10.1093/geront/gnt161

26. Centers for Medicare & Medicaid Services. *Quality Improvement Organizations: Sharing knowledge, improving health care* 2014: available at media.mcknights.com/documents/82/qio_fact_sheet_20390.pdf.

27. Centers for Medicare & Medicaid Services, Nursing Home Quality Initiative, available at www.cms.gov/Medicare/Quality-Initiatives-Patient-Assessment-Instruments/NursingHomeQualityInits/index.html (last accessed Jan. 27, 2015).

28. Kaplan, RL. Analyzing the impact of the new health care reform legislation on older Americans. *Elder Law Journal* 2011;*18*:213–245.

29. Li Y, Spector WD, Glance LG, Mukamel DB. State "technical assistance programs" for nursing home quality improvement: Variations and potential implications. *Journal of Aging and Social Policy* 2012;*24*:349–67. doi: 10.1080/08959420.2012.735157

30. www.amda.com/strategic-initiatives/competencies.cfm (last accessed Jan. 27, 2015).

31. APIC. Infection Preventionist's Guide to Long-Term Care 2013, www.apic.org (last accessed Jan. 27, 2015).

32. www.medicare.gov/nursinghomecompare (last accessed Jan. 27, 2015).

33. Castle NG,Ferguson JC. What is nursing home quality and how is it measured? *Gerontologist* 2010;**50**(4):426–442. doi: 10.1093/gerontol/gnq052

Chapter 49

Palliative and end-of-life care for the elderly

Molly M. Hanson, CRNP, Kristine Swartz, MD, and Brooke K. Worster, MD

Introduction to palliative care

The last century in the United States has seen a cultural shift in the way that people experience illness and care at the end of life. Tremendous technologic advances in health care have increased life expectancy and ushered in a new era of caring for patients with increasingly complex acute and chronic illnesses. As a call for greater quality in end-of-life care has emerged, the specialty of palliative care has developed to better address the specific needs of patients and families coping with serious illness.

Defining palliative care

The World Health Organization defines palliative care as:

> An approach that improves the quality of life of patients and their families facing the problem associated with life-threatening illness, through the prevention and relief of suffering by means of early identification and impeccable assessment and treatment of pain and other problems, physical, psychosocial and spiritual.[1]

Palliative care specialists should also be skilled in facilitating communication, advance care planning, discussion of patient and family goals of care, quality improvement efforts, and in caring for the dying and bereaved.[2] Palliative care is optimally delivered throughout the disease trajectory by an interdisciplinary team made up of palliative care physicians, nurses, social workers, and chaplains.

Although the specialty of palliative care maintains its roots in the hospice movement, a distinction must be made between palliative care and hospice. Whereas palliative care can be integrated into the care of any patient with serious illness at any stage of their disease process, hospice care is typically provided during the last six months of the patient's life, when the decision to forego curative treatment has been determined to be appropriate. Palliative care can be provided along side curative or disease-directed therapy to maintain quality of life and patient-centered care. This is often achieved in collaboration between the patient's primary medical team consisting of primary care providers, subspecialty providers, and palliative medicine interdisciplinary teams.

The growth of palliative care and improvements in quality care at the end of life

According to the Center to Advance Palliative Care (CAPC) the United States has seen a substantial rise in the prevalence of hospital-based palliative care programs, with 85% of hospitals with greater than 300 beds reporting the presence of an interdisciplinary team.[3]

There has been compelling evidence to suggest that palliative care interventions are associated with improved outcomes in areas such as symptom control, quality of life, mood, less aggressive treatment at the end of life, and, notably in one study, longer median survival.[4–6] Palliative care consultation for seriously ill hospital patients is associated with a reduction in overall health-care costs,[8–13] decreased ICU length of stay,[11–13] and improved patient, family, and provider satisfaction and perception of patient care outcomes.[7, 9, 14]

Specialist versus generalist palliative care

As the need for improvement in care for those coping with serious illness has been recognized, the demand

Reichel's Care of the Elderly, *7th Edition*, ed. Jan Busby-Whitehead *et al.* Published by Cambridge University Press.
© Cambridge University Press 2016.

for palliative care specialists and programming has grown significantly. Although the existence of hospital-based palliative care consultation teams has become more prevalent, gaps in funding and work force resources present barriers to meeting the complex needs of patients.[15–17] Furthermore, it has been suggested that this reliance on specialist care can, in some cases, add another layer of complexity and expense to the care of the seriously ill.[18]

Some essential aspects of the delivery of palliative care can be successfully provided by the patient's primary care provider or existing specialist. Since this relationship is often times developed over the course of years spent caring for the patient, an opportunity exists to drawn on this therapeutic relationship in such activities as advance care planning and discussion of patient and family goals. If the needs of the patient begin to take on greater complexity, such as in instances of refractory pain and symptom management or with management of truly complex decision making or conflict, then the palliative care specialist can work in collaboration with the generalist provider to address these issues. With this collaborative model, needs of a greater number patients can be met, while supporting the essential role of both generalist and specialist palliative care providers.

It is important to recognize the importance of ongoing professional education to help foster competency in the provision of generalist palliative care. Programs such as Education in Palliative and End-of-Life Care (EPEC), Oncotalk and End-of-Life Nursing Education Consortium (ELNEC) were developed to teach and reinforce basic skills needed for the delivery of primary level palliative care.[19–21] These courses have been used to teach both students and practicing clinicians such subjects as pain and symptom assessment and management, goals of care discussion, advance care planning and care for the imminently dying patient.[21] Increasing access to educational programs such as these, coupled with the continued growth of access to palliative care specialists, will best serve to promote quality in palliative care.

Navigating communication at the end of life

Successful communication with patients and families about issues surrounding serious illness and end-of-life care is an essential skill for all health-care providers. However, research has consistently shown that clinicians feel inadequately prepared in the provision of end-of-life care. This is particularly true surrounding the delivery of bad news and discussion of death and dying.[22–24] It is important to note, however, that patients and families often expect to be well informed about their diagnosis, and to act as active participants in collaborative decision making with their health-care provider.[25, 26] An important step in establishing a relationship with patients can be to determine how much and what type of information they would like to receive by asking them about their preferences.

Communication with patients and families who are facing serious or life-threatening illness can be challenging, but can be achieved using a systematic approach that encourages active listening, clear language surrounding medical information and discussion of patient- and family-centered goals (see Table 49.1). When discussing medical information with patients or with their families, it is important to first establish their current understanding of the illness. This can help to clarify misperceptions and inform the direction of the conversation. Once the clinician has a good understanding of the patient perspective, the current medical status and options can be reviewed with careful attention to avoid medical jargon and overly technical information. At this point, it can be helpful to discuss prognosis in terms of an expected range of hours to days, days to weeks, weeks to months, and so on. Although uncertainty should be acknowledged, prognostication provides the patient and family the opportunity to set their goals and expectations according to their own values and preferences.

As the patient and family take time to assimilate information and state their own goals, take a moment to respond to expressed emotion or allow for brief silence. After mutual understanding is established and questions are answered, relevant options and plans can be discussed. It is often helpful to make specific recommendations regarding interventions that will work to achieve the patient stated goals. For example, the clinician may make recommendations regarding resuscitation, artificial nutrition/hydration, returning to the hospital, or continuation of specific disease directed therapies. Supportive statements such as "I have seen caring families choose this option, and have also seen caring families choose this other option," can help to facilitate trust for further discussion at a

Table 49.1 The family meeting or goal-setting conference: approach to successful communication

1. **Preparation**
   - Review chart: know treatment course, prognosis, treatment options
     - Coordinate medical opinions among consultant physicians
     - Decide what tests/treatments are medically appropriate
   - Clarify goals for the meeting
   - Decide who you want to be present from the medical team

2. **Establish proper setting**

   Private, comfortable; everyone sitting in a circle

3. **Introductions/goals/relationship**
   - Allow everyone to state name and relationship to patient
   - State meeting goals; ask family to state their goals
   - Build relationship: ask nonmedical question about patient: *Can you tell me something about your father?*

4. **Family understanding of condition**
   - *Tell me your understanding of the current medical condition.*
   - For patients with a chronic illness, ask for a description of changes over the past weeks/months (activity, eating, sleep, mood): *How have things been going the past three months?*

5. **Medical review/summary**
   - Summarize "big picture" in a few sentences – use "dying" if appropriate
   - Avoid jargon or organ-by-organ medical review

6. **Silence/reactions**
   - Respond to emotional reactions
   - Prepare for common reactions: acceptance, conflict/denial, grief/despair; respond empathetically to conflict/denial (see Item 10)

7. **Present broad care options/set goals**
   - Provide prognostic data using a range
   - Present goal-oriented options (e.g., prolong life, improve function, return home, dignified death)
   - Make a recommendation based on knowledge/experience
   - *What is important in the time you have left?*

8. **Translate goals into care plan**
   - Review current and planned interventions – make recommendations to continue or stop based on goals
   - Discuss DNR, hospice/home care, artificial nutrition/hydration, future hospitalizations
   - Summarize decisions being made

9. **Document and discuss:**
   - Write a note: who was present, what decisions were made, follow-up plan
   - Team debriefing

10. **Managing conflict**
    - Listen and make empathetic statements: *This must be very hard.*
    - Determine source of conflict: guilt, grief, culture, family dysfunction, trust in medical team, etc.
    - Clarify misperceptions; explore values behind decisions
    - Set time-limited goals with specific benchmarks (e.g., improved cognition, oxygenation, mobility, etc.)

Source: Information adapted from the *Family Goal Setting Conference Pocket Card* and used with permission from the Medical College of Wisconsin.

later time. At the close of the conversation, a clear summary of decisions made and subsequent plans for next steps and follow-up should be discussed. It is also important to review and debrief with participating health-care providers; this will help to encourage continuity and cohesion within the interdisciplinary team.

Even as this approach to communication is designed to for the semi-formal discussion of specific goals of care, the principles can be applied in difficult conversations throughout the relationship with the patient. Skill in responding empathetically, in delivering prognostic information, and in using clear language surrounding medical information should be practiced and applied to daily patient interactions.

Symptom management

Patients often have a significant symptom burden at the end of life; pain, nausea, delirium, and dyspnea are among the most common. Frequently, patients have untreated symptoms in the last days to hours of life, with up to 90% of patients experiencing pain during the last week of life.[27] Recognizing and aggressively treating these symptoms provide both patient and family with a "good death." The following is a brief review of assessment and treatment of common symptoms at the end of life.

Pain

Assessment

Assessment of pain is critical at the end of life. This varies based on whether the patient is responsive at the time of assessment or not. If able to communicate, the initial evaluation of any patient's pain needs to take into account the current pain symptoms as well as any prior history of pain. Manifestations of chronic or acute pain in elderly, seriously ill patients are often complex and multifactorial. For example, age-related osteoarthritis may often obscure complaints of new bony or joint pain that may be from metastatic malignancy. A thorough pain assessment must include, via patient self-report if able, a description of the location, quality, onset, and exacerbating and relieving factors. Most mistakes in diagnosing and effectively treating pain in severely ill patients come from neglecting some aspect of the pain assessment.[28] The Agency for Health Care Policy and Research (AHCPR)

guidelines describe pain as "an unpleasant sensory and emotional experience associated with actual or potential tissue damage or described in terms of such damage."[29] Thus, one important aspect of effective pain control in seriously ill patients is to believe the patient or family member's report of pain.

The quality of a patient's pain can commonly be described in terms such as sharp, stabbing, throbbing, shooting, or tingling. This assessment helps in the determination of the type of pain the patient experiences. Nociceptive pain, which is derived from pain receptors, is either visceral or somatic. Visceral pain is often described as deep, aching and colicky, is poorly localized, and often is referred to cutaneous sites, which may be tender to palpation. In cancer patients, this pain often results from stretching of viscera by tumor growth. Somatic pain is often reported as constant, aching, or gnawing. Neuropathic pain affects peripheral nerves, spinal cord, or the central nervous system (CNS).[30] It is often described as burning, aching, or shooting in quality and can be persistent or spontaneous.[31]

Assessment of pain should include, when able, some objective measure of severity. Various scales exist to document pain, such as the Visual Analog Scale (VAS) or the numerical pain distress scale. An important aspect of severity of pain and degree of relief is to assess what patient goals and expectations are. Because many elderly adults underreport pain, engaging with the patient about what to expect from therapy is critical to the success of treatment.[32]

In nonverbal patients, the assessment of pain has added complexity. Observation of patient behaviors is recommended in non-verbal, seriously ill patients. [33] Behaviors that are commonly considered pain related include facial grimacing, moaning, or rubbing a body part. Some behaviors are less obvious. These include agitation, restlessness, irritability, or confusion. Various assessment tools are available to guide assessment of pain in elderly patients such as the pain assessment in advanced dementia scale (PAIN-AD) or the checklist of nonverbal pain indicators (CNPI). As a patient becomes nonverbal during the dying process, previous pain should be assumed still present and must continue to be effectively treated.[27]

Management

Although older patients are often at higher risk of drug-related adverse effects, appropriate treatment of pain in seriously ill patients is crucial to improve quality of life. Undertreatment of pain in elderly patients is associated with significant adverse outcomes, including functional impairment, falls, anxiety and depression, and greater health-care costs.[34] Opioid and nonopioid adjuvants should be the cornerstone of treatment in all severe, persistent pain. For most patients with cancer-related or other severe pain, the use of opioids is necessary and the benefits vastly outweigh the risks. Often, elderly patients' pain is undertreated because of concern of use of opioids.[36] Selection of opioids should take into account end-organ function, availability, cost, ease of use, and patient's past experiences. A combination of short- and long-acting opioids is crucial to successfully treating patients with persistent pain. Often, the use of immediate-release opioids is a first step in pain control, especially in previously opioid-naïve patients.

There are various age-related changes associated with the effectiveness and pharmacodynamics drug properties, including changes in metabolism, distribution, and excretion.[35] Decreases in hepatic and renal function are often present in healthy elderly patients, let alone in the seriously ill elderly cohort. Decreased metabolism and excretion can result from poor end organ function, and should be taken into account when dosing opioids. Ultimately, very effective and safe pain relief can be achieved with individualized monitoring and titration. In the absence of obstruction or problems with absorption, an alert elderly patient can tolerate oral medications. There is no change in oral bio-availability in elderly patients.

Considerations for selection of opioid

Morphine is the most commonly prescribed opioid because of cost and availability.[37] There are long-acting and immediate-release oral tablets, elixir, suppositories, and intravenous or subcutaneous dosing options. Elderly patients with impaired renal or hepatic function should be monitored closely. In patients with renal failure, the metabolites of morphine may accumulate and ultimately cause neurotoxicity.[38] Oxycodone, a semisynthetic opioid similar in bioavailability to morphine, is available in oral preparations. Oxycodone is hepatically metabolized and renally excreted as well.[39] Hydromorphone (Dilaudid) is a semisynthetic derivative of morphine which is available as oral tablets, liquid, suppository,

Table 49.2 Equianalgesic conversions

Drug	PO/PR (mg)	Subcutaneous/IV (mg)
Morphine	30	10
Oxycodone	20	n/a
Hydrocodone	20	n/a
Hydromorphone	7.5	1.5
Oxymorphone	10	1
Fentanyl	n/a	0.1 (100 mcg)

and parenteral formulations. The metabolite of hydromorphone is renally excreted and associated with neurotoxicity at increasing doses as well.[40] Fentanyl is a synthetic opioid and estimated to be 80 times more potent than morphine. In patients with true opioid allergies, fentanyl is a safe alternative because it is completely synthetic. Because of its high lipid solubility, fentanyl is available as a transdermal patch. This is a safe alternative in elderly patients who cannot swallow, but should never be used first-line in opioid naïve patients. Fever increases the rate of absorption of transdermal fentanyl.[42] Intravenous fentanyl is also available and is a safe alternative in patients with compromised renal function. Both ketamine and methadone can be safely used in elderly individuals, but because of their variable half-life, unpredictable side effect profile and high risk of accumulation without careful monitoring and titration, these medications should be managed by pain and palliative medicine specialists.

Understanding equianalgesic conversions is the cornerstone to safely starting, maintaining or converting patients with serious illness on any opioids. (See Table 49.2 for equianalgesic conversions.)

Dosing and titration

Opioid therapy must be selected on an individual bases, taking into account both medication of choice and route of administration. Intravenous and subcutaneous dosing is often required at the end of life for various reasons. Patient-controlled analgesia (PCA) pump use is often beneficial in elderly patients with severe pain. Indications for PCA pump include: unable to tolerate oral route, escalating pain that needs to be managed rapidly, severe incident pain, and dose-limiting side effects with other routes of

675

administration. Contraindications to the use of a PCA pump are primarily centered on concern for delirium or patient ability to participate in their own care. Titration of opioids is often required frequently in patients nearing the end of life. Escalation of both long-acting and immediate release formulations may be necessary to maintain adequate pain relief. The immediate release formulation should be between 10% and 20% of the total daily dose of the long-acting opioid. Increases in opioids, via all routes of administration, can be done safely every 24 hours. To effectively control pain, the minimum increase should be 25% of the total daily dose and can be as much as 100% increase, depending on the frequency of the use of the breakthrough opioid and the severity and circumstances of the pain syndrome. The dose should be increased until adequate pain control is achieved or intolerable side effects occur.

Although there is no specific maximum dose of any one opioid, if pain is no longer controlled on a specific regimen or dose titration yields treatment-limiting toxicities, opioid rotation may be necessary. This helps achieve a favorable balance between analgesia and side effects.[43, 44] The principle of incomplete cross-tolerance is important to the successful rotation from one opioid to another. Cross-tolerance occurs when continued use of one opioid leads to tolerance of another substance with similar pharmacologic properties. Incomplete cross-tolerance occurs with opioids, and thus dose decreases are needed. The percentage of decrease required is variable; the amount of pain the patient is currently experiencing, end organ function and other comorbidities may force a greater or lesser percentage decrease. The usual range of dose decrease is between 25% and 50%.[45]

Adjuvant analgesics

In patients with serious illness, many nonopioid medications are useful as adjuvants in the treatment of severe pain. Adjuvant analgesics may be used alone or in combination with opioids. These include anticonvulsants, antidepressants, corticosteroids, and topical anesthetics. Neuropathic pain is often best treated with nonopioid medications. Current guidelines recommend tricyclic antidepressants (TCA) or dual reuptake inhibitors of both serotonin and norepinephrine as the first line treatment, along with calcium channel binding agents (gabapentin and pregabalin) for neuropathic pain.[46] Side effects of TCAs primarily limit their use in elderly patients. Common side effects include urinary retention,

constipation, and delirium. As with most drugs in elderly patients, starting at a low dose with a slow titration is helpful to monitor and avoid serious side effects or drug–drug interactions.

Corticosteroids are useful in various types of pain syndromes. They are the standard of care in malignant spinal cord compression. In addition, bony pain from malignant metastasis and inflammatory pain from invasion of abdominal viscera also respond well to the anti-inflammatory effects of corticosteroids. Dexamethasone is commonly the preferred agent because of its duration of action as well as its limited effects on blood glucose levels.[37] The evidence on the benefit of steroids in cancer patients is not high quality, but corticosteroids have a lower side effect profile than NSAIDs in elderly terminal cancer patients and can be useful in the management of nausea and vomiting as well.[47]

Additionally, interventional procedures to manage pain are, at times, very valid options in patients at the end of life. Specifically in cancer patients, nerve blocks (celiac plexus, superior hypogastric, lumbar) are effective in relieving severe visceral and neuropathic pain from malignancy.[48]

Nonpharmacologic approaches to pain management

Although there is not a large body of evidence, many nonpharmacologic, complimentary therapies can provide pain relief in elderly patients nearing the end of life. Various sources recommend trials of acupuncture for pain as well as other cancer-related symptoms owing to the minimal side effects of treatment. Although no high-quality data is available, a 2011 meta-analysis showed no significant side effects of acupuncture, but they were unable to recommend acupuncture for adults with cancer pain due to lack of evidence of benefit.[49] Additional complimentary approaches to pain management include Reiki massage, meditation, therapeutic massage, physical therapy, as well as art and music therapy. Many of these are often employed through hospice programs. All of these can be used alone or in combination with pharmacotherapy.

Nausea and vomiting

Mechanisms

Nausea and vomiting are common symptoms during the end of life. These cause significant physical and

Table 49.3 Common pathways stimulated in nausea and vomiting

Pathway	Input	Neuroreceptor
Vestibular system	Motion, labyrinth disorders	Acetylcholine, histamine
Chemoreceptor trigger zone	Drugs, metabolic disturbances, bacterial toxins	Dopamine, serotonin, neurokinin
Peripheral pathways	Mechanical stretch, GI mucosal injury, local toxins and drugs	Mechanoreceptors and chemoreceptors (serotonin) in GI tract and viscera
Cortex	Anxiety, sensory input, increased intracranial pressure, meningeal irritation	Acetylcholine, histamine, serotonin

psychological distress for both patients and their families. Understanding the pathophysiology of nausea and vomiting is important in selecting the most beneficial therapy as well as avoiding polypharmacy. Various pathways mediate nausea and vomiting. See Table 49.3 for common pathways stimulated in nausea and vomiting.[50–53] These pathways provide input to the vomit center in the brain, resulting in either nausea or vomiting when a specific, minimum threshold is met.[50]

Assessment

A thorough history and physical exam is the first step in determining cause and subsequent treatment for nausea and vomiting. Once the most likely cause is established, determination of the specific mechanism and neuroreceptors involved will aid in targeted therapy and avoiding poly-pharmacy, a common complication in elderly patients. Various mnemonics exist to help guide a targeted physical exam and understanding of the likely cause. See Table 49.4 for one specific mnemonic useful in nausea and vomiting.[50–53]

Management

Once a determination of the likely cause of nausea and vomiting is deduced, a mechanism-based treatment strategy is effective. Using the most potent antagonist to the indicated neurotransmitter receptor has been effective in up to 80% of cases of nausea and vomiting at the end of life.[51] Although a mechanism-based treatment strategy is very effective, there is some evidence that starting with an empiric regimen consisting of a dopamine antagonist is also successful. See Table 49.5 for common antiemetics, site of action, and starting doses.

Table 49.4

V	Vertigo, vestibular
O	Obstruction of gut
M	Motility dysfunction within gut
I	Inflammation of gut
T	Toxins, drugs
I	Intracranial – increased intracranial pressure
N	Nerves – anxiety, depression
G	Gums, mouth, oropharynx – thrush, mucositis, etc.

Generally, the best method of treatment involves choosing one antiemetic with the desired receptor site of action and increasing that medication until a maximum dose is achieved or intolerable side effects occur. If a second antiemetic is needed, choosing one with a different site of action is more effective with less risk of adverse events.[50]

Corticosteroids are often effective in refractory nausea and vomiting. They have an unknown mechanism of action, but are thought to be effective via a decrease in gut edema. Although rarely necessary, refractory nausea and vomiting may require palliative sedation. The use of propofol has been investigated for its known antiserotonergic activity.[53]

Dyspnea

Assessment

Dyspnea, the subjective sensation of breathlessness, is a frightening symptom at the end of life. It can be either acute or chronic and is associated with

677

Table 49.5 Common antiemetics

Drug	Brand name	Receptor site of action	Dose/route
Metoclopramide	Reglan	Dopamine and serotonin (only at high doses)	5–20mg PO or IV before meals and at bedtime
Haloperidol	Haldol	Dopamine	0.5–4mg PO, SQ, IV q4–6 hours
Prochlorperazine	Compazine	Dopamine	5–10mg PO, IV q6 hours (also available in suppository form)
Chlorpromazine	Thorazine	Dopamine	10 25mg PO, IV q6 hours (also available in suppository form)
Promethazine	Phenergan	Histamine, acetylcholine, dopamine	12.5–25mg PO, IV q6 hours (also available in suppository form)
Diphenhydramine	Benadryl	Histamine	25–50mg PO, IV q6 hours
Ondansetron*	Zofran	Serotonin	4–8mg PO, IV q4–8 hours
Aprepitant	Emend	Neurokinin	125 mg PO ×1, then 80mg PO daily × 2–3 days
Olanzapine	Zyprexa	Dopamine, serotonin	2.5–5mg PO daily
Scopolamine	Transderm scop	Acetylcholine	1.5mg transdermal patch q3 days
Meclizine	Antivert	Acetylcholine	12.5–50mg PO q8 hours

* One example of medication in this class.

many end-stage pulmonary, cardiac, renal, and malignant diseases. Greater than 90% of patients with chronic lung disease suffer from dyspnea in the last year of life.[54]

The perception of dyspnea should be considered analogous to the perception of pain in patients with end stage illness: these are subjective findings. Clearly, both pain and dyspnea can cause tremendous suffering and should be aggressively managed. The pathophysiology behind dyspnea is complex, with many various pathways. Increases in $PaCO2$ or decreases in $PaO2$ or pH can stimulate either central of peripheral chemoreceptors. Additionally, activation of mechanical receptors in either the chest wall or respiratory musculature may stimulate breathlessness. Some patients may feel breathless with a normal arterial blood gas while others may feel comfortable with marked abnormalities on blood gas.[55]

Management

Asking patients to rate the severity or distress of their dyspnea is suggested to assess both its impact and allow a baseline value to evaluate effectiveness of therapy.[54] This assessment should be routinely documented in medical records to guide management and interdisciplinary care.

Therapeutic interventions should be based on underlying etiology whenever possible. Potentially reversible causes of dyspnea include pulmonary edema, bronchospasm, severe anxiety, and infection. Pharmacologic (bronchodilators, steroids, antibiotics), interventional (thoracentesis, chest tube placement), and nonpharmacological (fan, relaxation therapy, music) options should be explored.[54]

Supplemental oxygen is the standard of care for patients who are hypoxemic, however, minimal literature exists on its benefits in patients who do not have hypoxemia. Given its ease of use, minimal side effects, and rapid onset of action, a trial of supplemental oxygen should be used in any patient with subjective complaints of breathlessness.

At the end of life, the use of opioids, benzodiazepines, and steroids are still the cornerstone of treatment. Often patients are not in a hospital setting or may no longer want invasive procedures nearing the end of life. Morphine is often prescribed oral, intravenous, or nebulized. A Cochrane review comparing nebulized morphine to placebo revealed no evidence to support its use in the treatment of breathlessness.[56] However, both oral and intravenous morphine, or other opioids, can be very effective in treating dyspnea at the end of life. Although trials have shown variable results, the dosage and intervals have been called into question in the trials that showed little effect.[54] Additionally, multiple studies have shown that use of palliative morphine has no effect on survival time.[57]

Benzodiazepines have been shown to reduce dyspnea in patients. These are believed to work via reductions in the perception of breathlessness and should be considered when there appears to be a large anxiety component.[58] However, these medications may increase drowsiness or exacerbate delirium. Thus, they should be used only when dyspnea is not controlled with opioids and other less psychoactive options.[59]

Care for the imminently dying

Almost all primary care clinicians will participate in the care of a patient that is imminently dying. Unfortunately, few providers report having received adequate training on end-of-life care and struggle with recognizing the dying process, treating symptoms, and advising family (see earlier section Navigating Communication at the End of Life).[60] Patients and families all desire a "good death" often defined as "free from avoidable distress and suffering for patients, families, and caregivers,"[60] although there may be differences on how we get there.[62]

Most Americans want to die at home. A survey of oncology patients showed almost 90% preferred to die at home. Currently almost 50% of Americans die in the hospital, 25% in a nursing home, and 25% at home. The trend is toward more deaths occurring at home or in a nursing facility. The strongest predictor of dying at home is living in a locality with fewer hospital beds per capita.[63]

Of those dying in hospitals, end-of-life care is often less than adequate. Of families of patients dying in the hospital, 50% thought communication was a problem, 51% wanted more physician contact, and 80% thought the patient was not always treated with respect.[64] Hospice services are designed to provide end-of-life symptom management and guidance for families but have been historically underutilized. This has been changing and as of

2012, 44% of all deaths in America were under the care of hospice. Unfortunately, patients are often referred late in their disease, with a median length of stay of 17.4 days in 2014, which can lead to suboptimal utilization of resources.[65]. Criteria for admission to hospice are generally based on a physician certifying a patient may have a prognosis of six months or less if the disease runs its natural course and the patient elects hospice services. Further disease specific criteria are beyond the scope of this chapter but can be found at the National Hospice and Palliative Care website (www.nhpco.org).

Because many people still die in the hospital, it is important for physicians to be comfortable managing their care. There are several physiologic changes that occur in the last hours or days of life that need to be recognized. Weakness and fatigue gradually increase until the patient is bed bound. Care should be focused on preventing skin breakdown and alleviating pain. Patients often eat less and may stop drinking. This can be very distressing for families who are concerned their loved one is "starving" or is thirsty. Multiple studies have shown parenteral or enteral feedings do not alleviate symptoms or extend life for patients in the dying process.[66, 67] Studies have shown patients experience very little hunger and it is thought the resulting ketosis and dehydration may create a sense of well-being.[68] Occasionally intravenous fluids may be tried to reverse delirium; however, the evidence is mixed on its effectiveness.[69] It is important to recognize intravenous fluids can increase adverse effects such as pain, worsened fluid overload, breathlessness, excessive oropharyngeal secretions, and prolongation of the dying process. Providing guidance and education to loved ones about a patient's lack of hunger or thirst is often very effective in decreasing caregiver distress. Families should be instructed to provide good oral and nasal hygiene, which can provide the patient comfort and minimize thirst.[70]

It is important to recognize respiratory changes common at the end of life to appropriately educate family and to control symptoms. Tidal volumes diminish, often there are apneic periods, increased accessory muscle use, and Cheyne-Stokes respirations usually develop. As discussed earlier in the section on dyspnea, the sensation of dyspnea may be independent of oxygen saturation and should be treated as a subjective symptom like pain.

As the patient becomes more unconscious and the gag reflex diminishes, respiratory secretions often accumulate in the back of the throat leading to gurgling respirations. This "death rattle" occurs in one-fourth to one-half of all patients and predicts most will die within 48 hours.[73] It is important to reassure families this is not distressing to the patient. Non-pharmacologic interventions such as discontinuation of parental fluids and repositioning to ensure postural drainage can be quite effective. Aggressive suctioning is not recommended as it is ineffective and can be uncomfortable. The majority of patients respond to treatment with antimuscarincs such as scopolamine, glycopyrrolate, or hyoscyamine.[68] Glycopyrrolate is the only medication in this class that does not cross the blood-brain barrier and therefore does not cause an increased risk of delirium. This should be taken into account when choosing a medication from this class.

Terminal delirium occurs in 28%–83% of patients at the end of life and may be hypoactive, hyperactive, or mixed.[74] There has been "two roads to death" described in the literature to describe the neurologic changes that occur at the end of life.[75] Most people will take the "usual road" with decreasing levels of consciousness that progresses to coma and death. The less common, "difficult road," is often characterized by agitated hyperactive delirium that can be very distressing for the patient and family. Often the symptoms of delirium may be misinterpreted as physical pain, but it is important to recognize that uncontrolled pain rarely develops at the end of life if it had not been a problem prior. It may be reasonable to try an increase in opioids, but if symptoms do not improve, escalating doses may contribute to worsening delirium.[69] Review has shown best evidence for haloperidol and chlorpromazine but conclude benzodiazepines, other antipsychotics, and phenothiazines are effective as well.[76]

Pain should be managed aggressively with opioids at the end of life utilizing the tools and guidelines described earlier. Concerns about opioids hastening death have been refuted in the past by using the ethical principle of double effect. This principle states that an action with potential bad effects (respiratory sedation) is ethically permissible if the good effect (pain relief) is the intention. Furthermore, emerging evidence supports the fact that appropriate and aggressive pain management with opioids at the end of life does not cause respiratory depression or change survival.[77–79]

A small number of patients may have symptoms that are not well controlled with maximal medical interventions. In these cases patients may require controlled palliative sedation. Medications such as midazolam, propofol, or barbiturates are often used because they can be rapidly titrated to effect.[80] Palliative sedation should not be mistaken for physician assisted suicide and is ethically acceptable in cases of intractable suffering. Showing similar evidence regarding the use of opioids at the end of life, a study of patients undergoing palliative sedation found it did not shorten overall survival.[81] Decision for palliative sedation requires thorough discussion with all members of the care team, family, and patient if possible to ensure all are comfortable with the plan. Consultation with expert palliative medicine or anesthesia specialists is recommended.

There is good-quality evidence emerging that there is a beneficial relationship between overall patient well-being and religious commitment or practice. Many physicians still think it is inappropriate for them to discuss spirituality with their patients, feeling it is out of their range of expertise or is too intrusive. Studies have shown that patients with life-threatening illnesses use religion to sustain hope and help them cope.[82] Spiritual well-being has also been shown to be protective from end-of-life despair, defined as feelings of hopelessness, wishes for hastened death, and suicidal ideation.[83] Support of this is well within the scope of a clinician's practice and is critical to providing comprehensive care at the end of life. Several screening tools exist and are simple to complete, for example, the American College of Physicians – American Society of Internal Medicine End-of-Life Care Consensus Panel paper, "What are your hopes (your expectations, your fears) for the future?"[84] Addressing spiritual concerns can ensure appropriate referrals to chaplaincy services when indicated.

Anticipatory guidance is crucial to helping families with the dying process. It is difficult to predict exactly when a person may die and the clinician should avoid giving specific numbers. It is more appropriate to give ranges such as hours or hours to days. One study showed patients developed respirations with mandibular movements eight hours, acrocyanosis five hours, and radial pulselessness three hours prior to death but there was a wide individual variation. Eighty-four percent of patients had decreased consciousness twenty-four hours prior to death.[73] Basic information on the signs of death is appropriate to be relayed to family. Experts recommend reviewing the process, the signs of death, and death notification arrangements with caregivers to reduce stress at the time of death. The clinician should also inquire about cultural or religious preferences.[69] Families have identified improved communication as the single most important means of improving end-of-life care.[62]

Normal grief reactions may vary widely. It is thought people need to complete four tasks before the bereaved can effectively deal with the loss. First, they must recognize and accept that death has occurred. Second, they need to experience the pain caused by the loss. Third, they need to recognize the significance and changes to their life. Finally, they need to reinvest their energy in new relationships and activities. These tasks are interdependent but do not necessarily happen in order.[69] When grief is prolonged, very intense, or interferes with physical or emotional well-being, it is considered complicated. One study showed risk factors for complicated grief include age younger than 60, lack of perceived social support, history of or current depression, lower income, pessimistic thinking, and severity of stressful life events.[85] Consultation with someone skilled in bereavement care may be necessary. As a general resource, local hospice organizations provide bereavement counseling and support. If complicated issues with grief and bereavement are suspected, a referral to a hospice grief program is likely helpful.

Conclusion

As medical technology continues to both prolong life expectancy and alter the dying process, skilled palliative care continues to be a growing necessity for elderly patients and their families. Investments in education about communication and symptom management can drastically improve the dying process for patients, family, and providers.

References

1. World Health Organization. WHO definition of palliative care. Retrieved from www.who.int/cancer/palliative/definition/en. Published 2008.

2. National Consensus Project for Quality Palliative Care. *Clinical Practice Guidelines for Quality Palliative Care*, 3rd ed. Retrieved from www.nationalconsensusproject.org. Published 2013.

3. Center to Advance Palliative Care. *America's Care of Serious Illness: A State-by-State Report Card on Access to Palliative Care in Our Nation's Hospitals*. Retrieved from www.capc.org. Published 2008.

4. Bakitas M, Lyons KD, Hegel MT, et al. Effects of a palliative care intervention on clinical outcomes in patients with advanced cancer. *JAMA*, 2009; **302**(7): 741–749.

5. Jack B, Hillier V, Williams A, et al. Hospital based palliative care teams improve the symptoms of cancer patients. *Palliat Med.* 2003; **17**(6): 498–502.

6. Temel JS, Greer JA, Muzikansky A, et al. Early palliative care for patients with metastatic non-small-cell lung cancer. *N Engl J Med.* 2010; **363**(8): 733–741.

7. Armstrong B, Jenigiri B, Hutson SP, et al. The impact of a palliative care program in a rural Appalachian community hospital: A quality improvement process. *Am J Hosp Palliat Care.* 2012; **30**(4): 380–387.

8. Bendaly EA, Groves J, Juliar B, Gramelspacher, GP. Financial impact of palliative care consultation in a public hospital. *J Palliat Med.* 2008; **11**(10): 1304–1308.

9. Gade G, Venohr I, Conner D, et al. Impact of an inpatient palliative care team: A randomized control trial. *J Palliat Med.* 2008; **11**(2): 180–189.

10. Hanson LC, Usher B, Spragens L, Barnard S. Clinical and economic impact of palliative care consultation. *J Pain Symptom Manage.* 2008; **35**(4): 340–346.

11. Morrison RS, Penrod JD, Cassel JB, et al. Cost savings associated with US hospital palliative care consultation programs. *Arch Intern Med.* 2008; **168**(16): 1783–1790.

12. Norton SA, Hogan LA, Holloway RG, et al. Proactive palliative care in the medical intensive care unit: Effects on length of stay for selected high-risk patients. *Crit Care Med.* 2006; **35**(6): 1530–1535.

13. Penrod JD, Partha D, Luhrs C, et al. Cost and utilization outcomes of patients receiving hospital-based palliative care consultation. *J Palliat Med.* 2006; **9**(4): 855–860.

14. Cassarett D, Pickard A, Bailey FA, et al. Do palliative consultations improve patient outcomes? *J Am Geriatr Soc.* 2008; **56**: 593–599.

15. Goldsmith B, Dietrich J, Du Q. Morrison RS. Variability in access to hospital palliative care in the United States. *J Palliat Med.* 2008; **11**: 1094–1102.

16. Morrison RS, Maroney-Galin C, Kralovec PD, Meier DE. The growth of palliative care programs in United States hospitals. *J Palliat Med.* 2005; **8**: 1127–1134.

17. Weissman DE, Meier DE. Identifying patients in need of a palliative care assessment in the hospital setting: A consensus report from the Center to Advance Palliative Care. *J Palliat Med.* 2011; **14**(1): 1–7.

18. Quill TE, Abernethy AP. Generalist plus specialist palliative care – creating a more sustainable model. *N Engl J Med.* 2013; **368**(13): 1173–1175.

19. Back AL, Arnold RM, Baile WF, et al. Faculty Development to change the paradigm of

communication skills in oncology. *J Clin Oncol.* 2009; **27**: 1137–1141.

20. Kurz J, Hayes E. End of life issues action: impact of education. *Int. J. Nursing Educ. Scholarship.* 2006; **3**(1): 1–13.

21. Robinson K, Sutton S, von Gunten CF, et al. Assessment of the Education for Physicians on End-of Life Care (EPEC) Project. *J Palliat Med.* 2004; **7**(5): 637–645.

22. Sullivan AM, Lakoma MD, Block SD. The status of medical education in end of life care: A national report. *J Intern Med.* 2003; **18**: 685–695.

23. Khader KA, Jarrah SS, Alasad J. Influence on nurses' characteristics and education on their attitudes toward death and dying: A review of the literature. *Int J Nurs Midwifery.* 2010; **2**(1): 1–9.

24. Fallowfield L, Jenkins V. Communicating sad, bad, and difficult news in medicine. *Lancet.* 2004; **363**: 312–319.

25. Brown VA, Parker PA, Furbur L, Thomas AL. Patient preferences for the delivery of bad news – the experience of a UK Cancer Centre. *Eur J Cancer Care,* 2011; **20**: 56–61.

26. Jenkins V, Fallowfield L, Saul J. Information needs of patients with cancer: Results from a large study in UK cancer centres. *Briti J Cancer.* 2001; **84**: 48–51

27. Hermann C, Looney S. The effectiveness of symptom management in hospice patients during the last seven days of life. *J Hosp Palliat Nurs.* 2001; **3**(3): 88–96.

28. Abrahm JL. *A Physician's Guide to Pain and Symptom Management in Cancer Patients.* 2nd ed. Baltimore, MD: Johns Hopkins University Press; 2005.

29. Jacox A, Carr DB, and Payne R, et al. *Management of Cancer Pain: Clinical Practice Guideline No. 9.* Rockville, MD: Agency for Health Care and Policy Research, U.S. Department of Health and Human Services, Public Health Service, 1994: 23. AHCPR publication 94–0592.

30. Eisenberg E, McNicol ED, Carr DB. Efficacy and safety of opioid agonists in the treatment of neuropathic pain of nonmalignant origin: Systemic review and meta-analysis of randomized controlled trials. *JAMA.* 2005; **293**: 3043–3052.

31. Yarnitsky D, Eisenberg E. Neuropathic pain: between positive and negative ends. *Pain Forum.* 1998; 7: 241–242.

32. AGS Panel on the Pharmacological Management of Persistent Pain in Older Persons. Pharmacologic management of persistent pain in older persons. *J Am Geriatr Soc.* 2009; **57**: 1331–1346.

33. Herr K, Coyne PJ, Key T., et al. Pain assessment in the nonverbal patient: Position statement with clinical practice recommendations. *Pain Manag Nurs.* 2006; **7**(2): 44–52.

34. AGS Panel on Persistent Pain in Older Persons. The management of persistent pain in older persons. *J Am Geriatr Soc.* 2002; **50**: S205–S224.

35. Fine PG. Opioid analgesic drugs in older people. *Clin Geriatr Med.* 2001; **17**: 479–487.

36. Pergolizzi J, Boger RH, Budd K., et al. Opioids and the management of chronic severe pain in the elderly: Consensus statement of an International Expert Panel with focus on the six clinically most often used World Health Organization Step III opioids (buprenorphine, fentanyl, hydromorphone, methadone, morphine, oxycodone). *Pain Pract.* 2008; **8**: 287–313.

37. Derby S, O'Mahony S, Tickoo R. Elderly patients. In: Ferrell BR and Coyle N, eds. *Oxford Textbook of Palliative Nursing.* 3rd ed. New York, NY: Oxford University Press, 2010: 713–743.

38. Mercadante S, Arcuir E. Opioids and renal function. *J Pain.* 2004; **5**: 2–19.

39. Kirvela M, Lindgren L, Seppala T, Olkkola KT. The pharmacokinetics of oxycodone in uremic patients undergoing renal transplantation. *J Clin Anesth.* 1996; **8**: 13–18.

40. Paramanandam G, Prommer E, Schwenke DC. Adverse effects in hospice patients with chronic kidney disease receiving hydromorphone. *J Palliat Med.* 2011; **14**(9): 1029–1033.

41. Kornick CA, Santiago-Palma J, Khojainova N, et al. A safe and effective method for converting cancer patients from intravenous to transdermal fentanyl. *Cancer.* 2001; **92**: 3056–3061.

42. Varvel JR, Shafer SL, Hwang SS, et al. Absorption characteristics of transdermally administered fentanyl. *Anesthesiology.* 1989; **70**: 928–934.

43. Miller KE, Miller MM, Jolley MR. Challenges in pain management at the end of life. *Am Fam Physician.* 2001; **64**: 1227–1234.

44. Vadalouca A, Moka E, Argyra E, et al. Opioid rotation in patients with cancer: A review of the current literature. *J Opioid Manag.* 2008; **4**(4): 213–250.

45. Jage J. Opioid tolerance and dependence – do they matter? *Eur J Pain.* 2005; **9**: 157–162.

46. O'Connor AB, Dworkin RH. Treatment of neuropathic pain: An overview of recent guidelines. *Am J Med.* 2009; **122**: S22–S32.

47. Paulsen O, Aass N, Kaasa S, Dale O. Do corticosteroids provide analgesic effects in cancer patients? A systematic literature review. *J Pain Symptom Manage.* 2013; **46**: 96–105.

48. Wong GY, Schroeder DR, Carns PE, et al. Effect of neurolytic celiac plexus block on pain relief, quality of life, and survival in patients with unresectable pancreatic cancer: A randomized controlled trial. *JAMA.* 2004; **291**(9): 1092–1099.

49. Paley CA, Johnson MI, Tashani OA, Bagnall AM. Acupuncture for cancer pain in adults. *Cochrane Database Syst Rev.* 2011; **1**: CD007753. doi: 10.1002/14651858.CD007753.pub2.

50. Wood GJ, Shega JW, Lynch B, Von Roenn JH. Management of intractable nausea and vomiting in patients at the end of life: "I was feeling nauseous all of the time . . . Nothing was working." *JAMA.* 2007; **298** (10): 1196–1206.

51. Bentley A, Boyd K. Use of clinical pictures in the management of nausea and vomiting: A prospective audit. *Palliat Med.* 2001; **15**(3): 247–253.

52. Bruera E, Seifert L, Watanabe S, et al. Chronic nausea in advanced cancer patient: A retrospective assessment of a metoclopramide-based antiemetic regimen. *J Pain Symptom Manage.* 1996; **11**(3): 147–153.

53. Lundstrom S, Zachrisson U, Furst CJ. When nothing helps: Propofol as sedative and antiemetic in palliative cancer care. *J Pain Symptom Manage.* 2005; **30**(6): 570–577.

54. Mahler DA, Selecky PA, Harrod CG, et al. American College of Chest Physicians consensus statement on the management of dyspnea in patients with advanced lung or heart disease. *Chest.* 2010; **137**(3): 674–691.

55. Luce JM, Luce JA. Management of dyspnea in patients with far advanced lung disease: "Once I lose it, it's kind of hard to catch it . . ." *JAMA.* 2001; **285**: 1331–1337.

56. Jennings AL, Davies AN, Higgins JP, Broadley K. Opioids for the palliation of breathlessness in terminal illness. *Cochrane Database Syst Rev.* 2001; **4**: CD002066. PMID 11687137.

57. Thorns A, Sykes N. Opioid use in last week of life and implications for end-of-life decision-making. *Lancet.* 2000; **356**(9227): 398–399.

58. Smoller JW, Pollack MH, Otto, MW, et al. Panic anxiety, dyspnea, and respiratory disease: Theoretical and clinical considerations. *American Journal of Respiratory and Critical Care Medicine.* 1996; **154**(1): 6–17.

59. Man GC, Hsu K, Sproule BJ. Effect of alprazolam on exercise and dyspnea in patients with chronic obstructive pulmonary disease. *Chest Journal.* 1986; **90**(6): 832–836.

60. Barzansky B, Veloski JJ, Miller R, Jonas HS. Education in end-of-life care during medical school and residency training. *Acad Med.* 1999; **74**(10): S102–4.

61. Field M, Cassel C. Approaching death: Improving care at the end of life. In: Meier DE, Isaacs SL, and Hughes R, eds. *Palliative Care: Transforming the Care of Serious Illness.* Hoboken, NJ: Jossey-Bass; 2010: 79–91.

62. Steinhauser KE, Clipp EC, McNeilly M, et al. In search of a good death: Observations of patients, families, and providers. *Annal Intern Med.* 2000; **132**(10): 825–832.

63. Hansen SM, Tolle SW, Martin DP. Factors associated with lower rates of in-hospital death. *J Palliat Med.* 2002; **5**(5): 677–685.

64. Teno JM, Clarridge BR, Casey V, et al. Family perspectives on end-of-life care at the last place of care. *JAMA.* 2004; **291**(1): 88–93.

65. National Hospice and Palliative Care Organization. Retrieved from www.nhpco.org/sites/default/files/public/Statistics_Research/2015_Facts_Figures.pdf (accessed November 14, 2015).

66. Finucane TE, Christmas C, Traves K. Tube feeding in patients with advanced dementia: A review of the evidence. *JAMA.* 1999; **282**: 1365–1370.

67. Lipman TO. Clinical trials of nutritional support in cancer. *Parenteral and enteral therapy. Hematol. Oncol. Clin. North Am.* 1991: **5**: 91–102.

68. McCann RM, Hall WJ, Groth-Juncker A. Comfort care for terminally ill patients: The appropriate use of nutrition and hydration. *JAMA.* 1994; **272**(16): 1263–1266.

69. Plonk WM Jr, Arnold RM. Terminal care: The last weeks of life. *J Palliat Med.* 2005; **8**(5): 1042–1054.

70. Ferris FD, von Gunten CF, Emanuel LL. Competency in end-of-life care: Last hours of life. *J Palliat Med.* 2003; **6**: 605–613.

71. Jennings AL, Davies AN, Higgins JPT, et al. Opioids for the palliation of breathlessness in advanced disease and terminal illness. *Cochrane Database Syst Rev.* 2001; **4**: CD0020066. doi:10.1002/14651858.

72. Bruera E, Sweeney C, Willey J, et al. A randomized controlled trial of supplemental oxygen versus air in cancer patients with dyspnea. *Palliat Med.* 2003; **17**(8): 659–663.

73. Morita T, Tsunoda J, Inoue S, Chihara, S. Risk factors for death rattle in terminally ill cancer patients: A prospective exploratory study. *Palliat Med.* 2000; **14**(1): 19–23.

74. Casarett DJ, Inouye, SK. Diagnosis and management of delirium near the end of life. *Annal Intern Med* 2001; **135**(1): 32–40.

75. Freemon FR. Delirium and organic psychosis. In: *Organic Mental Disease.* Netherlands: Springer; 1981: 81–94.

76. Jackson KC, Jones L, Leurent B, et al. Drug therapy for delirium in terminally ill adult patients. *Cochrane Database Syst Rev.* 2012; **11**: CD004770. doi: 10.1002/14651858.

77. Grond S, Zech D, Schug SA, et al. Validation of the World Health Organization guidelines for cancer pain relief during the last days and hours of life. *J Pain Symptom Manage.* 1991; **6**: 411–422.

78. Thorns A, Sykes N. Opioid use in last week of life and implications for end-of-life decision-making. *The Lancet.* 2000; **356**(9227): 398–399.

79. Morita T, Tsunoda J, Inoue S, et al. *Effects of high dose opioids and sedatives on survival in terminally ill cancer patients. J Pain Symptom Manage.* 2001; **21**: 282–289.

80. Quill TE, Byock IR. Responding to intractable terminal suffering: the role of terminal sedation and voluntary refusal of food and fluids. *Annal Intern Med.* 2000; **132**(5): 408–414.

81. Sykes N, Thorns A. Sedative use in the last week of life and the implications for end-of-life decision making. *Arch Intern Med.* 2003; **163**(3): 341–344.

82. Post SG, Puchalski CM, Larson DB. Physicians and patient spirituality: Professional boundaries, competency, and ethics. *Ann Intern Med.* 2000; **132**: 578–583.

83. McClain CS, Rosenfeld B, Breitbart W. Effect of spiritual well-being on end-of-life despair in terminally-ill cancer patients. *The Lancet.* 2003; **361**(9369): 1603–1607.

84. Lo B, Quill T, Tulsky J. Discussing palliative care with patients. ACP-ASIM End-of-Life Care Consensus Panel. American College of Physicians–American Society of Internal Medicine. *Ann Intern Med.* 1999; **130**: 744–749.

85. Tomarken A, Holland J, Schachter S, et al. Factors of complicated grief pre-death in caregivers of cancer patients. *Psychooncology.* 2008; **17**(2): 105–111.

Chapter 50

The mistreatment of older adults

Laura Mosqueda, MD, and Elizabeth O'Toole, MSPH

Introduction

Elder mistreatment encompasses activities that include abuse, neglect, and exploitation of older adults. Although we know that it is a common and disturbing phenomenon, there is much we don't know. For example, there is a lack of agreement on terms: is it elder abuse or mistreatment of older adults? Do we call those who have been abused/mistreated victims or survivors? Do we call those who do the abuse stressed caregivers or perpetrators? One of the challenges for clinicians when confronted with this topic is in understanding the myriad of terms, types, contexts, systems, and people involved in this pervasive problem.

Elder mistreatment includes physical, sexual, or psychological abuse, as well as neglect, abandonment, and financial exploitation. It occurs in the context of a relationship in which there is an expectation of trust. Thus there are many categories of abusers: family members, paid caregivers, service providers, and others. A landmark report from the National Academies entitled *Elder Mistreatment: Abuse, Neglect, and Exploitation in an Aging America* was published in 2003.[1] This report stressed the importance of developing operational definitions in the context of research and we clearly need to do the same in the context of clinical practice. A good working definition is provided by the United States Department of Health and Human Services: "any knowing, intentional, or negligent act by a caregiver or any other person that causes harm or a serious risk of harm to a vulnerable adult."[2]

The breadth and depth of elder abuse

The statistics on elder abuse are sobering. Two national studies showed high rates of abuse in community-dwelling elders (i.e., they did not live in residential or licensed facilities). Acierno et al. conducted a national study of 5,777 community-residing adults aged 60 and older who had the capacity to consent and participate in a telephone interview. They found that 11.4% of respondents had experienced emotional, physical, or sexual abuse or potential neglect in the past year.[3] Prevalence rates within each category of abuse were 4.6% for emotional abuse, 1.6% for physical abuse, 0.6% for sexual abuse, 5.1% for potential neglect, and 5.2% for current financial abuse by a family member. The study's authors found that low social support significantly increased the risk for nearly all types of reported mistreatment.

Another national study, by Laumann and colleagues, looked at more than 3,000 community-dwelling elders between the ages of 57 and 85 years who had the capacity to give consent.[4] The instruments were administered by in-home interviewers or paper surveys that the participants filled out on their own. Although no formal cognitive testing was done, those who were deemed too impaired to give consent were excluded from the study. The past year prevalence rates of abuse were as follows: 9% verbal mistreatment, 3.5% financial mistreatment, and 0.2% physical mistreatment by a family member.

Studies that have specifically looked at abuse in minority communities also show alarmingly high rates of abuse and neglect. A study of Latino adults ($n = 198$) aged 66 and older living in low-income communities in the Los Angeles area found that 40.4% had experienced at least one type of abuse or neglect within the preceding year, with 21% reporting multiple types.[5] Door-to-door interviews were conducted by promotores, and all of the participants had capacity to provide their own consent. Of the respondents, 25% reported psychological abuse, 10.7%

Reichel's Care of the Elderly, 7th Edition, ed. Jan Busby-Whitehead *et al.* Published by Cambridge University Press.
© Cambridge University Press 2016.

physical abuse, 9% sexual abuse, 16.7% financial exploitation, and 11.7% caregiver neglect. According to Dong and colleagues, elder mistreatment was found in 15.0% of community-dwelling US Chinese older adults ($n = 3,159$) aged 60 and above in the Greater Chicago area.[6] Positive correlates included poorer overall health status, poorer quality of life, worsening health status over the past year, higher levels of education, and fewer children.

It is also of note that underreporting is a significant problem. The New York State Elder Abuse Prevalence Study found that the actual rate of abuse was nearly 24 times greater than the number reported to agencies such as Adult Protective Services.[7] Physicians are among the least likely people to make a report, even though we are mandated reporters in most states. A report based on analysis of a 2004 survey of Adult Protective Services agencies revealed that only 1.4% of abuse reports were from physicians.[8]

Why are older adults vulnerable to becoming victims?

There is good reason to consider elder abuse as its own special category in the spectrum of family violence. The normal and common changes that accompany aging create a new and special vulnerability to becoming victimized. These changes also mask and mimic markers of elder abuse, thus creating a conundrum: many injuries can be explained by innocent causes. For example, older adults bruise more easily due to thinning epidermis, capillary fragility and less subcutaneous fat. An older adult might also be on medications such as aspirin or warfarin which inhibit the coagulation pathway. It is then unsurprising when an elder appears in the office with bruising on the forearms or shins. However, one should ask questions if there are bruises in locations such as the upper arm, head, neck, or torso.[9] A simple "What caused you to have a bruise on your shoulder?" is a worthwhile question. Although people tend not to remember the cause of bruises in common locations, the clinician should expect to hear a reasonable explanation to understand why a bruise appeared in an unusual location. If the answer does not make sense, perhaps because it does not correspond with the location of the bruise, a further question such as "Has anyone hit you or treated you roughly?" should be asked.

Mrs. T comes into your office for a follow-up on her hypertension, atrial fibrillation, and diabetes (the HbA1c from two days prior was 8.9; her office blood pressure is 178/82 and heart rate is 80/min). She is on enalapril/hydrochlorothiazide, warfarin, and metformin. You, her primary health care provider, have known her for eight years, and in the past few months her previously well-controlled blood pressure and diabetes have been difficult to control. Today she has bruises on her left cheek, just in front of her ear, and on the right upper shoulder/base of the neck. You ask her how she got the bruises and she said, "I fell when I got up to go the bathroom in the middle of the night. You know me ... I bruise so easily! Next time I'll pay more attention and make sure I put a light on." You ask a follow-up question: "Mrs. T, I'm concerned because it's unusual to get a bruise on your head and neck from a fall such as this. I know there's been a lot of stress at home. Is anyone hurting you?" She breaks down in tears, explaining that her son moved in about six months ago and has been taking her money, first with her hesitating permission and now with impunity. More recently he has been physically threatening and two days ago, when he was inebriated, he grabbed her shoulder and hit her on the side of her face.

Had the clinician accepted her initial answer and not asked a follow-up question, the abuse would have likely continued and escalated. In fact, there are many examples of abuse that have been ongoing for months or years that, with the benefit of hindsight, reveal missed opportunities for intervention by medical providers.

Mrs. P is a 76-year-old woman with moderately advanced Parkinson's disease, poor vision, and diabetes. Her 51-year-old son lives with her because he was recently laid off and agreed to take on the role of caregiver as she needs an increasing amount of help with instrumental activities of daily living and activities of daily living. She had several falls in a six-month period and was noted to have bruises in many locations on her trunk and face. She was seen several times by her primary care doctor who accepted the idea that people with Parkinson's disease are likely to fall and never questioned her about the falls or her injuries. At the time of her hip fracture, it was learned that her son had been shoving her in anger and occasionally punching her if she asked for help at an inopportune time. This had been going on for the past eight months. She never told her doctor because "he never asked me."

Dementia and abuse

Cognitive changes create a special vulnerability to becoming victimized. We know that people with dementia are at significantly higher risk of being abused, yet we also understand that caregivers are often in difficult and demanding situations.[10, 11] For the person with dementia, however, abuse is abuse. The cause or motivation matters little.

Mr. J is an 86-year-old man with mild-to-moderate Alzheimer's disease. As it became unsafe for him to continue living independently, he was welcomed into the home of his son and daughter-in-law and their three children, aged 14–19 years. He had always been a fastidious person, but after the first few months of the move was often disheveled and unconcerned. When the family encouraged him to bathe, he would get angry and yell at them. They yelled back. When they tried to help him get undressed and put on clean clothes, he would resist their efforts and sometimes hit them. They hit him back.

This is a scenario that many of us have seen and understand. Despite our empathy and appreciation for what the family is trying to do with the best of intentions, this is still elder abuse. As we have learned from colleagues in domestic violence, it can be easy to blame the victim and thus miss our opportunity to protect and intervene. The fact that an older adult may be "difficult" or "hard to take care of" or "demanding" does not excuse an abusive act. It does, however, allow us to understand the dynamics and provide appropriate support for both the elder and the family. Asking questions at an early stage of this scenario could have allowed a clinician to identify the stress and anger that was brewing for the family.

There are some characteristics known to be associated with abuse of people with dementia. Recognizing these characteristics can help the clinician identify high-risk situations and prevent abuse or at least intervene at an early stage. People with dementia who have agitated, combative, resistive behaviors are more likely to be physically abused. Caregivers with mental health problems such as depression, anxiety, or substance abuse disorders are more likely to abuse. Those who have a higher perceived burden associated with their caregiving activity are also more likely to be abusive. The context in which the relationship exists is also important. For example, those who are socially isolated and/or have poor social support are more likely to be in an abusive relationship.

Mrs. U's three adult children (two daughters, one son) had been observing her memory problems for about a year. They had escalating concerns and brought her to the office for an assessment. In the past few months, she had two minor car accidents, gotten lost when walking in her neighborhood, and put a paper plate on top of the gas stove to heat a meal, which started a kitchen fire that was quickly extinguished by her visiting son. A thorough examination by an interdisciplinary team resulted in a diagnosis of probable Alzheimer's disease. At the time of the family conference, the psychologist and physician assistant explained the diagnosis to the family and discussed prognosis and the need for more assistance. Concerns regarding her behaviors, which included agitation especially when trying to convince/help her get into clean clothes, and a volatile temper, were discussed. The family explained that they had discussed some of these issues and had an idea: one of the daughters volunteered to move in with mom. She didn't work, was unmarried, and had no children. Further inquiry about this 42-year-old daughter revealed that she has bipolar disorder, which has been adequately treated for a few months. She has a long history of cyclical problems related to going on and off her medications. Knowing that the equation of a daughter with poorly controlled bipolar illness plus a demented mother with agitation could add up to an abusive situation, the team explained that it would be best to work on an alternate plan. The social worker provided counseling and assistance with the alternatives, and a high-risk-for-abuse situation was avoided.

Two studies, one in the United Kingdom and one in the United States, on abuse of community-dwelling dyads of people with dementia and their caregivers showed remarkably similar results. In interviews of 220 caregivers of people with dementia in the United Kingdom, Cooper et al. found that 52% reported some type of abusive behavior had ever occurred.[10] When asked specifically about the preceding 3 months, 34% reported abusive behavior toward the person with dementia. In the United States, Wiglesworth et al. studied a convenience sample of community-living adults ($n = 129$) aged 50 and older with a diagnosis of Alzheimer's disease or a related dementia and an adult caregiver willing to participate in the research.[11] Home interviews were conducted with caregiver-care recipient dyads and an expert panel made a determination about mistreatment of the care recipient. The study authors found that 47.3% had been mistreated and of these respondents, 88.5% experienced psychological abuse, 19.7% physical abuse, and 9.5% neglect. The caregiver's anxiety, depressive symptoms, social contacts, perceived burden, emotional status, and role limitations due to emotional problems were associated with different kinds and combinations of mistreatment types. The care recipient's psychological aggression and physical assault behaviors were also associated with mistreatment. Importantly, the study authors also concluded that caregivers of patients with dementia would admit to mistreatment when asked. This last finding is of particular relevance to clinicians and shows us that caregivers can and should be asked about being abusive to the person with dementia.

The fact that a primary care clinician often has a longstanding relationship with the family makes it even more important for clinicians to routinely ask caregivers about abuse. Ask in a way that is empathetic, straightforward, and clear: "I see that this is a very difficult situation for you. Many people in your shoes feel overwhelmed and end up doing things they wouldn't normally do. Have you ever hit your mother, or are you worried that you might?"

Inquiring about mistreatment

Knowing that elder abuse is a common and underreported phenomenon, it behooves the clinician to incorporate questions about abuse as a routine part of our practice. Even when there are no markers of abuse, questions such as "Are you afraid of anybody?" and "Is anybody using your money without your permission?" are reasonable ways to detect abuse and to open a dialogue with an elder that indicates it is both safe and appropriate to talk about this with you.

The assumptions made by a clinician influence the way our patients answer questions.

Mrs. O: My grandson is moving in with me next week.

Dr. M: That's very nice!

Mrs. O: Yes, doctor, it will be very nice.

If the clinician's response is more neutral, the patient may feel empowered and less embarrassed to provide a realistic glimpse into her situation:

Mrs. O: My grandson is moving in with me next week.

Dr. M: That's interesting. What do you think about that?

Mrs. O: Well ... actually I'm kind of worried. He is getting out of jail and has nowhere else to live, so I *agreed he could stay with me for a while. The last time he stayed with me, he took my ATM card and got over a thousand dollars from my account. I'm worried that he'll do that again.*

A small shift in what we ask and how we ask our patients about their home situation will provide information that may save their bank accounts, well-being, and even their lives.

Capacity

One of the most common types of elder mistreatment is financial abuse. In the majority of cases the elder's capacity to make a decision is in question. All of us have a right to make a bad decision, so at what point does one transition from the right to have autonomy to the need to be protected?

The ability to make a decision is rarely an all-or-none phenomenon. In the early stages of an illness such as Alzheimer's disease, a person may lack capacity to make decisions regarding complicated financial transactions that have important consequences, such as transfer of property, but may retain capacity to make other decisions with important consequences, such as where they want to live. Clinicians should be cautious when asked by family members or others to provide written statements that trigger the use of powers of attorney or to complete forms that declare a person to be incapacitated. Although this may be done in the spirit of helping a stressed family member, the request may signal the reemergence of a simmering family conflict or even nefarious conduct.

You are the primary care provider for Mr. B, an 86-year-old man with early Alzheimer's disease whom you have known for 11 years. As his cognition has steadily declined, his daughter Lynn has become more involved in his life. She drives him to appointments and accompanies him in the office, which he welcomes and appreciates. As you get to know her, Lynn seems respectful, appropriate, and loving. You are aware that there are two other children, a son who lives an hour away and a daughter who lives on the other side of the country. One day Mr. B tells you that he wants to transfer title on his house to Lynn and have her take over the supervision of his bank accounts. Lynn asks you to sign a form that she can take to the bank which states her father is too impaired to handle his accounts and that he wants her to assume control. He concurs that this is what he wants to do and asks for your help. You perform the Montreal Cognitive Assessment (MoCA) and find that Mr. B scores 17, indicating he's on the border of mild/moderate impairment. He has difficulty with delayed recall, abstraction, and the clock draw (an indicator of executive function), so it seems reasonable to comply with the daughter's request.

Brief mental status examinations used by primary care providers deliver helpful information when assessing cognition and diagnosing impairment but rarely are the sole determinant of one's capacity to make a decision. Geropsychologists and neuropsychologists utilize lengthy standardized tests to assess many domains of cognition. They measure and compare the elder's performance against others of similar age, education, and (sometimes) culture. In addition to assessing domains such as memory, language, intelligence, and personality, these specialized psychologists measure executive function (i.e., those abilities that are critically important to high-level decision making). Capacity assessments help both to make a determination regarding abuse potential and to assist with appropriate services and support that may help the older adult remain reasonably safe in the environment of their choosing. These psychologists will contact family members to help gain an understanding of the dynamics that may be influencing the decision.

The daughter is unhappy when you refer Mr. B to a geropsychologist rather than acquiescing to her request at the time of the visit. "I don't understand why you won't help us. You know how busy I am, and this is just an unnecessary roadblock." You insist, silently noting her strenuous objections are cause for concern. The geropsychologist performs a standardized battery of cognitive tests and obtains collateral information from all of his children. Using the framework for capacity assessment endorsed by the American Bar Association and the American Psychological Association,[12] she finds that Mr. B is significantly impaired in multiple domains. When she contacts his other two children, they are alarmed by Lynn's plan and say that Lynn has been making it harder and harder for them to see their dad or talk to him on the phone. She frequently tells them he doesn't want to talk or is taking a nap. The geropsychologist finds that Mr. B is vulnerable to undue influence; Lynn has been isolating him and telling him that the other children never call and that she is the one who will always be there for him. The testing confirms that he lacks the ability to make most financial decisions.

When the other children regain connections with their father, they learn that Lynn spent over $100,000 of his savings on purchases for herself during the past year.

In this case, the primary care provider's insistence on further testing and analysis identified a case of financial abuse and stimulated protection for Mr. B's remaining assets.

Systems and reporting

In the United States, state laws vary relating to elder abuse, neglect, and financial exploitation, so it is important to refer to the laws applicable in your state of practice. Helpful resources include the National Center on Elder Abuse's "State Resources" webpage, [13] the American Bar Association's Commission on Law and Aging,[14] and the National Adult Protective Services Association (NAPSA) "Help in Your Area" webpage.[15] For state regulations regarding nursing homes, visit the University of Minnesota's "Nursing Home Regulations Plus" website.[16]

In most states in the United States, health care providers are mandated to report any suspicion of elder abuse, neglect, or exploitation. The clinician does not need to investigate or be certain that abuse has occurred; if a reasonable suspicion is present, there is a duty to report. For suspicion of abuse in the community setting, Adult Protective Services (APS) is the agency to which a report is made. Although there is variability regarding the configuration and composition of the agency depending on local factors, APS is the investigatory, protective, and social services agency that is charged with serving elders who may have been abused or neglected in the community. As each state has its own definition regarding who is a mandated reporter and what is a mandated report, it is important for the clinician to know the state, tribal, and territorial requirements in the area where you practice.

In the United States, a separate system is in place for reporting suspected abuse in licensed facilities. The Long-Term Care Ombudsman is the agency that receives these reports. If there is a reasonable suspicion of abuse in a nursing home, board and care facility, or assisted living facility, the local Ombudsman office should be contacted. Although the contact information should be posted in a clearly visible location in every facility, one can also visit the National Consumer Voice for Long-Term Care's website to locate an ombudsman in your area.[17]

In the rare instance that an older adult's safety is at immediate risk and/or you believe a crime has occurred, call 911 or your local law enforcement agency (i.e., police, sheriff, or other peace officers). Document any quotes, injuries, and behaviors along with the reasons for your concerns and write a clear statement diagnosing abuse or neglect in your assessment.

Conclusion

An astute clinician has the ability to prevent and intervene in cases of elder abuse. This can only be done if the possibility of elder mistreatment is unfailingly on the differential diagnosis in many circumstances. The elder who has frequent falls, injuries, a sudden change in behavior or demeanor, who starts missing appointments, or who is not taking medications as expected – all of these may be indicators of mistreatment. Although we do not want to accuse unfairly, it is important that we ask questions when a suspicious injury or event occurs and then assess whether the response is appropriate and believable. Our patients may have no one else who will look, ask, and listen with compassion, and who will have the skill and knowledge to make a diagnosis that ends up preserving their health and well-being and, perhaps, saving their lives.

References

1. National Research Council. *Elder mistreatment: Abuse, neglect, and exploitation in an aging America.* Washington, DC: The National Academics Press; 2003.

2. United States Department of Health and Human Services; 2014. How can I recognize elder abuse? Available from: www.hhs.gov/answers/programs-families-children/prevent-abuse/recognize-elder-abuse.html (accessed December 10, 2014).

3. Acierno R, Hernandez, MA, Amstadter B, et al. Prevalence and correlates of emotional, physical, sexual, and financial abuse and potential neglect in the United States: The national elder mistreatment study. *Am J Public Health* 2010; **100**: 292–7.

4. Laumann EO, Leitsch SA, Waite LJ. Elder mistreatment in the United States: Prevalence estimates from a nationally representative study. *J Gerontol B Psychol Sci Soc Sci* 2008; **63**: S248–S254.

5. DeLiema M, Gassoumis ZD, Homeier DC, Wilber KH. Determining prevalence and correlates of elder abuse using promotores: low-income immigrant Latinos report high rates of abuse and neglect. *J Am Geriatr Soc* 2012; **60**: 1333–9.

6. Dong X, Chen R, Fulmer T, Simon MA. Prevalence and correlates of elder mistreatment in a community-dwelling population of U.S. Chinese older adults. *J Aging Health* 2014; **26**: 1209–24.

7. Lifespan of Greater Rochester, Inc., Weill Cornell Medical Center of Cornell University & New York City Department for the Aging. Under the Radar: New York State Elder Abuse Prevalence Study. 2011. Available from: www.nyselderabuse.org/documents/ElderAbuse PrevalenceStudy2011.pdf (accessed December 10, 2014).

8. The National Committee for the Prevention of Elder Abuse and The National Adult Protective Services Association. *The 2004 Survey of State Adult Protective Services: Abuse of adults 60 years of age and older report.* Washington, DC: National Center on Elder Abuse; 2006 Feb 45 p. Available from: www.napsa-now.org/wp-content/uploads/2012/09/2–14-06-FINAL-60+RE PORT.pdf.

9. Wiglesworth A, Austin R, Corona M, et al. Bruising as a marker of physical elder abuse. *J Am Geriatr Soc* 2009; **57**: 1191–6.

10. Cooper C, Selwood A, Blanchard M, et al. Abuse of people with dementia by family carers: Representative cross-sectional survey. *BMJ* 2009; **338**: b155.

11. Wiglesworth A, Mosqueda L, Mulnard R, et al. Screening for abuse and neglect of people with dementia. *J Am Geriatr Soc* 2010; **58**: 493–500.

12. American Bar Association Commission on Law and Aging and American Psychological Association. Assessment of older adults with diminished capacity: A handbook for psychologists. 2008. Available from: www.apa.org/pi/aging/programs/assessment/capacity-psychologist-handbook.pdf (accessed December 10, 2014).

13. National Center on Elder Abuse. State resources [Internet]. 2014. Available from: www.ncea.aoa.gov/Stop_Abuse/Get_Help/State/index.aspx (accessed December 10, 2014).

14. American Bar Association. Commission on Law and Aging [Internet]. 2014. Available from: www.americanbar.org/groups/law_aging.html (accessed December 10, 2014).

15. National Adult Protective Services Association. Get help in your area [Internet]. 2014. Available from: www.napsa-now.org/get-help/help-in-your-area (accessed December 10, 2014).

16. University of Minnesota. NH Regulations Plus [Internet]. 2013. Available from: www.hpm.umn.edu/NHRegsPlus (accessed December 10, 2014).

17. The National Consumer Voice for Long-Term Care. Locate an ombudsman. 2014. Available from: http://theconsumervoice.org/get_help (accessed December 10, 2014).

Driving and the older adult

David B. Carr, MD, Joanne G. Schwartzberg, MD, and Alice K. Pomidor, MD, MPH, AGSF

Introduction

Driving is an essential instrumental activity of daily living, but it becomes increasingly difficult to maintain with age-related comorbid medical conditions. Prevention, detection, and treatment of impaired driving ability may be challenging due to multiple comorbid illnesses, polypharmacy, unfamiliarity with assessment techniques, and time constraints. Clinicians may be reluctant to address this issue due to the potential impact on the relationship with the patient and legal/ethical concerns. However, assessment and intervention are important to prevent injury and the potential loss of driving privileges, the latter which may have a negative impact on quality of life.

Driving characteristics

There are more than 30 million drivers over the age of 65 in the United States, and approximately 200,000 are injured in motor vehicle crashes each year.[1] A total of 4,079 people aged 70 and older died in motor vehicle crashes in 2012.[2] There is an excess risk of injury and death in older adult motor vehicle crashes in comparison to middle-aged drivers possibly a result from older adults' fragility, limited physiologic reserves, and greater susceptibility to impact based on the types of crashes.

The number of older adults in the United States is expected to double within the next 40 years, resulting in a dramatic increase in the number of older adult drivers and average miles driven per year.[3, 4] The average older adult over age 70 years has approximately 11 years left to drive a car, and approximately 25% of drivers will be over age 65 by the year 2030.[5] It is essential to help older adults drive safely for as long as possible and, when necessary, determine satisfactory alternative means of transportation.

Even though many older persons self-restrict their driving to compensate for age-related changes and disease,[6, 7] crash rates per mile traveled start increasing for drivers 75 and older and increase markedly after age 80. Increased crash rates per mile traveled may be inflated since older driver mileage is more frequently city driving, which typically has higher crash rates than freeway driving.[8] Most traffic fatalities involving older drivers in 2005 occurred during the daytime (79%), on weekdays (73%), and involved other vehicles (73%). In two-vehicle fatal crashes involving an older driver and a younger driver, the vehicle driven by the older person was nearly twice as likely to be the one that was struck (60% vs. 33%, respectively).

Functional changes and medical risk factors

Functional abilities essential for driving can decline due to normal physiologic changes of aging, increased comorbid illness, or both.[9] Impairments in vision, neuromuscular strength and speed, cognitive function, and select medical conditions have been linked to crash risk for older adults.[10] Diseases such as cataracts, glaucoma, and maculopathy are the most prevalent visual concerns for older adults and the subsequent loss of contrast sensitivity, impaired visual fields, or impaired peripheral detection have all been noted to be associated with impaired driving.[11–13] These diseases can diminish useful field of view (UFOV), a measure of selective and divided attention that evaluates the visual area where information can be acquired in a brief glance without eye or head movements. Computerized UFOV testing measures the ability to identify objects and pay attention to them, as opposed to simple confrontational visual

Reichel's Care of the Elderly, *7th Edition*, ed. Jan Busby-Whitehead *et al.* Published by Cambridge University Press.
© Cambridge University Press 2016.

Table 51.1 Medications associated with crash risk

Alcohol
Muscle relaxants
Antidepressants
Benzodiazepines
Nonsteroidal anti-inflammatory drugs
Opioid analgesics
Sedating antihistamines

Table 51.2 Medical risk factors for driving

Chronic diseases	Acute illness
Vision	Stroke or transient
Glaucoma	ischemic attack
Macular degeneration	Brain injury
Cataracts	Alcohol
Diabetic retinopathy	Spinal cord
Cognitive	Hypoclycemia
Dementia	Syncope
CNS sedating medications	
Multiple sclerosis	
Depression	
Psychosis	
Parkinson's disease	
Motor	
Osteoarthritis	
Myopathy	
Falls	
Amputation	

field testing. Evaluating UFOV impairment appears to be much more accurate than static visual acuity in predicting crash risk: a 40% decline more than doubles the likelihood of a crash.[14, 15] More recently, this test has been adopted by PositScience and marketed as a tool to improve reaction time and reduce crash risk.[16] Neuromuscular factors such as reduced neck rotation, slowed foot reaction time, an orthostatic drop in blood pressure, and the history of a fall in the past year have all been shown to increase crash risk, particularly in women.[17–19]

Use of certain medications is also linked to increased risk, including benzodiazepines, opioid analgesics, alcohol, muscle relaxants, sedating antihistamines, and nonsteroidal anti-inflammatory drugs (Table 51.1).[20] Depression and the use of antidepressant medications may also impair driving performance in older populations.[21] In a sample of patients referred for medical fitness to drive, those that failed a road test were more likely to have polypharmacy and higher ratings of daytime drowsiness on the Epworth Sleepiness Scale (ESS),[22] a screen that has been linked to motor vehicle crash risk.[11]

Many medical conditions associated with impaired driving performance have been the subject of recent reviews (Table 51.2) [23, 24] and have been associated with increased crash risk.[25] Medical illnesses and treatments which may be linked to driving difficulty in self-report, case-control, and retrospective population studies include a history of falls, coronary artery disease, stroke or transient ischemic attack, kidney disease, and – in women – arthritis. [26–28] Since the odds ratios for crash prediction from a single medical condition are small, several guides have been developed to assist clinicians with determining the functional impact of medical conditions on driving ability.[29–31] These

recommendations are usually based on clinical consensus, clinical experience, expert medical opinion, or best practices even though the evidence may be limited. Cases of multiple comorbidities and polypharmacy make evaluation extremely difficult.

Alzheimer's dementia and Parkinson's disease have been linked to lower driving performance and greater crash risk due to their adverse impact on cognitive skills, including memory, visual-spatial skills, attention, reaction time, processing speed, and executive function.[32–35] The consensus among several professional organizations is that persons with moderate to severe dementia should stop driving.[36, 37] Two evidence-based recent reviews in the literature propose algorithms based on the recent evidence which may be useful to the clinician in managing and assessing older adults with dementia who would like to continue to drive.[38, 39] These approaches include rating dementia severity, assessing functional status, obtaining a driving history, and focused physical examination and referral when appropriate. Additional driving simulator or on-the-road assessments are likely to be needed.[40–42]

Driving assessment

The American Medical Association (AMA), in collaboration with the National Highway Safety Transportation Administration (NHTSA), created an advisory panel which developed the *Physician's Guide to Assessing and Counseling Older Drivers*, in

Table 51.3 Driving history red flags

Acute or unstable medical events: acute myocardial infarction, angina, hypoglycemia, stroke or transient ischemic attack, traumatic brain injury, syncope, vertigo, seizure, surgery, delirium, sleep apnea

Any expression of concern: about driving safety, from patient or caregiver

Medications: any psychoactive, cardiovascular, neurologic, or potentially sedating agents

Chronic medical conditions:

Vision – field cuts, cataracts, glaucoma, macular degeneration, hypertensive or diabetic retinopathy, retinitis pigmentosa

Cardiovascular disease – unstable angina, arrhythmia, valvular disease, congestive heart failure

Neurologic disease – dementia, Parkinson's disease, multiple sclerosis, peripheral neuropathy, stroke

Psychiatric disease – depression, anxiety, psychosis, alcohol or substance abuse

Musculoskeletal disability – arthritis, foot abnormalities, previous fractures, cervical disease

Respiratory disease – obstructive sleep apnea, chronic obstructive pulmonary disease, asthma, disease requiring oxygen supplementation on a daily basis

Metabolic disease – diabetes, renal failure, thyroid disease

2003 [43], updated in 2010 and revised in 2016.[29] Some studies suggest the Assessing Driving Related Skills (ADReS) battery of tests from the guide (see Figure 51.1) may be helpful in identifying unsafe drivers, although not all.[44–46] Several studies have shown that clinicians exposed to this curriculum revealed changes in knowledge, confidence, attitudes, and behavior.[47, 48] Canada (CanDRIVE) and individual expert authors have also released recommendations and protocols for driving evaluations.[49–51]

History

The first step of a medical assessment for driving ability is a targeted history. Be alert for acute and chronic medical conditions, medications or symptoms that may impair driving skills when taking the patient's history (Table 51.3). These "red flags" deserve further evaluation and follow-up.[29]

A general driving history should include questions such as those noted in Tables 51.4 and 51.5, which give the patient and caregiver the opportunity to express concerns that might otherwise be too embarrassing to discuss or which might be forgotten. Some providers may wish to provide these questions or use the *Physician's Guide to Assessing and Counseling Older Drivers* questionnaire "Am I a Safe Driver?" as a written handout for self-evaluation prior to initiating an assessment.[29] There are additional questionnaires available

that are recommended by expert consensus such as the those available online from the Hartford Guide [52, 53] and the Alzheimer's Association. However, it should be noted that few of these questionaires, except possibly the Driving Behavior Questionnaire,[54] have been validated in the literature as an effective method of identifying unsafe drivers.

Targeted physical examination

In addition to the general physical exam maneuvers needed to investigate any positive history items found above, the *Physician's Guide to Assessing and Counseling Older Drivers* recommends special items recorded on their Assessment of Driving-Related Skills (ADReS-Figure 51.1) to evaluate vision, motor, and cognitive function.

Far visual acuity should be assessed with the traditional Snellen E chart and visual fields can be checked by confrontation testing. Motor function is gauged through assessments of walking, range of motion, and strength. The rapid-pace walk is based on the time (in seconds) it takes the patient to walk a 10-foot path, turn around, and return with a score of 10 seconds or longer scored as abnormal. Range of motion testing using normative tables and/or a goniometer and manual motor strength testing (using a 0–5 scale) are also assessed.

Cognitive screening is performed in part using the clock-drawing test (CDT), where the patient is verbally

693

Table 51.4 Patient driving history questions

1. Do you now drive a car?
2. How many days did you drive this past week?
3. Have you noticed any change in your driving habits in the past year? Please check all that apply.

   _____Do not drive at night.
   _____Do not drive on freeways.
   _____Do not drive in rain/snow, bad weather.
   _____Do not drive during rush hour.
   _____Do not drive as far.
   _____Only drive when I absolutely must.
   _____Prefer for others to drive.
   _____Have cut back because of being too sick/tired.

4. In the past year, have you had any of the following events? Please check all that apply.

   _____Accidents
   _____Fender-benders
   _____Near-misses
   _____Tickets
   _____Discussions/warnings

5. Have you ever forgotten where you were going?
6. Do others honk at you or act irritated?
7. Have you ever gotten lost while driving?
8. Have others said they are worried about your driving, criticized you, or refused to ride with you?

Table 51.5 Caregiver driving history questions

1. Does the patient drive?
2. Have you noticed any unsafe driving?
3. Do you feel uncomfortable riding with the patient?
4. Has the patient gotten lost?
5. Does the patient rely on a co-pilot?
6. Does the patient rely on passengers?
7. Do others worry about the patient's driving?
8. Does the patient forget where they are going?
9. Do others have to drive defensively?
10. Have others refused to ride with the patient?
11. Has the patient changed their driving habits?
12. In the past year, has the patient had any of the following? Please check all that apply.

    _____ Accidents
    _____ Fender-benders
    _____ Near-misses
    _____ Tickets
    _____ Discussions/warnings

instructed to draw the face of a clock and to place the hands at 10 minutes past 11 using a blank sheet of paper and a pencil (see Table 51.1).[55] Memory, visual spatial skills, attention, and executive skills are some of the cognitive domains that are tapped during the clock drawing task. Greater than two errors on the CDT is associated with unsafe driving behaviors based on driving simulation performance.[55] The Trail Making Test part B is also recommended, with a time for performance over 180 seconds considered abnormal and meriting intervention. Patients are asked to connect dots in a path in sequence that alternates between numbers and letters, such as "1-A-2-B." Poor performance has been prospectively linked to crash risk in two studies of older adults who came in for their license renewals.[43, 45] A recent review also noted that there was a strong association with Trail Making B and road test performance validating the 3-or-3 rule (180 second cut-off or three errors).[56] The Trail Making B form and directions for its use are available for free in the *Clinician's Guide to Assessing and Counseling Older Drivers, 3rd Edition* which can be downloaded from the NHTSA website.[29]

Interventions

Driving self-assessment and education programs as a prevention strategy

The *Driving Decisions Workbook* is a self-assessment instrument designed to include medical content, and

Patient's Name: _____ Date: _____

1. **Visual fields:** Shade in any areas of deficit.

Patient's R   **L**

2. **Visual acuity:** _____ OU
Was the patient wearing corrective lenses? If yes, please specify:
_____

3. **Rapid pace walk:** _____ seconds
Was this perfomed with a walker or cane? If yes, please specify:
_____

4. **Range of motion:** Specify 'Within Normal Limits' or 'Not WNL.' If not WNL, describe.

	Right	**Left**
Neck rotation		
Finger curl		
Shoulder and elbow flexion		
Ankle plantar flexion		
Ankle dorsiflexion		

5. **Motor strength:** Provide a score on a scale of 0-5.

	Right	**Left**
Shoulder adduction		
Shoulder abduction		
Shoulder flexion		
Wrist flexion		
Wrist extension		
Hand grip		
Hip flexion		
Hip extension		
Ankle dorsiflexion		
Ankle plantar flexion		

6. **Trail-Making Test, Part B:** _____ seconds

7. **Clock drawing test:** Please check 'yes' or 'no' to the following criteria.

	Yes	No
All 12 hours are placed in correct numeric order, starting with 12 at the top		
Only the numbers 1-12 are included (no duplicates, omissions, or foreign marks)		
The numbers are drawn inside the clock circle		
The numbers are spaced equally or nearly equally from each other		
The numbers are spaced equally or nearly equally from the edge of the circle		
One clock hand correctly points to two o'clock		
The other hand correctly points to eleven o'clock		
There are only two clock hands		

Figure 51.1 Assessment of driving-related skills (ADReS).

Trail-Making Test, Part B
Patient's Name: _____ Date _____

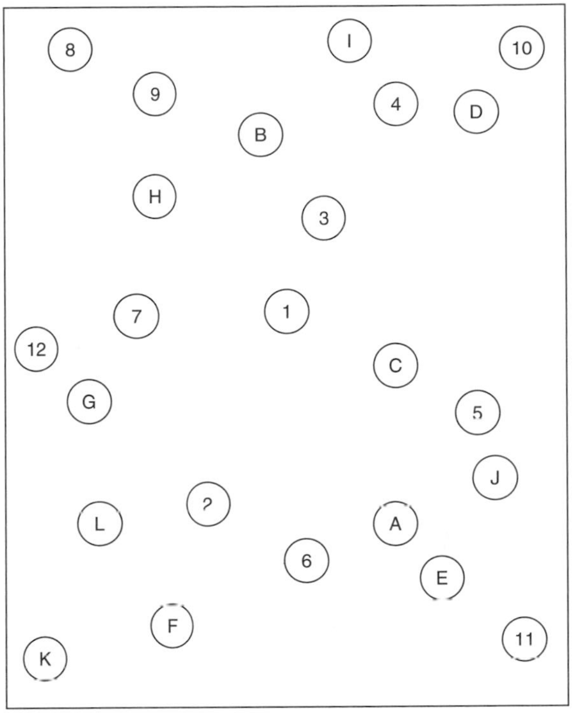

Figure 51.2 Trail Making Test B.

it has been studied against road test outcomes.[57] Health-care clinicians can recommend driving refresher courses, driving self-assessment, and self-education programs that include the Automobile Association of America's SeniorDriver program,[58] and the AARP Driver Safety Program.[59] A feature of the AAA program is the Roadwise Review,[60] a CD-ROM or online computer-based home assessment program that includes assessment of leg strength and general mobility, head/neck flexibility, high- and low-contrast visual acuity, working memory, visualization of missing information, visual search, and UFOV. AAA also offers a program to review medications that have the potential to impair driving,[61] in addition to DriveSharp,[16] a CD-ROM or online program to improve visual search and reaction time. ADEPT (Accurate Drivers Education and Professional Training) driver also offers a CD-ROM program to improve traffic safety awareness in older adults.[62] All of these programs could benefit by further validation to determine their efficacy to reduce crash risk.

Referral

Clinicians should try to minimize or compensate for the presence of impairments, so that the patient may continue to drive safely. Additional clinicians who may assist the primary care clinician in assessment of driving skills include ophthalmologists, neurologists, psychiatrists, neuropsychologists, and physical therapists. If the patient's deficits cannot be medically

Table 51.6 Older driver resources

1. Consider driving (function) in the context of your patient with medical illness(es)
   - Older Driver curriculum on AGS website http://geriatricscareonline.org/events/free-product-now-available-the-clinicians-guide-to-assessing-and-counseling-older-drivers/61
   - CMA fitness to drive www.cma.ca/En/Pages/drivers-guide.aspx
   - Austroads fitness to drive www.onlinepublications.austroads.com.au/items/AP-G56-13

2. For difficult cases, consider referring to a driving rehabilitation specialist
   - American Occupational Therapy Association http://myaota.aota.org/driver_search/index.aspx
   - Association of Driver Rehabilitation Specialists: ADED http://aded.site-ym.com/search/custom.asp?id=1984

3. For refractory cases, consider referral to your state licensing authority
   - Know the laws in your state www.iihs.org/iihs/topics/laws/olderdrivers?topicName=older-drivers

4. Consider Web resources and/or office handouts
   - We Need to Talk and at the Crossroads www.thehartford.com/mature-market-excellence/publications-on-aging
   - Alzheimer's Association: Dementia and Driving Resource Center http://www.alz.org/care/alzheimers-dementia-and-driving.asp

5. Self-help assessment or education
   - AAA SeniorDriving products http://seniordriving.aaa.com
   - DriveSharp from Posit Science www.drivesharp.com/aaaf/index
   - AARP traffic safety course www.aarpdriversafety.org
   - CogniFit senior driver https://www.cognifit.com/
   - ADEPT lifelong driver www.adeptdriver.com/products/lifelong-driver

6. Transportation alternatives
   - Social workers or local area on aging http://www.eldercare.gov/Eldercare.NET/Public/Index.aspx

7. Office tools
   - Driving health inventory http://drivinghealth.com/screeningassessment.html
   - DriveABLE www.driveable.com

corrected and do not have further potential for improvement with medical intervention, referral to a driver rehabilitation specialist (DRS) may be necessary. A DRS is often an occupational therapist who undergoes additional training in driver rehabilitation. A DRS should be able to do either driving simulation and/or on-road performance-based testing to specifically determine the patient's level of driving safety. In addition, the DRS may be able to suggest adaptive equipment (e.g., spinner nob, enlarged side view mirrors, hand controls, left foot accelerator) or training techniques (e.g., enhanced visual search in patients with visual field cuts). A list of certified driver rehabilitation specialists can be obtained from the Association for Driver Rehabilitation Specialists. Patients and health-care providers need to be aware, however, that DRS services are often not covered by health insurance other than state worker compensation and vocational rehabilitation programs.

Also, DRS specialists are often located in urban areas, which may impede referral from rural locations. A local driving school referral or driver education specialist may not be the equivalent of a medical DRS specialist, but may be helpful in the absence of these resources. Health-care clinicians may be called upon to document and verify the presence of impairment to help obtain access and financial support for adaptive equipment, driving rehabilitation, or restricted driving privileges. A list of resources for driving interventions and referrals is listed in Table 51.6.

Driving cessation

Clinicians should try to limit the adverse consequences for the patient if loss of the ability to drive cannot be prevented, and the patient must stop driving entirely – a circumstance termed driving retirement or cessation. Similarly to work retirement, helping the patient to plan in advance by discussing the eventual need for driving cessation can minimize negative effects and facilitate a smooth transition. The multiple adverse consequences of driving cessation for older adults are well documented and include depression, dependency, caregiver strain, social withdrawal, increased risk of entry into long-term care facilities, and restricted mobility.[63–69]

The health-care clinician's recommendation for driving retirement should emphasize concern for the patient's safety and the safety of others as the primary reason for driving retirement. Even so, many patients are understandably upset or angry upon receiving the recommendation, and in the case of cognitive impairment, some may lack the insight necessary to understand the consequences. In addition to allowing adequate time for discussion, it may be helpful to reinforce the recommendation by asking the patient to repeat back to you the reasons for driving retirement, to provide a prescription on which "Do Not Drive" is written, and to help the patient create a plan for alternative transportation. Some patients may also benefit from identifying peer driver behaviors that they consider to be unsafe, and using those examples to set their own threshold for when they would consider themselves unsafe to drive. Identifying a trusted friend or family member whose opinion is honored by the impaired driver may also help to support the recommendation. Keep in mind that a spouse who depends on the patient for transportation may find it difficult to support a recommendation for driving retirement. If the clinician does not have the time or expertise to address this important aspect, then referral to a social worker or gerontological care manager should be considered.

A follow-up letter documenting the recommendation for driving retirement should be sent to the patient, and – if the patient consents – to involved family members. A copy should also be kept in the chart for documentation. Referral to the state department of motor vehicles can be considered in refractory cases.

Clinicians should attempt to see their patients for whom driving is no longer possible soon after driving retirement, both to monitor for compliance with the recommendation to stop driving, and also to check for signs and symptoms of depression and anxiety. Extra care should be taken to assure that travel can be arranged for those who may have difficulty obtaining food, medications, and medical office visits. Finding alternative means of transportation is difficult for older adults, in both rural and metropolitan settings that lack well-developed systems of mass transportation that can accommodate frail older adults. The burden of meeting transportation needs will mostly likely fall on family, friends, and neighbors, some of whom may also suffer from undiagnosed driving impairment. Social agency and volunteer organization referrals for meeting transportation needs are an important part of the patient care plan for driving retirement, often beginning with the area agency on aging.[30] For patients who lack capacity and insight, it is essential for the appointed guardian or caregiver to help the patient comply with the recommendation to stop driving. Many strategies have been employed from placing reminder signage on doors to removing the vehicle altogether.

Legal and ethical issues

The AMA's official ethical opinion E-2.24 regarding impaired drivers and their physicians as issued in June of 2000 lists many of the issues faced by health-care clinicians who find themselves caring for older adult drivers. In particular, clinicians often find themselves in an ethical conflict between the standard of patient confidentiality and the duty to protect public safety. Many primary care clinicians may also be reluctant to report impaired drivers to their local drivers licensing authority for fear of jeopardizing their relationship with the patient. However, this concern must be weighed against state requirements for reporting unsafe drivers. It is essential for providers to know and comply with their state's reporting laws and to document all activities in the patient's chart. All conversations and efforts to communicate with the patient and caregiver, recommendations, referrals for further testing, direct observations, counseling, formal assessment, medical interventions, patient education handouts, and referral reports related to your recommendations regarding driving should be clearly documented, and copies should be kept in the patient's chart for future reference and possible protection in the event of third-party litigation. Policies in clinics regarding referral to the state should include consideration of obtaining local legal advice.

697

It is important to keep in mind that the health-care clinician cannot suspend or remove the right to drive. Only the state department of motor vehicles has the authority to perform a legal action regarding licensure. Requirements and reporting laws can be found at the Insurance Institute for Highway Safety (www.iihs.org/iihs/topics/laws/olderdrivers).

For the health-care clinician, the detection, prevention and treatment of driving impairment captures the classic problem of the needs and priorities of the individual versus the needs and priorities of society. The clinician must help to negotiate a delicate balance between the two.

Conclusion

There will be more older adult drivers over the next few decades and the majority will be safe based on overall crash statistics. However, clinicians will be faced with both acute and chronic medical conditions that impact driving in older adult patients and/or hasten driving retirement. Clinicians need to know the evidenced-based assessment tools and steps in the evaluation and management process.

In summary, here are the key points of this chapter.

- There will be more medically impaired drivers over the next few decades.
- Older adults are at increased risk for a crash based on exposure or miles driven and are at increased risk of a motor vehicle injury and death when compared to middle aged adults.
- Clinicians should consider driving as a key activity of daily living task and similar to falls, and thus realize that they can play an important role in the assessment and management of personal and public safety.
- Clinicians should know the evidence-based tools and steps in the evaluation of driving abilities and in counseling driving remediation or retirement.
- There are other health professionals that may be able to assist in driving assessment and/or remediation including driving rehabilitation specialists.
- Online/CD/DVD/classroom educational offerings for older adult drivers remain promising methods to maintain and/or improve driving skills, but they are in need of further evidence.
- Most older adults spend about seven to eight years without the ability to drive a car, and clinicians can

provide resources or referrals to social workers/ gerontological care managers to assist with alternate transportation.

References

1. Center for Disease Control. Older Adult Drivers: Get the Facts: Centers for Disease Control and Prevention, National Center for Injury Prevention and Control, Division of Unintentional Injury Prevention. 2014. Available at: http://www.cdc.gov/motorvehiclesafety/older_adult_drivers/index.html (accessed March 29, 2016).

2. Insurance Institute for Highway Safety, Highway Loss Data Institute. Older People 2014. Available at: http://www.iihs.org/iihs/topics/t/Older%20drivers/bibliography/bytag (accessed March 29, 2016).

3. National Highway Transportation Safety Administration. Traffic Safety Facts: 2005 Data Available at: www-nrd.nhtsa.dot.gov/Pubs/810623.pdf (accessed March 29, 2016).

4. D. O'Neill. The older driver. *Reviews in Clinical Gerontology*. 1996; **6**(03): 295–302.

5. D. J. Foley, H. K. Heimovitz, J. M. Guralnik, et al. Driving life expectancy of persons aged 70 years and older in the United States. *Am J Public Health*. 2002; **92**(8): 1284–9.

6. K. Ball, C. Owsley, B. Stalvey, et al. Driving avoidance and functional impairment in older drivers. *Accid Anal Prev*. 1998; **30**(3): 313–22.

7. D. R. Ragland, W. A. Satariano, K. E. MacLeod. Reasons given by older people for limitation or avoidance of driving. *The Gerontologist*. 2004; **44**(2): 237–44.

8. Insurance Institute for Highway Safety, Highway Loss Data Institute. Q&A: Older People 2006. Available at: www.iihs.org/iihs/topics/t/older-drivers/topicoverview (accessed March 29, 2016).

9. K. J. Anstey, J. Wood, S. Lord, et al. Cognitive, sensory and physical factors enabling driving safety in older adults. *Clin Psychol Rev*. 2005; **25**(1): 45–65.

10. K. K. Ball, D. L. Roenker, V. G. Wadley, et al. Can high-risk older drivers be identified through performance-based measures in a Department of Motor Vehicles setting? *J Am Geriatr Soc*. 2006; **54**(1): 77–84.

11. J. P. Szlyk, D. P. Taglia, J. Paliga, et al. Driving performance in patients with mild to moderate glaucomatous clinical vision changes. *Journal of Rehabilitation Research and Development*. 2002; **39**(4): 467–82.

12. J. P. Szlyk, C. L. Mahler, W. Seiple, et al. Driving performance of glaucoma patients correlates with peripheral visual field loss. *J Glaucoma*. 2005; **14**(2): 145–50.

13. L. Staplin, K. W. Gish, E. K. Wagner. MaryPODS revisited: updated crash analysis and implications for screening program implementation. *J Safety Res.* 2003; **34**(4): 389–97.

14. C. Owsley, K. Ball, G. McGwin Jr, et al. Visual processing impairment and risk of motor vehicle crash among older adults. *JAMA.* 1998; **279**(14): 1083–8.

15. O. Clay, V. Wadley, J. Edwards, et al. Cumulative meta-analysis of the relationship between useful field of view and driving performance in older adults: current and future implications. *Optometry & Vision Science.* 2005; **82**(8): 724–31.

16. Posit Science. Drivesharp. clinically proven software program to help drivers. Available at: www.drivesharp.com (accessed March 29, 2016).

17. R. A. Marottoli, E. D. Richardson, M. H. Stowe, et al. Development of a test battery to identify older drivers at risk for self-reported adverse driving events. *J Am Geriatr Soc.* 1998; **46**(5): 562–8.

18. K. L. Margolis, R. P. Kerani, P. McGovern, et al. Risk factors for motor vehicle crashes in older women. *J Gerontol A Biol Sci Med Sci.* 2002; **57**(3): M186–91.

19. R. B. Isler, B. S. Parsonson, G. J. Hansson. Age related effects of restricted head movements on the useful field of view of drivers. *Accid Anal Prev.* 1997; **29**(6): 793–801.

20. A. Hetland, D. B. Carr. Medications and impaired driving. *Annals of Pharmacotherapy.* 2014; **48**(4): 494–506.

21. A. Brunnauer, G. Laux, E. Geiger, et al. Antidepressants and driving ability: results from a clinical study. *J Clin Psychiatry.* 2006; **67**(11): 1776–81.

22. A. J. Hetland, D. B. Carr, M. J. Wallendorf, et al. Potentially driver-impairing (PDI) medication use in medically impaired adults referred for driving evaluation. *Ann Pharmacother.* 2014; **48**(4): 476–82.

23. B. M. Dobbs. Medical Conditions and Driving: Current Knowledge, Final Report. Association for the Advancement of Automotive Medicine. NHTSA Publication: 2005 Contract No.: DTNH22-94-G-05297.

24. J. Charlton, S. Koppel, M. Odell, et al. Influence of chronic illness on crash involvement of motor vehicle drivers: 2nd Edition: Monash University Accident Research Centre, Report #300. 2010. Available at: http://www.monash.edu/__data/assets/pdf_file/0008/216386/muarc300.pdf (accessed March 29, 2016).

25. Medical Fitness to Drive Guidelines: Royal College of Physicians Ireland. Available at: http://www.rsa.ie/Documents/Licensed%20Drivers/Medical_Issues/Sl%C3%A1inte_agus_Tiom%C3%A1int_Medical_Fitness_to_Drive_Guidelines.pdf (accessed March 29, 2016).

26. J. M. Lyman, G. McGwin Jr, R. V. Sims. Factors related to driving difficulty and habits in older drivers. *Accid Anal Prev.* 2001; **33**(3): 413–21.

27. R. Sims, G. McGwin, R. Allman, et al. Exploratory study of incident vehicle crashes among older drivers. *J Gerontol Med Sci* 2000; 55(A): M22–7.

28. G. McGwin, R. Sims, L. Pulley, et al. Relations among chronic medical conditions, medications, and automobile crashes in the elderly: a population-based case-control study. *Am J Epidemiol.* 2000; **152**(5): 424–31.

29. D. Carr, J. Schwartzberg, L. Manning, et al. *Physician's Guide to Assessing and Counseling Older Drivers,* 2nd Edition. Washington, DC: National Highway Traffic Safety Administration. 2010. Available at: http://www.nhtsa.gov/staticfiles/nti/older_drivers/pdf/811298.pdf (accessed March 29, 2016). American Geriatrics Society & A. Pomidor, Clinician's guide to assessing and counseling older drivers, 3rd edition (Report No DOT HS 812 228) Washington, DC, National Highway Traffic Safety Administration. Available at http://www.nhtsa.gov/Driving+Safety/Older+Drivers.

30. Austroads. Assessing Fitness to Drive 2012. Available at: http://www.austroads.com.au/drivers-vehicles/assessing-fitness-to-drive (accessed March 29, 2016).

31. Canadian Medical Association. CMA Driver's Guide: Determining Medical Fitness to Operate Motor Vehicles, 8th Edition Ottawa, Canada 2012. Available at: www.cma.ca/En/Pages/drivers-guide.aspx (accessed March 29, 2016).

32. E. Uc, M. Rizzo, S. Anderson, et al. Impaired visual search in drivers with Parkinson's disease. *Annals of Neurology.* 2006; **60**(4): 407–13.

33. J. Grace, M. Amick, A. D'Abreu, et al. Neuropsychological deficits associated with driving performance in Parkinson's and Alzheimer's disease. *Journal of the International Neuropsychological Society.* 2005; **11**(6): 766–75.

34. J. Stutts, J. Stewart, C. Martell. Cognitive test performance and crash risk in an older driver population. *Accid Anal Prev.* 1998; **30**(3): 337–46.

35. D. B. Carr, P. P. Barco, M. J. Wallendorf, et al. Predicting road test performance in drivers with dementia. *J Am Geriatr Soc.* 2011; **59**(11): 2112–7.

36. L. B. Brown, B. R. Ott. Driving and Dementia: A Review of the Literature. *Journal of Geriatric Psychiatry and Neurology.* 2004; **17**(4): 232–40.

37. G. Adler, S. Rottunda, M. Dysken. The older driver with dementia: An updated literature review. *J Safety Res.* 2005; **36**(4): 399–407.

38. D. B. Carr, B. R. Ott. The Older Adult Driver with Cognitive Impairment: "It's a Very Frustrating Life." *JAMA.* 2010; **303**(16): 1632–41.

39. D. J. Iverson, G. S. Gronseth, M. A. Reger, et al. Practice parameter update: Evaluation and management of driving risk in dementia: Report of the Quality Standards Subcommittee of the American Academy of Neurology. *Neurology*. 2010; **74**(16): 1316–24.

40. L. B. Brown, B. R. Ott, G. D. Papandonatos, et al. Prediction of on-road driving performance in patients with early Alzheimer's disease. *J Am Geriatr Soc*. 2005; **53**(1): 94–8.

41. B. R. Ott, D. Anthony, G. D. Papandonatos, et al. Clinician assessment of the driving competence of patients with dementia. *Journal of the American Geriatrics Society*. 2005; **53**(5): 829–33.

42. F. J. Molnar, A. Patel, S. C. Marshall, et al. Clinical utility of office-based cognitive predictors of fitness to drive in persons with dementia: A systematic review. *J Am Geriatr Soc*. 2006; **54**(12): 1809–24.

43. C. C. Wang, C. J. Kosinski, J. G. Schwartzberg, et al. *Physician's guide to assessing and counseling older drivers* Washington, DC: National Highway Traffic Safety Administration. Available at: http://www.nhtsa.gov/People/injury/olddrive/OlderDriversBook/pages/Contents.html (accessed March 29, 2016).

44. D. P. McCarthy, W. C. Mann. Sensitivity and specificity of the assessment of driving-related skills older driver screening tool. *Topics in Geriatric Rehabilitation*. 2006; **22**(2): 139–52.

45. B. R. Ott, J. D. Davis, G. D. Papandonatos, et al. Assessment of driving-related skills prediction of unsafe driving in older adults in the office setting. *J Am Geriatr Soc*. 2013; **61**(7): 1164–9.

46. A. Woolnough, D. Salim, S. C. Marshall, et al. Determining the validity of the AMA guide: A historical cohort analysis of the assessment of driving related skills and crash rate among older drivers. *Accid Anal Prev*. 2013; **61**: 311–6.

47. T. M. Meuser, D. B. Carr, M. Berg-Weger, et al. The instructional impact of the American Medical Association's Older Drivers Project online curriculum. *Gerontol Geriatr Educ*. 2014; **35**(1): 64–85.

48. T. M. Meuser, D. B. Carr, C. Irmiter, et al. The American Medical Association older driver curriculum for health professionals: changes in trainee confidence, attitudes, and practice behavior. *Gerontol Geriatr Educ*. 2010; **31**(4): 290–309.

49. F. J. Molnar, A. M. Byszewski, S. C. Marshall, et al. In-office evaluation of medical fitness to drive: practical approaches for assessing older people. *Can Fam Physician*. 2005; **51**: 372–9.

50. R. A. Murden, K. Unroe. Assessing older drivers: a primary care protocol to evaluate driving safety risk. *Geriatrics*. 2005; **60**(8): 22–5.

51. G. L. Odenheimer. Driver safety in older adults: The physician's role in assessing driving skills of older patients. *Geriatrics*. 2006; **61**(10): 14–21.

52. The Hartford Financial Services Group. Dementia and Driving. Available at: www.thehartford.com/mature-market-excellence/dementia-driving (accessed March 29, 2016).

53. The Hartford Financial Services Group. We Need to Talk. Available at: www.thehartford.com/mature-market-excellence/family-conversations-with-older-drivers (accessed March 29, 2016).

54. J. Reason, A. Manstead, S. Stradling, et al. Errors and violations on the roads: a real distinction? *Ergonomics*. 1990; **33**(10–11): 1315–32.

55. B. Freund, S. Gravenstein, R. Ferris, et al. Drawing clocks and driving cars: use of brief tests of cognition to screen driving competency in older adults. *Journal of General Internal Medicine*. 2005; **20**(3): 240–4.

56. M. Roy, F. Molnar. Systematic review of the evidence for Trails B cut-off scores in assessing fitness-to-drive. *Canadian Geriatrics Journal*. 2013; **16**(3): 120–42.

57. D. W. Eby, L. J. Molnar, J. T. Shope, et al. Improving older driver knowledge and self-awareness through self-assessment: the driving decisions workbook. *J Safety Res*. 2003; **34**(4): 371–81.

58. American Automobile Association. Tools & Additional Resources. Available at: http://seniordriving.aaa.com (accessed March 29, 2016).

59. AARP. Driver Safety Program. Available at: www.aarp.org/home-garden/transportation/driver_safety (accessed March 29, 2016).

60. American Automobile Association. Interactive Driving Evaluation. Available at: http://seniordriving.aaa.com/evaluate-your-driving-ability/interactive-driving-evaluation (accessed March 29, 2016).

61. American Automobile Association. How Medications Can Affect Driving. Available at: http://seniordriving.aaa.com/medical-conditions-medications/how-medications-can-affect-driving-ability-roadwise-rx (accessed March 29, 2016).

62. Life Long Driver LLC. ADEPT Driver Available at: www.lifelongdriver.com (accessed March 29, 2016).

63. D. R. Ragland, W. A. Satariano, K. E. MacLeod. Driving cessation and increased depressive symptoms. *The Journals of Gerontology*. 2005; **60A**(3): 399–403.

64. R. A. Marottoli, C. F. M. de Leon, T. A. Glass, et al. Consequences of driving cessation: decreased out-of-home activity levels. *Journal of Gerontology Social Sciences*. 2000; **55B**(6): S334–40.

65. L. P. Kostyniuk, J. T. Shope. Driving and alternatives: older drivers in Michigan. *J Safety Res.* 2003; **34**(4): 407–14.

66. E. E. Freeman, S. J. Gange, B. Muñoz, et al. Driving status and risk of entry into long-term care in older adults. *Am J Public Health.* 2006; **96**(7): 1254–9.

67. B. D. Taylor, S. Tripodes. The effects of driving cessation on the elderly with dementia and their caregivers. *Accid Anal Prev.* 2001; **33**(4): 519–28.

68. U.S. Department of Health and Human Services, Administration for Community Living. Area Agency on Aging Finder. Available at: www.aoa.gov/AoA_pr ograms/OAA/How_To_Find/Agencies/find_agencies .aspx?sc=FL (accessed March 29, 2016).

69. Insurance Institute for Highway Safety, Highway Loss Data Institute. December 2014. Available at: http://www.iihs.org/iihs/topics/t/older-dri vers/topicoverview (accessed March 29, 2016).

Chapter 52

Integrative medicine in the care of the elderly

Susan Gaylord, PhD

Introduction

A large and growing percentage of Americans use complementary and alternative medicine (CAM): therapeutic modalities, practices, and products that either supplement or substitute for conventional approaches and are not conventionally used or taught in mainstream Western medicine.[1–3] These modalities can be broadly grouped under the categories of mind-body therapies, manipulative/body-based therapies, biologically based therapies, and alternative medical systems, and include such practices as meditation, chiropractic, herbal medicine, acupuncture, homeopathy, and energetic healing.[3, 4] In the United States, separation of CAM practices from mainstream medicine is often rationalized as being due to lack of evidence regarding safety or efficacy, but other factors, including historical trends, unfamiliarity with philosophies and approaches, financial disincentives, and strong influence of the pharmaceutical and insurance industries, are also responsible.[5] Whereas mainstream health care has been slow to incorporate CAM practices or education, the public has forged ahead in combining CAM use with conventional care, usually without communicating about CAM with their conventional care providers.[2] With upward trends in CAM use among all subgroups of aging populations, including the large cohort of aging baby boomers, the demand for CAM-savvy health-care providers is urgent.[6]

Fortunately, increasing numbers of conventionally trained health-care providers and institutions are recognizing the value of becoming familiar with CAM philosophies, techniques, and practitioners, both for enhancing patient communication as well as for improving clinical practice. Many are taking steps toward integrating CAM into care of their patients.[7]

The terms "integrative medicine" or "integrative health care" refer to the selective incorporation of CAM diagnostic and healing approaches into mainstream health practices and systems.[4, 7] Ideally, integrative medicine draws on the formidable strengths of biomedicine and the benefits of holistic and natural healing modalities in an individualized, patient-centered approach that utilizes and enhances the patient's self-efficacy and self-healing capabilities.[7] Integration of CAM approaches into care of older people can be of significant benefit to their well-being and health outcomes, throughout the continuum of care.

This chapter begins with an overview of the demographics of CAM use in the US aging population, describes consumers' rationales for use of CAM therapies, then reviews CAM modalities and uses for common conditions impacting health and function in the geriatric population. The chapter concludes with a discussion of the role that integrating CAM can play in enhancing health care of older people, the challenges of integration, and the steps that conventional practitioners can take to successfully integrate such approaches into their practices.

CAM use among older people

In 2007, the most recent national survey of CAM use confirmed the growing popularity of all CAM modalities, with approximately 40% of all adults reporting use of one or more types of CAM in the last twelve months.[3] Subgroups of high CAM users included those with higher education and income, those with greater numbers of chronic conditions, and cultural subgroups such as Native Americans and Native Hawaiians. Older people made up a substantial proportion of CAM users, with 41% of those aged 60–69, and 32% of those aged 70–84, reporting CAM use in

---

Reichel's Care of the Elderly, 7th Edition, ed. Jan Busby-Whitehead *et al.* Published by Cambridge University Press.
© Cambridge University Press 2016.

the last twelve months.[3] When responses from baby boomers were compared with those from the previous generation of older people (the so-called silent generation), using data from the 2007 survey, striking findings emerged: while 35% of those born between 1925 and 1946 (aged 62–82) used CAM, a younger group aged 43–61 (the baby boomers, born between 1946 and 1964) reported CAM use of 43%. Overall, twice as many baby boomers reported accessing alternative medical systems (5.4% vs. 2.2%), massage (9.6% vs. 4.8%), and mind-body medicine (21% vs. 13.7%), while use of biologically based therapies was similar between groups (23.3% vs. 22.3%).[6] While not surprisingly the older group reported a substantially higher prevalence of chronic conditions (51% vs. 26%) and a slightly higher prevalence of painful conditions (56% vs. 52%), CAM use was higher for baby boomers than for the older generation, both for those with chronic diseases (45% vs. 38%) and for those with painful conditions (52.9% vs. 43.1%). [6] CAM use was particularly high for baby boomers with diabetes, cancer, and heart disease.[6] These data substantiate expectations that CAM use will continue to rise in parallel with aging of the baby boomer cohort, fueled by CAM's growing popularity as well as baby boomers' relatively higher rates of obesity and projected increased prevalence of chronic and painful conditions.[6]

Why are consumers using CAM?

Growing global consciousness and increased access to information have brought heightened awareness and acceptance of other systems of health care as well as increased knowledge of CAM options. A primary motive for CAM use – whether alone or with conventional care – is philosophical, and includes congruence with holistic beliefs, attraction to natural/organic products and treatments, placing a high value on preventing illness, and being motivated to treat the cause of illness rather than merely eliminating symptoms. For example, in one national survey, those who agreed with the statement that "the health of my body, mind and spirit are related, and whoever cares for my health should take that into account" were more likely to use CAM (46%) than those who did not endorse this item (33%).[8] Population subgroups whose health beliefs and philosophies differ from those of mainstream medicine, whether or not they are cultural minorities, have long been major users of traditional or alternative therapies.[9–13]

A common reason given for utilizing CAM therapies is their emphasis on prevention or to maximize well-being. For example, there is a growing popularity of mind-body approaches such as meditation and yoga for managing stress. Another common rationale is to provide a non-pharmaceutical or surgical alternative for a particular condition. For example, a patient may choose to avoid gallbladder surgery or diabetes by changes in diet, adding a mindful exercise regimen, and managing stress. An AARP survey of CAM use by people aged 50 and older, in which 53% reported CAM use, found that for CAM users, 66% used CAM to treat a specific condition, 65% for overall wellness, 45% to supplement conventional medicine, and 42% to prevent illness.[14]

Those who seek to recover from life-threatening diseases are often highly motivated to use CAM treatments, usually as complements to conventional care. For example, patients diagnosed with cancer use CAM in greater percentages than the general population, including for management of conventional-treatment side effects.[15] Those who suffer from chronic diseases, including those with symptoms that are either poorly understood, treated with only partial success by conventional medicine, or whose treatments include unwanted side effects, often investigate CAM treatments. Many patients with arthritis, Alzheimer's disease, diabetes, hypertension, cardiovascular disease, chronic fatigue, fibromyalgia, insomnia, irritable bowel syndrome, autoimmune syndromes, chronic pain, and a range of stress-related disorders have sought benefit from CAM.[16–20] Additionally, high CAM users include those wishing to enhance the likelihood of success of a particular health care encounter. For example, patients undergoing surgery may choose to incorporate particular CAM therapies, such as herbs, hypnosis, visualization, homeopathic remedies, or energetic therapies.

Those dissatisfied with conventional treatment, providers, practice settings, or the health-care system also are regular users of CAM services.[8] Some consumers report concerns about the safety or efficacy of specific conventional therapies; many are dissatisfied with the high costs of technological medicine. For others, there is a reduced tolerance for conventional medicine's paternalism and dissatisfaction with the conventional doctor-patient relationship.

Finally, those who use mainly alternative forms of health care may do so because they desire control over health matters and place a high value on their inner life and experiences.[8] These values and attitudes are supported by most alternative care providers and are in alignment with the philosophies undergirding their treatments. Providers of integrative medicine, to varying degrees, are also supportive of this philosophical perspective.

Patient-provider disconnect about CAM in conventional health care

One striking finding in research on use of complementary modalities is that, although 95% of US patients are using alternative as well as conventional care, often for the same condition, the vast majority of patients – about 70% [2, 14] – do not tell their conventional practitioners about their use of alternative modalities. Reasons given by patients for not discussing alternative therapy use with their physicians include the belief that physicians would not understand or be knowledgeable about the therapy; that they are not asked; fear of disrespect or disapproval; and their belief that the physician is uninterested.[2] This lack of communication may result in increased medical errors, noncompliance, and possible duplication of services, as well as greater health-care costs and undocumented outcomes. Integrative medicine offers a patient-centered approach to care that recognizes the need to understand and respect the patient's beliefs and values, thereby enhancing trust, cooperation in care, and skillful utilization of the powerful role that beliefs play in illness and health. Continuity and quality of care is enhanced when health professionals can communicate knowledgeably, and even coordinate care, with other members of the patient's health-care team, who may include chiropractic physicians, acupuncturists, massage therapists, or homeopaths. An integrative health-care perspective, whether through an individual provider or a health-care system, could facilitate such communication.

Overview of CAM and use for specific conditions

Following is a brief overview of CAM therapies in use in the United States, with examples of those shown to have therapeutic value in the care of older people. Texts and in-depth reviews of CAM therapies and research provide much greater detail.[21–25]

Mind-body therapies

Mind-body therapies incorporate an understanding of the inseparability and interaction of cognitive and emotional processes with the body organ-systems, and the underlying psychobiological mechanisms by which communication occurs, including immune and neurotransmitter substances. Examples are biofeedback, hypnosis, guided imagery, mindfulness meditation, and various forms of mindful exercise.

Biofeedback

Through training in biofeedback and a subset, neurofeedback, the older patient can learn to modify his or her own vital functions (such as breathing, skin temperature, heart rate, or even EEG brain waves), preventing, controlling, and treating a range of syndromes, including back and neck pain, pelvic floor dysfunction, difficulty swallowing, migraine and tension headaches, asthma, stress-related symptoms, hypertension, and palpitations related to arrhythmias.[26–37]

Hypnosis and guided imagery

Hypnosis uses the power of suggestion to induce trance-like states so as to access deep, often unconscious, levels of the mind to effect positive behavioral change. It has been used effectively to treat symptoms of asthma, irritable bowel syndrome, acute and chronic pain, sleep disorders, anxiety, phobias, and substance abuse.[38–42] Guided imagery involves auditory suggestions, either given by another individual or through a recording device, for purposes of relaxation and stress management. For example, one might imagine being on a beach or another favorite, safe place to facilitate a peaceful, relaxed, or receptive state of mind. Guided imagery is often incorporated in to hypnotic inductions. Important uses of hypnosis and guided imagery in a geriatric population include their substitution for or supplementation of anesthesia during surgery and in pain control.[39, 41, 43]

Mindfulness meditation

Meditation has been used and taught since its roots in ancient India and is increasingly popular in the United States. In mindfulness meditation, the practitioner usually focuses on an image, a sound, or simply the breath as an anchor to being in the present moment, noticing whenever the mind becomes distracted by thoughts of past or future, gently letting go of the distracting thoughts, and bringing the attention back to the present moment. Mindfulness and other meditation techniques can be useful in lowering stress responses and regulating emotional reactivity,[44] and have been shown to reduce such stress markers as heart rate, pulse rate, and plasma cortisol as well as to enhance electroencephalogram (EEG) alpha state, inducing deep relaxation.[22] Meditation also has been shown to enhance immune function and decrease anxiety, hypertension, and chronic pain.[45–64]

Mindful exercises

Mindful exercises includes such practices as yoga, tai chi, qigong, Alexander Technique, Pilates, and Feldenkrais – some thousands of years old, others developed only recently. These practices are adaptable for use by older people in varying states of health and can be used to improve mental and physical function. For example, tai chi has been found to improve sleep, to reduce pain in people suffering from osteoarthritis, to enhance balance in frail older people, and to improve symptoms of Parkinson's disease.[65–79] Yoga has been adapted for older people with varying degrees of fitness, including wheelchair-bound elders, and has been shown to improve risk factors for heart disease, diabetes, side effects of cancer, and musculoskeletal pain.[24, 25, 80–90]

Manipulative/body-based therapies

Manipulative and body-based therapies range from traditional to contemporary techniques, usually performed by a skilled practitioner, emphasizing physical touch, manual manipulation of tissues or energetic systems, and often involving movement. Examples are chiropractic (described under Alternative Health Systems), massage, other forms of bodywork (such as reflexology, functional integration, structural integration, and kinesiology) as well as various touch therapies.[21–25]

Massage and bodywork

Massage and bodywork involve many subcategories and techniques and can easily be individualized based on clients' needs and preferences. Research has shown that massage can promote relaxation, relieve muscle pain and headaches, and alleviate a range of stress-related conditions, thus lessening the need for pharmacological therapies.[91–102] This therapy can reduce swelling and increase lymphatic circulation, thus alleviating chronic inflammatory conditions,

facilitating the removal of toxins from the body, and enhancing recovery from illness.[103] Massage has been used effectively in hospitals, nursing homes, and hospice settings.[104–117] Another example of bodywork, functional integration, involves individualized hands-on touch and movement in which the practitioner directs the client's body through movements tailored to the client's needs. Structural integration, also known as Rolfing, was founded by Ida Rolf in 1970, and is based on the philosophy that proper alignment of body segments (head, torso, pelvis, legs, feet) via manual manipulation and stretching of the body's fascial tissues improves body movement and function. Reflexology is a form of acupressure, which is based on the same system as acupuncture. It originated in ancient China and was also used in ancient Egypt. Introduced to the United States early in this century by William Fitzgerald, MD, and further developed by physiotherapist Eunice Ingham, it involves applying precise pressure to points of the hands and feet that correspond to organs, glands, and other parts of the body to relieve tension, increase circulation, and stimulate deep relaxation. Applied kinesiology, a diagnostic system recently developed by George Goodheart, a chiropractic physician, involves determining imbalances in the body's organs and glands by identifying weaknesses in specific muscles. Once imbalances have been identified, various techniques may be used to strengthen the muscles involved in the underlying dysfunction. More research on these forms of bodywork could determine their application to specific conditions in the elderly.

Touch therapies

Touch therapies are energy-based healing systems that include laying on of hands, Reiki, and therapeutic touch. In laying on of hands, an ancient art found in various spiritual traditions, the practitioner directs healing energy, purported to come from a universal force, to the patient or to the site of illness. Reiki, which traces its origins from Tibet, is one form of this therapy. Therapeutic touch, another variation, was developed by Dolores Krieger, PhD, RN, and Dora Kunz, a healer, and is now being used in hospitals in the United States, particularly by the nursing profession. Therapeutic touch may be useful in reducing pain and anxiety and promoting healing, and can be particularly applicable to the elderly who need gentle and loving care.[100, 118–122]

Biologically based therapies

Biologically based therapies encompass a diverse array of approaches including dietary therapies, herbal medicines, and dietary supplements, and they comprise the most popular CAM category used in the United States.[3] Although many of these are utilized by conventional medicine, they are much more central to the care plans of CAM practitioners such as naturopathic physicians, chiropractic physicians, and homeopathic practitioners, as well as integrative medicine providers, such as physicians trained in functional medicine.[21, 23] A few of these include the following.

Dietary therapies

Conventional and alternative medicine agree on the optimizing effects on function of a diet high in fresh fruits and vegetables and the protective effects of phytochemicals, but beyond that, there are many variations in diet espoused, both within conventional medicine and within CAM.[123] CAM therapies and integrative health care are allied with the natural foods movement, which emphasizes the importance of whole, organic foods and the elimination from food products of pesticides, antibiotics, hormones, and food additives (such as preservatives, dyes, and artificial flavors) – substances that may play a role in decreased immune function, increased food allergies, increased chemical sensitivities, and other disorders. Individualized nutritional prescriptions that take into account the health and preferences of the older person are essential, and can be helpful in preventing disease, restoring function, and controlling pain.[21, 23]

There are a variety of nutritional prescriptions for preventing illness and promoting healing. The simplest is an organic, plant-based, whole-foods diet, which decreases the body's burden of chemical additives, maximizes natural vitamin and mineral intake, decreases fat and sugar, and increases fiber. Macrobiotics is a dietary prescription formulated by Michio Kushi based on the ancient Chinese philosophy and practice of balancing yin and yang, and emphasizing whole foods. A vegetarian diet calls for the elimination of all meat; a vegan diet eliminates all animal products, including milk and eggs. Raw food diets, on the other hand, do include animal products, but stress the importance of their being organic as well as uncooked. Juice therapies provide supplementary nutrients, particularly vitamins and minerals, both to prevent illness (i.e., during times of stress) and to restore the body to health. Fasting is a time-tested ritual, used for centuries in all societies to purge the body of toxic substances, enhance immune function, and increase spiritual awareness. Extreme fasts (not recommended for vulnerable people) may involve drinking only pure water; modified juice fasts include fresh organic vegetable juices and sometimes fruit juices. Ayurvedic medicine practitioners make dietary recommendations based on constitutional types, and traditional Chinese medicine practitioners prescribe diets based on both constitutional and illness characteristics.[22]

Herbal medicines and nutraceuticals

Using herbs and other plants as remedies can be traced back to prehistoric times. Often gathered from surrounding environments and prepared by knowledgeable laypeople, these medicines have long been used as tonics for preventing illness and as remedies for most functional disorders known to humankind (i.e., dyspepsia, respiratory disorders, menstrual disorders, anxiety, and depression) as well as treatments for more serious organic disorders such as cancer. Until the late nineteenth century, physicians prescribed herbal preparations extensively, but with the growth of manufactured drugs, the medical profession's knowledge and use of herbs declined and practically ceased in the United States.

Meanwhile, there has been a major resurgence of interest and use of herbals and a growing consumer awareness of the roles played by various nutraceuticals in health and illness. Raw herbs and a wide variety of nutraceuticals are available in health food stores, and many nutraceutical products can be purchased over the counter in pharmacies. CAM practitioners and integrative care providers, as well as many pharmacists, have been trained to advise on consumption of these products, including their interactions with pharmaceuticals, but conventional medicine continues to lag behind in education and training regarding uses and drug interactions. Although effective use of many herbal preparations has been established by tradition, increasingly, randomized controlled clinical trials are showing efficacy of certain herbal preparations in specific conditions. For example, research has established the efficacy of St. John's Wort for mild to moderate depression.[124] With the widespread use of herbals and supplements for self-care among elderly people, it is essential that care providers facilitate good, open communication with their patients about their use. As noted above, the majority of older persons do not communicate about CAM use with their providers [14]. Moreover, in one study, 80% of hospitalized patients reported use of a dietary supplement, with 52% reporting use of nonvitamin/nonmineral dietary supplements, while inquiry by providers about dietary supplement use was documented only 20% of the time.[125] It is essential that care providers incorporate knowledge about herbals and nutraceuticals into their continuing medical education to avoid harm and optimize care. There are excellent online reference sources to consult, such as the Natural Medicines Comprehensive Database, to stay abreast of the ever-changing science.

Aromatherapy; use of essential oils

Plant essences, including essential oils, have been used therapeutically for thousands of years in numerous cultures. "Aromatherapy," a term coined in 1937 for this ancient practice by the French chemist Rene Maurice Gattefosse, has been used for the treatment of such conditions as immune deficiency, bacterial and viral infections, and skin disorders, and as a tool for stress management.[22, 126] The oils transmit their healing properties not only by inhalation but also by absorption through the skin, exerting much of their effect through their pharmacological properties and small molecular size. Aromatic molecules interacting with the cells of the nasal mucosa transmit signals to the limbic system through which they connect with parts of the brain controlling heart rate, blood pressure, breathing, memory, and hormone balance. Research has shown that inhalation of particular essential oils can have either a calming or stimulatory effect on brain waves.[127] Aromatherapy, often combined with massage, has been used for pain, dementia symptoms, and anxiety in elderly patients in hospitals, nursing homes, and hospice care.[93, 115, 128–130]

Alternative healing systems

Traditional Chinese medicine/traditional Oriental medicine

Acupuncture and acupressure are part of a complete system of healing developed in China over 5,000 years ago. Both within China and in other oriental cultures such as Korea and Japan, variations in philosophy and techniques have developed. In general in this system,

health is dependent on the balanced flow of chi or qi, the vital life energy, throughout the body, and illness is due to a disturbance of chi. Acupuncture treatment balances the chi by inserting needles at points on the body where the chi flows, through one of twelve channels or meridians. Diagnosis involves inspection (visual assessment of the patient, particularly the spirit, form, and bearing), feeling the pulse, observing the tongue and eyes, and questioning the patient about physical and social environment. Acupuncture treatment can be useful for pain management (e.g., back pain, knee pain, and migraine), cancer-related symptoms (including nausea and vomiting), substance abuse treatment, depression, dementia symptoms, and stroke.[131–141]

Homeopathic medicine

Since ancient times, in India and Greece, it has been known that a remedy can have a curative effect if it produces, in a healthy person, symptoms similar to those of the disease. Samuel Hahnemann, a German physician disheartened with the medical practice of his day, in the early 1800's formally tested this principle – *similia similibus curentur*, "like is cured by like" – and subsequently established it as the basis of a system of medicine.[21, 22] Central to homeopathic therapeutics is the infinitesimal dose, the smallest dose necessary to produce a healing response. Through experimenting with lower and lower doses of drugs in efforts to minimize side effects, Hahnemann developed a technique called potentization, in which the original substance is repeatedly diluted and succussed (shaken vigorously after each dilution) to produce a medicinal substance diluted in many cases beyond Avogadro's number (6.23×10^{-23}), the point at which there is unlikely to be a single original molecule left.

Homeopathic treatment involves selection of a homeopathic preparation that produces symptoms in a healthy person similar to that of the patient's complete symptom picture. Even for acute conditions, prescribing takes into account the individualized response to illness. Particularly in chronic conditions, it may incorporate the person's entire symptomatology not only with regard to the present complaint, but over the course of a lifetime. The latter is termed constitutional prescribing. Although the mechanism by which the similar remedy acts is unknown, homeopathic theory maintains that in some way it stimulates the organism's own innate healing capacities. Illness is viewed as a disturbance of the vital force, as

707

manifested in physical, mental, and emotional responses that are unique to each individual. Symptoms are viewed as the organism's expression of its life energy, and care is taken not to suppress them, but to use them to guide healing.

Although homeopathic remedies can be purchased at health food and drug stores, they are best prescribed under the care of professional homeopaths, skilled integrative medicine physicians, or naturopathic physicians, since much training is required to be able to accurately prescribe an effective remedy or series of remedies, particularly for older people with complex life and treatment histories and often fragile constitutions. Homeopathy may be a useful and gentle healing modality for a wide range of acute and chronic ailments found in older people, including respiratory infections, allergies, insomnia, gastric upsets, fatigue, prolonged grief, anxiety, depression, and palliative care.[142–145]

Naturopathic medicine

Founded by Benedict Lust in the latter part of the nineteenth century, naturopathic medicine is a distinct primary health-care profession that emphasizes prevention and the self-healing capability of the individual. Naturopathic physicians focus on identifying and removing obstacles to healing and recovery, and treating the underlying causes of illness rather than merely eliminating or suppressing symptoms. Naturopathic physicians strive to use the gentlest healing methods possible, educating their patients and encouraging the patient's responsibility. The healing methods emphasize treating the whole person, including physical, mental, emotional, genetic, environmental, social, and spiritual factors. Therapeutic modalities include nutritional and botanical medicine, homeopathy, acupuncture, and hydrotherapy.[21, 22] Interviews with older people who utilized naturopathic practitioners found that patients sought naturopathic medical care because it was aligned with their values, including an emphasis on prevention, self-care, and healthy aging.[146]

Chiropractic medicine

Chiropractic, founded in 1895 in Iowa by D. D. Palmer, a self-educated healer,[22] is based on the understanding that structural distortions can cause functional abnormalities. Vertebral subluxation of the spine is an important structural distortion that disturbs body function primarily through neurologic pathways. Chiropractic adjustment is a specific and definitive system for correcting vertebral subluxation, harmonizing neuronal function, and stimulating the body's innate healing potential, focusing primarily on manual adjustment or manipulation of the spine. Chiropractic is the third largest independent health profession in the western world, following allopathic medicine and dentistry, with more than 65,000 licensed practitioners in the United States, trained in four-year post-baccalaureate programs and seeing over 20 million patients per year.[22] Patients visit chiropractic physicians particularly for the prevention and treatment of neuromusculoskeletal conditions of low back pain, neck pain, and headaches.[22, 147–149]

Prevalence of chiropractic use among Medicare beneficiaries aged 70 and older ranges from 4.1% to 5.4%; in younger beneficiaries it ranges from 6% to 7%.[147] Research comparing outcomes between users of chiropractic and users of medical care for treatment of uncomplicated back care suggests that chiropractic care may provide a protective effect on decline in function and self-rated health, as well as provide higher satisfaction with follow-up care.[148]

Spiritual healing practices

Spirituality is a powerful component of the healing process and is particularly important in the care of older people.[150–153] Faith healing is one prevalent form of spiritual healing.[154, 155] Shamanism is another manifestation and is one of the oldest healing traditions known to humans.[22, 156] A shaman is a man or woman trained to journey outside time and space via an altered state of consciousness, often to perform healing rituals. Traditionally, shamans have been called upon to diagnose and treat illnesses, perform divinations, and communicate with the spirit world. Recently in the United States, due particularly to the work of Michael Harner and his students, there has been a revival of the study of shamanic rituals and journeying for those needing spiritual healing.[156]

Rationales for integrating CAM therapies into the care of older people

There are several important reasons to consider incorporating the use of complementary therapies into the care of older individuals and patient populations. These include enhanced communication with patients and their caregivers, patient empowerment and its positive impact on health-care outcomes, research evidence of therapeutic effectiveness of many CAM therapies, increased therapeutic options for both patient and caregiver, and the potential for positive impacts on therapeutic environments and synergistic effects on therapeutic outcomes. Specific benefits for the geriatric population include an emphasis on non-pharmacological therapies, prevention, and self-care. These rationales will be discussed below.

Expanded options for patient care

By its nature, an integrative clinical practice provides an expanded array of health-care options. Conventional therapies are often limited by significant negative side effects, high cost, physiologic vulnerability, or patients' preferences. Although therapies such as prescription drugs may effectively address a particular condition, not every individual will respond well to a particular protocol, and many older people would prefer nonpharmaceutical options. For example, for mild to moderate depression, a practitioner may suggest aerobic exercise, acupuncture, or St. John's wort as an alternative or complement to an antidepressant.[157 162] Another example is an approach to management of hypertension that includes a combination of diet modification, a mind-body therapy (e.g., hypnosis, biofeedback, tai chi, or mindfulness), and medication.[74, 90, 163]

Enhanced patient and provider communication and satisfaction

CAM practices, while varied, in general share a holistic perspective on healing, one that emphasizes an individualized approach to diagnosis and treatment. Although many good health practitioners spend ample time with patients and provide a multifactorial assessment, it is often the disease, rather than the person, that guides the approach to treatment. CAM and integrative-care providers generally spend more time getting to know the patients' individual needs and desires, providing a patient-centered approach to diagnosis and treatment that may improve both patient and caregiver satisfaction.[23] Importantly, an integrative approach to patient care may improve communication among health-care providers and their patients. As described earlier, patients' lack of communication about their CAM practices is due in part to providers' perceived lack of knowledge, interest, time, or respect for patients' choices. Increased physician knowledge of CAM and respect for patients' choices could result in improved communication and satisfaction with care. Integration can also improve a patient's personal decision making and enhance physical and emotional well-being by increasing knowledge of a broader range of health-promoting practices. Furthermore, integration of complementary treatments such as mind-body therapies may increase patients' conscious participation in the healing process and feelings of empowerment. Health-care providers may also experience greater satisfaction through learning about integrative treatment strategies and developing skill in implementing them.

Decreasing dependency and overuse of pharmacological therapies

Increased use – and misuse – of pharmaceuticals is a significant motivator for integrating CAM with conventional medicine, particularly in caring for older persons. The conventional clinician-patient dyad is often content to passively employ multiple medications in the name of symptom reduction, efficiency, and convenience. With the proliferation of medical specialties, each with its own cadre of medicines, polypharmacy and adverse drug interactions have become the rule rather than the exception, particularly for the elderly patient with chronic illnesses. [164–166] Substituting non-pharmacologic therapies may reduce potential iatrogenic effects of multiple medications, including the potential for drug dependency and negative side effects, and could lower costs while maintaining positive health outcomes. For example, in a comparative outcome study in which older patients with major depression were randomized to an aerobic exercise regimen, or treatment with sertraline, or a combination of exercise and sertraline, all three groups showed equivalent improvement after four months. The aerobic exercise group significantly improved in respiratory capacity, and showed a marked reduction in relapse rate, compared with the sertraline-alone group.[167]

Enhancing health-care outcomes

There is evidence that the combination of conventional and complementary treatments often produces better outcomes than conventional therapies alone, particularly when outcomes include reduction of negative side effects of treatment. The synergy of integrative care in many clinical situations offers a variety of benefits, including, for example, decreased presurgical anxiety, accelerated recovery from surgery, decreased reliance on medications, reduction of side effects, and better outcomes.[168–170]

Added emphasis on disease prevention, wellness, and self-care

Although conventional medicine, including medical education, still emphasizes disease diagnosis and management over prevention,[171] CAM philosophies and CAM and integrative medicine practitioners tend to place greater emphasis on prevention, wellness, and self-care, and these philosophies and practices are attractive to many elders.[146, 172] Examples of preventive and self-care approaches emphasized in CAM and integrative medicine practices include dietary management, exercise, stress reduction, biofeedback, and the use of supplements. Many alternative therapies require for their use a large degree of self-determination, self-motivation, and self-efficacy – attitudes associated with enhanced healing. For example, mind-body and bodywork therapies require discipline of both mind and body over a long period of time, working to change habitual patterns of behavior or learn a new skill. The philosophy of many alternative therapies encourages self-education through reading books, listening to recordings, searching the Internet, and attending workshops and seminars that emphasize stress management and optimizing well-being.

Principles and practices of integrative medicine

Improving and sustaining function in elderly people is a multifactoral process, involving physical, cognitive, and social elements. The use of CAM therapies is compatible with a holistic healing perspective that recognizes the self-healing capacity of the organism and provides mechanisms to enhance those abilities. Many CAM and integrative health-care practices subscribe to a holistic model of health and healing, emphasizing the following principles and processes:

1. emphasizing self-care and empowerment;
2. preventing ill health by strengthening homeostatic balance and remaining in harmony with the psychosocial and physical environment;

3. enhancing wellness with optimal diet, exercise, and stress-reducing regimens;
4. stimulating and nourishing the body's self-healing abilities, recognizing that healing can be a gentle and gradual, developmental process;
5. individualizing treatment to the particular patient, rather than focusing on the disease condition;
6. addressing the underlying causes of illness, including emotional, environmental, and spiritual factors, rather than simply eliminating (suppressing) its surface manifestations;
7. using natural, nonpharmaceutical substances or techniques, while avoiding use of prescription medications (particularly those that might suppress symptoms or compromise the body's self-healing abilities);
8. viewing the mind, body, and spirit as interactive and inseparable;
9. acknowledging the electromagnetic nature of the human organism and the role of vitality in healing;
10. appreciating the importance of intuitive awareness in both the patient and provider.

As well as enhancing function, some CAM therapies, such as tai chi and meditation, which are often practiced in groups, promote socialization with other individuals. This socialization is particularly important, as many elderly people may have lost a spouse, close siblings, or friends, and are therefore at increased risk of becoming isolated and depressed.

Approaches to integrative health care

For the conventional practitioner, becoming educated about integrative health care may involve first becoming familiar with CAM by purchasing a textbook or taking a survey course so as to simply feel comfortable talking to patients about their CAM use. Learning about CAM providers who are practicing in the surrounding community is a second step toward integration. Later, the practitioner may be inspired to acquire specific knowledge and skills about one or more complementary/alternative modalities sufficient to practice at some level as well as to network with CAM providers, perhaps even joining a group practice. Many models of integrative care delivery are possible. While at one end of the spectrum there is the solo provider, at the other end of the spectrum are more complex models such as multidisciplinary practices, where a mix of complementary and conventional practitioners share space, and interdisciplinary practices, which involve various levels of integrated patient management through a partnered arrangement. One type of practice does not necessarily evolve into other, more elaborate, arrangements. The initial form and subsequent development depend on practitioner interests, resources, experience with integration, motivation, skills, and the ability to adapt within the culture of integration.

The challenges and promise of integrative medicine in the care of the elderly

Despite considerable interest on the part of health-care consumers and many practitioners, and the perceived and documented benefits, CAM integration with mainstream medicine is occurring relatively slowly. Reasons include simple inertia, financial disincentives, differences in beliefs about healing, lack of access to education about CAM, and limited information on clinical outcomes about complementary and alternative therapies. The challenge to health-care practitioners is to understand and address the key issues that are raised as conventional, complementary, and alternative healing systems interact and perhaps converge.

For the conventional practitioner who treats older people, the most compelling factor in the movement toward integrative health care may be the continually growing use of complementary and alternative therapies and practitioners by their patients, including the upcoming generations of older people. There is consumer demand for CAM, and future health-care providers must keep pace, if only to become knowledgeable about CAM, including risks, benefits, and comparative effectiveness of CAM and conventional care. Moreover, since patients' reason for not discussing CAM with their providers is partially because they perceive lack of knowledge or interest, and this lack of communication is to the detriment of patient-provider relationships and care outcomes, it becomes a matter of professional responsibility to become more conversant about CAM options. That includes staying current with the burgeoning medical literature on CAM efficacy and comparative effectiveness with conventional medicine.

Another compelling reason to make steps toward integrative medicine for the care of the elderly is that, in many cases, it is simply "good medicine" for older patients – particularly when use of a CAM therapy promotes self-care, preventive self-maintenance, lower health-care costs, or reduction in inappropriate use of pharmaceutical medicine. Finally, joining or leading an integrative medicine team may bring with it the personal and professional satisfaction that many providers of integrative health care enjoy, as they care for their patients in a patient-centered, humanistic atmosphere that emphasizes healing of mind, body, and spirit while enhancing care.

An integrative approach to caring for the elderly, throughout the continuum of care, could be a win-win-win solution – for the older patient, the care provider, and the health-care system.

References

1. D. M. Eisenberg, R. C. Kessler, C. Foster, et al., "Unconventional medicine in the United States. Prevalence, costs, and patterns of use" (1993) **328** *N Engl J Med* 246–52.

2. D. M. Eisenberg, R. B. Davis, S. L. Ettner, et al., "Trends in alternative medicine use in the United States, 1990–1997: Results of a follow-up national survey" (1998) **280** *JAMA* 1569–75.

3. P. M. Barnes, B. Bloom and R. L. Nahin, "Complementary and alternative medicine use among adults and children: United States, 2007" (2008) *National health statistics reports* 1–23.

4. National Center for Complementary and Alternative Medicine, "Complementary, alternative, or integrative health: What's in a name?" 2014, (2014).

5. S. A. Gaylord and J. D. Mann (eds.), *Understanding the convergence of complementary, alternative and conventional care in the United States*, vol. **1**, (Chapel Hill, NC 2004), pp. 1–24.

6. T. F. Ho, A. Rowland-Seymour, E. S. Frankel, et al., "Generational differences in complementary and alternative medicine (cam) use in the context of chronic diseases and pain: Baby boomers versus the silent generation" (2014) **27** *Journal of the American Board of Family Medicine: JABFM* 465–73.

7. J. D. Mann, S. A. Gaylord and S. K. Norton, Integrating complementary and alternative therapies with conventional care. In S. Gaylord, S. K. Norton and P. Curtis (eds.), *The convergence of complementary, alternative, and conventional health care: Educational resources for health professionals*, vol. 7, (Chapel Hill, NC 2004), pp. 1–35.

8. J. A. Astin, "Why patients use alternative medicine: Results of a national study" (1998) **279** *JAMA* 1548–53.

9. R. M. Becerra and A. P. Iglehart, "Folk medicine use: Diverse populations in a metropolitan area" (1995) **21** *Soc Work Health Care* 37–58.

10. W. S. Pearl, P. Leo and W. O. Tsang, "Use of Chinese therapies among Chinese patients seeking emergency

department care" (1995) **26** *Annals of Emergency Medicine* 735–8.

11. A. M. Marbella, M. C. Harris, S. Diehr, et al., "Use of Native American healers among Native American patients in an urban Native American health center" (1998) **7** *Arch Fam Med* 182–5.

12. C. Cook and D. Baisden, "Ancillary use of folk medicine by patients in primary care clinics in southwestern West Virginia" (1986) **79** *South Med J* 1098–101.

13. M. Planta, B. Gundersen and J. C. Petitt, "Prevalence of the use of herbal products in a low-income population" (2000) **32** *Fam Med* 252–7.

14. AARP and National Center for Complementary and Alternative Medicine, *What people aged 50 and older discuss with their health care providers*, (Bethesda, MD 2011).

15. E. Ernst and B. R. Cassileth, "The prevalence of complementary/alternative medicine in cancer: A systematic review" (1998) **83** *Cancer* 777–82.

16. T. A. Arcury, S. L. Bernard, J. M. Jordan, et al., "Gender and ethnic differences in alternative and conventional arthritis remedy use among community-dwelling rural adults with arthritis" (1996) **9** *Arthritis Care Res* 384–90.

17. J. A. Astin, K. R. Pelletier, A. Marie, et al., "Complementary and alternative medicine use among elderly persons: One-year analysis of a Blue Shield Medicare supplement" (2000) **55** *J Gerontol A Biol Sci Med Sci* M4–9.

18. L. M. Coleman, L. L. Fowler and M. E. Williams, "Use of unproven therapies by people with Alzheimer's disease" (1995) **43** *J Am Geriatr Soc* 747–50.

19. D. F. Foster, R. S. Phillips, M. B. Hamel, et al., "Alternative medicine use in older Americans" (2000) **48** *J Am Geriatr Soc* 1560–5.

20. H. H. Krauss, C. Godfrey, J. Kirk, et al., "Alternative health care: Its use by individuals with physical disabilities" (1998) **79** *Arch Phys Med Rehabil* 1440–7.

21. J. E. Pizzorno and M. T. Murray (eds.), *Textbook of natural medicine*, Fourth ed., (St. Louis, MO 2013).

22. M. S. Micozzi (ed.), *Fundamentals of complementary and alternative medicine*, Fourth ed., (St. Louis, MO 2011).

23. D. Rakel (ed.), *Integrative medicine*, Third ed., (Philadelphia 2012).

24. R. Lindquist, M. Snyder and M. F. Tracy (eds.), *Complementary/alternative therapies in nursing*, Seventh ed., (New York 2013).

25. C. M. Davis (ed.), *Complementary therapies in rehabilitation: Evidence for efficacy in therapy, prevention, and wellness*, Third ed., (Thorofare, NJ 2009).

26. F. Andrasik, E. B. Blanchard, D. F. Neff, et al., "Biofeedback and relaxation training for chronic headache: A controlled comparison of booster treatments and regular contacts for long-term maintenance" (1984) **52** *Journal of Consulting and Clinical Psychology* 609–15.

27. G. Bassotti and W. E. Whitehead, "Biofeedback as a treatment approach to gastrointestinal tract disorders" (1994) **89** *Am J Gastroenterol* 158–64.

28. S. P. Buckelew, R. Conway, J. Parker, et al., "Biofeedback/relaxation training and exercise interventions for fibromyalgia: A prospective trial" (1998) **11** *Arthritis Care & Research* 196–209.

29. K. L. Burgio, P. S. Goode, J. L. Locher, et al., "Behavioral training with and without biofeedback in the treatment of urge incontinence in older women: A randomized controlled trial" (2002) **288** *JAMA* 2293–9.

30. P. A. Burns, K. Pranikoff, T. H. Nochajski, et al., "A comparison of effectiveness of biofeedback and pelvic muscle exercise treatment of stress incontinence in older community-dwelling women" (1993) **48** *J Gerontol* M167–74.

31. J. R. Davis, M. G. Carpenter, R. Tschanz, et al., "Trunk sway reductions in young and older adults using multi-modal biofeedback" (2010) **31** *Gait & Posture* 465–72.

32. J. Greenhalgh, R. Dickson and Y. Dundar, "Biofeedback for hypertension: A systematic review" (2010) **28** *Journal of Hypertension* 644–52.

33. S. Haggerty, L. T. Jiang, A. Galecki, et al., "Effects of biofeedback on secondary-task response time and postural stability in older adults" (2012) **35** *Gait & Posture* 523–8.

34. A. McGrady, "The effects of biofeedback in diabetes and essential hypertension" (2010) **77 Suppl 3** *Cleveland Clinic Journal of Medicine* S68–71.

35. S. J. Middaugh and K. Pawlick, "Biofeedback and behavioral treatment of persistent pain in the older adult: A review and a study" (2002) **27** *Applied Psychophysiology and Biofeedback* 185–202.

36. S. D. Tadic, B. Zdaniuk, D. Griffiths, et al., "Effect of biofeedback on psychological burden and symptoms in older women with urge urinary incontinence" (2007) **55** *J Am Geriatr Soc* 2010–5.

37. A. Zijlstra, M. Mancini, L. Chiari, et al., "Biofeedback for training balance and mobility tasks in older populations: A systematic review" (2010) **7** *Journal of Neuroengineering and Rehabilitation* 58.

38. A. Alladin, "Mindfulness-based hypnosis: Blending science, beliefs, and wisdoms to catalyze healing" (2014) **56** *The American Journal of Clinical Hypnosis* 285–302.

712

39. J. A. Astin, "Mind-body therapies for the management of pain" (2004) **20** *Clin J Pain* 27–32.

40. R. Lea, L. A. Houghton, E. L. Calvert, et al., "Gut-focused hypnotherapy normalizes disordered rectal sensitivity in patients with irritable bowel syndrome" (2003) **17** *Alimentary Pharmacology & Therapeutics* 635–42.

41. J. Marcus, G. Elkins and F. Mott, "The integration of hypnosis into a model of palliative care" (2003) **2** *Integr Cancer Ther* 365–70.

42. P. J. Whorwell, "Hypnotherapy in irritable bowel syndrome" (1989) **1** *Lancet* 622.

43. E. V. Lang, J. S. Joyce, D. Spiegel, et al., "Self-hypnotic relaxation during interventional radiological procedures: Effects on pain perception and intravenous drug use" (1996) **44** *International Journal of Clinical and Experimental Hypnosis* 106–19.

44. J. A. Astin, "Stress reduction through mindfulness meditation. Effects on psychological symptomatology, sense of control, and spiritual experiences" (1997) **66** *Psychother Psychosom* 97–106.

45. I. Nyklicek, P. M. Mommersteeg, S. Van Beugen, et al., "Mindfulness-based stress reduction and physiological activity during acute stress: A randomized controlled trial" (2013) **32** *Health Psychol* 1110–3.

46. "Mindfulness may rival medication at preventing depression relapse" (2011) **27** *The Harvard Mental Health Letter / from Harvard Medical School* 7.

47. S. R. Andersen, H. Wurtzen, M. Steding-Jessen, et al., "Effect of mindfulness-based stress reduction on sleep quality: Results of a randomized trial among Danish breast cancer patients" (2013) **52** *Acta Oncologica* 336–44.

48. F. Asare and M. Simren, "Mindfulness-based stress reduction in patients with irritable bowel syndrome" (2011) **34** *Alimentary Pharmacology & Therapeutics* 578–9; author reply 79–80.

49. S. Asmaee Majid, T. Seghatoleslam, H. Homan, et al., "Effect of mindfulness based stress management on reduction of generalized anxiety disorder" (2012) **41** *Iranian Journal of Public Health* 24–8.

50. R. Branstrom, P. Kvillemo and J. T. Moskowitz, "A randomized study of the effects of mindfulness training on psychological well-being and symptoms of stress in patients treated for cancer at 6-month follow-up" (2012) **19** *International Journal of Behavioral Medicine* 535–42.

51. J. Cacciatore and M. Flint, "Attend: Toward a mindfulness-based bereavement care model" (2012) **36** *Death Studies* 61–82.

52. A. Chiesa, R. Calati and A. Serretti, "Does mindfulness training improve cognitive abilities? A systematic review of neuropsychological findings" (2011) **31** *Clin Psychol Rev* 449–64.

53. J. Kabat-Zinn, L. Lipworth and R. Burney, "The clinical use of mindfulness meditation for the self-regulation of chronic pain" (1985) **8** *J Behav Med* 163–90.

54. J. Kabat-Zinn, "An outpatient program in behavioral medicine for chronic pain patients based on the practice of mindfulness meditation: Theoretical considerations and preliminary results" (1982) **4** *General Hospital Psychiatry* 33–47.

55. A. J. Fiocco and S. Mallya, "The importance of cultivating mindfulness for cognitive and emotional well-being in late life" (2015) **20** *Journal of Evidence-Based Complementary & Alternative Medicine* 35–40.

56. A. S. Moss, D. K. Reibel, J. M. Greeson, et al., "An adapted mindfulness-based stress reduction program for elders in a continuing care retirement community: Quantitative and qualitative results from a pilot randomized controlled trial" (2015) **34** *Journal of Applied Gerontology: The Official Journal of the Southern Gerontological Society* 518–38.

57. E. Cash, P. Salmon, I. Weissbecker, et al., "Mindfulness meditation alleviates fibromyalgia symptoms in women: Results of a randomized clinical trial" (2015) **49** *Annals of Behavioral Medicine: A Publication of the Society of Behavioral Medicine* 319–30.

58. C. Eyles, G. M. Leydon, C. J. Hoffman, et al., "Mindfulness for the self-management of fatigue, anxiety, and depression in women with metastatic breast cancer: A mixed methods feasibility study" (2015) **14** *Integr Cancer Ther* 42–56.

59. E. Larouche, C. Hudon and S. Goulet, "Potential benefits of mindfulness-based interventions in mild cognitive impairment and Alzheimer's disease: An interdisciplinary perspective" (2015) **276** *Behav Brain Res* 199–212.

60. K. A. Schonert-Reichl, E. Oberle, M. S. Lawlor, et al., "Enhancing cognitive and social-emotional development through a simple-to-administer mindfulness-based school program for elementary school children: A randomized controlled trial" (2015) **51** *Developmental Psychology* 52–66.

61. J. W. Hughes, D. M. Fresco, R. Myerscough, et al., "Randomized controlled trial of mindfulness-based stress reduction for prehypertension" (2013) **75** *Psychosom Med* 721–8.

62. K. Reiner, L. Tibi and J. D. Lipsitz, "Do mindfulness-based interventions reduce pain intensity? A critical review of the literature" (2013) **14** *Pain Medicine* 230–42.

63. L. E. Carlson, "Mindfulness-based interventions for physical conditions: A narrative review evaluating levels of evidence" (2012) **2012** *ISRN Psychiatry* 651583.

64. A. K. Niazi and S. K. Niazi, "Mindfulness-based stress reduction: A non-pharmacological approach for

chronic illnesses" (2011) **3** *North American Journal of Medical Sciences* 20–3.

65. M. S. Lee, J. H. Jun, H. Lim, et al., "A systematic review and meta-analysis of tai chi for treating type 2 diabetes" (2015) **80** *Maturitas* 14–23.

66. S. L. Wolf, H. X. Barnhart, G. L. Ellison, et al., "The effect of tai chi quan and computerized balance training on postural stability in older subjects. Atlanta ficsit group. Frailty and injuries: Cooperative studies on intervention techniques" (1997) **77** *Physical Therapy* 371–81; discussion 82–4.

67. S. L. Wolf, H. X. Barnhart, N. G. Kutner, et al., "Reducing frailty and falls in older persons: An investigation of tai chi and computerized balance training. Atlanta FICSIT group. Frailty and injuries: Cooperative studies of intervention techniques" (1996) **44** *J Am Geriatr Soc* 489–97.

68. S. L. Wolf, R. W. Sattin, M. Kutner, et al., "Intense tai chi exercise training and fall occurrences in older, transitionally frail adults: A randomized, controlled trial" (2003) **51** *J Am Geriatr Soc* 1693–701.

69. L. Wolfson, R. Whipple, C. Derby, et al., "Balance and strength training in older adults: Intervention gains and tai chi maintenance" (1996) **44** *J Am Geriatr Soc* 498–506.

70. A. M. Wong and C. Lan, "Tai chi and balance control" (2008) **52** *Medicine and Sport Science* 115–23.

71. A. M. Wong, Y. C. Pei, C. Lan, et al., "Is tai chi chuan effective in improving lower limb response time to prevent backward falls in the elderly?" (2009) **31** *Age* 163–70.

72. Y. Zeng, T. Luo, H. Xie, et al., "Health benefits of qigong or tai chi for cancer patients: A systematic review and meta-analyses" (2014) **22** *Complement Ther Med* 173–86.

73. G. Y. Yeh, M. J. Wood, B. H. Lorell, et al., "Effects of tai chi mind-body movement therapy on functional status and exercise capacity in patients with chronic heart failure: A randomized controlled trial" (2004) **117** *Am J Med* 541–8.

74. G. Y. Yeh, C. Wang, P. M. Wayne, et al., "The effect of tai chi exercise on blood pressure: A systematic review" (2008) **11** *Preventive Cardiology* 82–9.

75. G. Y. Yeh, C. Wang, P. M. Wayne, et al., "Tai chi exercise for patients with cardiovascular conditions and risk factors: A systematic review" (2009) **29** *Journal of Cardiopulmonary Rehabilitation and Prevention* 152–60.

76. C. Wang, CH. Schmid, R. Rones, et al., "A randomized trial of tai chi for fibromyalgia" (2010) **363** *N Engl J Med* 743–54.

77. S. Amano, J. R. Nocera, S. Vallabhajosula, et al., "The effect of tai chi exercise on gait initiation and gait performance in persons with Parkinson's disease" (2013) **19** *Parkinsonism & Related Disorders* 955–60.

78. S. Du, J. Dong, H. Zhang, et al., "Taichi exercise for self-rated sleep quality in older people: A systematic review and meta-analysis" (2015) **52** *International Journal of Nursing Studies* 368–79.

79. R. Lauche, J. Langhorst, G. Dobos, et al., "A systematic review and meta-analysis of tai chi for osteoarthritis of the knee" (2013) **21** *Complement Ther Med* 396–406.

80. B. K. Bose, "Mindfulness, meditation and yoga: Competition or collaboration?" (2011) *International Journal of Yoga Therapy* 15–6.

81. M. S. Garfinkel, H. R. Schumacher, Jr., A. Husain, et al., "Evaluation of a yoga based regimen for treatment of osteoarthritis of the hands" (1994) **21** *J Rheumatol* 2341–3.

82. T. Schmidt, A. Wijga, A. Von Zur Muhlen, et al., "Changes in cardiovascular risk factors and hormones during a comprehensive residential three month kriya yoga training and vegetarian nutrition" (1997) **640** *Acta Physiol Scand Suppl* 158–62.

83. M. S. Garfinkel, A. Singhal, W. A. Katz, et al., "Yoga-based intervention for carpal tunnel syndrome: A randomized trial" (1998) **280** *JAMA* 1601–3.

84. A. S. Mahajan, K. S. Reddy and U. Sachdeva, "Lipid profile of coronary risk subjects following yogic lifestyle intervention" (1999) **51** *Indian Heart J* 37–40.

85. S. C. Manchanda, R. Narang, K. S. Reddy, et al., "Retardation of coronary atherosclerosis with yoga lifestyle intervention" (2000) **48** *J Assoc Physicians India* 687–94.

86. R. Murugesan, N. Govindarajulu and T. K. Bera, "Effect of selected yogic practices on the management of hypertension" (2000) **44** *Indian Journal of Physiology and Pharmacology* 207–10.

87. G. S. Birdee, A. T. Legedza, R. B. Saper, et al., "Characteristics of yoga users: Results of a national survey" (2008) **23** *J Gen Intern Med* 1653–8.

88. K. Curtis, A. Osadchuk and J. Katz, "An eight-week yoga intervention is associated with improvements in pain, psychological functioning and mindfulness, and changes in cortisol levels in women with fibromyalgia" (2011) **4** *Journal of Pain Research* 189–201.

89. A. Lazaridou, P. Philbrook and A. A. Tzika, "Yoga and mindfulness as therapeutic interventions for stroke rehabilitation: A systematic review" (2013) **2013** *Evid Based Complement Alternat Med* ID 357108.

90. K. Blom, B. Baker, M. How, et al., "Hypertension analysis of stress reduction using mindfulness meditation and yoga: Results from the harmony randomized controlled trial" (2014) **27** *American Journal of Hypertension* 122–9.

91. T. Field, "Massage therapy research review" (2014) **20** *Complementary Therapies in Clinical Practice* 224–29.

92. D. Trivedi, "Cochrane review summary: Massage for promoting mental and physical health in typically developing infants under the age of six months" (2014) *Primary Health Care Research & Development* 1–2.

93. K. Cino, "Aromatherapy hand massage for older adults with chronic pain living in long-term care" (2014) **32** *J Holist Nurs* 304–13; quiz 14–5.

94. P. Peungsuwan, P. Sermcheep, P. Harnmontree, et al., "The effectiveness of Thai exercise with traditional massage on the pain, walking ability and QOL of older people with knee osteoarthritis: A randomized controlled trial in the community" (2014) **26** *Journal of Physical Therapy Science* 139–44.

95. N. Sritoomma, W. Moyle, M. Cooke, et al., "The effectiveness of Swedish massage with aromatic ginger oil in treating chronic low back pain in older adults: A randomized controlled trial" (2014) **22** *Complement Ther Med* 26–33.

96. T. Field, M. Diego, G. Gonzalez, et al., "Neck arthritis pain is reduced and range of motion is increased by massage therapy" (2014) **20** *Complementary Therapies in Clinical Practice* 219–23.

97. J. G. Anderson, A. G. Taylor, A. E. Snyder, et al., "Gentle massage improves disease- and treatment-related symptoms in patients with acute myelogenous leukemia" (2014) **4** *Journal of Clinical Trials* 1–8.

98. M. Eriksson Crommert, L. Lacourpaille, L. J. Heales, et al., "Massage induces an immediate, albeit short-term, reduction in muscle stiffness" (2015) **25** *Scandinavian Journal of Medicine & Science in Sports* e-490–6.

99. S. L. Yuan, L. A. Matsutani and A. P. Marques, "Effectiveness of different styles of massage therapy in fibromyalgia: A systematic review and meta-analysis" (2015) **20** *Manual Therapy* 257–64.

100. F. Musial and T. Weiss, "The healing power of touch: The specificity of the 'unspecific' effects of massage" (2014) **21** *Forschende Komplementarmedizin* 282–3.

101. J. Rodriguez-Mansilla, M. V. Gonzalez Lopez-Arza, E. Varela-Donoso, et al., "The effects of ear acupressure, massage therapy and no therapy on symptoms of dementia: A randomized controlled trial" (2015) **29** *Clin Rehabil* 683–93.

102. W. Moyle, J. E. Murfield, S. O'Dwyer, et al., "The effect of massage on agitated behaviours in older people with dementia: A literature review" (2013) **22** *J Clin Nurs* 601–10.

103. V. Bayrakci Tunay, T. Akbayrak, Y. Bakar, et al., "Effects of mechanical massage, manual lymphatic drainage and connective tissue manipulation techniques on fat mass in women with cellulite" (2010) **24** *Journal of the European Academy of Dermatology and Venereology: JEADV* 138–42.

104. N. J. Rodgers, S. M. Cutshall, L. J. Dion, et al., "A decade of building massage therapy services at an academic medical center as part of a healing enhancement program" (2015) **21** *Complementary Therapies in Clinical Practice* 52–6.

105. F. M. Ardabili, S. Purhajari, T. Najafi Ghezeljeh, et al., "The effect of shiatsu massage on pain reduction in burn patients" (2014) **3** *World Journal of Plastic Surgery* 115–8.

106. B. B. Kahraman and L. Ozdemir, "The impact of abdominal massage administered to intubated and enterally fed patients on the development of ventilator-associated pneumonia: A randomized controlled study" (2015) **52** *International Journal of Nursing Studies* 519–24.

107. M. Adib-Hajbaghery, A. Abasi and R. Rajabi-Beheshtabad, "Whole body massage for reducing anxiety and stabilizing vital signs of patients in cardiac care unit" (2014) **28** *Medical Journal of the Islamic Republic of Iran* 47.

108. G. MacDonald, "Massage therapy in cancer care: An overview of the past, present, and future" (2014) **20 Suppl 2** *Altern Ther Health Med* 12–5.

109. S. S. Najafi, F. Rast, M. Momennasab, et al., "The effect of massage therapy by patients' companions on severity of pain in the patients undergoing post coronary artery bypass graft surgery: A single-blind randomized clinical trial" (2014) **2** *International Journal of Community Based Nursing and Midwifery* 128–35.

110. G. Martorella, M. Boitor, C. Michaud, et al., "Feasibility and acceptability of hand massage therapy for pain management of postoperative cardiac surgery patients in the intensive care unit" (2014) **43** *Heart & Lung: The Journal of Critical Care* 437–44.

111. M. Ucuzal and N. Kanan, "Foot massage: Effectiveness on postoperative pain in breast surgery patients" (2014) **15** *Pain Management Nursing: Official Journal of the American Society of Pain Management Nurses* 458–65.

112. W. Moyle, M. L. Cooke, E. Beattie, et al., "Foot massage and physiological stress in people with dementia: A randomized controlled trial" (2014) **20** *J Altern Complement Med* 305–11.

113. T. Thanakiatpinyo, S. Suwannatrai, U. Suwannatrai, et al., "The efficacy of traditional Thai massage in decreasing spasticity in elderly stroke patients" (2014) **9** *Clinical Interventions in Aging* 1311–9.

114. A. Mitchinson, C. E. Fletcher, H. M. Kim, et al., "Integrating massage therapy within the palliative care of veterans with advanced illnesses: An outcome study" (2014) **31** *Am J Hosp Palliat Care* 6–12.

115. K. Soden, K. Vincent, S. Craske, et al., "A randomized controlled trial of aromatherapy massage in a hospice setting" (2004) **18** *Palliative Medicine* 87–92.

116. G. Gorman, J. Forest, S. J. Stapleton, et al., "Massage for cancer pain: A study with university and hospice collaboration" (2008) 10 *Journal of Hospice and Palliative Nursing: JHPN: The Official Journal of the Hospice and Palliative Nurses Association* 191–97.

117. A. S. Dain, E. H. Bradley, R. Hurzeler, et al., "Massage, music and art therapy in hospice: Results of a national survey" (2015) 49 *J Pain Symptom Manage* 1035–41.

118. E. Kryak and A. Vitale, "Reiki and its journey into a hospital setting" (2011) 25 *Holist Nurs Pract* 238–45.

119. R. Toms, "Reiki therapy: A nursing intervention for critical care" (2011) 34 *Critical Care Nursing Quarterly* 213–7.

120. S. L. Pocotte and D. Salvador, "Reiki as a rehabilitative nursing intervention for pain management: A case study" (2008) 33 *Rehabilitation Nursing: The Official Journal of the Association of Rehabilitation Nurses* 231–2.

121. L. M. Bossi, M. J. Ott and S. DeCristofaro, "Reiki as a clinical intervention in oncology nursing practice" (2008) 12 *Clin J Oncol Nurs* 489–94.

122. B. Daley, "Therapeutic touch, nursing practice and contemporary cutaneous wound healing research" (1997) 25 *J Adv Nurs* 1123–32.

123. L. M. Steffen, "Eat your fruit and vegetables" (2006) 367 *Lancet* 278–9.

124. T. Varteresian and H. Lavretsky, "Natural products and supplements for geriatric depression and cognitive disorders: An evaluation of the research" (2014) 16 *Current Psychiatry Reports* 456.

125. L. A. Young, K. R. Faurot and S. A. Gaylord, "Use of and communication about dietary supplements among hospitalized patients" (2009) 24 *J Gen Intern Med* 366–9.

126. S. Y. Roh and K. H. Kim, "[Effects of aroma massage on pruritus, skin pH, skin hydration and sleep in elders in long-term care hospitals]" (2013) 43 *Journal of Korean Academy of Nursing* 726–35.

127. J. J. Wu, Y. Cui, Y. S. Yang, et al., "Modulatory effects of aromatherapy massage intervention on electroencephalogram, psychological assessments, salivary cortisol and plasma brain-derived neurotrophic factor" (2014) 22 *Complement Ther Med* 456–62.

128. S. Wilkinson, J. Aldridge, I. Salmon, et al., "An evaluation of aromatherapy massage in palliative care" (1999) 13 *Palliative Medicine* 409–17.

129. T. Satou, M. Chikama, Y. Chikama, et al., "Effect of aromatherapy massage on elderly patients under long-term hospitalization in Japan" (2013) 19 *J Altern Complement Med* 235–7.

130. C. Y. Fu, W. Moyle and M. Cooke, "A randomised controlled trial of the use of aromatherapy and hand massage to reduce disruptive behaviour in people with dementia" (2013) 13 *BMC Complement Altern Med* 165.

131. C. A. Paley, O. A. Tashani, A. M. Bagnall, et al., "A Cochrane systematic review of acupuncture for cancer pain in adults" (2011) 1 *BMJ Supportive & Palliative Care* 51–5.

132. R. Konno, "Cochrane review summary for cancer nursing: Acupuncture-point stimulation for chemotherapy-induced nausea or vomiting" (2010) 33 *Cancer Nursing* 479–80.

133. M. S. Lee and E. Ernst, "Acupuncture for pain: An overview of Cochrane reviews" (2011) 17 *Chinese Journal of Integrative Medicine* 187–9.

134. C. M. Martin, "Complementary and alternative medicine practices to alleviate pain in the elderly" (2010) 25 *The Consultant Pharmacist: The Journal of the American Society of Consultant Pharmacists* 284–90.

135. F. Liu, Z. M. Li, Y. J. Jiang, et al., "A meta-analysis of acupuncture use in the treatment of cognitive impairment after stroke" (2014) 20 *J Altern Complement Med* 535–44.

136. J. H. Zhang, D. Wang and M. Liu, "Overview of systematic reviews and meta-analyses of acupuncture for stroke" (2014) 42 *Neuroepidemiology* 50–8.

137. A. Mooventhan and L. Nivethitha, "Effects of acupuncture and massage on pain, quality of sleep and health related quality of life in patient with systemic lupus erythematosus" (2014) 5 *Journal of Ayurveda and Integrative Medicine* 186–9.

138. J. Rodriguez-Mansilla, M. V. Gonzalez-Lopez-Arza, E. Varela-Donoso, et al., "Ear therapy and massage therapy in the elderly with dementia: A pilot study" (2013) 33 *J Tradit Chin Med* 461–7.

139. S. Kumar, K. Beaton and T. Hughes, "The effectiveness of massage therapy for the treatment of nonspecific low back pain: A systematic review of systematic reviews" (2013) 6 *International Journal of General Medicine* 733–41.

140. X. F. Zhao, Y. Du, P. G. Liu, et al., "Acupuncture for stroke: Evidence of effectiveness, safety, and cost from systematic reviews" (2012) 19 *Topics in Stroke Rehabilitation* 226–33.

141. G. C. Zhang, W. B. Fu, N. G. Xu, et al., "Meta analysis of the curative effect of acupuncture on post-stroke depression" (2012) 32 *J Tradit Chin Med* 6–11.

142. K. Boehm, C. Raak, H. Cramer, et al., "Homeopathy in the treatment of fibromyalgia – a comprehensive literature-review and meta-analysis" (2014) 22 *Complement Ther Med* 731–42.

143. E. J. Peckham, E. A. Nelson, J. Greenhalgh, et al., "Homeopathy for treatment of irritable bowel

syndrome" (2013) **11** *Cochrane Database Syst Rev* CD009710.

144. K. I. Cooper and C. Relton, "Homeopathy for insomnia: A systematic review of research evidence" (2010) **14** *Sleep Medicine Reviews* 329–37.

145. K. Pilkington, G. Kirkwood, H. Rampes, et al., "Homeopathy for anxiety and anxiety disorders: A systematic review of the research" (2006) **95** *Homeopathy: The Journal of the Faculty of Homeopathy* 151–62.

146. E. B. Oberg, M. S. Thomas, M. McCarty, et al., "Older adults' perspectives on naturopathic medicine's impact on healthy aging" (2014) **10** *Explore* 34–43.

147. P. A. Weigel, J. M. Hockenberry and F. D. Wolinsky, "Chiropractic use in the medicare population: Prevalence, patterns, and associations with 1-year changes in health and satisfaction with care" (2014) **37** *J Manipulative Physiol Ther* 542–51.

148. P. A. Weigel, J. Hockenberry, S. E. Bentler, et al., "The comparative effect of episodes of chiropractic and medical treatment on the health of older adults" (2014) **37** *J Manipulative Physiol Ther* 143–54.

149. B. F. Walker, S. D. French, W. Grant, et al., "A Cochrane review of combined chiropractic interventions for low-back pain" (2011) **36** *Spine (Phila Pa 1976)* 230–42.

150. H. G. Koenig and J. J. Seeber, "Religion, spirituality, and aging" (1987) **35** *J Am Geriatr Soc* 472.

151. J. M. Stolley and H. Koenig, "Religion/spirituality and health among elderly African Americans and Hispanics" (1997) **35** *J Psychosoc Nurs Ment Health Serv* 32–8.

152. W. Gesler, T. A. Arcury and H. G. Koenig, "An introduction to three studies of rural elderly people: Effects of religion and culture on health" (2000) **15** *J Cross Cult Gerontol* 1–12.

153. H. G. Koenig, "Religion, spirituality, and health: The research and clinical implications" (2012) **2012** *ISRN Psychiatry* 278730.

154. D. E. King, J. Sobal and B. R. DeForge, "Family practice patients' experiences and beliefs in faith healing" (1988) **27** *J Fam Pract* 505–8.

155. D. E. King and B. Bushwick, "Beliefs and attitudes of hospital inpatients about faith healing and prayer" (1994) **39** *J Fam Pract* 349–52.

156. M. J. Harner, *The way of the shaman*, 10th anniversary ed., (San Francisco 1990), pp. xxiv, 171.

157. J. A. Blumenthal, A. Sherwood, M. A. Babyak, et al., "Exercise and pharmacological treatment of depressive symptoms in patients with coronary heart disease: Results from the upbeat (understanding the prognostic benefits of exercise and antidepressant therapy) study" (2012) **60** *J Am Coll Cardiol* 1053–63.

158. J. A. Blumenthal, M. A. Babyak, C. O'Connor, et al., "Effects of exercise training on depressive symptoms in patients with chronic heart failure: The HF-action randomized trial" (2012) **308** *JAMA* 465–74.

159. J. A. Blumenthal, M. A. Babyak, P. M. Doraiswamy, et al., "Exercise and pharmacotherapy in the treatment of major depressive disorder" (2007) **69** *Psychosom Med* 587–96.

160. W. J. Zhang, X. B. Yang and B. L. Zhong, "Combination of acupuncture and fluoxetine for depression: A randomized, double-blind, sham-controlled trial" (2009) **15** *J Altern Complement Med* 837–44.

161. E. Ernst, M. S. Lee and T. Y. Choi, "Acupuncture for depression? A systematic review of systematic reviews" (2011) **34** *Eval Health Prof* 403–12.

162. S. Kasper, M. Gastpar, H. J. Moller, et al., "Better tolerability of St. John's wort extract WS 5570 compared to treatment with SSRIs: A reanalysis of data from controlled clinical trials in acute major depression" (2010) **25** *International clinical psychopharmacology* 204–13.

163. I. C. Liao, S. L. Chen, M. Y. Wang, et al., "Effects of massage on blood pressure in patients with hypertension and prehypertension: A meta-analysis of randomized controlled trials" (2016) **31** *The Journal of Cardiovascular Nursing* 73–83.

164. C. Gomez, S. Vega-Quiroga, F. Bermejo-Pareja, et al., "Polypharmacy in the elderly: A marker of increased risk of mortality in a population-based prospective study (nedices)" (2015) **61** *Gerontology* 301–9.

165. C. Hein, A. Forgues, A. Piau, et al., "Impact of polypharmacy on occurrence of delirium in elderly emergency patients" (2014) **15** *Journal of the American Medical Directors Association* 850 e11–15.

166. C. Tannenbaum, "How to treat the frail elderly: The challenge of multimorbidity and polypharmacy" (2013) **7** *Canadian Urological Association Journal = Journal de l'Association des urologues du Canada* S183–5.

167. M. Babyak, J. A. Blumenthal, S. Herman, et al., "Exercise treatment for major depression: Maintenance of therapeutic benefit at 10 months" (2000) **62** *Psychosom Med* 633–8.

168. K. Armstrong, S. Dixon, S. May, et al., "Anxiety reduction in patients undergoing cardiac catheterization following massage and guided imagery" (2014) **20** *Complementary Therapies in Clinical Practice* 334–8.

169. F. Buyukyilmaz and T. Asti, "The effect of relaxation techniques and back massage on pain and anxiety in turkish total hip or knee arthroplasty patients" (2013) **14** *Pain Management Nursing:*

Official Journal of the American Society of Pain Management Nurses 143–54.

170. L. R. Brand, D. J. Munroe and J. Gavin, "The effect of hand massage on preoperative anxiety in ambulatory surgery patients" (2013) **97** *AORN Journal* 708–17.

171. D. R. Garr, D. T. Lackland and D. B. Wilson, "Prevention education and evaluation in U.S. medical schools: A status report" (2000) **75** *Acad Med* S14–21.

172. K. Votova and A. V. Wister, "Self-care dimensions of complementary and alternative medicine use among older adults" (2007) **53** *Gerontology* 21–7.

Chapter 53

Implications of an aging society

Daniel Swagerty, MD, MPH, AGSF, and Jonathan Evans, MD, MPH

Introduction

Understanding the changing demography of the older adult population is essential to providing quality medical care to older adults. With the growing numbers of adults older than 65, almost every medical specialty will be impacted. The fastest growing population cohort in the United States is adults older than 85. Understanding the differences in older adult care for the young-old and old-old provides an important basis for the study of geriatrics. In fact, individual variation is more pronounced in the older adult population than in any other age group. This chapter aims to explain the urgent and growing need for health professionals to be skilled in the care of older adults.

Over the last century the world has dramatically aged. Life expectancy has steadily increased, particularly in the developed world. There are many reasons for this significant increase in life expectancy including improvements in hygiene, sanitation, and medical advances. At the same time, birth rates have declined. The net effect on society as a whole is an older population.[1]

This aging of our society is expected to have many far-reaching consequences on the US and world culture, economy, social relationships, health-care delivery, and governmental responsibilities. An aging population will have an impact on everyone in society, regardless of age. Moreover, population aging, most notably in developed countries, is also occurring to a significant extent in the developing world. It is difficult to predict all of the ways in which our nation and the world will be challenged in the next several decades as a result of the aging population. Although many of the effects, such as increased health-care costs and demand for health care and social services are already evident, there is still a great deal of uncertainty because this phenomenon has not previously occurred. Our historical experience will be a very limited guide as we confront unprecedented acceleration in the growth and complexity of an aging population.[1–3]

The impact of aging on individual seniors must be considered in the context of the aging population. An individual's needs, preferences, goals, resources, and abilities change throughout the lifespan. As one grows, matures, and ages, there is a change in one's living situation, finances, functional independence, and self-reliance. Of particular concern to almost everyone is how much we must rely on others (such as family members, friends, the local community, and government) for our instrumental and basic activities of daily living. As the age of an entire society increases, more people reach advanced age without a proportional increase in the number of younger people to care for them. This shift in population demographics will likely cause fundamental changes in the nation's economy, labor force, the role of government, and the ability of government to provide needed services. There is also a fundamental shift in the ability, and perhaps willingness, of the younger members of society to provide for the needs of older generations, including the fact that the children of seniors are increasing seniors themselves.[4–9]

As described in other chapters in this book, it is well known what happens to the human body with normal aging. It is therefore possible to anticipate and extrapolate those changes to groups of individuals; however, a society is more than the sum of all of the individual members. Some of the consequences of an aging society will be obvious and predictable whereas others will be more obscure and unpredictable. The following sections will explore how the effects of individual aging can be extrapolated to predictable social

Reichel's Care of the Elderly, 7th Edition, ed. Jan Busby-Whitehead *et al.* Published by Cambridge University Press.
© Cambridge University Press 2016.

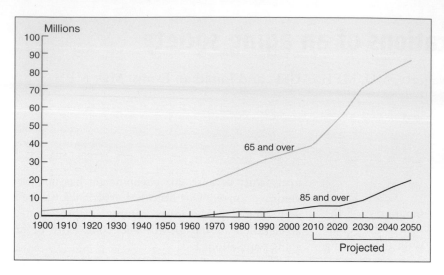

Figure 53.1 Number of people aged 65 and over, by age group in selected years 1900–2010. *Note:* Data for 2020–2050 are projections of the population. *Reference population:* These data refer to the resident population. *Source:* US Census Bureau, Decennial Census and Projections. (A black-and-white version of this figure will appear in some formats. For the color version, please refer to the plate section.)

impacts and how such impacts can also be difficult to predict for many reasons.

This chapter will discuss the impact of an aging society on health-care delivery, government, the economy, and on family relationships. It will explore some of the difficulties in anticipating future changes and needs, as well as some of the dilemmas that our and other aging societies face now and in the future. Population aging will be examined in an effort to understand better what the implications are for both older adults and the rest of society.

Current and projected size of the US older adult population

The post–World War II baby boom generation in the United States is now entering the 65-and-older age group; thus, this portion of the population is growing more quickly than the rest. Between 2000 and 2010, those over 65 years of age grew by 15.1% whereas the total US population increased by just 9.7%. There are more people 65 or older alive today in the United States, as well as the world, than have ever reached that age throughout our history. In the United States alone, the population aged 65 and older currently exceeds 40 million or 13% of the overall population. Figure 53.1 shows how, as the baby boom generation ages, those older than 65 will double in number by the year 2030 to 72 million or 20% of the US population. Particularly rapid growth is anticipated in the older-than-85 age group. The elderly population is also expected to become more ethnically diverse.

Consequently, we are entering a completely new era, with little in our past to guide our future.[1, 2]

Life expectancy

In the United States, improvements in health over the past century have resulted in increased life expectancy and contributed to the growth of the older population. As shown in Figure 53.2, Americans are living longer than ever before. Life expectancies at both age 65 and 85 years have increased. Current life expectancy is approximately 86 years for women and 78 years for men. Under current mortality conditions, men who survive to age 65 can expect to live an average of 17 years and for women, the life expectancy at 65 is currently 20 years. The life expectancy of people who survive to age 85 today is 6 years for men and 7.2 years for women. The further one progresses beyond age 65 years, the longer one is expected to live. Although life expectancies have improved dramatically over the last decade in the United States, individual life expectancies vary based on existing comorbidities, quality of life, race, and socioeconomic status.[10, 11]

Life expectancy at age 65 in the United States is lower than that of many other industrialized nations. The longest life expectancies are for Japanese women. Within the United States, the longest life expectancies are in Hawaii. This is due to the influence of a larger proportion of ethnic Japanese. Life expectancy also varies by race, but the differences change with age. In the United States, life expectancy at birth and at age 65 is higher for white people than for black people. At

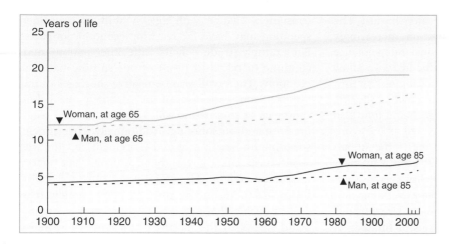

Figure 53.2 Life expectancy at ages 65 and 85 years, by gender, in selected years 1900–2009. *Reference population:* These data refer to the resident population. *Source:* Centers for Disease Control and Prevention, National Center for Health Statistics, National Vital Statistics System. (A black-and-white version of this figure will appear in some formats. For the color version, please refer to the plate section.)

older ages, however, the life expectancy among black people is slightly higher than among white people. This has been attributed to a "healthy survivor" effect, more social support, and other factors. Not surprisingly, differences in life conditions of older persons with inadequate income and those above the median income in the United States have led to the conclusion that there is a major discrepancy of one to two-and-a-half years in active life expectancy between the poor and the nonpoor.[10, 11]

Active life expectancy

The concept of active life expectancy is useful in thinking about functional status and independence in older adulthood. In life expectancy, the end point is death. In active life expectancy we are also concerned with the loss of independence or the need to rely on others for assistance with daily activities. Simplistically put, the remaining years of life for a group of persons can be "active" or "dependent," or some combination thereof. Active life expectancy answers the question "Of the remaining years of life for this cohort of persons, what proportion is expected to be spent with little or no disability?" The answer has implications for individuals, families, and societies. As one oft-quoted line states, "And in the end, it's not the years in your life that count. It's the life in your years."

The impact of death rate on society

The impact of an aging population on death rates and the subsequent broad social impact illustrate the complex consequences of an aging society. Currently, three-fourths of all deaths in the United States occur among those aged 65 years and older. Consequently, the overall number of deaths per year is expected to increase as the population increases in age. A predictable consequence will be an increased demand across the spectrum of health-care services for the quality and quantity of end-of-life care. It can also be expected that the new demand for end-of-life care services will require increases in specific health-care education for multiple disciplines, the number of individual and organizational providers, and the financing of this health-care service. The broader social impact is less predictable. More deaths may increase demand for the number and types of funeral services. Growth in funeral services will require a commensurate growth in the mortuary sciences as well as an increased demand for land for cemeteries. An additional social impact could be in greater tension over land use and zoning in certain municipalities and neighborhoods. This is just one instance in which the effects of an aging society will have broad, and not always predictable, effects on our local, regional, national, and global communities.[2–4, 6–8, 12–18]

Crossing the street

Among the myriad changes of normal aging are a decrease in stride length and a consequent reduction in gait speed. That is, older pedestrians walk slower. Studies of ambulatory community-dwelling elderly individuals have found that the time allotted at a crossing signal (i.e., how long the "walk" sign remains illuminated) is inadequate to allow many older adult pedestrians to cross the street before traffic resumes, thus creating a potentially serious safety hazard. The obvious solution to accommodate an increasingly older populace and promote functional independence is to change the timing of the traffic lights to allow more time for crossing the street. Changing the timing of traffic lights, however, has an obvious slowing effect on traffic flow. Any change in traffic flow also has a significant effect on safety, as well as the economy. In fact, controlling and linking traffic signals across large metropolitan areas has been a primary means by which an increase in cars has been accommodated over several decades without building new roads. In some areas, even changing a single traffic signal can have a major effect. Thus, a number of difficult choices confront society in the coming years as the older adult population grows. This is but one example of the unintended social consequences of one decision to accommodate the needs of an increasing number of older adults; others may not be as obvious as changing a stoplight.[19–21]

Consumer spending, work, and the economy

Our economy has undergone tremendous change over the last few decades for a multitude of reasons such as new technology, globalization, and a shift from manufacturing to service sector jobs. Although these changes have little to do with population aging, the increasing age of a population has dramatic effects on the economy. As the population ages, the labor market changes: it becomes older and decreases in size. It is likely that the retirement age will increase for many people, particularly professionals. Similarly, it is likely that the service sector will continue to grow, particularly in health care, financial services, travel, and generally in the professions. The kind of work that older workers desire and are able to do, particularly those who remain in the workforce beyond retirement age, is different from the kind of work done by young people just entering the work force. In particular, the transition of jobs to more service and less production includes less reliance on physical strength, making it possible for older workers in those areas to stay employed longer. This shift in the available workforce will have a tremendous economic impact.[3, 8, 17, 22]

Consumer spending is also largely dependent on the age of consumers. The demand for goods and services will change as the needs and preferences of consumers change with age. A shift in consumer spending may have far-reaching economic impacts. For example, trade deficits with other nations may continue to rise as a result of our shifting national economy. There will also be relative shortages in the number and expertise of our labor pool. Labor shortages of this nature will result in upward wage pressure and outsourcing. Additionally, government spending on health care and retirement benefits will significantly affect government priorities, tax policy, the federal debt burden, and the government's ability to impact the economy through public policy. It is quite possible that the size of the overall economy could shrink, if the numbers and types of workers decrease without significant increases in individual productivity.[1–3, 5, 8, 13, 22–25]

Housing

The housing needs and preferences of seniors are different from younger homeowners. After retirement, many people opt to downsize to a smaller home or apartment to access home equity, to reduce the time and expense of housekeeping and maintenance, to accommodate disabling medical conditions, or to relocate to another community. If a large number of people in a particular real estate market were to make similar decisions at the same time, real estate prices would be expected to change. Regardless of such an abrupt market change, it is likely that demand will change significantly over a long period of time, resulting in changing prices and supply. Increasingly, newer homes are built incorporating the principles of "universal design," or architectural features to accommodate lifelong aging as well as the occurrence of disability. Because retrofitting (involving redesign and construction on) older homes is expensive, this has been a welcome change in home design; however, affordable housing is currently in short supply in many communities, regardless of age. Affordable housing that is also accessible for adults with disabilities is in even shorter supply. Moreover, affordable housing coupled with assistance for activities of daily living (i.e., assisted-living facilities) for low-income older adults is nonexistent in many communities.

The default for many poor older adults who require even limited assistance with activities of daily living is long-term nursing facility placement because Medicaid pays for it. Figure 53.3 shows the increasing reliance on long-term care facilities to provide a residence for older adults who require

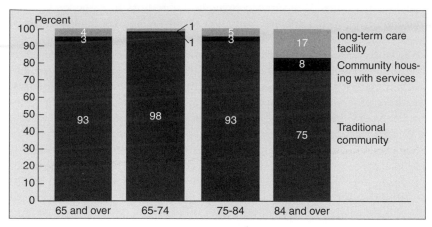

Figure 53.3 Percentage of Medicare enrollees aged 65 and over residing in selected residential settings, by age group, 2010. *Note:* Community housing with services applies to respondents who reported they lived in retirement communities or apartments, senior citizen housing, continuing care retirement facilities, assisted-living facilities, staged living communities, board-and-care facilities/homes, and other similar situations, *and* who reported they had access to one or more of the following services through their place of residence: meal preparation, cleaning or housekeeping services, laundry services, help with medications. Respondents were asked about access to these services but not whether they actually used the services. A residence is considered a long-term care facility if it is certified by Medicare or Medicaid, or it has three or more beds and is licensed as a nursing home or other long-term care facility and provides at least one personal care service, or provides 24-hour, 7-days-a-week supervision by a caregiver. *Reference population:* These data refer to Medicare enrollees. *Source:* Centers for Medicare and Medicaid Services. Medicare Current Beneficiary Survey. (A black-and-white version of this figure will appear in some formats. For the color version, please refer to the plate section.)

assistance with their activities of daily living. Although only 1.5% of all individuals aged 65–74 live in long-term care, this rises to nearly 25% for those older than 85. While the absolute numbers of people living in long-term care facilities is declining slowly, the level of disability of residents is significantly increasing. These older adults often enter long-term care facilities on a short-term basis following acute care hospitalization. They cannot, however, be discharged to the community, despite clinical improvement, because their care needs cannot be affordably met elsewhere. To avoid the demand for significant increases in nursing facility construction in the future, there must be much greater availability of affordable housing with services for older adults who require assistance with their activities of daily living. This will likely require the concerted cooperation between government at all levels and the private sector.[2–9]

Changes in government policies

If government does indeed serve the people, then the role, size, scope, and priorities of government will surely change as an aging society's needs change. Just as older consumers have different preferences and needs, so do older voters, and the adult children who serve as caregivers for older family members. Attitudes toward taxation and spending priorities vary by age. As already evidenced in our society, an older voter on a fixed income may be both particularly concerned about paying increasing taxes and about any threatened cuts to government programs from which they benefit. Younger voters may likewise be concerned about shouldering an even bigger burden of higher taxes to support retirement programs, particularly if they do not trust that those same programs will be available for them in the future. Additionally, funding for schools and roads compete with funding for health care and housing for older adults. To the extent that families have become smaller and geographically separated, many more older adults need to rely on all levels of government to meet their basic needs of health, nutrition, safety, and security.[3–5, 9, 23, 25–27]

Federal and state entitlement programs

A large and growing proportion of federal government spending goes to the large-scale entitlement programs that provide a variety of essential benefits to older adults – namely Social Security, Medicare, and Medicaid. As the number of Americans aged 65 and older increases, the cost of each of these programs also increases. Meanwhile, the proportion of younger Americans aged 65 and younger contributing to these three programs through payroll taxes is decreasing. Additionally, the amount of money paid out in benefits has grown faster than overall tax revenues or the economy has grown. Consequently, these programs represent an increasing percentage of the federal budget, and an increasing percentage of the national gross domestic product. Each of these three programs will now be discussed in greater detail.

Social Security

When the Social Security program was developed in the 1930s, the population of the United States was much younger, and life expectancy was much shorter. Relatively few people were expected to live long enough to collect any retirement benefits, and even fewer retirees would live to collect benefits for many years. In addition, for every one person collecting retirement benefits, there were more than 20 younger, working Americans paying into the system through payroll taxes. Subsequently, life expectancy has increased by more than 15 years, and the number of retirees has dramatically increased. In 1960, there were only five workers paying Social Security taxes for every Social Security beneficiary. Currently there are a little more than three workers for every beneficiary. By 2020, the number will be reduced to fewer than three workers, and by 2040 to just two workers. In the next half century, barring any changes to taxes or benefits, the Social Security Trust Fund will be depleted.[2, 3, 8]

To prevent or forestall future insolvency of the Social Security program, a variety of proposals to raise the minimum retirement age, reduce benefits, and/or raise payroll taxes have been debated. Others have proposed partially or completely privatizing Social Security. It should be noted, however, that Social Security income represents a large proportion of overall income for most retirees. Consequently, any reduction in benefits or any threat to the stability of the program is expected to have a major and broad societal impact.[2, 3, 6, 8, 22]

Medicare

Medicare is *the* health-care insurance program for Americans aged 65 and older and for the disabled. The Medicare program was developed to provide insurance coverage for seniors in response to what many economists termed a "market failure." That is, prior to Medicare's inception in the 1960s, many older Americans with chronic illnesses found themselves uninsurable in the private insurance market, despite their ability to pay insurance premiums. Consequently, Medicare was developed as a program for all older adults, regardless of income or wealth. Despite concerns about the inefficiency of the large bureaucracy of the federal government, Medicare is very efficiently run compared with most private insurance companies, virtually all of which spend a substantially larger proportion of premiums on overhead compared with Medicare. In addition, Medicare has controlled costs better than the private sector. Consequently, the rate of increase in health-care inflation has been much lower over the last two decades within the Medicare program when compared with the private sector. Because Medicare is very effective in controlling costs, projections about large increases in overall program costs (with the exception of Medicare Part D drug coverage) have been related more to the growth in the number of beneficiaries resulting from population aging rather than to runaway health-care costs. One way in which Medicare has effectively controlled spending has been to reduce and limit payments to hospitals, physicians, and other health-care providers. In recent years, however, many private insurers reduced payments or eligibility for covered services even further, such that hospitals generally regard Medicare as a reliable, if not preferred payer.[13, 24, 25, 28, 29]

Changes implemented by Medicare since the late 1980s, such as the Diagnosis-related Group Prospective Payment System for hospitals have fundamentally changed health-care delivery in this country, resulting in reduced hospital duration-of-stay patterns, a shift of care away from hospital settings, and tremendous growth in home health care and skilled nursing facility utilization. How much Medicare pays for a given service in a given site of care affects access to care, the location where care is provided, and even health-care quality. Moreover, although Medicare has sometimes taken its lead from the private sector, such as in offering managed care coverage, private insurance coverage for patients of all ages is also affected by coverage decisions made by Medicare. In many respects, Medicare has served as a model that private insurers have subsequently followed. Medicare also pays to train resident physicians at teaching hospitals throughout the nation. As a result, any changes made to Medicare have the potential to affect health-care delivery for everyone. As the largest of the federal entitlement programs, and with significant programmatic cost increases projected, an increase in revenues through taxation, premium increases, copayment increases, or a reduction in benefits is inevitable.[25, 28–30]

The Medicare Part D drug coverage program has extended prescription drug coverage to many and has partially privatized the Medicare program for others. The federal laws that created this program also restricted the ability of Medicare administrators to control costs by specifically prohibiting price controls on prescription drugs. Due to these restrictions, there is little doubt that the cost of the Medicare program will increase dramatically in the coming decades. The impact and fate of the Medicare Part D prescription drug program in the future are more uncertain. Some sources predict that the Medicare Part D prescription drug program will threaten the integrity of the entire Medicare program.[25, 28–30]

In addition to the impact of population aging on Medicare, the future of this program will also be affected substantially if coverage is extended to younger Americans. Extending Medicare eligibility or offering Medicare-style benefits to the working uninsured is one of many ideas that has been suggested by legislators, policy makers, business leaders, and others under the Affordable Care Act to deal with the dual crises of uninsurance affecting more than 41 million Americans, most of whom work, as well as a crisis in the current employee-sponsored insurance system, which is insufficient to provide coverage to tens of millions of uninsured working Americans. The employee-sponsored insurance system is expensive and burdensome to employers, adds to the cost of goods and services produced in this country, and is consequently seen as a threat to economic competitiveness in the global marketplace. American producers are competing with producers from other nations, virtually all of which have some sort of government-sponsored universal health-care coverage.[23, 24, 28, 31]

Medicaid

Medicaid is funded jointly by the federal and state governments. Each state has its own Medicaid program, with slightly different eligibility criteria and covered services. Medicaid pays for health services for the poor of all ages. Currently approximately 10% of older adults live in poverty with the remainder equally divided among high, middle, and low incomes. Rates of poverty vary considerably by education level, race, and gender. Approximately half of all elderly black women who live alone are poor. The projected financial status of baby boomers in old age is highly controversial and likely to show a wide range of financial status.[10]

Although Medicare is intended entirely for the aged and/or the disabled, Medicaid provides health-care benefits to eligible Americans of all ages, and disability is not an eligibility requirement for younger beneficiaries. Medicaid programs and services for children are among the most celebrated successes since Medicaid's inception 45 years ago. Like Medicare, Medicaid programs have been very effective in controlling costs per beneficiary. Medicaid also pays for long-term nursing facility care for poor older adults. Considering that nursing facility care costs $220 per day or more, it does not take long for most Americans to become impoverished as a result of nursing facility placement. As a consequence, Medicaid has effectively become long-term nursing facility insurance for many, if not most Americans. Therefore, it is not surprising that over the last several decades as the population has aged, the fastest-growing segment of Medicaid expenditures in every state is long-term facility care for older adults, often exceeding 70% of the Medicaid budget in most states. As the postwar baby boom generation ages and develops diseases or impairments over the coming decades, the need for long-term nursing facility placement is expected to increase further. Medicaid spending is therefore expected to increase, affecting government spending in all 50 states as well as the federal government, unless benefits are reduced or eligibility is limited. Without a substantial increase in Medicaid spending, and perhaps even with such an increase in funding, there is the real possibility of erosion in the quality of care to nursing facility Medicaid recipients. The quality of care would suffer due to the increased number of residents and complexity of care presenting to nursing facilities, which would also have increasing limitations in the number of available staff, adequately trained staff, and financial resources.

Moreover, many expect that there will be a significant increase in the number of poor older adults with inadequate housing, care, and assistance in the community, who are unable to find or afford residential long-term care. Within the Medicaid program itself, providing long-term care to a growing older adult population will affect the provision of services to younger beneficiaries, unless overall spending increases. To continue the same Medicaid benefits for a growing older adult population will likely require increased taxation at the state and federal level or a reduction in government spending elsewhere.[3, 8, 23, 28, 32]

Caregiver shortages

Not only are Americans living longer, they are also healthier overall and are generally living longer before disabling medical illness occurs. Increases in health have a modifying effect on the need for assistance with daily activities as well as on hospital utilization and other aspects of health-care delivery. Improvements in health and a reduction in disability rates are not of sufficient magnitude to counter the overall effects of population aging on the need for health-care services or the need for paid caregivers to assist with activities of daily living such as bathing, dressing, grooming, toileting, and ambulation.[2, 3, 13, 33]

At present, there is an overall national shortage of both nurses and physicians. There is even a greater shortage of nurses and physicians who have been specifically trained to serve the needs of older adults. There are wide geographical variations as well as more acute shortages in some communities compared with others in the same area. Likewise, the shortages are greatest among some medical specialties compared with others. In general, primary care specialties are in shortest supply, and these shortages are expected to be exacerbated substantially in the future as society ages.

It is estimated that 36,000 geriatricians will be needed in the United States by 2030. There are currently approximately 7,000 certified geriatricians and 1,500 certified geriatric psychiatrists. The current training output of geriatricians is inadequate to reach the goal of 36,000 geriatricians by 2030. Family medicine, internal medicine, and general psychiatry are the sources of applicants for geriatric fellowship programs. Since 2003, the number of US medical school graduates selecting these careers has declined. With an insufficient number of geriatricians and geriatric psychiatrists to provide direct care to all older adults, it is generally agreed that the future role

of these providers will be to train other physicians and health-care providers. Given the recent decline in the primary specialties providing geriatrics fellowship applicants, it is unlikely that there will be enough geriatric specialists to fulfill the training role. Unfortunately, it is also unlikely that there will be enough non-geriatrician primary care physicians for the geriatricians to train. Because of the expense involved in training health-care professionals as well as a shortage of all health-care faculty, especially those teaching the care of older adults, schools of nursing and medicine are not expected to expand enough in the future to reduce disparities in health-care delivery to older adults below current levels.[34–40]

Access to care is particularly problematic for older adult patients with cognitive or functional impairment who have difficulty seeking care. This population is increasing so rapidly that our current system of "complaint"-based health care with an emphasis on the provision of care in ambulatory clinics is expected to be even more inadequate for a growing number of older adult patients who are unable to ambulate, recognize medical concerns, and/or communicate their complaints to an appropriate health-care provider.[13–16]

Notwithstanding society's ability or willingness to pay for more physicians, nurses, and other caregivers such as nursing assistants, it is unlikely that there will be enough professional care providers to meet the needs of all older adults who require care. This creates a number of difficult issues for society. Given the limited availability of paid caregivers, the quality of care will suffer as care providers are increasingly burdened by workload. Avoiding this degradation in health-care quality will be very difficult under such circumstances. Many have asked who should be responsible for addressing this pressing societal issue. Some have suggested that immigration laws should be relaxed to allow an influx of relatively low-skilled foreign workers to fill entry-level jobs as nursing assistants. It is difficult to imagine in the current political climate that immigration laws will be substantially changed in this manner. Moreover, as the shortage of paid caregivers worsens, raising or merely attempting to maintain standards through regulation, such as minimum staffing requirements for long-term care facilities will likely mean raising the quality of care for a relatively few, while limiting access to care for many others. Also there will be a shifting of the burden away from the public sector onto individuals and families, irrespective of their ability to provide or to pay for care. Placing additional burdens on families will mean that some family members will have to leave the workforce, and the productivity of others will suffer as family members miss work for caregiving emergencies. There will be a substantial effect on the economy as a whole.[3–7, 9, 13, 33]

Health-care delivery

Health-care needs are changing, and these changes will be amplified as the population continues to age. Aging is associated with an increase in the prevalence of chronic conditions. In addition, modern medicine has succeeded in transforming what were once fatal illnesses (such as human immunodeficiency virus) into chronic diseases. The societal effect has been a significant increase in health-care costs due to greater prescription drug use and costs, health-care utilization, the complexity of medical care, and an expansion of the health-care continuum. A health-care system built around a model of acute management of single illnesses in isolation, either in the ambulatory or hospital setting, is now obsolete. Most acute care hospitalizations and deaths are now caused by acute exacerbations or complications of chronic disease. Much more health care is needed and must be provided in settings other than the ambulatory and hospital care settings. It is increasingly rare for the care of a single episode of illness to take place in only one site of care. Newer sites of post-acute care have been developed and expanded, such as subacute and long-term acute care hospitals. Consequently, care and communication is increasingly fragmented across multiple sites and multiple providers, creating new and greater challenges for care delivery. Hospital care is shifting toward more invasive, expensive, high-technology care in an increasingly more intensive care setting. The traditional services of the general hospital are increasingly provided in sites outside of the hospital. In the future, these services may not be provided in the hospital at all. Acute care hospitals may effectively become towers of intensive care units and complex surgery centers. Thus, the shifting of sites of care will continue. Hospital care will be deemphasized for all but the most critically ill patients.

As the nursing shortage becomes more critical, the trend toward task segmentation and off-loading of historically nursing responsibilities will continue to shift toward lower-skilled and lower-paid employees.

Likewise, the growing number of midlevel care providers is expected to increase as the physician shortage increases; however, increasing the number of nurse practitioners will decrease the number of nurses. Similarly, adding more medical schools or increasing medical school class size in an effort to increase the number of physicians will likely decrease the number of prospective nurses, physical therapists, and other health-care providers. One example of the impact of health-care provider supply on society is found in the significant shortage of pharmacists. The shortage of pharmacists has been made especially acute in recent years due to the relative explosion in prescription drug use, a trend that is expected to continue for the foreseeable future. Substituting pharmacy technicians and technological solutions, such as robots, to ease the burden on pharmacists has played an increasingly important role in delivering more pharmacy care with a limited number of trained professionals. Legitimate concerns about patient safety exist, however, as the role of the best-trained health-care provider (pharmacist) changes and their ability to provide direct oversight of care is potentially compromised.[2, 3, 13–16, 18, 30, 31, 33]

Family relationships

It has often been said that as a result of population aging, the family tree is getting taller, not wider. That is to say, more and more children now and in the future will have the experience of knowing their grandparents as well as their great-grandparents but will have fewer siblings and cousins than in past generations. The opportunity to share the collective wisdom of generations, the experience of having healthy, older relatives as role models, and the added attention that a child might experience as a result of having more older relatives and fewer age peers to compete with for their attention are all potentially positive aspects of aging families. On the other hand, the relationships within families change as individuals age and as the demands on younger family members increase while their numbers decrease.[2–4, 9, 13]

More than 65% of those aged 65–74 live with their spouse. Single and widowed individuals also overwhelmingly live in the community. Families and others provide a tremendous amount of support to the elderly. Role reversals occur when adult children become caregivers for aging parents, particularly those with Alzheimer's disease and other conditions resulting in cognitive impairment. Significant emotional and financial stress related to care giving or financially supporting older relatives will take a heavy toll on many. Moreover, the necessity of attending to medical emergencies or other health-related crises for older family members will affect attendance at work for younger family members, which could negatively affect productivity as well as job security. Although intergenerational family groups living together in one home will likely become more common, this will increasingly require some family members to move great distances from their home or work, causing significant stress, the loss of social support, and/or income disruption, because many parents do not currently live in the same community as their adult children.

More and more adult children will experience the stress and/or joy of watching widowed parents or grandparents remarrying or entering into significant personal relationships with others, causing the perception of one's own family to change as well. Thus there is the potential for richer family relationships, strengthened family bonds, a greater respect for older generations, and a more fulfilling life through family interaction. There will, however, also be excruciatingly painful decisions for many, related to caregiving, finances, and threats to one's ego and identity as roles, relationships, needs, and abilities change throughout life.

Summary

The aging of America, as well as the entire world, will have wide-ranging consequences on our society, economy, government, and our own lives, irrespective of our age. Everyone will be affected in some way by this demographic change. Untold opportunities and challenges will present themselves. A shortage of clinicians and paid caregivers will put greater strain on a health-care system that many feel is already broken. Ensuring the health and welfare of our nation, including those who are most vulnerable, will require a reassessment of personal and governmental priorities. It is likely that more of the caregiver burden will be shifted to families and informal caregiving networks, and more of the financial burden for long-term care will shift away from government onto the private sector. Necessary increases in government spending on Social Security, Medicare, and Medicaid, even if individual benefits decrease, will result in decreased discretionary spending by the federal and state governments. There will also be a

greater burden on local governments and communities to meet the needs of a growing number of older adults. Cultural attitudes toward the aged will likely change. Hopefully, this will be for the better, but that remains to be seen. Nevertheless, the opportunity for many to live longer, better lives is a real possibility. People will continue to enjoy the company of loved ones, to learn from elders, and impart that wisdom to younger generations. This is an invaluable gift that many more of us will experience and benefit from in the years to come.

References

1. Kinsella K, Wan H. *An Aging World: 2008*. November 2009. Washington, DC: U.S. Census Bureau, International Population Report; P95/01–1.

2. Werner C. The Older Population: 2010. *2010 Census Briefs*. Washington, DC: United States Census Bureau; November 2011. C2010BR–09.

3. Reznik GL, Shoffner D, Weaver DA. Coping with the demographic challenge: fewer children and living longer. *Soc Secur Bull*. 2007;**66**:37–45.

4. Eckert JK, Morgan LA, Swamy N. Preferences for receipt of care among community-dwelling adults. *J Aging Soc Policy*. 2004;**16**:49–65.

5. Golant SM. Political and organizational barriers to satisfying low-income U.S. seniors' need for affordable rental housing with supportive services. *J Aging Soc Policy*. 2003;**15**:21–48.

6. Newman S. The living conditions of elderly Americans. *Gerontologist*. 2003;**43**:99–109.

7. Oswald F, Wahl HW. Housing and health in later life. *Rev Environ Health*. 2004;**19**:223–252.

8. Pritchard RE. Creating Social Security incentives for older workers to remain in the workforce. *The J of Applied Bus Res*. 2011;**27**(3):1–8.

9. Kelman HR, Thomas C, Tanaka JS. Longitudinal patterns of formal and informal social support in an urban elderly population. *Soc Sci Med*. 1994;**38**:905–914.

10. General Interagency Forum on Aging-related Statistics. *Older American Update 2012: Key Indicators of Well-Being. Federal Interagency Forum on Aging-Related Statistics*. Washington, DC: US Government Printing Office; 2012.

11. Health Status. Available at: www.agingstats.gov/aging statsdotnet/Main_Site/Data/2012_Documents/Health_Status.pdf (accessed October 29, 2014).

12. Murphy SL, Xu J, Kochanek KD. Deaths: final data for 2010. *Natl Vital Stat Rep*. 2013;**61**(4):1–117.

13. Bragg, EJ, Warshaw GA, Petterson SM, et al. Refocusing geriatricians' role in training to improve care for older adults. *Am Fam Phy*. 2012;**85**(1):59.

14. Warshaw GA, Modawal A, Kues J, et al. Community physician education in geriatrics: applying the assessing care of vulnerable elders model with a multisite primary care group. *J Am Geriatr Soc.* 2010;**58**(9):1780–1785.

15. Boult C, Counsell SR, Leipzig RM, Berenson RA. The urgency of preparing primary care physicians to care for older people with chronic illnesses. *Health Aff (Millwood).* 2010;**29**(5):811–818.

16. Cooper RA, Getzen TE, McKee HZJ, Laud P. Economic and demographic trends signal an impending physician shortage. *Health Affil.* 2002;**21**:140–151.

17. Stewart SD. Effect of changing mortality on the working life of American men and women, 1970–1990. *Soc Biol.* 1997;**44**:153–158.

18. Centers for Disease Control and Prevention. *The State of Aging and Health in America 2013.* Atlanta, GA: Centers for Disease Control and Prevention, US Dept of Health and Human Services; 2013.

19. Hoxie RE, Rubenstein LZ. Are older pedestrians allowed enough time to cross intersections safely? *J Am Geriatr Soc.* 1994;**42**:241–244.

20. Langlois JA, Keyl PM, Guralnik JM, et al. Characteristics of older pedestrians who have difficulty crossing the street. *Am J Public Health.* 1997;**87**:393–397.

21. Koepsell T, McCloskey L, Wolf M, et al. Crosswalk markings and the risk of pedestrian-motor vehicle collisions in older pedestrians. *JAMA.* 2002;**288**:2136–2143.

22. Ozawa MN, Yeo YH. The effect of disability on the net worth of elderly people. *J Aging Soc Policy.* 2007;**19**:21–38.

23. Rudowitz R, Snyder L, Smith VK, et al. Implementing the ACA: Medicaid Spending & Enrollment Growth for FY 2014 and FY 2015. The Kaiser Family Foundation. Available at: kff.org/medicaid/issue-brief/implementing-the-aca-medicaid-spending-enrollment-growth-for-fy-2014-and-fy-2015 (accessed October 29, 2014).

24. Foster RS, Clemens MK. Medicare financial status, budget impact, and sustainability – which concept is which? *Health Care Financ Rev.* 2005–2006;**27**:127–140.

25. Davis K, Collins SR. Medicare at forty. *Health Care Financ Rev.* 2005–2006;**27**:53–62.

26. Johnson KJ. The emergence of a positive gerontology: from disengagement to social involvement. *The Gerontologist.* 2014;**54**(1):93–100.

27. Pew Research Center for the People and the Press. The Generation Gap and the 2012 Election. Available at: www.people-press.org/2011/11/03/about-the-surveys-13 (accessed on October 29, 2014).

28. Blendon RJ, Benson JM. The public and the conflict over future Medicare spending. *N Engl J Med.* 2013; **369**:1066–1073.

29. The Kaiser Family Foundation. The Facts on Medicare Spending and Financing 2014. Available at: http://kff.org/medicare/fact-sheet/medicare-spending-and-financing-fact-sheet (accessed October 29, 2014).

30. Zhang Y, Donohue JM, Lave JR, et al. The effect of Medicare Part D on drug and medical spending. *N Engl J Med.* 2009; **361**:52–61.

31. Cohen RA, Martinez ME. Health insurance coverage: Early release of estimates from the National Health Interview Survey, January–March 2014. National Center for Health Statistics. September 2014. Available at: www.cdc.gov/nchs/nhis/releases.htm (accessed November 1, 2014).

32. MetLife Mature Market Institute. The MetLife Market Survey of Nursing Home and Home Care Costs, 2012. Available at: www.metlife.com/WPSAssets/210528722 11163445734V1F2012NHHCMarketSurvey.pdf (accessed November 1, 2014).

33. Dwyer LL, Harris-Kojetin LD, Branden L, Shimizu IM. Redesign and operation of the National Home and Hospice Care Survey, 2007. National Center for Health Statistics. *Vital Health Stat.* 2010;**1**(53).

34. Warshaw GA, Bragg EJ, Brewer DE, et al. The development of academic geriatric medicine: progress toward preparing the nation's physicians to care for an aging population. *J Am Geriatr Soc.* 2007;**55**(12):2075–2082.

35. Bragg EJ, Warshaw GA, Meganathan K, Brewer DE. National survey of geriatric medicine fellowship programs: comparing findings in 2006/07 and 2001/02 from the American Geriatrics Society and Association of Directors of Geriatric Academic Programs Geriatrics Workforce Policy Studies Center. *J Am Geriatr Soc.* 2010;**58**(11):2166–2172.

36. Reuben DB, Bachrach PS, McCreath H, et al. Changing the course of geriatrics education: an evaluation of the first cohort of Reynolds geriatrics education programs. *Acad Med.* 2009;**84**(5):619–626.

37. Warshaw GA, Bragg EJ, Fried LP, Hall W. Which patients benefit the most from a geriatrician's care? Consensus among directors of geriatrics academic programs. *J Am Geriatr Soc.* 2008;**56**(10):1796–1801.

38. Boult C, Christmas C, Durso SC, et al. Perspective: transforming chronic care for older persons. *Acad Med.* 2008;**83**(7):627–631.

39. Association of Directors of Geriatric Academic Programs and the American Geriatrics Society Geriatric Workforce Policy Studies Center 2010 survey of US allopathic and osteopathic medical schools geriatrics academic programs. Available at: www.adgapstudy.uc.edu (accessed October 29, 2014).

40. Graduate medical education tables. *JAMA.* 2012;**308**(21):2264–2279.

Chapter 54

Retirement

A contemporary perspective

Barret Michalec, PhD

Within this chapter the term "retirement" is used to refer to an individual's departure (in some form) from the workforce (i.e., "retiring"), as well as the imprecise and indefinable span of time from when the individual disengages from the workforce until later in their life (i.e., being "in retirement"). The concept of retirement is primarily associated with aging and older adults, and is therefore riddled with assumptions, stereotypes, and misconceptions regarding its purposes and practices. Furthermore, the contemporary conceptualizations of retirement are in flux, and there is little consensus regarding what retirement is (or what it *should* be), what it means to be retired, or the socially acceptable role(s) of the retiree.

Retirement: a concept in flux

Whereas the traditional conceptualizations of retirement as an institutional practice in managing the labor force and as a particular stage of transition in the life-course still linger, the processes and practices related to retirement are evolving in the twenty-first century. Once believed to be an all-or-nothing event, retirement is now more ambiguous and indefinite in nature. While some individuals may still voluntarily (or involuntarily) completely exit the workforce at a specific time, more and more are choosing to engage in bridge jobs, partial employment, and/or flexible or phased retirement.[1] Regarding these practices, the "departure" from the workforce is not immediate but progressive, deliberate, and often calculated. During the period of time we have come to know as retirement some individuals indeed enhance their leisure-related activities, but others may disengage from social and physical activities for a variety of reasons. Put simply, "retirement," in the contemporary sense, is no longer as structured or fixed as it once was.

Scholars suggest that retirement in the traditional sense could actually be becoming obsolete.[2] In fact, one could argue that retirement is now thought of as just as much an idea or consideration as it is a certain goal or specific ending. Therefore, health-care providers and others interested in elder care would do well to question what may be stereotypical understandings of retirement and retirees (e.g., the "Golden Years," a time to rest, etc.) and focus more intently on learning an *individual* patient's own understanding and perceptions of retiring and retirement.

Much like college, marriage, and parenthood, retirement has traditionally been viewed as a specific stage of the life course and human aging process. But similarly to these other "stages," the socio-economical and cultural landscape as well as national- and organizational-level events and shifts have impacted not only retirement-related trends, but also how individuals view and engage in retirement. Significant influences specific to retirement include (but are certainly not limited to): the shift from an industrial to a post-industrial economy, the elimination of mandatory retirement, the recent Great Recession (and the impacts on employment rates and pension plans), the size and aging of the baby boomer generation, and the ever increasing life expectancy.[3–6] For example, during the tech-boom of the 1990s, there was a surge of what could be considered "early" (younger than 65) retirees voluntarily exiting the workforce. However, the financial impact of the Great Recession in the early 2000s pushed many older workers (55+) out of the workforce, whether they were encouraged to leave their jobs or simply let go, but also forced many older workers to clamor to stay within their current employment and forgo retirement for more income-earning and pension-building/rebuilding years.[7] Furthermore, with

Reichel's Care of the Elderly, 7th Edition, ed. Jan Busby-Whitehead *et al.* Published by Cambridge University Press.
© Cambridge University Press 2016.

baby boomers turning 65 at a rate of about 8,000 a day there is no doubt that this cohort will transform the institutions of aging, including the process of retiring and what it means to be retired.[8] Moreover, the changing statutes and regulations regarding Medicare, Medicaid, and Social Security substantially impact current and future retirement planning and retirement living for a number of generations. And as the life expectancy (at birth and post-65) continues to increase for men and women, it is likely that older individuals will spend more time out of the workforce and therefore more time in retirement than ever before. Unfortunately, at this time we know very little about the time frame of retirement or the various facets of retirement for the older and oldest old.

Although there is little disagreement that retirement refers to some type or form of departure from the workforce, given the flux and evolution of the notion of retirement, and what it means to be retired, an effective way to explore the various meanings and conceptualizations of retirement is to briefly examine prominent theoretical standpoints and perspectives that are frequently discussed in the retirement and aging literature.

Retirement: theoretical approaches and perspectives

Life-course perspective

Within the life-course perspective, development is seen as a series of transitions and choice points that are influenced both by the immediate social context and the larger socio-historical period.[9] In this sense, retirement is a transition and life-stage that is shaped by the context in which one ages and prepares to retire as well the socio-cultural milieu of that era. Hence, "retirement" will be viewed and experienced differently by a baby boomer than a millienial (Gen-Y) given the different norms, values, and general culture of the time periods in which they developed and how these shaped their perceptions, choices, and practices. From this perspective, you cannot extract the individual from their socio-historical context and the cultural nuances that they were exposed to and engaged with during the course of their life.

Modernization theory

Modernization theory suggests that the social status, or social value, of the elderly declines as societies become more modern (i.e., more technologically advanced).[10] Therefore, as technological progress increases, the social value of the elderly (those that are assumed to be less knowledgeable and/or comfortable in this arena) declines. This significantly impacts the employment opportunities for older adults, not merely in terms of the timing of retirement or the voluntariness of retirement, but also the opportunities for bridge jobs or part-time work. This perspective also argues that modernization reflects increased social mobility and dispersing of families – which could significantly impact retirement planning (in terms of location) as well as retirees' social network and the availability of various forms of support.

Activity theory

Activity theory argues that the more active people are, the more likely they are to be satisfied with life, in that how people think of themselves is based primarily on the roles or activities in which they engage and partake.[11] Activity theory recognizes that most elderly individuals continue with the roles and life activities established earlier because they continue to have the same needs and values. Hence, activity theory is an excellent lens to examine phased retirement, bridge employment, sustained social networks, productivity aging, and even retirement planning in general.

Disengagement theory

Although somewhat discounted, disengagement theory examines old age as a time when both the older person and society engage in mutual separation – such as retirement from work.[12] It is related, to some extent, to modernization theory in that according to disengagement theory, the status of older adults must decline as society becomes more modern and efficient; therefore, it is natural for older adults to disengage with the society with which they no longer feel active and participating members. The key to this particular approach is that it is a *mutual* disengagement – both sides purposefully withdraw from one another – and that this separation is natural and a normal tendency reflecting biological rhythms of life. It has been argued that disengagement can be functional. Regarding retirement, individuals disengaging from the work force *functions* to create opportunities for younger workers. However, it is difficult to understand the meso or macro functions of disengaging from core relationships and or social groups. Hence, whereas this perspective can clearly be used to better understand retirement planning and perhaps timing of retirement, it falls short when exploring activities and behaviors associated with contemporary notions of retirement.

Continuity theory

Similar to activity theory, continuity theory notes that people who grow older are inclined to maintain as much as they can regarding their habits, personality, and style that they developed in earlier years.[13] From this approach, any decrease in social engagement or role activity/fulfillment is better explained by poor health or disability than by some functional need for society to disengage older individuals from their roles. In terms of understanding retirement, this perspective would suggest that even if an individual has departed "formally" from their worker role, they may still very well desire to maintain and continue particular practices, relationships, and exercises associated with that role, as it reflects their identity.

Optimization with compensation

The fundamental tenets of the theory of optimization with compensation are parallel to the standard cost-benefit analysis approach. Within this context, older individuals seek to minimize losses and maximize resources (and potential gains) by maintaining engagement in activities with the highest rewards (emotional, psychological, physical, and financial), thereby optimizing the benefits of participation and compensating for limitations that may increase with age.[14] Regarding retirement, individuals may decrease their consumption (i.e., monetary spending) and compensate this with more leisure related and social activities. Socio-emotional selectivity theory fits well within this perspective.[15] Put simply, this approach argues that as individuals perceive their time "left" as short they shift in terms of what they value and desire from their social relationships from information (about themselves and the social world) to the positive emotions fostered from and within the connection. In turn, individuals tend to focus more intently on their core social network (the connections that tend to provide this emotional "good stuff"), spending less effort with peripheral ties – "trimming the fat" of their social network so to speak. Therefore, taking optimization with compensation and socio-emotional selectivity theories together, older

individuals, as they age and during retirement specifically, facing time, accessibility, and physical constraints may focus more intensely on family and close friends to optimize their emotional and social well-being. It is often erroneously suggested that because social networks decrease as one ages that an individual's emotional and social well-being is therefore negatively impacted. What socio-emotional selectivity theory (and perhaps optimization with compensation) propose, however, is that although the number of connections may wane, particular connections are given more effort and attention and therefore may bolster well-being and social connectivity in older age.

Role theory

Role theory has primarily been utilized to explore how preretirement roles will affect postretirement adjustment, the role transition (from worker to retiree), and role stressors associated with that transition.[16, 17] Minimal attention has been paid however, to the norm-based expectations of responsibilities and behaviors of retirees. In other words, although there has been much research on perceptions of and adaptations (or lack thereof) to role loss, examinations of what could be termed the "retirement role" (i.e., norms and behaviors regarding how one *should* be and act when they retire/as a retiree) has been absent from the literature. Scholars interested in aging and gerontology will be forced to explore how the role of retirees and even the role of retirement is shifting and evolving.

Retirement: the impact of social status

Although there are variations in the conceptualizations, perceptions, and experiences of retirement, it is imperative to understand that these perceptions and experiences are shaped not only by institutional and national-level policy and practices, but also by the race, gender, and socio-economic status (SES) of the individuals themselves. Put simply, retirement does not exist in a vacuum. Such social statuses impact individuals' experiences and opportunities throughout the life course, so it should be of no surprise that because they affect opportunities and privileges regarding education, employment, and social networks they will have substantial cumulative and immediate impacts on retirement planning and living in retirement in general. We often understand retirement (in the traditional sense) from the *privileged* life course perspective, one that includes educational attainment, consistent and stable employment (perhaps even with retirement benefits), and a supportive social network. In this sense, retirement can appear welcoming, pleasurable, and certain. But not everyone has access to these resources; some (i.e., racial and ethnic minorities, women, those of low SES) may face persistent and enduring hurdles and barriers throughout their life course, especially in old age, from micro-, meso-, and even macro-level practices and policies steeped in discrimination and inequity, which can significantly impact their perceptions of, planning for, resources available for, and experiences in retirement.

Retirement and health

Given that retirement represents a departure (of varying sorts) from the workforce and labor-related responsibilities, this transition and phase of the life course could reflect a window for health-care providers to promote physical, cognitive, and social health status. Strong predictors of well-being in retirement are voluntariness of entering retirement, pension characteristics, and health.[18] Yet there are still varying results as to whether physical and/or cognitive health improves or declines after retirement, and confusion regarding possible causal mechanisms and forces behind these potential changes.[19] Although it is likely that such confounding issues will continue to be identified and examined through various projects utilizing data from the expansive Health and Retirement Study (HRS),[20] it is important to note that the variations in findings related to retirement and health could be, in part, due to the individualistic nature of contemporary retirement, preexisting cognitive and physical conditions, perceived and available social support, as well as the significant and perpetual impact of socio-cultural factors. For instance, it has been shown that exercise and leisure-time physical activity may increase after the transition to retirement, yet it was found that SES moderated the association between the retirement and physical activity – with low SES being associated with a decrease and high SES being associated with an increase in physical activity.[21]

Although the traditional notion of retirement is proposed and advertised as a time of relaxation, self-reflection, and enhanced social engagement,

retirement, and the transition to retirement, can have negative impacts on self esteem and self-identity. As discussed earlier, individuals maintain particular roles and these roles constitute their identity. The sudden or abrupt loss of a valued role, such as the loss of the role of "worker" or "earner," due to retirement could therefore be quite debilitating to an individual's sense of self and psychological well-being. This role loss could then lend to increased unhealthy behaviors, anxiety, and even depression.[22] However, some older adults may be relieved to relinquish their worker role, and some may even seek new roles of interest in volunteering, other types of employment, caregiving, through social connections, and/or leisure related activities. In this sense the loss of the worker role, and retirement in general, may have a salutary effect on retiree's sense of self and psychological, emotional, and even physical well-being.

Given the wide variation of perceptions of and experiences in retirement, health-care providers engaged in care for the elderly and interested in how retirement may impact their patients should simply ask their patients their own personal thoughts on retirement, and what retirement means to them. Discussing formal and informal planning (financially, emotionally, psychologically, and socially) for a healthy and happy departure (of some sort) from the workforce, and/or intentions and desires for their time during this undefined period of time is not outside the realm of the health-care provider.

Although individuals' narratives regarding their perceptions of and attitudes toward retirement will vary greatly, there are a few principal "markers" that providers can assess from their patients considering or embarking on retirement. These could include the patient's perception of their financial stability/planning (including health insurance and long-term care insurance), preexisting and forecasted physical and mental health conditions as well as their planning for general age-related physical decline, available social support networks/connections, and their current activities and social roles. Doing so will not only provide a better understanding for the provider of their patient, but will also lend to more patient-centered care, help to develop individualized treatment/care plans, and perhaps even boost patient activation and participation in self-care.

References

1. Ruhm CJ. Bridge Jobs and Partial Retirement. *Journal of Labor Economics*. 1990;**8**:482–501.

2. Moody HR, Sasser JR. *Aging: Concepts and Controversies*, 8th ed. Thousand Oaks, CA: Sage Publications, Inc.; 2015.

3. Costa D. *Evolution of Retirement: An American Economic History, 1880–1990*. Chicago, IL: University of Chicago Press; 1998.

4. Munnell AH, Rutledge MS. The Effects of the Great Recession on the Retirement Security of Older Workers. *The Annals of the American Academy of Political and Social Science*. 2013;**650**:124–142.

5. Szinovacz ME, Martin L, Davey A. Recession and Expected Retirement Age: Another Look at the Evidence. *The Gerontologist*. 2014;**54**:245–257.

6. Gilleard C, Higgs P. The Third Age and the Baby Boomers: Two Approaches to the Social Structuring of Later Life. *International Journal of Ageing and Later Life*. 2007;**2**:13–30.

7. Goda GS, Shoven JB, Slavov SN. What Explains Changes in Retirement Plans during the Great Recession? *American Economic Review: Papers & Proceedings*. 2011;**101**:29–34.

8. American Association of Retired Persons [Internet]. Boomers @ 65: Celebrating a Milestone Birthday; 2014 [cited 2014 July 20]. Available at: www.aarp.org/personal-growth/transitions/boomers_65 (accessed 14 November 2015).

9. Elder GH. The Life Course Paradigm: Social Change and Individual Development. In P Moen, GH Elder & K Luscher (eds.), *Examining Lives in Context: Perspectives on the Ecology of Human Development*. Washington, DC: American Psychological Association; 1995: 101–139.

10. Aborderin I. Modernisation and Ageing Theory Revisited: Current Explanations of Recent Developing World and Historical Western Shifts in Material Family Support for Older People. *Ageing & Society*. 2004;**24**:29–50.

11. Longino CF, Kart CS. Explicating Activity Theory: A Formal Replication. *Journal of Gerontology*. 1982;**37**:713–722.

12. Achenbaum WA, Bengtson V. Re-engaging the Disengagement Theory of Aging: On the History and Assessment of Theory Development in Gerontology. *The Gerontologist*. 1994;**34**:756–763.

13. Atchley RC. A Continuity Theory of Normal Aging. *The Geronologist*. 1989;**29**:183–190.

14. Baltes PB, Baltes MM. Selective Optimization with Compensation. In PB Baltes & MM Baltes (eds.), *Successful Ageing: Perspectives from the Behavioral Sciences*. New York: Cambridge University Press; 1990: 1–34.

15. Carstensen LL. Social and Emotional Patterns in Adulthood: Support for Socioemotional Selectivity Theory. *Psychology and Aging*. 1992;**7**:331–338.

16. Ashforth B. *Role Transitions in Organizational Life: An Identity-Based Perspective*. Mahwah, NJ: Lawrence Erlbaum; 2001.

17. Wang M, Shultz K. Employee Retirement: A Review and Recommendations for Future Investigation. *Journal of Management*. 2010;**36**:172–206.

18. Bender KA. An Analysis of Well-Being in Retirement: The Role of Pensions, Health, and 'Voluntariness' of Retirement. *The Journal of Socio-Economics*. 2012;**41**:424–433.

19. Curl AL, Townsend AL. A Multilevel Dyadic Study on the Impact of Retirement on Self-Rated Health: Does Retirement Predict Worse Health in Married Couples? *Research on Aging*. 2014;**36**:297–321.

20. Juster FT, Suzman R. An Overview of the Health and Retirement Study. *The Journal of Human Resources*. 1995;**30**: S7–S56.

21. Barnett I, van Sluijs E, Ogilvie D. Physical Activity and Transitioning to Retirement: A Systematic Review. *American Journal of Preventive Medicine*. 2012;**43**:329–336.

22. Oliffe JL, Rasmussen B, Bottorf JL, et al. Masculinities, Work, and Retirement Among Older Men Who Experience Depression. *Qualitative Health Research*. 2013;**23**:1626–1637.

Cultural competence and health literacy

55

Gwen Yeo, PhD, AGSF, Joanne G. Schwartzberg, MD, and Stacy Cooper Bailey, PhD, MPH

In providing effective geriatric care, it is crucial to consider the background and abilities older patients bring to the clinical encounter. In this chapter, two of the most important considerations are explored.

Cultural competence

Our ethnogeriatric imperative

Although it is important to recognize that all older patients and all providers have cultural backgrounds that affect their clinical interactions, the diversity of cultures older patients bring to their clinical encounters increases the complexity of geriatric care. All elders have cultural beliefs and identities that need to be respected; however, most discussions of cultural competence in ethnogeriatric care relate to the populations that are defined as ethnic minorities. (See Box 55.1.) Based on the projected growth of the populations of ethnic and racially diverse older adults in the United States, the heterogeneity of cultures American geriatric practitioners see will increase dramatically. As

---

BOX 55.1

Cultural competence is a set of congruent behaviors, attitudes, and policies that come together in a system, in an agency, or among professionals that enables effective work in cross-cultural situations.

Source: Based on a definition by Cross TL, Bazron, BJ, Dennis, KW, and Isaacs, MR. *Towards a culturally competent system of care: A monograph of effective services for minority children who are severely emotionally disturbed.* Washington, DC: CASSP Technical Assistance Center, Georgetown University Child Development Center, 1989.

---

illustrated in Figure 55.1, elders in populations categorized as ethnic minorities are expected to reach 40% of all older Americans by midcentury, with the largest growth occurring among Latino and Asian populations.[1] These categories, however, drastically underrepresent the cultural diversity that geriatric providers see, because within each population, including the white majority, are elders and families from dozens of different countries of origin and distinct religious and regional subcultures. Adding to the complexity are individual differences in levels of acculturation, as the large number of elders who have immigrated at older ages to be with adult children are less likely to speak English or to be familiar with norms of US society, especially the health-care system.[2]

The series of National Health Disparities Reports confirm that disparities resulting in poorer health status and poorer health care exist for elders from many minority backgrounds. The 2012 report indicated that "health care quality and access are suboptimal, especially for minority and low income groups" and that while overall quality is improving, "access is getting worse, and disparities are not changing".[3, p.2] Some specific examples for those aged 65 and over include the following: female Medicare recipients reporting being screened for osteoporosis were significantly lower among Hispanics, Asians, Native American/Alaska Natives, and blacks; pneumococcal vaccine rates were lower among Hispanics, Asians, and blacks; colorectal cancer screening was lower among blacks and Asians; lower extremity amputations were higher among blacks; pressure sores in nursing homes were more prevalent among Native Americans/Alaska Natives, Hispanics, and blacks.[3] Although there are many more examples and numerous reasons for disparities, miscommunication, lack of cultural understanding, and lack of trust in

---

Reichel's Care of the Elderly, 7th Edition, ed. Jan Busby-Whitehead *et al.* Published by Cambridge University Press.
© Cambridge University Press 2016.

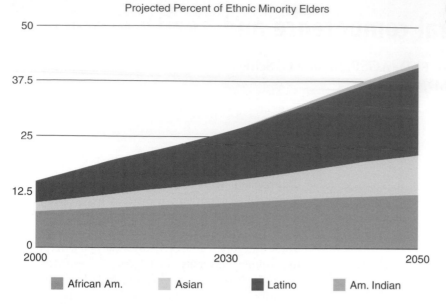

Projected Percent of Ethnic Minority Elders

Figure 55.1 Projected percent of ethnic minority elders.

Legend: African Am., Asian, Latino, Am. Indian

cross-cultural clinical encounters are frequent root causes of poor health outcomes.[4]

So, how are geriatric clinicians to deal with the complexity of cultural expectations, health beliefs, health practices, and preferences with which they are confronted, knowing that there may be negative consequences if there are culturally based misunderstandings? An important place to begin is the conscious development of both individual and organizational cultural competence.[5]

Organizational cultural competence

For physicians and other providers to be culturally competent, they need to practice in, and be supported by, a culturally competent environment. The Office of Minority Health has developed an important set of 15 culturally and linguistically appropriate standards (CLAS) for clinics, hospitals, and health-care systems to advance health equity,[6] some of which are guidelines, and others mandates (see Box 55.2).

The first standard is a general statement of the goal of the standards for health equity. Standards 2, 3, and 4 are important statements of major considerations needed to achieve the goal – commitment of the leadership of the organization, diversity of the workforce, and education for everyone in the system.

Standards 5 through 8 have been interpreted as mandates for health-care organizations based on Title VI of the 1964 Civil Rights Act (see Box 55.3) and court decisions that equate language access with discrimination in national origin.[6] They require that free-of-cost, timely language access (interpreting and translation services) be offered to all limited-English-language patients; that everyone be informed that services are available; that providers of services be trained and competent; and that materials and signage be translated to commonly used languages in the community.

Standards 9 through 13 specify the methods for implementing prior standards, including using goals, demographic information, and assessments in the organization, and using assessments, collaboration, and information in the community. "Think Cultural Health" at the Office of Minority Health's website includes information on CLAS standards and suggestions for implementation.

In geriatric care, it is crucial for health-care organizations to provide adequate language access. Since immigrant older adults are the most likely to have limited English proficiency (LEP), having trained interpreters available is critical to patient-centered geriatric care. Trained interpreters versus ad hoc interpreters (e.g., friends or family) have been found to decrease communication errors, increase patient comprehension, improve clinical outcomes, increase patient satisfaction, reduce errors of potential consequence, reduce length of stay, and reduce readmission rates.[7–9] Even if younger members of families are available to interpret for their elders, they may not have the vocabulary in one or both languages to

736

BOX 55.2 National standards for culturally and linguistically appropriate services in health and health care

The national CLAS standards are intended to advance health equity, improve quality, and help eliminate health care disparities by establishing a blueprint for health and health-care organizations to:

Principal standard

1. Provide effective, equitable, understandable, and respectful quality care and services that are responsive to diverse cultural health beliefs and practices, preferred languages, health literacy, and other communication needs.

Governance, leadership, and workforce

2. Advance and sustain organizational governance and leadership that promotes CLAS and health equity through policy, practices, and allocated resources.
3. Recruit, promote, and support a culturally and linguistically diverse governance, leadership, and workforce that are responsive to the population in the service area.
4. Educate and train governance, leadership, and workforce in culturally and linguistically appropriate policies and practices on an ongoing basis.

Communication and language assistance

5. Offer language assistance to individuals who have limited English proficiency and/or other communication needs, at no cost to them, to facilitate timely access to all health care and services.
6. Inform all individuals of the availability of language assistance services clearly and in their preferred language, verbally and in writing.
7. Ensure the competence of individuals providing language assistance, recognizing that the use of untrained individuals and/or minors as interpreters should be avoided.
8. Provide easy-to-understand print and multimedia materials and signage in the languages commonly used by the populations in the service area.

Engagement, continuous improvement, and accountability

9. Establish culturally and linguistically appropriate goals, policies, and management accountability, and infuse them throughout the organization's planning and operations.
10. Conduct ongoing assessments of the organization's CLAS-related activities and integrate CLAS-related measures into measurement and continuous quality improvement activities.
11. Collect and maintain accurate and reliable demographic data to monitor and evaluate the impact of CLAS on health equity and outcomes and to inform service delivery.
12. Conduct regular assessments of community health assets and needs and use the results to plan and implement services that respond to the cultural and linguistic diversity of populations in the service area.
13. Partner with the community to design, implement, and evaluate policies, practices, and services to ensure cultural and linguistic appropriateness.
14. Create conflict and grievance resolution processes that are culturally and linguistically appropriate to identify, prevent, and resolve conflicts or complaints.
15. Communicate the organization's progress in implementing and sustaining CLAS to all stakeholders, constituents, and the general public.

BOX 55.3 Title VI, Civil Rights Act of 1964

No person in the United States shall, on ground of race, color or national origin, be excluded from participation in, be denied the benefits of, or be subjected to discrimination under any program or activity receiving Federal financial assistance.

communicate medical issues adequately, and they may have their own ideas about the elder's health condition so that perspectives of the elder may not be available to the clinician (which is crucial in assessing pain or other symptoms the elder might want to keep private from family members). It is especially critical not to use children as interpreters even though they may have the best knowledge of English of any

737

family members. Not only are they less likely to have adequate vocabulary, but the responsibility can be traumatic for them. When trained onsite interpreters are not available, it is extremely important for organizations to provide telephonic or video interpreting. (For discussion of provider skills needed in working with interpreters, see the following section.)

In addition to the very important CLAS standards, another important issue for organizational cultural competence in geriatrics includes making available cultural guides for providers to access in cases of cultural questions or misunderstandings. Cross-cultural interactions in health care often include contradictory expectations or judgments about best management decisions when the Western biomedical model collides with long-held cultural health beliefs.[10] Having a consultant from the patient's cultural background who also understands the US health-care system is an important resource for clinicians to understand the older patient's perspective. These cultural guides with cross-cultural understanding could be from faith communities or hospital pastoral care departments; interpreters; nurses or other clinicians from the patients' background; patient navigators; *promatores;* or community health representatives.

Provider cultural competence

There is growing evidence that clinician-patient interaction in cross-cultural encounters impacts patient adherence, clinical decision making, patient satisfaction, health outcomes, and the overall quality of care. [4, 5] So how does a geriatric clinician develop the competence to provide effective care for older patients from cultural backgrounds with which s/he is not familiar? Ideally there would be cultural competency training in health professions schools, but a survey of 2,047 medical residents in their final year of residency from a variety of primary and specialty disciplines indicated that, while 96% felt it was important to consider the patient's culture when providing care, many reported receiving little or no training in cultural competency skills while they were in residencies.[11] The percentage who had little or no training in specific cultural competency skills included: determining how to address patients from different cultures (50%), assessing patients' understanding of their illness (36%), identifying mistrust (56%), negotiating treatment plans (33%), identifying relevant cultural (48%) and religious beliefs (50%),

understanding decision-making roles (52%), and working with interpreters (35%).[11] Aspects of provider cultural competence can be considered in the context of attitudes, knowledge, and skills.

Attitudes: cultural humility and unconscious bias

The geriatric clinician's journey to becoming culturally competent needs to begin with a broad base of cultural humility. It is impossible to be an expert in the hundreds of cultures and subcultures that might be represented among one's patients, so it is important to let the patients become the teachers and the clinician the learner in culturally related issues. It is always important to ask older patients their own perspective, even if the provider is "sure" he or she knows. According to Tervalon and Murray-Garcia, cultural humility incorporates a commitment to self-evaluation and self-critique, and to redressing the power imbalances in the patient-physician dynamic.[12] The self-evaluation and self-critique referred to includes reflecting on one's own background and what conscious or unconscious biases might lead to assumptions about individuals from different cultures that could affect clinical interactions. Shulman and others showed that physicians made different clinical decisions for patients of different races and/or genders even when they presented with the same clinical symptoms. Authors suggest that different decisions might result from unconscious assumptions held by physicians.[13] Unconscious or implicit clinician bias is increasingly being studied in relation to clinical decision making and to patients' satisfaction and their perceptions of clinicians.[14] For example, Green et al. found clinicians' implicit bias was related to their decisions about thrombolysis (15); Oliver et al. found that, while physicians had implicit and explicit biases, those biases did not predict decisions about total knee replacements.[16] Blair and colleagues found that clinicians with greater implicit bias were rated lower in patient-centered care by their black patients.[17]

Developing cultural humility and being aware of one's biases, however, does not relieve the provider of the need to learn as much as possible about the older patient's native culture to use as background for the encounter without making the assumption that that particular elder adheres to any of that culture's specific values and health beliefs. This tension between what is traditionally considered "culturally

738

competent" care when the provider makes an effort to recognize the elder's cultural needs and preferences and what is usually considered patient-centered care when the elder is treated as a unique individual is one of the most difficult challenges in effective ethnogeriatric care. The Ethnogeriatrics Committee of the American Geriatrics Society (AGS) has emphasized the importance of incorporating cultural information in working with diverse elders in their three-volume series, *Doorway Thoughts: Cross-cultural Health Care for Older Adults*, based on the assumption that clinicians need to be somewhat familiar with the cultural background of elders before they open to door to the encounter.[18–20] This does not preclude individualizing the interaction, however. One the AGS editors of the *Doorway Thoughts* series teaches clinicians to check out the cultural information with each older patient with questions such as, "Some people have found it helpful to [e.g., balance their diets between foods that are considered cold or *yin* and those that are considered hot or *yang*. What beliefs do you have about balancing your diet?]"

Knowledge: cultural health beliefs, cohort experiences, and epidemiology

Cultural health beliefs and values In an early classic description of clinical cultural competence, geriatrician Risa Lavizzo-Mourey and colleague identified knowledge of "population-specific health-related cultural values" as the first component.[21] These cultural values and beliefs include unique definitions of diseases common to some cultures that are not familiar in the biomedical model used by most American clinicians. Examples geriatric providers might encounter would be the concept of "susto," or fright, among some traditional Mexican-American elders that may be believed to cause a variety of symptoms; "high blood" in some traditional Southern African-American families, referring in most cases to high blood pressure believed to be caused by too much blood; or the traditional experience of depression in many parts of Chinese society as physical rather than emotional, so that depressed elders might report pain, dizziness, or fatigue rather than feeling sad.[22]

Other manifestations of health-related cultural values include attitudes about diagnosis and treatment, such as: the heavy stigma associated with mental illness and dementia among some traditional families from Korean, Vietnamese, and other Asian

backgrounds that make it less likely an elder would have cognitive symptoms evaluated; the belief that if an elder is told she has cancer, she will give up, which may lead many adult children from Middle Eastern or Filipino backgrounds to urgently request the physician not to tell their older parent the diagnosis; the reticence of some families from Mexican-American backgrounds to use hospice for elders because of the hope for a miracle cure; and the preference of some Native American elders to have healing ceremonies in their tribal home communities rather than Western pharmaceutical treatment. The belief from classical traditional Chinese medicine that health is a matter of balance of the elements, such as "hot" (yang) or "cold" (yin), has influenced similar beliefs in many other Asian countries so that herbal medicine or food choices to restore balance might be preferred over Western medicine. Background knowledge of health beliefs and values among populations in the community the geriatric clinician sees is a crucial step to cultural competence, but it is imperative that the clinician never assume a particular older patient has those beliefs or values.

Cohort experiences Another important component of the knowledge base for culturally competent geriatricians is knowing significant historical experiences that elders from specific ethnic backgrounds are likely to have had. Experiences that influence elders' trust in American health care, such as the common knowledge among African Americans of the Tuskegee Experiment, in which African-American men in a research study were not treated for syphilis, are extremely important to understand. The discrimination African-American, Native American, Latino, Filipino, Chinese, and Japanese communities experienced may present a barrier to trusting cross-cultural health care relationships. Other examples that may have affected elders' health or their attitude toward health care are the forced internment of Japanese Americans on the West Coast during World War II, and Native Americans' forced attendance in boarding schools where they were punished for speaking their native language and forced to cut their hair and dress and behave like mainstream American children. Periods and circumstances of immigration are also important parts of background knowledge about a patient population that can be used in taking the health and social history of an immigrant elder. For example, understanding the chaotic circumstances of the sudden evacuation of the first wave of Vietnamese

BOX 55.4 Questions to elicit patients' explanatory models

What do you think caused your problem?

Why do you think it started when it did?

What do you think your sickness does to your body? How does it work?

How severe is your sickness?

Will it have a short or long course?

What kind of treatment do you think you should receive?

What are the most important results you hope to receive from this treatment?

What are the chief problems your sickness has caused for you? What do you fear most about your sickness?

Note: There are different published versions of these "Kleinman Questions," some that include up to 12 questions. These nine are those from the original 1978 article.
Source: Kleinman A, Eisenberg L, Good B. Culture, illness, and care: Clinical lessons from anthropologic and cross-cultural research. *Annals of Internal Medicine.* 1978;88(2):251–8.

immigrants at the end of the Vietnam War, or the difficult life in refugee camps and the dangerous voyages encountered by later waves of Vietnamese immigrants, provides the basis for targeted questions that help providers establish rapport and understand health-related experiences of older Vietnamese Americans. A resource for clinicians to learn the cohort experiences of elders in US ethnic populations – *Cohort Analysis as a Tool in Ethnogeriatrics: Historical Profiles of Elders from Eight Ethnic Populations in the United States* – is available from Stanford Geriatric Education Center.[23]

Epidemiology of disease risks A second component of cultural competence identified by Lavizzo-Mourey and MacKenzie is knowledge of special risks of diseases and conditions populations face. Knowing what conditions are prevalent in older adults from specific backgrounds can make clinicians more aware of needed assessments and preventive health recommendations for particular elders. An important example is the excess risk of type 2 diabetes among elders from Latinos, African Americans, Native Americans, the Chinese, Asian Indians, the Japanese, Koreans, Filipinos, and Native Hawaiians.[24] Given the potentially devastating consequences of uncontrolled diabetes for so many conditions, including dementia, it is critical for providers to be aggressive in case finding and treatment, especially in older patients who are not overweight, as many with diabetes from many Asian backgrounds are not. A list of conditions that have been found to be more prevalent among older Americans from specific backgrounds is found in the article, "How Will the U.S. Healthcare System Meet the Challenge of the Ethnogeriatric Imperative?"[24]

Skills: eliciting explanatory models, showing respect, assessment, and working with interpreters

Eliciting explanatory models Understanding older patients' perception of their conditions (their explanatory models) can help clinicians make recommendations that are consistent with patients' views and are more likely to increase their adherence to clinical recommendations. A widely recommended strategy for eliciting the explanatory models is to use questions similar to those developed by Kleinman and colleagues.[25] (See Box 55.4.)

Then the question becomes, what should the provider do with the information that was elicited? Various models to incorporate patients' perspectives into recommended management of geriatric conditions have been suggested (see the LEARN model [26] in Box 55.5 as an example), but they all have in common the importance of negotiating an agreeable plan that allows clinicians to provide their best evidence-based care while recognizing and incorporating if possible their older patients' culturally influenced knowledge of their own health – the epitome of patient-centered geriatric care.

Showing culturally appropriate respect One way a geriatric clinician can help to establish an immediate relationship with an older patient from a different cultural background is to greet the elder in a culturally appropriate way. How would one know whether to shake hands, bow, or look the elder in the eye – all of which differ culturally? This is where a cultural guide from the elder's background can be very helpful to give a short lesson in greeting etiquette. In general, touching, especially across genders, is not considered

BOX 55.5 The LEARN Model of cross-cultural communication

- *Listen* with sympathy and understanding to the patient's perception of the problem
- *Explain* your perceptions of the problem
- *Acknowledge* and discuss the differences and similarities
- *Recommend* treatment
- *Negotiate* agreement

Source: Berlin E, Fowkes WA. A teaching framework for cross-cultural health care. *Western Journal of Medicine.* 1983;139:934–8.

appropriate in many Middle Eastern and Asian populations, especially among Muslims. In other cultures, such as many Latino cultures, shaking hands and gentle touching are expected and considered reassuring. Sustained eye contact can be interpreted as confrontational or disrespectful among some cultures such as some Native American or some parts of Asia, so providers may find older patients looking down during an encounter. If unsure about appropriate cultural greetings, asking the elder to provide a lesson would be acceptable. Older patients can also be helpful in instructing providers about their desired form of address and the name they prefer. In general it is usually considered most respectful to use "Mr." or "Mrs." and the family name until instructed otherwise; in some cases, however, it may not be clear which name is the appropriate family name, so asking the elder is always safest. A particularly important part of showing appropriate respect is always to greet the elder first before other family members even if he or she doesn't speak English. Because elders are held in much higher esteem in most other cultures than in the United States, both the older patient and other family members will expect deference to the elder.

Respect can also be conveyed by being careful not to use disrespectful movements or gestures. Showing the sole of one's shoe to someone is very insulting in many Middle Eastern cultures, and there are many hand gestures that are offensive in other cultures, such as several used by many Americans to express "OK" or "Come here, please." Again, being careful to follow cultural guidelines regarding touching is important.

Assessment In addition to language issues, cross-cultural geriatric assessments need to take into consideration other issues such as appropriate respect, relevant health histories in the context of elders' cohort experience, asking permission to examine parts of the body and being aware of cultural taboos that prohibit touching some areas, and using linguistically and culturally validated formal assessment measures.[27] If cognitive status is assessed, for example, there are many translations of the most common measures [e.g., Montreal Cognitive Assessment (MOCA) has been translated into 36 different languages, 21 of which have been validated],[28] and there are numerous original measures validated to be accurate in specific populations. Similarly, it is important to use culturally appropriate measures to assess depression. Mui and colleagues found that some of the items in the Geriatric Depression Scale (GDS) were not appropriate for the six different ethnic populations of Asian elders they studied and made suggestions for modifications.[29]

Many elders use herbal and other remedies common in their countries of origin, and in most cases they do not volunteer that information to their physicians unless asked. It is important, then, to explore their use, especially in cases where there is a potential interaction with prescribed medications, as in the case of diabetes drugs. (For more information of ethnogeriatric assessment, see http://geriatrics.stanford.edu/culturemed/overview/assessment.)

Working with interpreters As discussed previously, it is vital for clinicians to insist on using trained interpreters with elders who are limited English proficient rather than family members, especially children. Skills in working appropriately with interpreters include having them sit slightly behind patients so the patient faces the clinician, speaking in short phrases using lay terminology, recognizing that interpreters are obligated to interpret everything that is said so that they cannot be engaged in a side conversation, and not asking interpreters to perform tasks outside of their role, such as independently obtaining consent for a procedure. See an excellent example of appropriate clinical skills in using interpreters in the video developed by the Cross Cultural Health Care Program.[30]

Summary

In our increasingly diverse society, it is essential to promote the conscious development of both individual and organizational cultural competence. Accounting for the cultural background and identities of older patients is a crucial step toward improving patient-provider communication, reducing health disparities and improving health outcomes. We now turn our attention to another important consideration when communicating with older adults: health literacy.

Health literacy

Health literacy is defined by the Institute of Medicine as "the degree to which individuals can obtain, process, and understand the basic health information and services necessary to make appropriate health decisions."[31] A multifaceted concept, health literacy reflects a range of individual skills and abilities needed to navigate a complex and demanding health-care system. Patients with limited health literacy are likely to face considerable difficulty with health-related tasks – for example, describing symptoms to their provider, determining the correct amount of medicine to take, and understanding information provided in patient education materials. Although such tasks are routinely expected, if not required, of patients in order to effectively manage their health, estimates indicate that more than 90 million US adults are likely to struggle with these everyday health-care tasks.[31]

According to the 2003 National Assessment of Adult Literacy (NAAL), more than a third of US adults have *basic* or *below basic* health literacy and are unlikely to have the skills necessary to effectively obtain, process, and understand essential health information.[32] Individuals with low educational attainment, members of racial/ethnic minority groups, and those living in poverty are disproportionately affected. [32] Additionally, elderly persons are more likely to have poor health literacy skills than younger adults, with NAAL results indicating that 71% of older adults have difficulty reading and interpreting print materials, 80% have trouble navigating information provided in tables or charts, and 68% have difficulty performing basic arithmetic or interpreting quantitative information.[32, 33] The natural processes of aging and cognitive decline are likely to play a role in age-related literacy disparities.[33] In addition, multiple comorbidities, multiple physicians, multiple treatment plans, and polypharmacy further exacerbate challenges elderly patients are likely to face.

As elders use disproportionately more medical services and are burdened with greater chronic disease than younger adults, it has become increasingly important to determine how best to address the problem of limited health literacy among this population.

Current estimates suggest that low health literacy costs the United States from $106 to $238 billion each year; this economic burden is likely to increase as the US population ages.[34] Consequently, Healthy People 2020 identified addressing limited health literacy as a national priority.[35] Gaining an understanding of health literacy, its impact on health outcomes, and how best to address patients' health literacy limitations is therefore crucial for clinicians seeking to improve care of older patients.[31]

A health literacy primer

Health literacy encompasses a diverse collection of skills, including reading, writing, listening, speaking, and performing basic arithmetic, among others. How patients utilize this skill set within the health-care setting – as well as how providers and the health-care system deliver health information – is instrumental in determining an individual's ability to make sense of health information and to translate this information into action. Reducing the gap between individual literacy skills and the demands placed on patients by the health-care system is therefore a key goal of many health literacy interventions.

An individual's health literacy is inextricably influenced by a number of factors, including demographic characteristics (e.g., race, age, education), physical and mental capabilities (e.g., vision, hearing), and social and economic attributes (e.g., income, language spoken, culture), among others.[31, 36] Although the exact causal mechanisms through which health literacy affects health outcomes are unknown, health literacy is thought to influence a number of mediating processes, such as patients' ability to effectively access and use health care, interact with clinicians, or self-manage chronic conditions.[36, 37]

Health literacy and outcomes

Despite a limited understanding of causal pathways, evidence supports an association between health literacy and patient outcomes.[31, 38, 39] Recent systematic reviews have concluded that limited health literacy is associated with less health-related knowledge and comprehension, increased rates of emergency department use and hospitalizations, lower rates of mammography screening, worse understanding and use of medications, poor interpretation of health messages, worse health status, and higher all-cause mortality rates.[38, 39]

Although the relationship between health literacy and these outcomes is well substantiated, for other outcomes such as access to care, disease management and control, and quality of life, evidence is mixed.[39] Limitations and variations in how health literacy is measured may partially explain inconsistent study results.[39] In particular, the complexity of the health literacy concept makes it difficult to measure comprehensively in a short period of time. Assessments such as the Rapid Estimate of Adult Literacy in Medicine, the Test of Functional Health Literacy in Adults, and the Newest Vital Sign, which are routinely used in research settings, measure mostly patient reading and/or numeracy skills and do not address the broad constellation of skills that the health literacy concept encompasses.[40–43] Furthermore, these tests differ from one another in terms of their focus and the skills they measure; research has shown that they often perform differently even when used in the same study sample.[42, 44]

Strategies for addressing limited health literacy

Increasing health literacy skills on a population level is likely to require substantive improvements to the US educational system, health-care system, and society at large. However, there are a number of concrete steps that providers can take to help address the problem of limited health literacy in clinical practice. These include adopting clinical communication strategies, improving print materials, and optimizing modalities for patient education.

Clinical communication strategies

In 1998, the American Medical Association's House of Delegates adopted a policy recognizing limited literacy as a barrier to diagnosis and treatment.[45] Missed or inaccurate diagnoses can arise when physicians communicate poorly with the patient, for example, by using medical jargon or by failing to ask the right questions. They can also occur when patients misunderstand questions asked by clinicians, fill out office-based health questionnaires incorrectly, or are unable to articulate symptoms. Following are communication skills and tips offered to clinicians to ensure that (1) you understand the patient and (2) the patient understands you.

To ensure that you understand the patient:

- Encourage patient participation during the medical encounter by eliciting patient questions,

actively listening to patient concerns, and engaging in a conversation with the patient. Do not interrupt; remember that silence can be helpful.

- Ask, "What other questions do you have for me today?" or "What else may I answer for you today?" and provide a long, expectant pause to elicit patient concerns.
- Ask, "What have you tried already?" and "What do you think is happening?" to gain further insight into the patient's perspective on his or her condition.
- Summarize what the patient has told you in order to (1) reassure the patient that you have listened and understood, and (2) model the behavior you will later ask the patient to perform to confirm his or her own understanding of information discussed (i.e., "teach back").[46]

To ensure that the patient understands you:

- Speak slowly, clearly, and at an appropriate volume to ensure that patients are able to hear and follow the conversation.
- Avoid the use of medical jargon. If medical terminology is necessary, clearly describe all terms, providing examples or a definition that uses easy-to-understand language.
- Limit the amount of new information provided to patients. Studies suggest that most patients can only process three to five points of information during a single encounter.[47]
- Consider using graphics or visual aids to support learning.
- Verify patient understanding of information via *teach back, guided imagery*, or another interactive communication strategy.[48–50]

Teach back has emerged as a provider communication strategy that is well suited for patients of all literacy levels and may be particularly important for communicating with patients with limited literacy. The teach back method ensures that patients have correctly heard, processed, and retained information communicated to them by their physician. This is important, as studies indicate that 40%–80% of information provided to patients is forgotten immediately, and information that is remembered is often recalled incorrectly.[47] To perform teach back, physicians should ask patients to confirm that they understand the information provided to them by "teaching it back" to the physician. If the patient is unable to correctly communicate the information, then the physician should clarify the content again and ask once more for the patient to confirm understanding. This process should be repeated until the patient is able to demonstrate comprehension.

Providers often have the perception that performing teach back will be time-intensive and of limited utility. A seminal study by Schillinger and colleagues demonstrated, however, that utilizing the teach back method can have a positive impact on patient outcomes and only minimally increases the duration of clinic visits.[50] In this study, diabetic patients whose providers utilized teach back were significantly more likely to have lower hemoglobin A1c levels. Findings also indicated that visit duration did not differ significantly between providers who used teach back versus those who did not (22.1 minutes vs. 20.3 minutes, $p = .50$). In multivariate models, the only variables independently associated with glycemic control were higher literacy skills and provider use of interactive communication strategies. Teach back has thus become a recommended communication strategy by the American Medical Association, the Joint Commission, and the Agency for Healthcare Research and Quality, among others.[47, 51, 52]

Another useful technique to ensure patient understanding is the *guided imagery* approach.[49] In this approach, patients are asked to visualize and describe how they will carry out a health-related activity. For example, patients struggling with medication adherence may be asked to imagine and describe all steps related to their medication use, such as what time of day they will take their medicine, where they will store medication, and how they will remind themselves to take it each day. This approach has thus been referred to as a cognitive "dress rehearsal" where patients are given the opportunity to problem-solve and plan in detail how they will accomplish a specific health task.

Improving print materials

Early health literacy research focused primarily on assessing and improving the readability of print documents. This is essential, as print materials continue to be a predominant source of patient education. At clinic visits, patients routinely receive print materials covering a range of topics, from preventive screening recommendations to disease self-management support. At pharmacies, patients are given patient information leaflets, medication guides, and other

documents that they are expected to read and understand to support safe medication use.[53] Yet research has repeatedly shown that these materials are written at a reading grade level that is too high for the average patient; they are also often organized in a manner that is difficult for patients to navigate.[54, 55] In response to this common problem, a set of health literacy "best practices" have been developed for use in the design of print materials.[47, 53, 56] These best practices are based upon research in the fields of health literacy, adult education, and cognitive science:

- Use simple, easy-to-understand language whenever possible. Avoid jargon and define any medical terminology used.
- Provide patients with essential, "need-to-know" information only. Do not include lengthy biomedical explanations, but focus instead on necessary background information or context.
- Write in the active voice, in short and clear sentences.
- Consider "chunking" information so that it is grouped in a meaningful way. Use subject headings or other visual devices to signal the introduction of a new group of information.
- Use a large, easily readable font (12 point, serif font is recommended).
- Present information in sentence format, capitalizing only the first word in the sentence.
- Include adequate white space surrounding text by using appropriate margins and spacing.
- Use meaningful graphics that are relevant to the text, and provide labels for any graphs, illustrations, or visual aids.
- Use color sparingly, and ensure that there is adequate contrast between the text and paper – this is especially important for elderly readers.

When developing materials, providers should attempt to incorporate these best practices whenever possible. Currently used print materials should also be reviewed and changes made as necessary to ensure patient understanding. Health-care professionals should consider involving patients in the design and evaluation of print materials to ensure that they can be easily understood by their target audience.[48] Additionally, tools such as the Suitability Assessment of Materials (SAM) and the Patient Education Materials Assessment Tool (PEMAT) can be used to help guide revisions and identify areas of concern.[56, 57]

Optimizing modality

The adoption of new technologies has introduced novel ways to communicate with patients, promote healthy behaviors, and facilitate health-care delivery. Patient education materials are no longer provided solely in print; many are available online or in a multimedia format. Clinicians can also now communicate with patients via patient portals and email. Similarly, mobile technology – specifically text messaging and mobile applications – have been utilized for numerous health purposes, from reminding patients to take medications to providing weight loss support.[58]

Whereas technology offers clear benefits and can enhance patient care, it is important to remember that disparities exist in terms of access and use. Research indicates that elders and those with limited literacy may be less likely to access and utilize technology, particularly for health-related purposes.[59–61] Relying heavily on health information technology for health promotion and communication activities could further exacerbate literacy-related disparities. Similarly, abandoning print materials in favor of multimedia formats may not necessarily lead to greater comprehension and adoption of healthy behaviors. A 2012 systematic review by Wilson et al. examined the effect of modality (multimedia vs. print) on a number of patient outcomes.[62] Results from 30 studies included in the review were mixed, with little guidance available on which modality is best, particularly for patients with limited literacy skills. Overall, it is likely that providing patient education in multiple formats and at repeated intervals is necessary to promote learning, especially for older adults with limited literacy.

The need for universal precautions

Clinicians are sometimes tempted to use communication strategies and health literacy best practices only for those patients whom they believe are affected by limited literacy skills. This is problematic, as studies have shown that providers overestimate the literacy skills of their patients.[63, 64] Moreover, research demonstrates that even patients with adequate literacy skills are at risk for misunderstanding health information and that they also prefer health-literacy-informed health materials.[65–67] For example, Davis and colleagues found that 38% of patients with adequate literacy skills misunderstood at least one out of five common prescription medication instructions.

[65] Focus groups conducted with patients of various literacy levels revealed that incorporating health literacy best practices into the design of such instructions would help all patients better understand directions for use.[67] While providers are sometimes concerned that patients will be offended by the use of oversimplified or "dumbed down" communication, findings from these studies and others indicate that patients prefer the use of easy-to-understand language and will not be offended if providers communicate with them in this manner.

In 2010, AHRQ issued the Health Literacy Universal Precautions toolkit, which describes communication techniques that should be used with *all patients* to reduce the risk of misunderstanding.[47] This universal precautions approach was further supported by Dr. Koh, the Assistant Secretary for Health, in the 2013 Health Literate Care Model.[68] This model recommends that clinicians assume that all patients are at risk of misunderstanding health information; the model stipulates that providers should communicate health concepts clearly and subsequently verify patient understanding via teach back or interactive communication strategies. Utilizing a universal precautions approach will help ensure that all patients receive information in a clear manner, promoting patient safety.

Conclusion

Research has found that many patients, even those with adequate literacy skills, routinely misunderstand simple medical information. Such problems are magnified among older patients with multiple comorbidities, multiple physicians, and multiple medications and treatment plans. The complexity of communication is further multiplied among older patients from diverse backgrounds with limited English proficiency, especially when family members try to interpret the clinical interaction.

Evidence-based, person-centered geriatric care requires clinicians to incorporate cultural competence and health literacy techniques into practice, even though doing so may take additional planning and effort. As the value of the universal precautions approach is clear, making such effort is essential to promoting high-quality care for older patients.

References

1. Federal Interagency Forum on Aging-Related Statistics. *Older Americans 2012: Key Indicators of Well-Being.*

Washington, DC: Federal Interagency Forum on Aging-Related Statistics, 2012.

2. Stevens, G. Age at immigration and second language proficiency among foreign-born adults. *Language in Society.* 1999;**28**:555–78.

3. Agency for Health Care Research and Quality. *2012 National Healthcare Disparities Report.* Rockville, MD: US Department of Health and Human Services, 2012; May 2013.

4. Smedley BD, Stith, AY, Nelson, AR, ed. *Unequal Treatment: Confronting Racial and Ethnic Disparities in Health Care.* Washington, DC: The National Academies Press; 2003.

5. Betancourt JR. Becoming a physician: cultural competence – marginal or mainstream movement? *New England Journal of Medicine.* 2004;**351**(10):953–5.

6. Office of Minority Health USDoHHS. National Standards for Culturally and Linguistically Appropriate Services (CLAS) in Health and Health Care. 2013.

7. Karliner LS, Pérez-Stable E, Gildingorin, G. The language divide: the importance of training in the use of interpreters for outpatient practice. *Journal of General Internal Medicine.* 2004;**19**:175–83.

8. Flores G, Abreu M, Barone CP, et al. Errors of medical interpretation and their potential clinical consequences: a comparison of professional versus ad hoc versus no interpreters. *Annals of Emergency Medicine.* 2012;**60**(5):545–53.

9. Lindholm M HJ, Ferguson WJ, Reed G. Professional language interpretation and inpatient length of stay and readmission rates. *Journal of General Internal Medicine.* 2012;**27**(10):1294–9.

10. Fadiman A. *The Spirit Catches You and You Fall Down: A Hmong Child, Her American Doctors, and the Collision of Two Cultures.* New York: Farrar, Straus, & Giroux;1997.

11. Weissman JS, Betancourt J, Campbell EG, et al. Resident physicians' preparedness to provide cross-cultural care. *JAMA.* 2005 Sep 7;**294**(9):1058–67. PubMed PMID: 16145026.

12. Tervalon M, Murray-Garcia J. Cultural humility versus cultural competence: a critical distinction in defining physician training outcomes in multicultural education. *Journal of Health Care for the Poor and Underserved.* 1998 May;**9**(2):117–25.

13. Schulmlan KA, Berlin JA, Harless W. The effect of race and sex on physicians' recommendation for cardiac catheterization. *N Engl J Med.* 1999;**340**(8):618–26.

14. Chapman E, Kaatz, A, Carnes, M. Physicians and implicit bias: how doctors may unwittingly perpetuate health care disparities. *Journal of General Internal Medicine.* 2013;**28**(11):1504–11.

15. Green AR, Carney DR, Pallin DJ, et al. Implicit bias among physicians and its prediction of thrombolysis decisions for black and white patients. *J Gen Intern Med.* 2007 Sep;**22**(9):1231–8. PubMed PMID: 17594129. Pubmed Central PMCID: 2219763.

16. Oliver MN, Wells KM, Joy-Gaba JA, et al. Do physicians' implicit views of African Americans affect clinical decision making? *Journal of American Board of Family Medicine.* 2014;**27**(2):177–88.

17. Blair IV Steiner JF, Fairclough DL, et al. Clinicians' implicit ethnic/racial bias and perceptions of care among black and Latino patients. *Annals of Family Medicine.* 2013;**11**(1):43–52.

18. Adler R, Kamel H, ed. *Doorway Thoughts: Cross Cultural Health Care for Older Adults, Volume 1.* From the Ethnogeriatrics Committee of the American Geriatrics Society. Sudbury, MA: Jones & Bartlett; 2004.

19. Adler R, Brangman S, Pan C, Yeo G, ed. *Doorway Thoughts: Cross Cultural Health Care for Older Adults, Volume 2.* From the Ethnogeriatrics Committee of the American Geriatrics Society. Sudbury, MA: Jones & Bartlett; 2006.

20. Grudzen M, Brangman S, Pan C, Yeo G, ed. *Doorway Thoughts: Cross Cultural Health Care for Older Adults, Volume 3.* From the Ethnogeriatrics Committee of the American Geriatrics Society. Sudbury, MA: Jones & Bartlett; 2009.

21. Lavizzo-Mourey R, MacKenzie E. Cultural competence – an essential hybrid for delivering high quality care in the 1990s and beyond. *Transactions of the American Clinical and Climatological Association.* 1995;**105**:226–37.

22. Kleinman A. Culture and depression. *New England Journal of Medicine.* 2008;**351**(10):351–3.

23. Yeo G, Hikoyeda N, McBride M, et al. *Cohort Analysis as a Tool in Ethnogeriatrics: Historical Profiles of Elders from Eight Ethnic Populations in the United States.* Stanford, CA: Stanford Geriatric Education Center; 1998.

24. Yeo G. How will the U.S. healthcare system meet the challenge of the ethnogeriatric imperative? *Journal of the American Geriatrics Society.* 2009 Jul;**57**(7):1278–85. PubMed PMID: 19558479. Epub 2009/06/30.

25. Kleinman A, Eisenberg L, Good B. Culture, illness, and care: clinical lessons from anthropologic and cross-cultural research. *Annals of Internal Medicine.* 1978;**88**(2):251–8.

26. Berlin E, Fowkes WA. A teaching framework for cross-cultural health care. *Western Journal of Medicine.* 1983;**139**:934–8.

27. Yeo G, Gallagher-Thompson D. *Ethnicity and the Dementias,* 2nd Ed. New York: Taylor & Francis/Routledge; 2006.

28. Nasreddine ZS. The Montreal Cognitive Assessment [5/23/2014]. Available at: www.mocatest.org/default .asphttp://www.mocatest.org/default.asp (accessed May 2014).

29. Mui AC, Kang SY, Chen LM, Domanski MD. Reliability of the Geriatric Depression Scale for use among elderly Asian immigrants in the USA. *International psychogeriatrics / IPA.* 2003 Sep;**15** (3):253–71. PubMed PMID: 14756161.

30. Cross Cultural Health Care Program. *Communicating Effectively Through an Interpreter: An Instructional Video for Health Care Providers: Barriers to Communication.* Seattle, WA.

31. Nielsen-Bohlman L, Panzer A, Kindig DA, ed. *Health Literacy: A Prescription to End Confusion.* Washington DC: National Academy Press; 2004.

32. Kutner M, Greenberg E, Jin Y, Paulsen C. *The Health Literacy of America's Adults: Results from the 2003 National Assessment of Adult Literacy* (NCES 2006–483). Washington, DC: National Center for Education Statistics; 2006.

33. Centers for Disease Control and Prevention. *Improving Health Literacy for Older Adults: Expert Panel Report 2009.* Atlanta: U.S. Department of Health and Human Services; 2009.

34. Vernon JA, Trujillo A, Rosenbaum S, DeBuono B. Low health literacy: implications for national health policy; 2007 October. Available at: http://publichealth .gwu.edu/departments/healthpolicy/CHPR/down loads/LowHealthLiteracyReport10_4_07.pdf (accessed October 2007).

35. US Department of Health and Human Services, Office of Disease Prevention and Health Promotion. Healthy People 2020 Washington, D.C. [cited 2011 April 17]. Available at: www.healthypeople.gov (accessed April 2011).

36. Paasche-Orlow MK, Wolf MS. The causal pathways linking health literacy to health outcomes. *Am J Health Behav.* 2007 Sep–Oct;**31**(Suppl 1):S19–26. PubMed PMID: 17931132.

37. Von Wagner C, Steptoe A, Wolf MS, Wardle J. Health literacy and health actions: a review and a framework from health psychology. *Health Educ Behav.* 2009 Oct;**36**(5):860–77. PubMed PMID: 18728119. Epub 2008/08/30. eng.

38. Berkman ND, DeWalt DA, Pignone MP, et al. *Literacy and health outcomes.* Rockville, MD: Agency for Healthcare Research and Quality, 2004.

39. Berkman ND, Sheridan SL, Donahue KE, et al. Low health literacy and health outcomes: an updated systematic review. *Ann Intern Med.* 2011;**155**(2):97–107.

40. Davis TC, Crouch MA, Long SW, et al. Rapid assessment of literacy levels of adult primary care patients. *Fam Med.* 1991;**23**(6):433–5. PubMed PMID: MEDLINE:1936717. English.

41. Parker RM, Baker DW, Williams MV, Nurss JR. The Test of Functional Health Literacy in Adults (TOFHLA): a new instrument for measuring patients' literacy skills. *J Gen Intern Med.* 1995;**10**:537–42.

42. Baker DW. The meaning and the measure of health literacy. *J Gen Intern Med.* 2006;**21**(8):878–83.

43. Weiss BD, Mays MZ, Martz W, et al. Quick assessment of literacy in primary care: the newest vital sign. *Annals of Family Medicine.* 2005 Nov–Dec;**3**(6):514–22. PubMed PMID: 16338915. Pubmed Central PMCID: 1466931.

44. Wolf MS, Curtis LM, Wilson EA, et al. Literacy, Cognitive Function, and Health: Results of the LitCog Study. *J Gen Intern Med.* 2012 Oct;**27**(10):1300–7. PubMed PMID: 22566171. Pubmed Central PMCID: 3445686. Epub 2012/05/09. eng.

45. Ad Hoc Committee on Health Literacy – American Medical Association. Health literacy: report of the Council on Scientific Affairs. *J Am Med Assoc.* 1999;**281**:552–7. PubMed PMID: 321.

46. Makoul G. Essential elements of communication in medical encounters: the Kalamazoo consensus statement. *Acad Med.* 2001 Apr;**76**(4):390–3. PubMed PMID: 11299158.

47. DeWalt DA, Callahan LF, Hawk VH, et al. Health Literacy Universal Precautions Toolkit. (Prepared by North Carolina Consortium, The Cecil G. Sheps Center for Health Services Research, The University of North Carolina at Chapel Hill, under Contract No. HHSA290200710014. AHRQ Publication No. 10– 0046-EF.). Rockville, MD: Agency for Healthcare Research and Quality; 2010.

48. Sudore RL, Schillinger D. Interventions to improve care for patients with limited health literacy. *J Clin Outcomes Manag.* 2009 Jan 1;**16**(1):20–9. PubMed PMID: 20046798.

49. Park DC, Gutchess AH, Meade ML, Stine-Morrow EA. Improving cognitive function in older adults: nontraditional approaches. *J Gerontol B Psychol Sci Soc Sci.* 2007 Jun;**62**(Spec No 1):45–52. PubMed PMID: 17565164. Epub 2007/08/03. eng.

50. Schillinger D, Piette J, Grumbach K, et al. Closing the loop: physician communication with diabetic patients who have low health literacy. *Arch Intern Med.* 2003 Jan 13;**163**(1):83–90. PubMed PMID: 12523921. Epub 2003/01/14. eng.

51. Joint Commission. "What did the doctor say?": improving health literacy to protect patient safety. Health Care at the Crossroads report. 2007.

52. American Medical Association. The 2007 Health Literacy and Patient Safety: Help Patients Understand Kit: AMA Foundation; 2007.

53. Institute of Medicine. *Standardizing Medication Labels: Confusing Patients Less: Workshop Summary.* Hernandez LM, ed. Washington DC: National Academy Press; 2008.

54. Shrank W, Avorn J, Rolon C, Shekelle P. Effect of content and format of prescription drug labels on readability, understanding, and medication use: a systematic review. *The Annals of Pharmacotherapy.* 2007 May 1;**41**(5):783–801.

55. Shrank WH, Agnew-Blais J, Choudhry NK, et al. The variability and quality of medication container labels. *Arch Intern Med.* 2007 Sep 10;**167**(16):1760–5. PubMed PMID: 17846395. Epub 2007/09/12. eng.

56. Doak CC, Doak LG, Root JH. *Assessing Suitability of Materials: Teaching Patients with Low Literacy Skills.* 2nd ed. Philadelphia: JB Lippincott; 1996.

57. Shoemaker SJ, Wolf MS, Brach C. Development of the Patient Education Materials Assessment Tool (PEMAT): a new measure of understandability and actionability for print and audiovisual patient information. *Patient Educ Couns.* 2014 Sep;**96**(3):395–403. PubMed PMID: 24973195.

58. Patrick K, Griswold WG, Raab F, Intille SS. Health and the mobile phone. *Am J Prev Med.* 2008 Aug;**35**(2):177–81. PubMed PMID: 18550322. Pubmed Central PMCID: 2527290.

59. Bailey SC, O'Conor R, Bojarski EA, et al. Literacy disparities in patient access and health-related use of Internet and mobile technologies. *Health Expectations.* 2014. doi: 10.1111/hex.12294

60. Duggan M. Cell Phone Activities 2013. Pew Research Center. Available at: www.pewinternet.org/2013/09/19/cell-phone-activities-2013 (accessed 16 March 2014).

61. Sarkar U, Karter AJ, Liu JY, et al. The literacy divide: health literacy and the use of an internet-based patient portal in an integrated health system-results from the diabetes study of northern California (DISTANCE). *J Health Commun.* 2010;**15**(Suppl 2):183–96. PubMed PMID: 20845203. Pubmed Central PMCID: 3014858.

62. Wilson EA, Makoul G, Bojarski EA, et al. Comparative analysis of print and multimedia health materials: a review of the literature. *Patient Educ Couns.* 2012 Oct;**89**(1):7–14. PubMed PMID: 22770949.

63. Bass PF, Wilson JF, Griffith CH, Barnett DR. Residents' ability to identify patients with poor literacy skills. *Acad Med.* 2002 Oct;**77**(10):1039–41. PubMed PMID: 12377684. Epub 2002/10/16. eng.

64. Dickens C, Lambert BL, Cromwell T, Piano MR. Nurse overestimation of patients' health literacy. *J Health Commun.* 2013;**18**(Suppl 1):62–9. PubMed PMID: 24093346. Pubmed Central PMCID: 3814908.

65. Davis TC, Wolf MS, Bass III PF, et al. Literacy and misunderstanding prescription drug labels. *Ann Intern Med.* 2006;**145**(12):887–94.

66. Sudore RL, Landefeld CS, Barnes DE, et al. An advance directive redesigned to meet the literacy level of most adults: a randomized trial. *Patient Educ Couns.* 2007;**69**(1):165–95.

67. Webb J, Davis TC, Bernadella P, et al. Patient-centered approach for improving prescription drug warning labels. *Patient Educ Couns.* 2008 Sep;**72**(3):443–9. PubMed PMID: 18644691. Epub 2008/07/23. eng.

68. Koh HK, Brach C, Harris LM, Parchman ML. A proposed "health literate care model" would constitute a systems approach to improving patients' engagement in care. *Health Aff (Millwood).* 2013 Feb;**32**(2):357–67. PubMed PMID: 23381529.

Chapter **56**

Caregiving

Susan Parks, MD, Laraine Winter, PhD, and Danielle Snyderman, MD, CMD

A caregiver's story

Jane, 59 years old, has been a patient of yours for the past nine years. Her mother, Josephine, who has severe dementia, is also your patient. You have supported them both through the diagnosis and progression of Josephine's dementia. Jane, a nurse at the local emergency department, has had to scale down to part-time status over the past year because of her mom's increasing care needs. Determined to care for Josephine in her home, Jane has coordinated a schedule of 24-hour care that includes not only hired companion care but also her own time as direct caregiver to her mom.

The issue of caregiving has moved into the public spotlight in the past decade as our country and society grapple with how to care for an aging population. Caregiving is defined as "assistance provided to individuals who are in need of support because of a disability, mental illness, chronic condition, terminal illness or who are frail."[1] This can include "attention to any of the needs of the person, including hands on care."[1] This chapter focuses on informal caregivers – friends and family members – who care for chronically ill older adults.

Epidemiology

In 1900, only 4.1% of the population was 65 or older and only 0.2% was 85 or older. By 2050, an estimated 20.2% will be at least 65 years old and 5.0% at least 85. [2] Thus, the population aged 65 or older increased from approximately 3 million in 1900 to nearly 35 million in 2000 and is projected to reach nearly 90 million in the year 2060.[3]

Seventy-three percent of caregivers are spouses or children.[3] Adult daughters make up 29% of caregivers and wives another 23%.[3] Thus, the overwhelming majority of family caregivers are women.

Future cohorts of elderly people may have a different experience, based on trends in the structure of the American family. Household structure has been altered especially by trends in marriage and fertility. Divorce is a particular concern because of its potential to undermine effective bonds between parents and children, especially fathers and children.[7] Future cohorts of older adults may therefore be less able to rely on spouses and children.[2]

Chronic conditions increase the risk of functional limitations that threaten independence and increase dependence on family caregivers. In 2000, more than 100 million Americans had a chronic condition, and that number is expected to increase to 158 million by 2040. Chronic conditions are more disabling for the elderly than for younger adults. Nearly 45% of older adults are functionally limited as a result of chronic conditions, the most common being arthritis, hypertension, hearing loss, heart disease, and cataracts.[3]

Trends in disability are encouraging, however. Surveys have consistently documented declines in disability and improvements in instrumental activities of daily living and function in the elderly population.[8] Lower rates of disability portend a better quality of life, greater independence for elders, and lower demands on families and government programs.

Caregiving and caregiver burden

Even in the best-case scenarios of improving health, decreasing disability, and available family caregivers, the projected increase in the older adult population will inevitably place demands on both American families and government programs for the elderly.[3]

The cohort of family caregivers – defined as people who live with and care for a relative with physical or cognitive limitations – in the United States will continue to increase. A wide variety of physical and

---

Reichel's Care of the Elderly, 7th Edition, ed. Jan Busby-Whitehead *et al.* Published by Cambridge University Press.
© Cambridge University Press 2016.

cognitive disabilities affecting the elderly, including dementias, advanced cancers, and end-stage congestive heart failure, can require the assistance of a caregiver.

The term "caregiver burden" was coined in the early 1980s. It has been defined as the "physical, emotional, social, and financial toll of providing care,"[9] or the extent to which caregivers perceive their emotional or physical health, social life, and financial status as suffering as a result of caring for their relative.[10] The term is used in both the medical and lay communities to describe the stress felt by those in the caregiving role.

Despite the abundant literature on caregiver burden, some authors think that the term too broadly tries to encapsulate the stresses associated with this role. In addition, the degree of physical and emotional stress associated with caregiving is very individualized. Thus, we will outline individual components of health and well-being that are affected by caregiving.

Jane comes to your office today to discuss her worsened back pain. You take note that she is 15 minutes late, which is unusual for her. You notice she seems more distracted than usual as she begins to describe her pain. She attributes it to her sciatica and reports feeling like her back is "acting up" more now that she participates in more of the hands-on care for Josephine.

Impact of caregiving

Family caregiving and its effects on health and well-being have been topics of a large body of research since the caregiving was introduced. Some caregivers report high satisfaction with their role. Work by Donelan found that 89% of caregivers feel appreciated by their care recipient, and 71% report that the relationship between them and their care recipient has improved.[11]

Nevertheless, caregiving has well-documented negative effects on mortality, morbidity, and emotional and financial well-being. Higher caregiver burden has been associated with multiple ill effects on the caregiver, the care recipient, and the family as a whole.

Becoming a caregiver can have a significant economic and lifestyle impact.[12] Many caregivers are forced to leave their jobs to provide adequate care for their relative. This can have far-reaching effects on caregivers' financial status and sense of worth. Likewise, many caregivers feel a sense of isolation as their new role does not allow them the time to

participate in social or self-care activities. Marital and family conflict may also emerge from the stress of providing care.[13]

The health impact of caregiving has been well studied and widely reported. A landmark study documented increased mortality, especially in spousal caregivers.[6] In this study, spousal caregivers who experienced burden had a 63% higher mortality rate compared with caregivers who did not experience burden during a four-year study period.[6] More recent work has determined that mortality rates after the hospitalization of a spouse varied according to the diagnosis requiring admission.[14] The highest mortality rates among both men and women spousal caregivers occurred when hospitalization was for psychiatric disease or dementia.[14]

Many caregivers experience symptoms of depression and anxiety. Studies have found that the incidence of depression among caregivers ranges from 31% to 46%.[15–17] A large epidemiological study in Ontario, California, revealed an increase in any psychiatric diagnosis among caregivers compared with noncaregivers, 20.6% compared with 14.9%. Specifically for anxiety disorders, the increase among caregivers was 17.5% compared with 10.9% for noncaregivers.[18] The only category not higher among caregivers was substance abuse.[18] Two other studies showed equal or less alcohol use among caregivers.[15, 19]

Caregiver burden is also associated with increased risk of institutionalization of the care recipient.[20] Institutional placement is more closely associated with family support system collapse rather than with the patient's own health deterioration.[21] Also, increased use of formal in-home services is seen in cases of high caregiver burden.[20]

Because caregiving is often a protracted experience, and the health conditions that afflict care-recipients have changing trajectories, caregiving has been conceptualized as a career.[12] Some researcher have investigated psychological trajectories in the caregiving career, documenting decreasing sense of mastery and competence among many family caregivers.[22]

Dementia caregiving

Caregiving for dementia patients carries a unique set of stressors. For many dementia caregivers, the strongest predictors of burden, depression, and health issues are behavior problems, day/night reversal, wandering, and inappropriate behaviors.[23] Likewise, an important factor is fewer perceived positive or uplifting experiences.[23] Larger social networks can often have a protective effect against the development of caregiver burden.[23]

End-of-life caregiving

There are distinct issues related to caring for someone at the end of life, which have been explored in the medical literature. The issues of complex bereavement, loss of identifying role, and mental health concerns have been identified. Authors have called for "future study on how and whether providing care for a dying family member is different from providing care for a chronically ill family member."[1]

Identifying family caregivers and assessing burden

Family caregivers have long been recognized as "hidden patients."[24] Assessment of their physical and mental health status represents an emerging topic in health-care literature. It has been suggested that primary care physicians are in the unique position to discover patients who may be in the caregiving role by asking about caregiving while obtaining a social history.[25] Caregivers, however, have multiple other entry points into the health-care community, such as when applying for social services. The best time and place for caregiver assessment has been debated; however, it is universally agreed on that some form of caregiver assessment is a good practice. An expert panel on caregiving at the 2005 National Consensus Development Conference for Caregiver Assessment: Translating Research into Policy and Procedure developed a consensus report on caregiver assessment. Their extensive recommendations included identification, assessment of stressors, and current and needed resources.[26] One author described some of the outcomes of caregiver assessment as maintaining caregivers' health and well-being, preventing social isolation of caregivers, and providing appropriate support to caregivers.[27]

Researchers have developed several instruments with which to describe and quantify the degree of burden felt by caregivers. One such instrument, the Zarit Burden Interview (ZBI), has become widely used by researchers studying caregivers.[28] The original form of the ZBI has 22 questions (ZBI-22). Researchers have studied several shorter versions of

Table 56.1 Screening questions for health-care providers to assess degree of caregiver burden

Are you taking care of a relative at home?
Do you feel that you are currently under a lot of stress because of your caregiving responsibilities?
Are there family or friends who help you care for your loved one?
Do you have time to take care of yourself on a daily basis?

the ZBI.[29] The ZBI-1, which has only one question, has been shown to be effective when rapid screening is needed: "Overall, how burdened do you feel in caring for your relative?" (adapted from reference 29). However, some limitations with cancer caregivers were noted with the ZBI-1. See Table 56.1 for additional screening questions that can be used to better clarify the degree of burden perceived by a caregiver. Although the ZBI questionnaire was developed for research purposes, primary care providers should screen their patients for the overall degree of burden perceived by their patients who are caring for a relative.

Health-care providers should screen patients for depression if they are providing care to a relative. The 15-item Geriatric Depression Scale is a useful clinical tool for elderly caregivers;[30] however, simply asking, "Are you often sad or blue?" is also an effective screening question.

In response to your questioning of how her caregiving has impacted her, Jane confides in you the challenges of witnessing her mom's decline: "As a health-care provider, I've been able to see the toll dementia takes on a patient and their family, but I have a whole new appreciation now that it's happened to my family." She says several times, "It is just so hard." She describes that although she knows she is "doing right by her mom," it takes away from time she spends with her husband, plus her own health care needs seem to "be on the back burner." She reports sleeping less and often worrying about what is to come and whether she will have enough finances to support her mom's continued aging in place.

Caregiving interventions

One of the large caregiving intervention trials in the past decade was the REACH Study.[31] The original study developed and tested two 24-month primary care interventions to alleviate caregiver burden. The interventions were behavior management and the addition of caregiver stress management. Both arms resulted in patient behavior improvement. However, only the stress reduction component helped caregiver burden.[31]

Psychoeducational interventions have been shown to lead to decreased burden and increased overall well-being and satisfaction.[23] Importantly, these effects have only been demonstrated if the intervention includes active participation and skills building for the caregivers.[23] Psychoeducational interventions such as skills training and counseling showed improved burden, but these effects decreased over time.[32] Support groups had modest effect on decreasing burden.[32] Pharmacologic intervention for the patient did help lessen caregiver burden.[32]

Support for family caregivers

A variety of support services are available to assist caregivers, including information and assistance services, technology (including assistive devices and home modifications), education and training, support groups and counseling, respite care, and financial support (see Table 56.2).[5] There is evidence that support groups can improve the psychological well-being of caregivers.[33] Some evidence suggests that support groups can be most beneficial when they have an educational focus, such as helping with behavior management issues for those caring for a loved one with dementia. Support groups had modest effect on decreasing burden.[34] Other benefits of support groups include sharing difficult issues, sharing coping strategies, and lessening the feelings of isolation.[5]

Table 56.2 Practical interventions to aid caregivers

Encourage caregiver as a member of the care team
Proactively explore possible caregiving challenges
Emphasize importance of caregiver's self-care and well-being
Offer resources for Education and On-line support
Utilize other members of care team (teamlet models, social workers, area network for aging)
Validate strain and encourage caregivers to access respite care when appropriate

Source: Adapted from reference 32.

Respite services provide family caregivers with much needed rest from their caring responsibilities. Respite can be provided either inside or outside the home. Adult day-care programs are considered a form of respite care. Such care has been shown to have a varied effect on caregiver burden.[35–37]

Financial support may have a profound effect on those in the full-time caregiving role. On the federal level, the National Family Caregiver Support Program (NFCSP) exists under the Older Americans Act programs administered by the Administration on Aging and state and local aging agencies. The NFCSP had its first year of funding in 2001. This program is earmarked for caregivers of those who are 70 years or older to provide information about existing services, assistance to access these services, counseling, support groups, and training around issues of problem solving, respite care, and other services such as home modification.[5] In 2002, the NFCSP provided information on services to 4 million people, counseling to 182,000 people, and respite services to 76,000 people.[5, 38] Table 56.3 details national resources for caregivers.

Cross-cultural perspectives

Caregiving experiences vary across different countries and cultures. Recent work by Belle et al. has shown that a multicomponent intervention improves quality of life and depression among caregivers across different ethnic and racial groups within the United States.[39] Outside the United States, some cultures consider family caregiving as a key component of their long-term care. Germany, Australia, and the United Kingdom are examples of countries where caregivers are considered integral to the functioning of their long-term care systems. Legislation has dictated this. In other cultures, however, caregiving is considered the cultural norm. The provision of care by families is expected, not considered the exception. In those societies, nursing homes are few, and families provide care to their elder relatives in the home setting.

You make some recommendations to Jane for the management of her back pain but also take some time to further explore caregiver strain. You recognize the importance of Jane's role as a caregiver for her mom, but also let her know the impact of caregiving is a concern of yours. You tell Jane you are committed to supporting her and will do so by taking time at future

Table 56.3 Caregiver resources

Online resources	
AARP	www.aarp.org/families/caregiving
American Society on Aging	http://asaging.org/node/1459
Family Caregiver Alliance	www.caregiver.org
National Alliance for Caregiving	www.caregiving.org
National Family Caregivers Association	www.nfcacares.org
Next Step In Care, United Hospital fund	www.nextstepincare.org
National Transitions of Care Coalition	www.ntocc.org/WhoWeServe/Consumers.aspx
Disease-specific caregiving	
Cancer	
American Cancer Society	www.cancer.org/Treatment/Caregivers
National Cancer Institute	www.cancer.gov/cancertopics/copingfamilyfriends
Dementia	
Alzheimer's Association	www.alz.org/living_with_alzheimers_caring_for_alzheimers.asp
Heart failure	
American Heart Association	www.heart.org/HEARTORG/Caregiver/Caregiver_UCM_001103_SubHomePage.jsp
Stroke	
American Stroke Association	www.strokeassociation.org/STROKEORG/LifeAfterStroke/ForFamilyCaregivers/CaregivingResources/Caregiver-Resources_UCM_463834_Article.jsp
Resource locators	
ARCH National Respite Network	www.archrespite.org
Eldercare Locator, Administration on Aging	www.eldercare.gov
Meals on Wheels	www.mowaa.org
Medicare	www.medicare.gov
Paying for Senior Care	www.payingforseniorcare.com
Training and education	
AssistGuide Information Services	www.alz.org/care/alzheimers-dementia-care-training-certification.asp
Family Caregiver Alliance	https://caregiver.org/classes-events
Dementia Caregiver Center	www.alz.org/care/alzheimers-dementia-care-training-certification.asp
Video Caregiving	http://www.videogcaregiving.org

visits to address this specifically. You share with her the website for the Family Caregiver Alliance and ask her to schedule a follow-up with you in one month.

Conclusion

As our country faces an enormous increase in the number of older Americans, the role of family caregivers will become increasingly important. It is the role of many health-care professionals, especially primary care physicians, to identify people in the caregiving role and to screen for caregiving stress or burden. It is likewise important to screen for health effects including depression, anxiety, and substance abuse. It is also important to link caregivers to local resources. These include the area agencies on aging, the Alzheimer's Association, support groups, individual counseling, respite services, and adult day-care services. Occupational and physical therapy may also be useful services for family caregivers of frail or demented elders. Caregivers should also be assisted in applying for services through available financial resources, especially through the NFCSP or other organizations that exist in most communities.

References

1. Stajduhar K, Funk L, Toye C, et al. Part I: home-based family caregiving at the end of life: a comprehensive review of published quantitative research (1998–2008). *Palliative Med* 2010;24:573–593.

2. Agency on Aging. 2015. Available at: www.aoa.acl.gov/Aging_Statistics/future_growth/future_growth.aspx#age (accessed on 14 November 2015).

3. Wilmoth JM, Longino CF. Demographic trends that will shape US policy in the twenty-first century. *Res Aging.* 2006;28:269–288.

4. Stone R., Cafferata GL, Sangl J. Caregivers of the frail elderly: A national profile. *Gerontologist.* 1987;27:616–626.

5. Thompson L. Long-term care: support for family caregivers. Georgetown University Long-term Financing Project. 2004. Available at: http://ltc.georgetown.edu (accessed June 28, 2008).

6. Shultz R, Beach SR. Caregiving as a risk factor for mortality. The Caregiver Health Effects Study. *JAMA.* 1999;282:2215–2219.

7. Amato P, Booth A. A prospective study of divorce and parent-child relationships. *J Marriage Fam.* 1996;58:356–365.

8. Freedman VA, Martin LG, Schoeni RF. Recent trends in disability and functioning among older adults in the United States: a systematic review. *JAMA.* 2002;288:3137–3146.

9. George LK, Gwyther LP. Caregiver well-being: a multidimensional examination of family caregivers of demented adults. *Gerontologist.* 1986;26:253–259.

10. Zarit, SH, Todd PA, Zarit JM. Subjective burden of husbands and wives as caregivers: a longitudinal study. *Gerontologist.* 1986;26:260–266.

11. Donelan K, Hill CA, Hoffman C, et al. Challenged to care: informal caregivers in a changing health system. *Health Aff.* 2002;21:222–231.

12. Aneshensel C, Pearlin L, Mullan J, et al. *Profiles in Caregiving: The Unexpected Career.* New York: Academic Press; 1995.

13. Semple SJ. Conflict in Alzheimer's caregiving families: its dimensions and consequences. *Gerontologist.* 1992;32:648–655.

14. Christakis NA, Allison PD. Mortality after the hospitalization of a spouse. *N Engl J Med.* 2006;354:719–730.

15. Baumgarten M, Hanley JA, Infante-Rivard C, et al. Health of family members caring for elderly persons with dementia. *Ann Intern Med.* 1994;120:126–132.

16. Rosenthal CJ, Sulman J, Marshall VW. Depressive symptoms in family caregivers of long-stay patients. *Gerontologist.* 1993;33:249–256.

17. Williamson GM, Schultz R. Coping with specific stressors in Alzheimer's disease caregiving. *Gerontologist.* 1993;33:747–755.

18. Cochrane JJ, Goering PN, Rogers JM. The mental health of informal caregivers in Ontario: an epidemiologic survey. *Am J Pub Health.* 1997;87:202–207.

19. Kiecolt-Glaser JK, Dura JR, Speicher CE, et al. Spousal caregivers of dementia victims: longitudinal changes in immunity and health. *Psychosoc Med.* 1991;53:345–362.

20. Brown LJ, Potter JF, Foster BG. Caregiver burden should be evaluated during geriatric assessment. *J Am Geriatr Soc.* 1990;38:455–460.

21. Lowenthal MF, Berkman P. *Aging and Mental Disorders in San Francisco.* San Francisco: Jossey-Bass; 1967.

22. Lawton MP, Moss M, Hoffman C, et al. Two transitions in daughters' caregiving careers. *Gerontologist.* 2000;40:437–448.

23. Sorensen, S, Conwell Y. Issues in dementia caregiving: effects on mental and physical health, intervention strategies, and research needs. *Am J Geriatric Psychiatry* 2001;19:491–496.

24. Andolsek KM, Clapp-Channing NE, Gehlbach SH, et al. Caregivers and elderly relatives: the prevalence of caregiving in a family practice. *Arch Intern Med.* 1988;148:2177–2180.

25. Parks SM, Novielli KD. A practical guide to caring for caregivers. *Am Fam Physician.* 2000;62:2613–2620.

26. National Consensus Report on Caregiver Assessment. Vols. I and II. Available at: www.caregiver.org/care

giver/jsp/content node.jsp?nodeid=1630 (accessed June 28, 2008).

27. Nicholas E. An outcomes focus in carer assessment and review: value and challenge. *Br J Soc Work*. 2003;**33**:31–47.

28. Zarit SH, Reever KE, Bach-Peterson J. Relatives of the impaired elderly: correlates of feelings of burden. *Gerontologist*. 1980;**20**:649–655.

29. Higginson IJ, Gao W, Jackson D, et al. Short-form Zarit Caregiver Burden Interviews were valid in advanced conditions. *Journal of Clinical Epidemiology*. 2010;**63**(5):535–542.

30. Yesavage JA, Brink TL, Rose TL, et al. Development and validation of a geriatric depression screening scale: a preliminary report. *J Psych Res*. 1982–1983;**17**:37–49.

31. Burns R, Nichols LO, Martindale-Adams J, et al. Primary care interventions for dementia caregivers: 2-year outcomes from the REACH study. *Gerontologist* 2003;**43**:547–555.

32. Adelman RD, Tmanova LL, Delgado D, et al. Caregiver burden: a clinical review. *JAMA*. 2014;**311**(10):1052–1060.

33. Mittleman M, Ferris SH, Shulman E, et al. A comprehensive support program: effect on depression in spouse-caregiver of AD patients. *Gerontologist*. 1995;**35**:792–802.

34. Haley WE. The family caregiver's role in Alzheimer's disease. *Neurology*. 1997;**48**:S25–S29.

35. Lawton MP, Brody EM, Saperstein AR. A controlled study of respite service for caregivers of Alzheimer's patients. *Gerontologist*. 1989;**29**:8–16.

36. Forde OT, Pearlman S. Breakaway: a social supplement to caregiver's support groups. *Am J Alz Dis*. 1999;**14**:120–124.

37. Feinberg LF, Whitlach C. *Family Caregivers and Consumer Choice*. San Francisco: Family Caregiver Alliance; 1996.

38. Administration on Aging. *The Older Americans Act: National Family Caregivers Support Program (Title III-E and Title VI-C): Compassion in Action*. Washington, DC: US Department of Health and Human Services, Administration on Aging; 2004.

39. Belle SH, Burgio L, Burns R, et al. Enhancing the quality of life of dementia caregivers from different ethnic or racial groups. *Ann Intern Med*. 2006;**145**:727.

Chapter

57

Performance improvement in a changing health-care system

Albert G. Crawford, PhD, MBA, MSIS, John F. McAna, PhD, and Matthew Alcusky, PharmD, MS

Overview

Along with other aspects of the US health-care system, we are now witnessing rapid change in the area of health-care performance improvement. Accordingly, this chapter reviews the history and current state of health-care performance improvement. The key sections of this chapter include:

- Developments in the history of health-care performance improvement
- Main approaches to performance improvement
- Key organizations promoting performance improvement and their products
- Evolving incentives for performance improvement and participation in quality measurement and reporting programs
- The role of health information technology
- Details on key organizations

A prominent 2012 article by Blumenthal provides a valuable framework for this chapter:

> The guiding vision should also be based on the understanding that performance improvement requires that clinicians and patients be enabled to make better health care decisions by giving them the best available information when and where they need it and making it easy to do the right thing. Clinicians and patients need information about patients' personal health and health care and about medical evidence relevant to their decisions. Clinicians need environmental supports and financial incentives to choose diagnostic and therapeutic pathways that maximize the value of care. Organizational arrangements must support collaboration, teamwork, and coordination of care.[1]

Accordingly, this chapter will highlight the two levers identified by Blumenthal: environmental supports and financial incentives.

Key developments in the history of health-care performance improvement

Although a comprehensive review of the history of health-care performance improvement is beyond the scope of this chapter, reviewing some key developments will be instructive.

Donabedian: structure, process, and outcome

Donabedian's model sees health care quality as having three components: structure, process, and outcomes.[2, 3] *Structure* refers to the context in which care is delivered (i.e., buildings and equipment, staff and organization, and financing). *Process* refers to transactions between patients and providers, especially services provided. *Outcomes* refer to the effects of health care on the health of patients and populations. While other frameworks have been developed since Donabedian's time, his model remains a key paradigm for assessing health care quality.

Institute of Medicine reports

Two key publications by the Institute of Medicine (IOM) helped to produce a paradigm shift in public perception of the quality and safety of US health care. In 1999, the first, "To Err is Human: Building a Safer Health System" opened with this striking paragraph:

> Health care in the United States is not as safe as it should be–and can be. At least 44,000 people, and perhaps as many as 98,000 people, die in hospitals each year as a result of medical errors that could have been prevented, according to estimates from two major studies. Even using the lower estimate,

Reichel's Care of the Elderly, 7th Edition, ed. Jan Busby-Whitehead *et al.* Published by Cambridge University Press.
© Cambridge University Press 2016.

preventable medical errors in hospitals exceed attributable deaths to such feared threats as motor-vehicle wrecks, breast cancer, and AIDS.[4]

In 2001, the IOM followed up with "Crossing the Quality Chasm: A New Health System for the 21st Century," which began with a similarly bleak picture and stern warning:

> The U.S. health care delivery system does not provide consistent, high-quality medical care to all people. Americans should be able to count on receiving care that meets their needs and is based on the best scientific knowledge–yet there is strong evidence that this frequently is not the case. Health care harms patients too frequently and routinely fails to deliver its potential benefits. Indeed, between the health care that we now have and the health care that we could have lies not just a gap, but a chasm.[5]

Main approaches and methodologies of performance improvement

The plan-do-study-act cycle

The plan-do-study-act cycle (PDSA cycle) is a series of steps for gaining knowledge for the continual improvement of a process. Logically enough, the steps are as follows:

Plan: This step involves identifying a goal or purpose, formulating a theory, defining success metrics and putting a plan into action.
Do: Implementation of the plan.
Study: In this step, outcomes are assessed to validate the plan, specifically identifying good-versus-bad outcomes and/or areas for improvement.
Act: In this final step, the team integrates learning generated by the process in order to adjust goals, change methods, and/or even reformulate the theory itself. There is not necessarily just one cycle; ideally, the steps are repeated as needed to promote continuous improvement.[6]

Six Sigma

Six Sigma is another methodology for process improvement, originally developed and elaborated in industry, but recently adopted to promote health care quality and safety as well. Six Sigma seeks to improve the quality of process outputs by identifying and removing the causes of defects (errors) and minimizing variability in manufacturing and business processes. It uses a set of quality management methods, including statistical methods, and creates a special infrastructure of people within the organization ("champions," "black belts," etc.) who are experts in these methods. Each Six Sigma project carried out within an organization follows a defined sequence of steps and has quantified value targets (e.g., reduce process cycle time and/or costs, increase customer satisfaction, increase profits). The term "Six Sigma" originated in statistical modeling of manufacturing processes, and the maturity of a manufacturing process can be described by a sigma rating reflecting the percentage of defect-free products it creates.[7]

Lean

Lean manufacturing, or simply "lean," is a systematic method for the elimination of waste within a manufacturing process. Lean also takes into account waste created through overburden and waste created through unevenness in workloads. Working from the perspective of the client who consumes a product or service, "value" is any action or process for which the consumer is willing to pay. Essentially, lean is centered on making obvious what adds value by reducing everything else.[8]

Key organizations promoting performance improvement, and their products

Public sector organizations

Agency for Healthcare Research and Quality

The Agency for Healthcare Research and Quality (AHRQ) provides "tools, recommendations, and resources for clinicians and providers and hospitals and health systems."[9] Specifically regarding quality and patient safety, AHRQ provides "tips for preventing medical errors and promoting patient safety, measuring health care quality, consumer assessment of health plans, evaluation software, report tools, and case studies."[9] The following are some of the AHRQ programs and tools:

- AHRQ's Healthcare-Associated Infection Program
- Comprehensive Unit-based Safety Program (CUSP)

- Partnership for Patients
- Patient Safety Measure Tools & Resources
- Pharmacy Health Literacy Center
- Surveys on Patient Safety Culture
- Quality Measure Tools & Resources [9]

Among the most important AHRQ quality measure tools and resources is its National Quality Measures Clearinghouse (NQMC), "a public resource for evidence-based quality measures and measure sets."[10] NQMC also hosts the HHS Measure Inventory."[11] The HHS Measure Inventory is a repository of measures separate from the NQMC which are currently being used by the agencies of the US Department of Health and Human Services (DHHS) for quality measurement, improvement, and reporting. Not all measures in the HHS Measure Inventory meet criteria for inclusion in the NQMC.[11]

An AHRQ initiative parallel to the NQMC is its National Guideline Clearinghouse™, "a publicly available database of evidence-based clinical practice guidelines and related documents. Updated weekly with new content, the NGC provides physicians and other health professionals, health care providers, health plans, integrated delivery systems, purchasers, and others an accessible mechanism for obtaining objective, detailed information on clinical practice guidelines and to further their dissemination, implementation, and use."[12]

Centers for Medicare and Medicaid Services

The Centers for Medicare and Medicaid Services (CMS), despite its long history of implicitly rewarding volume rather than quality or value, has recently developed a new strategy to reward value, including two key programs, among others, the Physician Quality Reporting System (PQRS) and Meaningful Use (MU). The PQRS program is described briefly in the next section, whereas the description of the Meaningful Use program follows under "Meaningful Use Incentives" in the section on health IT and performance improvement. As will be discussed in more detail under "Evolving Incentives for Performance Improvement by Providers," CMS has developed PQRS, "a reporting program that uses a combination of incentive payments and payment adjustments to promote reporting of quality information by eligible professionals."[13]

Private sector organizations

Institute for Healthcare Improvement

As it states on its website, the Institute for Healthcare Improvement (IHI) "is a nonprofit organization focused on motivating and building the will for change, partnering with patients and health care professionals to test new models of care, and ensuring the broadest adoption of best practices and effective innovations."[14] IHI was officially founded in 1991, but its groundwork began in the late 1980s as part of the National Demonstration Project on Quality Improvement in Health Care, led by Dr. Don Berwick and a group of individuals committed to redesigning health care to become a system without errors, waste, delay, and unsustainable costs. Originally supported by a collection of grant-supported programs, it is now a self-sustaining organization with worldwide influence. IHI believes there is a need to view health care as a complete social, geopolitical enterprise.[15] In order to establish better models of health care, IHI created the Triple Aim, a framework for optimizing health system performance by simultaneously focusing on improving both the health of a population, and the experience of care for individuals within that population, and reducing the per capita cost of providing that care. A goal of IHI has been to use their framework to develop specific, practical initiatives to bring about change. The process of accomplishing this usually combines components focused on the individuals, families, and the population served; the restructuring of primary care services; cost control; and system integration and execution.[16]

National Committee for Quality Assurance and the Healthcare Effectiveness Data and Information Set

According to its website, "The National Committee for Quality Assurance [NCQA] is a private, 501(c)(3) not-for-profit organization dedicated to improving health care quality. Since its founding in 1990, NCQA has been a central figure in driving improvement throughout the health care system, helping to elevate the issue of health care quality to the top of the national agenda."[17]

A major function of NCQA is the management of voluntary accreditation programs for individual physicians, health plans, and medical groups. It also offers dedicated programs targeting vendor certification, software certification, and compliance auditing, and it provides an evidence-based program for case-management accreditation for payer, provider, and community-based organizations.[17]

Two major tools used by NCQA to evaluate health plans seeking accreditation are the Healthcare Effectiveness Data and Information Set (HEDIS) and the Consumer Assessment of Healthcare Providers and Systems (CAHPS) survey. More than 90% of America's health plans use HEDIS to measure their performance on important dimensions of care and service, (81 measures across 5 domains of care). Because this set of standard, tightly defined measures is collected by the vast majority of health plans in the United States, HEDIS provides a means of comparing the performance of health plans on an "apples-to-apples" basis. The CAHPS surveys were developed to provide useful information from patients' perspectives on their experiences and satisfaction with health care received. There are four versions that can be administered to adults and children in commercial and Medicaid plans. The surveys include a core set of questions; composite or summary scores developed from sets of these questions are used to evaluate key areas of care and service.[18]

The Leapfrog Group

Rapidly increasing health insurance costs were the major factor influencing several large US companies to meet in 1998 to explore ways to influence quality and affordability. The Leapfrog Group was formed and its members agreed to base their purchase of health care on principles that "encourage provider quality improvement and consumer involvement."[19] The group was officially launched in November 2000 with the initial focus provided by the 1999 Institute of Medicine report.[4] That initial focus was on reducing preventable medical mistakes by having members leverage their purchasing. The concept was to encourage large advances by rewarding hospitals that show significant improvements. The group selected practices that offered computerized physician order entry (CPOE), evidence-based hospital referral, intensive care unit (ICU) staffing by physicians experienced in critical care medicine, and use of a "Leapfrog Safe Practices Score," based on the National Quality Forum–endorsed Safe Practices. [20] More recent initiatives include public reporting of health care quality and outcomes to influence

consumers' choices. Originally funded by the Business Roundtable, Leapfrog is now supported by its members and major corporations, business coalitions, public agencies that purchase health care benefits, and from products and services it provides to support value-based purchasing.

Quality improvement organizations

According to the CMS website, a quality improvement organization (QIO) is a group of health quality experts, clinicians, and consumers organized to improve the care delivered to people with Medicare. [21] QIOs work under the direction of CMS to assist Medicare providers with quality improvement and to review quality concerns for the protection of beneficiaries and the Medicare Trust Fund. The QIO program is one of the largest federal programs dedicated to improving health care quality for Medicare beneficiaries and is an integral part of the US DHHS' National Quality Strategy for providing better care and better health at lower cost. The mission of the QIO program is to improve the effectiveness, efficiency, economy, and quality of services delivered to Medicare beneficiaries. "CMS identifies the core functions of the QIO Program as:

1. Improving quality of care for beneficiaries;
2. Protecting the integrity of the Medicare Trust Fund by ensuring that Medicare pays only for services and goods that are reasonable and necessary and that are provided in the most appropriate setting; and
3. Protecting beneficiaries by addressing individual complaints, such as beneficiary complaints; provider-based notice appeals; violations of the Emergency Medical Treatment and Labor Act (EMTALA); and other related responsibilities as articulated in QIO-related law."[21]

American Medical Association Physician Consortium for Performance Improvement

The American Medical Association (AMA) Physician Consortium for Performance Improvement* (PCPI*) is a national, physician-led program dedicated to enhancing quality and patient safety. Its ongoing mission is to align patient-centered care, performance measurement, and quality improvement. It develops evidence-based performance measures that are clinically meaningful, meet the current and future

759

needs of the PCPI membership, and are used in national accountability and quality improvement programs.[22] PCPI measures (encompassing structure, process, and outcome) can be used for evaluating quality of care for a wide range of clinical topics. The current performance measures portfolio includes measurement sets in 47 clinical areas and preventive care and more than 300 individual measures (www.ama-assn.org/apps/listserv/x-check/qmeasure.cgi?submit=PCPI).[23]

National Quality Forum

The National Quality Forum (NQF) is a nonprofit organization based in Washington, DC, dedicated to improving the quality of health care in the United States.[24] The NQF has a three-part mission: to set goals for performance improvement, to endorse standards for measuring and reporting on performance, and to promote educational and outreach programs. NQF members include purchasers, physicians, nurses, hospitals, certification bodies and fellow quality improvement organizations. The NQF is known for having developed a list of 28 medical errors it deemed serious reportable events, more commonly referred to as "never events" (www.qualityforum.org/Topics/SREs/List_of_SREs.aspx) because they are largely preventable medical events and, as such, should never happen. The NQF classifies these events according to six categories: surgical, product or device, patient protection, care management, environment, or criminal. Examples include operating on the wrong patient, leaving a foreign object in a patient after surgery, and sending a newborn home with the wrong parents.[25] One of the criteria for the meaningful use of electronic health record (EHR) technology is the ability to report health quality measures to the CMS. To that end, the NQF has introduced several health IT initiatives, such as "The Critical Paths for Creating Data Platforms" project to assess the readiness of electronic data to support selected innovative measurement concepts and others (www.qualityforum.org/HealthIT) to develop the infrastructure to support this reporting requirement.[26]

Evolving incentives for performance improvement by providers

The National Strategy for Quality Improvement in Healthcare (National Quality Strategy) unites federal agencies, health-care payers, providers, consumers, and other stakeholders in a common pursuit of improved health through quality health care for all Americans.[27] Originally published in March 2011, the National Quality Strategy specified three aims: better care, healthy people/healthy communities, and affordable care. These three aims were accompanied by six priorities: making care safer, engaging patients and families as partners in care, promoting coordination of care, implementing the most effective preventive and treatment practices, collaboration with communities to enable healthy living, and expanding access to affordable quality care through new health-care delivery models.[27] Numerous reporting initiatives and accompanying quality measures are presently in use across the public and private health-care domain, representing a concentrated effort to strengthen infrastructure for performance evaluation and improvement. In the context of a complex and evolving quality environment, the US DHHS has recognized the importance of measure harmonization to ensure consistent and meaningful reporting. Specifically, the National Quality Strategy emphasizes "an aligned focus on outcomes for children, adolescents, and adults and for the retirement of unnecessary, redundant measures that will reduce the reporting burden and will allow the remaining quality measures to send a stronger signal about where and how better care is achieved."[28]

Participation in quality measurement and reporting systems: CMS

The CMS has taken a central role in the initiation and proliferation of incentivized quality reporting and measurement programs. Several of CMS's most influential programs include value-based purchasing (VBP),[29] PQRS,[30] and the Meaningful Use initiatives.[31] Each program is composed of multiple components or levels which provide flexibility to reporting providers or institutions, with incremental parallel incentives for achieving advanced reporting or performance capabilities. The VBP program is used by CMS to hold institutions accountable for the quality of care provided, rewarding hospitals providing high-quality care with increased payments, and adjusting payments for underperforming hospitals.[29] These initiatives have undergone multiple revisions and updates to optimize effective implementation and continued performance improvement.

Table 57.1 Provider groups eligible for participation in the EHR Incentive Program [32, 33]

Medicaid EHR Incentive Program	Medicare EHR Incentive Program
Physician	Doctor of medicine or osteopathy
Dentist	Doctor of oral surgery or dental medicine
Certified nurse-midwife	Doctor of podiatric medicine
Nurse practitioner	Doctor of optometry
Physician assistant practicing in a RHC or FQHC	Chiropractor

The EHR Incentive Program: meaningful use

The Electronic Health Record (EHR) Incentive Program provides payments to eligible providers who utilize EHR technology in ways that positively impact patient care.[31] The program also provides payments to eligible hospitals and critical access hospitals meeting criteria for meaningful use of EHR technology.[31] The program does not make funds directly available to practitioners for purchase of an EHR, but instead provides incentive payments if specified requirements are met. Incentive programs exist for both Medicare and Medicaid, with non-overlapping requirements for each and differential eligibility criteria for participation.[32, 33] (See Table 57.1.) Although certain providers may be eligible for participation in both programs, providers must select and participate in only one. Hospital-based professionals providing greater than 90% of services in the inpatient setting are not eligible for either program. The maximum cumulative EHR incentive payments available to first-year participating providers is greater for Medicaid ($63,750); the maximum amount available to Medicare participants has gradually decreased from $44,000 for participating providers who began in 2011, the first implementation year, to $24,000 for providers initiating in the last incentivized year, 2014. Penalties will begin in 2015 for eligible Medicare providers who choose not to participate.[32]

The Medicaid and Medicare EHR Incentive Programs for eligible professionals consist of a three-stage process for demonstrating meaningful use of EHR technology.[29] Stage 1 involves data capturing and sharing, stage 2 requires advanced clinical processes, and stage 3 requires demonstration of improved clinical outcomes. Each stage has requisite objectives, as well as minimum measures within each objective, that must be met in order to be considered meaningful users of EHR technology. All Meaningful Use stage 1 participating providers must meet measure thresholds for 13 core objectives and 5 of 9 menu objectives in order to qualify for an incentive payment.[32, 33] Reporting of Clinical Quality Measures (CQMs) is also necessary to meet meaningful use requirements. There are no thresholds associated with reporting for the CQM, although the number of measures to be reported increased from 6 to 9 (of a possible 64) in 2014. Providers are able to select CQM appropriate for their patient population and practice, but CMS has issued recommended sets of 9 measures each for adult and pediatric populations. To achieve Meaningful Use stage 2 requirements, 17 mandatory core objectives must be met and at least 3 of 6 possible menu objectives must be fulfilled. In addition to growth in the number of objectives, the minimum thresholds for each measure have increased beyond the stage 1 requirements. The timeline for progression through the multiple stages of Meaningful Use depends upon when participation was initiated, and elements of stage 3 (planned to begin in 2016) remain to be fully defined.[29]

Physician Quality Reporting System

CMS is shifting from a policy of pay-for-reporting to one of penalizing nonreporting. The Physician Quality Reporting System (PQRS) has provided incentive payments to eligible professionals since 2007 for reporting of specified measures, with payment adjustments planned for 2015.[30] The data reported to CMS by eligible professionals is made available to providers for assessment of performance and peer comparison. Provider cost and quality information is derived from attribution of individual patients to a single provider through an attribution rule. In CMS programs, the plurality rule typically assigns patients to the provider from whom the largest quantity of ambulatory care was received in the preceding year.[34]

Multiple reporting methods are accepted by CMS, with distinct options for individuals and group practices. Since its introduction in 2010, group practices have been able to report through the group practice reporting option (GPRO). Payment incentives associated with the PQRS program began at 1.5% in 2007, increasing to 2.0% for 2009 to 2010 before decreasing to 1.0% in 2011 and subsequently 0.5% through 2014. Beginning in 2015, practices who fail to satisfy requirements for reporting during the 2013 program year will be subject to a 1.5% payment reduction on billed services for 2015, with a 2% reduction scheduled to begin in 2016 and continue thereafter. The list of eligible professionals for PQRS is expansive and includes all professionals paid based upon the Medicare Physician Fee Schedule. This list is categorized by physicians, practitioners (i.e., physician assistant, clinical social worker, registered dietician, etc.), and therapists (i.e., physical and occupational therapists, speech/language pathologists).[34]

Medicare value-based modifier

Implementation of the Medicare value-based modifier (VM) is based on participation in PQRS.[35] The VM incorporates cost and quality data to compare individual practice performance with a benchmark group of similar providers. Quality and Resource Use Reports (QRURs) are confidential feedback reports provided to PQRS and GPRO participating practitioners nationwide.[34] These reports contain cost and efficiency data, as well as information on the VM payment adjustment to be applied for the upcoming year. QRURs present beneficiary costs, standardized by region and risk adjusted using the CMS-hierarchical conditions category model and subsequently a QRUR adjustment model. This standardization and risk-adjustment process allows for a fair peer comparison among similar providers and an appropriate VM payment adjustment.[34]

The first phase of the VM was implemented in 2015 and applied to voluntarily participating practices of 100 or more eligible professionals based upon the practice's performance in 2013, with a possible upward, downward, or neutral payment adjustment. Payment adjustment is determined based upon an analytical method termed "quality tiering." Participation is mandatory in 2016 for practices with 10 or more eligible professionals, and full implementation is applicable to all eligible professionals planned for 2017.[35]

Reporting hospital quality data for annual payment: Medicare

The specifications for reporting of hospital quality data were promulgated in the Medicare Prescription Drug, Improvement, and Modernization Act (MMA) of 2003[36] and subsequently updated in the Deficit Reduction Act (DRA) of 2005.[37] The MMA clause defined for fiscal years 2005 to 2007 a 0.4% point reduction in the scheduled increase in Medicare reimbursement for hospitals that failed to report quality data to DHHS for a set of 10 specified indicators for an applicable year.[36] The clause was amended in the DRA to increase the penalty associated with failure to report quality data, resulting in a 2.0% point reduction for 2007 and all subsequent years.[37] The penalty changes in 2015 to one-quarter of the applicable percentage increase in Medicare reimbursement for that year. Furthermore, the DRA empowered the secretary of the DHHS to expand the set of measures beyond the 10 specified under the MMA. The measures would be deemed appropriate by the secretary and should reflect agreement among affected parties and ideally encompass measures built by consensus generating quality agencies.[37] Measures in which all hospitals were in compliance and those that did not represent best clinical practice were eliminated. Finally, the secretary was instructed to establish procedures for making reported quality data on measures of process, structure, outcome, patients' perspectives, efficiency, and costs of care available to the public.[37]

The Hospital Quality Alliance (HQA) was created as a public-private partnership to foster quality improvement in US hospitals.[38] Specific goals of the HQA include providing useful and valid information about hospital quality to the public, giving hospitals a clear sense of public reporting expectations, and standardizing data collection. The first publicly reported hospital data were made available by the HQA in November 2004 for the core set of 10 validated measures which represented three conditions (acute myocardial infarction, heart failure, pneumonia) identified by CMS.[38] For fiscal year 2015, the Inpatient Quality Reporting (IQR) Program requires hospitals to submit clinical process measure data through the only CMS-approved website (qualitynet. org).[29] In 2015, complete data must be submitted for an additional seven conditions beyond the original three in order to receive the full Annual Medicare Payment Update as specified in the DRA.[39] Beyond the clinical process measures, hospitals are required to report Hospital Consumer Assessment of Healthcare Providers and Systems (HCAHPS) data to reflect patients' perspectives of care, as well as data on health care–associated infections and structural measures for the hospital. Using Medicare claims, CMS calculates outcome rates without need for further data submission from the hospital (e.g., 30-day risk standardized mortality by condition, hospital wide all cause unplanned readmission).[39]

Medicare hospital value-based purchasing

The Medicare hospital value-based purchasing (VBP) program broadly encompasses the majority of US hospitals (more than 3,000 in 2012) and provides payment incentives for high-quality care.[29] Initial pay-for-performance projects have largely focused on process of care measures, although future efforts should aim to measure clinical and patient centered outcomes. Evaluations of hospital pay-for-performance initiatives have yielded mixed but promising results. Value-based purchasing was found to have a positive impact on composite quality scores in hospitals participating in the large CMS-funded demonstration project that was used to inform the structure of the VBP program.[40–42]

On the CMS website (www.cms.gov/Medicare/Medicare.html), current selections available under the heading "Quality Initiatives/Patient Assessment Instruments" include:

Quality Initiatives – General Information

ASC Quality Reporting

Electronic Prescribing Incentive Program

Home Health Quality Initiative

Hospital Quality Initiative

Hospice Quality Reporting

Hospital Value-Based Purchasing

IRF Quality Reporting

LTCH Quality Reporting

Measures Management System

Nursing Home Quality Initiative

Outcome and Assessment Information Set (OASIS)

Physician Compare Initiative

Physician Quality Reporting System

Quality Improvement Organizations

Quality Measures

ESRD Quality Incentive Program

Post-Acute Care Quality Initiatives

Commercial Pay-for-Reporting and Pay-for-Performance Initiatives: HEDIS

The National Committee for Quality Assurance updates the Healthcare Effectiveness Data and Information Set (HEDIS) measures annually, and HEDIS is widely used by health plans to report quality results.[43] In 2013, 171 million Americans were enrolled in plans reporting quality measures using HEDIS, consisting of all Medicare Advantage members, most Medicaid enrollees, and many commercial members.[43] Similar to PQRS, professionals are provided with performance data for comparison with local and national peers. The process for HEDIS measure development is rigorous, taking approximately 28 months. The process begins with identification of priority areas for measure development, then progresses through numerous intermediary steps including creation of technical subgroups, field testing and analysis, public comment, and ultimately addition of the measure to HEDIS. Measure domains for commercial plans in 2015 include Effectiveness of Care (33 measures), Access/Availability of Care (6 measures), Experience of Care (3 measures), Utilization and Relative Resource Use (17 measures), and Health Plan Descriptive Information (6 measures).[44]

Health information technology and performance improvement

The crucial role of health information technology

There is an emerging understanding that humans are inherently fallible, and that part of the solution to the problems of high cost and inadequate quality and safety of health care lies in redesigning systems of care to improve the effectiveness and efficiency of care and reduce the likelihood of errors. Health information technology (HIT) can play a key role in facilitating clinicians' memory, information processing, and decision making.

In 1997, the Institute of Medicine produced a landmark report called *The Computer-based Patient Record: An Essential Technology for Health Care*. A major conclusion of the report was that "computerization can help to improve patient records and that improved patient records and information management of health care data are essential elements of the infrastructure of the nation's health care system."[45] Nearly 20 years later, use of electronic health records (EHRs) and computerized decision support has rapidly increased over time, but is far from universal. In 2010, 15% of hospitals reported having and using what would be defined as at least a basic EHR system, and by 2013, the percentage rose to 59%; among office-based physicians the percentages were 51% and 78%, respectively.[46] Current objectives for HIT are to move from simply implementing the technology to actually using it in ways that improve the quality and efficiency of care.

The importance of HIT in both the conduct of day-to-day health care and in the continued improvement of its effectiveness, efficiency, and cost has been recognized legislatively at the national level. Two major pieces of legislation have been passed: the Health Information Technology for Clinical and Economic Health (HITECH) provision of the American Recovery and Reinvestment Act,[47] and the Affordable Care Act.[48] These provisions have given unprecedented levels of financial support for the adoption and implementation of HIT, primarily in the form of financial incentives for providers, and have emphasized the importance of this technology in delivery system reform.

Patient registries

The AHRQ handbook, *Registries for Evaluating Patient Outcomes: A User's Guide*, defines a patient registry as "an organized system that uses observational study methods to collect uniform data (clinical and other) to evaluate specified outcomes for a population defined by a particular disease, condition, or exposure, and that serves one or more predetermined scientific, clinical, or policy purposes."[49] Although registries can serve many purposes, three areas where they can provide useful information for performance improvement are determining clinical effectiveness or cost-effectiveness of health-care products and services, measuring or monitoring safety and harm, and measuring quality of care.

Registries are usually classified by how their populations are defined. These classifications include product registries for patients who have used certain biopharmaceutical products or medical devices; health services registries for patients who have had a common procedure or clinical encounter (e.g., office visit or hospitalization): or disease or condition registries for patients having the same or similar diagnoses (e.g., diabetes or congestive heart failure).

A recent report developed by the Quality Alliance Steering Committee identified some limitations with the use of registries for performance measurement and improvement, as well as potential solutions.[50] Although patient registries can play a vital role in measuring quality and cost, their role is often limited by significant shortcomings in their design and function; and their structure, size and scope must be adapted to meet changing needs. This report also identifies challenges that exist in leveraging registries to achieve better performance measurement, in particular, the time and expense of linking administrative and clinical data. Most currently endorsed measures that would use a new, hybrid database require elements from only one of the datasets. There is still a significant lack of measures that require both clinical and administrative data elements.

Finally, according to the report, using registries for performance measurement and improvement will involve finding solutions to several common registry limitations. These include:

- standardizing data elements and definitions across registries that address the same disease or treatment areas;
- developing a uniform method of patient identity management;
- helping registries actively interoperate with electronic health records systems;
- standardizing methodologies for sampling, data quality assurance, and risk adjustment;
- standardizing linkage methods;
- ensuring high provider participation across these programs; and
- guaranteeing that providers and data users are confident registries are sustainable.[50]

Electronic health records; reporting based on EHR data

EHRs have long been promoted as central to the solution of the problems of high cost, inefficiency, and inadequate quality and safety in the US healthcare system. Most define an EHR as a digital version of a patient's paper chart. HealthIT.gov describes EHRs as "real-time, patient-centered records that make information available instantly and securely to authorized users. While an EHR does contain the medical and treatment histories of patients, an EHR system is built to go beyond standard clinical data collected in a provider's office and can be inclusive of a broader view of a patient's care."[51] EHRs are capable of containing a patient's medical history, diagnoses, medication and treatment plans, immunizations, allergies, imaging, and laboratory test results; providing access to evidence-based tools to help providers make better decisions about a patient's care; and automating and streamlining provider workflow.

A major feature of an EHR is that "health information can be created and managed by authorized providers in a digital format capable of being shared with other providers across more than one health care organization."[51] EHRs should allow the sharing of information with other health-care providers and related providers (e.g., laboratories, specialists, imaging facilities, pharmacies, emergency facilities, and clinics) so that they can have a complete picture of a patient's care.

How to evaluate and select ambulatory EHR systems

Federal incentive programs provide payments to eligible providers as they "adopt, implement, upgrade or demonstrate meaningful use of certified EHR technology."[52] A key element of these programs is the use of "certified" EHRs. The HealthIT.gov website provides "the authoritative, comprehensive listing of Complete Electronic Health Records (EHRs) and EHR Modules that have been tested and certified under the ONC HIT Certification Program, maintained by The Office of the National Coordinator for Health Information Technology (ONC)."[48]

Reporting

As Lord Kelvin said, "If you cannot measure it, you cannot improve it."[53] To that end, federal quality measurement and reporting initiatives have been established in hopes of facilitating the improvement of the quality of care provided to patients. Measurement for these initiatives relies on the standard data and data formats required of EHRs under the "meaningful use" EHR Incentive Program.

The PQRS uses a combination of incentive payments and payment adjustments to promote reporting of quality information. The program provides an incentive payment to practices that satisfactorily

report data on quality measures for services provided to Medicare Part B fee-for-service beneficiaries. To encourage the use of EHRs, eligible professionals could qualify to earn a PQRS incentive through the EHR-based reporting method. Beginning in 2014, group practices could qualify to earn a PQRS incentive through the EHR-based reporting method.

The burden of PQRS reporting is reduced by using a qualified EHR. Participation in EHR-based PQRS reporting requires using a qualified EHR for the entire reporting period, although a provider can upgrade at any point during the reporting year. The EHR must contain all eligible encounters, along with all diagnosis, service, and procedure data, and all data elements must be recorded as structured data. "Missing data or improperly recorded data may affect both reporting and performance rates for the measures, and in turn, jeopardize the incentive payment."[54]

Meaningful Use incentives

As discussed earlier under "Evolving Incentives for Performance Improvement by Providers," the Medicare and Medicaid EHR incentive programs provide financial incentives for the meaningful use of certified EHR technology to improve patient care.[55]

Summary

This chapter began with a review of key developments in the history of health-care performance improvement, including Donabedian's model based on structure, process, and outcome, and the two Institute of Medicine reports highlighting serious gaps in US health care quality and safety. Three main methodologies of performance improvement were reviewed: the plan-do-study-act cycle, Six Sigma, and lean. The overview of key organizations promoting performance improvement considered both the public and private sectors. Key public agencies featured were the Agency for Healthcare Research and Quality and the Centers for Medicare and Medicaid Services. Private organizations included the Institute for Healthcare Improvement, National Committee for Quality Assurance and its Healthcare Effectiveness Data and Information Set, the Leapfrog Group, quality improvement organizations, and the American Medical Association Physician Consortium for Performance Improvement. The review of evolving incentives for performance improvement included Medicare and Medicaid incentives and disincentives,

BOX 57.1 Key organizations and resources

Agency for Healthcare Research and Quality
 General: www.ahrq.gov/workingforquality

 National Guideline Clearinghouse: www.guideline.gov

 National Quality Measures Clearinghouse: www.qualitymeasures.ahrq.gov

Centers for Medicare and Medicaid Services
 Physician Quality Reporting System: www.cms.gov/Medicare/Quality-Initiatives-Patient-Assessment-Instruments/PQRS/index.html?redirect=/PQRS

Meaningful Use:
 www.cms.gov/Regulations-and-Guidance/Legislation/EHRIncentivePrograms/Meaningful_Use.html

 www.healthit.gov/policy-researchers-implementers/meaningful-use-regulations

Value-based modifier:
 www.cms.gov/Medicare/Medicare-Fee-for-Service-Payment/PhysicianFeedbackProgram/ValueBasedPaymentModifier.html

EHR incentive programs:
 www.cms.gov/Regulations-and-Guidance/Legislation/EHRIncentivePrograms/index.html?redirect=/ehrincentiveprograms

Hospital Quality Initiative:
 www.cms.gov/Medicare/Quality-Initiatives-Patient-Assessment-Instruments/HospitalQualityInits/index.html

Quality improvement organizations:
 www.cms.gov/Medicare/Quality-Initiatives-Patient-Assessment-Instruments/QualityImprovementOrgs/index.html?redirect=/qualityimprovementorgs

National Committee for Quality Assurance and Healthcare Effectiveness Data and Information Set:
 www.ncqa.org/HEDISQualityMeasurement.aspx

US Department of Health and Human Services, HHS measure inventory:
 www.qualitymeasures.ahrq.gov/hhs/index.aspx

including the Physician Quality Reporting System, Meaningful Use, and the Value-based Modifier, and also commercial pay-for-reporting/pay-for-performance initiatives, especially the National Committee for Quality Assurance Healthcare Effectiveness Data and Information Set. The chapter concludes with a discussion of the role of HIT, including patient registries, and EHRs and reporting based on EHR data. For readers' reference, Box 57.1 provides contact information (e.g., URLs) for key organizations and resources.

References

1. Blumenthal D. Performance Improvement in Health Care – Seizing the Moment. *N Engl J Med* 2012;**336**:1953–1955.

2. Donabedian A. *Explorations in Quality Assessment and Monitoring*. Ann Arbor, MI: Health Administration Press; 1985.

3. Donabedian A. Evaluating the Quality of Medical Care. *Milbank Qtrly* 2005;**83**(4):691–729.

4. Institute of Medicine of the National Academies. *To Err Is Human: Building a Safer Health System*. Washington, DC: Institute of Medicine; 1999.

5. Institute of Medicine of the National Academies. *Crossing the Quality Chasm: A New Health System for the 21st Century*. Washington, DC: Institute of Medicine; 2001.

6. The W. Edwards Deming Institute. The Plan, Do, Study, Act Cycle. Washington; 2014, Available at: www.deming.org/theman/theories/pdsacycle (accessed Nov. 9, 2014).

7. Kubiak TM, Benbow DW. *The Certified Six Sigma Black Belt Handbook*. 2nd ed. Milwaukee, WI: ASQ Quality Press; 2009.

8. Womack JP, Jones DT. *Lean Thinking: Banish Waste and Create Wealth in Your Corporation*. New York, NY: Free Press; 2003.

9. Agency for Healthcare Research and Quality. For Professionals: Tools, Recommendations, and Resources for Clinicians and Providers and Hospitals and Health Systems; 2014. Available at: www.ahrq.gov/professionals/index.html (accessed Nov. 9, 2014).

10. Agency for Healthcare Research and Quality. National Quality Measures Clearinghouse; 2014. Available at: www.qualitymeasures.ahrq.gov (accessed Nov. 9, 2014).

11. US Department of Health and Human Services. Measure Inventory; 2014. Available at: www.quality measures.ahrq.gov (accessed Nov. 9, 2014)

12. Agency for Healthcare Research and Quality. National Guideline Clearinghouse. Available at: www.guideline .gov (accessed Nov. 9, 2014).

13. Centers for Medicare and Medicaid Services. Physician Quality Reporting System; 2014. Available at: www.cms.gov/Medicare/Quality-Initiatives-Patient-Asse ssment-Instruments/PQRS/index.html?redirect=/PQRS (accessed Nov. 9, 2014).

14. American Nurses Association. Institute for Healthcare Improvement (IHI); 2014. Available at: www.nursing world.org/MainMenuCategories/ThePracticeofProfes sionalNursing/PatientSafetyQuality/Quality-Organiza tions/IHI.html (accessed Nov. 12, 2014).

15. Institute for Healthcare Improvement. Institute for Healthcare Improvement: History; 2014. Available at: www.ihi.org/about/pages/history.aspx (accessed Nov. 11, 2014).

16. Beasley C. The Triple Aim. *Healthcare Executive* 2009;**24**(1):64–66.

17. National Committee for Quality Assurance. About NCQA; 2014. Available at: www.ncqa.org/AboutNCQ A.aspx (accessed Nov. 12, 2014).

18. National Committee for Quality Assurance. HEDIS & Quality Measurement; 2014. available at: www.ncqa.org/ HEDISQualityMeasurement.aspx (accessed Nov. 12, 2014).

19. Leapfrog Group. The Leapfrog Group Fact Sheet; 2014. Available at: www.leapfroggroup.org/about_us/leap frog-factsheet (accessed Nov. 12, 2014).

20. National Quality Forum. Hospital Care: Outcomes & Efficiency Measures Phase I; 2014. Available at: www .qualityforum.org/projects/hospital_outcomes-and-eff iciency_I.aspx.aspx (accessed Nov. 11, 2014).

21. Centers for Medicare & Medicaid Services. Quality Improvement Organizations – Centers for Medicare & Medicaid Services; 2014. Available at: www.cms.gov/ Medicare/Quality-Initiatives-Patient-Assessment-Inst ruments/QualityImprovementOrgs/index.html?redir ect=/qualityimprovementorg (accessed Nov. 12, 2014).

22. American Medical Association. Physician Consortium for Performance Improvement; 2014. Available at: www.ama-assn.org/ama/pub/physician-resources/phy sician-consortium-performance-improvement.page (accessed Nov. 12, 2014).

23. American Medical Association. PCPI and PCPI-Approved Measures; 2014. Available at: www.ama-assn .org/ama/pub/physician-resources/physician-consor tium-performance-improvement/pcpi-measures.page (accessed Nov. 12, 2014).

24. National Quality Forum. NQF-Home: Good Measures Improve Quality Care; 2014. Available at: www.quali tyforum.org/Home.aspx (accessed Nov. 11, 2014).

25. Rouse M. What Is National Quality Forum (NQF)? 2010. Available at: http://searchhealthit.techtarget.co m/definition/National-Quality-Forum-NQF (accessed Nov. 11, 2014).

26. SearchHealthIT. NQF Leader on Using EHR Technology to Report Health Quality Measures; 2010. Available at: http://searchhealthit.techtarget.com/vide o/NQF-leader-on-using-EHR-technology-to-report-h ealth-quality-measures (accessed Nov. 11, 2014).

27. United States Department of Health and Human Services. National Strategy for Quality Improvement in Health Care: Report to Congress. March 21, 2011.

28. United States Department of Health and Human Services. Working for Quality: Achieving Better Health and Healthcare for All Americans. September 24, 2014.

29. 42 CFR § 412, 413, 424, 476 (2012). CFR 2012.

30. Centers for Medicare and Medicaid Services (CMS), HHS. Physician Quality Reporting System Overview; 2014. Available at: www.cms.gov/Medicare/Quality-I nitiatives-Patient-Assessment-Instruments/PQRS/ind ex.html?redirect=/PQRS (accessed Nov. 1, 2014).

31. 75 CFR § 412, 413, 422 (2010). CFR 2010.

32. Centers for Medicare and Medicaid Services (CMS), HHS. An Introduction to the Medicare EHR Incentive Program for Eligible Professionals; 2014.

33. Centers for Medicare and Medicaid Services (CMS), HHS. An Introduction to the Medicaid EHR Incentive Program for Eligible Professionals; 2014.

34. Centers for Medicare and Medicaid Services (CMS), HHS. Physician Quality Reporting System (PQRS) List of Eligible Professionals; 2013.

35. Centers for Medicare and Medicaid Services. Summary of 2015 Physician Value-based Modifier Policies; 2014.

36. Medicare Prescription Drug, Improvement and Modernization Act; 2003:108–173.

37. Deficit Reduction Act of 2005. 2006 February 8;109–171 (109th Congress).

38. Jha A, Li Z, Orav E, et al. Care in U.S. hospitals – the Hospital Quality Alliance program. *N Engl J Med.* 2005 Jul 21;353(3):265–274.

39. Centers for Medicare & Medicaid Services (CMS), HHS. Hospital Inpatient Quality Reporting Program FY 2015 Reference Checklist; 2013.

40. Lindenauer PK, Remus D, Roman S, et al. Public reporting and pay for performance in hospital quality improvement. *N Engl J Med* 2007 Feb 1;**356**(5):486–496.

41. Werner RM, Kolstad JT, Stuart EA, Polsky D. The effect of pay-for-performance in hospitals: lessons for quality improvement. *Health Aff (Millwood)* 2011 Apr;30(4):690–698.

42. Ryan AM, Blustein J, Casalino LP. Medicare's flagship test of pay-for-performance did not spur more rapid quality improvement among low-performing hospitals. *Health Aff (Millwood)* 2012 Apr;31(4):797–805.

43. National Committee for Quality Assurance. The State of Healthcare Quality 2014; 2014.

44. National Committee for Quality Assurance. Summary Table of Measures, Product Lines and Changes, HEDIS 2015; 2014.

45. Institute of Medicine of the National Academies. Rewarding Provider Performance: Aligning Incentives in Medicare, 2006; September 2006.

46. DesRoches CM, Painter MW, Jha AK. Health Information Technology in the United States: Progress and Challenges Ahead, 2014. Available at: www.rwjf.org/en/library/research/2014/08/health-info rmation-technology-in-the-united-states.html (accessed 14 November 2015).

47. Health Information Technology for Economic and Clinical Health (HITECH) Act, Title XIII of Division A and Title IV of Division B of the American Recovery and Reinvestment Act of 2009. Pub L No 111–5, 123 Stat 226. February 17, 2009(codified at 42 U.S.C. §§300jj et seq.; §§17901 et seq).

48. Office of the National Coordinator for Health Information Technology, Department of Health and Human Services. Health information technology: initial set of standards, implementation specifications, and certification criteria for electronic health record technology. Final rule. Federal Register 2010;75 (144):44589–44654.

49. Agency for Healthcare Research and Quality. *Registries for Evaluating Patient Outcomes: A User's Guide*. 3rd ed. Rockville, MD: Agency for Healthcare Research and Quality; 2014.

50. Engelberg Center for Health Care Reform at Brookings Institution. How registries can help performance measurement improve care. Robert Wood Johnson Foundation; 2010. Available at: www.rwjf.org/en/librar y/research/2010/06/latest-from-aligning-forces-for-qual ity-communities/how-registries-can-help-performance-measurement-improve-care.html (accessed 14 November 2015).

51. HealthIT.gov. What is an electronic health record (EHR)? | FAQs | Providers & Professionals | www.He althIT.gov. Available at: www.healthit.gov/providers-professionals/faqs/what-electronic-health-record-ehr (accessed Nov. 11, 2014).

52. Centers for Medicare & Medicaid Services (CMS), HHS. Medicare and Medicaid programs; electronic health record incentive program. Final rule. Fed Regist 2010 Jul 28;75(144):44313–44588.

53. Dolin RH, Goodrich K, Kallem C, et al. Setting the Standard: EHR Quality Reporting Rises in Prominence Due to Meaningful Use. *Journal of AHIMA* 2014;88(1):42–48.

54. Primaris. PQRS Reporting based on EHR. 2013. Available at: http://primaris.org/pqrs-reporting-base d-on-ehr (accessed Nov. 12, 2014).

55. HITECH Answers. Meaningful Use, Meaningful Use definition, EHR Technology; 2014. Available at: www.hitechanswers.net/ehr-adoption-2/meaningful-use (accessed Nov. 12, 2014).

Chapter 58

Health-care organization and financing

Peter Hollmann, MD

An understanding of the organization of the health-care system enables the clinician to better navigate the system on behalf of the patient. It provides important insights that improve the ability of health-care professionals to continue to operate in their chosen profession, increasing the likelihood of succeeding and surviving financially. The US health-care system is frequently described as "broken." To understand how it can be improved, it is useful to have an appreciation of how it presently is configured and how it evolved. The purpose of this chapter is to provide an overview of fundamental principles of financing health care and insurance. The most relevant programs for the elderly, Medicare and Medicaid, are addressed. There are multiple complex and interacting segments that comprise the health-care delivery and financing system. Where the money comes from, where it goes, and why so much is spent will be examined. Possible responses to a system under stress that is facing the challenges of changing demographics and relentless cost trends are presented.

The health-care "system"

It is useful to remember that the care of the elderly patient occurs in a system that is complex and provides and finances care for well children, disabled adults, the uninsured, that is, the entire population. The many elements of the financing and delivery system are interdependent. Cross-subsidization occurs. This results in all elements being relevant to the elderly patient. It is Medicare, however, that has come to symbolize the health-care system for the geriatric patient. Medicare is far more complex than a governmental insurance company paying claims for persons older than 65 years of age. Medicare also pays for care provided to the disabled and those on dialysis; it contracts with private health plans and drug plans

to provide required and supplemental benefits to beneficiaries. It has a major role in financing medical education, researching the impact of system change through demonstration projects, and shaping the delivery system. Private insurance often mimics Medicare payment and benefits policies. Medicare is a financing system, not the delivery system. Health care is delivered by providers such as doctors and hospitals. There are suppliers such as drug and device manufacturers who not only provide important tools for improving health and preventing disease, but also significantly impact the cost and politics of health care. The system includes private and governmental payers other than Medicare. These payers ostensibly act on behalf of and respond to demands of employers and the voting populace and finance a greater dollar volume of health care than does Medicare. Their impact on the system is substantial. Private insurance is important for the elderly too, as most have some form of coverage beyond traditional Medicare, whether it is employee or retiree coverage, a Medicare Advantage plan, or "gap" coverage. Medicaid is critical for low-income seniors and those in long-term care institutions. The Veterans Administration plays an important role in funding and delivery of care. The most important parts of the health-care system are the patients and their families. The elderly, although just a population subset, are patients of great diversity in employment status, cultural, behavioral, financial, educational, health, and functional attributes.

There is general popular agreement that our system is seriously flawed. It is often stated that aligning incentives will improve the likelihood that the system will better serve the needs of society. A common goal of achieving a healthy population is agreed on (assuming providers of goods and services believe they will still be needed), but the uniformity of viewpoints

Reichel's Care of the Elderly, 7th Edition, ed. Jan Busby-Whitehead *et al.* Published by Cambridge University Press.
© Cambridge University Press 2016.

stops there. Complex systems also have great inertia because any change in one part of the system tends to affect another. The ripple from any change may be predictable, based on study of the past, such as service volume increasing in response to price reduction, or dauntingly unknown, such as the use of services by a baby boom cohort that may be of improved health status, yet accustomed to aggressive consumption of new technologies. The health-care system also exists within a social milieu in which health care consumes resources that might otherwise be used for education or housing and income equality, housing and education may have greater effects on health than medical care. Health-care professionals may not naturally operate on an assumption that the growth rate of the economy is as relevant to health-care organization and financing, and therefore their practice of medicine, as is the latest treatment innovation for a condition of interest. Furthermore, the financing and delivery system often seems to be no system at all with conflicting interests, as hospitals compete with doctors for fee updates and payers seek to avoid any updates in the face of increased utilization of services. Yet clinicians impact the system one patient at a time and have a unique potential to lead system change: a potential that comes with the experience of operating daily at the interfaces of finance, delivery, and caring for our patients.

International perspectives

This chapter focuses on the US system. Much can be learned from other countries. The United States spends more per capita and a greater portion of its GDP than other nations, yet is generally considered to have lower health status than our peer nations.[1, 2] Social factors, universal coverage, the balance of regulation and entrepreneurial liberty, per capita wealth, age of the population, diversity and homogeneity, national budget policy, delivery system, payment amounts, and benefits/coverage policy are all factors in this equation. For many of these factors there are significant differences between the United States and our fellow developed nations. However, there are also many consistent issues such as human behavior and economic principles and the need for political will to change.

Insurance basics

Health insurance serves two fundamental goals: prepay predictable expenses and provide financial protection against the cost of infrequent but very costly events. It is well established that the uninsured and underinsured do not receive recommended and necessary services. Traditionally, health insurance allowed the individual to obtain treatment for an acute illness that could otherwise not be purchased due to limitations of personal financial resources. The reason to prepay predictable expenses is a newer insurance phenomenon related to payment for prevention. It is intended to encourage appropriate use of services that will prevent disease, disability, and future medical expenses. It is also a mechanism to provide services at a contracted amount as compared with charges and to fund care for persons with essentially no resources, such as those with poverty-level incomes. A growing share of insurance finances go to health care for chronic illness. Insurance also finances the delivery system infrastructure.

Insurance is foremost a pooling or spreading of risk across a large population. It works by everyone paying a little into a pool that few will use. Those few who use it will exhaust the pool, less administrative costs and some reserves for unexpected variation. The reserves, besides being a cushion, produce investment income, lowering the amount needed to be collected from each person, known as the premium. In this manner, health insurance is no different than automobile, homeowners, or professional liability insurance. According to the Kaiser Family Foundation, in 2010, 10% of all Medicare beneficiaries accounted for approximately 60% of Medicare spending, but 12% incurred no Medicare expenses at all.[5] In younger populations where the prevalence of chronic illness is lower, the contrast between the few who spend a great deal and those who use little to no services is more stark. The high-use population is composed of different types of people. Some have one time high-cost events, such as those who survive major trauma without disability or those who die after an expensive course of care. Others have chronic illness punctuated with rare high-cost events such as coronary artery disease with bypass surgery or chronic illness with recurrent costly events such as congestive heart failure and recurrent inpatient care. According to the *CMS Chronic Conditions Chartbook 2012*, in 2010, the 14% of Medicare beneficiaries with six or more chronic conditions accounted for roughly half of the program expenditures.[3] Those with multiple chronic conditions and functional limitations are the most costly.[4]

The effect of spreading risk works best when it is spread over the largest possible population. Any segmentation creates the potential for the effects of what is known as "adverse selection" or "cherry picking." The United States does not have a system in which the entire population is enrolled in one insurance program. Although most payments are a form of fee for service, many provider groups receive payment that is at least partially based on some form of prepayment per person or "capitation," and therefore the provider assumes some insurance function or risk. This is expected to grow as Medicare seeks to move away from fee-for-service payment methods. Therefore, adverse selection is very relevant. Consider two health plans: plan A has 5% of its members with a serious chronic illness; plan B has 6% of its members with the same condition. The difference at first appears trivial; however, because the 5% account for 50% of all expenses in plan A, that means that each 1% change in the sick population will result in a 10% difference in total expenses. If plan B is to make ends meet, it will raise its premiums to cover its greater costs. This may lead people who do not use services and thus see less value in health insurance to leave to a lower premium plan, which then only decreases the pool of healthier people over which to spread the risk. Plan B spirals into insolvency. Risk or case mix–adjusted premiums might work, but the high-risk people may not be able to afford the higher premium. Adjusting premiums to risk also defeats the principle of pooling risk, unless the risk level is under the control of the insured, for example by using tobacco or not, or the premiums are paid from a pool, such as premium support programs in a federal health exchange under the Affordable Care Act. It also is the case that the risk adjustors account for a relatively limited amount of the per person variance because there remains a significant degree of unpredictability in expenses. Most insurance today has some form of risk adjustment. Large employer groups may be rated (have their premiums priced) by historical use experience. Small groups may be rated by age or sex adjustments. Medicare risk adjusts payments to Medicare Advantage plans based on factors such as age, diagnoses (high-cost conditions), and whether the person is institutionalized. One of the largest challenges in a voluntary health insurance system is setting premiums for well young adults at a level at which they will purchase coverage. They are indeed low risk and often see little value in insurance that they perceive as inadequately

risk adjusted, thus incentives or mandates are used to create the largest pool.

"Benefits" are what insurance covers or pays for. Benefit design is a critical element in understanding health-care financing, as it defines what is being financed through insurance. If hospital care is covered by insurance, then the price and volume of hospital services must be calculated and spread over the population paying premiums. If long-term nursing home care is not covered, then its cost and volume is irrelevant. Because insurance is a legal contract between the insurer and the insured, careful definition is critical. Certain services may be essential to the health of the patient, but that fact does not make them covered. Until Medicare created a prescription drug plan, there was no coverage for medications, yet medications were more important than many covered services to the health of most Medicare patients. Medicare does not cover long-term care in a nursing facility yet it is necessary for many. Benefit design may create or minimize adverse selection risk. Presume our example plan B had a different mix of member complexity from plan A not by random chance but because plan B had slightly different benefits that made it much more attractive to people with chronic illness. Perhaps coverage for a certain drug important to a person with the illness was slightly better. By providing better benefits plan B created its problem. Provider network may also create selection risk for a health plan. This same type of issue can affect physicians or physicians groups who accept some of the risk by becoming paid by capitation. Group A has no geriatricians and has a typical complexity patient panel mix. Group B has geriatricians who attract complex patients. If the two groups are paid the same amount per patient, group B will have to do a far superior management job to make ends meet. There is a great deal of unexplained variation or waste in health-care services utilization, but the disease burden of the patient, not the management skill of the clinicians, will dictate most of the cost of caring for the patient. It is unlikely that group B will succeed financially.

Long-term care provides a good example for two other important points: calculating cost offsets or "savings" and behavior change. Insurance coverage of a service will make it more accessible. This will expand its use and create a market for providers who will seek to expand it further. If home care is paid fully out of pocket, some will utilize it. If it is insured, the use will grow. Behavior changes with coverage. It is almost certain that some nursing home residents can be cared for more cost-effectively at home with home care services supporting other caregivers. If $50 per day on home care would prevent $150 per day of nursing home care, it would seem a good buy. It is a gross miscalculation, however, to base savings on the experience expected for one person. Insurance covers populations. In structuring the home-care benefit to cover that nursing home patient who could be cared for at home, it might be that five people at home who need home care, but are presently paying out of pocket, now become eligible for insurance to pay. The $150 per day "saved" results in $300 per day of home care for six patients, not $50 per day for one. Perhaps five caregivers missed less work, saving their employer costs and boosting productivity and society was better off. The health-care insurance costs were not reduced, however.

This brings us to the point of total costs, insurance costs, cost shifting, and returns on investment. Whether the insurance is provided by a for-profit company or the government, there is a budget of sorts. One way to control the budget is to shift costs to the patient by limiting the benefit. Medicare Part D drug coverage has beneficiary cost sharing so that it could be affordable to society (at least to the degree that Congress determined). States and the federal government have different programs that have unique budgets, but a single patient may be a beneficiary of both programs. Ideally, such shifting and fragmentation does not create unintended or harmful gaps or increase total costs, but too frequently it does. Multiple programs also create multiple administrative processes and added expense. More significantly, one payer may take actions to save a little for itself, even if it results in higher total costs and higher cost to the other payer and patient. Costs may also be shifted over time periods by making an investment. A diabetes program that delays diabetic morbidity may save an employer-sponsored private insurance company money if an upfront investment in the member's care can be amortized over years of membership premiums and the most costly episodes are prevented or deferred to an age of Medicare eligibility and thus shifted to the Medicare program. The insurance company will see a return on the investment assuming the member remains with them long enough. One of the ironic consequences of Medicare programs helping a person survive to

another year is that there will be another year of Medicare expenses. Medicare is not funded primarily by annual beneficiary premiums; therefore, if Medicare is to have a return on investment, it must reduce lifetime expenditures, which is very difficult to accomplish. For Medicare, a smaller population is less costly. Private insurance has a per member premium. Reducing membership reduces income and is not financially desirable.

An insurance company can control costs in limited ways. It can reduce the price of a service or it can reduce the frequency of a service: pay less or buy less. One way to reduce the price is to shift some cost to the member or to not cover the service at all. Price reductions may stimulate providers to increase volume to make up for lost income. Price reductions may make a service unavailable due to provider drop out. If the reduction is achieved by shifting the cost to the member, the member may forego the service. If the service was particularly cost-effective, this would be deleterious. The price change could result in substitution with a more costly service or result in disease progression to more costly stages due to lack of the service. If the service was not cost-effective, the frequency reduction achieved is positive. Attempting to reduce frequency by means other than price can have the same risk/benefit calculus. Administrative costs may be incurred implementing programs designed to reduce volume of services. Seemingly simple actions can have complex unanticipated results.

Financial principles

In a system in which there are issues such as cost shifting and adverse selection, it may appear that standard business principles do not apply; however, the delivery system is a business and fundamentals generally do apply. The financing system may contribute to confusion over fundamentals. For example, payments may be based on historical charges and not based on current true costs or competitive pricing. That said, every business has income and expenses. It has a product that it provides and makes money per some unit of product. It can have loss leaders or provide charitable services, but it cannot lose money on every service and survive. Inappropriate payment can affect service availability, by over stimulating growth of a highly profitable service and causing undervalued services to wither.

A solo practitioner running his or her office must have a good sense of these realities. There is the rent, the utilities, the employees and their benefits, professional liability insurance, and supplies. Then there is income that is typically fee for service. Each patient is a little different, but overall there is a predictable gross income per unit of patient service. Income must exceed expenses. There are also variable and fixed costs to consider. One more patient on the schedule will not change the rent or staffing, which are the fixed costs. That patient may use another paper gown as a variable cost, but mostly the patient is pure net income. At some number of additional patients, more staff will need to be added or another doctor asked to join the practice. At that point there might need to be a subsidy of the new doctor's salary. The practice founder will assess the value of the investment in the new doctor by estimating the cost today as compared with what a similar investment would generate over time and decide whether to bring on the associate or to purchase mutual fund shares for a better return on investment. Of course, there are also estimates of intangibles such as reduced on-call schedule, ability to better manage unexpected surges in patient demand, and other nonfinancial calculations that will occur.

The same principles apply for health-care systems. A hospital-employed geriatrician may directly produce income that exceeds his expenses and salary plus benefits. In such a case, that single unit is profitable. The geriatrician might be using only variable costs, if the clinic space and staffing is fixed anyway, but it is likely that fixed costs would be proportionally allocated to all users of facility and staff. The geriatrician may be a feeder of patients to the specialists and hospital. Hospitals have huge fixed costs. A few extra admissions incur few variable costs and are usually highly desirable. If the hospital believes that the geriatrician's patients would not have been at the hospital were it not for his employment, this might be recognized as his contribution to another cost or profit center. The geriatrician's patients may also give generously to the hospital capital campaigns. A geriatrics service acute and post-acute care may reduce hospital readmissions and complications and be of increasing importance in the emerging value-based payment world. On the other hand, if the hospital concludes that the geriatrician's patients always incur costs of care exceeding the reimbursement the hospital receives, the hospital may wish to no longer employ the doctor even if he earns his salary based on the office/clinic income. A geriatrician may work for a nursing facility–based special needs health plan that employs physicians and receives Medicare capitation payments. The plan may determine that a skilled geriatrician results in markedly fewer transfers to the hospital, better drug and laboratory usage, more appropriate specialty care, and lower costs. The number of patients seen per day is only relevant to the extent that it results in better, more cost-effective care; payment generated per nursing home visit is not relevant. The bottom line is that regardless of the setting, there is a calculation of productivity or income by some measure. There is a calculation of costs or resources used. There is either profit and sustainability, or loss and eventual demise. These calculations may be complex and involve assumptions that are controversial or flawed. If profit margins of a larger organization are good, the effect of a small unit may not be calculated or be worth the attention, but ultimately real income and real expense exist in any endeavor and are likely to be a factor.

Other basics warrant mention. The most salient is that in the financing and delivery dyad, costs to one party is income to another. Any cost reductions for payers result in income loss for the providers in the aggregate, although not necessarily for an individual provider. The tension is obvious.

Efficient provider units lower health-care costs without losing profitability of the unit. They can maintain the same profit margin by reducing expenses even while lowering the price of their services. This is the typical economic paradigm in competitive markets; however, health-care markets are distorted by many factors. A cost-effective provider is not the same as an efficient provider as described previously. Cost-effective providers could reduce their income because fewer of their services are used or increase their incomes because they shared in the cost savings, or because the more cost-effective services were the more profitable services for them.

Another important point concerns growth rates and compounding. In a mortgage, a lower principal will save great sums when interest is applied over time, but the interest rate can be more significant. Baseline expenditures and the growth trend are principal and interest in another setting. An extremely high trend in a service that accounts for a minute portion of total expenditures has an insignificant effect compared with modest growth in services that are responsible of a high proportion of total costs. Sustained high growth rate can, however, make a service that was once an inconsequential expense become very significant. An example of this in health care is the projected costs of high-cost "specialty" drugs such as the biological agents.

Medicare

Medicare was established in July 1966 by Title XVIII of the Social Security Act for people 65 and older regardless of income or health status. It has played a major role in reducing poverty rates among the aged and increasing access to care. It has funded infrastructure development, education and training, and been a major part of the social transformation of changing health care from a service paid by cash or barter to one paid by insurance. It accounts for one in five dollars spent on health care in America and 14% of the federal budget. It only pays for two-thirds of the health-care expenditures of the Medicare beneficiary, with 2010 out-of-pocket expenditures being $4,734 and average Medicare payments being $9,738.[5–8] It has been surpassed by Medicaid as the biggest governmental program by enrollment. Nonetheless, the impact of Medicare on the health-care system and the lives of the elderly would be difficult to overstate. Medicare is an "entitlement" program, contrasted to Medicaid, which is "welfare" or a needs-based program. Medicare benefits and costs were historically the same regardless of beneficiary income or wealth. In 2007, Medicare introduced a variable premium for Part B services based on income. Part D, the pharmacy benefit, which originated in 2006, is supported by income-adjusted beneficiary premiums.

There are four parts to Medicare, and each has different funding and benefits. They are: Part A (hospital insurance); Part B (medical insurance); Part C (Medicare Advantage); and Part D (prescription drug plan). In 1972, Medicare added eligibility for the disabled. People with end-stage renal disease (ESRD) are also eligible. People are entitled to Medicare if they or a spouse are eligible for Social Security, Railroad Retirement, or equivalent federal benefits due to age, or they are eligible due to disability [i.e., receive Social Security Disability Income (SSDI)], or if they have ESRD. The aged are eligible the first day of the month of their sixty-fifth birthday. SSDI recipients are eligible after two years of Social Security eligibility. ESRD and people with amyotrophic lateral sclerosis are eligible at the time of initiating dialysis or Social Security payment eligibility, respectively. There are approximately 54 million people covered by Medicare. Of these, 9 million are not elderly, but are disabled. Ten million are also eligible for Medicaid and half had incomes below $23,500 (roughly 200% of the federal poverty level). Forty-five percent of the beneficiaries have four or more chronic conditions, one-third limitations in activities of daily living, 31% have cognitive or mental impairments, 13% are older than age 85, and 16% are younger than age 65.[6] The population is varied and as expected age, gender and life-long socioeconomic status are factors.

Medicare has benefits that have deductibles, co-payments (set dollar amounts), and coinsurance (percent dollar amounts); that is, the beneficiary pays part of the bill or cost shares for any specific service. Some benefits have limits so that the beneficiary pays for all the service at some point. Parts B and D of Medicare have premiums; that is, the beneficiary must pay to enroll in that part of Medicare, whereas this is generally not the case for Part A. The "payment gap" created by deductibles, coinsurance, and benefit limits is often covered by "gap" insurance. Many beneficiaries purchase "gap" coverage offered by private insurers. Those eligible for Medicaid have coverage for this liability from Medicaid. The benefits structure for private insurance gap coverage is regulated by Medicare, but there are variations allowed.

Medicare Part A

Part A is hospital insurance, but it also covers skilled nursing care and hospice. It covers home health care following an inpatient stay. One-fourth of Medicare spending is on inpatient services, though through funding Medicare Advantage plans the number is higher. Part A is mostly funded by a payroll tax of 2.9% of earned income, with additional income from interest on savings in the trust fund and taxes on high-income earners' Social Security checks. The funds are held in the Hospital Insurance Trust Fund and may not be used for other purposes. Expenses are anticipated to outstrip income and savings so that around 2030 the Hospital Insurance Trust will be insolvent (2014 estimate).[5] The trust fund has frequent calculations of solvency and has had adjustments made in taxes and other income sources. Like Social Security, it is payroll based at present and therefore meeting the burden of rising expenditures falls to working people. Part A has benefits and deductibles in a given benefit period. The benefit period is defined by a 60-day continuous break without hospital or skilled nursing care. In 2015, there is a $1,260 deductible per benefit period for a hospital stay. There is a $157.50 per day co-payment for days 21–100 of a skilled nursing facility (SNF) stay. There is no co-payment for SNF days 1–20, and days over 100 are entirely the responsibility of the beneficiary. Hospice covers those with a terminal illness who are expected to live six months or less. It provides drugs, medical care, and support for those enrolled in an approved program. It accounts for 2% of Medicare expenditures, has seen a growing use, and serves over 1.5 million beneficiaries annually. Many think it is underused due to misconceptions such as being limited to care for terminal cancer, when actually less than half of the hospice enrollees have this condition. It covers and has eligibility criteria for conditions such as Alzheimer's disease, pulmonary disease, heart disease, and general debility. It covers services typically not covered by Medicare such as respite and grief counseling. Care in the home has no beneficiary cost sharing. Forty-seven percent of Medicare decedents used hospice care in 2013.[9]

Medicare Part B

Part B covers medically necessary services furnished by physicians in settings such as the hospital, office, or ambulatory surgery center. Home health (not following an inpatient stay), ambulance, durable medical equipment and surgical supplies, clinical laboratory and diagnostic services, and services by certain practitioners (e.g., nurse practitioners, clinical psychologists, and physical therapists) are paid by Part B. It covers the facility and professional components of outpatient services as well as drugs and biologicals that are not self-administered or otherwise part of Part D. Physician payments account for 12% of Medicare expenditures with hospital outpatient departments receiving 6%. Part B is funded mostly by the general treasury, with premiums from beneficiaries accounting for 25% of program support. Premium payments in 2015 are $105 per month for 94% of beneficiaries. Premiums are adjusted annually. Premiums vary for higher-income individuals. (In 2015, monthly premiums are between $147 and $336 per month for the 6% of beneficiaries who are higher income.) Funding for Part B is through the Supplemental Medical Insurance Trust Fund. The Supplemental Medical Insurance Trust has a Part B and a Part D fund within it. Part B services have an annual deductible ($147 in 2015) and a coinsurance of 20% of the allowance. This means the beneficiary is responsible to pay 20% of the allowed charge (Medicare's fee for a provider). For certain preventative services there is no cost sharing. Note that the allowed charge is made up of the amount that Medicare pays and the amount that the beneficiary (or the gap insurance) pays.

Medicare Part C

Part C is the Medicare Advantage (MA) program. These are private health plans that receive Medicare payments to provide actuarially equivalent benefits. The Part A and Part B benefits are both provided and the deductible, co-payments, and coinsurance are typically covered by a premium charged by the MA plan. In addition, the beneficiary must continue to pay their Part B premium. Although MA plans cover the Medicare deductibles, co-payments, and coinsurance, they typically have their own forms of cost sharing, such as office visit co-payments, which can be substantial in the aggregate for high utilizers. Most MA plans include Part D. Therefore, these plans are typically A, B, D, and gap coverage all rolled up into one product. Covered benefits must include all services covered by Medicare, but typically additional services such as more extensive preventive care are added. Part C accounted for 25% of Medicare spending in 2013. MA and the predecessor Medicare + Choice (M+C) plans have had variable membership and regional distribution over the years, in part affected by profitability based on federal payment schedules. Some regions have had a strong and durable presence of MA or M+C plans, whereas other areas have seen plans leave the market. With the advent of Part D and other factors, plans have grown and approximately 30% of the Medicare population is in an MA plan. For some high service use beneficiaries, out-of-pocket costs may be higher than traditional Medicare in these plans. Because MA plans represent a subset of the population, adverse selection or the converse "cherry picking" becomes a concern. This is worsened if beneficiaries can move freely back and forth between plans and traditional Medicare. If the MA plan is restrictive but less costly, patients may move into the traditional program when they become ill and the loss of premium savings is outweighed by ease of service use found in traditional Medicare. For this reason, the Centers for Medicare and Medicaid Services (CMS) has created lock-in provisions restricting movement.

Medicare Part D

Part D is the prescription drug benefit that 38 million Medicare beneficiaries have. Other Medicare enrollees have coverage through plans such as retiree or employee benefits so that more than 90% of Medicare beneficiaries now have drug coverage. It is funded with premiums (averaging $39/month, varying by plan selected), general revenues, and state revenues that previously were used for Medicaid prescription drug coverage. Part D coverage is provided by private insurers approved by CMS. There is a low-income subsidy for premiums. Part D was not optional for Medicaid enrollees who are also Medicare beneficiaries (the dual eligibles). The standard plan for 2015 has a $320 deductible and 25% coinsurance for the first $2,960 after the deductible. For the next segment of expenditures, the beneficiary pays 45% of the cost of brand drugs and 65% of the cost of generics. This is commonly labeled the "donut hole." Beneficiaries may receive help on the out-of-pocket expenses from family or state assistance programs, but not the Part D plan. After $7,062 of total drugs costs ($4,700 in out-of-pocket spending), there is a 5% coinsurance. However, in 2015 no plans use this standard design. About half have a deductible and use tiered co-payments, and most retain the coverage gap. Part D plans have formularies with preferred drugs having different coverage than other drugs or noncoverage for some drugs. CMS requires certain drugs to be on all formularies and designated classes must have a representative drug. Physician-administered drugs remain on Part B. The Part D benefit is costly with 11% of Medicare expenditures, very nearly the same as physician payments, going to Part D.

What Medicare does not cover

Medicare does not cover acupuncture, routine vision care and eyeglasses, dental services, hearing examinations and aids, and long-term custodial care. Care outside the United States is generally not covered. It does not cover all preventive care, specifically an annual physical examination for preventive purposes other than one for new enrollees. Claiming a routine preventive examination as a condition-related medically necessary visit is prohibited. In recent years, however, Congress has added selective preventive services to the benefits and with the advent of the Affordable Care Act, the recommendations of the US Preventive Services Task Force now affect coverage. Because Medicare covers skilled nursing care and skilled home care, the greatest misconception of the public regarding coverage relates to these services. Many beneficiaries believe long-term non-skilled or "custodial" nursing home care is covered. That is incorrect. Benefits are set by statute. This means Congress defines the coverage, not CMS. CMS may provide greater detail but is not able to add benefits outside an existing category of covered service. Medicare beneficiaries spent an average $4,734 in 2010 for health-care costs because of premiums, cost sharing, and services that are excluded from coverage.

Medicaid

Medicaid was begun in 1965 as a state and federal shared program to help the poor with medical expenses. It is Title XIX of the Social Security Act. The program was established so that it would be funded by state funds with federal matching monies. States could determine eligibility (with some restrictions set by the federal government) and select the covered services, payment rates, and administer the program. It is "needs based" with eligibility determined by income and assets limits; that is, it is a welfare program. Over time, the program has changed and the federal government has placed some further requirements on the states for them to receive matching funds, but fundamentally it remains state specific. Therefore, eligibility and benefits do vary, and a beneficiary who moves from one state to another may be at risk for losing coverage. Medicaid covers poor women and their children, the blind or disabled, and the medically needy, and it funds the Programs for All Inclusive Care of the Elderly along with Medicare. The medically needy elder is typically a nursing home resident who was always poor or who has exhausted his or her savings and "spent down" to eligibility. The Programs for All Inclusive Care of the Elderly participants receive all their services through the program, require a nursing facility level of care, but are managed in an alternative setting by using flexible benefits not typically provided by Medicare. Seventy million Americans have Medicaid. It funds 16% of all personal health-care spending. Fourteen percent of all Medicaid recipients are "dual eligibles" who also have Medicare. Medicaid funds 40% of all nursing home and home-based long-term care. It provides gap coverage for deductibles, co-payments, and coinsurance for Medicare benefits, and prior to 2006, paid for prescription drugs. Because of the high per person costs for the elderly nursing home resident and the disabled, the aged and disabled comprise only 25% of the Medicaid population, yet account for two-thirds of Medicaid spending.[10]

Delivery system financing and organization

There are multiple components of the delivery system, but we will describe only a few key provider types.

Hospitals

There are approximately 5,500 hospitals in the United States. In the past two decade, the number of inpatient days per 1,000 persons has steadily dropped.[11] Over the same period, the outpatient hospital services growth has been strong. Hospitals have also consolidated, giving them much greater market power in negotiating rates with private payers. This has been useful as they have seen their profit margins from Medicare decline. Since the 1980s, hospital inpatient services have been paid by Medicare with a prospective payment system called Diagnosis-Related Groups (DRG). A hospital receives a single payment for an inpatient admission based on the diagnosis that caused the admission. Procedures and complications affect the DRG selection and there are special allowances for extreme outlier stays. The goal of such a system is to create incentives for the hospital to improve efficiency. Hospitals also receive payment updates or penalties based on quality performance measures. Private payer inpatient payment methodologies vary by payer and hospital.

Physicians

Physician supply has steadily increased; however, most of the increase has been in non–primary care specialties. The growth in larger group practices that could support infrastructure investments such as electronic health records is significant. The physician workforce is changing; women now outnumber men in medical schools, and more physicians are employees than in the past. Physicians are paid by Medicare on a modified fee for service or "piece-work" basis. The modification consists of surgical procedures being paid with one fee for all related services within

a "global" time period and for reductions when multiple surgical procedures are performed on the same day. Related services in the global period include the office visit services called "evaluation and management." These are the history, examination, assessment, and plan "cognitive" services. In general, the physician payment methodology by CMS has a financial incentive to perform more services. Since 1992, all Medicare fees are determined by a conversion factor and relative value units (RVUs). This is called the resource-based relative value system (RBRVS). Services of all types (procedural and evaluation and management) are ranked in a relative manner based on physician work. Work is determined by time, technical skill and effort, mental effort and judgment required, and stress due to risk to the patient. RVUs are assigned using a previously valued service as the reference or comparator. Valuation based on relativity to a reference service is the origin of the term "relative value." Practice expenses are then calculated based on the expenses incurred for clinical staff, supplies, and other costs associated with a specific procedure, and converted to RVUs by using a mathematical formula. Finally, professional liability costs related to a specific procedure are estimated and given a RVU amount. The three components of the RVUs are added up and converted to dollars by using a conversion factor (CF). For example, five RVUs with a CF of $30 would result in an allowance of $150. Practice expenses vary by whether a procedure is done in a facility, whereby the facility incurs the expense, or whether the service was nonfacility, that is, in the doctor's office.

A committee of physicians representing multiple specialties (including primary care–oriented specialties) is convened by the American Medical Association (AMA) to oversee the valuation process and make recommendations for RVUs to CMS. CMS can accept the recommendations or not, but the acceptance rate is high. The RBRVS methodology replaced a physician charge-based system and was intended to rationalize payment and reduce a disparity favoring procedure-oriented specialties. Congress defined the basics and CMS determines significant details. The ultimate valuations are based on work, practice expense, and liability costs, which is the basis for it being called "resource based." It is noteworthy, and a source of some criticism, that the current methodology does not create payment based on concepts such as cost-effectiveness, quality,

777

value to society, or the need to support a primary care infrastructure. Other payers do not necessarily use the Medicare payment methodology, but the majority uses some variant.

The highest volume and highest total cost service in medicine is the office visit. The cost per service is relatively low, but the volume is staggering. RBRVS values office visits and other evaluation and management services based on different levels defined by the amount of history, examination, and medical decision making required. Included in the valuation is some amount of work before the face-to-face service, such as reviewing a record sent in advance, and some amount of work after the service, such as dictating a consult note or following up on a laboratory result with the patient. The growing sentiment and evidence base that the valuations inadequately recognized the work and practice expense of care coordination required for the medically complex, chronically ill patient has led to some payment changes such as Medicare paying for chronic care management on a monthly basis starting in 2015.

The process by which a physician is paid starts with the reporting of that service to a payer by using a Current Procedural Terminology (CPT) code. CPT is the nomenclature system maintained by the AMA. Payers (in Medicare, CMS) assign each code a coverage determination (covered, not covered, or included in the payment of another service) and a fee. The claim a physician submits will be processed through an electronic claims system that may look for or have "edits" based on multiple factors such as diagnoses to indicate whether the service is medically necessary or covered. There are typically edits to be sure that one service may be paid with another service on the same day, or not because reporting both is incorrect. The rules for correct procedure code selection, knowing what Medicare covers, and payment processing steps can be confusing and require education.

CMS assigns an allowance for every procedure. Physicians who participate in Medicare (i.e., agree to the Medicare fee as payment) are paid the allowance, less coinsurance and deductibles, directly by Medicare. Physicians who do not participate in Medicare may bill the patient, but only up to 109.25% of the allowance, and then the physician must collect from the patient who is the recipient of the Medicare payment. Physicians may "opt out" of Medicare. In this case, the physician privately contracts with the patient, is not bound by any allowance,

and neither the patient nor the doctor may receive Medicare funds for the doctor's service. The physician who opts out is completely out of Medicare. The patient who sees such a physician may still receive services paid by Medicare from other providers. Medicare physician participation rates and rates of physicians willing to see new Medicare patients remain high and steady despite Medicare physician fee updates not keeping up with practice cost inflation. Whether Congress interprets this as professionalism or sufficient satisfaction with the program is uncertain. Physician payment is likely to undergo significant change in the years ahead as Medicare seeks to move away from a fee-for-service method. Quality metrics are being applied increasingly. Demonstrations in advance primary care practices (patient-centered medical homes) and accountable care organizations are harbingers of different incentives to organize and transform.

Nursing facilities

Approximately 5% of all Medicare payments were for skilled nursing facility (SNF) care. SNF reimbursement is based on a variation of the DRG. Facilities receive a global per diem payment that covers all services such as nursing, therapies, room and board, and medications. The payment is based on a resource utilization group that is determined from information provided as part of the Multidisciplinary Resident Assessment process.

Perspectives on health-care costs

Health-care costs have outpaced inflation and the growth of the economy so that an increasing percentage of the GDP is devoted to health care. If the GDP pie grows sufficiently, the non–health-care portion or slice in absolute size may be larger in successive years, even if it is a smaller portion of the pie. Consumption of health care does correlate with wealth, in international comparisons and by socioeconomic class in America. All of the GDP will be used for something, why not health care? Increased life years, including when adjusted for quality of life (function), have resulted from the health-care system and almost certainly not just from other effects such as secular dietary changes and no smoking policies. A part of the reason for increased volume of services is that more meaningful care can be provided for an expanding group of patients. We now do better controlling diabetes and hypertension and detecting breast cancer in early stages. Costly drugs really do help people with rheumatoid arthritis. The cost of health-care insurance, however, is rising at a rate that is suppressing wages and leading employers to discontinue or reduce coverage. Many elderly are using a growing portion of their income for health care. The federal budget is strained by cost trends that are independent of demographic change, which itself will further stress the budget. Health is determined by more than health care. Spending on housing, education, and nutrition may be much more effective in promoting the next advance in function or longevity than spending on, for example, a new drug to treat advanced malignancy. Studies on regional variation on spending in health care indicate that higher expenditures are inversely correlated with measurable quality. Concerns about quality, value, and sustainability indicate that the cost trend warrants critical review.

Many have examined costs in America. Although there may not be unanimity of opinion, there are some summary conclusions that can be reasonably made. It is useful to note that there are likely many factors and an improvement in any one area should not be cast away as irrelevant. No magic bullet is likely. Demographics account for a relatively small aspect of the trend. Care at the end of life does consume a large percentage of total expenditures, but this is true at all ages. The costs are growing at the same rate as other services and the costs for the very old are not due to futile intensive care unit days, but due to long-term and palliative care. Competition has had mixed effects. When payers with market clout forced hospitals and others to compete for patients by price, there was a period of trend reduction. More typically competition has resulted in one facility trying to outdo the other in technology arms races that fuel the fire of cost growth. Price is a factor with drugs and devices costing more than in other international systems that negotiate better with industry. Physicians earn more relative to the rest of the population when compared with western European countries. Our employer-based insurance system that became the model for our governmental programs was created by providers, presumably for providers, although that seems a distant memory to those battling with these payers today. Administrative costs are significant, typically described as the low single digits for Medicare and 10%–15% for commercial insurance. This has been fairly stable, is not the bulk of costs,

and may include investments in technology and services that will improve efficiency and quality. There is still an opportunity to create savings from better administrative efficiency and reduced marketing costs. Disease frequency, some of which is preventable by lifestyle interventions, may account for significant differences in per capita spending in international comparisons. Most agree that the biggest factor is the use and rapid diffusion of new technology, typically without a strong evidence base of utility established at the time of diffusion. Cost-effectiveness is rarely assessed.

Attempts to reign in costs have had mixed effects. Fraud, although rare, exists and must be rooted out continuously. Fraud reduction programs generally more than pay for themselves. Payer-created price reductions often resulted in cost shifting to other payers or increased volume of services to maintain gross income. Copayments or deductibles designed to moderate patient demand obviously shift cost to the patient, but the sickest patients account for most of the costs. Their services are typically the least discretionary, so savings from reduced utilization may not result. Removing some cost insulation may lead to consumers being more aware of and engaged in solving a national social problem. A forceful control on technology diffusion does forestall costs for a while but requires a political will that is currently lacking. Systems that operate within a budget such as an integrated delivery system that also provides financing or assumes financial risk do best in cost control. In our pluralistic payment system, budgets are not like those of single-payer systems in other countries and accordingly are harder to enforce. Furthermore, the delivery system is not a system organized with the capacity, authority, and information systems necessary to control expenditures within a national or regional budget. A primary care focus has had success, although restrictions by "gatekeepers" have not.

It is hoped that costs can be controlled by reducing duplication of care, errors, and other waste through use of an electronic health record and other delivery system changes. The same information systems can facilitate more effective use of evidence-based medicine. In an example of misaligned incentives, the cost of the system changes may be borne by a provider, but the benefit may accrue to the financing system. Changing payment from one that favors new procedures and volume of services to one that supports chronic disease care using teams, non–face-to-face interventions, and community resources [Edward Wagner's Chronic Care Model (CCM)] may be effective, if not in saving money, in improving care.[12] Disease management programs that properly target the most at risk and use effective interventions do save money by reducing hospitalization and, ergo, serious morbidity. Identification of at risk persons who are about to cross the threshold from average utilizer to high-cost utilizer may be possible. There needs to be a substantial investment into better understanding comparative cost-effectiveness of medical interventions. Only now, after years of resistance, are we developing ways to measure quality and efficiency and make them transparent and actionable for the provider and consumer alike. However, the notion of "value-based payment," although an admirable concept that is growing in real dollar relevancy, has significant needs in proving validity. Ideally, it will fund transformation and stimulate positive change rather than just be used as a reward for a nice report card. There will be stumbling along the way as this process matures. The financing and payment system must support a transformation in health care, even while there is legitimate concern about the predictability of the result of many interventions. There will be those who are adversely affected by change and will oppose it. Ultimately, all these efforts to improve our system will still require a social calculation of value. The transformational process is underway. All members of our society must make it work for the patient.

References

1. http://kff.org/global-indicator/health-expenditure-per-capita (accessed Apr 26, 2015).

2. http://data.worldbank.org/indicator/SH.XPD.TOTL.ZS (accessed Apr 26, 2015).

3. www.cms.gov/Research-Statistics-Data-and-Systems/Statistics-Trends-and-Reports/Chronic-Conditions/Downloads/2012Chartbook.pdf (accessed Apr 26, 2015).

4. www.thescanfoundation.org/sites/default/files/Georgetown_Trnsfrming_Care.pdf (accessed Apr 26, 2015).

5. https://kaiserfamilyfoundation.files.wordpress.com/2014/07/7305–08-the-facts-on-medicare-spending-and-financing.pdf (accessed Apr 26, 2015).

6. https://kaiserfamilyfoundation.files.wordpress.com/2014/09/1066–17-medicare-at-a-glance.pdf (accessed Apr 26, 2015).

7. http://kff.org/medicare/report/how-much-is-enough-out-of-pocket-spending-among-medicare-beneficiaries-a-chartbook (accessed Apr 26, 2015).

8. http://files.kff.org/attachment/report-a-primer-on-medicare-key-facts-about-the-medicare-program-and-the-people-it-covers (accessed Apr 26, 2015).

9. www.medpac.gov/documents/publications/jun14databookentirereport.pdf?sfvrsn=1 (accessed Apr 26, 2015).

10. http://files.kff.org/attachment/issue-brief-medicaid-moving-forward (accessed Apr 26, 2015).

11. www.aha.org/research/reports/tw/chartbook/2014/chapter3.pdf (accessed Apr 26, 2015).

12. Wagner EH, Austin BT, Von Korff M. Organizing care for patients with chronic illness. *Milbank Qrtly* 1996;**74**(4):511–44.

Chapter 59

Advance care planning
Using values and orders in end-of-life care

Stephen S. Hanson, PhD, and David J. Doukas, MD

This chapter focuses the reader's attention on using *written* preventive ethics tools in geriatric practice in planning for end-of-life care. Since an oral expression for future care may not lead to the intended consequence,[1] clinicians must guide their patients more toward written mechanisms. However, as nonwritten communication remains essential to patients' discovering and describing their advance care preferences, the clinician must regularly and often repeatedly converse with patients in order to present and complete those written documents, just as patients must converse with their proxy decision makers. Advance care planning is not a singular event; it is a process of ongoing conversation that may change as preferences and goals change over the course of time. This chapter highlights the ethical significance of the living will and durable powers of attorney for health care, examines some of the ethical conflicts that can be associated with the use of written advance directives, and considers a stepwise preventive ethics approach to these advance directives in clinical practice.

The beginnings of advance directives

Although the concept of living wills began in the 1960s, the legal beginnings of what we now call "advance directives" arose from a grassroots response to *In Re Quinlan*, decided by the New Jersey Supreme Court in 1976.[2] Ms. Quinlan, a 21-year-old woman, suffered two prolonged anoxic episodes of unknown origin, was resuscitated by a rescue team, hospitalized, and subsequently was in a persistent vegetative state (PVS). Her father petitioned the court for guardianship of her person for the purpose of requesting that respirator support be discontinued, with the understanding that the higher probability was that his daughter would die. His request was eventually granted by the court.

The Quinlan case established the legal basis to (a) allow patients to make written or oral advance declarations regarding their own end-of-life treatment (i.e., the living will); (b) allow patients to appoint proxy decision makers (i.e., the durable power of attorney for health care); and (c) encourage a meaningful discourse on values and the role of family and loved ones in future end-of-life treatment decisions (relevant later in the concepts of the *values history* and the *family covenant*). Today, advance directives are used by health-care providers as evidence of a patient's preferences to help guide medical care for those incompetent to make their own medical decisions.[3] In this way, advance directives are an extension of the well-recognized ability of individuals to exercise self-determination through informed consent or refusal.

The living will

An individual exercises self-determination with advance directives that make, and then project into the future, decisions regarding medical interventions. These health-care decisions to accept or refuse treatment are binding on physicians and institutions. The living will, then, is an expression of informed choice in advance of the time in which the patient is terminally ill (or persistently vegetative depending on the relevant statute) and has lost decision-making capacity. The latter is a clinical judgment, to be made according to prevailing standards of reasonable clinical judgment. States vary according to whether the patient's declaration or living will must be written, or whether a written or oral declaration must take a particular form. Living will laws also provide for criminal and civil immunity for physicians and institutions that carry out a valid living will in which no malpractice occurs.

Reichel's Care of the Elderly, 7th Edition, ed. Jan Busby-Whitehead *et al.* Published by Cambridge University Press.
© Cambridge University Press 2016.

Readers should familiarize themselves with the details in relevant statutes for each reader's jurisdiction. Many states allow surrogate decision making for patients who have not named a surrogate decision maker, which allows treatment refusal for those patients without living wills. States usually delineate who has legal standing as a surrogate in a hierarchy of guardians, family members, and so on, in a rank ordering determined state by state.

Regardless of where a patient's advance directive is written, an advance directive is a tool for patients to continue to exercise self-determination after their capacity to make their wishes known has ceased. Even if a directive does not comply with the state's statutory requirements (as may be the case when a document has been created in a different state than the one in which patient now resides) it may still serve as evidence of a patient's preferences to assist in guiding medical treatment.[4]

Many advance directives are aimed at refusing unwanted types of treatments when prognosis is poor, but some persons who wish to continue treatments have also executed advance directives to that effect, sometimes known as an "affirmation of life." Such directives may be valid in guiding care, depending upon the state; however, if a therapy is not beneficial or palliative in nature (i.e., per evidence-based medicine criteria or credible physiologic reasoning), it may still be morally acceptable for a physician or health-care facility to refuse to provide it and seek to transfer the patient's care to another physician or facility.

The durable power of attorney for health care

As experience was gained with living wills, a concern arose that the scope of advance informed refusal in living wills was not broad enough. Living wills often refer only to circumstances where patients are terminally ill or persistently vegetative; often, these conditions are not met even though a patient may not have decision-making capacity. The preferences indicated in an advance directive that applies to one diagnosis and prognosis likely do not apply to different circumstances. In such cases, patients' preferences would best be represented by family members or other loved ones.

For many years, common and statutory law have allowed individuals to appoint an agent through a durable power of attorney. A *power of attorney* is the assignment of certain legal powers to others, for example, to dispose of property in the physical absence of the owner. A simple power of attorney may not be *durable*; that is, it may not persist beyond that individual's loss of decision-making capacity. The *durable* power of attorney was developed to permit the conveyance of one's legal powers to another upon one's loss of decisional capacity. The durable power of attorney for health care (DPAHC), also called a health-care proxy, permits a named individual to make one's health-care decisions upon one's loss of decision-making capacity of any type. An important distinction between the DPAHC and the living will is that the DPAHC takes effect with any form of a loss of decision-making capacity, while living wills often apply directly only in cases of terminal illness or persistent vegetative states. Also, proxy decision makers can generally request or refuse *any* intervention, while living wills typically discuss only life-prolonging interventions.

Regardless of the form of advance directive, either living will or DPAHC, the use of the "substituted judgment" standard is preferable to that of the "best interest" standard. Substituted judgment requires a knowledge of the patient's values and preferences of what they would or would not want done using values- or scenario-based constructs that the patient has articulated in the past to their agent and other loved ones. A best interest standard is a weaker inference of what would be best for the patient who may not have had the opportunity to vocalize her or his values or preferences for life-sustaining treatments.

The learning point for clinicians is to illustrate the need for their patient to articulate (a) what treatments they would or would not want done in the future and (b) why. These preferences should be made clear both to their doctors and to their trusted loved ones, who may be placed in the position of making future decisions. By extension, patients should also be actively encouraged to appoint a proxy under a DPAHC and asked to consider a living will (if that is their wish) so that their future incapacitated selves will be protected from ambiguity due to insufficient information regarding end-of-life care treatment. These conversations should be revisited over time as patient goals and wishes can change as diseases progress.

The Patient Self-Determination Act

A major legal development in advance care planning was the Patient Self-Determination Act (PSDA) of

782

1990, which took effect in December of 1991.[5] The PSDA aims to reduce the number of situations in which patients do not have written advance directives by requiring institutions that receive federal funds and HMOs to notify their patients on admission (or enrollment in the case of HMOs) about their relevant rights under relevant state law to execute an advance directive. In addition, patients are to be notified about their rights of informed consent generally. Finally, among other provisions, the law also requires hospitals to have policies on these matters, to notify patients that there are such policies, and to provide information to patients about these policies.

Although the PSDA has increased patient awareness of advance health-care planning, it has not solved the problem of patients not having advance directives. [6, 7] Regrettably, the PSDA often does not get carried out by health-care professionals, but instead is usually a single query to the patient or family by admissions personnel or is in a raft of documents mailed to a new patient joining an HMO. It takes time, discussion, and patient education to effect an increased usage of advance directives.[8, 9] The clinician should assume that she or he bears significant responsibility for discussing advance directives with patients in the outpatient setting and for anticipating and seeking to prevent ethical conflicts that can arise in association with advance directives.

MOLST/POLST advance directives

A newer form of advance directive is the medical (or physician) orders for life-sustaining treatment (MOLST or POLST, although other similar acronyms – MOST, POST, COLST – are used in different states), a directive designed to guide emergency medical personnel in a crisis. MOLST directives are generally meant for persons who have serious health conditions, who wish to avoid some or all life-sustaining treatments, and who reside in long-term care facilities or otherwise outside of a hospital. The MOLST is a directive created by a patient and a physician, and signed by a physician or other clinician as a standing medical order, meant to follow the patient to whatever residence or facility he or she might access. As these are medical orders, they are to be followed in nursing homes, by emergency medical personnel, and in other circumstances where emergency decisions about life-sustaining care might have to be made outside of the hospital setting. Because these orders are in a concrete and portable form, and are often stored in an online

registry as well, they are available to help guide treatment in many cases where a living will or durable power of attorney might not help.

MOLST forms differ from state to state, but they generally include a statement about preferences regarding CPR in the case of a cardiac arrest, and a statement about preferences regarding other life-sustaining treatments versus comfort-care-only treatment in a life-threatening circumstance, including intubation, feeding tube placement, antibiotic use, and so on. They may also have a section regarding patient preferences about transfer to hospital or even contacting emergency care in a crisis.

The purpose of the MOLST is, in most cases, to enable patient wishes regarding avoiding unwanted treatment in an emergency. Since, in the absence of a clear order to the contrary, emergency personnel are obligated to provide every possible treatment to preserve life, a MOLST directing aggressive treatment is possible but not necessary. Although all but three states (Arkansas, Alabama, and South Dakota) at the time of publication either have a MOLST program or are developing one, the stage of development of the program and the acceptance of MOLST forms as valid orders in various health-care institutions vary widely. [10] Readers should familiarize themselves with their local state and institutional policies, but they should not assume that those policies are stable and unchanging. Indeed, interested readers in many states may be able to act so as to change their state or institutional policies. A guide to states with programs, and contact information for persons seeking to develop programs, can be found at www.polst.org/programs-in-your-sta te/#.

Ethical challenges with advance directives

Living wills, MOLST forms, and DPAHCs have a number of structural challenges that can limit their utility in guiding a patient's health care, especially if they are not addressed before a crisis arises.

1. Patients may not realize that having an advance directive is important to their own future.[11] Without one, decisions may be made contrary to those the patient might make. Decisions might not be made by those the patient would prefer or would want to trust with such decisions.

2. In some states a standard living will lacks detail. Typically, statutes refer to the withdrawal of

mechanical or other artificial means of sustaining life without adequate specification of what this might entail. However, many states' forms are now more explicit that all life-sustaining treatment (which is defined in the statute) should be withheld or discontinued. These states may also allow patients to choose which categories of treatment they wish continued and which withheld, specifically regarding cessation of nutrition and hydration.

It is important at this point to note that specificity in an advance directive is valuable to indicate what the directive covers and what it does not. For example, a do not attempt resuscitation (DNAR) order means that resuscitation ought not be attempted for a patient in the case of cardiac arrest. It does not mean that the patient chooses to refuse other therapies for other life-threatening conditions, nor does it even necessarily mean that the patient refuses intubation for a potentially reversible pulmonary condition, for example. Specificity in living wills, however, is often not possible because the document may be completed prior to the onset of the condition that is now requiring decisions for treatment. For this reason, more general discussions of values and discussion with family or loved ones (who may not be relatives) who know the patient well are of great value when creating a more generally useful advance directive. Few of the forms provided by the state have any mechanism for this sort of documentation, which is why it is often very important to go beyond the forms to have fuller conversations over time with a patient.

3. A patient may fail to provide future health instructions to his proxy. This lapse may occur because the patient trusts the agent named to make decisions and believes that trust is sufficient, or because the patient has not been provided the opportunity to make such decisions. Patients may also write instructions or make oral statements in association with a living will or durable power of attorney for health care that strike the physician as unreasonable (e.g., "Do everything – he's a fighter"), or as unhelpfully vague (e.g., "Don't keep me alive if I'm a vegetable"). These may be requests either for treatment or against treatment. Aggressive management does not make sense in all cases any more than nonaggressive

management makes sense in all cases. Instructions by patients that may be problematic (e.g., instructions for non-beneficial treatments that are also without palliative benefit) need to be identified when they are made and discussed with the patient, *before* they lead to ethical conflict.

4. Patients or their families can inaccurately assess what their religious traditions require of them in resisting death and fighting illness, and their religious advisor can rectify these erroneous beliefs.[12] However, religious advisors can sometimes influence patients or families, even if the advisor is not well informed about the patient's condition and its prospects; this makes it important to ensure that the advisor is clear about the details of the particular patient in question.

5. Some health-care professionals may have difficulty with some strategies for permitting patients to die, the withdrawal of nutritional therapy in particular. Some take the view that withdrawal of artificial nutritional therapy is tantamount to starvation and suicide. The US Supreme Court has held that nutritional therapy is legally the same as any other medical intervention and that its withdrawal is like that of a ventilator, not a killing.[4] Some state statutes also make this clear. However, this can be an emotionally charged issue for both providers and patients. Persons with a strong belief that there is a moral difference, such as that indicated by the Roman Catholic Church in their *Ethical and Religious Directives*, fifth edition, may be less interested in the legal status of withdrawing artificial nutrition and hydration and more concerned with whether it is consistent with their moral views.[13] It may also be the case that some facilities (e.g., Catholic-owned or operated) may have policies that prohibit withdrawal of artificial nutrition and/or hydration in some cases, even though this could violate a patient's stated preferences. It should not be assumed that any given patient, provider, or institution agrees with this position, as there is significant variance of viewpoints within persons of any faith. At the time of this printing, it is not clear whether there will be legal challenges to such policies or what the result of such challenges might be. The reader will have to assess her or his own positions and consider (ideally well ahead of time) how she or he will respond if colleagues or institutional policies are such that they may come

into conflict with the appropriately stated preferences of patients for cessation of nutritional therapy.

6. The patient's family and loved ones may object to the patient's decisions expressed in advance directives. Family members may disagree about how to interpret a living will or a DPAHC based on differing perceptions of prognosis and realistic treatment. The worst time for family conflicts about differing views of what treatment is appropriate is *after* the patient has lost decision-making capacity. It is far better to help the patient (prior to the loss of capacity) identify the best advocate for their values and preferences, and who may not serve those interests well. Often, as necessary, palliative care providers can act as a facilitator in these discussions.

7. Living wills and DPAHCs are not a physician's order. These advance directives need to be translated directly into physician's orders upon entry into the health-care system. These orders should be explicit, comprehensive, and timely. No professional caring for the patient should have any doubt about just what is and is not to be done when life-threatening events occur. The physician's obligations do not end with writing orders for nonaggressive management and comfort care measures. There are substantive ethical obligations to the dying and their families. The patient is owed appropriate palliative management of pain and suffering and threats to dignity. The family is owed assurance and support that the patient's wishes are being carried out and that, therefore, everything that ought to have been done was indeed done.

A response to these ethical challenges: the values history

These ethical challenges of advance directives led investigators to develop an explicitly value-based advance directive instrument called the values history to address prospectively the above challenges.[14–17] The term "value history" was first used by Dr. Edmund Pellegrino in the 1980s to describe the interactive discussion and narrative of values that should take place between patient and physician.[18] The values history is an attempt to catalyze this conversation about the patient's values and beliefs regarding advance directives, thereby promoting patient autonomy through a value-based discourse. These collected values, and the narrative of their discussion, can then be utilized in future medical scenarios in ways that cannot readily be addressed by means of a standard advance directive.

Documenting the patient's values helps to contextualize these preferences for future use (in the absence of a known illness). The values contained in the values history can indicate the medical therapies that patients would wish to forgo if they were terminally ill. Specifically, there is a high degree of correlation between financial, emotional, and physical burden avoidance and the desire to forego end-of-life treatment.[19–21] Patient values can help the patient and the patient's family and physician better understand how to invoke the patient's specific directive preferences in future, unforeseen medical circumstances. This approach allows for greater flexibility in the physician's response to the patient's future incapacity by heightening awareness of *why* patients would prefer or not prefer treatment modalities, which then assist the family and physician in writing orders when the need for them later arises. Almost all jurisdictions and the Department of Veterans Affairs policy allow specific directive statements to be added to a living will as well as the DPAHC, when their intent is in concordance with the advance directive.

The values history contains two parts: (a) the values section, which identifies values, and (b) the directives section, which offers specific preference statements based on the patient's values. The values section elicits from the patient his values regarding end-of-life care. The patient is first asked to evaluate his future life in the context of duration of life versus quality of life. The patient is then asked to identify the end-of-life values that are most important to him. The physician is encouraged to discuss the patient's values at length to allow for their elaboration or for the addition of other values that more completely reflect the individual's concerns or beliefs about end-of-life treatment. The directives section invites the patient to select specific treatment directives in light of those values and beliefs. The goal of this two-part approach is to encourage patient–physician discussion on the use of medical treatments at the end of life (particularly when they may be most relevant, or most concerning to them), which may assist the patient to understand better and articulate his values. In turn, the physician can better respect the patient's autonomy by clarifying misconceptions that could hinder the informed consent process.[22]

The values history's directives section list of treatment preferences should focus first on those that are most likely to be used for the patient, given their current medical problems. The directives section begins with treatment preferences in acute care situations: consent for or refusal of cardiopulmonary resuscitation, ventilator use, and endotracheal tube use. Preferences regarding treatments in chronic care follow, such as use of intravenous fluids, enteral feeding tubes, and total parenteral nutrition, medication, and dialysis. During this part of the values history process the physician explains the treatment modalities, their beneficial effects, short-term and long-term consequences, and possible harms in the contexts of terminal illness, irreversible coma, and PVS. During conversations on discontinuing treatment, the patient should be reassured that the administration of medications for symptom relief (including treatment for pain, nausea, and shortness of breath) would not be withheld if required for comfort care, even if such therapy may involve an incremental increase of the risk of mortality.

The values history is different from the living will and DPAHC in that "trials of intervention" can be more easily articulated for specific treatments.[23] This concept of trials of intervention is important in critical care, replacing the "all or nothing" approach. [24] The clinical reality is that aggressive management is often undertaken in a trial to see if it will benefit the patient with either (or both) physiological or palliative goals. Trials of intervention also create the possibility of openly discussing the patient's values and the physician's values to find common ground.

For all of the preceding directives (except cardiopulmonary resuscitation), the patient may choose wanting an intervention, a trial of intervention (limited by time or medical judgment), or nonintervention. The patient may decide that after a set time trial attempting an intervention, if no benefit of the therapy were apparent, the intervention should be discontinued. The patient can instead decide to have a treatment continued as long as it benefits the patient, in the physician's best medical judgment (and if possible, in coordination with the proxy). Benefit-based trials require a significant level of trust among the patient, the proxy, and the physician. The task for the physician is to allow adequate time for a therapy

to benefit the patient before considering stopping it. The parameters the physician will use should be discussed with the patient. Benefit-based trials more accurately convey how the DPAHC agent may approach intervention in an unforeseen future medical condition. Trials thereby allow for assignment of treatment as a trial with subsequent decisions made on the basis of benefit (or lack of it), time, or a later decision by the patient's proxy. Identifying common ground of values is the core strategy of preventive ethics.

The values history also offers several unique directives: refusal of intensive care treatment, autopsy, a "proxy negation" directive to exclude a specific potential decision maker (due to differing values) and "do not call 911" for patients in long-term care facilities or home care.[15] In states or institutions without MOLST statues or policies, this may allow persons to guide caregivers about their preferences for emergency treatments in the case of a crisis. However, it does not replace a MOLST, as it is not a medical order, nor does a MOLST replace a values history. The MOLST can translate the values and preferences in a Values History into medical orders that can be followed. The values history can help one glean the values and reasons behind the selection of the preferences in the MOLST.

The end of the directive section allows the patient to add consent, refusal, or trials of intervention to other specific directives not otherwise addressed (e.g., specific types of surgery).

The family covenant in advance care planning

In a series of publications, the *family covenant* has been proposed as an effective means to negotiate the place of family and significant others in the patient's health decisions.[25, 26] The family covenant is a health-care agreement that can facilitate proactive discourse on advance care planning. The family covenant articulates the roles of the patient, family or loved ones, and physician, as *they define them* in an interactive conversation. An initial health-care agreement delineates boundaries of information sharing and proxy consent, with the physician serving as facilitator in potential future times of conflict. This is a process-based approach, intended to provide a richer context of values and preferences through interactive discussion, as voiced by the participants.

The family covenant's open health-care agreement is predicated on a promise among the patient, physician, and those loved ones designated by the patients who agree to participate (including the patient's health-care surrogate/proxy). The initial promise is then reinforced by time and trust in the ongoing bond between the parties, with the physician serving as facilitator if conflict arises. The family covenant's construct determines the level and scope of persons who have informational access to the patient's future health affairs, both when able and incapacitated, and designates which loved ones may participate in future decision making on behalf of the incapacitated patient. The family covenant helps to clarify the values of each participant at its outset by articulating parameters concerning information sharing and surrogate decision-making in end-of-life care. These parameters are defined by those participating in the covenant. It promotes communication, collaboration, and transparency while being pragmatic in understanding that loved ones sometimes can benefit from the facilitative assistance of the patient's physician.

The family covenant adds two important aspects to advance care planning – articulating the role of loved ones, and the discourse among them in forging an ongoing health agreement. This advance directive model can therefore help with the difficulties of health-care proxies when a loved one is not sure what the patient would want done and turns to other family members for assistance.[27] It also would help when a living will's original premises are found to be too vague, and would reinforce the decisions articulated in one's values history. Very importantly, it explicitly identifies those loved ones who are *included* in the covenant – such that those outside of the covenant do not have standing in the sharing of information or decision making for the patient.

A preventive ethics strategy for advance directives

The ethical challenges discussed previously often occur because the physician waits too long to involve the patient (and his or her loved ones) in decision making in the outpatient setting, well in advance of hospitalization or admission to a nursing home. Primary care physicians are uniquely well positioned to discuss goals of care because of their ongoing relationship with the patient and deeper appreciation of their patient as a whole person. Regular discussion of advance directives with all geriatric patients should be regarded as the

ethical standard of care. These discussions should take place at hospital admissions – and the response of the reader's institutions to the PSDA should not be presumed to be sufficient – but should also take place in other potentially less stressful settings.

Ideally, advance directives should be discussed in the relative comfort of the outpatient setting.[28] Discharge planning should also be utilized as an additional setting in which decision-making discussions can be initiated, in anticipation of readmission. If a potential problem that may occur upon or before a patient's next hospital admission can be foreseen, do not let the patient be discharged without discussing that likely outcome, and ideally documenting patient preferences in such a case. The primary clinical task is preventive, aimed at foreseeing what kinds of decisions about treatment might need to be made if a known condition progresses or escalates, and asking patients about those decisions.

When possible, a patient should complete advance care planning over several visits. Such a methodology has two advantages over precipitous consent to an advance directive.[29, 30] First, treating this as an ongoing decision-making process enables time for this to be a reflective process by the patient; thus decisions are made thoughtfully. With discussion occurring over time, the physician can distribute the time required for these discussions over several medical visits. Second, the family and other loved ones can be part of this process when the patient consents to their involvement. The patient's loved ones, and specifically the DPAHC agent, should receive a copy of the completed living will, DPAHC, values history, and family covenant. Any MOLST directives should be shared with any facilities providing long-term care, as well as family or loved ones who are regular care providers. Any misunderstandings can be clarified at a meeting of family members, agent, patient, and care providers, including homecare workers and/or agencies. The authors urge that all advance directives be reviewed with the patient periodically (every 6–12 months), especially if there is a significant deterioration in the patient's health status or change in family dynamics. This way, changes in values or preferences that may occur over time can be documented, as well as discussed. Orders could then be updated as necessary.

The authors propose the following eight steps as a preventive ethics strategy for advance directives. Although these steps take time, they will be cost beneficial in the time, stress, and ethical conflicts that they can prevent for the reader, for patients, for patients' families and loved ones, for institutions, and for society.

1. Explain that there are different forms of advance directives and that they serve different purposes and take effect under different conditions. The living will can be used by the patient only to refuse (or request) certain types of treatment in advance of the time that the patient is both terminally ill (as defined in relevant state or federal statute) and found in reasonable clinical judgment to have lost the capacity for making his own decisions. The reader should be clear with the patient about whether the applicable law permits an advance directive to be implemented only when a person is terminally ill or if it may also be implemented when a person is in a PVS. If the state law narrowly restricts the types of situations in which a living will may be implemented, the patient is well advised to consider executing a DPAHC that can be implemented in a broader range of health circumstances.[31] The DPAHC can be used to assign to someone else the power to make decisions for the patient when in reasonable clinical judgment the patient has lost the capacity to make his own decisions. The patient need not also be terminally ill, as is the case for living wills. If relevant statutes exclude from the agent's authority the right to authorize certain types of treatment (e.g., electroshock therapy), these exclusions should be made clear to the patient. Patients' instructions on their DPAHC document should be reviewed. If the patient's instructions could in some circumstances be reliably judged to be not beneficial or difficult to implement, this should be explained to the patient, so that the patient can clarify his intent and preferences. For example, a request that everything be done may not make sense for a patient who is irreversibly dying despite aggressive management that results, on balance, only in unnecessary pain and suffering. Such an outcome is justifiably regarded as unreasonable in beneficence-based clinical ethical judgment, and this should be explained to the patient. All alternatives should be reviewed so that potential conflicts between the patient's preferences and beneficence-based clinical ethical judgment are understood and satisfactorily addressed. For patients who have executed both documents, the living will and DPAHC should be reviewed for potential areas of conflict. For example, a statement requesting CPR be attempted in case of

cardiac arrest will be hard to interpret if another statement requesting comfort care only exists on another document (or the same one). For patients for whom a MOLST is possible and appropriate, the MOLST should also be compared with the living will and DPAHC for conflicts. These should be pointed out to the patient and the patient's preference for the management of such conflict elicited. The patient should be asked to make note of such preference in the documents and the reader should record such preferences in the patient's record. Patients should also be made aware of the possibility of a values history or family covenant, or similar advance directive, as an adjunct to state-form-based living wills. Although such amendments are not defined by statute, almost all states do allow for modifications to an official living will or DPAHC. As such, they can also be of great help in guiding treatment when the patient's condition does not fall into the limited set of conditions that trigger a specific state's living will, or when questions arise that are more complex than whether or not to attempt life-sustaining therapies in cases of terminal illness or PVS. Although proxy decision makers are ideally there to decide in just those sorts of cases, they can often make better decisions with guidance from the patient. These may also be an effective way to clarify preferences beyond the too-vague or unreasonable-to-implement stage previously discussed.

2. The patient should be provided with a frank description of the kinds of interventions that are employed in aggressive management of life-threatening events, especially critical care interventions. The patient should be provided a brief but accurate description of such interventions as intubation and support by mechanical ventilation, cardiopulmonary resuscitation, admission to the critical care unit, the administration of medication, fluid, and nutrition by peripheral and central lines, and so on.[32] Both the short- and the long-term consequences should be discussed, including reliable estimates of the probability of successfully implementing the patient's preferences given the patient's present and future expected health status. [33] Patients with chronic diseases need to appreciate that life-threatening events usually accelerate the process of decline, and aggressive management followed by survival usually leaves

the patient with a lower baseline than before the event; more importantly, patients with known chronic conditions can more specifically plan for what diagnoses are possible or probable with their condition and execute specific directives, including MOLST documents if available.

It is especially important that the concept of trial of intervention be discussed with the patient.[34] A trial may be (and is often) stopped when it is no longer benefiting the patient. In particular, the patient should understand that in contemporary critical care, an admission to the intensive care unit is also a trial of intervention. This trial usually is undertaken to know whether it will benefit the patient, because it is still quite difficult to reliably predict which patients will and which patients will not benefit from intensive care admission. This trial, too, can be ended if the intended effect is not forthcoming – and the patient should articulate what such an endpoint would be.

3. Many patients make health-care decisions on the basis of their religious beliefs, traditions, and convictions. Patients often turn to religious advisors for help in making decisions about advance directives. When they do, the religious advisor should not be offering advice in a vacuum. With the patient's permission, therefore, the religious advisor should be provided with the information described in the previous two steps. In addition, the reader should be aware that most faith communities do not make it obligatory to continue aggressive life-sustaining treatments at all costs. Rather, moral theological views tend to recognize limits to what medicine can accomplish.[35] As noted previously, patients sometimes may not be aware of this and so may overestimate what their faith requires of them. If a patient or a religious advisor insists that the patient's faith requires that everything be done, this should be discussed with the patient and advisor in a frank way, apprising them of the prospects of success and the resulting cost in unnecessary morbidity, pain, and suffering. It may be appropriate to ask them to reconsider.

4. The patient should be asked whether the patient anticipates someone in the patient's family having concerns, problems, or objections to the patient's decisions in her advance directives. For example, a patient may prefer to name an adult child as agent with DPAHC, rather than her spouse. The patient's spouse may be unaware of this preference. Offer the patient the opportunity to meet with family members so that the patient's preferences and decisions can be explained. Adult children, especially, need to be made aware of the role reversal that can occur with aging parents. Now, the children may need to take over decision making – as if the patient were now a child, and the adult children were now parents of the patient. Family members, especially those named as a DPAHC, should be included in discussions about the patient's health-care preferences, when possible. Family members have an ethical obligation to respect the patient's choices, but do not face legal penalties for failing to do so. Clinicians may be required to remind family members of their loved one's choices and values and, in extreme cases, may even need to try to overrule decisions being made.

5. A semantic note: Beware of ever using the language of withdrawing or withholding "care." Treatments may be withheld or withdrawn, while *caring* for patients never stops. Caring for patients also includes diligent attention to, and palliative management of, pain and suffering and protection of the patient's dignity.

6. Ask the patient where the patient keeps or will keep originals of his advance directives and who has or will have copies. The reader should be sure that there are copies of the patient's directives in the patient's office records, the hospital records, and the nursing home's records. In particular, the reader should be certain that the emergency department of the patient's hospital has copies of the patient's directives. The patient's DPAHC agent, if one is named, should also have copies. For patients who live at home, the locations of advance directive documents should be known by family, loved ones, and DPAHC agents.

7. Ask yourself and your colleagues – especially nursing colleagues, as well as trainees – if any of them have concerns, problems, or objections to the patient's advance directives. When possible, you should plan for these contingencies. For example, as noted above, some individuals may object to withdrawal or withholding of nutrition or hydration.[13]

Two responses to this can be considered. First, if the patient is being supported by other interventions (e.g., a ventilator, or antibiotics, or pressor drugs), one or more of these could be discontinued to allow the patient to die comfortably. For patients on

789

multiple life supports, this may provide a resolution acceptable to all.

The second response applies when nutritional therapy is the main or sole intervention that is prolonging the patient's life. This is frequently the case for patients in a PVS. It is arguably a right in conscience for health-care professionals who disagree with withdrawal of artificial nutrition and hydration to withdraw from the care of the patient from whom nutritional support will be withheld or withdrawn provided sound transfer of medical care to another physician is facilitated. The reader's practice and institutional policy where the reader practices should recognize and respect such a right and the conscientious views that lead to its exercise. Interventions such as an ethics consult or a palliative care consult may help to resolve these difficulties. If not, sound transfer of care must be facilitated, as rights of refusal to provide treatment due to conscience become much more difficult to sustain ethically when that refusal provides a legitimate barrier to treatment for a patient. As professionals, individuals who hold these views must respect the patient's preference as also being reasonable and in conscience they are free to withdraw from the patient's case only after ensuring that the patient will not suffer any loss of care by their withdrawal.

8. Having undertaken the previous seven steps, the reader is in a position to write an order that implements the patient's advance directive(s). The reader's orders should be comprehensive and clear. The goal is the following: no professional with responsibility for the patient, upon reading the orders, should be unclear or uncertain in any way about what should and should not be done in the case of a life-threatening event. These orders should be readily accessible in the patient's chart, that is, as a face sheet. When a patient is to be discharged, the physician should, where applicable, write a relevant MOLST document to implement these orders and values.

As noted previously, there are serious beneficence-based and autonomy-based obligations to dying patients. Chief among these obligations are adequate pain and suffering control and maintenance of dignity. Seriously ill patients can tolerate high doses of analgesics, if the level is titrated appropriately. This approach minimizes the risk of mortality from aggressive pain and suffering management. Because the patient's death can be acceptable in both beneficence-based and autonomy-based clinical judgment, an increased risk of mortality for the sake of adequate pain and suffering control does not violate beneficence-based clinical ethical judgment. Quality assurance mechanisms should be extended to cover review of pain and suffering management for dying patients, so that these matters can be addressed openly and with institutional sanction.

Special considerations

Implementing advance directive orders for patients in nursing homes, for patients electing to die at home, and for surgery involves special considerations. For nursing home patients, the order written in step eight, in addition to pain and suffering control, might simply be "do not call 911." This strategy avoids all forms of aggressive management in nursing homes without resuscitation equipment and personnel trained in its appropriate use. For states with the option of a MOLST, this order may take the form of a MOLST; but even where a MOLST per se is not possible, a physician may write an order in a patient chart to not call 911 when that is a patient's wish. Lines of communication are very important when such advance directive orders are utilized. Caregivers, both formal and informal, need to be informed about these decisions. It is also important, in such a case, that families have someone to contact to discuss symptom management and for reassurance, as in the absence of this 911 is often a family's only other option.

This strategy may meet some institutional resistance. Some managers of nursing homes want to avoid any mortality in the nursing home and so may resist the "do not call 911" order. The authors know of no reported cases against physicians or hospitals that have implemented valid advance directives in accordance with the patient's wishes, and nursing homes can develop policies that respect and implement living wills. Done well, this process will be self-educating for the institution's personnel and leadership.

For patients at home, some states allow "do not call 911" orders by statute; even where no statute exists, a joint patient and physician decision not to call 911 can be reached.[36] However, a patient does not have an unlimited, autonomy-based positive right to impose unreasonable care burdens on family members, including the obligation to care for a loved one dying at home.[37]. To prevent future ethical conflict, a "do not call 911" order or decision should be conducted with a frank and mutually respectful discussion of the sense of family members' obligations and an articulation of their limits.

Patients with advance directive(s) including DNR orders may require surgery to reduce the patient's pain and suffering. The patient may be a reasonable, albeit high, risk for surgical intervention; surgeons and anesthesiologists often, if not always, request that DNR orders be rescinded during and perhaps for a period after surgical procedures. They reason that administration of anesthesia or intraoperative technique can result in life-threatening events from which the patient has a reasonable probability of recovering and then going on to enjoy the benefits of the surgery. In most cases, patients making a DNR decision were not discussing reversible iatrogenic events in the conduct of requested medical procedures.[38]

The preventive ethics strategy here is not surprising: negotiation with the surgical team. The reader and the surgical team should undertake a frank appraisal of the patient's surgical risk. The reader should also negotiate with the surgical team when the reader's orders for nonaggressive management of life-threatening events will again take effect (i.e., essentially a postoperative trial of intervention). The reader needs to be aware of surgeons' understandable sensitivities about mortality rates. The reader and surgical colleagues should work with their institutions and payers to ensure that death subsequent to surgery and reinstatement of the reader's orders for nonaggressive management of life-threatening events is an acceptable form of postoperative mortality.

To summarize an optimal means to address advance care planning, Table 59.1 depicts this process in brief. The family can be part of this process when the patient consents to their involvement. At its completion, the patient's loved ones, and specifically the

Table 59.1 Advance care planning from documents to orders

1. After patient execution of either or both the living will and DPAHC (as part of well elder care), the physician asks the patient which loved ones he/she would want as part of his/her own family covenant to share information, as well as to help the proxy (or clarify the living will) in future circumstances of incapacity. The members of this family covenant then meet (in person or by phone) to determine the boundaries that the patient and each member hold as a promise to each other.
2. The physician discusses with the patient values regarding quality of life versus duration of life, as part of the values history.
3. The physician reviews the patient's quality-of-life values with the patient and requests that the patient select those most important to him/her, while exploring other alternative patient values as well.
4. Using the patient's values as a framework, the patient and physician discuss the various therapeutic options in the directive section, especially examining "why" a therapy is accepted or refused.
5. The physician facilitates the consent process:
   a. By framing the process in relation to known patient values.
   b. By exploring other values that may emerge in the process.
   c. By clarifying for the patient inconsistencies between values and directives in a nonpaternalistic fashion, by removing reversible constraints to consent.
   d. By framing treatment options in terms of known patient conditions and diseases as well as high-risk activities and genetic propensities.
6. Other specific advance directive preferences concerning surgery, and calling 911 from home or the nursing home should be discussed. When possible and appropriate, the physician should also create a MOLST document to enact patient preferences outside the hospital.
7. The directives individually should be initialed and dated. The patient signs, dates, and has witnessed the completed values history, with copies placed in the medical chart (i.e., doctor's office, hospice, and/or extended care facility). The original should be placed in a readily available place in the patient's home (known to family and friends). The family covenant members should be participants in reviewing these values and preferences (as consented to in the covenant).
8. Periodically, these values and preferences should be reviewed among physician, patient, and family covenant members.

DPAHC agent, should receive a copy of the completed living will, DPAHC, MOLST, values history, and family covenant.

Conclusion

The moral weight of future treatment refusal should not be left to oral statements. Written advance directives, the living will, the DPAHC, and the MOLST (where possible and appropriate) are essential tools in advance care planning. The values history and family covenant are powerful supplementary documents that can add clarity and meaning to these advance directives by facilitating patient conversation on end-of-life care with family and physicians. Taken together, these advance directives allow the physician to respect patient autonomy and to understand better his or her patient's values and preferences regarding end-of-life care.

My advance directive for future medical treatment

Patient's name: _____
I currently have signed _____
[] My living will
Date signed: _____
Location: _____
Discussed with:
[] My doctor
Name _____ Date _____
[] My proxy/health surrogate
Name _____ Date _____
[] My other family members
Name _____ Date _____
Name _____ Date _____
Name _____ Date _____
Name _____ Date _____
Name _____ Date _____
[] My durable power of attorney for health care
Proxy name _____
Address _____ Phone _____
Date signed: _____
Location: _____

Discussed with:
[] My doctor
Name _____ Date _____
[] My proxy/health surrogate
Name _____ Date _____
[] My other family members
Name _____ Date _____
Name _____ Date _____
Name _____ Date _____
Name _____ Date _____

Name _____ Date _____
[] My organ donation card
Date signed: _____
Location: _____
Discussed with:
[] My doctor
Name _____ Date _____
[] My proxy/health surrogate
Name _____ Date _____
[] My other family members
Name _____ Date _____
Name _____ Date _____
Name _____ Date _____
Name _____ Date _____
Name _____ Date _____

My family covenant

I have entered a family covenant with my doctor, _____, and the following family members and friends:
Name _____
Name _____
Name _____
Name _____
Name _____

If other family members or friends are not included above, they are not to be consulted about my health, given medical information without my consent or that of my proxy, and they are not to be part of any medical decision making on my behalf.

My family covenant directs members to carry out my autonomous values and preferences in the following way, in conjunction with my living will and/or durable power of attorney for health care:

[Potential areas for consideration:

[] Who has access to my health-care information (confidentiality)?

[] Who else may participate in my health-care decisions?

[] Who is my proxy and whom else should he or she consult (or not)?]

Describe here:

_____
_____
_____

Signature _____ Date _____

Witness/address _____
Witness signature _____ Date _____
Witness/address _____
Witness signature _____ Date _____

Source: Doukas, DJ and Reichel, W. *Planning for Uncertainty.* 2nd ed. Baltimore: Johns Hopkins University Press, 2006. Reprinted with permission from Johns Hopkins University Press.

The values history

Patient's name: _____

This values history serves as a set of my specific value-based directives for various medical interventions. It is to be used in health-care circumstances when I may be unable to voice my preferences. These directives shall be made a part of the medical record and shall be used as supplements to my living will and/or durable power of attorney for health care if I am terminally ill and unable to communicate, if I am in an irreversible coma or persistent vegetative state, or if I am in end-stage dementia and unable to communicate.

I. Values section

There are several values important in decisions about end-of-life treatment and care. This section of the values history invites you to identify your most important values.

A. Basic life values

Perhaps the most basic values in this context concern length of life versus quality of life. Which of the following two statements most accurately reflects your feelings and wishes? Write your initials and the date next to the number you choose.

_____ 1. I want to live as long as possible, regardless of the quality of life that I experience.

_____ 2. I want to preserve a good quality of life, even if this means that I may not live as long.

B. Quality-of-life values

There are many values that help us to define for ourselves the quality of life that we want to live. The following values appear to be those most frequently used to define quality of life. Review this list and circle the values that are most important to your definition of quality of life. Feel free to elaborate on any of the items in the list, and to add to the list any other values that are important to you.

1. I want to maintain my capacity to think clearly.
2. I want to feel safe and secure.
3. I want to avoid unnecessary pain and suffering.
4. I want to be treated with respect.
5. I want to be treated with dignity when I can no longer speak for myself.
6. I do not want to be an unnecessary burden on my family.
7. I want to be able to make my own decisions.
8. I want to experience a comfortable dying process.
9. I want to be with my loved ones before I die.
10. I want to leave good memories of me for my loved ones.
11. I want to be treated in accord with my religious beliefs and traditions.
12. I want respect shown for my body after I die.
13. I want to help others by making a contribution to medical education and research.
14. Other values or clarification of values above:

_____
_____
_____

II. Directives section

The following directives are intended to clarify what you want and do not want if one day you are terminally ill and unable to communicate, you are in an irreversible coma or persistent vegetative state, or you are in end-stage dementia and unable to communicate. Some directives involve a simple yes or no decision. Others provide for the choice of a trial of intervention. Write your initials and the date next to the number for each directive you complete.

Initials/date

_____ 1. I want to undergo cardiopulmonary resuscitation.
_____ YES
_____ NO
Why?

_____ 2. I want to be placed on a ventilator.
_____ YES
_____ TRIAL for the TIME PERIOD OF _____
_____ TRIAL to determine effectiveness using reasonable medical judgment.
_____ NO
Why?

_____ 3. I want to have an endotracheal tube used in order to perform items 1 and 2.
_____ YES
_____ TRIAL for the TIME PERIOD OF _____
_____ TRIAL to determine effectiveness using reasonable medical judgment.
_____ NO
Why?

_____ 4. I want to have total parenteral nutrition administered for my nutrition.
_____ YES
_____ TRIAL for the TIME PERIOD OF _____
_____ TRIAL to determine effectiveness using reasonable medical judgment.
_____ NO
Why?

_____ 5. I want to have intravenous medication and hydration administered. Regardless of my decision, I understand that intravenous hydration to alleviate discomfort or pain medication will not be withheld from me if I so request them.
_____ YES
_____ TRIAL for the TIME PERIOD OF _____
_____ TRIAL to determine effectiveness using reasonable medical judgment.
_____ NO
Why?

_____ 6. I want to have all medications used for the treatment of my illness continued. Regardless of my decision, I understand that pain medication will continue to be administered including narcotic medications.
_____ YES
_____ TRIAL for the TIME PERIOD OF _____
_____ TRIAL to determine effectiveness using reasonable medical judgment.

_____ NO
Why?

_____ 7. I want to have nasogastric, gastrostomy, or other enteral feeding tubes introduced and administered for my nutrition.
_____ YES
_____ TRIAL for the TIME PERIOD OF _____
_____ TRIAL to determine effectiveness using reasonable medical judgment.
_____ NO
Why?

_____ 8. I want to be placed on a dialysis machine.
_____ YES
_____ TRIAL for the TIME PERIOD OF _____
_____ TRIAL to determine effectiveness using reasonable medical judgment.
_____ NO
Why?

_____ 9. I want to have an autopsy done to determine the cause(s) of my death.
_____ YES
_____ NO
Why?

_____ 10. I want to be admitted to the intensive care unit.
_____ YES
_____ NO
Why?

_____ 11. *For a patient in a long-term care facility or for a patient receiving care at home who experiences a life threatening change in health status:* I want 911 called in case of a medical emergency.
_____ YES
_____ NO
Why?

_____ 12. Other directives:

_____

_____

_____

I consent to these directives after receiving honest disclosure of their implications, risks, and benefits from my physician, being free of constraints, and being of sound mind.
Signature _____ Date _____
Witness/address _____
Witness/address _____
13. Proxy negation: I request that the following persons NOT be allowed to make

decisions on my behalf in the event of my disability or incapacity:

Name _____ Date _____

Name _____ Date _____

Source: Reprinted by permission of Appleton & Lange, Inc. Adapted from Doukas D and McCullough L. The values history: the evaluation of the patient's values and advance directives. *J Fam Pract.* 1991;32:145–53.

References

1. *Schiavo v. Schiavo*, No. 8:05-CV-530-T-27TBM (M.D. Fla. Mar. 22, 2005), aff'd, No. 05–11556 (11th Cir. Mar. 23, 2005).

2. *In Re Quinlan*, 70 N.J. 10, 355 A.2d 647 (1976).

3. www.ag.ny.gov/sites/default/files/pdfs/bureaus/healt h_care/EOLGUIDE012605.pdf, last accessed June 9, 2014.

4. *Cruzan v. Director, Missouri Department of Health*, 497 U.S. 261 (1990).

5. *Omnibus Budget Reconciliation Act of 1990.* Pub L. No. 101–508.

6. Robinson M, Dehaven M, Koch K. Effects of the patient self-determination act on patient knowledge and behavior. *J Fam Pract.* 1993;37:363–368.

7. Silverman H, Tuma P, Schaeffer M, Singh B. Implementation of the patient self-determination act in a hospital setting: an initial evaluation. *Arch Intern Med.* 1995;155:502–510.

8. Bailly D, and DePoy E. Older people's responses to education about advance directives. *Health Soc Work.* 1995;20:223–228.

9. Hoffman LJ, Gill B. Beginning with the end in mind. *Am J Nurs.* 2000;Suppl:38–41.

10. www.polst.org/programs-in-your-state (last accessed July 21, 2014).

11. Sulmasy DP, Terry PB, Weisman CS, et al. The accuracy of substituted judgments in patients with terminal diagnoses. *Ann Intern Med.* 1998;128:621–629.

12. Brett AS. "Inappropriate" treatment near the end of life: conflict between religious convictions and clinical judgment. *Arch Intern Med.* 2003;163:1645–1649.

13. United States Conference of Catholic Bishops. Ethical and Religious Directives for Catholic Health Care Services, 5th ed. 2009. Available at www.usccb.org/ab out/doctrine/ethical-and-religious-directives (last accessed July 21, 2014).

14. Doukas DJ, Reichel W. *Planning for Uncertainty: Living Wills and Other Advance Directives for You and Your Family.* 2nd ed. Baltimore: John Hopkins University Press; 2007.

15. Doukas DJ, McCullough LB. The values history: the evaluation of the patient's values and advance directives. *J Fam Pract.* 1991;32:145–153.

16. Doukas DJ, McCullough LB. Assessing the values history of the aged patient regarding critical and chronic care. In: Gallo JJ, Reichel W, Andersen L, eds. *Handbook of Geriatric Assessment.* 1st ed. Rockville, MD: Aspen Publishers, Inc.; 1988:111–124.

17. Doukas DJ, Lipson S, McCullough LB. Value history. In: *Clinical Aspects of Aging.* 3rd ed. Baltimore: Williams & Wilkins; 1989:615–616.

18. Pellegrino ED. Personal communication, 1981.

19. Doukas DJ, Gorenflo DW. Analyzing the values history: an evaluation of patient medical values and advance directives. *J Clin Ethics.* 1993;4:41–45.

20. Doukas DJ, Antonucci TA, Gorenflo DW. A multigenerational assessment of values and advance directives. *Ethics Behav.* 1992;2:51–59.

21. Doukas DJ, Gorenflo DW, Venkateswaran R. Understanding patients' values. *J Clin Ethics.* 1993;4:199–200.

22. Ackerman T. Why doctors should intervene. *Hastings Center Rep.* 1982;12:14–17.

23. Wear S. Anticipatory ethical decision-making: the role of the primary care physician. *HMO Pract.* 1989;3:31–46.

24. Civetta J, Taylor R, Kirby R, eds. *Critical Care.* Philadelphia:J. B. Lippincott; 1988.

25. Doukas DJ. Autonomy and beneficence in the family: describing the family covenant. *J Clin Ethics.* 1991;2:145–148.

26. Doukas DJ, Hardwig J. Using the family covenant in planning end-of-life care: obligations and promises of patients, families, and physicians. *J Am Geriatr Soc.* 2003;51:1155–1158.

27. Upadya A, Muralidharan V, Amoateng-Adjepong Y, Manthous CA. Patient, physician, and family member understanding of living wills. *Am J Respir Cri Care Med.* 2002;166:1430–1435.

28. Emanuel LL, Barry MJ, Stoeckle JD, et al. Advance directives for medical care – a case for greater use. *N Engl J Med.* 1991;324:889–895.

29. Scissors K. Advance directives for medical care. *N Engl J Med.* 1991; 325:1255.

30. Forrow L, Gogel E, Thomas E. Advance directives for medical care. *N Engl J Med.* 1991;325:1255.

31. Emanuel LL, Danis M, Pearlman RA, et al. Advance care planning as a process: structuring discussions in practice. *J Am Geriatr Soc.* 1995;43:40–46.

32. Moore KA, Danks JH, Ditto PH, et al. Elderly outpatients' understanding of a physician-initiated advance directive discussion. *Arch Fam Med.* 1994;3:1057–1063.

33. Uhlmann RF, Pearlman RA. Perceived quality of life and preferences for life-sustaining treatment in older adults. *Arch Intern Med.* 1991;**151**:495–497.

34. Reilly R, Teasdale T, McCullough LB. Option of trial in advance directives. *Gerontologist.* 1992;**32**:69.

35. Grodin MA. Religious advance directives: the convergence of law, religion, medicine, and public health. *Am J Public Health.* 1993;**83**:899–903.

36. Stollerman G. Decisions to leave home. *J Am Geriatr Soc.* 1988;**36**:375–376.

37. Jecker NS. The role of intimate others in medical decision making. *Gerontologist.* 1990;**30**:65–71.

38. Cohen CB, Cohen PJ. Required reconsideration of "do-not-resuscitate" orders in the operating room and certain other treatment settings. *Law Med Health Care.* 1992;**20**:354–363.

Chapter 60

Ethical decision making in the care of the elderly

G. Kevin Donovan, MD, MA

One might ask, if the ethics of medicine is meant to represent common and immutable truths, why would we need any special attention to ethics in the geriatric patient, above and beyond that which applies to everyone? The fact is that even though ethics may concern itself with universalizable rights and wrongs, its proper application must vary with the clinical situation and therefore with the individual patient. It is not irrelevant that a patient may be aged, but this alone will not justify a universalized approach, because the effects of age may range from nil in the independent and competent elderly patient, to being the most important factors, ethically and medically, in the patient with age-related disability or dementia.

General principles

It would be good, therefore, to start with some general principles, and from there consider particular applications. A variety of approaches to ethical analysis exist; one of the most recognized is based on prima facie principles.[1] These include *autonomy, beneficence, nonmaleficence, and justice*. "Autonomy" (from the Greek for "self rule") requires both liberty and the capacity for intentional action. "Nonmaleficence" is the avoidance of doing harm, and "beneficence" is the obligation to do good. "Justice" in this context is usually concerned with the fair distribution of resources. In applying these principles to ethical analysis, they prove most helpful in characterizing an ethical dilemma as a conflict between two principles, both of which we would wish to honor. Therefore, a wish to honor a patient's autonomy, for instance, could conflict with our wish to provide beneficent treatments or minimize avoidable harms. Because autonomy in particular can weigh heavily in moral dilemmas with elderly patients whose capacity may

become impaired, it is useful to remember that autonomy means not only "self rule" but is also based on "respect for persons." Thus we may be able to find ways to respect an individual's autonomy even as their capacity for decision making may diminish.[2]

Although principles are very useful for framing an ethical problem, they may be less effective for determining a proper resolution. Other philosophical systems, such as *deontology, consequentialism*, or *virtue-based ethics*, may prove useful here. Deontology proposes to search for the right rules, which, if followed, will lead to inevitably right outcomes. Another approach, consequentialism, will look to a good outcome as the indicator of a morally good action, and is often formulated as doing the greatest good for the greatest number. In recent years, a revitalization of virtue-based ethics places the focus on the character (and virtues) of the one doing the action, as well as the intention underlying that action. This is far from an exhaustive list; other methodologies are often employed, ranging from feminist, care-based, narrative, communitarian, to theological ethics, all having their uses, as well as their strengths and weaknesses. In reality, most individuals other than philosophers, when approaching an ethical dilemma, do not typically employ a single methodology for every case, but may adapt their thinking to the case at hand, often using a somewhat blended approach.

The patient as decision maker

When faced with the need to make decisions that are both medically and morally challenging, the ideal situation would involve a patient who is an autonomous adult with full decision-making capacity. In many cases the patient's full decision-making capacity seems self-evident. For doubtful cases a variety of

---

Reichel's Care of the Elderly, 7th Edition, ed. Jan Busby-Whitehead *et al.* Published by Cambridge University Press.
© Cambridge University Press 2016.

evaluative instruments have been proposed.[3] It should be remembered that capacity varies not only with age and state of health, but also is specific for certain types of decision making. Therefore, one might have capacity (a medical judgment) for making treatment decisions for oneself, even after the same patient has been declared incompetent by a court (a legal determination) for handling his or her own financial affairs. Unfortunately, patients' capacity to make their own decisions is often not called into question until and unless they disagree with the recommendations of their physicians. A determination that a patient no longer has decision-making capacity should follow the procedures prescribed by hospital policy or state law. Most frequently the determination may require the concurrence of two physicians, and may even require that one of them be a psychiatrist.

For those patients who are deemed nonautonomous (i.e., with diminished or absent capacity), there are still methods to honor their autonomy. Foremost among these is the application of their previously indicated wishes. These may be no more than verbal declarations, but in the best case they would come in the form of a legally binding *advance directive*. Advance directives typically come in two categories, a *living will*, specifying in advance those interventions that the patient would reject or accept, or a proxy appointment. A living will may have the disadvantage of too much specificity, such as listing specific medications or even dosages, or too much generality, listing interventions that are irrelevant to the patient's present circumstances, while not accounting for those that are. Either in conjunction with this or standing separately may be the *appointment of a surrogate decision maker*, sometimes in the legal form of a *durable power of attorney for healthcare*. More recently patients have been filling out a Physician Orders for Life-Sustaining Treatment (POLST) or Medical Orders for Life-Sustaining Treatment (MOLST) form where state law permits it. These forms are an approach that takes the items often found in a living will, puts them in the form of signed physician orders, and mandates their acceptance in the hospital or nursing home charts and therefore are immediately in force. Other patients may fill out a *values inventory* as part of their advance care planning. (See Chapter 59 on advance care planning.)

When a proxy decision maker has been appointed by the patient, his or her obligation is to use the patient's values in determining a proper course of action. When a surrogate or proxy has not been appointed by the patient, some state jurisdictions list a legally binding hierarchy of relatives who would be empowered to make decisions on behalf of the patient. Unfortunately, nothing about a legally mandated hierarchy ensures that a specifically ordered relative would have knowledge of the patient's values and preferences or even be inclined to employ them. In those less common cases where there is no morally or legally valid proxy and no indication of the patient's prior preferences or values, decisions can only be made using a "best interest" standard, frequently after the appointment of a guardian by the court. Attempting to apply such a standard can be particularly problematic. Some have suggested an actuarial approach to predict patient preferences;[4] others suggest that the patient's apparent acceptance and comfort with their current status should be considered more determinative than their previously stated wishes, as a truer reflection of respect for persons.

Goals of care

All medical decision making should focus on, and be in accord with, goals of care that have been determined by the treatment team, and agreed to by the patient or the patient's surrogate. These discussions should be routinely triggered when discussing prognosis or treatments with low probability of success, or patient's hopes and fears, or any time the physician can anticipate a remaining lifespan likely limited to 6–12 months. A model for this decision-making interaction has been described as "Beneficence in Trust."[5] In this model, the physician and patient work together for an outcome that is mutually beneficial, and is both right (the medically appropriate action) and good (the desirable action, according to the patient's values). The physician's expertise is crucial in determining what is medically right, and therefore making an appropriate recommendation. Yet, we must remember that nothing about a medical education makes the physician's judgment about what constitutes a good outcome for a particular patient take precedence over the patient's own values. Although focus must remain on the patient's good, the locus of the conversation may vary widely. Ideally such conversations would be included in some fashion in every outpatient encounter. In reality, a detailed discussion rarely takes place in this setting, even when the patient has a progressive, potentially terminal disease.

It is a difficult conversation at best, made more problematic by the time constraints in an outpatient setting, and unfortunately represents uncompensated time when many physicians are held responsible for all their billable minutes. A less desirable location is in the lawyer's office; although patients should be encouraged to have a last will and testament and any other necessary financial arrangements, this is not the optimal setting for discussions about their end-of-life care. In this setting, conversations which are primarily medical not legal may result in an advance care document that is more legally than medically appropriate. When a patient is admitted to the hospital or a nursing home, especially when they had been recently hospitalized for a severe progressive illness, a discussion of end-of-life care becomes more urgent. If the patient is facing a poor prognosis with the prospect of severe suffering or imminent death, or themselves have brought up hospice, palliative care, or a desire to die, such a conversation is crucial. Inexplicably, even these conditions do not always trigger timely discussions.

Actions and intentions

A discussion of goals may lack clarity when the motives or intentions behind certain actions are not made explicit, either by the physician or the patient. It is true that not every bad outcome is associated with bad intentions; in fact, this is not usually the case. Good actions can also lead to a bad outcome that may be foreseeable but unintended, and can be justified by applying the Principle of Double Effect. According to this, a morally good or neutral act may be justifiable even when a bad outcome can be foreseen, if certain conditions are met. Only the good outcome must be intended; the bad outcome, even if foreseeable, must be unintended, and the bad act cannot be the means to the good outcome. This must take place in a situation where the risks are proportional to the good that can be achieved. (See Box 60.1.) The classic example is the use of morphine in sufficiently high doses for pain relief in a terminal patient, even when there is a foreseeable risk of an earlier death to the patient due to respiratory suppression. The intention here is pain relief for the patient, but not pain relief by means of terminating the patient's life. The true intention is made clear when escalation of the morphine dose is stopped at the point of pain relief, but at a point that does not necessarily result in an accelerated death to the sufferer.

BOX 60.1 Double effect

Act – Morally good or neutral
    Intention – Only the good effect desired
    Means –The bad effect is not the means to the good effect
    Proportionality – The good effect outweighs the bad effect

---

Other axioms can also prove useful in seeking appropriate goals, such as those regarding quality of life, and withholding and withdrawing treatments. The first guideline is that quality-of-life judgments should be made according to the individual's own value of their life and is not to be a judgment made by a third-party. This will have a great bearing and even change the nature of discussions about the benefits and burdens of a particular treatment. Although it is not uncommon to hear someone say, "I wouldn't want to live like that," the important point is not whether *you* would want to live like that, but whether the *patient* is willing to do so. We are notoriously bad at predicting the tolerability of conditions experienced by others; only they can ultimately make a proper judgment about whether their life is worth living and medical interventions are worth enduring. Also, it is routinely accepted that both the withholding and withdrawing of life-sustaining treatments are morally equivalent. Although they may at times *feel* different to the involved parties, the comparability of such actions in a dying patient is found not only in their similar outcomes, but also in their equivalent intentions. Both are aimed at allowing the patient to die without an unwanted prolongation of their dying by burdensome but ineffective life-sustaining interventions.

Actions that result in death

Finally, the question must be asked: Are there goals or intentions that should be considered morally impermissible? Most commonly, these would arise in a discussion of killing versus allowing to die. Most recently, the discussion has extended to the morality of euthanasia and physician-assisted suicide. Let us consider each of these in turn. The distinction between killing and allowing to die has enjoyed a long tradition in medical morality. The direct and intentional killing of one's patient has been discouraged or forbidden in the Hippocratic and Judeo-Christian traditions throughout the centuries. Some confusion or even denial regarding the difference has played a significant role in the discussions of legalization of euthanasia and physician-assisted suicide (PAS). It is important, therefore, that if the distinction is real it should be understood clearly for what it is and what it is not. Some would argue that the difference is based on active versus passive "killing." This will not take us far, because the act of turning off the respirator in a terminally ill patient, a classic instance of allowing to die, is clearly active and not passive. Causation and intentionality have also been considered important, where the death is expected to be the result of an underlying illness. In order to clarify the differences, these definitions have been offered: "Killing is an act in which an agent creates a new lethal pathophysiological state with the specific intention of causing a person's death" and "Allowing to die is an act in which an agent removes an intervention, which is opposing a pre-existing fatal condition, or does not begin that intervention."[6] The second definition was phrased in that way to acknowledge that allowing to die could occur with the intention of causing the death (passively) or without directly intending the person's death. Under this concept, all killing would be wrong, but also some allowing to die could be wrong, when it is done with the intention of making the individual die. For those who do not intend the death of the patient in a withdrawal of support (which allows them to die), there may be no discernible difference in the action itself. If I unplug the ventilator, how does anyone know what my intentions were? I might be intending a patient's death or I might not. It is in this ambiguity between concrete actions and discernible or opaque intentions that the confusion about the real difference is found. It might even be difficult for the physician performing an "unplugging" to be certain of his or her own motives. Nevertheless, there are some indicators that may clarify the different intentions. For instance, if the patient is taken off the ventilator but then begins to spontaneously breathe, does this make the participants think it was a failure? If the life-sustaining treatment is withdrawn without the subsequent death of the patient, is the next question asked, "Well, now what can we do next?" Wouldn't these reactions be indicators of an intention not to simply remove an unwanted burdensome or ineffective intervention? Doesn't it begin to look like the burden to be removed is the burden of the patient or the patient's life?

In traditional medical ethics, intentionally killing our patients is considered morally wrong, and therefore the distinction between killing and allowing to die has been important. In the present era, the challenge lies not only in maintaining the distinction, but in countering a proposed refutation of the immorality of killing itself. Although the traditional proscriptions against directly killing patients (euthanasia) or supplying them the means to kill themselves (PAS) are still maintained in most locales and by most physician groups,[7] this is no longer universally true. Following practices first started in the Netherlands and Belgium, at least three states in the United States have legalized PAS through a popular referendum or legislative activity, and others through judicial opinions. The stated justification is usually one of compassion (i.e., relieving a patient of the burden of their suffering), which then extends to relieving them of the burden of their life. In the United States, only PAS has been practiced legally, as is the case in Switzerland. In Belgium and the Netherlands, both PAS and euthanasia are now options. At the present time, these options are limited to actions by physicians. Although this may be seen as an attempt to maintain societal control, no serious discussions have taken place as to why these acts should be restricted to physicians. In fact, in venues where these actions are not legalized, they still have been done by nonprofessionals, sometimes with the guidance of publications from the Hemlock Society or Compassion and Choices. These groups may provide detailed instructions about medications to use, doses to ingest, and even supplementary actions to ensure completion of the desired effect (i.e., tying a plastic bag around one's head).[8] Some physicians who are willing to participate in PAS are less willing to take an active role in directly euthanizing a patient, with objections that are not restricted to its illegality in the United States. However, with growing acceptance of PAS, there may be growing demands for direct euthanasia by physicians. This is almost inevitable, not only because of some reports of messy attempts by non-physicians, but also because not everyone can maintain the capability to participate in PAS as a patient. In fact, if members of the public and the profession come to see this as a benefit, as a good thing, to be offered by the profession, then its extension from PAS for the terminally ill, to euthanasia or PAS for a variety of nonlethal conditions in other patients is logically inevitable. In fact, this is no longer conjecture; there are multiple examples already of this sort of "mission creep" – the Swiss organization Dignitas has assisted in suicides already for patients whose problems ranged from uncomplicated old age to loss of good looks. In the Lowlands, deaths have been arranged for depression, hearing loss, and anticipated bad prognoses for infants and children.[9, 10]

This has inevitably resulted in reaction from those members of the profession who do not see this as a good thing.[11] Those arguing against it point out that euthanasia/PAS are not normally required for beneficent care. Pain relief is almost always possible, and suffering which may be psychological, emotional, or existential is not best treated by causing the patient's death. Moreover, what appears to be an autonomous action on the patient's part could easily devolve into a sense of obligation or expectation, if one's continued life is sensed to be burdensome to others, either financially or emotionally. Such a shift in traditional medical practice diminishes the value of palliative care, as it diminishes the self-worth of the patient as well, at a time when their declining capabilities may make them question their continued purpose in life.[12] Moreover, assuming such a role may do irreparable harm to the profession itself. Patients may justly be concerned if the physician pledged to safeguard their life and health is the same one offering to usher them out of it. If support for PAS and euthanasia grows, and with it the expectation that this will become the responsibility of the medical profession, it may lead to one of the most crucial ethical and moral dilemmas facing the profession in the near future.

Case 1: Disclosing a diagnosis of dementia

An 82-year-old woman is brought into your office by her daughter. The daughter tells you about her mother's gradually worsening memory loss with increasing forgetfulness over the past few years. In addition, the patient has expressed paranoid thoughts that her daughter wants to put her in a nursing home and that people are stealing her possessions. The patient lives alone, but nearby, her daughter. The patient is adamant about continuing to live on her own and has expressed that living in a nursing home is a fate worse than death. She currently dresses, feeds, and bathes herself. The daughter conducts most of her

mother's finances, arranges and administers her medications, and also does her shopping. There had been no significant accidents or incidents in which the mother is wandering or becomes lost. After a thorough evaluation, you feel this patient most likely has dementia caused by Alzheimer's disease. When you expressed this to the patient's daughter, she requests that you not tell her mother, as it would only anger, depress or worry her. The daughter would like you to start a medication for dementia but asks you not to tell the patient the real purpose of the medication.

Discussion

The primary professional obligation of physicians is to the patient's good. How is this good to be determined and carried out? The doctor must offer beneficent treatment and care options, avoid harm, and respect the autonomy of the patient. These principles cannot be adequately followed without employing certain specific virtues. Along with virtues such as competence, fidelity, and compassion, this situation calls for honesty. Unless patients are treated with the respect due them, they can't be expected to respond appropriately and be capable of autonomous decision making. Therefore, patients have a right to be told the truth about their condition. This right cannot be abrogated by third parties, even loving family members, whose own anxiety may cause them to make an error in judgment about the patient's capabilities.

For the same reason, a beneficent physician is not allowed to make a paternalistic and unilateral decision to withhold potentially troubling information. Both ethics and the law support this approach; however, it is not without exceptions. A patient may decide to waive her right to information. This may be prompted by cultural, psychological, or emotional aspects of an individual patient. Such a waiver, however, must be explicit, and can be determined in advance. When a physician suspects that a patient may prefer not to hear unpleasant or troubling medical facts, the patient should be asked, "How much do you want to know?" And then "Who should I tell, and what should they be told?" Such an explicit waiver should then clearly be documented in the medical record.

An additional and more common exception occurs when a patient has such diminished capacity that she can't fully comprehend, or deal with, the information, or act on it in a fully autonomous way.

When this status is suspected, the evaluation of capacity should be formal, and typically doctors are required to determine that an advance directive (if available) should now be activated. Unfortunately, even after a predictable decline, too many patients have failed to indicate what their preferences might be or who a suitable proxy decision maker would be. One of our obligations as physicians should be to ensure these discussions take place when the patient is still capable of indicating their preferences. This should then obviate the need to seek legal guardianship.

What is not sufficient is the assertion by a family member, no matter how insistent, that a patient should not be told, and cannot deal with information. Nor should the doctor and loved ones go around or talk over the head of the patient. Age and state of health don't automatically impair the geriatric patient's autonomy. In fact, it may be a quarrelsome disposition of the patient that triggers such caregiver behaviors, ones that will likely be worsened if the patient feels that she or he is no longer treated with respect. The children do not automatically assume the parent's role, nor do they automatically have rights to information and decision making. It is imperative that these issues be fully discussed early in the course of diagnosis and treatment.

There may be good reasons for a patient to know their diagnosis of early dementia. These include the opportunity for further planning for legal, financial, and long-term care issues. Moreover, patients may then become free to decide how to spend their time with people and things that are most important to them and to reconcile themselves with others when necessary. Additionally, some patients may seek the opportunity to participate in treatment trials for their condition, but only if that condition has been made known to them. Reasons to avoid disclosure, in addition to those already discussed, often focus on concerns about depression and the fear of suicide. The best preventative for this may be the provision of emotional and spiritual support in addition to adequate health care and support for the tasks of daily life. It is crucially important that patients not be made to feel that they are a burden either to the system or to their families. Rather, it should be possible to focus on the positives that do exist, even as the patient's condition devolves from one stage to another.

Case 2: Substituted judgment and medical futility

An 89-year-old woman has a history of diabetes, hypertension, congestive heart failure, chronic obstructive pulmonary disease, and advanced dementia. She has been a resident in a nursing home for the last five years. You meet this patient and her family for the first time when she is hospitalized for a hip fracture. Soon after her hip repair, the patient develops pneumonia. She requires oxygen therapy to maintain appropriate oxygen saturation; however, the patient has become delirious and frequently takes off her oxygen mask. The house staff order restraints to keep the oxygen therapy in place. Furthermore, the patient's intake of fluids and nutrition has substantially decreased during this illness. She develops acute renal failure associated with dehydration. An intravenous catheter is placed to administer fluids, which, despite her restraints, is quickly torn out by the patient. Further attempts to place an intravenous catheter are unsuccessful.

You meet with the family to discuss this patient's complicated hospital course, her prognosis, and the goals of care for the patient. You ask the family about the patient's wishes regarding resuscitation and other life-sustaining medical therapies. The patient has not executed an advance directive. One daughter says that the patient did not previously express treatment wishes, but she believes that her mother would want everything done to keep her alive and would not want a DNR order. She requested the patient be transferred to the intensive care unit for progressive management.

Discussion

This clinical scenario is unfortunately all too common. In this case, the physician has no clear indication of the patient's wishes, no clear surrogate decision maker, and only an indirect estimation of the patient's probable values that might impact subsequent care. The estimations provided by family members regarding a patient's probable preferences have not been shown to be highly reliable,[13] and only the treating physician's estimations were shown to be less reliable. The first task will be to decide on the morally appropriate and legally valid surrogate decision maker. As we have seen, this might be designated by local law; however, even such laws do not typically help choose between proxies at the same level of hierarchy, such as children or siblings. The physician, sometimes with the help of an ethics consultant, can seek to determine who knows the patient best, and would have his or her best interests at heart. With a large number of family members who may be clamoring for information or a vote in the decision making, it is frequently helpful to ask them to designate a spokesperson. This family member can then be the conduit for delivering information to the rest of the family and giving feedback on decision making. Proxies or surrogate decision makers must be made to understand that decisions should not be made according to their preferences, but on the preferences of the patient only. This *substituted judgment* is often the most difficult aspect of surrogate decision making.

With the patient who has such multiple and chronic problems, and a predictably poor prognosis, physicians may be tempted to discourage certain treatment options on the basis of medical futility. Families, such as in this case, may be resistant to couching the problem in such terms. There is no common definition of futility that is likely to be universally accepted, other than that of strict physiological futility. If an intervention is completely incapable of achieving a desired goal, everyone can agree that it would be futile. However, this is not the case with most of those interventions that we think would be of dubious value and inadvisable. In fact, families often perceive that what we might describe as futility is in fact a disguised value judgment. It is not so much that an intervention would have no effect, but rather that we think its continued effect would not be worthwhile. It is these judgments that typically shape our recommendations to forgo ventilator support, dialysis, and other life-sustaining interventions near the end-of-life.

The problem at this juncture usually resides in differing concepts of futility.[14] If strict medical futility occurs when (a) there is a goal, (b) an intervention is aimed at achieving this goal, and (c) there is virtual certainty that the intervention will fail in achieving this goal, then the failure of agreement usually revolves around the acceptable goal. Hippocrates stated, "The physician must not treat the patient who is overmastered by his disease, realizing in such cases medicine is powerless."[15] Physicians often see futility in situations other than those that have no possible physiological benefit. Other goals of aggressive treatment, such as to prevent bodily death, may be thought to serve no useful purpose, when their idea of benefit is more oriented towards pain reduction or a peaceful death. If goals of care have not been explicitly agreed upon, conflict may well follow.

It is better to prevent than try to remedy conflicts with the proxy decision makers. Thorough and explicit discussions may help to redirect requests that "Everything be done." The treating physician should reassure the family that she or he wants everything done that can provide real benefit under the circumstances. Reasons why a possible intervention is not thought beneficial should be explained and alternatives detailed. Engaging in such a dialogue rather than giving an immediate refusal is more likely to be successful. Physicians must also remember that *nonmaleficence* is an important principle; physicians are not obligated to provide treatments they believe are ineffective or harmful. A patient or surrogate's right to participate in the decision-making process is a negative right (i.e., they can accept or reject proposed treatments). It does not constitute a positive right to demand treatments that are not medically indicated. The effort to avoid doing harm, while respecting the patient's values requires patience, humility and good communication skills. It may be rewarded by avoiding unnecessary intensive care, yet providing those interventions that may still prove beneficial, sometimes as a time-limited trial.

Case 3: Nutrition and hydration

A 77-year-old man with end-stage Alzheimer's and multi-infarct dementia is admitted to a geriatric psychiatric ward for worsening aggressive behavior, after physically attacking his wife. He lives at home with his wife, who is assisted by live-in nursing help. The patient's oral intake has substantially decreased, and he has lost approximately 15 pounds in the past three months. On admission, the patient's laboratory values indicate likely dehydration and malnutrition. You place a line intravenously to rehydrate him, and the nutrition consultant asserts that the patient requires a feeding tube to address malnutrition. On meeting with the patient's wife, she asks you not to give her husband fluids or a feeding tube. "What good would it do in the end? Can we just let him go?" she asks you.

Discussion

In the recent past, perhaps nothing has generated more controversy, headlines, or policy statements than issues regarding the provision of nutrition and hydration. When considering a decision to withhold (or withdraw) nutrition and hydration, candidate patients generally fall into three categories: the *unfeedable*, those with a short gut or bowel obstruction, the *terminal*, and the *stable*, but neurologically devastated. Controversy does not usually attach to the first two categories. There is no moral obligation to do the impossible, and there is little evidence that extraordinary measures to provide feedings to the terminally ill patient are actually beneficial. In fact, the evidence would point the other way. The third category has triggered the most discussion and controversy, and we will consider how it applies to patients with dementia.

The question becomes: Should patients with Alzheimer's and advanced dementia fit into the second or third category? It is anticipated that all patients who live long enough with Alzheimer's will experience difficulty with eating. There is a loss of appetite, as well as motor function, which then interferes with intake, chewing, and swallowing. This can be considered a normal part of the disease process as it is nearing its end. Although a feeding gastrostomy can be placed, the available evidence indicates that it would not serve the purpose of improving nutrition or prolonging life under the circumstances. Careful explanation of these facts to the patient and family long before the apparent need would arise can obviate difficult discussions and emotional angst when the time comes. Most families can accept that this is a normal and irreversible event at the end of a dementia patient's life. Moreover, when patients and physicians understand the limitations of tube feedings in this situation, enthusiasm fades. Although the most common diagnostic category for patients receiving tube feedings is dementia, tube feedings have not been shown to reduce the risk of aspiration, to maintain weight or nutritional status, to prevent pressure sores, or to delay mortality in such patients.[16–18]

The initial justifications given for withholding or withdrawing nutrition and hydration were that they were artificially supplied. Because this required a medical procedure, it was argued that it could be refused or discontinued as burdensome, like any other medical intervention. The fact of the matter is that the primary burden of the feeding tube, and its most important risks, occur in its placement, not in its maintenance. Moreover, further discussions about supplying nutrition and hydration have not focused on the presence of a feeding tube at all, but rather the provision of these by any route, including oral. It is certainly preferable to offer hand feedings orally to a dementia patient near the end of life rather than put in a feeding tube. Currently, arguments are being made that neither approach is necessary, that no feeding at all needs to be done. There are serious discussions about the voluntary stopping of eating and drinking (VSED). This is being proposed for those patients who still have the capacity to choose it, and also to be done to those who have lost capacity to accept that choice.[19] It should be noted that the examples given above are less controversial than the withholding or withdrawing of nutrition/hydration from neurologically devastated but stable patients. The concern revolves around the intention of such cessation. These patients are not dying, but it is the feedings that are keeping them alive. A decision to withdraw nutrition and hydration usually follows a decision that their lives are no longer worth sustaining. Therefore, such a withdrawal is rightly seen as intended to end their lives, rather than relieve them of any medical burdens involved in the feeding.[20] Because of this, individuals and institutions who see this withdrawal as an unacceptable act of euthanasia have chosen not to participate. Consequently, withdrawal of nutrition and hydration from medically stable patients will not be done in Catholic hospitals and nursing homes.[21] This restriction would not apply to the unfeedable patients, nor those who are imminently dying anyway, such as patients with advanced dementia.

Conclusion

Every interaction with a patient has an ethical component. In many cases, it is implicit and uncontroversial. Sometimes, it is explicit and becomes the central focus of activity. Resolution of ethical dilemmas can be aided by a systematic approach guided by principles and axioms. In all cases, the good of the patient is a foremost consideration, balanced by the realization that the physician is also a moral agent. This means that physicians are not mere servants to autonomy as they seek to balance the myriad factors involved but always must seek that which truly benefits the patient.

References

1. Beauchamp TL, Childress JF. *Principles of Biomedical Ethics*, 7th ed, New York: Oxford University Press, 2013.

2. Taking care: Ethical caregiving in our aging society, Report of the President's Council on Bioethics, Washington, DC, 2005.

3. Sessum LL, Zembrzuska H, Jackson JL. Does this patient have medical decision-making capacity? Clinician's corner, *JAMA*, July 27, 2011; **3006**(4):420–427.

4. Ditto PH, Clark CJ. Predicting end-of-life treatment preferences: perils and practicalities. *Journal of Medicine and Philosophy*, April 2014; **39**(2):196–204.

5. Pellegrino ED, Thomasma D. *For the Patient's Good: The Restoration of Beneficence in Health Care*. Oxford: Oxford University Press, 1987.

6. Sulmasy, DP. Killing and allowing to die: another look. *J Law Med Ethics*. 1998; **26**:55–64.

7. AMA Code of Medical Ethics 2010–2011, Chicago; WMA Resolution on euthanasia, 53rd World Medical Association General Assembly, Washington DC, October 2002, reaffirmed with minor revision by the 194th WMA Council Session Bali, Indonesia, April 2013.

8. Humphrey D. *Supplement to Final Exit: The Latest How-To and Why of Euthanasia/Hastened Death* (unabridged). Junction City, OR: Norris Lane Press, 2000.

9. Groenewoud JH, van der Maas PJ, van der Wal G, et al. Physician-assisted death in psychiatric practice in the Netherlands. Special Issue, *N Engl J Med*. 1997; **336**:1795–1801.

10. End-of-life decisions: "Exit" members vote to broaden assisted suicide services, Swiss News Information, May 24, 2014. Available at: www.swissinfo.ch/eng/end-of-life-decisions_exit-members-vote-to-broaden-assisted-suicide-services/38653642 (accessed 19 Jan 2016).

11. Pellegrino ED. Doctors must not kill. *J Clin Eth*. 1992;**3**(2):95–102.

12. Donovan GK. The disabled and their lives of purpose. *Linacre Quarterly*. Aug. 2009;**74**(5):265–269.

13. A controlled trial to improve care for seriously ill hospitalized patients: The study to understand prognosis and preferences for outcomes and risks of treatments (SUPPORT). The SUPPORT Principal Investigators. *JAMA* November 22, 1995;**274**(20):1591–1598.

14. Kasman DL. When is medical treatment futile: a guide for students, residents, and physicians. *J Gen Intern Med*. 2004;**19**:1053–1056.

15. Hippocrates, The Art. In: *The Loeb Classical Library: Hippocrates*. Vol **II**. Goold GB, ed. Jones WHS, trans., Cambridge, MA; Harvard University Press, 1995; 185–217.

16. Lazarus BA, Murphy JB, Culpeper L. Aspiration associated with long-term gastric versus jejunal feeding: a critical analysis of the literature. *Arch Phys Med Rehab*. 1990;**71**:46–53.

17. Ciocon JO, Silverstone FA, Graver LM, Foley CJ. Tube feedings in elderly patients. Indications, benefits, and complications. *Arch Intern Med*. 1988; **148**:429–433.

18. Mitchell SL, Kiely DK, Lipsitz LA. The risk factors and impact on survival of feeding tube placement in nursing home residents with severe cognitive impairment. *Arch Intern Med*. 1997;**157**:327–332.

19. Menzel PT, Chandler-Cramer MC. Advance directives, dementia, and withholding food and water by mouth, *Hastings Center Report*, May–June 2014:23–37.

20. Rady MY, Verheijde JL. Liverpool Care Pathway: life-ending pathway or palliative care pathway? *J Medical Ethics*. 2015; **41**(8):644.

21. Congregation for the Doctrine of the Faith. Responses to certain questions of the United States Conference of Catholic Bishops concerning artificial nutrition and hydration. August 1, 2007. Reprinted in *Ethics & Medics* Nov 2007; 32(11):1–3.

Additional references

Beauchamp, TL and Childress, JF. *Principles of Biomedical Ethics*, 7th edition, New York: Oxford University Press, 2009, 457 pages.

The President's Council on Bioethics, *Taking Care: Ethical Caregiving in Our Aging Society*, Washington, DC: Government Printing Office, September 2005, 309 pages.

Pellegrino, ED. Doctors must not kill, *J. of Clin. Ethics* 1992: **3**(2): 95–102.

Index

Italicized page numbers indicate a table, figure, or box on the designated page

Alzheimer's Disease (AD) (cont.)
immunization clinical trials, 136
incidence rates, 125, 126
marginalization of patients with, 7
Medicare Part A coverage for, 775
musculoskeletal injuries and, 462
neuroimaging in, 133–134
pharmacological treatment,
134–135
risk factors, 126
stages of, 126
trazodone for insomnia in,
271–272
urinary incontinence in, 386
amantadine
for cerebellar ataxia, 261
for influenza, 335–336
for PD, symptomatic treatment, 251,
253
AMDA. *See* Society for Post-Acute and
Long-Term Care Medicine
AMDR. *See* Acceptable Macronutrient
Distribution Range
American Academy of Clinical
Endocrinologists, 448
American Academy of Family
Physicians, 11, 50–51
American Academy of Hospice and
Palliative Medicine, 11
American Academy of Nursing, 11
American Association of Clinical
Endocrinologists, 415
American Association of Endocrine
Surgeons, 415
American Association of
Endocrinologists, 412
American Association on Intellectual
and Developmental Disabilities
(AAIDD), 640
American Board of Internal Medicine
Foundation, 10–11
American Cancer Society, 10, 11, 46
American College of Cardiology
(ACC), 47–48
American Dental Association, 587
American Geriatrics Society (AGS), 11,
409, 739
American Heart Association (AHA),
47–48
American Medical Association, 52
American Medical Association
Consortium for Performance
Improvement (AMA-PCPI),
759–760
American Medical Directors
Association, 11, 61
American Physical Therapy
Association, 11
American Recovery and Reinvestment
Act, 764

American Society of Consultant
Pharmacists, 61
American Society of Emergency
Physicians, 11
American Society of Nephrology, 11
American Thyroid Association, 412
Americans with Disabilities Act
(ADA), 667
aminoglycosides, 59
amiodarone, 163, 246, 412
amitriptyline, 63
for migraines/tension type headaches, *222*
for neuropathic pain, *215*
for postherpetic neuralgia, 338
amnestic mild cognitive impairment
(aMCI), 131, 135–136
amoxicillin
for acute bacterial sinusitis, 581
for erysipelas, 497
for otitis media, 578
for urinary tract infection, 368
amphetamines, 63, *247*, 324
ampicillin, for UTI, 368
amyloidosis, 211, 214, 529–531
amyotrophic lateral sclerosis (ALS,
Lou Gehrig's Disease), *205*, 206
amyotrophy, *212*
anabolic steroids, exogenous, 84
anal fissure, *322*
anastrazole, 542
Andres, R., 8
anemia
aplastic anemia, 218, *219*
approach to
classification, 523–524
initial evaluation, 524
autoimmune hemolytic anemias,
528
clinical consequences, 523
common etiologies, 523
Crohn's disease and, 320
definition/prevalence, 523
delirium and, *153*
dizziness and, 118
fall risks and, 53
fecal incontinence and, 388
gastric cancer and, 316
gastrointestinal bleeding and, *319*
GERD and, 311
heart failure and, 166, 167
HIV infection and, 347, 349
hyponatremia and, 360
hypoproliferative anemia, 531
hypothyroidism and, 410
immune thrombocytopenic purpura, 529
of inflammation, 523
kidney disease and, 358
macrocytic anemias, 523

myelodysplastic syndrome, 523,
527–528
vitamin B12 deficiency, 526–527
malnutrition and, 328
as medication side effect, *219*
microcytic anemias, 523
iron deficiency anemia, 524–525
thalassemia, 525
normocytic anemias, 328, 523
anemia of chronic kidney disease,
523, 526
anemia of inflammation, 523,
525–526
odynophagia and, 314
peptic ulcer disease and, 315
pneumonia and, 335
renal disease and, 358
thrombocytopenia, 347, 528–529
angina
beta blockers for, 191
exertional, 159
peripheral arterial disease and, 199
angiodysplasia, *320*
angiotensin receptor blockers (ARBs)
acute tubular necrosis and, 359
in albuminuria, 431
in heart failure, 168
for hypertension, 191
in MI, *161*, 162
angiotensin-converting enzyme (ACE)
inhibitors
acute tubular necrosis and, 359
in albuminuria, 431
in heart failure, 168
for hypertension, 190
in MI, *161*, 162
side effects, 190
angle-closure glaucoma, 571
Anglo-Scandinavian Cardiac
Outcomes Trial–Lipid-Lowering
Arm (ASCOT-LLA) program, 439
animal models of aging research,
18–19, 23
Animal Naming test, 133
ankle fractures, 470
Annual Wellness Visit, 32
anorectal disorders
colonic ischemia, 323–325, *324*
constipation/fecal incontinence,
321–323
anorexia nervosa, 88–89
bupropion contraindication, 292
depression and, 50
frailty and, 100, 101
antagonistic pleiotropy theory, 18
anthracyclines, 542
antiarrhythmics. *See also* amiodarone;
lidocaine; mexiletine;
procainamide
empiric, 163

medical house calls, 652–653
physician recommendation for, 4
problem-specific programs, 653
safety assessment, 37
home health agency, 32
homeopathy, 706, 707–708
HOPES program. *See* Helping Older
People Experience Success
(HOPES) program
hormone therapy (HT). *See also* estrogen replacement therapy; testosterone therapy
causative for headaches, 227
for frailty, 102–103
in hypopituitarism, 414–415
for post-menopausal symptoms,
402–403, *404*
in postmenopausal women, 448
risks and benefits, *404*
for urinary tract infection, 369
vaginal bleeding from, 399–400
hospice care programs
Alzheimer's care costs, 126
complementary pain management
in, 676
continuity of care issues, 3
description, 655–656
goals of, 2
for heart failure, 172
home hospice, 652
life expectancy considerations, 172
Medicare Home Hospice, 661
in nursing facilities, 661–662
palliative care comparison, 671
quality of life focus, 553
specialized teams in, 3
Hospital Elder Life Program, 150, *151*
Hospital Insurance Trust Fund, 774
Hospital Quality Alliance (HQA), 762
Hospital Readmission Reduction
Program (Affordable Care Act),
172
hospital-acquired pneumonia (HAP),
301, *302*
hospital-acquired pressure ulcers
(HAPUs), 509, 511
HPV. *See* human papilloma virus
infection
human lifespan (life expectancy), 1
centenarians, 21–22
childhood cancer survivors and, 22
HIV patients and, 22
strategies for increasing, 17
human papilloma virus (HPV) infection, 347, 400
hydralazine nitrates, for heart failure,
168
hydrocele, 377–378
hydrocephalus. *See* hydrocephalus *ex
vacuo*; normal pressure

hydrocephalus; obstructive
hydrocephalus
hydrocephalus *ex vacuo*, 260
hydromorphone, *554*, 675
hydroxychloroquine, for rheumatoid
arthritis, 455
hyperactive delirium/hypoactive delirium, 151
hyperaldosteronism, 188, 415
hypercalcemia of malignancy, 410
hypercholesterolemia
peripheral arterial disease and,
196–197
risk factors, 198
treatment algorithm, 436
hyperglycemia, 8
hyperhomocysteinemia, *235*, 236
hyperkalemia, 360
diuretic side effects, 190
electrolyte abnormalities in, 179
hyperkeratotic lesions, feet, 598
hyperlipidemia. *See also* lipid
management
cardiovascular disease and, 429
as dementia risk factor, *126*
exercise benefits, 424
hypertension and, 188, 429
as ischemic stroke risk factor, *235*
pancreatitis and, 328
retinal vein occlusion and, 574
statin therapy for, 48, 207, 326
hypernatremia, 360
hyperparathyroidism
bone mineral density and, 409, 450
osteoporosis and, *447*
primary, 408–409, 450
secondary and tertiary, 409–410,
450–451
hypertension, 187–191
in acute MI, 160
antihypertensive considerations, 429
atrial fibrillation and, 176–177
as CAD risk factor, 157
calcium channel blockers in, *161*
as CGA component, 30
classifications of levels, *188*, 188
comorbidities/end organ effects, 189
diagnosis, 188
epidemiology of, 187
exercise benefits for, 81
fixed-dose agents for, 64
heart failure and, 166
hemorrhagic stroke and, 235
HIV infection and, 349
hyperaldosteronism and, 188, 415
ischemic stroke and, *235*
JNC8 treatment guidelines, 47
pathophysiology of, 187–188
peripheral arterial disease and, 197,
199

polypharmacy and, 361
prevention and screening, 47
pseudohypertension, 188
pulmonary embolism and, 302
refractory hypertension, 188
renal disease and, 358
renal disorders and, 188, 358, 360
renal elimination and, 60
secondary causes, 188
sleep apnea and, 269
systolic, 157, 166, 360
treatment
algorithm, 436
benefits, 189
considerations, 190
nonpharmacologic, 189–190
targets, 189
treatment, pharmacologic, 190–191
ACE inhibitors, 190
angiotensin receptor blockers,
191
calcium channel blockers, 190
thiazide-type diuretics, 190
treatment targets, 47
vitamin D and, 91
hypertensive nephrosclerosis, 190
hyperthyroidism, 411–412
atrial fibrillation and, 176–177
hypertension and, 188
subclinical, 412
hypertrophic cardiomyopathy, 166,
191
hypnic headache, *222*, *224*
hypochondriasis, 6
hypoestrogenic atrophic vaginitis, *399*
hypoglycemic agents, 425–429, *426*
biguanides, 425–427, *426*
DPP-4 inhibitors, *426*, 428
falling risks, *62*
insulin therapy, 428–429
meglitinides, *426*, 427
sulfonylureas, *426*, 427
thiazolidinediones, *426*, 427
hypogonadotrophic hypogonadism,
414
hypokalemia
atrial fibrillation and, 176–177
causative for constipation, *322*
digoxin toxicity in, 169
as diuretic side effect, 190, 361
ectopic ACTH production and, 415
electrolyte abnormalities in, 179
hypomagnesemia, 169
causative for constipation, *322*
digoxin toxicity in, 169
as diuretic side effect, 190
electrolyte abnormalities in, 179
hyponatremia, 360
hypopituitarism, 413–415
clinical manifestations, 413–414

intellectual disabilities (ID). *See also* severe and persistent mental illness
  autism spectrum disorders, 642–643
  definition, 640
  dementia and, 641
  evidence-based interventions, 642
  family caregiving for, 646
  polypharmacy prevalence, 642
  population characteristics, demographic trends
    age-related changes, 641–642
    life expectancy, mortality, 640–641
    prevalence, 640
    social characteristics, 641
intensive care units, 3
INTERHEART Study, 437
interleukin-6 (IL-6), inflammatory factor, 2, 20, 89, 100, 348
intermittent claudication, in PAD, 192, 193, *194*, 196, 197
internal medicine, 2
interstitial lung diseases (ILD), 304
  diagnosis, 304
  treatment, 304
intertrigo, 502
intertrochanteric hip fractures, 466, 469
Interventions Testing Program (ITP), 23
intracerebral hemorrhage (ICH), 241
intracranial mass, 227
intracranial stenosis, 239
intravenous vasodilators, for heart failure, 169
ipilimumab, for melanoma skin cancer, 488
ipratropium bronchodilator, for COPD, 63, 299
IQCODE. *See* Informant Questionnaire for Cognitive Decline in the Elderly
irbesartan, *171*
iron deficiency anemia, 524–525
irritable bowel syndrome (IBS), 317
ischemic bowel disease, *320*
ischemic heart disease (IHD), 82. *See also* myocardial infarction
  clinical presentation, 158–159
  epidemiology/primary prevention, 157
  muscle weakness and, *207*
ischemic option neuropathy, 189
ischemic strokes
  acute, classification of subtypes, *234*
  blood pressure management, 237–238
  fatality risks, 233
  fibrinolytic therapy and, *163*

hypertension and, 189
neuroimaging and, 121
recovery variables, 241
risk factors, 234, *235*, 235
treatment of, 239–240
warfarin and, 178
isometric contraction, 85
isoniazid, for tuberculosis, 337
isoproterenol, *247*

Japanese people, lifespan, 22
Jeste, D. V., 643
joint replacement
  for knee/hip, osteoarthritis, 455
  post-surgery gait retraining, 619
  PRT benefits for, 84
  skilled nursing facility recovery, 618
Judeo-Christian traditions, 799
jugular venous distension, 175
JUPITER (Justification for the Use of statin in Prevention: an Intervention Trial Evaluating Rosuvastatin) trial, 439

Kaposi's sarcoma, *346*, 347, 600
Katz Index of Independence in Activities of Daily Living, 35
Kegel exercises (pelvic floor muscle training, PFMT), 30, 402
Kemoun, G., 110
keratoacanthoma, 485
keratolytic agents, for onychomycosis, 599
Kerrigan, D. C., 110
kidneys, effects of aging, 159. *See also* acute kidney injury; renal disorders
King's Health Questionnaire (for urinary incontinence), 36
Kingston Standardized Cognitive Assessment-Revised (mini-KSCAr), 52
Kirkwood, Thomas, 18
knee osteoarthritis, 454
Krieger, Dolores, 705
Kunz, Dora, 705

labyrinthitis, 121, 257
lacrimal system. *See* eyelids and lacrimal system
lagophthalmos, 565
lamotrigine
  for neuralgia-induced headaches, 226
  for seizure treatment, *219*
  tremors exacerbated by, *247*
lansoprazole (Prevacid), for GERD, *312*
large artery atherosclerosis, *234*
latanoprost, for glaucoma, 571–572

Laumann, E. O., 685
Lavizzo-Mourey, Risa, 740
Lawton, J. M., 36
laxatives
  fecal incontinence and, 393, 394
  lubiprostone as alternative, 323
  for obstipation, *322*
  types of, 555
  underuse of, 64
Leapfrog Group, 759
LEARN model of cross-cultural communication, *741*
Lee, L. W., 110
leflunomide, for rheumatoid arthritis, 455–456
left bundle branch block, 159
left ventricular assist devices (LVADs), 169–170
left ventricular dysfunction, 189
left ventricular hypertrophy (LVH), 159, 166, 173
Legionella pneumophila, 334
leiomyomas, 399–400
lentigo maligna melanoma, 487
letrozole, 542
leucopenia, in HIV infection, 347
leukemia, 531–532, *532*
  acute myelogenous leukemia, 531–532
  chronic lymphocytic leukemia, 529, 531
  chronic myeloid leukemia, 531
leukocytoclastic vasculitis, 495
leukocytosis, 159
levetiracetam, for seizures, 218, *219*
levodopa therapy, 129
  for multiple system atrophy, 250
  for Parkinson's disease treatment, 245, 248, 252
    dosage fluctuations, variations, 252–253
    reduced mortality effect, 255–256
levothyroxine, 59
lichen sclerosis, 376, *399*, 399
lidocaine, 163
  for herpes zoster, 500
  topical, for neuropathic pain, 214–215, *215*
life expectancy projections, U.S., 720–721
life-course perspective, of retirement, 731
lifespan (life expectancy)
  biomarkers of, 17
  caloric restriction research, 23
  centenarians, 18, 21–22
  disparities in the U.S., 22
  early theories of, 18
  gender differences, 22

massage, 221, 705
mastalgia (benign breast disease), 405
MAST-G (Michigan Alcohol Screening Test), 290
mastication muscles
  age-related changes, 590
  anatomy/characteristics, 590
  examination techniques, 590–591
MAT. *See* multifocal atrial tachycardia
matrix modeling factors, 20
Mayo Clinic Study of Aging (MCSA), 131
McGill Pain Scale, 516
McGurk, S. R., 645
McKibbin, C. L., 645
MDD. *See* major depressive disorder
MDRD. *See* Modification in Renal Disease (MDRD) equation
MDS. *See* Minimum Data Set
Medawar, Peter, 18
Medicaid
  annual caregiver funding, 4
  EHR Incentive Programs, 761
  eligibility and coverage, 776–777
  home healthcare coverage, 651, 652
  home-based waiver programs, 4
  Minimum Data Set assessment, 40
  origin, 660, 776
  support for non-medical community services, 655
Medicaid Waiver program, 660
medical history, 33
medical intensivist, 3, 610, 662
Medical (or Physician) Orders for Life Sustaining Treatment (MOLST/POLST) advance directives, 783, 786, 787, 788, 790, 798
Medicare, 774–776
  "bundle" payment system exploration, 618
  cochlear implantation coverage, 579
  CPT code system, 778
  EHR Incentive Programs, 761
  establishment of, 660, 774
  home healthcare coverage, 651, 652
  Independence at Home program, 653
  items not covered by, 776
  Minimum Data Set assessment, 40
  opting out, by physicians, 778
  Part A (hospital insurance), 617, 618, 660, 661, 662, 774–775
  Part B (medical insurance), 765, 775
  Part C (Medicare Advantage), 769, 771, 775
  Part D (prescription drug plan), 776
  post-acute care expenditures, 618
  pressure ulcer claims data, 510, 511
  prostatitis treatment data, 375

  role in quality improvement strategy, 10
  urology treatment data, 366, 370
  wellness visits support, 51
  wheelchair payment process, 619
Medicare Detection of Cognitive Impairment, 134
Medicare Hospice Benefit (MHB), 655–656, 662
Medicare Hospital VBP program, 760, 763
Medicare Prescription Drug, Improvement, and Modernization Act (MMA, 2003), 762
Medicare Quality Improvement Organizations (QIOs), 668
Medicare Value-based Modifier (VM), 762
meditation, 676
Mediterranean diet, 440
meglitinides, 426, 427. *See also* nateglinide; repaglinide
meibomian gland dysfunction, 566
melanoma, 487–488
  contributing factors, 487
  diagnosis, 487–488
  metastatic, prognosis, 488
  subtypes, 487
  treatment, 488
melatonin receptor agonists, 268. *See also* ramelteon
memantine, 135, 255
Ménière's disease, 117, 119, 257
meningitis
  bacterial, 347
  cryptococcal, 345
  headaches in, 228
  viral, 347
menopause. *See also* post-menopause
  endometrial cancer and, 401
  urinary tract infections and, 367–368
Men's AIDS Cohort Study (MACS), 348
mental illness. *See also* severe and persistent mental illness
  caregiving for people with, 749
  cultural/societal attitudes towards, 283, 739
  intellectual disabilities with, 642
  nursing facilities regulations, 662
mental status domain (of CGA), 32
mental status examination, 275–276
meperidine, 62
metabolic acidosis
  osteomalacia, 218
  renal disease and, 358
metabolic bone disorders. *See also* osteoporosis

hyperparathyroidism, 449, 450 (*See also* hyperparathyroidism)
osteomalacia, 448, 449, 463
Paget's disease, 449, 451
renal osteodystrophy, 449, 451
metabolic syndrome
  aging risk factor, 17
  caloric restriction benefits, 23
  description, 429
  insulin resistance factor, 70, 429 (*See also* insulin resistance)
  intellectual disabilities and, 641
  statin benefits for, 326
metformin, 23, 195, 425–427
methadone
  for cancer-related pain, 554
  for opioid dependence, 293
methicillin-resistant *S. aureus* (MRSA), 332, 338–339
  clinical presentation, diagnosis, 339
  community-acquired, 338–339
  hospital-acquired, 338
  management, 339, 340
methimazole, for Grave's disease, 412
methotrexate
  for atopic dermatitis, 493
  for autoimmune blistering disorders, 497
  for multiple sclerosis, 205
  for psoriasis, 491
  for rheumatoid arthritis, 455
metoclopramide
  for cancer related nausea, vomiting, 555
  causative for parkinsonism, 250
  for migraines with nausea, vomiting, 221, 223
metolazone, with loop diuretics, for HF, 168
metoprolol, 162
metronidazole
  for diarrhea, 318
  small fiber polyneuropathy and, 211
  topical, for rosacea, 489
  for vaginal discharge, 399
mexiletine, 247
MI. *See* myocardial infarction
miconazole nitrate, for tinea pedis, 599
microcytic anemias
  iron deficiency anemia, 524–525
  thalassemia, 525
micronutrients, 51, 102, 374
Middle East respiratory syndrome (MERS), 335
midfoot disorders
  pes planus (flatfoot), 601
  posterior tibial tendon dysfunction, 601–602
migraine headaches, 222–223

progressive resistance training and, 84–85
Sjögren's syndrome and, 459
musculoskeletal injuries
ankle fractures, 470
atypical femur fractures, bisphosphonate use, 464–465
distal radius fractures, 471–472
hip fractures, 466–469
diagnosis, 467
femoral neck, 466, 467–469
intertrochanteric, 466, 469
outcomes, 467
presentation, management, 466–467
principles, 466
subtrochanteric, 466
injury factors
comminution, 463–464
intra-articular fractures, 464
open fractures, 463
polytrauma, 463
long bone injuries, 463
metastatic disease, 464
patient factors
bone quality, 462–463
pre-injury status, 462
soft tissue quality, 463
systemic disease, 462
pelvic ring fractures, 463
periprosthetic fractures, 464
preoperative considerations, 465–466
proximal humerus fractures, 462, 470–471
vertebral compression fractures, 472–473
music therapy, 676
MUST. *See* Malnutrition Universal Screening Tool
mutation accumulation theory, 18
myasthenia gravis, *205, 206,* 206–207
mycophenolate mofetil
for atopic dermatitis, 493
for autoimmune blistering disorders, 497
for myasthenia gravis, 207
myelodysplastic syndrome (MDS), 523, 527–528
myeloid leukemia, 410
myeloma cast nephropathy, *358*
myelopathy/spinal cord compression, 256
myeloproliferative neoplasms, 532–533
myocardial infarction (MI), 157. *See also* acute ST-segment elevation myocardial infarction
acute, symptoms, 158–159
atrial fibrillation and, 176–177

beta blockers for, 191
clinical presentation, 159
complications of, 164–165
confusion in, 8
diagnosis, 159–160
differential diagnosis, 160
HIV infection and, 347
hypertension and, 189
management, acute, symptoms, *161*
peripheral arterial disease and, 199
pharmacologic management, 160–163
angiotensin/aldosterone inhibition, 162
antiplatelet therapy, 160, *161*
antithrombotic therapy, 161–162
beta blockers, 162
other agents, 163
statin therapy, 162–163
strokes and, 238
myocarditis, 166
myxedema, 10

nails, aging-related changes, 481
naltrexone
for alcohol dependence, 292
for opioid dependence, 293
narcissistic personality disorder, 280
Narcotics Anonymous, 292
narrow-angle glaucoma, 391
nasal cavity and sinus
age-related changes, 581
common pathologies, 581–582
anosmia, 582
epistaxis, 582
rhinitis, 581
sinusitis, 581–582
congestion, in cluster headaches, 223
nateglinide, 427
National Adult Protective Services Association (NAPSA), 689
National Adult Reading Test, 133
National Assessment of Adult Literacy (NAAL) report, 742
National Cholesterol Education Program Guidelines, 436
National Committee for Quality Assurance (NCQA), 758–759
National Consumer Voice for Long-Term Care, 689
National Core Indicators Adult Consumer Survey, 641
National Culturally and Linguistically Appropriate Services (CLAS) in Health and Health Care, *737*
National Demonstration Project Quality Improvement in Health Care (IHI), 758

National Epidemiologic Survey of Alcohol and Related Conditions (NESARC), 286
National Family Caregiver Support Program (NFCSP), 752
National Hospice and Palliative Care Organization (NHPCO), 656
National Institute on Aging, 23
National Institute on Alcohol Abuse and Alcoholism, 285
National Nursing Home Quality Care Collaborative (NNHQCC), 668
National Osteoporosis Foundation, 409, 446
National Patient-Centered Clinical Research Network, 430
National Pressure Ulcer Advisory Panel (NPUAP), 510, 511, 514–518
National Quality Forum (NQF), 760
National Quality Measures Clearinghouse (NQMC), 758
National Survey on Drug Use and Health (NSDUH), 286
Native Americans
community based services for, 655
diabetes prevalence, 421
life expectancy, 22
Native Hawaiians, 22
Natural Medicines Comprehensive Database, 707
naturopathic medicine, 706, 708
nausea and vomiting
in acute angle closure glaucoma, *226*
CAM mind-body therapies, 704, 707
in chemotherapy treatment, 554–555
corticosteroids for, 676
at end-of-life
assessment, *677,* 677
management, 677, *678*
mechanisms, 676–677, *677*
in intracranial mass, 227
management in cancer, 554–555, *555*
in migraines, *221,* 223
NSAIDs for, 676
in secondary headaches, *225*
NCEP ATP III panel, 438
NCQA. *See* National Committee for Quality Assurance
nebivolol, *171*
nephrolithiasis, 408
nesiritide, 169
neuraminidase inhibitors, 335–336. *See also* oseltamivir; zanamivir
neuroendocrine theory, 18
neurohumoral system, *159*
neuroimaging
in Alzheimer's disease, 126

833

neuroimaging (cont.)
in chronic vestibular syndrome, 122
in dementia, 122, 126, 128, 129, 133–134
for headaches, 229
in muscle weakness, 208
in normal pressure hydrocephalus, 260
in strokes, 234
neuroleptics, 282
neurologic problems, 203–229
evaluation considerations, 203–204
headaches, 220–229
evaluation, 228–229
primary types, 221–224, *224*
secondary types, 224–228
muscle weakness, 204–209
evaluation, 208–209
neurological causes, 204–207
non-neurological causes, 207–208
treatment, 209
seizure disorders, 215–220
causes, 216
differential diagnosis, *217*, 217
evaluation/risk factor assessment, *217*, 217–218
management/treatment, 218–220, *219*
pharmacologic treatment, *219–220*
presentation in the elderly, 216–217
prevalence rates, 215–216
sensory disorders/neuropathies, 209–215
alcohol-related neuropathy, 212–213
demyelinating neuropathies, 212
diabetic neuropathy, 11, 190, 210–211
evaluation, 213–214, *214*
monoclonal gammopathy, 213
post-herpetic neuralgia, 46–47, 211–212
related terminology, *213*
sensory peripheral neuropathy, 122
treatment, 214–215, *215*
vitamin B12 deficiency, 213
neuromuscular disease, 84
neuropathies. *See* sensory disorders/neuropathies
neurotrophic ulcers, feet, 598
New York City Almshouse, 659
New York State Elder Abuse Prevalence Study, 686
nicotine replacement therapy (NRT), 54, 292
nifedipine, for aortic insufficiency, 173
nitrates, 60, 163

nitrofurantoin, for urinary tract infection, 368
nitroglycerin, *161*
nizatidine (Axid), for GERD, *312*
NKI receptor antagonists, *555*
NKI receptor antagonists, for cancer-related nausea, vomiting, *555*
NMDA receptor antagonists (N-methyl-D-aspartate receptor antagonists), 135
nodular basal cell carcinoma, 485
nodular melanoma, 487
nonamestic mild cognitive impairment (naMCI), 131
nonarteritic ischemic optic neuropathy, 575
nonbenzodiazepines (z-drugs), 266. *See also* eszopiclone; zolpidem
non-dihydropyridine calcium channel blockers, *62*
non-Hodgkin's lymphomas, 347, 410
nonischemic dilated cardiomyopathy, 166
nonmaleficence principle (in ethical decision-making), 797
non-ST-elevation acute coronary syndromes (NSTEACS), 163–164, *164*
nontuberculous mycobacterium (NTM), 304–305
presentation, diagnosis, 305
treatment, 305
normal pressure hydrocephalus (NPH), 130, 250
gait patterns, 260
ventriculoperitoneal shunting for, 261
normocytic anemias, 328
anemia of chronic kidney disease, 526
anemia of inflammation, 525–526
North American Symptomatic Carotid Endarterectomy Trial (NASCET), 239
nortriptyline, 54
for major depression, 277
for migraines/tension type headaches, *222*
for postherpetic neuralgia, 338
nose valves, for sleep apnea, 270
nosocomial infections, 332, 338, 368. *See also* urinary tract infection
NQF. *See* National Quality Forum
NSAIDs nonsteroidal anti-inflammatory drugs (NSAIDs), 135
acute kidney injury and, 359
for acute pericarditis, 175
acute tubular necrosis and, 359
avoidance in HF patients, 169
for benign breast disease, 405

for cancer-related pain, *554*
causative for headaches, 227
GERD and, 311
for gout, 456
interaction cautions, 282
for migraines, tension headaches, *221*, 223
for osteoarthritis, 454
peptic ulcers and, 315
risk factors, 311
for tension type headaches, 221
NSTEACS. *See* non-ST-elevation acute coronary syndromes
NTM. *See* nontuberculous mycobacterium
nuclear medicine, 12
numeric rating scales, 39
nurse practitioner (NP), 2
as activists/sounding boards, for patients, 3
geriatric, 28
health maintenance emphasis, 9–10
in nursing facilities, 663
nursing facilities, 3
AMDA's improvement focus, 668–669
infection risk factors, 331
legal regulation/quality of care
civil litigation, 665
criminal prosecutions, 664
discrimination issues, 667
drug prescription, management, 667
elopement, 667
improvement opportunities, 667–668
informed consent, 665
overview, 663–664
restraints, 665–667
long-stay residents, 662
mental ill patients, regulations, 662
psychiatric problems of patients, 274
short-stay residents/patients
post-acute care, 660–661
respite care, 661
terminal care/hospice care, 661–662
structure of medical practice
full-time, facility-based physician, 663
nurse practitioner/physician assistant, 663
physician/continuity of care model, 662–663
post-acute/LTC practitioner, unassigned admissions, 663
nutrition
anorexia and, 88–89
BMI and, 92
cachexia and, 89

Parkinson's Plus syndromes, *249*
paroxetine (Paxil°), 138, 316
paroxysmal nocturnal dyspnea, 166
paroxysmal unilateral headache, 226
Partnership for Patients (AHRQ), 758
passive fecal incontinence, *387*, 387
patent foramen ovale (PFO), 238
Patient Education Materials Assessment Tool (PEMAT), 744
Patient Health Questionnaire-2 (PHQ-2), 50
Patient Health Questionnaire-9 (PHQ-9), 35, 40, 50
Patient Protection and Affordable Care Act (2010), 32
Patient Safety Measure Tools & Resources (AHRQ), 758
Patient Self-Determination Act (PSDA, 1990), 782–783
Patient-Centered Medical Home, 2
Patient-Centered Outcomes Research Institute, 430
PDE5 inhibitors, for erectile dysfunction, 635
PE. *See* pulmonary embolism
Peabody, F. W., 5
Pearl, Raymond, 19
pegloticase, for gout, 457
pelvic floor muscle training (PFMT, Kegel exercises), 30, 392, 402
pelvic organ prolapse, 402
Pelvic Organ Prolapse Quantitation (POPQ) system, 402
pelvic ring fractures, 463
pemphigoid, 496, *498*
pemphigus, 496, *498*
penile disorders, 376–377
 balanoposthitis, 376–377
 paraphimosis, 376
 Peyronie's disease, 377
 phimosis, 376
peptic ulcer disease, *315*, 315
 diagnosis/treatment, 315
 gastric bleeding and, 240
 MI and, 160
 presentation, 315
percutaneous coronary intervention (PCI)
 in acute MI, *161*, 161
 in acute STEMI, 163
percutaneous pericardiocentesis, 175
percutaneous tibial nerve stimulation treatment (PTNS), 391–392
performance improvement. *See* healthcare performance improvement
pericardial diseases
 pericardial constriction, 175–176
 pericardial effusion and tamponade, 175

pericarditis, 175
perindopril, *171*
periodic lateralizing epileptiform discharged (PLEDS), 217
periodic limb movement of sleep (PLMS), 248
periorificial dermatitis, 490
peripheral arterial disease (PAD), 192–199
 aspirin for, 169
 as CAD equivalent, 440
 clinical presentation, *194*
 comorbidities, 199
 complications, 199
 differential diagnosis, 196
 hypertension and, 189
 intermittent claudication in, 192, 193, *194*, 196, 197
 limb salvage recommendations, 198–199
 management, *196*
  antiplatelet/antithrombotic drugs, 197
  diabetes, 197
  exercise rehabilitation, 197–198
  hypercholesterolemia, 196–197
  hypertension, 197
  smoking cessation, 196
  vasodilators, 197
 screening, diagnosis, intervention, 194–196, *195*
peripheral neuropathy
 as ART therapy side effect, 351
 in HIV infection, 347, 351
peripheral vascular disease
 PRT benefits for, 84
 vitamin D and, 91
peroxisome proliferator-activated receptor-gamma (PPAR-γ) agonists, 427. *See also* pioglitazone; rosiglitazone
persecution delusions, 275
persistent vegetative state (PVS), 781, 790
personality disorders, 279–280
Personality Outlook Profile Scale, 14
personalized medicine, 12
pes planus (flatfoot), 601
Peyronie's disease, 377
Pfeiffer, Jules, 6
PFMT. *See* pelvic floor muscle training
Pharmacy Health Literacy Center (AHRQ), 758
phenobarbital, 245–246
phenothiazines, *247*
phenotype model of frailty, 97–98, *98*
phenytoin, 59, 218, 226
phenytoin/fosphenytoin, *219*
pheochromocytoma, *117*, 188, 415, 416
Philadelphia Almshouse, 659

phimosis, 376
PHN. *See* postherpetic neuralgia
phobias, 276
phosphodiesterase inhibitors, 393. *See also* sildenafil; tadalafil; vardenafil
photoaging mitigation role of skin, 480–481
photodynamic therapy
 for non-melanoma skin cancer, *486*
 for onychomycosis, 599
PHPT. *See* primary hyperparathyroidism
phymatous rosacea (PhR), 489
Physical Activity Guidelines Advisory Committee Report (2008), 69
physical barrier function of skin, 478
physical health domain (of CGA), *32*
physical performance assessment, 36
physical therapy
 for gait disorders, 261
 geriatric, 28
 in pain management, 676
physician assistant (PA), 663
Physician Quality Reporting System (PQRS, CMS), 758, 761–762, 765
physician-assisted suicide (euthanasia), 7
physician-assisted suicide (PAS), 7, 799–801
physicians. *See also* doctor-patient relationship
 as activists/sounding boards, for patients, 3
 attitude problems, U.S., 3
 communication skills, 1, 5–6
 compassionate care, 1, 12–13
 culturally sensitive care, 5
 health maintenance emphasis, 9–10
 as integrator of biopsychosocial-spiritual model, 1–3
 intelligent treatment, ethical decision-making, 10–11
 interprofessional collaboration, 11
 recommendations to caregivers, 4
 specificity in nursing home recommendations, 3
Physician's Guide to Assessing and Counseling Older Drivers (AMA/NHTSA), 692, 693, 694
Pilates, 261, 705
pill-induced esophagitis, 311
pimecrolimus, 491
PIMs. *See* potentially inappropriate medications
pioglitazone, 427
Pittsburg Sleep Quality Index, 265
pituitary gland disorders
 adenomas, 413